Teacher's Edition

Expanded Edition

HEALTH

Making Life Choices

Second Edition

Frances
Sizer • Eleanor
Noss • Linda
Kelly
Webb Whitney DeBruyne

Contributing Authors
*The Section Review and Chapter Review exercises
were written by high school teachers:*

Patricia Kosiba
P.D. Schreiber High School
Port Washington, New York

Rhonda Helgerson
Del Rio High School
Del Rio, Texas

National Textbook Company
a division of NTC/CONTEMPORARY PUBLISHING GROUP
NTC Lincolnwood, Illinois USA

T1

Production Credits

Editors	Lynda Kessler, Pam Starkey
Photo Research	Jan Seidel
Production Editor	Mario M. Rodriguez
Permissions	Elaine Arthur
Illustrators	Randy Miyake, Miyake Illustration; Matthew Thiessen; Precision Graphics
Copyediting	Mary Berry
Composition	Parkwood Composition Service, Inc.
Index	Jane Hilken
Cover design	Mario M. Rodriguez
Cover photos	The Stock Market
Proofreader	Bette Holzer, Carol Maurer
Prepress services	Clarinda Company

Teacher's Expanded Edition: ISBN 0-538-42986-0

Published by National Textbook Company, a division of
NTC/Contemporary Publishing Group, Inc., 4255 West Touhy Avenue,
Lincolnwood, Illinois 60712-1975 USA
© 2000 NTC/Contemporary Publishing Group, Inc.
Manufactured in the United States of America.

07 06 05 04 03 02 01 00   8 7 6 5 4 3 2 1

Teacher's Edition

The eighteen teachers listed below contributed most of the activities suggested in this Teacher's Edition:

Lee C. Ancona
Granbury High School
Granbury, TX

Kimberly Dawn Ballard
Walter Williams
High School
Burlington, NC

Deneise J. Crace
Meridian High School
Meridian, ID

Robin GrayBallard
Suva Intermediate School
Montebello Unified School District
Montebello, CA

Steve Guelff
Billings West High School
Billings, MT

Donna J. Ketchum
Frontier Central High School
Hamburg, NY

Susan E. Kurtin
Bleyl Junior High School
Cypress/Fairbanks I.S.D.
Houston, TX

Roxanna L. Laycox
West Carrollton
High School
West Carrollton, OH

Carol A. Martin
Pekin Community
High School
Pekin, IL

Tim McCormick
Wheeling Park High School
Wheeling, WV

Betzy L. Nelson
Orange Park
High School
Orange Park, FL

Donna S. Paris
Haywood County Schools
Waynesville, NC

Candace O. Purdy
Maine South High School
Park Ridge, IL

Kathleen M. Schaefer
Gates Chili High School
Rochester, NY

Linda Troolin
East High School
Duluth, MN

Todd V. Urbanek
Boswell High School
Fort Worth, TX

Kathleen Zammett Walter
Great Neck North
High School
Great Neck, NY

Constance P. Wood
Orange Park High School
Orange Park, FL

Overview of the *Health: Making Life Choices* Textbook Program

The *Health: Making Life Choices* textbook program consists of the following components:

- ▶ *Health: Making Life Choices,* Student Text, Expanded Edition
- ▶ *Health: Making Life Choices,* Teacher's Expanded Edition
- ▶ *Health: Making Life Choices,* Teacher's Resource Box (reproducible handouts, tests, worksheets, etc.)
- ▶ *Health: Making Life Choices,* Transparency Acetates
- ▶ *Health: Making Life Choices,* Video Library (up-to-date videos offered at reduced prices)
- ▶ *Health: Making Life Choices,* Nutrition Videodisc (live action, still photos, and text on videodisc)
- ▶ *Diet Analysis* (user-friendly software for analyzing diets)
- ▶ *Health: Making Life Choices,* computerized testing software

Each component listed above is described in the following pages. Making yourself familiar with the components and their relationships to each other will help you obtain maximum benefit from the individual components and from the program as a whole.

Health: Making Life Choices, Student Textbook, Expanded

Health: Making Life Choices is a new textbook, written for high school, comprehensive health courses. The text covers a broad range of topics, including areas of mental, physical, and social health. The text is divided into the following eight units:

 I. Introduction to Health
 II. Your Emotional and Mental Health
 III. Your Physical Health
 IV. Drug Use and Abuse
 V. Disease Prevention
 VI. The Life Cycle
 VII. First Aid and Safety
 VIII. Global Issues

Perhaps the full scope and intent of *Health: Making Life Choices* is best stated in its opening sentence: *"This book is about enjoying life."* Ten years ago, or even five years ago, to many people this sentence would have seemed completely inappropriate as a description of the content covered in a high school health course. Today, it says exactly what it should say, for the essence of contemporary health education is teaching self-responsibility and skills to promote a long and happy life for everyone.

How does *Health: Making Life Choices* help teenagers learn to enjoy life? To begin, as the title indicates, it focuses on the development of student decision-making skills. Two primary goals of the text are to give students the information they need to understand the different aspects of health and wellness, and to provide instruction and strategies to help students evaluate information so that they can make wise lifestyle choices—choices that will promote total wellness and inhibit the development of lifestyle diseases.

Another major goal of the text is to build all students' self-esteem. In almost every chapter of the text, students learn of the connection between self-esteem and the topic being discussed in that particular chapter. A full section is devoted to self-esteem in Chapter 3. Throughout the text, students read that it's okay to be different, to look the way they look, and to feel what they're feeling. It would be impossible for students to read through the text without developing a greater sense of their self-worth and a realization that they can achieve their goals.

Another theme woven throughout the text is that of abstinence—abstinence from sexual intercourse and the use of the drugs of abuse, alcohol, and tobacco. Students learn about the dangers and drawbacks involved with these choices and are provided with information about the various kinds of pressure to participate in sexual behaviors and to abuse substances such as drugs, alcohol, and tobacco. Students also learn strategies for resisting these pressures.

In addition to its emphasis on the goals and themes mentioned above, *Health: Making Life Choices* is different from the other high school health textbooks in several ways. Following is a brief mention of these differences.

Accuracy

You can count on each and every fact in *Health: Making Life Choices* to be scientifically accurate and current. The authors receive over 30 professional journals and publications each month and file the information in a computer retrieval system. Each fact is thoroughly checked and rechecked and the information is updated constantly. You will not find a more accurate, up-to-date text than *Health: Making Life Choices*.

More Thorough Coverage

If a topic is introduced in *Health: Making Life Choices*, it is thoroughly explained. Topics are not treated superficially. For most, if not all of the major topics included in the standard health course, *Health: Making Life Choices* contains more information than do the other available texts. On topics such as stress, mental and emotional problems, nutrition, weight control, drugs of abuse, alcohol, tobacco, and human sexuality—the topics health teachers around the country say are the most important—*Health: Making Life Choices* contains several more pages of in-depth information than do the other texts.

Increased Reading Comprehension

Several aspects of *Health: Making Life Choices* will help students increase their reading comprehension. As was previously mentioned, the topics covered in *Health: Making Life Choices* are explained fully and completely. Students are not left with vague impressions and unanswered questions.

If you have an opportunity to show the different texts you are considering for your health course to your students, notice that they will stop and read what they see in *Health: Making Life Choices* much more so than they will with any other text. This happens because *Health: Making Life Choices* passes the test that so many of today's textbooks fail—it's interesting. The author's writing style is concerned, personal, and relevant to today's teenagers.

Additional features to help increase comprehension include "Mini Glossaries" in the lower right-hand corner of every two-page spread, which provide students easy access to definitions that they are often reluctant to search for, and "Key Points" at the end of each heading, which will help students summarize what they have just read. You will find none of these reading enhancements in any of the other high school health textbooks.

High Student Appeal

It is doubtful that you will find another high school text that will appeal to high school students as much as *Health: Making Life Choices*. All of the texts are, of course, bright and colorful with lots of photos and art. In addition, however, *Health: Making Life Choices* has several text features that should capture students' attention and spark their curiosity and enthusiasm. Features such as the "Fact or Fiction" questions at the beginning of the chapters, the colorful cartoons that teach with humor, the "Straight Talks" that present a variety of topics in a conversational format that students will enjoy, the "Life Choice Inventories" that require students to deal with their favorite topic—themselves—and finally, the "Teen Views" features that give your students opinions about the key health topics straight from the mouths of their peers all across the country. All of these features are unique to *Health: Making Life Choices*. The last one mentioned, "Teen Views," should be of special interest to your students.

Illustrations

In research prior to the development of the text, many teachers said that the illustrations in a health book were of critical importance. Therefore, a special attempt was made to produce large, colorful, easy to understand drawings, charts, and tables. Quickly scanning the text should make it evident that *Health: Making Life Choices* contains many interesting and informative illustrations not found in any other text.

Cross References

Few high school textbook authors are as concerned with helping students make the best use possible of the. text as are the authors of *Health: Making Life Choices*. Therefore, throughout the text, students will find references to related information and special features located in other parts of the text. This gives students every opportunity to follow their interests and pursue further information at the appropriate times. Once again, you will not find this kind of careful construction and concern for the students in any other text.

To sum up, *Health: Making Life Choices* is a carefully designed, carefully crafted, thoroughly researched and written text that your students will enjoy reading. It deals with the issues that concern today's teens, and it gives them strategies to help them lead a productive, enjoyable life.

Sexuality Material

The sexuality material is divided into two parts: *Understanding Sexuality* and *Preventing Pregnancy and Sexually Transmitted Diseases.* The three major sections of *Understanding Sexuality* deal with sexual activity, sexual myths, and sexual orientation. *Preventing Pregnancy.and Sexually Transmitted Diseases* deals with the major contraceptive methods, sterilization, and contraceptive failure.

Teacher's Expanded Edition

The *Health: Making Life Choices* Teacher's Edition was designed to help you make the most effective use possible of the student text. This edition is similar to many others that you have seen. The pages from the student text have been reduced to 85% of their actual size, which allows space for the teacher notes that appear along both sides of the text and across the bottom.

While this Teacher's Edition is similar in many ways to others you have seen, it is also unique in several ways. The most obvious difference is found in the activities suggested down the side of the teacher's edition. Most of these activities were written by teachers who are currently teaching health in classrooms across the country. Compare these activities to those you will see in other texts. The differences are obvious. In the directions for conducting the activities in the *Health: Making Life Choices* teacher's edition, the teachers tell you such things as likely reactions from students to a certain question or instruction, specific directions for dividing students into groups and assigning different responsibilities to different group members, which props are needed to conduct an activity, and on and on. In short, you will find the kind of information you would expect from a teacher who has conducted that activity several times in a classroom much like your own. Although you might expect to find this sort of assistance in any teacher edition, it is unique to *Health: Making Life Choices.*

Another unique aspect of the activities in the *Health: Making Life Choices* teacher's edition is the attention given to students of different ability levels and learning styles. Whereas most of the activities in other teacher's editions are paper/pencil and discussion types of activities, here you will find many activities involving props and games. Students are constantly making things such as posters, bulletin boards, and audio visual aids for oral presentations, and playing games such as bingo and jeopardy. In short, they are doing the types of activities that most high school teachers must do to keep their students interested and motivated.

Following is a brief review of the many additional features of this teacher's edition that will help you teach your course with *Health: Making Life Choices.*

Chapter Opener Pages

Each chapter opens with a special two-page, chapter opener spread. Each of these chapter opener spreads contains several different features:

- ▶ **Key Points**—short summing up of the key points and themes of the chapter to enable you to get a quick feel for what's included in the chapter.

- ▶ **Activity to Introduce the Chapter**—one or two suggestions for activities to get students interested in the main points of the chapter before you make the first reading assignment.

- ▶ **Bulletin Board Ideas**—ideas to help you and/or students develop interesting chapter related bulletin boards.

- ▶ **Answers to "Fact or Fiction"**—answers to the true/false "Fact or Fiction" exercise that appears on the first student page. On some planner pages there was not enough space for these answers, in which case, a page reference directs you to the answers on a page toward the end of the student chapter.

- ▶ **Not Enough Time?**—Because research indicated teachers all across the country were having a difficult time including all of the information they wanted to include in their one-semester courses, suggestions have been made as to how you might want to teach each chapter of this text if you only have one day or two days to teach it. Obviously, all of the health texts available have much more information and activity suggestions than could possibly be incorporated into a one-semester course. The Not Enough Time? feature tries to help you make sure that you include the most important information and do the most effective activities.

Side Panels

Along the sides of your teacher's edition you will find objectives and activities for each section of the student text. The teaching suggestions for each section are divided into four parts: **Focus**, **Teach and Apply**, **Assess**, and **Close**.

Focus:
Under the Focus heading are the main learning objectives for that particular section and one or two activities to focus the students' attention on the topics covered in that section.

Teach and Apply:

Under the Teach and Apply heading, you will find a variety of activity suggestions for teaching that section.

Depending on the length of the section, there could be as few as one activity or as many as twenty activities. It is not expected that you will complete all of these activities. You should pick and choose those that you think will work best for you and your students.

All of the activities have been designated as to type. These types of the activities are:

▶ Interdisciplinary Activity
▶ Class Activity
▶ Class Debate
▶ Background Information
▶ Learning with Visuals
▶ Discussion
▶ Comprehension Check
▶ Group Activity
▶ Guest Speaker
▶ Role Play

In addition, **On Line with Health** provides teachers with health-related Web sites to share with students.

Assess:

For each section, following the Teach and Apply heading, you will find an activity or two to help you evaluate the students' comprehension of the material contained in that section. For variety, and in many cases for applicability reasons, some of the evaluations are subjective rather than objective. These include essays, role plays, and oral presentations. Answers to the Section Reviews are listed here also.

Close:

Under the Close heading, you will find one or two activities to sum up that section's lesson for the students. In many cases, the activity calls for the students to cite key points. In many other cases the activity is a different version of one of the Teach and Apply activities.

Bottom Panels

Across the bottom of the Teacher's Edition, you will find additional activity suggestions and background information. The notes at the bottom of the pages are slightly more general in nature than what you will find in the side columns. Following is a brief look at the bottom panel boxes.

► **Special Needs**—These activities focus on the seven intelligences proposed by Howard Gardner. Activities are developed in the following areas: linguistic, musical, logical-mathematical, spatial, bodily-kinesthetic, interpersonal, and intra-personal.

► **Multicultural Issues**—Background information and activity suggestions are presented to help the students become more aware and more understanding in their dealings with people from other cultures.

► **Critical Thinking**—Activities in this category call upon students to use higher-order thinking skills, such as comparing and contrasting, synthesizing, and evaluating.

► **Cooperative Learning**—Group activities and projects call upon students to use their interpersonal skills to interact with classmates to achieve a common goal.

► **Focusing on Self-Esteem**—The activities and ideas presented here will help bolster students' self-esteem.

► **Decision Making Activities**—These activities allow students to use their knowledge and background to make decisions pertaining to health issues.

► **Ability Levels**—Activities in this category are geared for different ability levels: basic, average, and advanced.

► **Pursuing Wellness**—The ideas presented here will give students practical ways to achieve wellness in their lives.

► **Enrichment**—Enrichment activities are connected with the text material but take students a little further in their thinking and understanding.

► **Healthy People 2000**—Includes some of the national health promotion and disease prevention objectives prepared and distributed by the U.S. Department of Health and Human Services, Public Health Service.

► **Quick Quiz**—For many sections throughout the text, a Quick Quiz of ten true/false questions has been provided for the teacher to use as an oral evaluation of students' understanding of the material covered.

Chapter Review Answers:

The chapter review answers are all the answers to the objective questions and exercises at the end of the chapter. You should note that the answers to the recall questions are divided into the sections to which they apply.

This will help you assign questions for a particular section should you be teaching one section in a chapter but not another.

Teacher's Resource Box

Accompanying the *Health: Making Life Choices* student text and teacher edition is an extensive package of already prepared, reproducible classroom material for you and your students. Here is a brief listing of what you will find in the supplementary material:

▶ **Detailed Daily Lesson Plans**—These lesson plans provide a complete semester's teaching plan for using *Health: Making Life Choices* and its accompanying material. While this is only one of many ways to teach the course, it may provide a helpful starting point, especially if you are new to the course or you are using *Health: Making Life Choices* for the first time.

▶ **Study Material**—For each chapter of the text you will find the following worksheets to help you teach the vocabulary and to reteach concepts that prove difficult for some students:

a) *Vocabulary Games*—includes crossword puzzles and other games for the key terms from the text.

b) *Reteaching Sheets*—for each section or two, a sheet that gives students an opportunity to relearn the most important concepts of that section, or sections.

c) *Study Outlines*—a sheet that lists the main heads of the chapter with space for students to write in either your lecture notes or the key points from the chapter.

d) *Reading Clozes*—reading comprehension exercises that call for students to fill in the blanks of a chapter summary. These exercises have been shown to increase student retention of the material studied and to improve students' overall reading comprehension skills.

▶ **Activities**—includes a variety of activity handouts, such as enrichment activities, self-assessment activities (including worksheets of the Life Choice Inventories contained in the student text), fully developed cooperative learning activities, multicultural activities, and an abundance of activity handouts related to specific concepts in the chapters.

▶ **Spanish Language Exercises**—Several activities have been translated into Spanish to help Spanish-speaking students learn the vocabulary and key concepts in *Health: Making Life Choices.*

▶ **Chapter Tests**—For each chapter of the student text, you will find two chapter tests. Version A is a lower-level test consisting only of objective-type questions. Version B is an average to higher-level test including some objective questions, at least four or five short-answer questions, and a couple of essay questions.

▶ **Teacher Information Sheets**—Also referenced in the teacher's edition are Teacher Information Sheets that give you background information on various topics to help you teach those topics.

▶ **Special AIDS Unit**—As an addition to Chapter 16, you will find in your supplementary material an AIDS unit that includes lesson plans, handouts, blackline masters, and teaching suggestions—all organized into a ready-to-teach unit on AIDS.

▶ **Transparencies**—over 100 full-color transparency acetates are included in the supplementary material. These are referenced in your teacher's edition to help you know when and where to use them.

Videos

The *Health: Making Life Choices* program includes videos on various topics. The video library makes a variety of titles available at greatly reduced prices. These titles will change as new topics and new videos become available.

Nutrition Laserdisc

The Nutrition laserdisc accompanying *Health: Making Life Choices* contains a wealth of material related to the nutrition and weight control chapters. Included on this disc are live action videos from CNN.

Diet Analysis Software

The Diet Analysis software is available for IBM PCs and Macintosh computers. Students use this software program to analyze their diets. After filling out a food recall form, students go through the step-by-step program to analyze their intakes of major nutrients. Results are printed out and the students can analyze the nutritional content of several days intake of as many as 30 foods for each day. Percentages of RDA, calories, fats, proteins, carbohydrates, vitamins and minerals for the individual are provided. There is also an exercise option that allows students to enter type and duration of exercise so that the program can alter the personal RDA recommendations accordingly.

Computerized Testing Software

This computerized testing software is available for the IBM PC, compatibles, and Macintosh, and includes all of the questions contained on the printed chapter tests in the supplementary material. The program allows you to create, edit, store, and print your own individual tests.

CNN Health and Fitness Update Videos

These exciting video updates consist of 15 to 20 short segments covering the most important news stories in the areas of health and fitness as covered by one of the world's leading news agencies, CNN. For each video segment you will find corresponding teaching material, which includes questions and teaching suggestions to help you prepare for and follow up on each segment.

Nutrition Interactive CD-ROM

This interactive multi-media experience lets your students explore nutrition concepts as never before. With *Nutrition Interactive*, your students will do more than just read about a topic—they will interact, watch, listen, and react to it! *Nutrition Interactive* is a multimedia tool that will excite your students' curiosity and desire to learn.

Student Review Software

This easy-to-use software contains hundreds of questions correlated to the text chapters. True/false, multiple-choice, and short answer questions challenge your students' knowledge, helping them prepare for chapter tests.

Multicultural Considerations in Teaching Health

. . . Among the Wodaabe of Niger, mothers are not allowed to speak directly to their first or second born children, and except for nursing, they aren't allowed to touch them. The grandmothers and aunts take care of these children. The Wodaabe feel that this child-rearing practice emphasizes loyalties throughout the entire clan.

. . . In years past, Chinese parents often adopted an infant girl to marry their son. They raised the girl, training her themselves so she would be more agreeable to them and more compatible with other members of the family. This custom is still practiced today in Taiwan.

. . . It is fairly common in the Middle East for a man to marry one of his father's brother's daughters.

The first sentence in Section 1 of *Health: Making Life Choices* says that "You make hundreds of choices every day—what to eat, whom to be with, how active to be, when to sleep, and more." This sentence introduces the major theme of the text—that each person is responsible for his or her own health and wellness and that each individual makes lifestyle choices that will determine to a great extent that person's level of health and wellness throughout life.

How your students make their choices will be deeply affected by their cultures, which may have been influenced by those as diverse as the ones described at the beginning of this essay. Even if two students were the same in every way—age, maturity level, personality, intelligence, etc.—and even if these two students read *Health: Making Life Choices* and tried to implement its strategies with equal enthusiasm and commitment, these two students would make very different choices in their lives if they came from different cultural backgrounds. Their most fundamental choices—the foods they eat, their friends, their social activities, their mates, and their values—would differ considerably because of their different cultures.

The fact that culture exerts a powerful influence on an individual's thoughts, motives, feelings, and behaviors is obviously something of which you are well aware. The problem that may not be as immediately obvious is how this awareness can and should affect the ways in which you teach your health course. The answer to this question will depend on many factors, including the cultural backgrounds of your students, your own personal beliefs as to the importance of broadening the cultural awareness of all your students, the resources you have available, and the amount of time that you can devote to multicultural issues.

For the most part, the content of *Health: Making Life Choices* is acultural—the information presented is scientific in nature and the strategies presented may be used by people of all cultures and races. Information about the drugs of abuse, alcohol, and tobacco, for example, and recommendations for the use or non-use of these substances is accurate and useful for all people, regardless of their culture. Certain topics, however, such as the emotional health issues discussed in Chapter 2 and the social behaviors discussed in Chapter 18 "Pairing, Commitment, and Marriage" could be treated differently if approached from different cultural perspectives. Unfortunately, the wide range of topics covered in today's typical health course make it impossible for the authors of any high school health textbook to deal with the different cultural aspects of the individual topics in the depth required to make the discussions meaningful and useful for students.

Of course you need to be aware of the fact the students may respond differently to different activities as a result of their cultural background. For example, suppose you were to try an exercise such as the following as you taught sections on self-knowledge and self-awareness in Chapter 2. Let's say that you asked the students to write 20 different statements in response to the question, "Who am I?" If, after students finished, you had them count the number of entries that related to a social identity, such as family ("I am a son/daughter"), religion ("I am a Roman Catholic"), or a group to which they belong ("I am a member of the basketball team"); and then you had them count the number of entries that related to individual characteristics ("I am intelligent" or "I am bashful"); the exercise would tend to evoke different patterns of response based on the respondent's dominant culture. People from individualistic cultures such as the United States and Canada would be more likely to define their self-identities primarily in terms of individual traits rather than in terms of social groups. In contrast, students who had grown up in collectivist societies such as in Japan and China, would be more likely to define their self-identities in terms of the social entities to which they belong. An example such as the one above makes it clear how important it is for today's teachers, especially those in areas serving students from a variety of cultures, to learn more about the cultures of the students they teach. The following reading list is by no means a comprehensive list of multicultural readings, but it does provide you with beginning sources in your attempt to become more knowledgeable about different cultures and how they might be dealt with in the classroom. It also provides some resources for materials that you could use in implementing multicultural education in your classroom.

Although the amount of material that must be covered in a one-semester health course does not allow time for examination of different cultural perspectives on health in the main body of content, the *Health: Making Life Choices* Teacher's Edition, does provide you with suggestions for supporting the student text in terms of multicultural issues. You will also find in your supplementary package several enrichment lessons, the purpose of which is to give all students a sampling of the health attitudes and practices from many different cultures. As time permits, distribution of these enrichment lessons will allow you to broaden your students' understanding of other cultures and thereby hopefully increase their tolerance of peoples of different colors and cultures so that tomorrow's world will be a more peaceful, harmonious world for all people.

Readings and Resources for Multicultural Education

Acuña, Rodolpho. *Occupied America: A History of Chicanos.* Glenview, IL: Harper Collins Publishers.

Allen, P. G. (1986). *The Sacred Hoop: Recovering the Feminine in American Indian Traditions.* Beacon Press.

American Ethnological Society, 1703 New Hampshire Ave. N.W., Washington, D.C. 20009.

Aptheker, H. (1973). *The Education of Black People: Ten Critiques, 1906-1960* by W. E. B. DuBois. New York: Monthly Review Press.

Asante, Molefi Kete. *The Afrocentric Idea.*

Asante, Molefi Kete. *Kemet Afrocentricity, and Knowledge.*

Banks, J. A. (1989). *Multicultural Education: Issues and Perspectives.* Boston, Mass.: Allyn and Bacon.

Banks, J. A. (1988). *Multiethnic Education: Theory and Practice.* 2nd ed. Newton, Mass.: Allyn and Bacon, Inc.

Banks, J. A. (1991). *Teaching Strategies for Ethnic Studies,* 5th ed. Boston: Allyn and Bacon.

Baringer, F. (February 4, 1990). "Africa's Claim to Egypt's History Grows More Insistent, " *New York Times,* p. 6E.

Barzun, J. (1965). *Race: A Study in Superstition.* New York: Harper.

Beard, M. R. (1972). *Women as Force in History.* New York: Collier Books.

Belenky, M., B. Clinchy, B. Goldberger, and N. Tarule. (1986) *Women's Ways of Knowing.* New York: Basic Books.

Benedict, R. (1959). *Race: Science and Politics.* New York: Viking.

Bernal, M. (1987). *The Afroasiatic Roots of Classical Civilization,* Vol.1: *The Fabrication of Ancient Greece 1785-1985.* London: Free Association Books.

Biddis, M. D. (1970). *Father of Racist Ideology: The Social and Political Thought of Count Gobineau.* New York: Weinright and Talley.

Brock-Utne, B. (1985). *Educating for Peace: A Feminist Perspective.* New York and Oxford: Pergamon Press.

Carlson, L. H. and Colburn, G. A. (1972). *In Their Place: White America Defines Her Minorities, 1850-1950.* New York: John Wiley and Sons.

Chase, A. (1977). *The Legacy of Malthus: The Social Costs of the New Scientific Racism.* New York: Alfred A. Knopf.

Clarke, J. H. (1990). "African People on My Mind." In *Infusion of African and African American Content in the School Curriculum: Proceedings of the First National Conference,* edited by A. G. Hilliard III, L. PaytonStewart, and L. 0. Williams, Morristown, N.J.: Aaron Press.

The Commission on Minority Participation in Education and American Life. (May 1988). *One-Third of a Nation.* Washington, D.C.: The American Council on Education.

Common Bonds: Anti-Bias Teaching in a Diverse Society. Wheaton: MD. Association for Childhood Educational International.

Cultural Survival, 11 Divinity Ave., Cambridge, Mass. 02138.

DeMott, Benjamin. (1990). *The Imperial Middle: Why Americans Can't Think Straight about Class.*

DePalma, A. (May 19, 1991). "Ethnic Diversity Brings Separate Worlds." *Montgomery Advertiser* (quotes Ernest L. Boyer).

D'Souza, D. (1991). *Illiberal Education: The Politics of Race and Sex on Campus.* New York: The Free Press.

Donald Duk. Minneapolis: Coffee House Press. A novel for young adults that explores Chinese culture from viewpoint of Chinese-American.

Downing, T. E., and G. Kusher, eds. (1988). *Human Rights and Anthropology.* Cambridge, Mass.: Cultural Survival, pp.21-26.

Drake, St. C. (1987). *Black Folk Here and There.* Vol. l. Los Angeles: Center for Afro-American Studies, University of California.

DuBois, W. E. B. (1969). *The Souls of Black Folk.* New York: Signet. (First published 1903).

Edelman, M. (1992). *The Measure of Our Success.* Boston: Beacon Press.

Elshtain, J. B. (1987). *Women and War.* New York: Basic Books.

"Everyone's Kids Books Newsletter" (71 Elliot St., Brattleboro, VT, 05301).

Gossett, T. F. (1973). *Race: The History of an Idea in America.* New York: Schoken.

Gould, S. J. (1981). *The Mismeasure of Man.* New York: W. W. Norton.

Grant, M. (1924). *The Passing of the Great Race: Or, The Racial Basis of European History.* New York: Charles Scribner's Sons.

Gray, P. (July 8, 1991). "Whose America?" *Time* 138:13-17.

Greene, M. (1988). *The Dialectic of Freedom.* New York: Teachers College Press.

Grumet, M. R. (1988). *Bitter Milk.* Amherst: University of Massachusetts Press.

Hall, E. T. (1981). *Beyond Culture.* Garden City, N.Y.: Anchor Press/ Doubleday.

Henry, J. (1965). *Culture Against Man.* N.Y.: Random House.

Hilliard, A. (1976). "Alternatives to IQ Testing: An Approach to the Identification of Gifted Minority Children." *Final Report to the California State Department of Education.*

Hilliard, A., and C. Leonard. (eds). (1990). *African American Baseline Essays.* Portland, Or.: Portland Public Schools, revised 1990.

Hilliard, A. G. III, L. Patyon-Stewart, and L. Obadele. (1990). *The Infusion of African and African American Content in the School Curriculum.* Morristown, N.J.: Aaron Press.

Hirsch, E. D. (1987). *Cultural Literacy: What Every American Needs to Know.* Boston: Houghton Mifflin. Howe, l. (February 18, 1991). "The Value of the Canon." *The New Republic*: 40-44.

Jones, S. M. (1972). "The Schlesingers on Black History," *PHYLON: The Atlanta University Review of Race and Culture* 33, 2:104-1 11.

Kamin, K. (1974). *The Science and Politics of I.Q.* Potomac, Md.: Lawrence Erlbaum Associates.

Keita, S. (1990). "Studies in Ancient African Crania." In *American Journal of Physical Anthopology* 83: 35-48, 1990.

Kinnear, M. (1982). *Daughters of Time: Women in the Western Tradition.* Ann Arbor: University of Michigan Press.

Kohn, A. (1986). *No Contest: The Case Against Competition.* Boston: Houghton Mifflin.

Lee, C. C. "Cultural Dynamics." In *Multicultural Issues in Counseling.* Alexandria, VA: American Association of Counseling and Development.

Marriott, M. (August 11, 1991). "As a Discipline Advances, Questions Arise on Scholarship." *The New York Times.*

Martel, E. (Spring 1991). "Teacher's Corner: Ancient Africa and the Portland Curriculum Resource. "*Anthro Notes: National Museum of Natural History* (Smithsonian) Bulletin for Teachers 13,2.

Martin, J. R. (1984). "Bringing Women into Educational Thought." *Educational Theory* 4, 34:341-354.

Minority Rights Group, 29 Craven St., London VC2N 5N5, England.

Montague, A. (1968). *The Concept of the Primitive.* New York: Collier-Macmillan.

"Multicultural Books for Children" (newsletter), The Boston Globe. P.O. Box 2378, Boston, MA 02107-2378.

Murray, N. (January/February 1991). "Is the Playing Field Really Level?" *Rethinking Schools*: 7. National Afrocentric Institute, Temple University, Philadelphia, PA 19122

The National SEED Project Center for Research on Women, Wellesley College, Wellesley, MA 02181

Nelson, L., and S. Kagan. (September 1972). "Competition—The Star Spangled Scramble." *Psychology Today* 53, 6:90-91.

Noddings, N. (1984). *Caring: A Feminine Approach to Ethics and Moral Education.* Berkeley: University of California Press.

Our Family, Our Friends, Our World: An Annotated Guide to Significant Multicultural Books for Children and Teenagers. New Providence, NJ: R. R. Bowker Co.

Pallas, A. M., G. Natriello, E. L. McDill. (June-July 1989). "The Changing Nature of the Disadvantaged Population: Current Dimensions and Future Trends." *Educational Researcher* 18, 2: 2.

Parekh, B. (1986). "The Concept of Multi-Cultural Education.", In *Multicultural Education: The Interminable Debate*, edited by S. Modgil, G. K. Verma, K. Mallick, and C. Modgil. Philadelphia: The Falmer Press, pp.19-31.

Pardo, W., B. S. Adams, and N. Schniedewind. (1988). "A Systemwide Program In Human Rights Education." *Educational Leadership* 45, 8: 48-50.

Parker, W. P. (1991). "Multicultural Education in Democratic Societies." Paper presented at the annual meeting of the American Educational Research Association, Chicago.

Rossiter, M. W. (1982). *Women Scientists in America: Struggles and Strategies to 1940.* Baltimore and London: Johns Hopkins University Press.

Ruddick, 5. (1989). *Maternal Thinking: Towards a Politics of Peace.* Boston: Beacon Press.

Schniedewind, N., and E. Davidson. (1983). *Open Minds To Equality: A Sourcebook of Learning Activities To Promote Race, Sex, Class, and Age Equity.* Englewood Cliffs, N.J.: Prentice Hall.

Schniedewind, N., and E. Davidson. (1987). *Cooperative Learning, Cooperative Lives: A Sourcebook of Learning Activities for Building a Peaceful World.* Dubuque, Iowa: W. C. Brown.

Schwartz, B. N. and R. Disch. (1970). *White Racism: Its History, Pathology, Practice.* New York: Dell.

Serfontein, J. H. P. (1978). *Brotherhood of Power: An Exposé of the Secret Afrikaner Broederbond.* Bloomington, Indiana: Indiana University Press.

Sertima, I. V., ed. (1984). (Ed). *Black Women in Antiquity.* New Brunswick, N.J.: Transaction Books.

Service, Elman. *Profiles in Ethnology.* Harper & Row, 1978.

Sherritt, C. (1990). "What Not to Do in the Name of Multiculturalism." *Contemporary Education* 61, 4:215-216.

Sirkin, G. (January 18, 1990). "The Multiculturalists Strike Again." *The Wall Street Journal,* p. A14.

Sleeter, C. (1991). *Empowerment Through Multicultural Education.* Albany: S.U.N.Y. Press.

Sleeter, C. E. (September 1990). "Staff Development for Desegregated Schooling." *Kappan*: 33-40.

Smith, P. (1970). *Daughters of the Promised Land.* Boston and Toronto: Little, Brown.

Stanton, W. (1960). *The Leopard's Spots: Scientific Attitudes Toward Race in America 1915-1959.* Chicago: University of Chicago Press.

Steele, S. (February 1989). "The Recoloring of Campus Life." *Harpers Magazine*: 47-55.

Stoddard, L. (1971). *The Rising Tide of Color Against White World Supremacy.* Westport, Conn.: Negro University Press. (First Published 1920).

Stotsky, S., P. Anderson, with D. Beierl. (Fall 1990). "Variety and Individualism in the English Class: Teacher-Recommended Lists of Reading for Grades 7-12." Pull-out section in *The Leaflet* 89, 3:1-11.

Sue, D., and Sue, D. W. *Counseling the Culturally Different: Theory and Practice.* New York: Wiley.

Takaki, Ronald. *Strangers from a Different Shore: A History of Asian-Americans.* New York: Penguin USA.

Teaching Tolerance, 400 Washington Ave., Montgomery, Alabama 36104, 1-205-264-0286. Publish a free semi-annual magazine that provides educators with ideas, resources, and techniques for teaching tolerance in a diverse society.

Teacher's Resource Guide: North American Indians. Anthropology Outreach & Public Information. National Museum of Natural History, Smithsonian Institution, Washington D.C. 20560.

Tetreault, M. K. (1986). "The Journey from Male-Defined to Gender-Balanced Education." *Theory Into Practice* 25: 227-234.

UNESCO. (1981). *General History of Africa.* Berkeley: University of California Press.

Van Sertima, I. (1976). *They Came Before Columbus.* New York: Random House.

Weatherford, J. (1988). *Indian Givers: How the Indians of the Americas Transformed the World.* New York: Fawcett Columbine.

Wilson, W. J. (1987). *The Truly Disadvantaged: The Inner City, the Underclass, and Public Policy.* Chicago: the University of Chicago Press.

Woodson, C. G. (1933). *The Miseducation of the Negro.* Washington, D.C.: Associated Publishers.

Yurco, F. (March 1991). "An Evaluation of the Portland Social Studies Baseline Essay." *Network News and Views* 10,25.

Yurco, F. (Sept.-Oct. 1989). 'Were the Ancient Egyptians Black or White?" *Biblical Archaeological Review* 15, 5:24.

SQ3R Study Method

The reading and study technique known as the **SQ3R method**, which has been acknowledged by educators for years as one of the most effective ways to improve student comprehension and retention is explained here. SQ3R stands for the five study steps of *survey, question, read, recite,* and *review.*

S = **Survey**—Students will get an overall idea of what a chapter is about by skimming through the chapter before reading it. Encourage students to read the introduction and look at the opening photograph for an idea of what the chapter is about. Also have students focus on chapter headings, pictures and illustration captions throughout the chapter before they begin reading the chapter. This step alone will improve comprehension.

Q = **Question**—Too often students fail to focus on the key concepts of the passages they are reading. Turning each topic heading into one or more questions will help them focus on the most important concepts.

R1 = Read—The first R in SQ3R refers to *read.* Students should read short sections, from one topic heading to the next, trying to understand the information presented.

R2 = Recite—The second R stands for *recite.* When students have finished reading a section, they should silently *recite* what they have learned. There's no point in going on until students understand and remember what they've already read. The "question-read-recite" cycle should be repeated for each heading throughout the chapter.

R3 = Review—When students have finished reading they should skim over the chapter again, questioning and quizzing themselves and reciting answers as they go. Use the Chapter Review at the end of the chapter to further help your students review.

Resource List

Chapter 1

*University of California Berkeley
Wellness Newsletter*
11 Commerce Boulevard
Palm Coast, FL 32142
1-904-445-6414

*Harvard Health Letter,
Harvard Heart Letter,
Harvard Mental Health Letter*
164 Longwood Avenue
Boston, MA 02115
email: jphillip @ warren.med.
harvard.edu

Johns Hopkins News-Letter
Box 1230
3400 North Charles Street
Baltimore,MD 21218
Web site:
http://www.jhu.edu/newslett/info/

Mayo Clinic Health Letter
To order: 1-800-678-5747, Ext. 45

U.S. Dept. of Health and
Human Services
5600 Fishers Lane
Rockville, MD 20857
1-301-443-2403

Hall of Health
2230 Shattuck Avenue
(Lower Level)
Berkeley, CA 94704
1-510-549-1564
(tours; cosponsored by Children's
Hospital, Oakland and Alta Bates
Medical Center)

Chapter 2

National Institute of Mental Health
U.S. Dept. of Health and
Human Services
5600 Fishers Lane, Rm. 7C02
MSC8030
Bethesda, MD 20892-8030
1-301-443-4513

Emotions Anonymous International
P.O. Box 4245
St. Paul, MN 55104-0245
1-612-647-9712
Fax: 1-612-647-1593
email: eaisc@mtn.org

Human Relations Media
175 Tompkins Avenue
Pleasantville, NY 10570
1-800-431-2050

The VOC Volunteer
Opportunities Catalog
600 S. Marion Parkway
Denver, CO 80209-2597
1-303-715-1010
Fax: 1-303-715-1212
email: voc@voc.org

Chapter 3

Stepfamily Association of America
650 J Street, Suite 205
Lincoln, NE 68508
1-800-735-0329

Health Education Services
10200 Jefferson Blvd.
P.O. Box 802
Culver City, CA 90232-0802
1-310-839-2436
email: access @ socialstudies.com

Chapter 4

American Institute of Stress
124 Park Avenue
Yonkers, NY 10703
1-914-963-1200
Web site: http://www.stress.org

Chapter 5

American Anorexia and
Bulimia Assoc., Inc.
165 West 46th Street, Suite 1108
New York, NY 10036
1-212-575-6200
email: amanbu@aol.com

National Eating Disorders Org.
(NEDO)
6655 S. Yale Avenue
Tulsa, OK 74136
1-918-481-4044

Related information:
Anorexia Nervosa and Related
Eating Disorders
(ANRED)
Web site: http://www.anred.com

American Association of
Suicidology
4201 Connecticut Avenue NW,
Suite 310
Washington, DC 20008
1-202-237-2280
Web site:
http://www.cyberpsych.org/aas.htm

American Mental Health
Counselors Association
801 N. Fairfax Street, Suite 304
Alexandria, VA 22314
1-800-326-2642

American Psychiatric Association
1400 K Street NW
Washington, DC 20005
1-202-682-6000

National Assoc. of Private
Psychiatric Hospitals
1317 F Street, Suite 301
Washington, DC 20004
1-202-393-6700
Web site: http://www.naphs.org

National Association of State
Mental Health
Program Directors
66 Canal Center Plaza, Suite 302
Alexandria, VA 22314
1-703-739-9333

National Council of Community
Mental Health Centers
12300 Twinbrook Pkwy., Suite 320
Rockville, MD 20852
1-301-984-6200

National Institute of Mental Health
U.S. Dept. of Health and
Human Services
5600 Fishers Lane, Rm. 7C02
MSC8030
Bethesda, MD 20892-8030
1-301-443-4513

National Mental Health Association
1201 Prince Street
Alexandria, VA 22314
1-800-969-6642

National Association of Anorexia
Nervosa and Associated Disorders
Box 7
Highland Park, IL 60035
1-847-831-3438

Depressive and Manic
Depressive Assoc.
730 N. Franklin, Suite 501
Chicago, IL 60610
1-800-826-3632

National Foundation for
Depressive Illness
P.O. Box 2257
New York, NY 10116
1-800-248-4344

Recovery, Inc.
802 N. Dearborn Street
Chicago, IL 60610
1-312-337-5661

American Self-Help Clearinghouse
Northwest Covenant Medical Center
25 Pocono Road
Denville, NJ 07834
1-973-625-7101
Web site:
http://www.cmhc.com/selfhelp
email: ASHC @cybernex.net

Childhelp USA
National Child Abuse Hotline
1-800-4-A-CHILD

Chapter 6

American Medical Association
Dept of Health Education
515 N. State
Chicago, IL 60610
1-312-464-5000

American School Health Association
7263 State Route 43
P.O. Box 708
Kent, OH 44240
1-330-678-1601

American Association for
Health Education
1900 Association Drive
Reston, VA 22091
1-703-476-3437

Chapter 7

American Dietetic Association
216 W. Jackson Blvd.
Chicago, IL 60606-6995
1-800-877-1600

American Meat Institute (AMI)
1700 North Moore Street, Suite 1600
Arlington, VA 22209
1-703-841-2400
Fax: 1-703-527-0938

Beech-Nut Nutrition Hotline
1-800-523-6633

Consumer Nutrition Hotline of the
American Dietetic Assoc.
1-800-366-1655

U.S. Dept. of Agriculture
Information Line
Washington, DC
1-202-720-2791

Food and Drug Administration (FDA)
Office of Consumer Affairs
Consumer Inquiries Information Line
5600 Fishers Lane
Rockville, MD 20857
1-301-827-4420

Alliance for Food and Fiber's
Food Safety Hotline
1-800-266-0200

Gerber Products Company
1-800-443-7237

U.S. Dept. of Agriculture
FNCS
Food and Nutrition Service
3101 Park Center Drive
Alexandria, VA 22302
1-703-305-2276

U.S. Dept. of Agriculture
Meat and Poultry Hotline
1-800-535-4555

Nutrition Hotline of the American
Dietetic Association
1-800-366-1655

National Dairy Council
1025 Higgins Road
Rosemont, IL 60018
1-847-803-2000

World Health Organization
525 23rd Street, NW
Washington, DC 20037
1-202-974-3000

Chapter 8

Nutrition Hotline of the American
Dietetic Association
1-800-366-1655

*The Facts about Weight Loss
Products and Programs*
Weight Loss, Federal Trade
Commission
Washington, DC 20580

Federal Trade Commission (FTC)
Consumer Response Center
Washington, DC
1-202-326-2222

Overeaters Anonymous
World Service
P.O. Box 44020
Rio Rancho, NM 87174-4020
1-505-891-2664

Chapter 9

American College of
Sports Medicine
P.O. Box 1440
Indianapolis, IN 46206
1-317-637-9200

American Running and
Fitness Association
4405 East-West Highway, Suite 405
Bethesda, MD 20814
1-800-776-2732

For large selection of exercise videos:
Collage Video—1-800-433-6769 and
Fitness Wholesale—1-800-537-5512

President's Council on Physical
Fitness and Sports
Room 738H Humphrey Building.
200 Independence Avenue, SW
Washington, DC 20201
1-202-690-9000
Fax: 1-202-690-5211

U.S. Bicycle Polo Association
P.O. Box 19424
Sacramento, CA 95819-0424
1-916-739-0724
Fax: 1-916-452-7857
email: usbikepolo@ aol.com

Chapter 10

The American Medical Hair
Restoration Directory
1-800-456-8090

National Headache Foundation
1-800-843-2256

National Organization of
Mall Walkers
P.O. Box 256
Hermann, MO 65041
1-573-486-3945

Chapter 11

Food and Drug Administration (FDA)
Office of Consumer Affairs
Consumer Inquiries Information Line
5600 Fishers Lane
Rockville, MD 20857
1-301-827-4420

Chapter 12

National Drug and Alcohol
Treatment
Referral Routing Service
1-800-662-HELP

Just Say No International
1-800-258-2766

National Association on Drug
Abuse Problems
355 Lexington Avenue
New York, NY 10017
1-212-986-1170

National Clearinghouse for Alcohol
and Drug Information
P.O. Box 2345
Rockville, MD 20847-2345
1-800-729-6686

National Helpline – Drugs
1-800-COC-AINE
National Drug and Alcohol
Treatment
Referral Routing Service
1-800-662-HELP

Chapter 13

Al-Anon World Service Office
1600 Corporate Landing Parkway
Virginia Beach, VA 23454
1-757-563-1600
1-800-344-2666
Fax: 1-757-563-1655

Alcohol and Drug Helpline
1-800-821-4357

Substance Abuse and
Mental Health Services Admin.
Info. Line
U.S. Dept. of Health and
Human Services
5600 Fishers Lane
Rockville, MD 20857
1-301-443-3783

Alcoholics Anonymous
General Services Office
Box 459, Grand Central Station
New York, NY 10163
1-212-870-3400

Covenant House "9-Line"
1-800-999-9999

National Council on Alcoholism and
Drug Dependence
New York, NY
1-800-NCA-CALL

Chapter 14

American Lung Association
1740 Broadway
New York, NY 10019
1-212-315-8700

Americans for Nonsmokers' Rights
2530 San Pablo Avenue, Suite J
Berkeley, CA 97402
1-510-841-3032

Centers for Disease Control
and Prevention
1600 Clifton Road, NE
Atlanta, GA 30333
1-404-639-3311

Tobacco Institute
1875 I Street, NW
Washington, DC 20006
1-202-457-4800

Chapter 15

American Medical Association
515 N. State Street
Chicago, IL 60610
1-312-464-5000

Centers for Disease Control
International Travelers Hotline
1-404-332-4555

National Foundation for
Infectious Diseases
4733 Bethesda Avenue, #750
Bethesda, MD 20814
1-301-656-0003

HIV/AIDS Treatment Information
Service 1-800-TRIALS-A

National Kidney Foundation
1-800-622-9010

Chapter 16

AIDS Action
1875 Connecticut Avenue NW,
Suite 700
Washington, DC 20009
1-202-986-1300
Fax: 1-202-986-1345

National AIDS Hotline
1-800-342-AIDS

AIDS Reference Guide
1100 17th Street NW, Suite 300
Washington, DC 20036
1-202-775-9008

American Foundation for
AIDS Research (AmFAR)
121 Wall Street, 13th Floor
New York, NY 10005
1-212-806-1600
and
American Foundation for
AIDS Research (AmFAR)
5900 Wilshire Blvd., 2nd Floor—
East Satellite
Los Angeles, CA 90036
1-213-857-5900

American Social Health Association
(Information on sexually-
transmitted diseases, etc.)
Web site:
http://sunsite.unc.edu/ASHA/

National Association of People
with AIDS
1413 K Street NW
Washington, DC 20005
1-202-898-0414

San Francisco AIDS Foundation
10 United Nations Plaza
San Francisco, CA 94102
1-415-487-3000

National Hemophilia Foundation
116 West 32nd Street, 11th floor
New York, NY 10001
1-212-328-3700

World Health Organization
525 23rd Street, NW
Washington, DC 20037
1-202-974-3000

Chapter 17

American Diabetes Association
1660 Duke Street
Alexandria, VA 22314
1-800-232-3472
1-703-549-1500

American Heart Association
7272 Greenville Avenue
Dallas, TX 75231-4596
1-214-373-6300

American Heart Association
Local Chapter: 1-800-242-8721

National Stroke Association
1-800-787-6537

High Blood Pressure Information
from the American Heart Assoc.
Website:
http://www.amhrt.org/Heart_and_St
roke_A_Z_Guide/hbp.html

National Cancer Information Center
of the American Cancer Society
P.O. Box 142302
Austin, TX 78714-2302
1-800-AC5-2345

American Cancer Society
Cancer Information and
Patient Services
2200 Lake Blvd.
Atlanta, GA 30319
1-404-816-4994

The Susan G. Komen Breast
Cancer Foundation
P.O. Box 97100
Dallas, TX 75397
1-800-IM-AWARE (1-800-462-9273)

National Alliance of Breast Cancer
Organizations (NABCO)
Information Services Department
9 East 37th Street, 10th floor
New York, NY 10016
1-888-806-2226 (toll-free)
email: nabcoinfo@aol.com

National Cancer Institute
Cancer Information Service
1-800-4-CANCER

National Cancer Association
1-800-601-9242

Chapter 18

Ask Dr. Gayle
Web site: http://www.parentsplace.
com/cgi-bin/objects/family/

Chapter 19

National Child Abuse Hotline
1-800-422-4453

National Council on Family Relations
3989 Central Avenue NE, Suite 550
Minneapolis, MN 55421
1-888-781-9331 (toll free)

Chapter 20

Child Care Information Service
National Association for the
Education of Young Children
(NAEYC)
1509 16th Street NW
Washington, DC 20036
1-800-424-2460

National Institute of Child Health and Human Development
Bldg. 31, Room 2A32
31 Center Drive, Mail Stop 2425
Bethesda, MD 20892
1-301-496-5133

Beech-Nut Nutrition Hotline
1-800-523-6633

Gerber Products Co.
1-800-443-7237

Chapter 23

Alzheimer's Disease and Related Disorders
Information and Referral Service
919 N. Michigan Avenue
Chicago,IL 60611
1-800-272-3900

American Association of
Retired Persons
601 E Street NW
Washington, DC 20049
1-202-434-2277

National Council on the Aging
409 Third Street SW, Suite 200
Washington, DC 20024
1-202-479-1200

National Hospice Organization
1901 N. Moore Street
Arlington, VA 22209
1-703-243-5900

National Osteoporosis Foundation
Washington, DC
1-202-223-2226

Chapter 24

National Capitol Poison Center
3201 New Mexico Avenue NW,
Suite 310
Washington, DC 20016
1-202-625-3333

National Safety Council
3300 N E Expressway, Suite 7A
Atlanta, GA 30341
1-800-441-5103

Chapter 25

The Alliance for Food and Fiber's
Food Safety Hotline
1-800-266-0200

American Red Cross
National Headquarters
202-737-8300

Chapter 26

U.S. Gov't. Consumer
Information Center
Pueblo, CO 81009
1-719-948-3334

EarthShare
1-800-488-8887

U.S. Environmental
Protection Agency
401 M Street SW
Washington, DC 20460
1-202-260-4600

Freedom from Hunger
P.O. Box 2000
1644 DaVinci Ct.
Davis, CA 95617
1-916-758-6200

Habitat for Humanity International
322 W. Lamar
Americus, GA 31709
1-912-924-6935

Kids for a Cleaner Environment
(Kids F.A.C.E.)
P.O. Box 158254
Nashville, TN 37215
1-800-952-3223

National Pesticide
Telecommunications
Network Hotline
1-800-858-PEST

U.S. Environmental
Protection Agency
Safe Drinking Water Hotline
1-800-426-4791

Chapter 27

CARE
650 First Avenue, 2nd floor
NewYork, NY 10016
1-212-686-3110

U.S. Gov't. Consumer
Information Center
Pueblo, CO 81009
1-719-948-3334

The U.S. Consumer Product
Safety Commission
1-800-638-CPSC

Consumers Union
101 Truman Avenue
Yonkers, NY 10703-1057
1-914-378-2000

Federal Trade Commission (FTC)
Consumer Response Center
Washington, DC
1-202-326-2222

National Council Against Health
Fraud, Inc.
P.O. Box 1276
Loma Linda, CA 92354
1-909-824-4690

Expanded Edition

HEALTH

Making Life Choices

Second Edition

Expanded Edition

HEALTH

Making Life Choices

Second Edition

Frances
Sizer
Webb

•

Eleanor
Noss
Whitney

•

Linda
Kelly
DeBruyne

Contributing Authors
*The Section Review and Chapter Review exercises
were written by high school teachers:*

Patricia Kosiba
P.D. Schreiber High School
Port Washington, New York

Rhonda Helgerson
Del Rio High School
Del Rio, Texas

National Textbook Company
a division of NTC/CONTEMPORARY PUBLISHING GROUP
NTC   Lincolnwood, Illinois USA

Production Credits

Editors	Lynda Kessler, Pam Starkey
Photo Research	Jan Seidel
Production Editor	Mario M. Rodriguez
Permissions	Elaine Arthur
Illustrators	Randy Miyake, Miyake Illustration; Matthew Thiessen; Precision Graphics
Copyediting	Mary Berry
Composition	Parkwood Composition Service, Inc.
Index	Jane Hilken
Cover design	Mario M. Rodriguez
Cover photos	The Stock Market
Proofreader	Bette Holzer, Carol Maurer
Prepress services	Clarinda Company

About the Authors

Frances Sizer Webb, MS, RD, FADA, received an Associate of Arts in Nursing from Miami-Dade Community college in 1977; she attended Florida State University's College of Human Sciences where, in 1980, she received her BS, and in 1982, her MS in nutrition. She has counseled clients in the University's stress-reduction clinic and served as consultant to schools and alcoholism programs in Florida. She coauthors the textbooks *Nutrition: Concepts and Controversies,* now entering its eighth edition; *Life Choices: Health Concepts and Strategies; Essential Life Choices;* and *The Fitness Triad: Motivation, Training, and Nutrition.* She has published in *Shape* magazine, in the health newsletter *Healthline,* and in the *Journal of Chemical Senses.* She is a member of the American School Health Association. She is vice-president and a founding member of Nutrition and Health Associates, an information resource center in Tallahassee, Florida, where she devotes full time to studying and writing on topics in health and nutrition.

Eleanor Noss Whitney, Ph.D. received her bachelor's degree in biology from Harvard University in 1960 and her doctoral degree in biology from Washington University in 1970. She taught biology and nutrition at Washington University, Florida A & M University, and Florida State University; taught community classes and workshops in weight control, stress-reduction, and addiction recovery; and served as counselor for people recovering from alcoholism until 1993. She now devotes full time to research, writing, and consulting in nutrition, health, and environmental health. As cofounder of Nutrition and Health Associates, she authors and coauthors numerous textbooks on nutrition, health, and environmental topics. She is the founder of an environmental education foundation, and a member of and contributor to many environmental organizations including the Union of Concerned Scientists, the National Resources Defense Council, the Nature Conservancy, the Worldwatch Institute, and Zero Population Growth.

Linda Kelly DeBruyne, MS, RD, received her BS in 1980 and her MS in 1982 in nutrition and food science at the Florida State University. She is also a founding member of Nutrition and Health Associates, where her speciality areas are fitness and life-cycle nutrition. Her other textbooks are *Life Span Nutrition: Conception through Life; The Fitness Triad: Motivation, Training, and Nutrition; Nutrition for Health and Healthcare* and *Nutrition and Diet Therapy.* She also serves as consultant to a group of Tallahassee pediatricians for whom she teaches infant nutrition classes to parents. She is a member of the American Dietetic Association and the American Alliance for Health, Physical Education, Recreation and Dance.

Dedication

To families everywhere—may our nation support them as it rests upon their shoulders. And to Philip, mon mari, for the nurturing love and guidance that you lavish on our own family.

—Fran

To my beautiful grandchildren: Max, Zoey, Emily, and Rebecca. And to everyone else's grandchildren, too.

—Ellie

To my husband, Tom, and our sons, Zachary and Tyler, with love and gratitude for the happiness they bring me.

—Linda

Acknowledgments

To our partner Sharon Rolfes, thanks for her support in many ways. To Pam Schmidt, for her excellent manuscript help and generous sharing of her educational expertise. Our families receive our deepest gratitude for their support throughout this project. We are grateful for the teenagers, especially Amanda Webb, Spencer Webb, and Zak DeBruyne, who inspired us with their questioning minds. We thank our editors, Bob Cassel, Mario Rodriguez, Jan Seidel, Lynda Kessler, and all of their associates. Many thanks go to Caroline Ann Sizer for her work on the first edition of *Making Life Choices.* Special thanks to Drs. Tara Wah and Paige Harbough, for their generous and helpful reviews of chapters concerning reproduction and first aid. Thanks also to Jeff Herring for reviewing the family chapter. We also appreciate the efforts of all our reviewers.

Second Edition Reviewers

Joel R. Barton, III, Ph.D.
Lamar University
Beaumont, TX

Terry Collins
Oxnard High School
Oxnard, California

Charlene Cook
Goshen High School
Goshen, IN

Sue Couch, Ed.D.
Texas Tech University
Lubbock, Texas

Marge Danielson, M.S., MFCC
Thousand Oaks, California

Joleen Eiklenborg
Education Service Center
Waco, TX

Lillian Goodman, R.N., M.Ed.
Consultant: Health Occupations
Education Div. of Adult and
Career Ed., Los Angeles Unified
School District, California

Paige Harbough, M.D.
Tallahassee, Florida

Dee Herman
Northside High School
Fort Wayne, Indiana

Jeff Herring, M.S., LMFT
Tallahassee, Florida

Dr. Gay James
Southwest Texas State University
San Marcos, TX

Elaine Jones
Kenwood Academy
Chicago, Illinois

Tim McCormick
Wheeling Park High School
Wheeling, WV

Judith McGuire
Boone County High School
Florence, Kentucky

Ron Meurer
West Mesa High School
Albuquerque, New Mexico

Timothy Mitchell
Bellaire High School
Bellaire, Texas

Betzy Nelson
Orange Park High School
Orange Park, FL

Kathleen Schaefer
Gates Chili High School
Rochester, NY

Dr. Roger Shipley
Texas Woman's University
Denton, TX

Elaine Stover, M.A.
Family Counselor
Thousand Oaks, California

Linda Troolin
East High School
Duluth, MN

Lori Turner
Northport, AL

Tara Wah, M.D.
Tallahassee, Florida

Connie Wood
Orange Park High School
Orange Park, FL

Jim Wussow
Health Coordinator/Plano ISD
Plano, TX

First Edition Reviewers

Cheryl Bower
Newberg High School
Newberg, Oregon

William K. Brookes
(Technical Review)
Florida

Deneise Crace
Meridian High School
Meridian, Idaho

Paul Dean
Pine Bluff High School
Pine Bluff, Arkansas

Thomas Dolde
Connellsville Area High School
Connellsville, Pennsylvania

Rick Ford
Carter High School
Strawberry Plains, Tennessee

Ira Gibel
Oceanside High School
Oceanside, New York

Rhonda Helgerson
Del Rio High School
Del Rio, Texas

Nancy Kidd
Oshkosh North High School
Oshkosh, Wisconsin

Patricia Kosiba
P.D. Schreiber High School
Port Washington, New York

Roxanna Laycox
West Carrollton High School
West Carrollton, Ohio

Charles Lee Libby
East Central High School
San Antonio, Texas

John Markham
Northbrook High School
Houston, Texas

Carol Martin
Pekin Community High School
Pekin, Illinois

Sandy Mayon
Robert E. Lee High School
Baytown, Texas

Bruce Miller
Heritage High School
Broadlands, Illinois

Betzy Nelson
Orange Park High School
Orange Park, Florida

Peter Olson
South Carroll High School
Sykesville, Maryland

Don Rogers
Richmond High School
Richmond, Indiana

Michael Smith
Wilson High School
Long Beach, California

Marlene Snyder
Sharon High School
Sharon, Pennsylvania

Steven Sykes
Harrison Central High School
Gulfport, Mississippi

Ron Topolinski
(Technical Review)
California

Linda Troolin
East High School
Duluth, Minnesota

Todd Urbanek
Boswell High School
Fort Worth, Texas

Laura Van Dellen
Bell High School
Los Angeles, California

Glenda Warner
Ferncreek High School
Louisville, Kentucky

Dennis Weisz
Sioux City West High School
Sioux City, Iowa

Teen Views

We would also like to take this opportunity to thank the teachers and principals at the high schools listed below who helped us obtain responses from the students who participated in the development of the Teen Views feature. Thanks also to the parents of all the teens whose responses appear in these features for giving us their consent to print their child's response. Finally, our sincere thanks to all the students who sent us their thoughtful, mature, and honest replies to the questions we posed. We regret that we didn't have space to print all the responses. We received literally hundreds of comments and found it quite difficult to choose from so many great replies. We hope that all teens benefited from this unique experience. We feel confident that these teens are representative of their peers around the country.

Connellsville High School, Connellsville, Pennsylvania

East High School, Duluth, Minnesota

Manzano High School, Albuquerque, New Mexico

Newberg High School, Newberg, Oregon

Northeastern High School, Elizabeth City, North Carolina

Orange Park High School, Orange Park, Florida

Poughkeepsie High School, Poughkeepsie, New York

South Carroll High School, Sykesville, Maryland

South High School, Fargo, North Dakota

West High School, Billings, Montana

Westside High School, Omaha, Nebraska

Wheeling Park High School, Wheeling, West Virginia

Woodrow Wilson High School, Long Beach, California

Contents in Brief

Contents

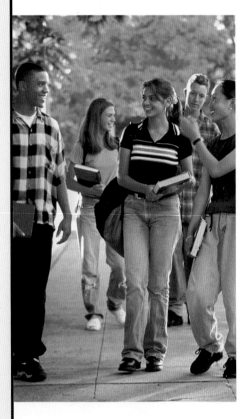

Unit 3 Your Physical Health

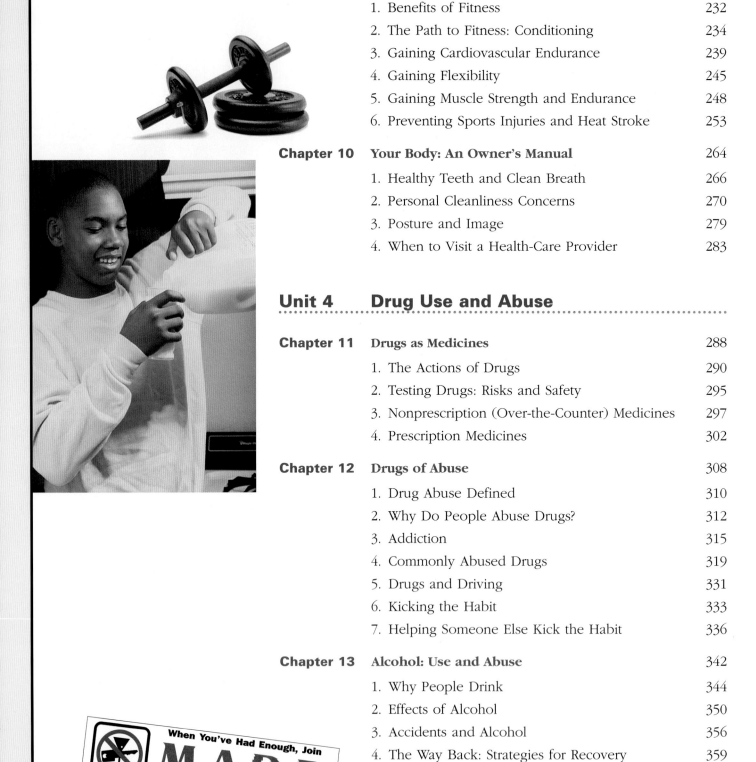

When You've Had Enough, Join

M A D D

Mothers Against Drunk Driving

Unit 7   First Aid and Safety

Life Choice Inventory

Consumer Skills

xx

Straight Talk

xxi

Teen Views

Health Strategies

Introduction

This book was written for you, the high school health student, to meet your needs for knowledge about health. As the millennium changes, a new day dawns in health education. Science has revealed that today's personal choices exert powerful influences on tomorrow's health and illness, and even on life and death. You are a member of the first generation in history to face so many choices of such lasting impact on your health. You are also among the first to be privileged with access to sound health information with which to make those choices.

Part of this book's title, *Making Life Choices,* tells you that our mission is to help you in making the choices that so deeply affect your life both today and in the future. Learning the facts about health (learning the concepts) is of first importance, but this alone is not enough. To truly benefit from your studies, you must develop ways of applying facts, (develop skills) and use them in your daily life. Therefore, this book emphasizes strategies for applying facts about health.

A note about our style: We present health concepts in a comfortable, informal style of writing, which makes concepts more easily understood. As scientists, we place a high value on accuracy, and we check and recheck our facts so that you can rely on them. Stay aware that facts change with time, and issues sometimes develop in unexpected ways.

We hold a positive attitude. Our emphasis is on what *to* do, not on what *not* to do, to gain the best quality of life. The chapters tell how to *prevent* disease, not how to cure it; how to eat well, not how to diet; how to give up destructive habits; and how to cultivate healthful habits in their place.

Some notes about the book's features: Here are the major features you can expect to find in the chapters:

▶ *Fact or Fiction* is the name of a for-fun quiz at each chapter's start that identifies and corrects common misconceptions about the topics in the chapter.

▶ *Mini Glossaries* are little glossaries that appear in the bottom corners of most right-hand pages to give you easy access to the definitions of key terms when you need them.

▶ *Key Points* follow the smaller sections within the chapters. They quickly review and reinforce the important concepts.

▶ *Life Choice Inventories* let you explore where you stand today with regard to health issues. These self-assessment questionnaires have been tested for validity in many classrooms across the nation.

▶ *Health Strategies* sections present skills and actions to help you apply the chapter material to daily life.

▶ *Consumer Skills* features can guide you in judging health information you may read or hear about, and in purchasing health products.

▶ *Teen Views* present the thoughts and opinions of teenagers in health classes across the country, written by them especially for you.

▶ *Straight Talk* sections ask and answer some interesting questions that may be on your mind about concepts related to the chapter topics.

America has seen a healthy trend toward eating right, exercising more, and making other lifestyle choices that support a better quality of life. These trends were not easily or quickly established, but resulted from the efforts of health educators, medical professionals, political figures, and consumers who demanded more health education and more health-supporting products. People's choices make trends, and it is up to you and all teens today to decide where we go from here—forward toward healthier lives, or backwards to greater risks.

We hope you enjoy learning from our book as we have enjoyed producing it. We will consider our book successful if it provides you with the knowledge you need to face today's world and to choose wisely in the years that lie ahead.

Frances S. Sizer Webb
Eleanor N. Whitney
Linda K. DeBruyne
June, 1998

Expanded Edition

HEALTH

Making Life Choices

Second Edition

OUTCOMES

CHAPTER 1

Health Choices and Behavior

- Explain the relationship between health and wellness.
- Describe how most of the lifestyle diseases of today are related to lifestyle choices.
- List the lifestyle habits that you can adopt to maximize your wellness.
- Describe how your mental, spiritual, physical, and social health are associated with wellness.
- Explain how you can use motivation to change your health behaviors.
- Define the steps in goal setting.

FEATURES

Health Strategies: Reading the News About Health (page 12)

Health Strategies: Steps to Goal Setting (page 16)

Life Choice Inventory: How Long Will You Live? (pages 8–9)

Consumer Skills: Understanding Health News (page 13)

Straight Talk: Suit Yourself (page 20)

TEACHING SUPPORT

- *Vocabulary:* Learning Key Terms, Crossword Puzzle, Fill in the Missing Term
- *Study Outline*
- *Reading Cloze*
- *Reteaching:* Lifestyle Diseases, Motivation, Wellness
- *Enrichment:* What Is Important?, Wellness Day
- *Career Briefs:* Sociologist

- *Life Choice Inventory:* How Long Will You Live?
- *Quizzes:* Sections 1–3
- *Tests:* Pre-Test, Chapter 1 Test A, Chapter 1 Test B
- *Transparencies:* Lifestyle Choices Affect Health, Invest in Learning

MULTIMEDIA SUPPORT

- Health Video Library
- CNN Health and Fitness Update Videos
- Westest
- Student Review Software
- Diet Analysis Software
- Nutrition CD-ROM

LESSON PLANNING

You will find detailed daily lesson plans for both **traditional scheduling** and **block scheduling** in your Teacher's Resource Box.

KEY POINTS

Chapter 1 is 22 pages long and divided into three sections. Briefly, this chapter introduces students to the concept of wellness and the different areas of health. It stresses the importance of the individual's daily choices in determining that person's level of wellness. It also gives students some key concepts and skills for changing their health behaviors for the better.

ACTIVITY TO INTRODUCE THE CHAPTER

This activity will serve to introduce the chapter as well as allow the students to begin getting to know each other. Follow these steps.

1. Introduce the definition of life management skills and the concept of wellness.

2. Divide the class into small discussion groups or have the students work individually on paper. Ask students:

  a. What do they expect to gain from this course? What information will help them manage their lives?

  b. How would students define wellness in their own words?

  c. What are two personal wellness goals they would each like to achieve by the end of the course?

CHAPTER
1

Contents

NOT Enough Time?

You could easily spend four or five days teaching this chapter if students read the entire chapter, do a fair number of the suggested activities in the Teacher's Wraparound Edition, and review a sampling of the worksheets from the Teacher's Resource Box accompanying this text. It is likely, however, that you will have only one or two days to devote to this chapter.

Following are some suggestions to help you make sure that you cover the key topics in this chapter if you have limited time. (Refer to the daily lesson plans in your Teacher's Resource Box for additional suggestions.)

DAY 1 Assign students to read Sections 1 and 2 prior to class. Also assign the Life Choice Inventory and the Fact or Fiction. During class have students do the Focus Activity for Section 1 on page 4 and the

Health Choices and Behavior

What do you think? Are the following statements true or false? If you think they are false, then say what is true.

1. People make hundreds of choices every day that affect their health.
2. The way adults contract most diseases is by catching them from somebody else.
3. You can make yourself physically younger or older by the ways you choose to live.
4. Accidents are among the major causes of death for teenagers.
5. To give up a harmful health habit, all you need is the motivation to do so.

(Answers on page 19)

Introduction

This book is about enjoying life. It challenges you to increase your knowledge, strengths, and skills in many areas—in emotional health, nutrition, and disease prevention, to name a few. The text aims to help you move forward in all these areas with confidence.

This is an ambitious goal, especially since everyone already has at least some experience in, and knowledge about, these subject areas. Most schoolwork ensures that people learn the basics of language and mathematics. However, people also need to learn **life management skills**, the skills people use to meet their own needs every day. If you apply yourself as you read and study this book, you can fill in important gaps in your own knowledge. You can also grow more successful at taking care of yourself.

BULLETIN BOARD IDEAS

Reproduce the Wellness Line in Figure 1–3 on page 7. Use the bulletin board as a teaching activity when studying the Wellness Line.

Answers to FACT or FICTION

1. **True.**
2. **False.** Today, most of the leading causes of death are primarily related to lifestyle, not infectious diseases.
3. **True.**
4. **True.**
5. **False.** To give up a harmful health habit, you also need commitment. It also helps to have support from others, as well as high self-esteem.

Learning with Visuals activity in Section 2 on page 12. Conclude the class with one or both of the Quick Quizzes for Section 1 (page 10) and Section 2 (page 14). You may want to assign some of the reteaching activities from the Teacher's Resource Box for those students who do not do well on the quizzes. Reteaching worksheets available in the Teacher's Resource Box include: Lifestyle Diseases, Motivation, and Wellness. The Study Outline and Reading Cloze will be of help in reteaching concepts to students.

DAY 2   Assign students to read Section 3, the Consumer Skills box on page 13, and the Straight Talk on page 20. During class do both Discussion activities on page 16, and the Interdisciplinary Activity: Creative Writing on page 18. Reproducible quizzes and two versions of the Chapter Test are available in the Teacher's Resource Box.

SECTION
1

FOCUS

OUTCOMES

In this section students will learn:

1. The correlation between wellness, life choices, and longevity.

2. Benefits of positive lifestyle choices.

FOCUS ACTIVITY

Place two sheets of poster board on the wall. Write the word *wellness* in the center of one poster board. Write the word *health* in the center of the other poster board. Circle each word.

Have students take turns writing definitions of the words on the poster boards outside the circles. Read the definitions aloud to the class.

With a bright marker, write the definitions you will be using in class inside the circles.

TEACH & APPLY

DISCUSSION

The first sentence of the introduction to Chapter 1 says "This book is about enjoying life." This sentence gives students the reason for studying and working through this health course. Ask students to list the courses they've taken in the past two years and the real-life applications for those courses. Have them do the same for health. After discussing all their reasons, direct their attention to the first sentence. Did anyone think that the personal advantages to studying health would be as broad as "enjoying life"?

SECTION
1

Wellness and Your Choices

Welcome to Life Choices

Today's Choices

✓ Exercise
✓ Relax
✓ Wear seatbelt
✓ Eat wisely
✓ Drink water
✓ Brush and floss teeth
✓ Stay smoke-free
✓ Stay alcohol-free
✓ Stay drug-free
✓ Enjoy life

You make hundreds of choices every day—what to eat, whom to be with, how active to be, when to sleep, and more. In making these daily choices, you change your **health**, whether you mean to or not. Today's choices will either improve you or harm you. Plus, their effects will multiply over time. Today's choices, repeated for a week, will have seven times the impact. Repeated every day for a year, they will have 365 times the effect on your health. Over years, the effects accumulate still further.

Today's choices affect not only your physical health, but also your **wellness**—all the characteristics that make you strong, happy, and able to function well with friends and family and in school. Consider, first, your physical health.

Physical Health Yesterday and Today

If you use the information presented in this book, you can make choices today that will improve your chances of living a long life. In the past, many children and teenagers, as well as older people, died helplessly of **infectious diseases**, such as polio and smallpox, that were poorly understood and unpreventable. Today, however, that rarely happens. Some infectious diseases do still threaten young people in our society and must be taken seriously. Their causes are known, though, and the great majority of

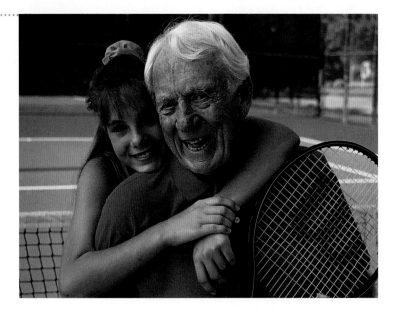

All the characteristics that make you strong, happy, and able to function well with family and friends add up to your wellness.

COOPERATIVE LEARNING

Divide the class into groups of three or four. Assign each group one of the lifestyle factors listed in the chapter. Have each group discuss and write down their views on the following.

1. What are all possible consequences to individuals who do not follow this lifestyle factor?

2. Are there any consequences that affect other people within your environment?

3. How do these consequences affect one's quality of life?
   a. Immediate effects (daily)
   b. Long-term effects (if the behavior continues for long periods of time)
   (Answers will vary but may include: Not getting enough sleep could cause difficulty staying awake during school, lower grades, long term—high levels of stress;

1890s	1990s
Flu	Heart disease
Pneumonia	Cancer
Tuberculosis	Stroke
Digestive diseases	Chronic lung disease
Bronchitis	Accidents
Scarlet fever	Pneumonia/flu
Stroke	Suicide
Kidney disease	Diabetes
	HIV infection
	Liver disease

Figure 1–1 The Leading Causes of Death. The lists to the left show, in order, the leading causes of death for the <u>whole</u> U.S. population. For <u>teenagers</u> today, accidents are the leading cause of death.

cases of these diseases are preventable. A later chapter shows how to prevent infectious diseases.

Most infectious diseases are under control today. As a result, people who are young today can expect to live longer lives than ever before. What do you want to be like when you are in your 80s? You can plan for those years now, and strive to make them a healthy, happy time of your life—or not.

Because people today are living longer than ever before, they are able to maintain better health far longer than in the past. By the same token, they are also able to harm their health more.

The daily choices that have the power to affect your health are called **lifestyle choices**. They are your choices of how to treat your body and your mind. People who consistently make poor lifestyle choices, on a daily basis, can expect to suffer from a set of diseases known as **lifestyle diseases**. These diseases include heart and lung diseases, cancer, diabetes, and liver disease. Figure 1–1 above contrasts the major causes of death 100 years ago with those today. It shows that while people used to "catch" most of their deadly diseases from disease agents ("germs"), they now are more likely to "contract" diseases because of the ways they choose to live.

When people neglect their own bodies, they become likely to suffer from lifestyle diseases. The choice to smoke, for example, is a major cause of lung disease. The choice to abuse alcohol is a major cause of liver disease. Poor choices in nutrition and physical activity can make heart disease and diabetes likely. Figure 1–2 on the next page shows that the vast majority of people affect their own health by the choices they make.

This is not to say that people who contract lung disease, liver disease, heart disease, or cancer are always solely responsible. Two causes, besides people's own choices, can bring on these diseases. One is heredity. Some people simply tend to develop certain diseases, while others do not. The other cause is factors in the environment—not only infectious disease agents but also pollution of air, water, and food.

Although you cannot avoid harmful hereditary and environmental factors, you can control them to some extent. Knowledge of your heredity can help you learn what steps to take to lessen your chances of developing diseases that run in your family. Knowing what effects your environment can

MINI Glossary

life management skills: the skills that help a person to realize his or her potential to be well and enjoy life. This book's Health Strategies sections give examples.

health: a range of states with physical, mental, emotional, spiritual, and social components. At a minimum, *health* means freedom from physical disease, poor physical condition, social maladjustment, and other negative states. At a maximum, *health* means "wellness."

wellness: maximum well-being; the top of the range of health states; the goal of the person who strives toward realizing his or her full potential physically, mentally, emotionally, spiritually, and socially.

infectious diseases: diseases that are caused by infecting organisms; they can be passed from person to person.

lifestyle choices: choices, made daily, of how to treat the body and mind. Examples are what to eat, and when to exercise.

lifestyle diseases: diseases that are made likely by neglect of the body. They cannot be passed from person to person. Examples are heart disease, cancer, and diabetes.

not getting enough exercise—reduced fitness level, not being able to physically meet the demands of daily life; smoking—bad breath, smelly clothes, long term—cancer or other respiratory diseases; using alcohol—accidents, relationship problems, long term—cirrhosis of the liver.

4. Make a list of ways in which teens can change these behaviors and what benefits they would receive if they did change their lifestyle behaviors.

Have the class share and discuss each group's answers. Students should realize that every behavior they exhibit will have positive and negative impacts on their own lives and the lives of those around them. They should realize that by following these basic lifestyle factors, they are making good decisions that will improve their level of health and their quality of life.

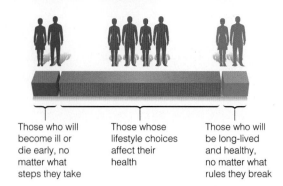

***Figure 1–2** Lifestyle Choices Made Today Affect Health in Later Life. The vast majority of people affect their health by the choices they make. Only a few people with excellent health habits have their lives cut short by disease. Only a few people who ignore all health warnings have long lives and remain healthy.*

Those who will become ill or die early, no matter what steps they take

Those whose lifestyle choices affect their health

Those who will be long-lived and healthy, no matter what rules they break

have on your health can help you decide where to live, what laws to vote for, and what causes to support.

The more you learn, the more control you can gain. Figure 1–3 on the next page shows that your wellness can exist anywhere along a line, from maximum wellness on the one end to total failure to function (death) on the other. Where would you like to be on this line? If you read the figure, you'll see that it also shows how your choices affect your position on the wellness line.

When people understand that they have some control over their health, they realize that the responsibility for their health is also theirs. People are not helpless victims of chance. They have power to change things. Furthermore, that power lies within themselves: *you* change your health. Taking responsibility lays the foundation for lifelong health. It is central to wellness, as Figure 1–4 on page 8 demonstrates.

 Deaths from diseases of the past were caused mainly by infections. Today's deaths from diseases, in contrast, are closely linked to lifestyle choices. It is possible to benefit your state of health by gathering information about positive choices and applying that information throughout life.

Age: A Matter of Definition

As fine, strong, and young as you may be, you already carry within you the older person you will become. Will that person, at 30, 60, or 90 years of age, be fine, strong, and young, too? You can choose the answer to that question and set your own goal.

Of course, chance may change your plans. Accidents or diseases may come along over which you have no control. Barring bad luck, though, you can choose your later health. In other words, you can tilt the odds in your favor, even in terms of *how old* you will be.

"Wait a minute," you may say. "When I've lived 60 years, I'll be 60 years old. No one can change *that*." That's true, but only on the calendar. Your **chronological age** after 60 years will be 60, but what about your **physiological age**?

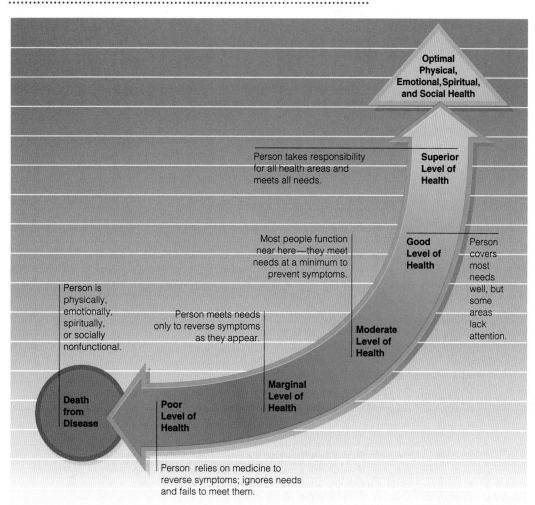

Figure 1–3 The Wellness Line—How Well Do You Meet Your Needs? This arrow points in both directions to form a continuum. This means that no matter how well you maintain your health today, you may still be able to improve tomorrow. Likewise, a person who is well today can slip down the scale in the future by failing to maintain health-promoting habits.

MINI Glossary

chronological age: age as measured in years from date of birth.

physiological age: age as estimated from the body's health and probable life expectancy.

Two scientists have shown that people can dramatically alter the age they seem to be. These scientists studied nearly 7,000 adults in California and noted that some people seemed younger, and others older, than their years.

To find out what made the difference, the scientists focused on the lifestyle habits of the people they were studying. Six practices seemed to have the most impact on the condition of these people's body systems—that

note that using a remote control to change the television channels can create "couch potatoes," which affects the physical aspect of a person's life.)

Then ask students to recommend changes each person could make to improve the physical, social, and mental aspects of their lives that have been affected by technology. (For

example, students could recommend that a person go to a gym to work out instead of sitting in front of the television with the remote control.)

Students should gain an understanding that advances in technology have both positive and negative effects on our lifestyles. (Students should be careful to retain the anonymity of the people they write about.)

them. Smokers don't smoke cigarettes hoping to contract cancer. They *know* the facts, but *deny* the possibility.

COMPREHENSION CHECK

The work *continuum* will be new to many students. Tell them that a continuum is something that changes gradually from one end to the other. For example, the range of temperatures of their tap is a continuum, especially if they have one handle that swivels from hot to cold and vice versa. There is no particular point at which the temperature changes from hot to cold. The main point for them to understand is that you cannot divide a continuum into two halves (good and bad, and so on). Health is shown on a continuum because you can't separate people into two groups and say the people on one side have good health and the people on the other side have bad health. Health and wellness are matters of degree.

CLASS ACTIVITY

Decide which day you will discuss the differences between physiological and chronological age. Two or three days prior to that day, ask the students to interview five people of varying ages over 30. They are to record answers to these questions.

1. How old are you?
2. How old do you feel physically? Mentally? Why?
3. How would you rate your lifestyle on a scale of 1 to 10 with 1 being excellent health habits?

(continued on next page)

(continued from previous page)

(Questions could be expanded to include what they regret, what they are thankful for, etc.) Then, before you collect this assignment, discuss with students what they found out. After the discussion, ask the students to write down any conclusions they can draw from their mini-survey.

Students should be sensitive to people who may not want to share personal information with them, and they should be careful to retain the anonymity of those surveyed.

Before you assign the inventory, ask students to talk about any centenarians they know of. What characteristics come to mind when they think of these people? Why do these people believe they lived (or have lived) longer than most?

A reproducible copy of the Life Choice Inventory is provided in the Teacher's Resource Box.

FAST FACTS

Seventy percent of all New Year's resolutions are health related.

Life Choice Inventory

How Long Will You Live?

No one can answer the "How long will you live?" question for sure, of course. But you can add to or shorten the probable length of your life by a good many years, depending on what choices you make. Your chances of dying younger or older are affected by how you live.

The Longevity Game illustrates this principle. To play the game, answer the ten questions that follow. For each question, add or subtract years as instructed. Use the scoring section on the next page as a guideline, and start with age 74 (the average life expectancy for adults in the United States today) on the top line. If a question doesn't apply, go on to the next one. If you are not sure what to add or subtract, make a guess.

1. *Physical activity.* If your routine activities require regular, vigorous activity or you work out each day, add 3 years. If you don't get much exercise at home, work, school, or play, subtract 3 years.
2. *Relaxation.* If you have a relaxed approach to life (you roll with the punches), add 3 years. If you're aggressive, ambitious, or nervous (you have sleepless nights, you bite your nails), subtract 3 years. If you consider yourself unhappy, subtract another year.
3. *Driving.* Drivers under 30 who have had traffic tickets in the last year or who have been involved in an accident, subtract 4 years. Other violations, minus 1. If you always wear seatbelts, add 1.
4. *Blood pressure.* High blood pressure is a major cause of the most common killers—heart attacks and strokes. However, most victims don't know they have it. If you know you have it, you are

Figure 1–4 Personal Responsibility is Central to Wellness. *These four broad areas of wellness are made up of many other health components. For example, the health of the environment contributes to both physical and social wellness; fitness contributes to physical and emotional/mental wellness; and so on.*

Pursuing Wellness

You may want to point out to students that medical researchers are learning more and more about the significant roles heredity, lifestyle, and environment play in contributing to the three main causes of death—diabetes, cancer, and heart disease—among Americans.

Diets, which vary from culture to culture, are among the lifestyle factors affecting incidence of disease.

For example, the American Diabetes Association reported in the mid 1990s a 9.6 percent rate of diabetes among the Hispanic and African American population and a 6.2 percent rate among the Anglo population. Diet and genetic combinations are believed to contribute highly to the disease.

likely to do something about it. If you *know* your blood pressure, add 1 year.

5. *Family history.* If any grandparent has reached age 85, add 2; if all grandparents have reached age 80, add 6. If a parent died of a stroke or heart attack before age 50, minus 4. If a parent, brother, or sister has (or had) diabetes since childhood, minus 3.

6. *Smoking.* Smoking seriously damages health. Cigarette smokers who finish more than two packs a day, minus 8; one or two packs a day, minus 6; and one-half to one pack, minus 3.

7. *Drinking.* The best plan is to abstain from drinking alcohol. Adults who drink two drinks a day on average, subtract 1 year. Those who drink more lose 1 more year for each additional drink in a day.

8. *Gender.* Women live longer than men. Females add 3 years; males subtract 3 years.

9. *Eating.* If you avoid eating fatty foods and don't add salt to your meals, your heart will be healthier. You're entitled to add 2 years.

10. *Weight.* Now, weigh in. If your doctor says you are overweight by 50 pounds or more, minus 8; 30 to 40 pounds, minus 4; or 10 to 29 pounds, minus 2.

SCORING

Add up the column of numbers, beginning with 74, to obtain the total number of years you can expect to live. Don't take the score too seriously. However, do pay attention to those areas where you lose years. They could point to choices you might want to change. Your answers to the Life Choice Inventory are personal and private. Share them with others only if you are comfortable doing so.

Example:

Start with:	74 years
1. Physical activity	−3
2. Relaxation	+3
3. Driving	−1, +1
4. Blood pressure	0
5. Family history	+2
6. Smoking	0
7. Drinking	0
8. Gender	+3
9. Eating	0
10. Weight	0
Your probable length of life	79 years

Source: Adapted for young people from "The Longevity Game" by Northwestern Mutual Life Insurance Company, copyright 1992, with permission. For older people, points are also given for age (already having lived a while) and for being 65 and working (that is, for being active at retirement age).

is, on their physiological age. The six factors were:

▶ Sleeping regularly and adequately.
▶ Eating regular meals, including breakfast.
▶ Engaging in regular physical activity.
▶ Not smoking.
▶ Not using alcohol, or using it in moderation.
▶ Keeping weight under control.

The effects of these practices tended to add together. The more of them that a person habitually chose, the younger the person seemed to be. Those who followed all six positive practices were in the best health, even if older in calendar years than some of the other people. In fact, the physical health of those who reported all six health practices was about the same as that of people *30 years younger* who followed few or none. Such findings demonstrate that although you cannot alter the year of your birth, you can, in effect, make yourself younger or older by the way you choose to live.

These effects are only beginning to be visible in people in their teen years, but are still noticeable. Think about people your age. Have you

Incidence and mortality rates for cancers of the lung, female breast, prostate, colon, and rectum are lower among Native Americans, Asian and Pacific Islanders, and Hispanics, than they are among whites. Because cancer risk is strongly associated with lifestyle and behavior, differences in cancer rates between ethnic and cultural groups can provide clues about factors involved in the development of cancer, such as dietary patterns and alcohol

use. Cultural values and belief systems can also affect attitudes about seeking medical care.

The American Heart Association also has identified a correlation between diet and disease. For example, in Japan, where fish, rice and vegetables are the dietary staples, the rate of heart disease is much less than in the American culture.

ASSESS

EVALUATE

Have students write a one-page essay on the six factors that have the most impact on the condition of people's body systems. (See page 9.) The essay should include how the students rate themselves in these areas. Is some improvement needed?

SECTION 1 Review Answers

1. **a.** chronological age; **b.** centenarians; **c.** physiological age; **d.** wellness
2. improve you or harm you
3. false
4. smallpox and polio
5. Answers will vary; could include: heart and lung diseases, cancer, diabetes, and liver disease.
6. Chronological age is measured in years from date of birth; physiological age is estimated from the body's health and probable life expectancy.
7. Answers will vary.

A reproducible quiz for Section 1 is provided in the Teacher's Resource Box.

CLOSE

Have the students make out a contract for change to improve or maintain a specific lifestyle pattern. Students may volunteer to share some of the changes they are making. You should also make a contract and volunteer some of the changes you will make.

---

noticed that the healthiest ones appear much more energetic, enthusiastic, and happier than the others? Have you noticed that those who appear healthiest are often considered to be the most attractive?

Lifelong health habits also affect the length of life. Evidence comes from the study of **centenarians**—people who are 100 years old or older. Scientists naturally are curious to know how these people's lifestyles differ from those of people who died earlier. Often, the same factors turn up. Centenarians are usually well nourished, but not overweight. They usually are nonsmokers and don't abuse alcohol or other drugs. They maintain regular patterns of eating and sleeping. Above all, they are usually physically active. Try answering the questions in this chapter's Life Choice Inventory on pages 8 and 9 to see the effects of your lifestyle choices on the probable length of your own life.

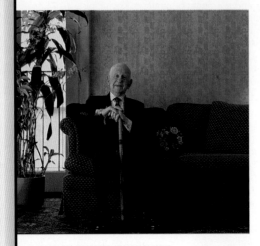

People who have lived a long time often say they have made wise life choices: not smoking, maintaining healthy body weight, staying physically active, and many others.

KEY POINTS *Lifestyle choices affect the condition of body systems, health in later life, and even length of life. Lifestyle choices also affect the apparent ages of people in their adult years.*

> ❝*May you live all the days of your life.*❞
>
> Jonathan Swift
> (1667–1745)
> English satirist

SECTION 1 Review

Answer the following questions on a sheet of paper.

Learning the Vocabulary

The vocabulary terms in this section are *life management skills, health, wellness, infectious diseases, lifestyle choices, lifestyle diseases, chronological age, physiological age,* and *centenarians.*

1. Match the following phrases with the correct vocabulary terms:
   a. age as measured in years from date of birth
   b. people 100 years old or older
   c. age as estimated from the body's health and probable life expectancy
   d. maximum well-being

Learning the Facts

2. Each choice you make today will do one of two things to your health. What are the two possibilities?
3. In general, infectious diseases do more harm today than they did 100 years ago—True or False?
4. Give two examples of uncontrollable infectious diseases of the past.
5. People who neglect their own bodies are likely to suffer from lifestyle diseases. List three examples of lifestyle diseases described in this section.
6. Explain the difference between chronological age and physiological age.

Making Life Choices

7. Let's say that right now you are happy with your state of wellness, and want to be healthy in the future, too. What daily choices can you make now that will enhance your future wellness? What choices should you *not* make?

Chapter 1, Section 1

The following quiz will help you assess your students' understanding of the material covered in this section of the chapter. You might use the quiz as an oral exercise, which will lead into a class discussion of the topics covered. Or, you might use it as a paper/pencil quiz to evaluate your students individually.

*If students have difficulty with the concepts covered in the Quick Quiz and the Section Review, you might suggest they review the material using the **S**urvey, **Q**uestion, **R**ead, **R**ecite, **R**eview (SQ3R) study method, which is described in detail in the introduction to this Teacher's Wraparound Edition.*

1. Heredity and factors in the environment are two causes of lifestyle illnesses. (True)

SECTION 2
Portrait of a Well Person

Wellness expresses itself in all parts of your life: not only physical, but also mental, emotional, spiritual, and social health. To show you what high goals you can aim for in your own life, the next sections describe a superbly well person. The descriptions are roughly in the order of the chapters to come.

Emotional, Mental, and Spiritual Health

A well person works on developing many emotional, mental, and spiritual strengths. Among other things, the person:

► Maintains a strong sense of self.
► Is willing to accept new ideas and try new behaviors.
► Handles setbacks without loss of self-esteem.
► Is aware of emotions, and manages and expresses them appropriately.
► Recognizes emotional problems in self or others, and seeks help when needed.
► Feels that life has meaning.
► Lives by cherished values.
► Manages stress with skill and enjoyment, not letting it become overwhelming.

You might wonder if *spiritual health* means belonging to any particular religious organization. It could, but it doesn't have to. It does mean having a feeling of purpose and a sense of values in life.

KEY POINTS *Emotional, mental, and spiritual health are a part of wellness.*

Well people enjoy outdoor play and relaxation.

MINI Glossary

centenarians: people who have reached the age of 100 years or older.

2. Chronological age is the same thing as physiological age. (False)
3. Wellness is a person's maximum state of well-being. (True)
4. The major causes of death are the same today as they were 50 years ago. (False)
5. A person has no control over his or her life expectancy. (False)
6. Physiological age is estimated from the body's health and probable life

expectancy. (True)
7. Lifestyle choices made early in life have no effect on health later in life. (False)
8. The term *health* refers only to the physical state of a person. (False)
9. A lifestyle disease can be passed from person to person. (False)
10. Wellness includes the physical, mental, emotional, spiritual, and social states of life. (True)

SECTION 2

FOCUS

OUTCOMES

In this section students will learn:

1. Three general areas of a person's health.
2. Qualities necessary to achieve optimum health in each of these areas.

FOCUS ACTIVITY

Divide the class into three subgroups in the following way: If there are 30 students in the class, put the words *Physical Health* on ten index cards; the words *Social Health* on ten cards; and the words *Mental Health* on ten cards. Shuffle the cards and have each student choose one. Students are then to find the other nine students with the same type of card to form the three groups. Direct them to brainstorm all the qualities necessary to maintain optimum wellness in the area indicated on their cards. Each group can review its list for the class. You can then display the lists for comparison with the lists in the book. This activity allows students to begin focusing on the specifics of wellness.

TEACH & APPLY

BACKGROUND INFORMATION

Students may ask how much sleep is enough. There is no one, easy answer to this question. Children need more than

(continued on next page)

(continued from previous page)

eight hours of sleep a night. Sleep needs vary for adults. Some, about 8%, are short sleepers and average five hours a night. Others are long sleepers, requiring up to 10 or 11 hours a night. Most, however, fall into the 6–8 hour range. People over the age of 50 do tend to sleep less—only 6 hours a night on the average.

CLASS DEBATE

Ask students to consider the following statement: *Maintaining an appropriate weight means that a person can't really enjoy food, and people who really enjoy food can't maintain an appropriate weight.* Do they agree or disagree, and why? Have those who agree stand on one side of the room. Have those who disagree stand on the opposite side of the room. Those who are undecided should stand in the center of the room. Allow students to tell why they agree or disagree with the statement. If students feel an explanation is convincing, they may change sides at any time. Continue until all who want to speak have had a chance to express an opinion.

LEARNING WITH VISUALS

Draw an equilateral triangle on the board. Label the sides with the components of wellness— physical, social, mental—one on each side. Ask students if they agree that optimum health needs equal amounts of the three components—that there needs to be balance between the three. Then, ask how weaknesses on one side would influence the other sides. (Examples: How would low self-esteem influence a person's social and

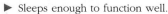

Health Strategies

Reading the News about Health

To develop your skills in reading health information, pick out an article on health news. As you read, answer the following questions:

▶ *What sort of language does the writer use?* Do the words try to shock or impress you, or imply a "final" decision? Alternatively, does the writer suggest the experimental nature of science, with words such as *may, might,* or *could?*

▶ *Does the report mention other studies?* Good reporters also describe other studies and findings that came earlier.

▶ *What methods did researchers use to perform the study?* These should be described in detail. For example, it matters whether the study had eight or eight thousand subjects, and whether the study ran for ten days or ten years.

▶ *Who is doing the reporting of the study?* Good reporters often have a science background, or they have followed the topic of their report for many years. Other reporters "drop in" for one story.

▶ *How meaningful is the finding? Are the study's subjects similar to you, so that you may apply the finding to yourself?* Were the subjects single cells, animals, or human beings? A study on amoebas is unlikely to apply directly to you without further research.

▶ *Does the finding make sense to you? Does it "fit" with the information you know about health?* You may not know enough to make this judgment yet. By the last day of this class, however, you should have developed a "feel" for identifying true information.

Beware especially of reports that seem to reverse common knowledge. Wait for more evidence before applying such reports.

Physical Health and Preventive Care

A well person also values physical health and works to maintain it. Among other things, the person:

▶ Sleeps enough to function well.
▶ Enjoys food and uses it to meet nutritional needs.
▶ Maintains appropriate weight.
▶ Works to achieve and maintain physical fitness; enjoys outdoor play.
▶ Uses over-the-counter drugs with respect; uses prescription drugs with care.
▶ Does not abuse any drugs, including alcohol and tobacco.

Since life's events are at times outside an individual's control, a well person is also alert to the chances of accidents and diseases. Thus a well person:

▶ Is aware that accidents are a real possibility and takes preventive measures.
▶ Is aware that infectious diseases (especially sexually transmitted diseases, including AIDS) are a real possibility and takes measures to prevent them.
▶ Knows what his or her disease risks are and takes whatever measures can help prevent them.
▶ Views health information and products realistically and is on the lookout for misinformation and fraud. (The Consumer Skills feature on the next page gives tips for understanding health news.)
▶ When necessary, can use the health care system wisely.

KEY POINTS *A well person attends to physical health and uses the health care system appropriately.*

Social Health

A well person realizes that other people and groups are an important part of life. Although the person doesn't forget to take care of his or her own wellness needs, the person also:

▶ Develops supportive friendships.
▶ Effectively resolves conflicts.
▶ Socializes well with others without the influence of alcohol or other drugs.
▶ Develops and maintains psychological intimacy with others.
▶ Can form a successful long-term partnership.
▶ Understands and accepts his or her sexuality.
▶ Understands the risks of sexually transmitted diseases and pregnancy and takes responsibility for his or her own behavior.
▶ Continues growing, learning, and facing new challenges throughout life.

Focusing ON Self-Esteem

Establishing an individual identity is one of the most important stages of social development during adolescence. Self-esteem is, of course, a key factor in establishing one's identity.

Research indicates there is a direct relationship between control over decisions and goals and level of self-esteem. Individuals who believe they are in control of their lives have higher levels of self-esteem than individuals who do not perceive themselves as being in control. Those with high self-esteem feel freer to make decisions and plan for the future.

Understanding Health News

Consumer SKILLS

A news reader who had stopped eating butter years ago for his heart's sake, complained after reading this headline: *Margarine Fat as Bad as Butter for Heart Health*. "Do you mean to say that I could have been eating butter all these years? That's it. I quit. No more health changes for me."

His response is understandable. Behavior changes, after all, take effort to make and are hard to continue. It feels awful when science appears to have turned its advice upside down, and meanwhile you've worked sincerely to make a change. Sometimes it's hard to know what is really true.

Our reader might have avoided confusion had he known some facts about the way health information is reported in the news. He isn't alone in not knowing. Most people are confused by today's health news, and especially by information from the Internet, but they needn't be. They can learn how to read any news based on information about science and reporting.

What most readers don't know is this: in science, the findings of a single study never prove or disprove anything. Many studies on the same topic are needed to confirm or disprove a finding. News media, however, report single findings as if they are much more important than they really are. Every study is presented as if it solved a mystery. The excitement of a "breakthrough" in the headlines makes for interesting reading, and so sells more magazines and newspapers.

To spot exaggerations of science, watch for phrases like these: "Now we know . . . ," "The answer has been found . . . ," "This study proves . . . ," "The truth is . . . , " or "In a startling finding . . . ." Real scientific reporting never uses such phrases, but instead sounds like this: "Our finding supports the idea . . . ," "The possibility is raised . . . ," or "More research will help to reveal. . . ."

Misinformed readers who wish for simple answers to complex health problems often believe headlines, and try to apply them right away. It is better to read the whole story with an educated eye. Then answer the questions presented in the Health Strategies box, "Reading the News about Health," on page 12.

In the end, use common sense. Even if it does turn out that the fat of margarine is damaging to the heart, for example, do you eat enough margarine to worry about its effects? Before making a decision, read more about the effects of fats on the arteries in Chapters 7 and 17. Then weigh any new reports against what you already know.

Information on the Internet should be read in the same ways as news. Many false reports there appear to be reliable. Logging onto the Internet is like walking into a bookstore—no one guarantees the truthfulness of the information you'll find there, and much is pure fiction. Sites with addresses ending in ".gov" are often reliable because government agencies approve their contents.

When a headline tries to shock you with a new "answer" to a health question, or the Internet tries to convince you something is true, read the whole story critically. It could indeed be an exciting breakthrough. More often, though, it is a sensational story whose goal is to sell newspapers and magazines, not to offer balanced health information.

Critical Thinking

1. Why are many studies needed to confirm or disprove a scientific finding?
2. Why do you think people are so anxious to believe news media reports about scientific "breakthroughs"?

---

physical sides? How would constant colds and flu affect a person's mental and social health?) The point should be made that unless all three sides are in a healthy balance, a person cannot be considered healthy.

Consumer SKILLS

Answers to Critical Thinking

1. One study cannot prove or disprove anything. Many studies are needed.
2. Answers will vary. People want to believe in scientific "breakthroughs" because they may offer a cure or an easy fix for a problem being suffered.

ASSESS

EVALUATE

Have students rank the factors that affect health according to their importance and explain why they chose one factor above another. See if the class can come to a consensus.

SECTION 2 Review Answers

(Section 2 Review begins on page 14.)

1. physical, mental, emotional, spiritual, social (p. 11)
2. Answers will include any three from each group:
  a. Maintains strong sense of self; is willing to accept new ideas and try new behaviors;

(continued on next page)

From a teaching viewpoint, this means that helping students take control of their lives should have a positive impact on self-esteem development.

Encourage students to choose their own goals for part of this course. Allow them to choose a specific number of the activities at the end of each chapter in this book.

Ownership of the learning process is one way to aid improved self-esteem in teens.

Effective development of one's identity is enhanced by high self-esteem. Students will have a clearer picture of self, and, therefore, be better able to deal with input from others if they have a strong sense of self-worth.

(continued from previous page)

handles setbacks without loss of self-esteem; is aware of emotions and manages to express them appropriately; recognizes emotional problems in self or others and seeks help when needed; feels life has meaning; lives by cherished values; manages stress with skill and enjoyment. (p. 11) **b.** Gets adequate sleep; enjoys food and uses it to meet nutritional needs; maintains appropriate weight; works to achieve and maintain physical fitness; enjoys outdoor play; does not abuse any drugs. (p. 12) **c.** Develops supportive friendships; effectively resolves conflicts; develops and maintains psychological intimacy with others; can form a successful long-term partnership; continues growing, learning, and facing new challenges throughout life; knows what is involved in facing death and accepts grief in all stages; relates to the larger environment and takes a share of responsibility for it. (pp. 12–14)

3. Answers will vary.

A reproducible quiz for Section 2 is provided in the Teacher's Resource Box.

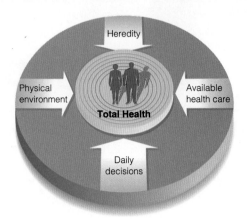

Figure 1–5 *The Factors That Affect Health. The figure shows that heredity, environment, and available health care affect your health. Daily choices do, too.*

▶ Knows what is involved in facing death (one's own or someone else's) and accepts grief in all of its stages.
▶ Relates to the larger environment (home, community, world) and takes a share of the responsibility for it.

KEY POINTS *Social health is a part of wellness.*

Figure 1–5 above sums up all that has been said so far. Outside factors affect health, but daily decisions do, too. The descriptions given here not only define wellness but imply actions to achieve it. The Health Strategies sections throughout this book are about taking action—they suggest what to do. The first of them appears on page 12.

SECTION 2 Review

Answer the following questions on a sheet of paper.

Learning the Facts

1. Wellness expresses itself in five parts of your life. Name these five parts.
2. List at least three ways to describe:
  a. Emotional, mental, and spiritual health.
  b. Physical health.
  c. Social health.

Making Life Choices

3. Social health has many parts. One part is the ability to socialize with others without being influenced to do unhealthy things. Recall how you have been tempted or influenced by others to do things that are not healthy. How would those things affect your wellness?

CLOSE

Ask students to list health goals that they would like to work toward in their own lives, and to set realistic time limits for accomplishing them.

QUICK QUIZ

Chapter 1, Section 2

The following quiz will help you assess your students' understanding of the material covered in this section of the chapter. You might use the quiz as an oral exercise, which will lead into a class discussion of the topics covered. Or, you might use it as a paper/pencil quiz to evaluate your students individually.

*If students have difficulty with the concepts covered in the Quick Quiz and the Section Review, you might suggest they review the material using the **S**urvey, **Q**uestion, **R**ead, **R**ecite, **R**eview (SQ3R) study method, which is described in detail in the introduction to this Teacher's Wraparound Edition.*

1. Keeping an open mind can contribute to your emotional, mental and spiritual health. (True)

SECTION 3
Making Behavior Changes

Health knowledge is of little value if people only use it to make "A"s on their health tests. It is valuable only when people use it to guide their behavior. If you are not making good health decisions, you may need to change your behavior. To do that, you need **motivation**.

Motivation to Change Health Behaviors

Motivation is the force that moves people to act. It may come naturally, or it may be learned. Whichever type it is, powerful motivation makes action almost a certainty.

The motivation that comes naturally is from instincts, or human **drives**—deep, physical urges such as hunger, thirst, fear, and tiredness. Drives are strong motivators that make you take the actions necessary to meet your needs for food, water, safety, and sleep. Drives may also urge you to act in situations involving other people. Aggression and the need to protect family members are examples.

The other kind of motivation, learned motivation, may also be powerful. Consider how some people are driven by the desire for possessions, recognition, or achievement. Others desire to shed their possessions and lead a simple life. Still others are driven to work extremely hard for things they believe in. These types of motivation are learned.

You can understand motivation from the example of a black box with a reward inside. Suppose you were told, "If you put a dollar in the slot, you can take $1,000 out." Most people would not hesitate for a moment. They would drop their dollar in. Suppose you were told, however, "If you put a dollar in the slot today, you can take $1,000 out 20 years from now." Now you might think a minute. Today's dollar may mean more to you than many more dollars years away. Still, you might decide to drop your dollar in. Now suppose you were told, "If you put a dollar in, you may take $1,000 out, but when you touch the box, you'll get an electric shock." Most people want to know, "How much will it hurt?" Now suppose you were told, "If you put a dollar in, there's a one in ten *chance* you can take $1,000 out."

People are motivated to act at times like these only if they think that the rewards or benefits are worth waiting for, outweigh the costs, and are pretty likely. That is, motivation is shaped by four factors:

▶ **The value of the reward**. (How big is the reward?)
▶ **Its timing**. (How soon will the reward come, or how soon will the price have to be paid?)
▶ **The costs**. (What will be the risks or consequences of seeking the reward?)
▶ **Its probability**. (How likely is the reward, and how certain the price?)

Now think about someone's health behavior—not your own, because it's easier to see someone else's behavior clearly. Pick a person who smokes a lot, or eats too much, or drinks a lot, or has some other negative health

The motivation to succeed helps you to meet your goals.

Glossary

motivation: the force that moves people to act. Motivation may be either instinctive (drives) or learned.

drives: motivations that are inborn, not learned, such as hunger, thirst, fear, and need for sleep. Also known as *instincts*.

SECTION 3
FOCUS

OUTCOMES

In this section students will learn:

1. Factors that influence the motivation to improve one's own health.
2. Steps to goal setting.
3. Factors needed to make the goal achievement successful.

FOCUS ACTIVITY

Put four dollar signs ($) on the board. Number each one. Tell the students they are going to choose one of the "prizes." Then explain each one:

1. $ = If you work every weekend, for a full year you will be guaranteed two free years of college (tuition, room, and board).
2. $ = If you work every day after school and weekends for one full month, you will receive a $1,000 bonus in addition to your paycheck.
3. $ = If you pay $5 a week for four weeks, you will receive $100 at the end of the month.
4. $ = If you work ten hours a week for one year, you might win a four-year scholarship.

Ask for a show of hands as to which one they would choose. Record the votes for each one. Then ask for volunteers to explain the reasons for their choices. Write abbreviated answers on the board: *value, timing, costs, probability*. Explain that students were probably motivated by one of these factors. Discuss the problems in motivation when it comes to improving health practices.

TEACH & APPLY

DISCUSSION

Use this as an introductory discussion to the section "From Awareness to Action." Ask the students to quickly list five things that they'd like to change about themselves. (The changes must be possible.) Then ask them to put a "+" next to each one that they know how to change. Tell them to put another "+" next to the ones they *really, really* want to change; then another "+" next to the ones they definitely will change, and finally another "+" next to those they are already changing.

DISCUSSION

Place the capital letters A T E D A on the board, one underneath the other. Begin a discussion/information session on the steps listed in the section "From Awareness to Action." Ask for examples of each step. (Example: A="I could change my weight." T="I could do this by decreasing my junk food intake." And so on.)

BACKGROUND INFORMATION

You might want to introduce students to the concept of short-term goals versus long-term goals. The short-term goals are more specific, more easily obtained goals. They should have dates assigned to some. For example, if most of your students are freshmen and sophomores, they could have a long-term goal of choosing and applying for admission to a college or university. Short-term goals would include discussing their career interests with a counselor this semester, taking an aptitude test the following semester, and so on.

habit. Probably, the person knows that the bad habit harms health, yet the person goes ahead and does it anyway. Why?

If people find it hard to get motivated to seek health, the reason is often because of the timing and probability factors. They have to wait too long to receive the reward, or they aren't sure they'll ever receive it.

Here's an example:

▶ If you enjoy ice cream now (immediate reward), you won't notice your weight gain (consequences) until next month (pay later).
▶ If you go without ice cream now, you can't expect to see any weight loss until next week (no immediate reward).

No wonder people sometimes fail to change their poor health habits! You have to know, and really believe, that you will benefit before you'll be willing to change your behavior. That's why health education is so important.

Since you are reading a whole book on your personal choices and your health, you are probably going to learn facts that will make you want to improve your health behavior. If you want to change, will you do it? The next section describes how awareness leads to action.

KEY POINTS *Motivation is the force that moves people to act. It is affected by the weights people give to the rewards and the consequences that will follow the action.*

From Awareness to Action

How does a person go about changing a health behavior? The question is important, because even people who are motivated, and who know how to improve their health, still fail to alter their behaviors. The steps that often lead to behavior change seem to be these:

▶ *Awareness*: "I could choose to change."
▶ *Thinking*: "I know how to change."
▶ *Emotion*: "I want to change (motivation)."
▶ *Decision*: "I will change."
▶ *Action*: "I am changing."

These steps don't always appear in the same order. However, they always seem to appear.

Do you think about your own behavior and possible changes? If so, you should realize that it is important to know when you are ready for change. A lot of thinking goes into changing behavior. No one can see this thinking but you. Others may push you to alter your behavior, but only you can actually do it. People outside you may think that nothing is happening if they don't see action. However, when you are thinking, something very important is happening. You are moving toward the decision point.

Much needless energy is wasted struggling with other people's saying "you should; you ought to; you must." Worse, you may waste energy with shame and guilt over "I can't; I failed again." You will make needed changes in your own time. People can push you, and this may help or it may not. In any case, only *you* can act.

> ❝*Well begun is half done.*❞
>
> Horace (65–8 B.C.)
> Roman poet and satirist

 Health Strategies

Steps to Goal Setting

1. Identify something you'd like to work on—your goal. Write it down in general terms.
2. State three or more specific behaviors that will help you achieve your goal. Write them down.
3. Identify steps you'll have to take to get ready.
4. Commit to a specific time to get your plan under way.
5. Set up a chart on which you can measure your progress in units.
6. Plan rewards for yourself that fit the goal you've chosen.

HEALTHY PEOPLE 2000

Healthy People 2000 is a government document setting forth numerous health goals for the nation. Some of these goals apply to teenagers and appear in these features.

In today's society, a supportive community can make a vital difference in the well-being of its members. Accordingly, there is evidence that community-based health programs can play a strong role in improving the health status of citizens. Multiple opportunities exist for community health promotion efforts on the part of government, voluntary and self-help groups, businesses, and schools. Such local community programs are often more efficient than centralized programs managed far from the point of delivery. Furthermore, indigenous programs maintain the sensitivity to family and neighborhood values that is vital to encourage change successfully towards healthier lifestyles within the community.

An important part of changing behavior permanently is the knowledge that success may require many practice runs. You should expect to stumble along the way. You don't have to succeed totally the first time. Be gentle with yourself.

KEY POINTS *People who change their behaviors go from aware-ness to action. Setbacks are normal and expected.*

Action: Setting Goals

To succeed in big ways, it's best to start small. Undertake manageable changes, one at a time. Suppose a person decides to give up smoking and drinking, and take up exercising, and get a job, and write more letters, and go to religious services every day, and spend at least two added hours each day on homework, and. . . . That person is in for a rude surprise. All these changes are possible, but not all at once. After only a few days, such a person will be exhausted and will give it all up. We congratulate the person on having identified many worthy goals, but we suggest the person plan realistically to achieve them. New behaviors require energy. They need to be taken up a few at a time—in fact, probably one by one. A major part of ensuring successful change is setting reasonable goals.

Experts suggest that a way to begin goal setting is to write down some areas you would like to work on. Then pick a goal to work on first. Perhaps you'd like to choose the goal that you know you could accomplish most quickly. Perhaps you'd choose the one that would bring you the most benefits. Maybe you'd start with a goal that just "feels right." If you can't think of any goal to work on right now, that's OK, too. You'll know when you are ready. The Health Strategies feature to the left, "Steps to Goal Setting," will start you on your way. Figure 1–6 gives examples of how to make your goals specific.

Following is an example of how to apply the Health Strategies steps:

1. My goal: I'd like to get in shape.
2. Three behaviors that will help me achieve my goal:
   a. I'll save $3 a week so that I can buy some hand weights.
   b. I'll read a good book on fitness.
   c. I'll join a walking club.
3. Preparation:
   a. I'll keep the money in my top drawer.
   b. I'll borrow the book from the library.
   c. I'll clean up my walking shoes.
4. My time commitment: I'll start on Tuesday, and I'll continue saving and walking for a month.
5. How I'll measure my progress:
   a. I'll record how far I walk each day.
   b. I'll graph my distances over a month.
6. My first reward: When I've collected $12 and walked for a month, I'll buy my hand weights.

Don't Say:	Do Say:
■ "I will get better at dancing."	"I will attend all my dance classes and practice as instructed."
■ "I will lose weight this week."	"I will write down everything I eat every day."
■ "I will prepare better for exercising."	"Each Saturday morning, I will wash, dry, and fold my exercise clothes for the week."
■ "I will do well on the test (in the game) Thursday."	"I will study (practice) for the test (game) in the library (gym) every evening from seven to eight o'clock."
■ "I will exercise with friends so that I'll enjoy it more."	"Each Sunday evening I'll call and make dates for at least three workouts the next week."
■ "I will make progress at my chosen activity."	"I will keep a daily log of my improvement."

Figure 1–6 How to Set Specific Goals

Schools have a special role in enhancing and maintaining the health of their community's children. School health education can foster healthful behaviors and help prevent hazardous ones, particularly in the areas of physical fitness, smoking, and nutrition. Standard course curricula can be modified to include health promotion, as, for example, through the addition of environmental health components to science classes. Provision of healthy meals, safe work and play areas, and physical education courses that stress the acquisition of lifetime exercise habits can be instituted as well. In partnership with parents and other community groups, schools can help to create health promotion programs and enhance health education curricula. Schools can, in addition, open their facilities and health curricula to the adults of the community, thereby serving as an even greater local resource.

TEACHER SUPPORT

Key Passage
You might help students remember and understand this concept by asking them "How do you eat an elephant?" (one bite at a time)

FAST FACTS

The average American teenager spends about 38 hours a week in class or studying; the average Japanese teenager spends 59 hours.

GROUP ACTIVITY

Your supplementary material contains a worksheet entitled "Steps to Goal Setting" that reinforces the Health Strategies on page 16. Make copies of this worksheet for each student. As homework, after you have discussed the steps in class, students are to fill out the worksheets based on their own personal goals. Remind students that the goals should be attainable. Be sure they know the homework will be discussed in class. Then, on the day the homework is due, have two large empty versions of the worksheet ready on newsprint. Tape these to the board. Ask the students to review the steps and check their homework to be sure it is complete. Then ask two volunteers to copy their worksheets on the newsprint (or you write while they recite their steps to you). Once both are done, ask the class to evaluate whether both goals are attainable. Would you make any suggestions or additions to make them stronger?

(continued on next page)

(continued from previous page)

Now, have the students get into groups of four. Once in groups, the students should take turns sharing their goals and steps. (Be sure students know they don't have to share their goals.) The others in the group should make suggestions and give affirmations. Group members sign each other's goals, indicating support for one another. These can then be collected for grading. You may want to put them up on a bulletin board for one week after you've graded them. At the end of the week, ask how people are doing—if possible, tune in to a few specifics.

INTERDISCIPLINARY ACTIVITY: CREATIVE WRITING

Have students invent an adult who is either very healthy or very unhealthy. They should then write a one- or two-page story describing this fictitious person's lifestyle. In the story they should be sure to describe the person's sleeping habits, eating habits for each meal and between meals, physical activity during a typical day, and any habits that the person might have that could affect the person's health either positively or negatively.

In the final paragraph or two, students should predict their character's ending years. They should tell how long their character will live and whether or not the character will be happy and healthy during those last years, or if the character would be ill and unhealthy during those years. Have the students read their papers in class, then discuss the common elements of both the healthy and unhealthy choices.

Meaningful, specific plans like these can carry you through the rough spots in a behavior change program. Therefore, it's worth putting some effort into thinking through your plans. A vague desire to improve is not enough. You must translate that desire into specific actions that you can achieve. It's OK to state a goal in general terms. However, be sure to translate it into specific, doable action behaviors.

 KEY POINTS *In taking action to change behavior, it helps to set goals. Try one at a time. Make it realistic, give yourself a time limit, measure your progress, and reward yourself.*

Commitment

To change a behavior, a person has to make a **commitment**—a decision not just for today, but for the long term. Commitment is a step in which the **will** is involved.

Sometimes, even after what seems to be a firm commitment to changed behavior, a person slips back. Why? Once you have made a change, you will maintain it only if you continue to feel rewarded by the change.

The Rule of Three   At the time of committing to a change, a "rule of three" seems to help people get through the early stages. This means trying a new behavior at least three times, or for at least three days, without rejecting it. This goes for every little piece of behavior change.

Take the decision to eat better, for example. One small change might be to drink milk every day, but suppose you don't much like milk. You could apply the rule of three as follows. Try milk once and you may not like it. Try it a second time and you may say to yourself, "This isn't as good as cola, but I can drink it." Try it a third time and you may say, "This is OK—I like it." At that point, the new choice has become easier. It may even become the preferred choice.

The Miracle of Hard Work   In reading about the way a person might try switching from cola to milk, notice the committed attitude you can take. You aren't just impulsively trying a new behavior, only to abandon it later. You are making the effort to install and maintain a behavior change for life.

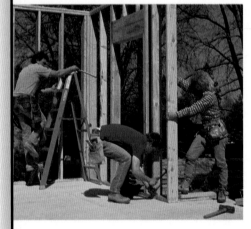
Permanent change takes effort—the miracle of hard work.

Notice, too, that you are willing to put in the necessary effort and practice for a permanent change. Now compare yourself with your friend Amy, who wants to go on a crash diet to get thin, but *not* to change any of her habits permanently. Amy has bought some diet pills to cut her appetite long enough to lose 10 pounds. She has no plans to change any of her eating habits, so she's going to regain the 10 pounds, plus some. You should have no trouble predicting which person will gain health and fitness: you will. Amy will be a yo-yo dieter, which means she will continue to lose weight and regain more. It will become a cycle.

Promises of instant health gains without effort are more inviting to consumers than plans suggesting that people have to work to get what they want. That's why diet pills and other quick fixes are advertised so often on TV. But diet pills are precisely that—quick fixes, not permanent solutions. Permanent behavior changes, like switching from cola to milk, take work, not miracles.

QUICK QUIZ

Chapter 1, Section 3

The following quiz will help you assess your students' understanding of the material covered in this section of the chapter. You might use the quiz as an oral exercise, which will lead into a class discussion of the topics covered. Or, you might use it as a paper/pencil quiz to evaluate your students individually.

*If students have difficulty with the concepts covered in the Quick Quiz and the Section Review, you might suggest they review the material using the **S**urvey, **Q**uestion, **R**ead, **R**ecite, **R**eview (SQ3R) study method, which is described in detail in the introduction to this Teacher's Wraparound Edition.*

1. A person can learn motivation. (True)
2. Happiness is a human drive. (False)
3. The potential for reward is the most

A factor that can help you maintain changed behavior is the approval of supportive family members or friends. Ask them to pat you on the back, or to join you.

The Changed Self-Image A final factor that people changing their behavior have to realize is that the way they think of themselves must change as well. Sometimes a behavior slips back because a person's view of self is slow to change. People have to do some psychological work along with their physical work in order to change through and through. A person who gives up smoking has to imagine, and really see, herself as a confirmed ex-smoker. A person who takes up swimming every day has to adopt a new identity: "I am a swimmer." In short, the person needs:

▶ A changed self-image.

Two additional factors help immensely if behavior change is to succeed. These factors may be more important than any others named in this chapter:

▶ A sense of **self-efficacy**.
▶ High self-esteem.

People who believe in their own abilities are most often the ones who succeed in changing their own behavior. People who prize themselves enough to invest energy and effort in their own wellness are most likely to maintain healthy behavior changes.

 KEY POINTS *Commitment to a behavior depends on continued rewards from it. To make a change or to maintain a positive new behavior, a person must receive support from other people, develop a new self-image, and cultivate high self-efficacy and high self-esteem.*

 Answers to FACT or FICTION Here are the answers to the questions at the start of the chapter.
1. **True.**
2. **False.** Today, most of the leading causes of death are primarily related to lifestyle, not infectious diseases.
3. **True.**
4. **True.**
5. **False.** To give up a harmful health habit, you also need commitment. It also helps to have support from others, as well as high self-esteem.

 SECTION 3 Review

Answer the following questions on a sheet of paper.

Learning the Vocabulary

The vocabulary terms in this section are *motivation, drives, commitment, will,* and *self-efficacy.*

1. Match the following phrases with the correct vocabulary terms:
   a. strong motivators that make you take the actions necessary to meet your needs.
   b. a firm decision to do something, not just for today, but for a long time.

Learning the Facts

2. What are the two basic types of motivation?
3. Motivation is shaped by four factors. What are they?
4. List the five steps that lead to behavior change.
5. In changing your health behavior, it's best to make several big changes at once rather than one at a time—True or False?
6. Explain the "rule of three." Tell why it is useful.

Making Life Choices

7. List a behavior that you would like to change in your life. How would you go about changing this behavior—what steps would you follow and why?

 MINI Glossary

commitment: a decision adhered to for the long term; a promise kept.

will: a person's intent, which leads to action.

self-efficacy (EFF-ih-kasee): a person's belief in his or her ability to succeed at the task at hand.

important factor in creating motivation. (True)
4. When trying to change your behavior, it is important never to experience setbacks. (False)
5. When trying to change a pattern of behavior, it is helpful to choose a specific goal and plot a specific course of action. (True)
6. A plan of action should include rewards for successful effort. (True)
7. Commitment to change should not require constant effort or will power. (False)
8. Temporary changes of behavior, such as a crash diet, can produce permanent results. (False)
9. The support of family and friends is not a useful motivating factor. (False)
10. Increased self-esteem is an essential part of a successful change in behavior. (True)

A reproducible quiz for Section 3 is provided in the Teacher's Resource Box.

CLOSE

Hand out an envelope to each student. Then hand back the "Steps to Goal Setting" worksheet they completed earlier. (See page 17.) On the back of the worksheet, the students are to write a short note to themselves explaining how far they expect to be on this goal in three months. They are then to put these in the envelope and address the envelope to themselves. Explain to the students that these will be given to them in three months for their own self-evaluation.

Reproducible Study Outline and Reading Cloze worksheets for Chapter 1 are provided in the Teacher's Resource Box.

Reproducible Chapter 1 Tests A and B are also provided in the Teacher's Resource Box.

CNN® You can update your coverage of health and fitness topics, as well as spark lively classroom discussion and deeper understanding, by using the **CNN Health and Fitness Updates.** These video updates are produced by Turner Educational Services, using the resources of CNN, the world's first 24-hour, all-news network.

With the introduction of the **CNN Health and Fitness Updates,** West Educational Publishing is proud to be the

Straight Talk

Suit Yourself

With all that people have to deal with during their teen years, does it make sense to make health a subject of study? Educators seem to think so. But how do teens themselves feel about it? These Straight Talk sections, which appear at the ends of all the chapters in this book, explore questions teens might honestly ask about subjects of interest to them. In this Straight Talk, the person asking the questions is a health educator. The person answering them is a teenager.

 A lot of states require that all students take a health course during high school. Do you agree that this is a good idea?

Of course it is. I have to say, though, that I don't expect to learn anything new. I take care of myself pretty well anyway, most ways, and the ways I don't take care of myself are my choices. I'll change my behavior when I choose to, and not when some parent or teacher tells me I should.

 Fair enough. Your health is absolutely your own, no one else's. No one can force you to change your health behavior.

I wish they wouldn't even try. I have enough to deal with, without some adult telling me to brush my teeth, or eat right, or not take drugs. What bothers me the most is that I already do the right things, pretty much, and I'm in good shape. Why is it that with all the things my friends and I do right, some people need to pick out the one thing we do wrong and focus on that?

 When someone tells you how to take care of yourself, does it ever make you feel like doing exactly the opposite?

It sure does. I hate it when people say, "It's for your own good." If it were for my own good, I'd do it, believe me. I'm doing something that's more important to me right now. And I hate it when my parents say, "That's bad for you." If it were bad for me, would I do it? With all the pressures I'm under, don't they see I don't need them telling me what to do?

Besides, they weren't perfect at my age, either. My uncle smoked until he was 40. Then he quit—and he didn't get cancer. Now he tells me not to start smoking. Also my parents tell me not to marry until I'm over 21. Well, they were married at 18 and had me when they were 19. Why do I have to be perfect, when they weren't?

 Surely you know one reason. They might choose to do differently, if they had it to do over again. They might be trying to spare you some grief they couldn't avoid for themselves.

OK, I know that's true. I know they care about me, but I still don't like them telling me what to do. Why don't they control their own actions, and let me control mine?

 OK, but suppose they just want you to know the facts about health? If they didn't make any judgments, but just laid out the facts for you to look at, would this be acceptable to you?

That sounds OK, but I think I pretty much know the facts. I know smoking and drugs are bad for

20

special needs

Seven Intelligences Overview

Students who have difficulty with the written word (i.e. students with learning disabilities or mildly mentally handicapped students) may require special consideration when instruction revolves around textbook content. Some students are auditory learners; they learn by hearing. Reading aloud is often effective with these learners. Some students are visual learners; they learn by seeing. Illustrations, charts, photos, and other visuals "stick with" these students best. Some students are kinesthetic learners; they learn by doing. Many students who display learning difficulties fall into this last category. Kinesthetic learners need active lessons, broken down into steps to assure learning takes place. They benefit most from role-playing activities and demonstrations *they* give. It's also important that these learners

Health is defined broadly in this book. It includes the ways you get along with important people in your life. Health is defined as "life management skills," which means how you manage your life in every area.

Some of those skills are important to me, I admit. You know what I'd like? I'd like a book or a course that answers my questions, not the questions of some adult who has forgotten what it's like to be a teenager. I'd like to talk about the things that really matter. Like how to deal with peer pressure. How to feel good about yourself without seeming conceited. How to get it across to your parents that you can be trusted. How to balance sports and schoolwork and dating and home responsibilities. How to not go crazy when people criticize you, how to please everybody else and still do some of what you want to do for yourself. How to figure out who you are and who you want to become.

Those are the important questions, and there are more. I'd like to get those questions answered.

 That's what this book is intended to do. Of course, it won't succeed totally (nobody's perfect). If you'll help, though, it may succeed in part. Ask the questions that are important to you. Get your classmates and teachers talking about them. The more you express your own interests and concerns, the better the chance that you'll get them met.

I don't want to be told how to behave, though. With that understanding, I'll participate in discussions.

OK, let's keep it that way. The facts are here, and you can apply the ones that seem important to you. Your body is your own. So are your mind and your relationships. So *you* choose. Pick the rewards you want. Go after them. And best wishes.

you, and exercise is good for you. I know to brush my teeth every day.

 Do you know how to get what you want without getting into an argument?

No, actually, I don't, but what does that have to do with health?

21

exclusive partner of CNN for textbook/video integration in high school health. By making use of the **CNN Health and Fitness Updates** you can bring the power of CNN, the network known for providing in-depth, live coverage and analysis of breaking news events, to your health class.

For assistance in using and incorporating the **CNN Health and Fitness Updates** into your classroom presentations, see the *Classroom Guide to the CNN Health and Fitness Updates*. The **CNN Health and Fitness Updates** are available with West Educational Publishing's *Health: Making Life Choices*.

ON LINE WITH HEALTH

You may want to have your students visit the following URL, where they will find information and additional web site resources to enhance their study of this chapter. As with all web sites, you should check this one out first to be sure the information found there is appropriate for your students.

American Medical Association Adolescent Health On-Line **http://www.ama-assn.org/adolhlth/adolhlth.htm**

This Web site is geared for adolescents aged 11–21. The links include Science Update, Adolescent Health Links, American Medical Association Adolescent Health Resources, and others.

successfully complete one step in the lesson before progressing to the next. Other learning styles to be considered as lessons are these: (1) Linguistic—The ability to use language to excite, please, convince, stimulate, or convey information; (2) Musical—The ability to enjoy, perform, or compose a musical piece; (3) Logical-mathematical—The ability to explore patterns, categories, and relationships by manipulating objects or symbols, and to experiment in a controlled, orderly way;

(4) Spatial—The ability to perceive and mentally manipulate a form or object, to perceive and create tension, balance, and composition in a visual or spatial display; (5) Bodily-kinesthetic—The ability to use fine and gross motor skills in sports, the performing arts, or arts and crafts production; (6) Interpersonal—The ability to understand and get along with others; (7) Intrapersonal—The ability to gain access to and understand one's inner feelings, dreams, and ideas.

VOCABULARY

1. Chronological age is measured in years from date of birth, while physiological age is estimated from the body's health and probable life expectancy.

2. Drives come naturally and are inborn. The need for food is an example of a drive. Learned motivation is driven by the desire for possessions, recognition, or achievement. Working hard for things you believe in is an example of learned motivation.

3. a. will **b.** lifestyle choices **c.** infectious diseases **d.** lifestyle diseases **e.** motivation **f.** health **g.** wellness **h.** life management skills **i.** centenarians **j.** commitment

RECALL

SECTION 1

1. enjoying life; increasing knowledge, strength, and skills in emotional health, nutrition, and disease prevention (p. 3)

2. 1890—five of the following: tuberculosis, digestive diseases, pneumonia, bronchitis, scarlet fever, kidney disease, flu, stroke; 1990—five of the following: accidents, suicide, cancer, chronic lung disease, pneumonia/flu, HIV infection, liver disease, heart disease, diabetes, stroke (p. 5)

3. heredity, environment (p. 5)

4. Answers will vary; could include: where to live, what laws to vote for, and what causes to support. (pp. 5–6)

5. sleeping regularly and adequately; eating regular meals, including breakfast; engaging in regular physical activity; not smoking; not using alcohol, or using it in moderation; keeping weight under control (p. 9)

6. The more good lifestyle choices (good sleep, eating, exercise, weight, etc.) you make, the younger you will be physiologically, while bad choices (smoking, excessive alcohol) will age you physiologically. (p. 9)

SECTION 2

7. Answers will vary; should include five of the following: maintains a strong sense of self; willing to accept new ideas and try new behaviors; handles setbacks without loss of self-esteem; aware of

CHAPTER 1 Review

Summarizing the Chapter

Your ability to respond correctly to the following statements ensures your understanding of the main concepts in the chapter.

1. Explain the relationship between health and wellness.
2. Describe how most of the lifestyle diseases of today are related to lifestyle choices.
3. List the lifestyle habits that you can adopt to maximize your wellness.
4. Describe how your mental, spiritual, physical, and social health are associated with wellness.
5. Explain how you can use motivation to change your health behaviors.
6. Define the steps in goal setting.

Learning the Vocabulary

life management skills	physiological age
health	centenarians
wellness	motivation
infectious diseases	drives
lifestyle choices	commitment
lifestyle diseases	will
chronological age	self-efficacy

Answer the following questions on a separate sheet of paper.

1. Explain the difference between chronological age and physiological age.
2. Explain the difference between learned motivation and drives, and give an example of each one.
3. *Matching*—Match each of the following phrases with the appropriate vocabulary term from the list above:
   a. a person's intent, which leads to action
   b. decisions made daily that have to do with how a person treats his or her body and mind

c. diseases that can be passed from person to person
d. diseases made likely by neglect of the body, not passed from person to person
e. the force that moves people to act
f. a range of states with physical, mental, emotional, spiritual, and social components
g. maximum well-being
h. skills that help a person realize his or her potential to be well and enjoy life
i. people who are 100 years old or older
j. a decision adhered to for the long term; a promise kept

Recalling Important Facts and Ideas

Section 1

1. According to the first page of the chapter, what is this book about?
2. What were five of the leading causes of death in the 1890s? in the 1990s?
3. Name the two causes, besides people's own choices, that bring on lifestyle diseases.
4. Knowing what effects your environment can have on your health, what decisions can you make about your environment to maintain or improve your health?
5. List the six lifestyle practices that greatly affect the difference between chronological and physiological age.
6. State how the lifestyle factors can affect a person's physiological age.

Section 2

7. Name five of the eight characteristics of mental, emotional, and spiritual health.
8. Briefly describe five ways a person can be alert to the chances of accidents and diseases.
9. List five ways a person can be socially healthy.

Section 3

10. Give two examples of learned behavior.
11. What are the six steps in goal setting?
12. How does high self-esteem enhance behavior changes?
13. What must a person continue to feel in order to maintain a change in his or her behavior?
14. What are two factors, in addition to the rule of three, that can help a person maintain a changed behavior?

22

Critical Thinking

1. After completing the Life Choice Inventory, are you satisfied with your results? What can you do to change the negative areas into positive ones? If all your areas are positive, what will you do to keep them positive?
2. Explain what the health and wellness line (continuum) is. Where do you think you are on that line right now? List five things you could do to move toward the positive end, and five things you could avoid doing to stay away from the negative end.
3. Many Americans are concerned with the treatment of diseases, but they neglect disease prevention. Discuss some of the barriers people might face in disease prevention. How can we promote prevention instead of waiting until treatment is needed? How would or could you do this in your school?

Activities

1. Keep a daily activity log of what you do. After a week write down changes you can make to improve your wellness. What do you need to do more? What should you do less?
2. Imagine a couple that fits the definition of wellness. What characteristics do you think they have? Brainstorm with your classmates to develop a complete picture of them.
3. You are asked to speak at a local elementary school about the importance of wellness. List some of the main points you would stress to the students. How would you help the students understand the importance of maintaining wellness throughout their lives? Since these students are younger than you, you may need to devise interesting and unique approaches to get their attention and get your points across.
4. Explain why it is important to balance your physical, mental, emotional, spiritual, and social health. Can you achieve wellness in only one area? Explain your answers.
5. Study your local environment. Is pollution a problem? Do you have an adequate number of health care professionals and facilities in your area? Summarize the negative environmental factors in your area and state what you can do to offset these factors.
6. Find advertisements in magazines or newspapers for devices that claim to increase your physical health. Write an editorial for the class newspaper discussing the claims these articles make and contradictions involved with each.
7. Make a video to promote health and wellness for the class. Include at least one aspect of each part of health: physical, social, spiritual, emotional, and mental.
8. List a goal you have for the future. Below your goal list specific steps that will help you reach your goal.
9. Consider the statement: "A major part of ensuring successful change is setting reasonable goals." Now separate into groups of three or four students. Decide on a behavior change that your group will role play. (Examples: cutting down on sugary foods, getting more sleep, and so on.) Role play the behavior change in two ways. First, role play an overly ambitious goal, such as determining never to eat sugary foods again. Next, role play a more reasonable goal, such as eating sugary foods only once every two days. Present your role plays to the rest of the class.
10. Write a lifestyle autobiography. First, think back over your life and write about the lifestyle choices you made or that were made for you. How have they affected your health? Next, write about your life now. What lifestyle choices are you making now? In what ways are they affecting your health now? Will they affect your health in the future? Finally, think about the lifestyle choices you are likely to make as you age. Will the choices support your health? Or, will they negatively affect your health? Why will you make these choices?

Making Decisions about Health

1. Imagine that a friend of yours has told you that she has developed some friendships that she is now afraid will lead to trouble. The new friends are engaging in some risky behaviors; some smoke and drink, and a few take drugs. Your friend says that she sees trouble ahead, but at the same time, she is enjoying the thrill of these new and somewhat dangerous activities. She wants advice on how to change her behavior before it's too late. Based on what you have learned in this chapter, what can you tell your friend?

23

emotions, and manages and expresses them appropriately; recognizes emotional problems in self or others, and seeks help with them when needed; feels that life has meaning; lives by cherished values; manages stress with skill and enjoyment. (p. 11)
8. The person is aware that accidents are a real possibility and takes preventative measures; is aware that infectious diseases (especially sexually transmitted diseases, including AIDS) are a real possibility and takes measures to prevent them; knows what his or her disease risks are and takes whatever measures can help prevent them; views health information and products realistically and is on the lookout for misinformation and fraud; uses the health care system wisely, when necessary. (p. 12)
9. Answers will vary; should include five of the following: develops supportive friendships; effectively resolves conflicts; socializes well without the influence of drugs/alcohol; develops and maintains psychological intimacy with others; forms successful long-term partnerships; understands and accepts his or her sexuality; understands the risks of sexually transmitted diseases and pregnancy and takes responsibility for his or her own behavior, continues growing, learning, and facing new challenges; knows what is involved in facing death (one's own or another's) and accepts grief in all stages; relates to the larger environment (home, community, world) and shares responsibility for it. (pp. 12, 14)

SECTION 3

10. desire for possessions, recognition, or achievement (p. 15)
11. identify what you want to achieve, state three or more specific behaviors that will help attain the goal, identify steps you will have to take to get prepared, commit to a specific time to start your plan, set up a chart on which you can measure progress, plan rewards that fit the goal chosen (p. 16)
12. when a person feels worthwhile, he or she will invest energy in themselves to maintain wellness and a healthy behavior (p. 19)
13. rewarded (p. 18)
14. Answers will vary; could include: hard work, support from others, a new self-image, high self-esteem. (pp. 18–19)

23

OUTCOMES

FEATURES

CHAPTER 2

Emotional Health

- Discuss the importance of self-acceptance, positive thinking, and values clarification to emotional health.
- Recognize that the acceptance and appropriate expression of feelings are important to emotional health.
- Discuss the advantages of assertive behavior, and identify assertive behavior strategies.
- Describe the role that fear of rejection plays informing new relationships, and discuss ways to overcome this fear.
- Outline the steps for making a decision.
- Discuss the need for developing a workable relationship with society.

Health Strategies: Think Positively (page 26)
Health Strategies: Dealing with an Emotion (page 32)
Health Strategies: How to Apply Constructive Problem Solving (page 36)
Health Strategies: Making Your Wishes Known (page 38)
Health Strategies: Tips for Overcoming Shyness (page 40)
Health Strategies: A Method for Making Decisions (page 41)
Life Choices Inventory: Do You Cultivate Emotional Well-Being? (page 28)
Consumer Skills: "Added-Value" Advertising (page 30)
Straight Talk: Teenagers and Violence (page 45)

CHAPTER 3

Your Changing Personality

- Describe the eight stages of life according to Erik Erikson.
- Discuss the importance of developing an identity during the teen years.
- Summarize Maslow's hierarchy of needs.
- Describe how sexual maturation and gender identity affect personality.
- Discuss how positive self-talk, positive body image, and self-acceptance help in the development of high self-esteem.
- Identify the value of positive peer groups. Identify the dangers of deviant peer groups.

Health Strategies: Improving Self-Esteem (page 62)
Health Strategies: Finding New Interests (page 68)
Health Strategies: Making New Friends (page 70)
Life Choice Inventory: How Well Do You Speak Up for Yourself? (page 64)
Life Choice Inventory: How Sharp Are Your Refusal Skills? (page 74)
Straight Talk: Dealing with Peer Pressure (page 72)
Teen Views: What Experiences Have You Had with Peer Pressure? (page 69)

CHAPTER 4

Stress and Stress Management

- Identify signs of stress and common stressors experienced by high school students.
- Describe how the nervous system, hormonal system, and immune system respond to stress.
- Describe the three phases of the stress response.
- Identify coping devices and defense mechanisms.
- Explain how to prevent and manage stress.

Health Strategies: Managing Stress (page 98)
Health Strategies: Steps to Relaxation (page 100)
Life Choice Inventory: How Well Do You Resist Stress? (page 91)
Consumer Skills: Claims Made about Stress Vitamins (page 94)
Straight Talk: Healing and the Placebo Effect (page 102)
Teen Views: In Your Opinion, What Causes the Most Stress in Teens? (page 93)

CHAPTER 5

Emotional Problems

- Describe the causes of emotional problems.
- Identify common emotional problems.
- Discuss the issue of teen suicide.
- Identify professionals who can offer help for emotional problems. Explain how to find competent psychological services.
- Discuss how to go about helping another person who has an emotional problem.

Health Strategies: Coping with Mild Depression (page 112)
Health Strategies: Dealing with Anxiety (page 114)
Health Strategies: Finding Help (page 122)
Straight Talk: Life in Overdrive: Attention-Deficit/Hyperactivity Disorder (page 125)

YOUR EMOTIONAL AND SOCIAL HEALTH

TEACHING SUPPORT

- *Vocabulary:* Learning Key Terms, Crossword Puzzle, Matching
- *Study Outline*
- *Reading Cloze*
- *Reteaching:* True or False
- *Enrichment:* John's Dilemma, Community Help, Allison's Problem, Describing Yourself
- *Career Briefs:* Recreational Therapists

- *Life Choice Inventory:* Do You Cultivate Emotional Well-Being?
- *Quizzes:* Sections 1–4
- *Tests:* Chapter 2 Test A, Chapter 2 Test B
- *Transparencies:* Negative Self-Talk, Positive Self-Talk

- *Vocabulary:* Learning Key Terms, Crossword Puzzle, Complete the Words
- *Study Outline*
- *Reading Cloze*
- *Reteaching:* Healthy Personality Circle Puzzle; Healthy Personality; Stages, Needs, Gender, and Self-Esteem
- *Enrichment:* Healthy Personality Gender Roles, Cooperative Learning

- *Career Briefs:* Counselors
- *Life Choice Inventory:* How Well Do You Speak Up for yourself?
- *Quizzes:* Sections 1–4
- *Tests:* Chapter 3 Test A, Chapter 3 Test B
- *Transparency:* Maslow's Hierarchy of Needs

- *Vocabulary:* Learning Key Terms, Crossword Puzzle, Fill in the Blanks
- *Study Outline*
- *Reading Cloze*
- *Reteaching:* Match the Mechanism
- *Enrichment:* Time Management Skills—Planning Ahead, What Creates Stress in Your Daily Life?, Decision-Making Tree—Coping Positively, Stress and Disease—Is There a Relationship?

- *Career Briefs:* Occupational Therapists
- *Life Choice Inventory:* How Well Do You Resist Stress?
- *Handouts:* Interventions to Manage Stress, Stress-Reducing Strategies
- *Quizzes:* Sections 1–5
- *Tests:* Chapter 4 Test A, Chapter 4 Test B
- *Transparency:* Stress Ending in Recovery or Exhaustion

- *Vocabulary:* Learning Key Terms, Fill-In Puzzle, Break the Code
- *Study Outline*
- *Reading Cloze*
- *Reteaching:* Phobia Matching, Reviewing the Chapter
- *Enrichment:* Being a Good Friend, Finding Emotional Health, Angel's Role
- *Career Briefs:* Psychologists

- *Handouts:* Performance During Past Year as Indicator of Severity of Mental Disorders, Developing Emotional Health Through Recovery
- *Quizzes:* Sections 1–4
- *Tests:* Chapter 5 Test A, Chapter 5 Test B

MULTIMEDIA SUPPORT

- Health Video Library
- CNN Health and Fitness Update Videos
- Westest
- Student Review Software
- Diet Analysis Software
- Nutrition CD-ROM

LESSON PLANNING

You will find detailed daily lesson plans for both **traditional scheduling** and **block scheduling** in you Teacher's Resource Box. Other suggested scheduling formats can be found in the supplemental Lesson Planning guide.

KEY POINTS

Chapter 2 is 26 pages long and divided into four sections. This chapter introduces the concept of self-understanding and how it relates to emotional and mental health.

A person's self concept is reflected in the person's relationships and the way the person fits into his or her environment. Healthy persons accept who they are and strive to adjust or change those factors that inhibit their successful progress in society. How one feels about oneself and others, and how one interacts with people, influence health in many ways.

This chapter helps students discover who they are, while examining the behaviors that will help them fit into society more successfully. This chapter will also help them learn a six-step decision-making strategy.

ACTIVITY TO INTRODUCE THE CHAPTER

Have students write an "About Me" poem. Write the following format on the board. Have the students write a poem about themselves using this format as a guide.

line 1—(first name only)

line 2—(four traits that characterize you)

line 3—(sister, brother) of (sister's or brother's first name only)

line 4—who loves (three things)

line 5—who fears (three things)

line 6—who feels (three things)

line 7—who would like to see (three things)

CHAPTER 2

Contents

STRAIGHT TALK
Teenagers and Violence

NOT Enough Time?

Following are some suggestions to help you make sure that you cover the key topics in this chapter if you have limited time. (Refer to the daily lesson plans in your Teacher's Resource Box for additional suggestions.)

DAY 1 Assign students to read Chapter 2 prior to Day 1. On Day 1 begin with the Activity to Introduce the Chapter, the "About Me" poem on page 24. During class have students do the Focus Activity on page 26 followed by the Class Activity on page 31. Then have students do the Class Activity at the bottom of page 29. If you have extra time at this point, you may wish to include the Discussion on page 34 and the Class Activity on page 36. Conclude with a review of the steps for making decisions (Health Strategies, page 41) and the Evaluate activity on page 42.

Emotional Health

FACT or FICTION

What do you think? Are the following statements true or false? If you think they are false, then say what is true.

1. Emotional health is not related to physical health.
2. Once a person adopts values, they remain firmly fixed for a lifetime.
3. It is best to reject illogical or unpleasant feelings.
4. The most emotionally healthy people do not need the help of others—they stand alone on their own two feet.
5. The primary problem people have in making new relationships is the fear of being rejected.
6. The best way to solve a problem is to think up a solution and to concentrate on making it work.

(Answers on page 44)

Introduction

If you possess **emotional health**, you seek, value, and maintain good relationships with yourself, with others, and with society. These relationships are a key part of total wellness. Emotionally healthy people like themselves. Therefore, they take care of themselves physically—they eat well, exercise, and get enough rest. Emotionally healthy people successfully develop personal relationships. They receive support from these relationships, which helps them feel secure. Emotionally healthy people have also found ways to fit in, or get along, with the larger society to which they belong. Thus emotional health benefits overall wellness and all areas of life.

In contrast, many people who are emotionally unhealthy are self-destructive. Emotionally unhealthy people often abuse alcohol, nicotine, or other drugs. They often overeat or undereat, overwork or work too little. They may take dangerous risks such as driving while intoxicated or participating in other illegal activities. These self-destructive behaviors can lead to drug addictions, cancer, obesity, heart disease, accidents and injuries, and other ills.

How can you know if you are emotionally healthy? How can you improve your emotional health? This chapter attempts to help you answer these questions, starting with the Life Choice Inventory on page 28.

---

line 8—resident of (town, state, country)

line 9—(last name only)

Collect the poems, save them, and ask students to read them aloud at the end of the chapter or unit.

BULLETIN BOARD IDEAS

Have students make collages from pictures depicting various emotions discussed on pages 31–33 (also see Life Choice Inventory, page 28 and Health Strategies, page 32). Have the students title their collages, label each picture with the emotion it depicts, and circle five emotions they have felt. Ask some students to tell about their collages. Display the collages on the bulletin board.

Answers to FACT or FICTION

1. **False.** Emotional health is closely tied to physical health.
2. **False.** Once a person adopts values, that person continues to test those values and can change them when necessary.
3. **False.** It is best to face and deal with all feelings as promptly as possible, even those that seem illogical or unpleasant.
4. **False.** Emotionally healthy people do need others for friendship and support. This helps them stand on their own two feet.
5. **True.**
6. **False.** The best way to solve a problem is to think up many possible solutions, select from among them, try out solutions, evaluate results, and move on to try other solutions if the problem remains unsolved.

DAY 2 Begin with the Focus Activity on page 34. (Be sure to set this up with the student ahead of time.) Review the SOFTEN technique on page 40 and have students do the Evaluate activity on page 39. Review steps for making decisions (Health Strategies, page 41) and have students complete the Group Activity on page 41.

DAY 3 Begin with the Group Activity on page 31. Then have students complete the Chapter Review on pages 48–49.

DAY 4 Conclude with the Life Choice Inventory, "Do You Cultivate Emotional Well-Being?" on page 28. Discuss the inventory with students. At this point, you may want to give students Chapter 2 Test A or Test B, which are provided in your Teacher's Resource Box.

SECTION 1

FOCUS

OUTCOMES

In this section students will learn that:

1. Self-knowledge is important for good mental health.

2. Replacing negative thoughts with positive ones can help improve a person's health.

3. The family's values have the greatest influence on the values of its children.

4. Emotions are okay, but it may not be acceptable to act on all feelings.

5. People who express their feelings appropriately are generally more mentally healthy than those who don't.

FOCUS ACTIVITY

Ask students, "How are you feeling right now? Put your thumb up for positive or down for negative." Get a general feel for the class. Ask some of the students to volunteer to tell why they are feeling/thinking this way.

TEACH & APPLY

CLASS ACTIVITY

Arrange the desks in one large circle around the room. Have each student put his or her name at the top of a blank piece of plain paper (best if paper has no lines). Pass the papers one person to the left or right every 20–30 seconds (you say "pass") until everyone has written something positive about each person. Remind them not to sign their names. After all the

Health Strategies

Thinking Positively

Here are some steps to changing negative thoughts into positive ones.

1. Recognize your own negative thoughts.

Examples: "I'm so dumb," or "I'm ugly," or "I'm low class."

Your own negative thoughts may be so familiar that you scarcely notice them. Pay close attention to identify the negative messages you are sending yourself.

2. Stop the negative thoughts.
Sometimes it helps to hold an image in your mind, to block out the negative self-talk. The image could be a check mark or a "positive" (plus) sign. This gives your mind time to switch tracks to a positive point of view.

3. Replace negative with positive thoughts.

Examples: "I'm learning," or "I'm becoming fit," or "I'm streetwise."

Your own positive traits are the best source for your positive-thought statements. If you have trouble coming up with good things to say about yourself, ask a parent or a guidance counselor to help you identify some positive statements.

SECTION 1

Self-Knowledge

One of the most important relationships in your life is the relationship you have with yourself. Your relationship with yourself must support you throughout your lifetime. Besides, it supports your relationships with others and with society.

To develop a good relationship with yourself, you first need to think about yourself. Get to know yourself as you are right now. The point is to develop a relationship with yourself that pleases you. Then when asked, you can honestly reply, "This is the way I am, and I feel OK about it."

This doesn't mean you should stop changing. You may want to improve yourself in a lot of ways; most people do. But you can still say, "This is the way I am—I am a person with faults and virtues, I am learning and growing, and I like myself."

Self-confidence is attractive. It's attractive to friends, to dating partners, to teachers, to everyone. The emotional warmth, energy, and enthusiasm that seem to radiate from a confident person set up a sort of chain reaction. Before long the people around that person start to feel good, too. Who wouldn't like someone who made them feel that way?

Being self-confident is not the same as being conceited. A person who is conceited has a falsely high opinion of himself or herself for traits that are imaginary or greatly exaggerated. Such a person constantly puts on a show of being smart, or tough, or physically attractive, or rich. Other people's opinions are overly important to such a person, because the person doesn't have a secure sense of self. When you are with conceited people, you can almost sense that they feel empty and insecure inside.

In contrast, a person who is confident may be smart, or tough, or attractive, or rich, or may not be. In any case the confident person feels OK about his or her traits without exaggerating them. When you are with confident people, you feel that they are comfortable with themselves.

Self-confidence starts with self-knowledge, which is not given at birth. Human beings normally are conscious of only a small part of themselves. To discover more takes learning and practice that, ideally, continue for a lifetime.

Self-knowledge begins when you ask yourself, "Who am I?" You may answer this question by just saying your name: "I am Leslie Owens." You may add that you are a young man or woman, an important aspect of yourself. You may go on to describe other outward traits, such as your height, weight, age, occupation, and race. Beneath these surface traits, though, who are you, really?

To become acquainted with yourself, you must learn about and manage three parts of your private, internal world—your thoughts, values, and emotions (feelings). Once

CRITICAL THINKING

Family plays a major role in developing a person's value system. Students probably have not even been aware of the ways in which they've acquired their parents' values.

Have the students discuss values with their parents and then report to the class.

One option would be to have students choose the ten values that mean the most to them from a list you have written on the board, and place them in order of importance. The students could then give their parents, either together or separately, the same list of values and have their parents prioritize the list. Students could then compare their own list to their parents' and identify similarities and differences.

you've discovered how you function in these areas, you can judge which parts serve you well and which you wish to change, now or later.

Thoughts, values, and emotions also play roles in the decisions you make. We all know what it's like to face a decision in which feelings pull us one way and values another. The process of making a decision involves weighing and evaluating what you think is true, what you believe is right, and how you feel about the situation. The best decisions from an emotional health point of view are those that are in line with all three aspects of the self.

 A first step toward emotional health is getting to know yourself. You can accept yourself as you are (imperfect, like everyone else), even though you may wish to change some things.

Thoughts

Your **thoughts** take place in the outermost layer of your brain—the brain's **cortex**. Your thoughts are conscious; you are always aware of them. They help you to gather information about yourself and your world, and to make sense of it.

Your thoughts shape your actions. If you think destructive, negative thoughts, you will act in destructive, negative ways. If you think constructive, positive thoughts, you will act in constructive, positive ways. In general, negative thoughts breed more negative thoughts, and can lead a person to think badly of everything. On the other hand, a person can acquire peace of mind, reduced stress, and improved health through simply learning to think positively.

The idea is simple, but training your mind to think positively is not easy. It requires effort, discipline, and practice. The rewards, however, are well worth the work. The Health Strategies feature, "Thinking Positively," shows how to change negative thoughts into positive ones.

 Thoughts help you gather information about yourself and the world. Positive thoughts are believed to set the stage for positive life experiences.

Values

Your **values** are your rules for behavior—or more simply, what you view as right and wrong. Values have been called *life's steering wheel*, because they guide the direction your life takes. You learn your first values from your family. You learn such statements as "We work hard," "We believe in education," or "We stick together."

A person's values change from time to time. Working them out remains a lifelong task. The teen years are a time when most people struggle to balance the values of their parents with those they observe in peers. Some teens reject their parents' values for a while. However, most return to them as proven rules for living.

Your values guide you in assigning positive and negative weights to behaviors. For example, you may value sports and reading positively, but

One of the most important relationships in your life is the relationship you have with yourself.

Glossary

- **emotional health:** the state of being free of mental disturbances that limit functioning; also the state of having developed healthy perceptions and responses to other people and life events, based on thoughts, emotions, and values. Also called *mental health*.

- **thoughts:** those mental processes of which a person is always conscious.

- **cortex:** the outer layer of an organ; in the brain, the outer, thinking portion—the gray matter.

- **values:** a person's set of rules for behavior; what the person thinks of as right and wrong, or sees as important.

papers have made their way around the circle, allow time for students to silently read what the others have written about them. This lets students know how others perceive them in a positive way. (Comments can include physical attributes, values, personality characteristics, academic ability, and so on)

 Vocabulary worksheets are provided in the Teacher's Resource Box.

BACKGROUND INFORMATION

The terms *emotional health* and *mental health* are often used to mean the same thing: freedom from mental illnesses and psychological disturbances that limit a person's functioning. Other times, the terms are differentiated. *Emotional health* may refer to the ability to appropriately react to the changing environment and to cope appropriately with feelings such as anger, compassion, sympathy, frustration, and so on. In this scheme, the term *mental health* also includes normal brain processes beyond the scope of this book, such as development of language and memory, control of body functions, normal awareness states, and other brain functions. We have chosen the term *emotional health* to mean not only freedom from mental disturbances, but also to describe healthy interactions with others, healthy personality development, and accurate interpretation and application of the emotions.

As another option, students could interview their parents about values, asking such questions as:

1. What are your five most important values?

2. Can you describe how your values changed as you were growing up? As you became an adult?

3. Have your values been much different

from *your* parents' values (students' grandparents)? If so, how?

4. What values, if any, are unique to your generation?

5. Did you consciously try to teach me any particular values? If so, which ones, and how did you do it?

6. Are you happy with my values? How would you change them?

Stress, which is discussed at length in Chapter 4, is mentioned in questions 4 and 10. You might want to ask students before they do the inventory if they know what stress is. (the effects of physical and psychological demands on a person)

When scoring, students shouldn't take the results of the inventory too seriously. They should remember, however, the emphasis on work in Chapter 1. Whatever the emotional state, it could probably be better, but they must work at it. If their scores are low, they might want to get to work on their emotions.

DISCUSSION

Ask students if they believe that conceited people are really insecure. Have them think about, but not name, people they think of as conceited. What actions indicate that the person is really insecure?

FAST FACTS

Spending time with people you care about can enhance your sense of self-worth. These people will help you feel good about yourself.

Do You Cultivate Emotional Well-Being?

Do you cultivate emotional well-being? On a separate paper, try answering these questions to get an idea. Don't take your score too seriously. Your answers to the Life Choice Inventory are personal and private. Share them with others only if you are comfortable doing so.

1. I spend time doing work that I enjoy.
   (a) Almost always. (b) Sometimes.
   (c) Almost never.
2. I find it easy to relax.
   (a) Almost always. (b) Sometimes.
   (c) Almost never.
3. In my spare time, I participate in activities that I enjoy.
   (a) Almost always. (b) Sometimes.
   (c) Almost never.
4. When I am about to be in a stressful situation, I realize it ahead of time, and I prepare for it.
   (a) Almost always. (b) Sometimes.
   (c) Almost never.
5. I handle anger: (a) By expressing it in ways that hurt neither myself nor other people.
   (b) By bottling it up so that no one knows I'm angry. (c) I am never angry, or I express anger aggressively.
6. I participate in group activities at school, in sports, in a religious organization, or in my community. (a) Quite often (b) Very seldom.
   (c) Never.
7. I find it easy to express my feelings.
   (a) Almost always. (b) Sometimes.
   (c) Almost never.
8. I can talk to close friends, relatives, or others about personal matters.
   (a) Almost always. (b) Sometimes.
   (c) Almost never.
9. When I need help with personal matters, I seek it out.
   (a) Almost always. (b) Sometimes.
   (c) Almost never.
10. When I am under stress, I make extra sure to exercise regularly, to work off my tension.
    (a) Almost always. (b) Sometimes.
    (c) Almost never.

SCORING

For each *a* answer, give yourself 2 points.
For each *b* answer give yourself 1 point.
For each *c* answer, give yourself 0 points.
Find where you are now on the emotional health line (continuum).

Where Are You on the Emotional Health Line (Continuum)?

Below 13 needs improvement	14 or 15 good but could be better	16–17 very good	18–20 excellent

Lowest level of emotional health   Highest level of emotional health

---

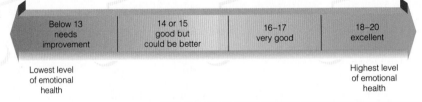

COOPERATIVE LEARNING

Developing Values

The following is an activity that will help students realize what their values are and what values are important to them.

Have students make a list of ten values they believe in. Have them rank them in order of importance to them. Follow this by having students pair up and compare their lists, and come to an agreement on five values that they believe are the most important. Lists will vary between groups but may include responses such as family, friends, their car, virginity, or relationship with God.

Instruct your students to cut one sheet into five smaller pieces, have them write the values on the small sheets, one value per sheet. After each group has completed this procedure have them pick one of the values and throw it on the ground. Go around to each

To discover how strong your values are, ask yourself some honest questions.

shopping and housework negatively (or the reverse). The weights that you assign then guide your thinking and actions.

Values are both conscious and unconscious. Sometimes you can state them in words, but many times they guide your behavior without your awareness.

People who know themselves well are keenly aware of their values. That awareness helps them to choose their behaviors without confusion. For example, a student who values honesty and is conscious of this value will choose without hesitation not to cheat on exams. Another student may have the same values but may not be aware of them. This student may suffer emotional distress in trying to decide whether or not to cheat.

Some sellers of products have learned that values can direct purchasing decisions. They try to "give" you some values concerning products they sell, as the Consumer Skills feature on the next page points out.

You can discover your own values by stating your beliefs. For example, you might say, "I believe it is best to be honest." This means you value honesty. Then, to discover how strong your values are, you can ask some questions about them. For each value that you state, ask the following questions:

▶ Would I be willing to state this value to others?
▶ How faithfully will I stand by this value when it is challenged, or when acting according to the value brings negative consequences?
▶ Do I act consistently and repeatedly in line with this value?

If the value you place on honesty is very strong, you will be honest even when it's hard to be honest, or when it's tempting to lie.

When two values a person holds conflict with each other, decisions and actions become difficult. At such points you may struggle to decide: Should I have fun (value: enjoying life) or study (value: good grades)? Should I tell

Sometimes your values pull you one way, and your feelings another.

group and pick one of the values and throw it on the ground, then have each group go to two other groups and have them take one value each and throw them on the floor.

Each group will have one value left. It may or may not be the value that they thought was the most important. Have each individual write a response to how they feel about the value that is left. Their responses may include how different they would rate some of their values especially after losing them. They

should view each value differently when they know that they don't have it anymore. They may also view differently the value that is left when they realize what things were given up. It may be more important or less important than some of the things that were given up.

Collect responses and have volunteers share their responses with the class.

CLASS ACTIVITY

Have students write a positive statement about themselves. They should look at this statement daily for one week. Have them reevaluate how they feel about themselves after one week of reading something positive everyday. Have their feelings about themselves changed? If so, how?

The transparencies Negative Self-Talk and Positive Self-Talk are available in your Transparency Acetate Binder.

TEACHER SUPPORT

Key Passage
Help students identify their values by listing *fame, helping others, leadership, friendship, honesty, wealth,* and so on, on the board.

GROUP ACTIVITY

Have students list at least ten positive qualities about themselves under the heading "I am ...." Then have them share their lists in pairs, small groups, or with the entire class. Ask for conclusions: What did they learn from this process? Discuss with entire class.

CLASS ACTIVITY

Have students bring two to five items that illustrate personal values (trophy, photo of someone special, souvenir, and so on) from home to share with the class. Ask students to show their items to the class and explain what values they depict.

Consumer SKILLS

Ask students to explain how value has two meanings in this feature. (value as an important rule for behavior; value as something having worth or benefit)

Discuss with students the difference between the real value of a product (shoes protect your feet) and the false value (you will be popular because you wear shoes endorsed by a star player). Ask students to list products in addition to those mentioned in the text and give both a real and a false value for each.

Answers to Critical Thinking:

1. Some examples are autos, beer, athletic shoes, jeans, perfume, and makeup.

2. An example is groups of attractive people socializing, having fun as they drink a certain beer.

3. One reason is to gain acceptance and approval from peers.

COMPREHENSION CHECK

Discuss with students how they can benefit from knowing their values. (prevents emotional distress resulting from being unable to decide what to do) Help them identify their own values by listing such values as fame, helping others, leadership, friendship, honesty, wealth, etc. on the board. When they have

"Added-Value" Advertising

Consumer SKILLS

Did you ever know someone who always "had to have" the latest gadget or fashion item on the market? Advertisers wish everyone felt this way. They use all sorts of gimmicks to convince you that you need what they are selling. One gimmick is to imply that your self-worth depends on your owning their product. Cars, sneakers, jeans, sports equipment, and many other products are sold by way of the concept of "added value."

Advertisers convey the idea that the products themselves are worthwhile. Cars deliver you where you need to go, sneakers cover and protect your feet, jeans clothe you, and sports equipment may help you become more fit.

Beyond these functions, advertisers suggest that their brand names also have an added value. You must have a *certain* basketball shoe or jacket to prove to others that you are worthwhile. Some people may even begin to feel unworthy if they do not possess the "in" brands, even if the brand they own is just as high in quality as the popular brand.

What happens to such people when their possessions go out of fashion? They scramble to replace them with the latest added-value items, because without them they feel diminished in **status**. Only people who value themselves for their own internal worth are protected from this effect. Their sense of worth is based on substance, not on symbols.

Critical Thinking

1. *What sorts of products can you think of that sellers try to tie to people's values?*
2. *What sorts of visual images are used in television and magazine ads to make the connection between a product and a certain status?*
3. *Why do some people spend money on products that are promoted in this way?*

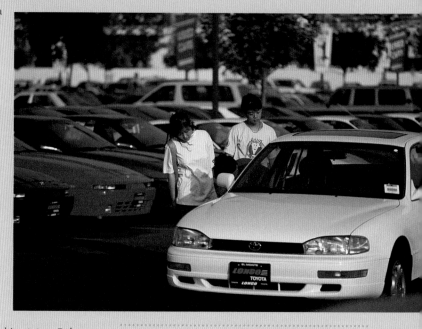

Emotionally healthy people value themselves for their own internal worth, not for the possessions they own.

special needs

Bodily-kinesthetic

Dealing with emotions in a reasonable way can be a real challenge because there first must be an understanding of just what is reasonable. You can help students build their own set of strategies for dealing with specific types of emotion-charged situations by taking advantage of their strengths.

Some of your students may have difficulty understanding the concept of displaced anger. A role-playing activity may help students with kinesthetic learning strengths grasp the concept. Establish very specific situations so that there's no doubt in their minds as to who or what they are really angry at, and to whom or what they express that anger. Here is an example of the type of situation you could present:

my friend a true but unpleasant fact (value: honesty) or keep quiet to protect the friend's feelings (value: friendship)?

Making such decisions becomes easier when you know which values you hold most dear. To find out, write a list of values that apply to you. Then, try ranking them in order of importance. If you clearly value honesty most, rank that as number one, and so on. Some values may share the same rank. When you make decisions with guidance from the values highest on your list, those decisions "feel right" and are easier to make.

Values keep on changing. One of the skills to develop in moving through life is to learn when to change to new values and when to stick by old ones.

 Knowing your values is a key part of self-knowledge. Learning to manage and live by your values is an important part of emotional health.

Emotions

An **emotion** is a feeling that occurs in response to an event as experienced by an individual. Some emotions are probably present in people from birth, such as affection, anger, and fear. Others, such as envy and prejudice, are learned. The terms *emotions* and *feelings* are often used to mean the same thing.

The emotions you feel in response to an event often depend on earlier experiences of the same kind. The experience of hearing the front door open, for example, may bring on the emotion of fear or happiness or interest, depending on what you are expecting. Failing to reach a goal may arouse a mixture of emotions, including impatience, anger, and irritation. Losing a loved one (the experience of grief) brings a series of emotions, including both anger and sorrow.

Sometimes a person has a feeling and cannot pinpoint its cause. When this happens, the person may try to ignore the feeling because it doesn't make sense. Even when feelings seem unreasonable, though, they are not "wrong." They are as natural as the wind. Feelings are acceptable and healthy—all of them.

The cartoon in the margin shows a shouting person who is angry but won't admit it. Anger is not accepted in many social settings, so people often deny it. Other emotions people often deny are hurt and loneliness—feelings that can reveal weakness and vulnerability.

It is acceptable to feel anything. It may not be acceptable to act on all feelings, but you must deal with them somehow.

Sometimes you must hold back an emotion for a moment (for example, if fear would prevent action needed to help a loved one in danger, you would hold back your fear and take action). It is fine to do so, and sometimes necessary for survival. However, it is usually best to face the feeling as soon as possible. Emotions can build up, making it difficult for a person to function. Generally, people who are aware of their feelings and who express them appropriately are more emotionally healthy than people who ignore them. Some psychologists now use the term **"emotional intelligence"** (shortened to EQ) to describe these qualities in people.

People may fear some feelings because the feelings could lead to unacceptable behaviors. It helps to keep in mind the difference between feelings

People deny anger because, in our society, it seems unacceptable or inappropriate.

status: a person's standing or rank in relation to others, many times falsely based on wealth, power, or influence. While desirable to many, these characteristics do not define human worth.

emotion: a feeling that occurs in response to an event as experienced by an individual. Examples are love, anger, and fear.

emotional intelligence (EQ): the ability to recognize and appropriately express one's emotions in a way that enhances living.

A teacher hands back a test. The student is angry with the teacher, who marked several problems wrong that the student thought were right. The student questions the teacher, but does not express anger. The student then walks out of the classroom and yells at her friend when her friend simply asks if she can borrow a couple of dollars for lunch.

Tell students to "go all out" when they express the anger. After a few students role

play the situation, point out to students that people who displace anger are often not aware of the fact that they are yelling at someone other than the person with whom they are angry. Also discuss the point of view of the person who is yelled at.

COMPREHENSION CHECK

Ask students if they ever become angry with their parents. How do they express their anger? Do they hold it inside sometimes? Has the anger they feel toward their parents ever affected their behavior toward other people? How could they benefit from using the strategies for dealing with emotions described in the text? (recognize it; own it; verbalize it; express it physically; think about the situation)

TEACHER SUPPORT

Key Passage

Here are some added facts about the physical aspects of emotion:

a. Physical reactions in the body accompany most emotions. Examples are a pounding heart, sweaty palms, "butterflies" in the stomach, dry throat and mouth, and trembling.

b. These reactions are involuntary, not under the individual's control. They are caused by the autonomic nervous system (ANS).

c. The lie detector (polygraph) is an example of a device that monitors the physical changes in the body associated with emotions. The machine records general emotional arousal; not truth or falsehood.

Vocabulary worksheets are available in your Teacher's Resource Box.

Friends and family members can be an important part of your support system.

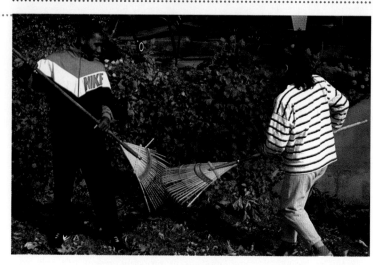

Health Strategies

Dealing with an Emotion

To deal with an emotion, you must:

1. Recognize it. What am I feeling?
2. Own it. Accept that you feel it.
3. Verbalize it. Express it in words to yourself or someone else:

I'm angry.	I'm frustrated.
I'm upset.	I'm afraid.
I'm hurt.	I'm thrilled.
I'm sad.	I'm stressed.
I'm excited.	I'm uneasy.
I'm resentful.	I'm touched.
I'm envious.	I'm nervous.
I'm anxious.	I'm lonely.

4. Express it physically. Take physical action to express emotions:

Pat yourself on the back.	Hug someone.
Sing a song.	Laugh.
Punch a pillow.	Dance.
Jump in the air.	Cry.
	Write about it.

5. If a negative emotion persists or returns, **think about the situation.** A confrontation may be necessary.

and actions. Some actions are not acceptable, of course, but feelings toward them are OK.

As an example, a young mother, listening to her baby crying, may have a sudden urge to hit the baby. That is natural. All mothers have such feelings. It is not OK to actually hit the baby, though. Instead, the mother should take a deep breath, pace around, or sit down and relax a minute.

As another example, a teen rejected by a steady date, in a flood of self-pity, may feel like committing suicide. That feeling, too, is natural. An appropriate action, though, would be to cry, to go for a walk, to release anger through physical activity, or to ask a friend for support.

In each example above, the emotion, while normal and OK, was not a reliable guide to action. More appropriate than to act on each emotion is to wait it out or express it in ways that are harmless to self and others.

When you can do the following, you have grown toward emotional health:

► Recognize all kinds of feelings in yourself.
► Admit that you have all sorts of feelings.
► Express all kinds of feelings in acceptable ways.

Expressing feelings is best done physically. That means doing something: speaking, writing, crying, shouting, laughing, or otherwise acting out emotions. Calmly saying "I'm angry" may not fully express the feeling of anger. It releases more of the emotion to speak angrily, or to pound the table, or to beat on a punching bag.

A person who feels anger but cannot express it holds it inside and builds **resentment** instead. It is healthier to admit and to express anger in appropriate ways than to **suppress** it and be consumed inwardly by resentment.

QUICK QUIZ

Chapter 2, Section 1

The following quiz will help you assess your students' understanding of the material covered in this section of the chapter. You might use the quiz as an oral exercise, which will lead into a class discussion of the topics covered. Or, you might use it as a paper/pencil quiz to evaluate your students individually.

*If students have difficulty with the concepts covered in the Quick Quiz and the Section Review, you might suggest they review the material using the **S**urvey, **Q**uestion, **R**ead, **R**ecite, **R**eview (SQ3R) study method, which is described in detail in the introduction to this Teacher's Wraparound Edition.*

1. Emotionally healthy people are good at forming and maintaining personal relationships. (True)

It is not acceptable to knock down another person with a blow to the jaw just to express your anger. However, doing nothing at all can be harmful to you. Once you have let off steam by yelling, crying, running, dancing, or whatever, you can relax again. Then you can calmly think about the event that triggered the emotion in the first place.

Sometimes you may find that expressing the feeling is all you need to do to cope with it. However, other times negative emotions return over and over again. If they do, they are a signal that you need to think about the situation. You may need to change something.

Take Tom, for example. Tom was furious at his parents. He recognized the anger, accepted it, and verbalized it. Tom also expressed it physically in a socially acceptable way every day after school—by digging a hole in the back yard. After a year the hole was big enough for a swimming pool, and Tom was a superb physical specimen—but still an angry person. He had to get to the bottom of the problem and change the situation. It was time for a **confrontation**. After Tom presented his parents with the reasons for his anger, the problem proved solvable. The Health Strategies feature on the opposite page, "Dealing with an Emotion," outlines steps you can take to live comfortably with your feelings.

 KEY POINTS *Recognizing, accepting, and expressing feelings are important to emotional health. Feelings sometimes need physical expression and sometimes indicate other needs for action.*

SECTION 1 Review

Answer the following questions on a sheet of paper.

Learning the Vocabulary
The vocabulary terms in this section are *emotional health, thoughts, cortex, values, status, emotion, emotional intelligence, resentment, suppress,* and *confrontation.*

1. Write a one-sentence description of *emotional health.*
2. the thinking portion of the brain
3. mental processes
4. Write a sentence using each vocabulary term.

Learning the Facts
5. What is the difference between being conceited and being confident?

6. What are the three parts of a person's private, internal world?
7. What is the danger of negative thinking?
8. Where do you learn your first values?
9. What happens when emotions build up and are not dealt with?

Making Life Choices
10. To gain self-knowledge, you need to be aware of your strengths and weaknesses. Knowing your strengths builds your self-esteem. Knowing your weaknesses helps you form a realistic self-concept. Take a personal inventory by making two lists—one that includes at least ten strengths, and one that includes at least ten weaknesses. List ways you can improve your weaknesses and build on your strengths.

 MINI Glossary

resentment: anger that has built up due to failure to express it.

suppress: to hold back or restrain.

confrontation: a showdown; an interaction in which one person expresses feelings to another. Managed aggressively, a confrontation may be a destructive fight. Managed assertively, a confrontation may be a constructive conversation in which one person makes his or her wishes known to another.

2. Self-knowledge involves assessing your thoughts, values, and emotions. (True)
3. Your pattern of thinking does not seriously affect your behavior. (False)
4. A person is frequently unaware of his or her thoughts. (False)
5. With effort a person can train her/himself to think positively. (True)
6. Once a belief in a particular value is acquired, it rarely changes. (False)
7. Values are abstract concepts which have

no effect on a person's actual behavior. (False)
8. A well person is open to reevaluating her or his values and opinions. (True)
9. Envy and prejudice are learned emotions. (True)
10. Emotional intelligence (EQ) refers to a person's ability to suppress his or her feelings. (False)

 ## ASSESS

EVALUATE

 SECTION 1 Review Answers

1. Answers will vary.
2. cortex (p. 27)
3. thoughts (p. 27)
4. Answers will vary.
5. A conceited person has a falsely high opinion of himself and puts on a show of being smart, tough, physically attractive, or rich. A confident person feels OK about himself whether or not he is smart, tough, physically attractive, or rich. (p. 26)
6. thoughts, values, and emotions (p. 26)
7. Negative thinking can breed more negative thinking until the person thinks only negative thoughts. Also, it can cause a person to act in destructive, negative ways. (p. 27)
8. from family (p. 27)
9. They can make it difficult for a person to function. (pp. 31–32)
10. Answers will vary.

 WORKSHEETS

A reproducible quiz for Section 1 is available in the Teacher's Resource Box.

CLOSE

Ask students to think of a negative thought they've replaced today—or identify one during the day. Remind students to practice replacing negative thoughts with positive ones whenever they occur.

SECTION 2

FOCUS

OUTCOMES

In this section students will learn:

1. Differences between passive, aggressive, and assertive behavior.
2. How support groups can be crucial to a person's sense of belonging and well-being.
3. That overcoming shyness may take practice.
4. That making wishes known through assertive behavior gets better results than passive or aggressive behavior.

FOCUS ACTIVITY

Ahead of time, set up a scenario in which a student will act a certain way when coming to class and you will respond passively and/or aggressively—then assertively. Have the student respond appropriately for each method used. Have the other students respond to what they saw. What were they thinking and feeling about the situation?

TEACH & APPLY

DISCUSSION

Discuss how people from different cultures and ethnic backgrounds might respond to or handle various situations because of tradition. Situations might include the death of a family member, a marriage, and so on.

SECTION 2

Relating to Others: Resolving Conflicts and Forming Relationships

Recall that the emotionally healthy person functions well in three areas—in relation to self, to others, and to society. So far, this chapter has been devoted to one of the most important relationships in anyone's life—the relationship with self. Now, what about relationships with others?

People who value themselves, because they are confident and happy, attract other people into friendships. A person's friends can form a strong **support system**, which can be a great help in time of need. The members of your support system may be family members, neighbors, school friends, members of a sports team, people in a religious organization, a **mentor** or advisor, or a therapy or self-help group. Of course, the person participating in such friendships and social groups stands ready to give, as well as to receive, and so does not need to be embarrassed about asking for support sometimes. You will learn some basic skills for getting along with others in this chapter. You'll learn more about peer groups in the next chapter.

Dealing with Conflicts

It's amazing how often people must deal with a **conflict**. Every day, at home, at school, at work, or out with friends, small situations occur and are settled without a fuss. Someone accidentally bumps into another, who good-naturedly steps aside. How is it, then, that a bump leads to a push, shoving becomes hitting, and a brawl erupts? The difference lies in people's reactions to annoyance. The question to ask, therefore, is not *whether* you will experience conflicts, but how to handle them when they come up.

It's important to learn how to keep your cool but still stand your ground when conflict arises. If you don't stay calm, the conflict could lead to **violence**. On the other hand, if you always give in to keep the peace, your needs may often go unmet. Or you may pretend to ignore the conflict, causing it to "go underground" and get worse.

A true tale shows the outcome of conflict handled badly. Two families, the Hatfields and the McCoys, lived in the mountains on opposite banks of the river that separates eastern Kentucky and West Virginia. Some claim the theft of a hog started it all, but whatever the first event, it ignited a 40-year **feud** that ravaged the two families, then their counties, and finally even their states.

Viewing the "Enemy" If you think a feud like the one between the Hatfields and the McCoys could never happen today, you are mistaken. The

The feud between the Hatfields and McCoys offers an example of what can happen when conflicts go on unresolved.

CRITICAL THINKING

Five conflict resolution strategies are presented in Figure 2–1 on page 37. Each method produces an effect, both on the conflict and on the person using it. Students may judge themselves and others based on the values they assign to the various methods. For example, a person who walks away from a fight could be viewed as "chicken" by some students, or "cool" by others. To help students identify and analyze how they feel about using each of the methods, ask students to

With honesty and assertiveness, people can resolve conflicts constructively.

story demonstrates a dangerous change that occurs in the minds of people in conflict. At some point, they begin to view one another as "enemies" and start searching for evidence of one another's villainy. The Hatfields were missing a pig, someone reported seeing an extra pig at the McCoy's place, the Hatfields retaliated, both sides heard rumors of other crimes, and the shooting started. Examples more likely today are these:

▶ Tomika thinks that Tom lied. Now Tomika is waiting to catch Tom in another lie.

▶ Tom thinks Tomika has spread a rumor about him. Now, whenever he sees her talking to another person, Tom imagines that Tomika is gossiping about him.

▶ Tom can see none of the good things that Tomika does. Tomika notices only bad things about Tom.

Problems quickly multiply. People embroiled in conflict stop communicating. Soon, they hate one another on vague general principles. Then others "pick sides," and more and more people become involved. You may know of examples like these:

▶ Your friends hate your "enemy's" friends.

▶ Members of this group don't speak with members of that group.

▶ People in his family cannot become friends with people in her family.

Trust or **tolerance** can be forever lost—unless someone stops the conflict.

Before the end of the Hatfields' and the McCoys' feud, deadly deeds were done by both sides. Even more horrifying, though, were the crimes each family *imagined* the other to have committed. Many friends and neighbors had also become involved. The governors of both states started bickering about the "crimes against their states" committed by the feuding neighbors. Incredibly, each of the two states armed its militia to do battle against the other, and the U.S. Supreme Court finally had to step in to prevent a war.

MINI Glossary

support system: a network of individuals or groups with which one identifies and exchanges emotional support.

mentor: a wise person who gives advice and assistance.

conflict: a struggle or opposition between people; especially, when people compete for something in the belief that only one can have what he or she wants, at the expense of the other.

violence: brutal physical force intended to damage or injure another.

feud: a bitter, continuing hostility, often involving groups of people.

tolerance: accommodation and acceptance of differences between oneself and others; being tolerant of people's age, body shape, gender, disabilities, race, religion, views, and other differences. (Another meaning of *tolerance* has to do with the body's adaptation to medicine and drugs, as defined in Chapter 11.)

give their opinions about the following statements.

1. A person who gives in when conflict arises is cooperative.

2. A person who walks away during an argument is afraid.

3. A person who does nothing about a con-

flict saves the other person's feelings.

4. A person who fights dirty usually wins.

5. A person who tries to understand the other's point of view can meet his or her own needs by doing so.

COMPREHENSION CHECK

Have students name the five steps in dealing with an emotion listed on page 32. (1—Recognize it; 2—Own it; 3—Verbalize it; 4—Express it physically; 5—If a negative emotion persists or returns, think about the situation and confront it if necessary.)

Ask students, "How would these steps be important when dealing with a conflict?"

GUEST SPEAKER

Invite students or community members who are in support groups to come into the class as guest speakers to discuss the value of the groups, how someone gets into a group, the purpose of the group, and so on. These groups are often listed in the phone book under headings like "Self-Help" or "Support Groups." They are also listed weekly in some newspapers.

CLASS ACTIVITY

Review the importance of support systems. List and explain the systems in your school and community, e.g., school support groups; aftercare for substance abuse; Alcoholics Anonymous; and special groups for depression, pregnant and parenting teens, children of dysfunctional families, eating disorders, chronic illness, children of alcoholics, grief, or others. Counselors can provide this information for you or may come in to explain the student support services available in your school district. Community support systems can be located through the mental health association, school counselors, treatment facilities, newspapers, or phone books.

FAST FACTS

People who are hostile are inclined to have more coronary artery blockage.

Health Strategies

How to Apply Constructive Problem Solving

When you find yourself in conflict with another person:

► Be honest and assertive. Say what you mean and what you feel.
► Use only "I" statements ("I don't like it when ...") rather than "you" statements ("Why don't you ..." or "You are a ...").
► Reflect. Repeat the other person's complaint in your own words, to be sure you understand—and wait for agreement.
► Ask, don't guess. You don't really know what is on the other person's mind until you ask. Wait silently for the whole answer.
► Take a "side-by-side" attitude. Put yourself in the other's shoes; respect the other; say that you don't wish to be enemies.
► Use humor. Laughter relieves stress.
► Choose a good time and place for working out issues. Agree to meet for a formal "gripe hour."
► Solve only one issue at a time. Other issues demand their own gripe sessions.
► Be sure that the issue at hand is the real issue and that some deeper, more personal problem is not hiding behind the complaint.
► Stand up for yourself. Ask for specific changes that will lead to an end to the conflict. Ask for only one or two changes at a time.
► Be open to change yourself.
► Don't try to win. If there's a winner, there's a loser. Both people should win—in terms of closeness, friendship, and self-esteem.
► If you fail, try again with a **mediator** present.

Eventually, the conflict eased and peace returned to the area. However, terrible damage had been done. Most members of the two families had been killed or jailed, their homes burned down, and their mountain lands lost to creditors. The moral of the story: conflicts tend to pick up steam unless somebody does something to release the pressure.

Luckily, most conflicts can end happily, or at least less disastrously. Resolving a conflict takes courage and work, but it can be done, as the next section describes. One warning: the earlier you take action, the better.

Is It Conflict, or Just an Acceptable Difference? The first task in resolving a conflict is to establish that true conflict exists. People naturally express different viewpoints, or react differently to the same events, and these differences are best tolerated. Also, some people waste energy dwelling on a past wrongdoing, but no one can go back and change the past. Some examples help to clarify these points:

► Different viewpoints: Person A says, "Baseball is the greatest of all sports." Person B says, "Ice skating is far superior."
► Different reactions: Person A says, "Wow, our team was terrible out there!" Person B says, "Our star player was sick, but we held our own in spite of it!"
► Past wrongdoings: Person A says, "You didn't come to my party. Why should I go to yours?" Person B says, "I didn't mean to miss it. I thought it was next week."

No one has anything to gain by struggling with these issues. Who can say whether baseball or ice skating is best? When issues like these arise, make it clear that you don't mind discussing them just for the fun of it, but solidly refuse to argue. In other words, agree to disagree, and forgive past wrongs.

True conflict, though, is another matter. Left unsettled, conflict can ruin relationships, interfere with work or school performance, and even lead to violent acts of revenge, especially when people believe their honor is at stake. This chapter's Straight Talk section takes up the issues of the violence that occurs in school and elsewhere.

Strategies for Resolving Conflicts Conflicts, if well-handled, can end constructively. People who face up to their disagreements with others are motivated to make things better. All sorts of ideas, innovations, and inventions have sprung from what were, at first, uncomfortable situations.

With the right attitude, people can break down barriers and create more trust—essential for resolving conflict. Both parties should adjust their attitudes to do the following:

► Desire resolution: have a genuine desire to solve the problem.
► Join in teamwork: be willing to work together toward finding a solution.
► Strive for win-win: know that if each person helps meet the other's needs, everyone's needs can be satisfied.

HEALTHY PEOPLE 2000

Increase to at least 50 percent the proportion of elementary and secondary schools that teach nonviolent conflict resolution skills, preferably as a part of quality school health education.

Schools provide a strategic setting for the prevention of violent and abusive behavior.

They contain a captive audience, many of whose members are at risk of becoming victims or perpetrators of interpersonal violence. Health-related knowledge, attitudes, and behaviors can be positively affected through school health education curricula. Curricula have been developed for various grade levels that seek to change knowledge about and attitudes toward violence and to instill interpersonal skills for resolving conflicts

1. GIVING IN One person yielding to the other person's wishes.

Good Uses: Use when issues are not critical to your needs. Use as a way to bargain—give in on an unimportant item in exchange for something you truly want and need. Giving in saves time and hassles. It lets people know you are flexible and willing to bargain.

Cautions: Your needs may be overlooked. Giving in to bullying or threats invites more of the same. If you give in too quickly, you may feel cheated, angry, manipulated, or resentful and so perpetuate the conflict.

2. WALKING AWAY One party physically or psychologically leaves the conflict.

Good Uses: Use when cooling off is needed—when your or another's anger rises—to avoid the threat of violence. Use when you need time to think about other options that are open to you.

Cautions: The conflict may continue unresolved, and may worsen if not addressed. A mediator, or a third person who wants to help resolve the conflict, can sometimes help to get problem solving back on track.

3. DOING NOTHING Both sides ignore the problem.

Good Uses: Use when time will cure the problem—for example, when one party is leaving town soon, or when classes will soon change. Use when the problem feels unimportant to both parties.

Cautions: Hostility can go "underground" to silently grow worse. The problem can compound. The parties may feel stress and discomfort in each other's presence.

4. FIGHTING DIRTY One party attempts to "win" by underhanded means, such as lying, manipulating (pouting or crying), threatening, blaming and calling names. These tactics press the other person's "hot buttons" and bring up sensitive issues to which the other person reacts defensively.

Good Uses: None.

Cautions: Fighting dirty clouds issues and often worsens conflicts.

5. CONSTRUCTIVE PROBLEM SOLVING Both parties understand that they have much to gain by resolving the conflict, and they work toward solutions.

Good Uses: Use when both parties are competing for the same resources. This is especially important when the issues are critical to your needs. The more important the issue, the more urgently you need to solve the problem. When the parties solve the issue together, it usually stays solved.

Cautions: Finding the solution takes work, and requires you to compromise. Both people must be willing to give up a little to come to an acceptable solution. Both parties must also agree to follow the ground rules and attitudes presented in this chapter.

CONFLICT RESOLUTION STRATEGIES

Figure 2–1 Five Conflict Resolution Strategies—Pros and Cons

▶ Honor the relationship: desire to maintain or improve the friendship, partnership, or community.
▶ Be flexible but firm: be flexible on *how* needs are met; be firm that one's needs *will* be met.
▶ Be sincerely apologetic when appropriate.
▶ Show courage: have courage to face the problem even while feeling threatened or afraid of hurting others' feelings.
▶ Be open-minded: be willing to brainstorm and listen to all ideas for new solutions, even if the ideas are later discarded.

With the attitudes described above, people can approach resolving their conflicts. Some methods of resolving conflicts are shown in Figure 2–1 above. Some work better than others, but all are shown for comparison. The Health Strategies section on page 36 gives details about one method that usually works best: constructive problem solving. To use it effectively, the parties express their wants and needs, but at the same time respect the feelings of other people.

MINI Glossary

mediator: a neutral third person who helps two people in conflict to communicate more effectively.

You can update your coverage of health and fitness topics, as well as spark lively classroom discussion and deeper understanding, by using the **CNN Health and Fitness Updates.** These video updates are produced by Turner Educational Services, using the resources of CNN, the world's first 24-hour, all-news network.

With the introduction of the **CNN Health and Fitness Updates,** West Educational Publishing is proud to be the exclusive partner of CNN for textbook/video integration in high school health. By making use of the **CNN Health and Fitness Updates** you can bring the power of CNN, the network known for providing in-depth, live coverage and analysis of breaking news events, to your health class.

For assistance in using and incorporating the **CNN Health and Fitness Updates** into your classroom presentations, see the *Classroom Guide to the CNN Health and Fitness Updates.* The **CNN Health and Fitness Updates** are available with West Educational Publishing's *Health: Making Life Choices.*

nonviolently. The principles underlying these curricula, already successfully applied to the prevention of substance abuse, include providing information about the medical and social consequences of individual behaviors and improving interpersonal and decision-making skills.

While effectiveness of such curricula in reducing violent and abusive behaviors is yet to be established, some study results seem

promising. At least one study has shown that a school curriculum can diminish attitudes that justify violent behavior and improve social problem-solving abilities.

GROUP ACTIVITY

Define assertive, passive, and aggressive behaviors, then have students work in groups to come up with examples of the difference between assertive and aggressive behavior. Then give groups the following situations and ask them to tell how an aggressive person and an assertive person would react: 1. a fellow worker is not doing his fair share of the work; 2. a classmate is disrupting class, making it hard for others to concentrate; and 3. a brother or sister is spending too much time listening to your radio in your room. (See Figure 2–2 on page 39.)

ROLE PLAY

Give students some situations in which they can role play assertiveness. Some possible situations are: someone cuts in front of the lunch line, someone walks into the room and changes the TV channel while you're already watching something, a friend who has stayed overnight pulled out almost all of your CDs from their cases and is about to leave without having put any of them back. Monitor the role plays, pointing out the advantages of assertive behavior versus aggressive or passive behavior.

Assertive, Not Aggressive, Communication Of great importance during a conflict is your style of **communication**. You have to perform a sort of balancing act between getting what you want and meeting the needs of others. The happy center between the extremes of never speaking out and verbally attacking others is **assertive** behavior, rather than **passive** or **aggressive** behavior.

To be assertive is to say what you mean—not to tiptoe around and drop hints, at the one extreme, and not to attack the other person, at the other. Assertiveness does not come naturally to many people. They may not even value it. They may think it's selfish. However, assertiveness has great value when problems must be worked out.

In Figure 2–2 on the next page, three conflict situations are described in which people are behaving nonassertively (passively or aggressively). The people are not succeeding in getting what they want. See if you can decide how they could get what they wanted by being assertive.

In the first example, Sarah is passive. She simply does not speak up for herself. In the second, Mom makes it clear to James that she feels overworked, tired, and grumpy. However, she doesn't say what she wants him to do about it. In the third example, Ken tells his little sister what their father had told her to do, which is assertive. However, he then goes on to insult her, which is aggressive and hurtful.

By contrast, notice how the appropriate responses differ in tone and content. They each express a single, specific, concrete request of the moment. Assertive statements are like that: "Please wash the dishes." "Please pay me the five dollars you owe me." Also, they speak of the action they want, not of the person. The person spoken to knows exactly what to do and does not have to feel attacked. To insist that someone change a behavior that has been bothering you for a long time, apply the Health Strategies on this page, "Making Your Wishes Known."

Assertiveness is the key to getting cooperation and resolving conflicts. It makes it easier, not harder, for people to get along with you.

The Mediator's Role Sometimes the help of a neutral third party can move people in conflict closer to resolution. In the Hatfield and McCoy story, a mediator—in this case, the U.S. Supreme Court—stepped in to help separate real issues from imaginary ones. Mediators can be guidance counselors, teachers, friends, or anyone who can lend a clear head.

A mediator meets with both parties, but stays neutral (that is, doesn't take sides). This gives each party time to tell its version of what happened, with no interruptions. The mediator then helps to identify the facts and issues that are common to both parties. Many times, a mediator can help the arguing parties to respect each other, to wait while the other talks, and to tell the truth. Once everyone agrees on the same set of facts, solutions become possible. In some high schools, trained students act as "peer mediators" to help settle conflicts among their fellow students.

Health Strategies

Making Your Wishes Known

To confront someone, express yourself assertively but not aggressively. These rules apply to minor annoyances or conflicts. Unacceptable behaviors, such as hitting or stealing should be dealt with by teachers, parents, or other authorities.

1. To decide whether to mention something that bothers you, ask yourself, "Does this bother me every time it happens, or is it an isolated incident?" If it happens often, mention it. If not, handle it yourself by walking it off or waiting it out.
2. Make feeling statements about yourself ("It hurts my feelings when you . . ."), not judgment statements about the other person ("You are insensitive").
3. Pair a resentment with an appreciation: "I appreciate (this), but resent (that)." It's easier for the other person to deal with a problem behavior if you indicate that the person's other behaviors are OK.
4. Focus on the one incident that bothers you. Don't discuss everything else that has made you mad for months.
5. Be specific. Identify the *behavior* you want. Don't just complain.

multicultural issues

Discuss with your students the importance of learning some techniques for bridging cultural gaps when forming new relationships. As they meet new people at school, in the shopping mall, at recreational activities, or in the workplace, now or in the future, they can begin to build bridges by expressing an interest in the other person's culture.

Asking questions about things that are public information is a good way to show interest and to begin a relationship. These are questions that are not too personal or sensitive. You may want to poll your students for their ideas as to questions and comments that are appropriate, as well as those that are inappropriate.

***Figure 2–2** Nonassertive versus Assertive Responses*

Situation	Nonassertive Responses	Assertive Responses
1. A person steps in front of Sarah, who has been standing in line for an hour.	*Sarah:* "Well, excuse me!" or *Sarah:* Says nothing aloud; mutters "Some people…"	*Sarah:* "Excuse me. I was here first. The end of the line is back there."
2. James comes home, pours some juice, sits down, and flips on MTV.	*James's mom (from kitchen):* "I sure wish I could rest like that at the end of the day. But no, I have to cook dinner, bathe the baby, wash up—I'm tired, too."	*James's mom:* "Would you please cook dinner while I bathe the baby?"
3. Ken notices that his little sister hasn't cleaned up her room even though their father told her to do so earlier.	*Ken:* "Sis, Dad told you to clean up your room. What's the matter with you? You're the laziest child I ever saw."	*Ken:* "Dad told you to clean up your room. Now do it." (And he sees that she does.)

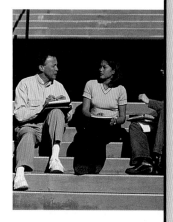

Sometimes a mediator can help people resolve conflicts.

People who lose their fear of conflict and use the techniques offered in this section can stop small problems from getting worse. With practice, problem solving becomes easier. The person who becomes known as a peacemaker gains a real sense of satisfaction. He or she also possesses a highly valued skill to use at home, at school, at work, and at leisure.

 KEY POINTS *Conflicts are normal in relationships. Assertive communication and conflict resolution strategies can often prevent escalation of conflicts.*

Forming New Relationships

Sometimes people need to make new friendships. Many people fear trying to make new friends at first. *Why Am I Afraid to Tell You Who I Am?* is the title of a book written by John Joseph Powell to help people overcome their fears about relationships. The title reveals the primary problems people have: the fear of making fools of themselves and the fear of being laughed at or rejected.

Reaching out to other people usually does not lead to rejection. To get started, though, you have to be willing to risk rejection and to handle it if it occurs. It helps to keep three things in mind. First, "If I'm rejected, I won't be any worse off than I am now." Second, "If it doesn't work out, it's no reflection on me, because I tried. The other person had other needs." Third, "If it does work out, both of us will have a new friend."

What most often happens when you reach out is that the other person is pleased to be approached. At best, a rewarding relationship has a chance to form.

Glossary
MINI

communication: a two-way exchange of ideas or thoughts.

assertive: possessing the characteristic of appropriately expressing feelings, wants, and needs while respecting those of others. Assertiveness is the key to obtaining cooperation.

passive: possessing the characteristic of not expressing feelings appropriately, of remaining silent.

aggressive: possessing the characteristic of being insulting or overly demanding to others or otherwise invading their territory; an inappropriate expression of feelings.

Because language reflects so much of the culture, students might want to ask how to say simple words and phrases such as *hello, good-bye, please,* and *thank you.* From this starting point they might move on to ask questions about holidays, foods, dress, recreation, and how one shows respect. Point out to students that they may find their cultures have many of the same goals and values, but the manner in which they are expressed may vary. Their interest in other people's cultures will not only help develop relationships with greater appreciation between themselves and people of other cultures, but will enrich their school environment and workplace as well.

SECTION 2 Review Answers

1. Answers will vary.
2. family members, neighbors, members of a sports team, people in a religious organization, advisor (p. 34)
3. Your needs may go unmet. (p. 34)
4. four of the following: decide whether to mention something; make feeling statements about self rather than judgmental statements about the other person; pair a resentment with an appreciation; focus on the one incident rather than accumulated annoyances; be specific about the behavior if problem is major (p. 38)
5. tell of your own feelings, ask about the other person's feelings, listen closely (p. 40)
6. Answers will vary.

A reproducible quiz for Section 2 is available in the Teacher's Resource Box.

CLOSE

Have students practice ways of saying things in an assertive manner. Have volunteers role play some ways to say things assertively. See pages 38–39 for suggestions.

Many people who know this can't act on it, though, because they don't know how or because they are too shy. A few suggestions can help. Each can be practiced, as suggested in the Health Strategies, "Tips for Overcoming Shyness," on this page. One expert suggests thinking of the word *soften* to remind you of what to do during actual conversations with new people:

S Smile.
O Open posture.
F Forward lean.
T Touch.
E Eye contact.
N Nod.

Here are some other helpful hints:

▶ Tell of your own feelings (people always find feelings interesting).
▶ Ask about the other person's feelings (people like you to be interested in them).
▶ Listen closely (people love to be listened to).

 KEY POINTS *People need other people to form a support network. Rejection is a risk in forming new friendships, but the risk is worth taking. The "SOFTEN" steps can help bridge the gap to others.*

Health Strategies

Tips for Overcoming Shyness

For many people, shyness takes the fun out of life. Psychologists who treat shyness say to:

▶ Rehearse what you have to say. Write down what you'd like to say. Read it out loud—first by yourself, then in front of a mirror, then with a friend, and finally in the setting you've been rehearsing for.
▶ Build your self-esteem by focusing on your strong points and praising yourself for good deeds or a good performance. Turn stumbling blocks into stepping stones.
▶ Talk into a tape recorder to improve your speaking voice.
▶ Observe and copy the behaviors of people you admire.
▶ Learn to laugh at yourself when things go wrong. Don't put yourself down.
▶ Remember that you are not alone. At least two out of every five people are as uncomfortable as you are.
▶ Do not try to hide your "true self." Accept who you are, with all your traits.
▶ Focus your attention on others and what they are saying. Do not focus on your own words, actions, and appearance.
▶ Before you enter a social setting, imagine yourself succeeding in it.
▶ Avoid using alcohol or other drugs to relax. They are not shortcuts to the social skills you desire. Also, using them can increase the chance that you will make a fool of yourself.

SECTION 2 Review

Answer the following questions on a separate sheet of paper.

Learning the Vocabulary

The vocabulary terms in this section are *support system, mentor, conflict, violence, feud, tolerance, mediator, communication, assertive, passive,* and *aggressive.*

1. Write a sentence using each vocabulary term.

Learning the Facts

2. In addition to friends, what other people can be part of a support system?
3. What could happen if you always give in to keep the peace?
4. List four strategies to become more assertive.
5. Give three helpful hints that could assist you when meeting someone for the first time.

Making Life Choices

6. Look over the Health Strategies feature, "Making Your Wishes Known," on page 38. Which strategies listed are you skilled in using? Which strategies listed do you need to improve on? How could you go about making each improvement?

QUICK QUIZ

Chapter 2, Section 2

The following quiz will help you assess your students' understanding of the material covered in this section of the chapter. You might use the quiz as an oral exercise, which will lead into a class discussion of the topics covered. Or, you might use it as a paper/pencil quiz to evaluate your students individually.

*If students have difficulty with the concepts covered in the Quick Quiz and the Section Review, you might suggest they review the material using the **S**urvey, **Q**uestion, **R**ead, **R**ecite, **R**eview (SQ3R) study method, which is described in detail in the introduction to this Teacher's Wraparound Edition.*

1. A person's friends and family frequently serve as a support system. (True)
2. Expressing a feeling of anger or distrust

SECTION 3
Making Decisions and Solving Problems

Some decisions—What shall I wear today?—are easy to make. Others are more weighty, such as "How can I tell my parents I don't want to be the person they want me to be?" In tackling tough decisions, it helps to follow a plan. One such plan is presented in the Health Strategies feature on this page, "A Method for Making Decisions." The discussion that follows offers help with the steps.

The first step, *naming the problem,* may be simple, but it may not be. Pinpointing the problem of what to wear usually is simple enough. Some problems, though, are so complex that they require years to figure out ("How can I straighten out my relationship with my parents?"). Whatever the problem is, the first step is to put it into words. Then you can begin seeking a solution.

Breaking a problem up into parts will make it more manageable. Say, for example, that you feel you don't fit in with your peers. Stated that way, the problem seems impossible to solve. Stated in its smallest units, though, it may look like this:

▶ I like to discuss world events. The group likes gossip.
▶ The group spends more money than I can afford to spend.

When you think about these smaller components, you can deal with them one by one. If they arouse emotions such as resentment, anger, or embarrassment, this may be a sign that the group's values are not in line with your own. This realization may help you to think up solutions that will meet your needs.

The brainstorming step involves thinking up many different solutions to the problem. During this step, don't try to solve the problem. Instead, exercise your imagination, and tap your creativity. This can be fun—and funny.

Brainstorming for the problem just described can bring out possibilities such as seeking other friendships, joining a club for people with more common interests, taking a class dealing in world events, and so on. Some ideas may be impractical. Some may be pure fantasy: move to another state; don't leave the house for a year; call the president of the United States. Writing down even impractical solutions is valuable, though. It could just be that a combination of answers is best. It helps to view them all.

In thinking about each solution, judge it based on your own values and feelings. Imagine and list the probable outcomes, both positive and negative. Compare the ideas. Then rank them in order from best to worst.

Consider the practicality of each solution. For example, a person who wanted to socialize with a group of

Health Strategies

A Method for Making Decisions

When you find yourself saying, "What should I do?" try this:

1. **Name the problem.** Be sure it's the real problem.
2. **Describe it specifically.** Name the problem's parts.
3. **Brainstorm.** Name all the solutions you can think of, no matter how crazy they may seem.
4. **Think about each solution and list its advantages and disadvantages:**
   ▶ How does it square with your values?
   ▶ Does it honor the values of your parents and others whom you respect?
   ▶ Would it solve the problem?
   ▶ Would it affect both you and others for better or worse?
   ▶ What are its possible consequences?
5. **Choose a solution, and act on it.**
6. **Evaluate the outcome:**
   ▶ Is the problem solved?
   ▶ What else happened?
   ▶ Would another solution work better?

SECTION 3

FOCUS

OUTCOME

In this section students will learn:

1. A six-step strategy for making decisions.

FOCUS ACTIVITY

Write a problem on the board for students to think about. (A local school issue is a good choice.) Ask, "What do you think should be done about this problem?" After getting several ideas, ask how they came up with their solutions. Discuss ways that people decide how to solve problems.

TEACH & APPLY

GROUP ACTIVITY

Brainstorm with students typical problems that teenagers encounter. (no money and want to go to the prom, boyfriend/girlfriend seems to be jealous all the time, people have been spreading untrue rumors, and so on) Divide the class into small groups and give each group one of the problems. Have them use the decision-making process to arrive at possible solutions. Then have them rank-order the proposed solutions. Discuss the results with the class. Each group can write its solutions on construction or butcher paper to hold up when explaining to the class. Post these ideas in the room. Discuss the problems of making joint decisions when different people have different values.

can cause it to intensify. (False)

3. Demonstrating flexibility while resolving a conflict is a sign of indecision. (False)

4. Assertiveness is generally very highly valued by society. (False)

5. Assertive behavior is neither passive nor aggressive. (True)

6. Assertiveness is the key to cooperation. (True)

7. A mediator is a person who takes sides in order to resolve a dispute. (False)

8. Good relationships are free from conflict. (False)

9. Discussing your feelings can be a good way to open a friendship. (True)

10. Body language is a way of expressing your feelings without words. (True)

GROUP ACTIVITY

Ask students to think about a problem they have had and what they did about it. Have them evaluate the effectiveness of their solutions using the three bulleted questions on this page.

ASSESS

EVALUATE

Without using the book, have students name the six steps in the decision-making process listed on page 41.

SECTION 3 Review Answers

1. Name the problem, describe it specifically, brainstorm, think about each solution, choose a solution and act on it, evaluate the outcome. (p. 41)
2. It begins the process of finding a solution. (p. 41)
3. Often a combination of solutions is the best. (p. 41)
4. Did the solution produce the results you expected? How did the solution fit with your feelings and values? Did the solution fail to meet your needs in any significant way? (p. 42)
5. Answers will vary.

A reproducible quiz for Section 3 is available in the Teacher's Resource Box.

CLOSE

Have students identify a current problem in their lives and make a plan to solve it.

Emotionally healthy people need others for friendship and support.

friends but who had money problems might consider helping the group plan some affordable but enjoyable activities, such as a potluck dinner or a hike. By helping plan, the person could assist the group without spending needed money. Then the person could participate because the activities would be low in cost.

Once you have thought all possible solutions through, you can pick one that fits your values and your personal circumstances. Try it out. Then answer the following questions to evaluate the solution:

► Did the solution produce the results you expected?
► How did the solution fit with your feelings and values?
► Did the solution fail to meet your needs in any significant way?

If the solution seems satisfactory, the decision was a good one. If the solution seems less than ideal, you can usually adjust it or discard it in favor of another. In that case, you begin the process of deciding all over again.

KEY POINTS *Problems can be solved by making decisions and taking action. A method that helps is to go through these steps: name the problem, describe it, brainstorm about it, and evaluate all possible solutions in view of your values. Then choose a solution, act on it, and evaluate the results.*

SECTION 3 Review

Answer the following questions on a sheet of paper.

Learning the Facts

1. List the six steps for making decisions.
2. Why is the first step in the process so important?
3. Why should you be sure to brainstorm all the possible solutions to a problem?
4. What are three questions you can use in the evaluating process?

Making Life Choices

5. List a problem you are facing right now. Work it through using the Health Strategies feature, "A Method for Making Decisions," presented on page 41.

Chapter 2, Section 3

The following quiz will help you assess your students' understanding of the material covered in this section of the chapter. You might use the quiz as an oral exercise or, you might use it as a paper/pencil quiz to evaluate your students individually.

Like the Quick Quiz, the Section Review can also be used as an assessment tool to spark class discussion or as an individual student evaluation. It can also be used as a review in preparation for this quiz.

1. Articulating a problem is the first step in resolving it. (True)
2. Emotional problems are always clear and easy to pinpoint. (False)
3. It is better to approach a problem in its entirety rather than try to break it down

SECTION 4

Finding a Place in Society

You and the other people with whom you have relationships fit into a larger circle—your society. Your society may consist of the community you live in, your school, and your ethnic or religious group. It may also include other circles. Societies have sets of values and expectations of their own that they impose on their members. Sometimes the fit is easy, sometimes not.

Our society has traditionally been steered by middle-class adults. Many adults of the middle class tend to put off enjoying today so that tomorrow there will be money or prestige or time to have fun. They also value doers—those devoted to action and achievement. In another culture, a mother may enjoy her child because he is sitting in her lap and laughing in her face. In our culture, a mother is more likely to be thinking of how well the child is preparing for tomorrow.

Not all societies uphold the same values for their members. Furthermore, in our society and many others, no law forces people to live by the values of the majority. However, if they don't go along, they lose approval and support. People whose values differ from society's may experience **alienation** and **ostracism**. A person who doesn't fit in is a **nonconformist**.

In any case, each person has to work out some relationship with the larger world. One person may choose to live totally in keeping with personal goals and values. Another may choose to live with a subgroup in society whose values differ from the majority's values.

Society is really a mosaic of many small societies, each a group of like-minded people. The important thing is to find a place that provides comfort and rewards and that respects your individuality. Be careful, though, not to get caught in a subgroup such as a gang, whose values and practices destroy your hopes for your future. Chapter 3 talks more about gangs.

For most people, an important part of finding a place in society is to discover a fitting job or career. A book written for people trying to find their place in the world of work is *What Color Is Your Parachute?* by R. N. Bolles. The title implies that the leap into a job is somewhat like jumping from an airplane. You have no guarantee of success. All you have is what you came

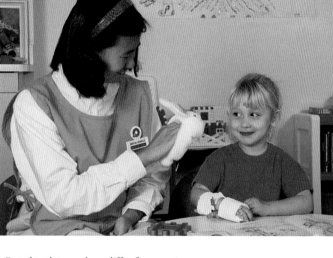

For most people, discovering a fitting job or career is an important part of finding a place in society.

MINI Glossary

alienation: withdrawing from others because of differences that cannot be resolved.

ostracism: rejection and exclusion from society.

nonconformist: a person who does not share society's values and therefore behaves in unconventional ways.

into small parts. (False)

4. When brainstorming, it can even be useful to come up with impractical solutions. (True)

5. Each potential solution to a problem should be judged according to your own values and feelings. (True)

6. Practicality is not an important consideration in deciding how to resolve a problem. (False)

7. If the solution to a problem is unsatisfac-

tory, it is sometimes necessary to start all over again. (True)

8. Steps for making a decision include: naming the problem, evaluating possible solutions, acting on a solution, and evaluating the results. (True)

9. It is not a good idea to list the probable outcomes of a solution. (False)

10. If a solution is practical it doesn't matter whether or not it agrees with your personal values. (False)

SECTION 4

EVALUATE

Assign students an essay in which they describe how they know they are accepted by a group or society.

SECTION 4 Review Answers

1. alienation
2. ostracism
3. nonconformist
4. the community you live in, your school, your ethnic or religious group, and others (p. 43)
5. loss of approval and support, alienation, ostracism (p. 43)
6. volunteer in different occupational fields (p. 44)
7. Answers will vary.

A reproducible quiz for Section 4 is available in the Teacher's Resource Box.

CLOSE

Discuss with students ways of getting people who are nonconformists to conform to society's expectations, or ways that society can better accept their differences. (don't put others down for being different, and so on)

Reproducible Study Outline and Reading Cloze worksheets for Chapter 2 are available in the Teacher's Resource Box.

Answers to FACT or FICTION

Here are the answers to the questions at the start of the chapter.

1. **False.** Emotional health is closely tied to physical health.
2. **False.** Once a person adopts values, that person continues to test those values and can change them when necessary.
3. **False.** It is best to face and deal with all feelings as promptly as possible, even those that seem illogical or unpleasant.
4. **False.** Emotionally healthy people do need others for friendship and support. This helps them stand on their own two feet.
5. **True.**
6. **False.** The best way to solve a problem is to think up many possible solutions, select from among them, try out solutions, evaluate results, and move on to try other solutions if the problem remains unsolved.

with—yourself. The better you know yourself, the better you can choose, and succeed at, a job or career.

Some experts believe that rewarding work is the single most important aspect of adult life relating to well-being. Many people who are unhappy at work wish they had explored more options, through courses and summer jobs, before specializing in one field. Such people may decide to change careers later in life. They may find it worth all the effort to finally be in the right career.

If you are uncertain about a career for yourself, you might try some volunteer work with a variety of industries. For example, some veterinarians may appreciate your help in their offices a few hours a week. A local theater might need people to usher the attending crowds. A hospital, nursing home, or other health care facility might welcome some afterschool help.

The best experience for glimpsing careers comes not from the typical paying jobs that teens take to earn spending money. Instead, the best experience comes from volunteer positions that allow teens a behind-the-scenes look at what life in those positions is really like. Take volunteering seriously. The experience and relationships with mentors are more valuable than the money you might earn elsewhere.

KEY POINTS *Each person must work out a relationship with society that is rewarding. Finding suitable work is a major task that supports emotional health. Efforts to discover your own interests and talents are well spent.*

SECTION 4 Review

Answer the following questions on a sheet of paper.

Learning the Vocabulary

The vocabulary terms in this section are *alienation, ostracism,* and *nonconformist.*
Match the following phrases with the correct vocabulary terms.

1. self-chosen withdrawal from society
2. rejection by society
3. a person who does not share society's values and therefore behaves in unconventional ways

Learning the Facts

4. What elements make up society?

5. What are the disadvantages of having values that differ from society's values?
6. Give some suggestions to a teenager who is unsure about a future career.

Making Life Choices

7. At this point in your life much of your time is spent in school, a type of self-contained society. The school staff has a set of values and expectations they impose on you. Which values and expectations do you accept? Are there any you reject? Give an example of a values confrontation you have experienced in school and how you handled it.

QUICK QUIZ

Chapter 2, Section 4

The following quiz will help you assess your students' understanding of the material covered in this section of the chapter. You might use the quiz as an oral exercise, which will lead into a class discussion of the topics covered. Or, you might use it as a paper/pencil quiz to evaluate your students individually.
Like the Quick Quiz, the Section Review can

also be used as an assessment tool to spark class discussion or as an individual student evaluation. It can also be used as a review in preparation for this quiz.

1. The values and expectations of society always reflect the values of individuals. (False)
2. The values of society frequently represent the values of middle-class adults. (True)

Straight Talk

Teenagers and Violence

The **violent crime** associated with some groups of teens today triggers fear in almost everyone near them, and rightly so. In most communities, the overall rate of murders and muggings has remained fairly constant over the past 20 years. In 1996, the rates even started creeping downward a bit. However, younger criminals are now committing a larger portion of these crimes, especially in lower-income neighborhoods.

 I often hear about teenagers and crime. How are teens connected with crime?

Most often, reports about teens and crime focus on teenage criminals. They may fail to report what most high school students already know: that teenagers are crime's most frequent victims. Teenagers suffer the effects of violent crime and theft at a rate of about twice that of adults.

Many teens grow up with fear of crime. Statistics show that hundreds of thousands of youths carry guns to school, at least occasionally. They feel they must protect themselves from fellow students. Closer to a million carry knives for that purpose. Many teens feel forced to cut classes or whole days of school to avoid violent classmates.

Homicide is now the leading killer of black males aged 15 to 24. Among causes of death of white youngsters, homicide is second only to auto accidents involving alcohol. Shooting and stabbing injuries that do not kill flood the emergency rooms of many communities. Disputes once settled with fists are now settled with guns. Every 100 hours, more youths die on the streets than were killed in the Persian Gulf War.

Who is committing all these violent crimes?

From the mid-80s to the mid-90s, the number of murders committed by adults past age 25 decreased by 20 percent. During the same period, murders committed by teenagers increased by 165 percent. Rates of other juvenile crimes also skyrocketed during that time.

In large part, adolescent crime tends to follow an increase in drug trafficking, as Chapter 12 explains. Drug abuse, especially involving marijuana, has been increasing among younger and younger children, as gangs lure them into their drug operations. Millions of adolescents, more than ever before, are confined in correctional institutions each year. This prompts some experts to declare the situation a national emergency.

MINI Glossary

violent crime: a crime that involves threat or uses force, including assault, murder, rape, or robbery.

45

Background Information
How you discuss this feature with your students will depend in a large part on the situation within your school. If violence is or has recently been a problem in your school or in the neighborhood surrounding your school, your students will have more input in and stronger feelings about the subject. If their area is fairly crime-free, they will feel more detached from the information. Try to bring up recent incidents of either local or wider importance for them to think about and discuss.

Class Activity
The feature lists several reasons for teen violence. (drug abuse and drug trafficking, gangs, legal system, music lyrics, television and movies, and so on) Ask students to name the reasons as you write them on the board. Then have students examine the list and rank the reasons, from strongest to weakest, in their view. What examples can they provide to support their ranking? If there are strong feelings within the class between different ideas, you might wish to have a class debate, but be sure to have the students support their opinions with examples and evidence.

3. Nonconformists can be ostracized from society. (True)
4. Society is actually composed of many small groups of like-minded people. (True)
5. Your career is not an important component of your social identity. (False)
6. Career choices do not affect your sense of personal well-being. (False)
7. Performing rewarding work can signifi-

cantly increase your sense of self-esteem. (True)
8. Volunteer work, though unpaid, can provide a rewarding learning experience. (True)
9. It is not worthwhile to pursue interesting work experience if it is unpaid. (False)
10. An individual's relationship to his society is an esential aspect of his wellness. (True)

Teenagers and Violence (continued)

 I only know a few kids who are into those things. Where do regular kids fit into the picture?

Luckily, the majority of teenagers are emotionally strong, socially healthy, and on a path that leads to a successful life. For example, three out of five teens volunteer at least a few hours every week for worthy causes. Overall, teen criminals constitute a small group of "repeat offenders." Teens in this minority are usually male and have long-standing social problems. These few are chronically in trouble at home, at school, and with the law.

Unfortunately, these offenders often victimize other teens as their targets. They disrupt schools and drain limited resources. Further, they create an atmosphere of fear that keeps innocent teenagers constantly under stress, on their guard. Some experts openly worry about lasting psychological damage to great numbers of adolescents who are growing up in an atmosphere that lacks the peace and security they need.

 What causes so much violence in our society?

One theory blames the legal system. The theory holds that our society is too soft on criminals, and calls for more police and longer jail times for offenders. This may sound like a simple solution, but the problems of crime and violence are complex. For example, the United States locks up more of its citizens for longer times than most other developed nations, yet its teenage crime rate continues to climb higher. Drug abuse, including alcohol abuse, almost certainly encourages delinquency. The great majority of young men arrested for such crimes as assault, burglary, or grand larceny test positive for drugs. Often, their victims do, too.

Some people blame the violent themes heard in music lyrics, viewed on television or in music videos, and seen in other media for violent behavior in teenagers. Study after study shows that children who watch violence on television become more aggressive and insensitive to violence in real life. The media may even glamorize violent criminals as clever, sexy, independent, and successful people who easily outfox the law. Some teens imitate the slick role models they see, sometimes even without their own awareness. By the way, real criminals most often score about 10 points below average on intelligence tests and are a far cry from the fictional characters of the movies.

Figure 2–3 When a Situation Gets Tense

Sometimes people feel forced to fight to defend their honor. They fear that their friends will think of them as cowards unless they fight. To defuse a situation that may lead to a fight, try these tactics.

- Commit yourself to maintaining peace. Make it your highest priority.
- Avoid people who are looking for trouble, or who have a history of violence. If you run into such a person, keep it brief and quiet. Anything you say may be taken as a challenge.
- If things become tense, say, "I don't want to fight with you about this."
- Speak calmly, without raising your voice.
- Take an attitude of friendliness (even though you don't feel friendly), smile (even though you're angry and frightened), and be ready to apologize (even if you did nothing wrong). Remember, your goal is to avoid a fight, not to prove your point. Later, you can resolve the issue with a mediator.
- Remember also that you may be dealing with someone who is out of control, or who can be violent without cause. Don't try to take a stand.
- Always give the person a way out of the argument; do not corner the person mentally, or yourself physically.
- If the situation recurs, get help later from teachers, parents, or school officers.

Source: Adapted from Safe Strategies for Saving Face, *Sex, etc.*, Spring 1997, p.6.

46

Class Activity

Video tape a daily news program for students to watch in class. Discuss the rise in teen violence and make a list of possible causes. Have students write essays on how they can help to decrease violence and crime in their own communities.

Group Activity

The feature mentions the use of rules and restrictions by schools to counter teen violence. Have the class name various rules and restrictions at your school, while you write them on the board. Then have the class rank the rules and restrictions from tolerable to intolerable. Once they have established a class list, have students come up with the reason for each rule. Then ask each student to write one argument for each of the five most intolerable rules. Divide the class into groups to discuss the reasons for the rules. Have each group arrive at an alternate method of dealing with the problem, using the six-step method for making decisions (listed on page 41). As a class, evaluate the solutions.

Class Activity

Reread the final paragraph of the feature with the students. Discuss the "avoidance" programs the students are familiar with. How effective do they consider them to be? What does it mean to focus resources on positive behaviors? Have students evaluate each of the possible solutions listed. (programs fostering parent-child closeness, community

Making wise decisions is one of the major challenges of the adolescent years. Decisions made too quickly or without adequate information can have long-term and serious outcomes. Adolescents require the proper knowledge and the opportunity to explore their choices in a safe environment, before attempting to implement or put their decisions into action. (Any acronym can be substituted for FACE)

FACE THESE EASY STEPS TO A DECISION
1. FIND & IDENTIFY
2. ALL POSSIBLE SOLUTIONS OF ALTERNATIVES
3. CONSEQUENCES
4. EVALUATE

Finding and identifying the problem or situation should be simple, but often other issues keep the situation from being clear.

I think someone needs to do something to take control and protect teenagers from violence. What can we do to help?

Sometimes, if enough people stand together on an issue and say, "Enough," the actions that result can change the whole picture. Some strategies people use to prevent violence include:

▶ Providing positive, caring adult role models for young people who have none.
▶ Teaching young people social skills, such as how to maintain self-control, how to form friendships, how to communicate and interact with others in positive ways, and how to resist peer pressure.
▶ Using students to teach their peers about violence prevention.
▶ Providing recreation, student work, or volunteer activities for young people so they have the chance to spend time in structured, purposeful environments.

Further, by protecting yourself, you can often reduce the likelihood of being crime's victim. For example, you can learn and use the conflict resolution strategies offered in Chapter 2. In addition, you can take an honest look at your friends. If they often fight or carry weapons, take yourself out of their crowd and find other buddies. More tips for what to do in tense situations are listed in Figure 2–3 on the opposite page.

Further, you can protect yourself from random violence by learning and using a few simple safety rules. Figure 2–4 on this page lists them for you.

 In my school, rules and restrictions make us mad. We have lockins, lockouts, drug tests, metal detectors—they even tell us that we can't wear some kinds of clothes and makeup! What's the point of all these rules?

Rules and restrictions reflect many schools' attempts to gain order and discipline, so that their students can learn in peace and safety. In districts with high rates of crime, testing and "zero tolerance" for drugs, guns, and knives have worked to reduce violence to some degree. Banning certain gang-related clothing or cosmetics is also believed to help keep the peace within school walls. Peer mediation programs, mentioned in the chapter, also go a long way toward ending arguments that could otherwise lead to fights.

Solutions such as these do work, but not perfectly. School administrators, teachers, and parents need more scientific information about how to reduce violence. One recent study of second and third graders

Figure 2–4 Ways to Avoid Being a Target of Violent Crime

At school:
■ Avoid carrying lots of cash.
■ Leave expensive jewelry at home.
■ Avoid areas with overgrown shrubbery.
■ Get involved in school crime watch.
■ Stay involved in school activities.
■ Be active in school drug prevention programs.

On the streets:
■ Determine the safest way to travel, and use it.
■ Walk in well-lighted areas.
■ Walk with friends rather than alone.
■ Don't pick up hitchhikers.

At home:
■ Check in with a parent when you get home.
■ Keep all doors and windows locked when you are inside.
■ Don't let anyone in without a parent's permission.
■ Know the quickest way out in case of fire.
■ Keep a list of key phone numbers (parents at work, a neighbor, the police and fire departments, and the local poison control center).
■ If things don't look quite right when you come home, don't go in. Go to a neighbor's home or a public phone, and call the police.

suggests that violent behavior can be "unlearned." Youngsters who were taught ways of solving problems, understanding others, and managing anger were much less likely to hit, kick, or shove classmates than were children who received no training. Researchers are hoping for a lasting effect as the children grow.

Meanwhile, a new idea is taking hold among researchers who study adolescents. Much attention and resources go to problem behaviors of teens, but parents want more for their children than just avoidance of drugs, violence, and other negative behaviors. More resources focused on positive behaviors could lead teens to lives rich with health, successes, and joyful experiences. Programs that foster parent-child closeness, community involvement, religion or spirituality, promotion of peace, protection of the environment, improving literacy, or commitment to stamping out inequality can be life-enhancing. Seek out these groups and become involved.

47

involvement, religion or spirituality, promotion of peace, protection of the environment, improving literacy, commitment to stamping out inequality) Are they involved in any of these? Do they feel these present a viable solution to teen violence? Why or why not? What would they add to the list?

Class Activity
Have students bring in a newspaper article about violence. Discuss ways that this situation could have been avoided; use Figure 2–3 and Figure 2–4.

ON LINE WITH HEALTH

You may want to have your students visit the following URLs, where they will find information and additional Web site resources to enhance their study of this chapter. As with all Web sites, you should check these out first to be sure the information found there is appropriate for your students.
National Foundation for Depressive Illnesses, Inc. **http://www.depression. org**
Mayo Clinic Health Oasis **http://www. mayohealth.org**
Both sites offer information about mental illnesses and how to get help. The Mayo Clinic site has vast amounts of information on many, many different health-related topics.

All possible solutions or alternatives must be considered in order to determine the best solution to the problem. (Brainstorming) Some of the possible alternatives may at first seem foolish, but may result in the best answer; so, include all possibilities.

Consequences can be positive or negative. Adolescents often overlook or ignore the consequences of a decision. Examining the outcomes before a decision is made will help prevent a short-sighted decision.

Evaluating and then reaching a decision is the goal of the FACE process. As information is measured and each step is considered, the best decision becomes more clear.

APPLICATION—Have students describe a situation or problem they or a friend have experienced recently and FACE it. **Examples (a)** a teenager is tempted to be an hour later than their midnight curfew, **(b)** a student encourages a friend to fight.

VOCABULARY

1. a. alienation **b.** thoughts
c. ostracism **d.** cortex
e. support system **f.** status
g. nonconformist **h.** emotional health
2. Answers will vary.
3. a. assertive, passive
b. emotion **c.** values
d. confrontation

RECALL

SECTION 1

1. relationship with one's self (p. 26)
2. The emotional warmth, energy, and enthusiasm of a self-confident person makes other people feel good. (p. 26)
3. peace of mind, reduced stress, and improved health (p. 27)
4. Answers will vary; could include: recognize your negative thoughts, stop them, or replace them with positive thoughts. (p. 26)
5. It makes choosing behavior less confusing (p. 29)
6. Would I state this value to others? Will I stand by this value when challenged? Do I act consistently and repeatedly in line with this value? (p. 29)
7. They are natural. (p. 31)
8. anger, hurt, loneliness (p. 31)
9. speaking, writing, crying, shouting, laughing (p. 32)
10. Not expressing emotions at all would be harmful. Physical expression allows you to think calmly about what triggered the emotion initially. (pp. 32–33)

CHAPTER 2 Review

Summarizing the Chapter

Your ability to respond correctly to the following statements ensures your understanding of the main concepts in the chapter.

1. Discuss the importance of self-acceptance, positive thinking, and values clarification to emotional health.
2. Recognize that the acceptance and appropriate expression of feelings are important to emotional health.
3. Discuss the advantages of assertive health behavior, and identify assertive behavior strategies.
4. Describe the role that fear of rejection plays in forming new relationships, and discuss ways to overcome this fear.
5. Outline the steps for making a decision.

Learning the Vocabulary

emotional health	violence
thoughts	feud
cortex	tolerance
values	mediator
status	communication
emotion	assertive
emotional intelligence	passive
resentment	aggressive
suppress	alienation
confrontation	ostracism
support system	nonconformist
mentor	violent crime
conflict	

Answer the following questions on a separate sheet of paper.

1. Matching—*Match each of the following phrases with the appropriate vocabulary term from the list above:*

a. withdrawing from others because of differences that cannot be resolved
b. conscious mental processes
c. rejection by society
d. the gray matter of the brain
e. individuals or groups that offer emotional help
f. a person's standing in relation to others
g. one who has values that are different from society's and behaves unconventionally
h. being free of mental disturbances that limit functioning
2. Create a story using ten vocabulary terms from the list above. Underline all the vocabulary terms in the story.
3. a. An _____ person expresses feelings appropriately, while a _____ person remains quiet.
b. Fear is an example of an _____.
c. _____ are what a person views as important.
d. An interaction in which one person expresses feelings to another is called _____.

Recalling Important Facts and Ideas

Section 1

1. Which relationship supports you throughout your life?
2. Why is self-confidence so attractive?
3. List three benefits of positive thinking.
4. Describe how to change a negative thought into a positive one.
5. What is the advantage of being aware of your values?
6. What three questions can you ask yourself about how strong your values are?
7. Why are all feelings considered acceptable?
8. Name three emotions people often deny.
9. What are some of the physical ways of expressing feelings?
10. Why is it helpful to express emotions physically?

Section 2

11. What are the problems with passive and aggressive behaviors?
12. Why does assertive behavior improve your relationships with people?
13. What is the most common fear people have when meeting someone new?
14. What is the "SOFTEN" technique?

48

Section 3

15. What are the six steps you should follow when faced with making a decision?

Section 4

16. What does the middle class tend to put off?

17. What are the advantages of having a career you enjoy?

Critical Thinking

1. Take the Life Choice Inventory on page 28. Then answer the following questions. Are you satisfied with your score? Why or why not? Why is it necessary to continually work towards improving your score? What do you have to gain by putting your efforts into improving your emotional health?

2. Think back over your recent experiences and identify a situation in which you did not act assertively.
   a. Write a description of the experience. Include the reason for the conflict as you perceive it, the verbal interchange that occurred, and the outcome of the situation.
   b. Analyze your behavior. According to the definitions provided in Section 2, were your responses passive or aggressive?
   c. Write a revised version of the incident in which you act assertively. Describe the feelings you would probably experience after such an exchange.

3. Maintaining emotional health is easier for a person with a strong, well-developed support system than for someone who remains isolated from others. Examine how extensive your support system is by making a list of all your supports. Be sure to include people you have relationships with in all areas of your life. Which people on your list would you consider to be the most valuable supports? Are you satisfied with the support system you have developed for yourself? Describe any changes or improvements you would like to make.

Activities

1. Create a collage of magazine illustrations of different emotions.

2. Make a list of activities in your school and community that enhance emotional health. Suggest other activities the school could offer.

3. Devise a list of community resources for people seeking help for emotional problems. Provide the name, address, and phone number of each agency.

4. Write a short report on how school has affected your emotional health in the past year.

5. Keep an emotion diary for two days. List the emotions you felt, the situations that prompted them, and the outlets you used to deal with them.

6. Select a popular song that depicts a particular emotion. Discuss the music and lyrics that portray emotion.

7. Think back through your day yesterday. Beginning with getting up, list every situation you can think of that caused an emotional response in you. Next to the situation, list the emotion you felt. For example, when your alarm rang you might have felt happiness because of something special you were going to do. Or, when the bell for third period rang, you might have felt dread because of a test. When you have finished the list, put a + by the emotions you consider to be positive. Put a − by the emotions you consider to be negative. Look at the emotions you marked as negative. Beside each, tell how you might have turned the negative into a positive. For example, when the bell for third period rang and you felt dread, maybe the feeling of dread could have been a more positive feeling if you had studied more. If you don't think it would have been possible to change the negative feeling into a more positive feeling, tell how you would have handled the negative feeling.

Making Decisions about Health

1. You have just been treated unfairly and are uptight and tense. You return to your room where you pace around, shaking your head, many unsaid remarks still tumbling in your thoughts. Several times you start to pick up the phone, but there's no one you want to bother with your problems. Several times you start towards the door, but there's no place you want to go, feeling so uptight. Finally, you settle down, still angry, and try to do some homework, but you end the day with a knot in your stomach. Describe how you could have handled this situation to reduce your distress.

SECTION 2

11. With passive behavior a person's wishes are never expressed, and with aggressive behavior a person's feelings are expressed at the expense of the feelings of another person. (p. 38)

12. It makes it easier, not harder, to get along with others, because you make your wishes and needs known to them. It is the key to cooperation. (p. 38)

13. fear of rejection (p. 39)

14. smile, open posture, forward lean, touch, eye contact, nod (p. 40)

SECTION 3

15. name the problem, describe it specifically, brainstorm, think about each solution, choose a solution and act on it, evaluate the outcome (p. 41)

SECTION 4

16. enjoying today so that there will be money or prestige for tomorrow (p. 43)

17. Rewarding work is the single most important aspect of adult life relating to well-being. (p. 44)

KEY POINTS

Chapter 3 is 28 pages long and divided into four sections. Briefly, this chapter introduces students to the concepts of human needs, personality development, self-esteem, peer groups, peer pressure, and deviant peer groups. It stresses the importance of having our needs met, but doing so in a constructive rather than destructive way. Special emphasis is given to peer pressure and selection of peer groups during the teen years. The chapter has a theme: all that we are and all that we become depend on the development of self-esteem and the choices we make in our attempts to satisfy our needs.

ACTIVITY TO INTRODUCE THE CHAPTER

Write these words on the board or an overhead: 1. friendly, 2. helpful, 3. honest, 4. funny, 5. responsible, 6. grateful, 7. patient, 8. good listener, 9. empathic, 10. inventive, 11. generous, 12. sensitive, 13. loyal, 14. kind. Now have the students remember a time when they displayed each of these qualities. On a piece of paper have them jot down their examples for each one. Don't let them give up until they have an example for each one. Give them ten points for each example. Then say, "If you have 140 points, you have a pretty good start on developing self-esteem. You are a fine human being. If you have less than 140 points you are still a fine human being, but your memory is shot!!" This activity will show the students

CHAPTER 3

Contents

STRAIGHT TALK
Dealing with Peer Pressure

NOT Enough Time?

Following are some suggestions to help you make sure that you cover the key topics in this chapter, if you have limited time. (Refer to the daily lesson plans in your Teacher's Resource Box for additional suggestions.)

DAY 1 Assign students to read Sections 1 and 2 prior to Day 1. Also assign the Focus Activity on page 52. On Day 1 have the students do the Focus Activity on page 57 and the Class Activity on page 59. Conclude the class with the Section 1 and 2 Reviews or Quick Quizzes. You may want to assign reteaching activities from the resource

Your Changing Personality

FACT or FICTION

What do you think? Are the following statements true or false? If you think they are false, then say what is true.

1. One of the most important tasks of the teen years is to work out an individual identity.
2. Human beings need the respect of others even more than they need shelter.
3. People with high self-esteem see only the good parts of themselves and ignore the bad parts.
4. People who imagine themselves as greater or more successful than they are need to get a grip on reality and stop dreaming.
5. A peer group is usually a negative and destructive force that changes good kids into bad kids.

(Answers on page 71)

Introduction

You may overhear someone say, "Leticia is so great to be around" or "I think Mr. Wood is awful." In each case, the speaker is reacting to Leticia's or Mr. Wood's personalities. Your **personality** is a large part of how people see the total "you," on the outside. There is much more to you than what's seen from the outside, but your personality, the way you think, feel, and behave, defines you to others.

Personalities are not fixed for life. Each person has certain tendencies, and these are inborn. Personalities can keep changing through life, however. A baby may be born shy or outgoing, but the future child, teen, or adult can become more outgoing or more quiet. You are continually molding your personality to fit the picture you have of who you really are, your **self-image**.

This chapter explains some influences that affect personality. It also guides you in developing a healthy sense of self.

that everyone has good qualities, but using them requires daily practice.

BULLETIN BOARD IDEAS

Write the following quote in large letters on a piece of paper, and place it in the center of the bulletin board. "What you do with your problem is far more important than what your problem does to you."—Robert Schuller

Ask students to write a paragraph on what the quote means to them. What is Schuller trying to say? How could they apply this statement to themselves and problems they have had in their lives? Post the student essays around the quote. At the end of the chapter, ask students to reread their paragraph and determine if they still agree with their earlier thoughts.

Answers to FACT or FICTION

1. **True.**
2. **False.** Human beings first need the essentials for survival—food, clothing, and shelter. Then they become free to notice other needs.
3. **False.** People with high self-esteem cherish their good parts, but also acknowledge and work on the areas that need improvement.
4. **False.** People who imagine themselves as greater or more successful than they are may be taking an important first step toward a more successful future.
5. **False.** Peer groups are usually positive forces that can help teens develop a sense of identity.

materials for those students doing poorly on the quizzes.

DAY 2 Assign students to read Sections 3 and 4. Lead students in the Class Activity on page 52. Continue with the Focus Activity on page 62, followed by the Class Activities on pages 65 and 68.

DAY 3 Assign students the Close Activity on page 71 prior to Day 3. Discuss student responses to that assignment on Day 3. As time allows do the Group Activity on page 63 and lead the Discussion activity on page 70. Use the Section 3 and 4 Reviews and the Quick Quizzes for evaluation.

FOCUS

OUTCOMES

In this section students will learn:

1. Two popular theories of personality, one developed by Eric Erikson, the other by Abraham Maslow.

2. Ways Erikson's developmental stages combine with Maslow's hierarchy of needs to help people understand how personality develops.

FOCUS ACTIVITY

Have students look up the word *need* in the dictionary. Then have them list the needs they feel they must have satisfied to live a happy and productive life. To start them thinking, ask the question, "When you were first born, what were your needs?" Then tell them to progress chronologically to where they are now, listing any needs they feel they had or have now, including fulfilled and unfulfilled needs. As a class, discuss the needs students listed and why they feel those needs are so important to them. Collect or have them keep the lists in their notebooks.

TEACH & APPLY

CLASS ACTIVITY

Have the students list traits that they feel best describe their own personalities. Give them two or three minutes and then put up an overhead transparency with the following traits listed:

SECTION 1

Life's Stages and Human Needs

Certain patterns of change take place during people's lives and affect their personalities. When people see the patterns of their lives, they can make conscious choices that would not be possible otherwise. In this section you will learn about two personality theories that may help you better understand your own development and behavior.

Erikson's Eight Stages of Life

A pioneer in **psychology**, Erik Erikson, has described how people become who they are. Erikson's widely accepted theory says that people move through eight stages in the course of their lives. In each stage they learn important things about themselves and about the world.

Each stage ideally consists of positive development, and each builds on the one before it. The one-year-old learns basic trust as an infant, for example, and then can progress toward becoming independent in the next year. Each stage also has, however, a negative side. The less well one task is achieved, the less successful will be the next. The eight stages are shown in Figure 3–1 on page 54.

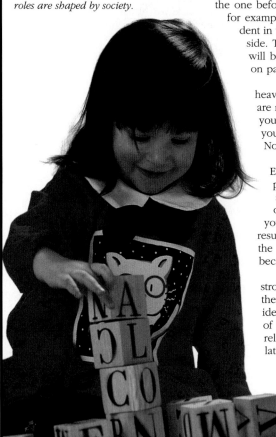

Early in life, children's gender roles are shaped by society.

Erikson's theory can be destructive if it is applied too heavy-handedly. It is not meant to be a grading scale. You are not "better" if you are higher on the scale or "worse" if you are lower. No one has had a perfect childhood—not your parents, your teachers, nor the authors of this book. No one moves perfectly through life's tasks.

The positive path of development, according to Erikson, might go like this. If, as an infant, toddler, and preschooler, you received mostly approval from the adults in your life, you progressed confidently from one stage to the next. By the time you started school, you were sure of your ability to master new tasks. As a result, you worked confidently and persistently through the school years, even in the face of frustrations. You became industrious.

A person who starts out strong like this develops a strong, positive self-image. By the end of the teen years, the successful person has achieved a positive sense of identity. From there, it is natural to move to the first stage of adulthood—the stage of building a mature, intimate relationship with another person. Intimacy and dating are later topics of this book.

Suppose, however, that a person's life story is primarily negative. Suppose the baby is neglected, frightened, beaten, or abused. The baby is already mistrustful and fearful of the environment. If faced with ridicule and punishment,

COOPERATIVE LEARNING

Developing Positive Self-Esteem

Explain to students that everyone has strengths that make them unique and different than others, and they also have weaknesses that separate them from others.

Most people tend to dwell on their weaknesses and this diminishes their self-esteem. There are some things that a person can do to improve self-esteem. Developing self-esteem is done through positive self-talk, acceptance of ourselves, and accepting how others view us or as we believe others view us. The following activity will help students develop positive self-esteem through messages they get from their peers.

Positive comment activity—Have the students place desks in one large circle facing in. Begin by making a positive comment about the student sitting nearest to you. Then ask the child will become unruly or afraid to try new things. The child develops guilt and a negative self-image ("I'm not OK"). This person may have trouble rising to challenges in school, sticking with demanding tasks, and forming a strong identity as a teenager. Such a person is unlikely to be ready to form a successful relationship with another person and may become an inadequate parent, later on.

If you see yourself at all in the negative description just given, you are not alone. Many people who cross your path in a day feel they are "not OK" to some extent, falling short of the standard they think has been set for them. It's normal to feel "not OK," but you can grow out of it.

 Erikson's theory divides the human life span into eight stages. Each stage presents different developmental tasks. One must successfully complete earlier tasks before moving on to later ones.

The Tasks of the Teen Years

The teen years present a demanding task to the developing person—that of working out an individual identity. To develop an identity means to partially move away from what is known and to explore the unknown. Teens try out new ideas, develop new words, and give new meanings to old phrases. "Cool," "awesome," or "dis" have had special meanings when spoken by some teens. Clothes, music, and art are other areas in which teens use their imaginations to explore and search for their identities.

At the same time that teens are searching for an individual identity, they may tightly associate with a group identity, especially in the early teen years. This may seem to work against the struggle for individuality. However, it is really a step toward independence, because joining a group is a way of joining the larger society outside the family.

Teens are also developing a new way of thinking. Children think only in concrete terms, relying on past experiences to predict the future. They experience things as they come. Teenagers, though, begin to think in more abstract terms. They can imagine what might happen "if this" or "should that" be the case.

Teenagers can consider **variables** and use logic to make predictions of what might happen. They can plan to achieve desired outcomes, and they spend hours with one another exploring "what ifs." (One caution: people develop on their own timetables. Although many people develop these high-level reasoning abilities in their teens, many others are still developing along these lines after entering college.)

The hours teenagers spend in each other's company permit them to practice reasoning, a skill that gives them a great advantage in working out relationships with others. Thinking develops considerably during adolescence.

Many teens feel emotions in extremes:

▶ Loving parents and then hating them.
▶ Feeling like total successes and then like total failures.
▶ Wanting freedom and needing safety.
▶ Being thrilled with new experiences and seeking comfort in familiarity.

Teens imitate others, yet search for a unique identity. They may be generous and unselfish one day, self-centered and greedy the next.

MINI Glossary

personality: the characteristics of a person that are apparent to others.

self-image: the characteristics that a person sees in himself or herself.

psychology: the scientific study of behavior and the mind.

variables: changeable factors that affect outcomes.

---

aggressive, caring, impulsive, confident, outgoing, cooperative, sincere, creative, curious, careless, blunt, courteous, tactful, narrow-minded, pessimistic, intelligent, realistic, selfish, humble, nervous, optimistic, sensitive, mature, proud, honest, humorous, and serious. Give them an additional two minutes to add to their lists. Then, after each trait they have listed, have them write a (P) if they think that trait is a positive one and an (N) if they think that the trait is a negative one. Have students put their papers in their notebooks to be used later in the chapter.

DISCUSSION

Remind students that the negative words we say to each other can be as destructive and damaging as a physical attack, and the effects are often more long lasting. There are positive words or phrases that make us feel good about ourselves and there are negative words or phrases that make us feel bad about ourselves. The *way* in which someone says something can affect us in a positive or negative manner. Have the students, during the next 24 hours, jot down every positive comment they hear about themselves or someone else. Also have them jot down every negative comment they hear.

Stimulate class discussion by asking: Where were most negative comments made—directly to the person or behind that person's back? Why do we handle negative things the way we do? Emphasize that making positive comments helps students develop self-esteem for themselves as well as others. Encourage them to make positive comments as often as possible.

---

each person in the class to make a positive comment about that student. Continue until each person in the class, including yourself, has received comments from the class. Comments will vary but might include great smile, nice dresser, smart, outgoing, funny, athletic, and so on.

Have students record the comments that classmates give them. Ask them to write about how the comments affected their self-esteem, as well as how it felt to give others compliments. Students will find that the comments they received from their peers make them feel better about themselves. Some of the comments may concern things about themselves that they believed to be weaknesses. Students will realize that their self-esteem improves when they compliment others or do something nice for other people.

HENSION CHECK

students summarize in
heir own words the positive
and negative sides of each of
Erikson's stages. Ask for volunteers to give their summaries.

BACKGROUND INFORMATION

Erikson said that each of the eight stages is characterized by a primary crisis or dilemma, which he called a *development task*. An individual's failure to resolve or succeed at these tasks throws off the individual's balanced development and makes life harder. Erikson considered that answering the question "Who am I?" is the most important task of the teen years.

FOCUS ACTIVITY

Ask students to consider how they're progressing through Erikson's fifth Stage of Life. A way to do this is by having them make posters or collages with pictures and words that answer the question, "Who Am I?"

COMPREHENSION CHECK

Review the meaning of the word *internalize* with your students. It means to make something such as a value, belief, or idea part of a person's permanent personality or mental makeup. The belief or idea that is inter-nalized becomes part of the per-son's guiding principles. It may be a conscious or unconscious decision to internalize the idea.

Figure 3–1 Eight Stages of Life According to Erikson. *The numbered paragraphs describe the tasks a healthy person will master at each stage.*

1 Infancy (0 to 1) To learn trust. The infant learns that needs will be met. (If neglected or abused, the person learns distrust that can last a lifetime.)

2 Toddler stage (1 to 2) To learn independence. The toddler learns self-will. (If thwarted in this development, the adult may remain dependent and feel inadequate.)

3 Preschool age (3 to 5) To learn initiative (the ability to think and act without being told to do so). The child explores with curiosity and imagination. (If discouraged in this development, the adult may avoid leadership and risks.)

4 School age (6 to 12) To develop industriousness (earnest, steady effort). The child has confidence to pursue self-chosen goals. (If this development fails, the adult will lack social confidence and will perform poorly.)

5 Adolescence (13 to 20) To develop an identity. The teenager develops a strong sense of self, goals, and timing and becomes busy learning how to fit into the social circle—as leader, follower, female, male. The adolescent picks out role models and grows with confidence. (The failure of this development produces a confused person without a secure sense of direction.)

6 Young adulthood (21 to 40) To develop intimacy (close, personal relationships). The young adult can commit to love, to work, and to a social group. (Failure leads to avoidance of intimacy, misuse of sexuality, isolation, and destructiveness.)

7 Adulthood (41 to 60) To develop generativity (giving yourself and your talents to others.) The mature adult moves through life with confidence, taking pride in accomplishments. (The negative side of this is stagnation, self-involvement, and failure to encourage others.)

8 Older adulthood (61 and older) To retain ego integrity (satisfaction with life). The person feels fulfilled and faces death with serenity. (The adult who has not moved positively through earlier stages experiences isolation, despair, and fears of death.)

COOPERATIVE LEARNING

You have probably been using group activities in your class for as long as you have been teaching. Your reasons might include the need for sharing limited equipment or your desire to help with the students' socialization.

Recently, more than ever before, the need for structured group work, or *cooperative learning* as it is frequently called, has become more evident.

In the workplace, it is becoming apparent that many young people have not learned the skills necessary for them to be successful. Among the unlearned skills are problem-

These extremes are all normal, and experimenting with them leads to the development of an identity. Teens need to keep their options open. At times almost anything they try may seem a possible way to pattern their lives.

Although it may sound as if the teen years are "out of control," they are not. The teen is in the driver's seat, steering a course to the future self. Wrong turns are everywhere, and mistakes are common. Luckily, few teens permanently damage themselves by their wrong turns. If they are harmed, it is usually by allowing their mistakes and false starts to damage their internal sense of self-worth, their self-esteem.

A person who emerges from the teen years feeling "OK" can move on to adult tasks without difficulty. The less fortunate teen who internalizes a sense of self-doubt and failure may have difficulty in performing the tasks of adulthood. Happily, much is known about enhancing even a sagging sense of self-esteem, as you will see in a later section.

 KEY POINTS *People develop their identities and their ability to reason during the teen years. This prepares them to accomplish the tasks of adulthood.*

Human Needs According to Maslow

Erikson saw life's tasks as associated with age groups. The theorist Abraham Maslow, in contrast, described a **hierarchy**, or a sort of ladder, of human **needs** that people of all ages experience. He linked these needs to life's accomplishments. Some people don't even know they have needs, but everyone does.

According to Maslow, people will struggle to meet their basic needs before they can begin to think about "higher" needs. Hunger is a basic need. People who are hungry may not be able to think about their need for love. Once the basic need for food is met, however, other needs naturally arise. In other words, needs build on one another. When you have met the most basic ones, you become aware of, and can strive to meet, the "higher" ones (see Figure 3–2 on the next page).

Most basic are needs related to survival—needs for food, clothing, and shelter (physiological needs). Next are the needs to feel physically safe and secure (safety needs). If safe and secure, people are free to notice their needs to be loved and to feel emotionally secure (love needs). If those needs are met, people can try to get in touch with their needs for respect and esteem. Given that, they can seek to achieve the ultimate: **self-actualization**. This is the realization of their full potential: becoming "all that they can be." Only a few people, perhaps 1 to 2 percent, ever develop that far.

Maslow believed that all self-actualizing people share some traits in common. Such people:

- ▶ Accept themselves and others, and accept imperfections.
- ▶ Are self-motivated, rather than externally motivated.
- ▶ Are problem solvers, rather than complainers.
- ▶ Have a strong set of values by which they live, and are sensitive to ethical issues.
- ▶ Believe in the power of people, holding that most are basically good.
- ▶ Are at peace with themselves and their world.

Such people also may have had "peak experiences"—emotional, often spiritual or religious experiences that helped to clarify their place and purpose in the world.

> 66 *When I was a boy of fourteen, my father was so ignorant I could hardly stand to have the old man around. But when I got to be twenty-one, I was astonished at how much the old man had learned in seven years.* 99
>
> Mark Twain
> (1835–1910)
> American writer

MINI Glossary

hierarchy: a ranking system in which each thing is placed above or below others.

needs: urgent wants for necessary things.

self-actualization: the reaching of one's full potential; the highest attainable state in Maslow's hierarchy of needs.

 TRANSPARENCIES The transparency, "Maslow's Hierarchy of Needs," is provided in the Transparency Acetate Binder.

COMPREHENSION CHECK

Ask students to explain a basic difference between Erikson and Maslow. (Erikson's theory says tasks progress primarily by age; Maslow's says they develop by needs.)

 WORKSHEETS Vocabulary worksheets are provided in the Teacher's Resource Box.

ASSESS

EVALUATE

 WORKSHEETS A reproducible quiz for Section 1 is provided in the Teacher's Resource Box.

FAST FACTS

Positive imaging can improve your athletic skills. In a recent study, one group of men practiced free throws every day for a month. A second group simply visualized themselves shooting successful free throws. The group that practiced boosted performance by 24%, while the group that visualized boosted their performance by 23%.

solving skills, creative-thinking skills, and skills to enhance teamwork. Cooperative learning is designed not only to encourage teamwork but also to teach the skills necessary for *effective* teamwork. In addition, it is a good way to give students practice with problem-solving and creative-thinking activities.

The main difference between unstructured group work and cooperative learning is *interdependence*. Interdependence means depending on one another. When group members are interdependent, the success of the group as a whole depends on the contribution of each individual member of that group.

Review Answers

1. Personality is how others see you; self-image is how you see yourself. (p. 51)
2. Self-actualization, hierarchy (p. 55)
3. Answers will vary.
4. eight (p. 52)
5. Children think in concrete terms, teenagers in more abstract terms. (p. 53)
6. Answers will vary; could include: complete success vs. complete failure, loving parents then hating them, wanting freedom and needing safety, and desiring new experiences vs. comfort in familiarity. (p. 53)
7. hunger; survival, including clothing and shelter (p. 55)
8. 1–2 percent (p. 55)
9. Answers will vary.

CLOSE

On an 8½ × 11-inch paper, have the students draw a pyramid and divide it into five horizontal sections. Beginning at the bottom, have them label each section in this order: physical needs, safety needs, love needs, esteem needs, and self-actualization needs. Review "Human Needs According to Maslow" on pages 55 and 56. Hand back, or have the students take out of their notebooks, their lists of needs (Focus Activity, p. 52) and ask them to copy those needs below the pyramid they drew. Now have the students look at each need and label it as a physical need (PN), a safety need (SN), a love need (LN), an esteem need (EN), or a self-actualization need (SA).

Assign a summary paragraph in which students explain why basic needs must be met before higher needs can be met.

Figure 3–2 Maslow's Hierarchy of Needs

Once basic needs are met, a person can aspire to meet higher needs.

Like all people, teens share the common need for respect and the esteem of others. Many people say that some of their best experiences as teenagers involved some sort of service to others. To be helpful, especially to those who really need help, fills a need to feel important and to be appreciated by others. Being helpful enhances self-esteem.

Performing needed service to others helps also in the development of identity. Teens who work together during disasters to assist other people may "find themselves" (develop part of their identities) in the process. Other teens who join service clubs that volunteer help in the community may find that this experience adds to self-understanding and identity.

No one ever arrives at the point of being completely finished with any level of needs. Needs at all levels surface every day. Still, at a given time in life, needs on one or two levels take center stage in importance.

Needs never end. As soon as one is met, another takes its place. It can be said that life is a series of needs to be satisfied or problems to be solved, but this is not a complaint. It gives us something to work on, which is itself a need we all seem to have.

KEY POINTS *Personality develops throughout life, according to Erikson. The development is propelled by the needs in Maslow's hierarchy.*

SECTION 1 Review

Answer the following questions on a sheet of paper.

Learning the Vocabulary

The vocabulary terms in this section are *personality, self-image, psychology, variables, hierarchy, needs,* and *self-actualization.*

1. What is the difference between personality and self-image?
2. _____ is the highest attainable state in Maslow's _____ of needs.
3. Write a sentence using each vocabulary term.

Learning the Facts

4. According to Erik Erikson, how many stages do people move through in their lives?
5. How does the thinking of teenagers differ from children's thinking?
6. What are some of the extremes in emotions that teens may feel?
7. What are some of the most basic human needs according to Maslow?
8. What percentage of people are able to reach self-actualization?

Making Life Choices

9. List in order Maslow's hierarchy of needs (refer to Figure 3–2 on this page if you need help). Identify what your specific needs are in each of Maslow's major categories. Try to come up with at least six items for each of the five areas. Make a list of some steps you could take that you believe would help to bring you closer to self-actualization.

QUICK QUIZ

Chapter 3, Section 1

The following quiz will help you assess your students' understanding of the material covered in this section of the chapter. You might use the quiz as an oral exercise, which will lead into a class discussion of the topics covered. Or, you might use it as a paper/pencil quiz to evaluate your students individually.

Like the Quick Quiz, the Section Review can also be used as an assessment tool to spark class discussion or as an individual student evaluation. It can also be used as a review in preparation for this quiz.

1. Erik Erikson's theory states that lessons improperly learned in infancy can affect an individual's ability to develop for the rest of her or his life. (True)
2. It is not possible to outgrow a feeling of

SECTION 2
Gender and Personality

Two parts of human development undergo rapid change during the teen years. One is the development of physical gender characteristics. Another, which goes along with the physical events, is the development of gender identity—a personality with maleness or femaleness.

Physical Maturation

Children grow and mature physically from birth to adulthood. However, not until some time around the early teen years do they enter the period of sexual maturation called **adolescence** or **puberty**. During these years, nature seems in a hurry to complete the final details needed for full adulthood. The adolescent growth spurt is a time of rapid growth and change (see Figure 3–3 on the next page). It includes the development of an identity that lasts a lifetime.

During adolescence, individual growth rates vary tremendously. Generally, girls begin an intensive growth spurt by age 10 or 11, while boys hit this time of rapid growth at 12 or 13. Two healthy, normal adolescents of the same age may vary in height by a foot. At this time in life, external standards such as growth charts and weight tables are all but useless. To take them too seriously is a mistake—a mistake that could lead to a damaged self-image.

As they grow toward adulthood, girls naturally develop more body fat than do boys. This normal fat is needed for breast formation and other normal development. Sadly, most normal-weight high school girls fear this fat and, when asked, report that they are overweight. Especially damaging are comparisons of their normal, living bodies with the super-skinny models seen in advertisements. The models starve themselves, and photographs are designed to make them look skinnier still.

In contrast to girls, boys naturally develop more muscle tissue. As is true in girls, this tissue grows in response to hormones.

The hormonal changes of adolescence greatly affect every organ, including the brain. Hormones also bring mood changes.

As the body improves in coordination, movements requiring control and skill become possible. Athletics, acting, dancing, and playing musical instruments all may now be in reach.

For some, the changes occur faster than the individuals can adjust to them. For others, the changes come so slowly that they fear being left behind. Most important is to accept and welcome your emerging identity. The teen years soon pass; you then join society's adults as an equal.

As boys and girls become young men and women, their social relationships must also change. They must develop new ways of dealing with their peers and work out new rules to govern their relationships. Physical maturity does not mean the end of growth and change—far from it. Mental, emotional, and spiritual growth and change can continue for a lifetime.

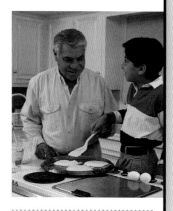

As gender roles change, more men are enjoying the peaceful tasks of the home.

MINI Glossary

adolescence: the period of growth from the beginning of puberty to full maturity. Timing of adolescence varies from person to person.

puberty (PYOO-ber-tee): the period of life in which a person becomes physically capable of reproduction.

inadequacy. (False)
3. The teen years are spent attempting to develop an individual identity. (True)
4. When a teen conforms to the expectations of a peer group, it is often a way of breaking away from the family. (True)
5. Teenagers, like children, think only in "concrete" terms. (False)
6. Teenagers frequently experience extreme and contradicting emotions. (True)
7. Experimentation is a normal part of developing an individual identity. (True)
8. An individual develops the ability to reason during the adult years. (False)
9. Abraham Maslow wrote that emotional, or "higher," needs can develop only after the basic human needs, such as hunger, have been met. (True)
10. According to Maslow, human development is propelled by a constant progression of needs. (True)

SECTION 2

FOCUS

OUTCOMES

In this section students will learn about the:

1. Two parts of human development that occur rapidly during the teen years—physical maturation and the development of gender identity.
2. Ways stereotypes can stifle individual development of your potential as a person.

FOCUS ACTIVITY

Tell students that within the human species we have male and female gender roles. Have students make a list, using one- or two-word answers, of personality traits they feel are considered feminine by our society. Ask them to make another list of the personality traits they feel are associated with masculinity. Students might identify some traits as both masculine and feminine. Lead a class discussion about how gender roles shape our society.

TEACH & APPLY

BACKGROUND INFORMATION

Tell students that:

a. Girls increase their strength by about 45% during puberty; boys by 65%.
b. Boys develop greater amounts of oxygen-carrying hemoglobin. This, along with the male's larger heart

(continued on next page)

(from previous page)

...nd lungs, gives him greater endurance.

c. Boys are only slightly stronger than girls before puberty. After puberty, the average male can bench press about 1.7 times as much as the average female.

d. Boys secrete about 30 to 200 micrograms of testosterone each day following puberty. Girls secrete from 5 to 20 micrograms. Because testosterone stimulates muscle growth, this difference means that girls do not develop as much muscle tissue as do boys in response to exercise.

CLASS ACTIVITY

Have each student write down the name of one role model important to them. Then give each student 60 seconds to tell the class who the person is and how that person has affected his or her life.

CLASS DISCUSSION

Have each student write down their definition of "human." What does it mean to be a "human being" as opposed to an animal? Have students share their definitions and work out a class definition. Ask students to

Females

Growth
Rapid gains peak around age 12, then growth slows to a stop at maturity.

Hair
Hair grows on underarm and genital areas, and other body hair may grow coarser and longer.

Skin
Acne may develop.

Body shape and composition
Hips widen, fat deposits collect, and breasts develop.

Hormonal changes
Ovaries produce more estrogens and progesterone.

Reproductive organs
Uterus and ovaries enlarge; genitals enlarge; ovum ripening begins; and monthly menstruation begins.

Males

Growth
Rapid gains peak around age 14, then growth slows to a stop at maturity.

Hair
Hairline of forehead begins to move upward (recede). Hair grows on face, in underarms, and around genitals. Other body hair grows coarser and longer.

Skin
Acne may develop.

Body shape and composition
Muscle tissue develops.

Hormonal changes
Testicles produce more testosterone.

Reproductive organs
Penis and testicles enlarge; sperm production begins.

Figure 3–3 Physical Changes of Adolescence. The organs, functions, and structures mentioned here are discussed in more detail in Chapter 6 and later chapters.

However, the changes that have taken place during adolescence do tend to become a permanent part of a person's identity.

 KEY POINTS *Adolescence is a time of rapid physical and mental change that makes possible the development of sexual and other forms of maturity.*

Gender Identity

Your personality is affected by your **gender**. You are male or female, and this helps mold your behaviors and your self-image.

•multicultural issues•

People from diverse cultures share similar concerns and participate in similar activities, such as getting an education, making a living, and interacting with friends. The ways people handle these concerns and perform these activities vary from culture to culture. Point out to students that as they meet new friends,

they invariably share a lot of information about themselves and how they live. As they share information, they often may find that they live in ways very different from the ways their new acquaintances live.

Ask students to imagine they have met someone their age over the Internet or through a pen-pal program. Have students write letters to this person that include the following information.

Not everyone accepts society's gender roles.

The male or female roles people play are known as their **gender roles**. A person's inherited genes probably play some part in development of a person's gender role. Clearly, though, society's expectations are powerful in their effects. Each society trains its individuals, from birth on, to act as it expects male or female people to act. Not everyone adopts all of society's gender roles. In fact, if enough people find them a bad fit, the roles themselves may change. The parts of the male or female role that a person accepts and lives by become that person's **gender identity**.

Society responds even to its newest members according to its gender roles. People can be overheard to say, when observing a newborn boy, "My, how big and strong he is!" If the baby is a girl, they might say, "She's so tiny and delicate!" Actually, newborns differ in size, strength, and activity not according to gender but according to their individual hereditary makeups.

Toddlers begin to learn gender roles before they can even talk. Two-year-olds show real understanding of these roles. By age 11, the patterns are deeply ingrained. They are virtually cast in concrete in adults. Young teens, with their newly maturing sexual bodies, often exaggerate these roles to make sure that those around them are aware of their **femininity** or **masculinity**.

Today, if you are male, you have probably grown up under pressure to "succeed"; to be strong, brave, and independent; and to hide emotions. You may have been encouraged to play rough games, to defeat others, and not to get too close emotionally.

If you are female, you have probably grown up with demands to be beautiful or attractive and sensitive to others' feelings. Perhaps you have been urged to be artistic, to avoid aggression, and to take care of others.

Complete acceptance of society's gender roles is not always easy or desirable. People are individuals. Roles that may fit one person perfectly may

MINI Glossary

gender: the classification of being male or female.

gender roles: roles assigned by society to people of each gender.

gender identity: that part of a person's self-image that is determined by the person's gender.

femininity: traits, including biological and social traits, associated with being female.

masculinity: traits, including biological and social traits, associated with being male.

list the things that a human can do that an animal cannot do. Discuss why animals can't do some things that a human can do.

CLASS ACTIVITY

Have students number their papers from 1 to 20. Read the following job titles and ask the students to write an F if they think it is a "female" job title, an M if they think it is a "male" job, or a B if they think "both," either male or female, could do that job. 1. welder; 2. nurse; 3. doctor; 4. lawyer; 5. construction worker; 6. telephone operator; 7. TV news anchor; 8. engineer; 9. president of a large company; 10. U.S. senator; 11. collegiate volleyball player; 12. data processor; 13. circuit judge; 14. officer in the armed forces; 15. principal of a high school; 16. kindergarten teacher; 17. high school physics teacher; 18. chef (cook); 19. plumber; 20. ballet dancer.

Discuss as a class why students classified each occupation as they did. Make the point that many of these jobs reflect traditional gender roles but that not everyone accepts gender roles. Some people find them a bad fit and change their roles. A woman who doesn't feel comfortable in a traditional role may become a truck driver and be very good at that trade. A male may succeed in a profession, such as nursing, that has in the past been seen by society as a predominately female profession.

COMPREHENSION CHECK

Ask students to explain the difference between gender roles and gender identity. (Gender roles are behaviors society expects; gender identity refers to each person's behavior. The roles are broader; identity is specific to each person—no two are identical.)

1. the length of their school day
2. the subjects they are studying in school and how much homework they have
3. how they get to school
4. where they eat lunch on school days and what foods they have
5. how responsibilities are shared in their families
6. how they manage their home chores and responsibilities
7. what they do when they are not in school
8. how long vacations are and what they do on vacations
9. what they plan to do after high school
10. what holidays they celebrate and how they celebrate them

Encourage students to exchange this information with someone from another culture.

Left Sidebar

...OUND ...MATION

...me societies demonstrate gender roles that seem opposite to those of our own society. Margaret Mead found that among the Arapish of New Guinea, men were passive, cooperative, peaceful, and nurturing—the father was said to "bear children"! Eighty miles away, the Mandugumor women were expected to be violent, competitive, sexually aggressive, and eager to solve disputes by fighting.

ASSESS

EVALUATE

A reproducible quiz for Section 2 is provided in the Teacher's Resource Box.

Review Answers

1. gender (p. 59)
2. Masculinity (p. 59)
3. Puberty (p. 57)
4. Gender roles are assigned by society, while gender identity includes traits that are determined by a person's gender. (p. 59)
5. 10 or 11 (p. 57)
6. Answers will vary, but could include any of the following. For females, rapid growth gains peak around age 12, hair grows on underarm and genital area and other body hair may grow coarser and longer, hips widen, fat deposits collect, and breasts develop, ovaries produce

Main Column

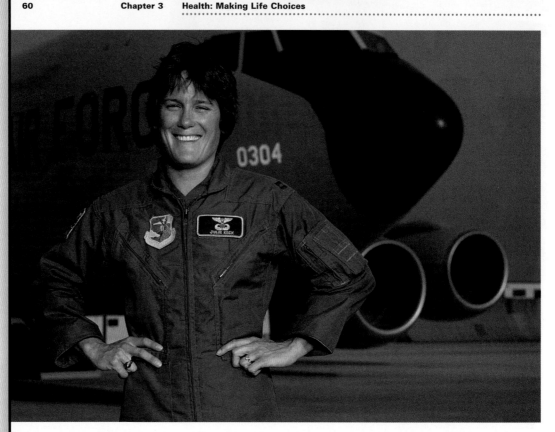

Gender identity is important, but even more so is the full realization of a person's potential.

be unsuitable for another. If everyone accepted roles without question, societies would never change. Furthermore, strict roles—**stereotypes**—may stifle individual development. No one is treated fairly when allowed only a limited space in which to grow toward personhood.

It takes generations to replace old gender stereotypes completely. Some that you may see changing during your lifetime are these:

▶ Men are active and independent; women are passive and dependent.
▶ Men hide their emotions; women show their emotions.
▶ Men discipline their children; women nurture them.
▶ A man's success is seen in his earnings or status; a woman's success is measured by the man she marries.

Evidence that these confining roles are breaking down can be seen all around us. The armed forces now accept women in their ranks. The nursing profession welcomes men into the field. Once-exclusive clubs are opening their doors to people of both genders.

One of the happiest outcomes of these recent changes in our society's gender roles is that men today can enjoy some of the roles formerly reserved

QUICK QUIZ

Chapter 3, Section 2

The following quiz will help you assess your students' understanding of the material covered in this section of the chapter. You might use the quiz as an oral exercise, which will lead into a class discussion of the topics covered. Or, you might use it as a paper/pencil quiz to evaluate your students individually.

Like the Quick Quiz, the Section Review can also be used as an assessment tool to spark class discussion or as an individual student evaluation. It can also be used as a review in preparation for this quiz.

1. Puberty begins during early childhood. (False)
2. Boys begin this period of rapid growth earlier than girls. (False)
3. Many girls regard normal and natural body fat as a sign that they are over-

for women only. Just as women can now work in politics, become corporate executives, or build bridges, so men can enjoy cooking, nurturing children, and performing other peaceful tasks in the home.

The process of breaking down old gender stereotypes has not been trouble-free, however. Strong female figures in politics and the military, for example, have been verbally attacked for being too aggressive or outspoken—traits that their attackers identify as male. Also, both men and women are speaking out against **sexual harassment** that was once endured silently. Sexual harassment amounts to sexual jokes; name calling; or unwanted sexual attention, touching, or threats. Harassment frequently involves a misuse of power, often from a person's superior. Workers may be sexually harassed by bosses, for example, but may keep quiet for fear of losing their jobs. According to one source, 85 percent of all teenagers have endured sexual harassment of one sort or another. Sexual harassment is illegal, and it shouldn't be ignored. If you experience it, tell the person to stop it. If it doesn't stop, report it to school or other officials.

Your gender identity is important, but it is only a part of your personality. More important still is the full realization of your potential as a person. The next section explains one of the key requirements for developing a healthy personality and, in fact, for all emotional health—self-esteem.

 In developing an identity, each person adopts characteristics that go with that person's gender. Gender roles are useful as long as they allow freedom for individual differences.

Society imposes gender roles on its members.

more estrogen and progesterone, uterus and ovaries enlarge, genitals enlarge, ovum ripening begins, and monthly menstruation begins; For males, rapid growth gains peak around age 14, hair of forehead begins to recede, hair grows on face, in underarms, and around genitals, and other body hair grows coarser and longer, muscle tissue develops, testicles produce more testosterone, penis and testicles enlarge, sperm production begins; for both females and males, acne may develop. (p. 58)

7. Answers will vary, but could include any of the following: men are active and independent while women are passive and dependent; men hide their emotions while women show theirs; men discipline their children while women nurture them; a man's success is seen in his earnings or status while a woman's success is measured by the man she marries. (p. 60)

8. Answers will vary.

9. Answers will vary.

CLOSE

Have the class list any people they know—famous or not—who have broken stereotyped roles and become very individualistic. Now have each student write a short paragraph on why it is important for each human being to become an individual, and how the differences in people benefit our society. Have the class members discuss their lists and the positive aspects they noted.

SECTION 2 Review

Answer the following questions on a sheet of paper.

Learning the Vocabulary

The vocabulary terms in this section are *adolescence, puberty, gender, gender roles, gender identity, femininity, masculinity, stereotypes,* and *sexual harassment.*

1. The classification of being male or female is called your _____.

2. _____ consists of the traits associated with being male.

3. _____ is the period of life in which a person becomes capable of reproduction.

4. What is the difference between a person's gender identity and gender role?

Learning the Facts

5. At approximately what age do adolescent girls begin a growth spurt?

6. List some changes that occur due to increased levels of hormones during puberty.

7. Name some common gender stereotypes.

Making Life Choices

8. The changes that take place during adolescence tend to become a permanent part of a person's identity. What do you think are some of the most common things boys and girls your age worry about most as their bodies show physical changes?

9. Besides puberty, what are some other things that influence a person's identity?

MINI Glossary

stereotypes: fixed pictures of how everyone in a group is thought to be; ideas that do not recognize anyone's individuality.

sexual harassment: unwanted sexual attention, often from someone in power, that makes the victim feel uncomfortable or threatened.

weight. (True)

4. The physical changes which occur during the teen years vary widely for each individual and have a profound effect on emotional development. (True)

5. A person's gender role is determined more by social expectations than by his or her biology. (True)

6. Gender roles are learned only during the teen years. (False)

7. Acceptance of society's gender roles always promotes emotional and physical well-being. (False)

8. Gender stereotypes are currently undergoing dramatic change. (True)

9. The breakdown of conventional gender roles is allowing men to experience behaviors typically reserved for women. (True)

10. What we now call sexual harassment has only existed for the past twenty years or so. (False)

SECTION 3

Developing Self-Esteem

How many people do you know who really believe in and respect themselves? Do you? People who know and like themselves are emotionally healthy. They have high **self-esteem**. People with high self-esteem do not think they are perfect. In fact, they know they are not, but they like themselves anyway. They not only cherish the positive sides of themselves, they have learned to accept the negative, even though they may be trying to improve. In contrast, a person who *claims* to be perfect probably has low self-esteem. Such a person cannot admit imperfections without feeling threatened by them, and so the person denies having any faults.

High self-esteem is crucial for emotional health. Poor self-esteem is closely linked with a wide range of problems: drug and alcohol abuse, addictions of all kinds, crime and violence, child and family abuse, teenage runaways, teenage pregnancy, prostitution, gang membership, and failure of children to learn. Poor self-esteem, therefore, diminishes not only individuals, but also society. Society spends billions of dollars in medical expenses, law enforcement, and education every year because of the problems caused by poor self-esteem.

People with high self-esteem, on the other hand, contribute to society's well-being. In return, they reap benefits from society in terms of emotional and financial support. They feel worthwhile, and so they do not hesitate to assert themselves to get what they want.

The Life Choice Inventory beginning on page 64 provides a way to measure your self-esteem. One way to improve self-esteem is by developing a positive view of your inner self, as described next.

Positive Self-Talk

A technique for viewing your inner self positively is to practice making positive statements about yourself. These statements, called **positive self-talk**, can be ones you think are true now or statements you plan to make true by means of practice. Positive self-talk gives you power—that is, it makes you feel effective. You give yourself the power to become the person you want to become and to do the things you want to do. Positive ideas replace self-defeating messages. The Health Strategies section on this page, "Improving Self-Esteem," lists some positive actions for developing a more successful you.

To practice positive self-talk, repeat to yourself an idea that you wish to become a reality. For example, a person who wishes to feel less anxious might think or say aloud, "I can relax when under stress." A person who wishes to feel less lonely might think, "I can be alone without being lonely" or

TEACHER SUPPORT

Key Passage

Ask students what *esteem* is. (to hold in high regard; to think of with respect; to prize) Esteem comes from a Latin word meaning "to estimate." Can they see the connection?

FOCUS

OUTCOMES

In this section students will learn:

1. The definition of self-esteem.
2. How important self-esteem is in developing emotional health.
3. Ways to evaluate self-esteem and raise their own personal self-esteem.

FOCUS ACTIVITY

Write *self-image* on the board. Ask the students for a definition. (the characteristics a person sees in himself or herself) Now write *self-esteem* on the board. Ask for a definition. (the value a person attaches to his or her self-image) Write *value* on the board. Ask for a definition. (relative worth, importance, degree of excellence) Discuss the value each of us places on the different parts of our self-image, and how these values relate to our self-esteem.

Health Strategies

Improving Self-Esteem

These actions can improve your self-esteem:

1. Write out positive statements about yourself.
2. Find activities that are related to your goals, and join in.
3. Be grateful. Remember to take count of and appreciate what you have.
4. Practice positive self-talk.
5. Seek out books and movies with positive themes.
6. Surround yourself with friends who believe in you.
7. Support others—believing in, supporting, and speaking positively about others help you become more positive and stronger.
8. Refuse to think negatively about yourself or others. Accept the fact that everyone is growing emotionally at their own pace.
9. Celebrate your successes.
10. Give and receive affection—hugs, for example.

CRITICAL THINKING

Eating disorders are critical problems in the United States, especially among teenage girls. Discuss with students why this is the case. How has society and our culture influenced people in such a way as to "pressure" them into experiencing eating disorders?

Have students write letters to the editor of the local newspaper describing what they think it would be like to be trapped in the destructive behaviors associated with anorexia and bulimia.

"I like people, and they like me." Other statements that can start a person's changing for the better are "I deserve success" and "I accept myself as I am."

You can also help yourself to succeed at whatever task you choose, or to develop whatever quality you desire, by mentally seeing yourself already there. Imagining a successful outcome in advance helps people battle diseases, win athletic contests, and overcome emotional problems.

Another suggestion for making desires become reality is "acting as if" you already have the quality you are seeking. This is often called "fake it 'til you make it." This technique is not only useful for personal growth. It is also used to teach salespeople how to sell products successfully, athletes to win sports competitions, and others to succeed in many other areas of life.

 To develop high self-esteem, use positive self-talk to turn ideas about what you'd like to be into realities. Act as if qualities you wish for were already yours.

Positive Body Image

Another part of self-esteem is a positive **body image**. Negative body image is a common problem in our society. Each year, millions of people try to change the way they look. Forty million go on diets. Half a million undergo cosmetic surgery. Multitudes try contact lenses, facials, and new cosmetics in hopes of becoming more attractive. People feel that they must be sexually attractive, and our society defines sexual attractiveness very narrowly.

A factor in the body image of teens is how early or how late an individual develops an adult-looking body. It might seem that the earlier developers would have an advantage in this regard, and this is so—but only for boys. Early-maturing boys report feeling positive about their bodies. Many early-maturing girls, though, report the opposite. They feel threatened by becoming different from their peers and may even try to hide their maturity under baggy clothing.

These gender differences in self-acceptance may be the result of a society that stresses individuality for males, but that values group behavior in females. The important thing is that each person is maturing normally on his or her own timetable, and each deserves respect and acceptance. Some are early to mature, some are later, but all eventually arrive.

As you might guess, a negative body image and the intense pressure from society for a sexier appearance make many people easy prey for advertisers who want to take advantage of consumers.

Improving your body's appearance by means of good nutrition and physical activity benefits your physical health. Chapters 7 through 9 offer many tips on how to develop nutritional health and fitness. Once you've attained a healthy body, though, let that be enough. Don't compare your body with the unrealistic, overly thin or overly developed standards for sexual attractiveness you see in advertisements or on television. Fitness is beautiful, but both thinness and bulkiness can be taken to extremes.

 A positive body image is part of self-esteem, but the bodies seen in advertisements and on television are unrealistic. Learn to see through insulting sales pitches. Aim for fitness, not for thinness or bulkiness.

> 66 *No man can make you feel inferior without your consent.* 99
>
> Eleanor Roosevelt
> (1884–1962)
> American humanitarian
> and writer

Mini Glossary

self-esteem: the value a person attaches to his or her self-image. Self-esteem is high in those who value themselves. It is a vitally important part of emotional health.

positive self-talk: the practice of making affirming statements about oneself to oneself, helpful in building self-esteem.

body image: the way a person thinks his or her body looks, which may or may not be the way it actually does look.

Share several of the best letters with the class. Now have students write letters from the editor in reply to the first letters. The emphasis of these letters should be on encouraging the person to accept himself or herself and on suggesting ways to maintain and achieve a healthy weight and outlook.

Encourage students to personalize this activity to help them understand the dangers of eating disorders and how to help people trapped by these disorders.

Eating disorders are discussed in more detail in Chapter 8.

TEACH & APPLY
Your Changing Personality

GROUP ACTIVITY

Divide the class into groups of six to eight students. Provide a piece of 24 × 36-inch paper for each student, along with masking tape and a broad-tip marker for each group. Choose one person in each group to be the recorder. Have each group sit in a semicircle facing a wall. Place a chair against the wall and tape a sheet of paper to the wall next to the chair. One student at a time volunteers to sit on the chair while each of the other students in the circle tells one *positive* trait about him or her. The recorder lists all these traits on the paper, then reads the list. The list can then be given to the student before a clean sheet is taped up for the next volunteer. Students can "pass" going to the chair if they choose. When all groups have finished, discuss as a class what was learned. Ask students for their observations about the body language of the person in the chair and the person telling the trait. Does the way others see us match the way we observe ourselves?

COMPREHENSION CHECK

Students learned about the differences between passive, assertive, and aggressive behaviors in the last chapter. For review, ask students to give examples of each type of behavior. Ask them why it is important to learn how to be assertive, rather than passive or aggressive.

Class Discussion

Use the Life Choice Inventory as a springboard for class discussion. Many students will be inclined to argue that the best or most idealistic answers are *a* and *c* rather than *b*. Try to get students who have answered *b* to explain the advantages of their choice. The more aggressive students should see the potential advantages of not alienating people, while the passive students should see the advantages for their emotional well-being in not harboring grudges or anger.

CLASS ACTIVITY

Have each student write a positive statement about himself or herself each Monday, then focus on the statement for a week by repeating it to themselves each day. You could set aside a minute of each class for them to reinforce the statements by practicing self-talk.

CLASS ACTIVITY

Have the students write answers to the following questions. If I were to die today, how would I want to be remembered? How would I define myself? In a nutshell, what is unique about me? What have I accomplished? What accomplishment brings me the greatest pleasure?

To reinforce the concept of positive self-talk and self-esteem ask student volunteers to read their essays to the class. Post all the essays on the bulletin board with the names covered.

How Well Do You Speak Up for Yourself?

If you have high self-esteem, you will find it easy to be assertive, rather than aggressive or passive, in speaking up for yourself. These questions offer a way to measure your assertiveness. Indirectly they measure your self-esteem. (Some items may not apply to you. Try to imagine that they do.)

1. Your mother has said that she wants you with the family at six o'clock today. At five o'clock, a friend invites you to a get-together you can't refuse. You:
   a. Go with your friend, stay through six, and explain to your mother later.
   b. Call your mother and explain that you must go with your friend.
   c. Complain to your mother that she is too demanding, but stay home.
   d. Tell your friend you can't go, and say nothing to your mother.

2. You studied with several of your friends for a test. They all got good grades. You wrote the same kind of answers but got a low grade. You think your work was just as good as theirs. You:
   a. Write an anonymous note to the principal saying that the test grades are obviously unfair.
   b. Take your test to the teacher, and ask why your grade was low.
   c. Complain to all your friends, and say nothing to the instructor.
   d. Keep your mouth shut so that the teacher won't be even more unfair to you the next time.

3. You have just cleaned the kitchen. Then someone puts a greasy pan on the countertop and starts to leave. You:
   a. Wait until you are alone, then put the greasy pan between the person's bedsheets.
   b. Tell the person, "Please wash your frying pan before you leave."
   c. Make a general remark about how inconsiderate people leave dirty dishes for others to clean up.
   d. Say nothing; wash the pan yourself later.

4. You are on your first date with someone you have admired from a distance for a long time. At the end of the evening, the other person gets much more physical than you want to be. You:
   a. Back off, and leave as quickly as you can without saying anything.
   b. Tell the other person that things are going too far for you.
   c. Keep pulling away, and let the other person guess the message.
   d. Say nothing and go along, because you want to date the person again.

5. You get home with a new cassette tape of your favorite music, only to find that the tape you just bought is already ruined in the package. You:
   a. Storm into the store and make a scene so that all the customers will know you were sold a messed-up tape.
   b. Go back to the store, ask to see the manager, and explain that the tape you just bought is ruined.
   c. Never shop in that store again.
   d. Do nothing.

COOPERATIVE LEARNING

Following are some suggestions to use with cooperative learning groups to help your students become "teammates."

Individually, each student must be responsible, not only for completing his or her individual part of a task, but also for learning the material necessary for the completion of the whole task. For example, if students are working in groups to learn the stages of progression, each group member should have an individual responsibility. Not only would each member be responsible for his or her own part of the task, but each member would also

6. You are in your room, studying for a big exam. Your sister is playing the stereo loudly. You:
  a. Knock on your sister's door, walk in, and switch off the stereo.
  b. Ask your sister to turn down the volume, and explain why.
  c. Go someplace else to study, and refuse to speak to your sister for the week.
  d. Give up trying to study.

7. Your friends like horror movies, but you don't enjoy them at all. Your friends are making plans to see the latest horror movie this Saturday night. You:
  a. Tell them you think horror movies are for mental midgets, and you're not going.
  b. Tell them you don't enjoy horror movies, and ask if they'd consider another movie.
  c. Go to the movie, then make humorous negative remarks about it, hoping they will get the message.
  d. Stay home Saturday night.

8. You occasionally babysit for Mrs. Harper's three children. Lately she has been making excuses when it comes time to pay you. You:
  a. Tell her that you're fed up and that you won't babysit for her anymore.
  b. Tell her that it's inconvenient for you to be paid late.
  c. Decide you won't work for her again.
  d. Say nothing.

9. You and your friend are in a pet store together. You see your friend slip a rubber dog bone into a coat pocket. You:
  a. Grab the dog bone, put it back on the shelf, and threaten to turn your friend in.
  b. Tell your friend how you feel about shoplifting, and recommend replacing the dog bone.
  c. Say nothing, but resolve never to go shopping with your friend again.
  d. Act as if nothing has happened.

10. Your parents have given you some money to spend on clothes. They have told you exactly what they want you to buy. You need clothes, but you disagree with the style they are urging you to buy. You:

  a. Buy what you want, and tell them they are way out of touch with today's styles.
  b. Tell them how you'd rather spend the money and why it's important to you.
  c. Buy what they want you to have, and try to trade it for something else later.
  d. Buy what they want you to have, wear it, and thank them for it.

SCORING

Give yourself 10 points for each *a* answer, 8 for each *b*, 6 for each *c*, and 4 for each *d*. Add them up. Your answers to the Life Choice Inventory are personal and private. Share them with others only if you are comfortable doing so.
If you scored:

85 to 100—You have no trouble asserting yourself, but your behavior borders on aggressiveness. You know what you want, but you have to give more thought to how you go about getting it.

75 to 84—You are assertive to the right degree. You have a good sense of what you want, and you speak your mind. People are not offended by your frankness, and they accommodate you when they can.

50 to 74—You need to practice voicing your opinions and speaking up for your rights. Get in touch with your needs, and speak up.

Below 50—You almost never voice an opinion. You are building up some resentments. Work on raising your self-esteem. Start practicing assertiveness—be honest with yourself and others.

Source: Adapted from S. Schlatner, Get smart, *Coed,* March 1981, p. 36b.

be responsible for knowing the information contained in the entire analysis and how it all fits together. Everyone in the group is responsible for making sure other members understand the material. Asking questions of different group members will let you know who understands the material.

While the students are working in groups,

communication skills are important. You need to set guidelines for the students' interaction and communication while they are in their groups. You must insist that they speak positively to each other, using encouragement rather than insult. It is important that you monitor their interaction while they are in groups.

CLASS ACTIVITY

Have the students take the following "Positive Inventory." On a piece of paper have each of them number 1–11, leaving three or four lines between numbers. Preface this activity by saying, "Everyone is good at something. That is part of what makes us unique. Take this positive inventory of yourself. List everything you can for each item of the inventory. No matter how small you think it might be, it is still important." You can now read the eleven items to the class or use an overhead transparency you have made in advance. The items are: 1. The things I like about myself are . . . 2. I once received an award for . . . 3. Something I can do that I am proud of is . . . 4. The last time someone gave me a positive comment was . . . 5. An accomplishment that made me feel good about my abilities was . . . 6. Something I am learning to do right now is . . . 7. Something I did today that I feel good about is . . . 8. Something I did this week that I feel good about is . . . 9. Something I did this month that I am proud of is . . . 10. Things I have learned to do are . . . 11. Something I will do this year that I will be proud of is . . .

Give students 10–15 minutes to work. Now have a class discussion about their answers. Stress how great it is that everyone is a one-of-a-kind, unique individual and that these differences bring us together and make us strong, rather than dividing us.

Self-Acceptance

Another way to acquire a positive view of your inner self is to appreciate your own uniqueness. Many unhappy people compare themselves with others and rate themselves low by comparison. Learn to see yourself as special and unique—as a person who is worthwhile and valuable.

Instead of making comparisons between yourself and others, celebrate the strengths you see in others and also those you know you possess. This is possible even in the "faking it" stage. Believe in yourself.

Part of developing self-esteem is to value who you *are*, and not just what you *do*. Society often focuses on achievements such as how much money people make, how many awards they win, the grades they earn, and the like. While these all are worthy goals, stay aware that they do not define the worth of a person. People who link their inner selves too tightly with outer accomplishments easily fall into the trap of defining themselves by their deeds. Then, when they fail or make mistakes, they think of themselves as failures or mistakes. They don't realize that the mistake is what they *did*, not what they *are*.

Know that you are unique and worthwhile aside from your achievements and accomplishments. You are important in spite of your failures and mistakes. Once you've developed high self-esteem, achievements and accomplishments follow naturally.

> *"He who undervalues himself is justly undervalued by others."*
>
> William Hazlitt
> (1778–1830)
> English essayist

KEY POINTS   *Enjoy your accomplishments and admit to your failures, but don't let them define you.*

SECTION 3 — Review Answers

1. Positive self-talk (p. 62)
2. Self-esteem (p. 62)
3. Body image (p. 63)
4. high—knows and likes themselves, does not think they're perfect, accepts the negative side of themselves; low—claims to be perfect, denies having any faults (p. 62)
5. self-esteem (p. 62)
6. The individual "acts as if" he or she already has the quality he or she is seeking. (p. 63)
7. People feel that they must be sexually attractive, and our society defines sexual attractiveness very narrowly. (p. 63)
8. Answers will vary.

CLOSE

Refer students to the quote by William Hazlitt on this page. Ask them to consider the meaning of the statement. Do they agree or disagree and why? Discuss or debate in class.

SECTION 3 — Review

Answer the following questions on a sheet of paper.

Learning the Vocabulary

The vocabulary terms in this section are *self-esteem, positive self-talk,* and *body image.*

1. _____ is the practice of making affirming statements to oneself about oneself.
2. _____ is the value a person attaches to himself or herself.
3. _____ is the way a person views his or her body.

Learning the Facts

4. Name two qualities of a person who has high self-esteem and two qualities of a person who has low self-esteem.
5. What is to be gained by using positive self-talk?
6. How does the "fake it 'til you make it" technique work?
7. Why is a negative body image so common in our society?

Making Life Choices

8. List ten things about yourself and your life that you really like. Beside each item you listed, write one way you can use these things you like to help others feel more positive about themselves. For example, if you think you have a nice smile, smile at friends and others more often.

QUICK QUIZ

Chapter 3, Section 3

The following quiz will help you assess your students' understanding of the material covered in this section of the chapter. You might use the quiz as an oral exercise, which will lead into a class discussion of the topics covered. Or, you might use it as a paper/pencil quiz to evaluate your students individually.

Like the Quick Quiz, the Section Review can also be used as an assessment tool to spark class discussion or as an individual student evaluation. It can also be used as a review in preparation for this quiz.

1. Self-esteem involves being aware of your personal shortcomings and liking yourself in spite of them. (True)
2. Poor self-esteem costs the state billions of dollars. (True)

SECTION 4

The Importance of Peer Groups

So far, this chapter has emphasized the individual. However, an important part of normal development in the teen years is an association with **peer groups**. A peer group is simply a group of friends similar to yourself in age and stage of life. For many adolescents, peer groups are a positive influence on development. Peer groups help to bridge the gap between the dependent state of childhood and the independent state of full adulthood.

You also hear about peer groups in a negative way when they apply **peer pressure**, or when they become **cliques**, **gangs**, or **cults**. Kids sometimes ignore their own values and do things just to fit in with the crowd.

Peer groups operate as many other organizations do. Each has a set of rules and expects certain behaviors from its members. For example, if the crowd expects sophisticated, "cool," or snobbish behavior, students who act otherwise may be treated with hostility. Although the pressure to belong can be fierce, individuals should remember that they are free to move from group to group to satisfy changing needs and interests.

The Formation of Peer Groups

Children have friends, but they still receive their initial sets of values and identities from their parents. Then, for most people in their early teens, peers become important in providing clues to each individual's identity. By observing the reactions of their peers, young teens learn valuable lessons about their own tendencies and how they interact with others.

Peer groups may form when individuals with similar backgrounds or interests get together. They naturally develop rules that govern the behavior of the members. Sometimes they go to extremes and become cliques that exclude most outsiders and that ridicule those who fail to conform.

Most peer groups, though, provide their members with benefits. A circle of friends offers a place to share ideas and opinions. These friends also provide support and strength in a sometimes threatening world. It's easier to be confident when you know others are on your side.

Some groups of young teens are easy to identify. They talk alike, dress alike, and do everything together. These tight groups help young people to find their places in the larger society. Within these groups, young teens begin to develop their identities. By the late teen years, associations with peers usually loosen to become less demanding. They still remain important, however, and evolve into more mature friendships that may last throughout life.

Some teens hesitate to try getting into new groups. They have trouble "breaking the ice" with new people—they are shy. Shyness is really a fear that if other people knew the person within, rejection would follow. Shy people can get over these fears by seeking comfortable settings in which to meet with others and by realizing that many other people feel the same way. Tips for shy people were offered in a Health Strategies feature in Chapter 2.

To find their identity, teens often experiment with different styles.

MINI Glossary

peer groups: groups of people who are similar in age and stage of life.

peer pressure: the internal pressure one feels to behave as a peer group does, in order to gain its members' approval.

cliques: peer groups that reject newcomers and that judge both their members and nonmembers harshly.

gangs: peer groups that exist largely to express aggression against other groups.

cults: groups of people who share intense admiration or adoration of a particular person or principle.

SECTION 4

FOCUS

OUTCOMES

In this section students will learn:

1. The definition of peer groups and their value in normal development.
2. Ways deviant peer groups can cause negative peer pressure and lead to rejection and punishment from society.
3. Ways peer groups help bridge the gap between the dependent state of childhood and the independent state of adulthood.

FOCUS ACTIVITY

Tell students that individual positive development is very important. However, a normal part of development, starting in the teen years, is an association with peer groups. Discuss this as a class. Ask for a definition of the term *peer group*. Ask them for the names of some peer groups they have been associated with since starting school. Examples they might mention are students, girls, boys, minorities, Boy Scouts, Girl Scouts, church groups, clubs, bands, speech teams, sports teams, and so on. Discuss in class the reasons they enjoyed these peer groups and stress that sometimes we outgrow certain peer groups and go on to others.

3. Positive self-talk is a series of statements designed to improve self-esteem. (True)
4. Visualization is not helpful in overcoming obstacles. (False)
5. Social values have a profound and often damaging effect on an individual's body image. (True)
6. Fashion models are realistic role models for young girls who are developing their own body images. (False)
7. Being fit means being as thin as possible. (False)
8. Self-esteem can be developed by constantly comparing yourself with others. (False)
9. Self-acceptance involves appreciating your own unique strengths and values. (True)
10. It is healthy to define yourself according to your achievements, such as grades or salary. (False)

Young teens tend to band together in tight groups. Peer groups of older teens may be more loosely defined. Peer groups can form whenever like-minded individuals get together.

TEACH & APPLY

CLASS ACTIVITY

On the left side of the board or an overhead transparency, write *Constructive Outcomes.* On the right, write the words *Destructive Outcomes.* Now have the students tell you all the constructive or good outcomes that can be experienced from being connected to peer groups. List their answers under *Constructive Outcomes.* Do the same thing for *Destructive Outcomes,* listing all the negative outcomes that can be experienced from being connected to peer groups. Have a class discussion of your lists. Are there any trends that can be seen? In the overall scheme of an 80-year life span, which outcomes would be the most desirable in allowing individuals to reach their full potential?

DISCUSSION

Ask students to think about what it means for a group to be *tight.* Can they think of examples of particularly *tight* groups? Do they feel that this is a positive or a negative aspect of a group? Do they think groups can be too tight? Do they think that belonging to such a group helps or hinders someone in developing his or her personal identity? How? Can they think of specific examples from such groups?

COMPREHENSION CHECK

Ask students what it means to conform. (to go along with agreed upon rules or customs) What word in the last chapter had an opposite meaning? (non-conformist)

The Value of Peer Groups

An important function of peer groups is to help lessen teenagers' natural fears. Young people often feel an exaggerated sense of uniqueness—"I'm the only one who feels this way!" or "Everyone is looking at me, and I must look awful!" These extreme feelings are natural, but of course, they are not based on reality. Most people feel the same emotions from time to time. As for the judging stares from the crowd—those people are all thinking about themselves and probably believing that everyone is staring at *them.*

Peer groups provide a shelter from these extremes. As part of the group that talks alike and looks alike, young teens have positive proof that others feel as they do. Numbers also provide safety and a degree of anonymity in which each person can try out a newly emerging identity.

Some peer groups serve other needs, too. A jogging club, for example, provides companionship and exercise. The important thing is to find people you can be comfortable with. The Health Strategies features, "Finding New Interests" on this page, and "Making New Friends" on page 70, offer some tips on finding people who share your interests and on making friends. Belonging to a wide variety of groups may help teens learn to get along with many kinds of people, a skill of great value in meeting the relationship demands of adult life.

Finally, peer groups can help teens through tough times. It's natural to share feelings with others. For example, a student whose parents were divorcing was constantly upset. She talked about her feelings to some friends and was surprised to learn how many had gone through similar experiences. As she listened to their stories, she came to realize that although her pain was significant, it was not permanent. She also found that talking with others made her feel better. It helped to know that she wasn't alone.

KEY POINTS *Peer groups tend to reduce the fears and emotional extremes that teenagers experience. These groups provide outlets for interests and can offer support through tough times.*

Parents Are Primary Influences

Although parents may fear that peer group values will replace parents' values, research shows otherwise. Along with a search for independence, most teens maintain strong relationships with their parents and permanently adopt many parental values. Teenagers are not simply blank pages awaiting scripts written by their peers. Teens are already close to maturity and are simply fine-tuning the lessons they've learned in life up to that point.

In general, teens adopt their parents' values on issues that matter—family, religion, work, morals, standards, and

Finding New Interests

Here are just a few ways to find new interests and friends who share them:

► Take a photography class.
► Learn to work in pottery.
► Try out for a school play.
► Sign up for a nature course.
► Learn a sport; join a team.
► Enroll in a fitness program.
► Volunteer your time.
► Work in a youth group.
► Work at a job.
► Call someone you admire but don't know well.
► Organize a group to attend concerts.
► Join the Reserve Officer's Training Corps (ROTC).

Peer Pressure Refusal Skills

The concept of refusal skills is an outgrowth of an idea that originated in chemical dependency treatment. This concept teaches teens to resist destructive peer influence or pressure (see pages 72–75). It provides them with the skills and techniques necessary to function effectively in tense social situations and main-

tain power and control for good decision-making.

One important skill is called the 30-second rule. This rule applies in all negative peer pressure situations. The longer the period of time a teen stays in contact with "the pressurer," the less probable an escape. A teen is probably most able to resist pressure in the first 30 seconds. A good indication to teens that a situation is likely to cause trouble is an uncomfortable or uneasy feeling.

What Experiences Have You Had with Peer Pressure?

It would be impossible to list and explain every encounter I have had with peer pressure. Experiences involving peer pressure occur every day. It deals with more than just drugs and alcohol. Peer pressure is anything that tries to make you stray from your uniqueness. In order to fall victim to it, all you have to do is adopt the ideas of another that do not coincide or are hypocritical to your own ideas.
Jordan Hedges, 17,
Orange Park High School, FL

One day my friends and I went down to this bridge. You are supposed to jump off the bridge and land in the water. I told them that I wouldn't jump. I was scared and I didn't want to get hurt. They started to call me names, so I just left. I wasn't going to do something I didn't want to do.
Andy Vartmann, 15,
East High School, MN

People are pressuring people to be on the same side of an issue as themselves. They have made me feel like a fool because I wouldn't take a side or because I disagreed with them.
Carrie Zimmerman, 16,
Newberg High School, OR

I witnessed a fight that happened because of peer pressure. The two people who were fighting did it because people told them to fight. These two people fought over a silly thing because they thought they would be cool. In the end, they both got into trouble.
Julie Zakara, 14,
Westside High School, NE

My experiences with peer pressure have been limited due to the type of people with whom I associate. They are the studious type and are inclined to be over-achievers. When I want to go out and have fun, they usually pressure me back into studying. This type of peer pressure is not bad, but it also does not allow me to do some of the things I enjoy.
Sean Niles, 17,
Orange Park High School, FL

I have had a lot of incidences dealing with alcohol and drugs. My friends were taking pills to make them hyper for a game coming up. They asked me if I wanted some. I kind of rejected them. They said they were only hyper pills made of caffeine. I almost gave in to the pressure, but I didn't. I wanted to see how they would react to the pill. Before the game they were shaking really bad and their hearts were beating hard and very fast. They thought it was neat, but I got scared.
Matt Stephenson, 15,
South Carroll High School, MD

the like. Teens most often adopt peer values concerning style and taste—dress, music, clothes, cars, and so forth. Teens also may turn to peers for attitudes on issues their parents may hesitate to discuss—sexuality, drugs, birth control, and dating. In this way, teens tend to blend family values with new values they've worked out for themselves. However, they usually end up with sets of values very like those of their parents.

 Parents remain important to changing, growing teens. Peer groups assist people in defining their identities, but parents provide the foundation.

Here are seven ways for teens to handle negative peer pressure. (Encourage your students to think of other creative ways.)

1. Ignore them.
2. Say, "No thanks, I'm not interested."
3. Leave.
4. Use flattery—"You're smarter than that."
5. Act shocked—"I can't believe you would ask me to do that."
6. Think of a better idea or plan.
7. Use parents as an excuse.

Application—(You may wish to add situations and invite student input.) Lead the class in a discussion of the consequences of any of these actions.

1. Cheating during an exam
2. Stealing/shoplifting
3. Cutting class or school

Following are some questions to help you promote discussion of the student views concerning peer pressure:

a. Do students feel that they encounter a lot of peer pressure? How often?

b. Do they agree with Jordan Hedges that peer pressure is anything that causes you to "stray from your uniqueness"?

c. What sorts of physical dares like the one described by Andy Vartmann have students received?

d. Are there times when it's right to fight, or is fighting always a poor choice?

e. We usually think of peer pressure as being negative. Can students cite positive examples, such as the one given by Sean Niles?

CLASS ACTIVITY

Ask students to explain the word *unique.* (one of a kind) Then ask them to explain what it means to have "an exaggerated sense of uniqueness." Can they see that it is unhealthy (although quite natural for teens) to imagine oneself to be more unique than one really is? Ask them to list their unique behaviors, those that only they possess. How much duplication is there when students compare their lists?

Some communities are taking action against destructive behaviors.

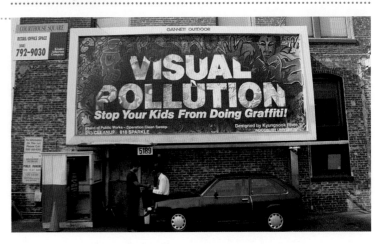

Health Strategies

Deviant Peer Groups—Gangs and Cults

A teenager's needs to develop an identity and to belong to a group are strong. These needs are so strong, in fact, that young teens can be led astray by groups that are not beneficial. Such **deviant** groups may provide an identity and meet a person's need to belong, but they do so at a high price. A positive-minded peer group may help a student stay in school. A deviant group, however, may influence the person to drop out.

A gang is one kind of deviant peer group that makes up its own rules and values—mostly negative. Gangs enforce their rules within their organization by their own authority. They remain outside of the larger society. The gang's rules may require committing serious crimes, taking or selling illegal drugs, or taking part in other harmful activities. The gang's activities are mostly related to obtaining money in illegal ways for the benefit of high-ranking gang members. Those who "follow the rules" of the gang, including committing crimes or performing dangerous stunts, are rewarded with praise and esteem from other gang members.

Gang members demonstrate conformity in the extreme. They often dress alike, talk alike, and use special symbols to identify themselves with their gangs. They struggle and even physically fight to develop a reputation within the gang. A gang can become a dangerous substitute for other institutions such as family or community.

Cults are related to gangs in that they are often money-making groups, with the top organization leaders profiting most. According to one group that monitors "mind control" cults, about 200 such organizations are active today. Some of them have enormous scope and power.

Cults may masquerade as religious groups, healing centers, addiction treatment centers, or even financial advisors. In reality, though, they may exist for the sole purpose of

Focusing ON Self-Esteem

amassing hundreds of millions of dollars for themselves. People who are drawn into cults are often convinced—through guilt, brainwashing, threats, or even legal actions—to hand over their worldly goods, and to work for the profit of the cult while living in poverty. Beware of religious organizations that require that you pay large sums for the promise of "spiritual cleansing" or "clearing out internal evils." The only thing they'll clear out is your wallet.

When people join groups that step outside of the rules of the larger society, they bring on themselves rejection and punishment from the majority. The people most drawn to such groups seem to be those who fail to fit in successfully with peer groups during young life, and for whom the larger society has little to offer as adults.

Peers are important. Make sure you choose them with care. People who get involved with deviant groups often find it difficult to get themselves out again. The Straight Talk section that follows offers tips on how to stand up to unwanted peer pressure.

 Deviant peer groups such as gangs exert negative influences on the people who join them. The rules of gangs are often in opposition to the rules of society. Cults often exist for the sole purpose of obtaining large sums of money from those who join them.

Review

Answer the following questions on a sheet of paper.

Learning the Vocabulary

The vocabulary terms introduced in the section are *peer groups, peer pressure, cliques, gangs, cults,* and *deviant.*
Fill in the blank with the correct answer.

1. _____ is the internal pressure a person feels to behave as a group does.

2. _____ are often interested primarily in making money.

3. Peer groups that reject newcomers and judge their members harshly are called _____.

Learning the Facts

4. What changes occur in peer groups from early teens to late teens?

5. What are some functions of peer groups?

6. What is the advantage of being able to get along with many types of people?

Making Life Choices

7. Peer groups can pressure teens toward positive or negative behaviors.
   a. Relate a positive personal experience with peer pressure. What did you gain?
   b. Describe a negative personal experience with peer pressure. If you had this situation to live over again, how would you do it?
   c. Has it become easier or harder to resist peer pressure as you have gotten older? Why do you think this is so?

Glossary

▷ **deviant:** outside the normal system.

 Review Answers

ASSESS

1. Peer pressure (p. 67)
2. Cults or gangs (p. 70)
3. cliques (p. 67)
4. Peer groups for early teens become important in providing clues to the individual's identity. By observing their peers, young teens learn valuable lessons and how to interact with others. By late teens, associations loosen to become less demanding. More mature friendships evolve that may last for a lifetime. (p. 67)
5. They help lessen teenagers' natural fears, provide proof that others feel as they do, and provide teens with a circle of friends to share ideas as well as for support. (p. 67)
6. Being able to get along with many different groups helps prepare teens to meet the relationship demands of adult life. (p. 68)
7. a. Answers will vary.
   b. Answers will vary.
   c. Answers will vary.

CLOSE

Have students evaluate the peer groups they are in now. On a piece of paper, for their eyes only, have them list the peer groups in which they are involved. The students should label each as positive or negative based on its rules, its controls, its punishments, and its outcomes. Have the students evaluate their dependency on the group. Have their choices in peer groups made them more or less independent?

Choosing to "hang around" with people who feel good about themselves can help raise our level of self-esteem. Knowing this, we should evaluate each of our friendships.

2. Goal-setting is an important component of self-esteem. Remember the three R's of goal-setting to increase self-esteem: goals should be *realistic, reachable,* and *revisable.* Again, choosing friends who set and accomplish goals will move you toward higher self-esteem.

3. Often gang membership is based on proving yourself to others. True friendship does not have an "entrance exam" to prove loyalty.

Comprehension Check
You might ask students which type of peer pressure is more common for them—the positive type or the more negative type.

Discussion
Discuss with students their need to belong to groups—to be with others. You might want to use the following quotation, along with the material on this page, to help students see both sides of the issue. "Some people fear finding themselves alone—and so they don't find themselves at all."—Andre Gide

Discussion
Ask students to brainstorm ways in which adults are caught by peer pressure. What are some adult peer groups? You may want to lead students to thinking about the workplace, and the desire to impress the boss or fellow workers. In what ways can these influences cause adults to set aside their values, or change their values? Points to consider include seeking acceptance with the boss or coworkers by heavy drinking, overlooking or participating in unethical behavior, and so on.

Dealing with Peer Pressure

Each day presents teenagers with new choices to weigh against personal values. Which choices are right? Which are wrong? While many choices lead to productive and positive experiences, other paths lead to destructive lifestyles that can set a negative course that lasts a lifetime. Teenagers don't make these choices alone. They are influenced by the behaviors of their peer groups.

 When people talk about peer pressure, they usually say that your friends are pushing you to do things you don't want to do—and that you can "say no." Are peers usually a bad influence?

No, they are not. In fact, a positive peer group can encourage individuals to achieve things they never thought possible. Group values can give individuals the strength to say no to temptations. A peer group can be a major influence in a student's decision to stay in school, for example.

Some groups are mostly negative, though. The inborn human need to belong is so strong that teens who lack either strong self-esteem or the skills needed to refuse peer pressure will do almost anything to fit in with some group. They seek approval from others, even at enormous personal cost. At the extreme, some teens may even risk their lives performing high-risk stunts required by some gangs for admission. Also, some may take up drinking alcohol or begin using other drugs to prove to a group that they can do as the members do. This may be especially destructive because it may set up lifelong patterns of behavior.

 How can kids fight against the urge to do self-destructive things in order to fit in?

Most important is to first decide for yourself, away from the group, what you will or will not do. In other words, the first person to say no to is yourself. Then, be prepared to say no to others.

 How, exactly, can I say "no" without losing friends?

A set of 20 skills, called **refusal skills**, can help. With practice, you can use these skills to handle almost any sort of uncomfortable situation, including refusal to engage in behaviors that run counter to your values or that are illegal. It does take practice to become good at all 20 skills, but the result is well worth the effort. You are probably using all of them right now, at least to some extent. The Life Choice Inventory on pages 74 and 75 can give you some idea about which of the 20 are your strongest and which could use more work.

For the most benefit, the user of refusal skills must practice using them until they feel natural even when peer interactions get sticky. A polished response requires both rehearsal and repetition. Rehearsal means that you should think up imaginary situations and then figure out ways of applying one or more skills to each one. Repetition means using the skills every time an opportunity to do so arises.

 Does peer pressure disappear as people mature?

People encounter the most peer pressure during early adolescence, but even adults experience some peer pressure. The phrase *keeping up with the Joneses* applies to adults who still feel a need to live as

72

special needs

Musical
Peer groups can be especially important to students with special needs. Sometimes, rather than being given an opportunity to choose their own peer group, disabled students are grouped together solely on the basis of their "handicaps." Ask students to brainstorm a list

of different groups they belong to. Examples might include: family, clubs, band or choir, church, scouting organizations, sports teams, and so on. Note that these groups are made up of members that have something in common.

One unifying factor in peer groups is often the type of music listened to. Put a list of different styles of music on the board. You may want to include rap, pop, rock, punk, classical, alternative, retro, gospel, folk, and so on.

others do. An immature "us against them" mentality leads young adolescents to behave cruelly to others. Unfortunately, some people get stuck in the "us against them" mentality of early adolescence. It expresses itself in adults in many forms of prejudice and bigotry, including racism, sexism, ageism, and others.

 I want to join a new peer group. What about the impression I make on people? Doesn't that matter?

It certainly does. People who do not know you may judge you on the surface only—just by your manners. Like it or not, first impressions are lasting in people's minds. Manners do make a difference.

Imagine this: You are invited to share a meal with someone's family. You want to impress them, but you arrive sloppily dressed, chew with your mouth open, make a mess at the table, and belch loudly as you finish your meal. How would they view you?

 Do you mean that to be part of a social group, I have to memorize a bunch of rules about which fork to use?

In the situation described above, you desire acceptance by people who have other customs. When you want to belong to a social group, you need to observe how they do things. Manners alone can open doors, sometimes—even the door to someone's positive impression of you. Where manners are concerned, remember the old saying "When in Rome, do as the Romans do."

Keep in mind, too, that the most important person in your life is you. Taking care of that person will ease the way to desired friendships and help you make right decisions.

A peer group that values achievement can help motivate its members to stay in school.

MINI Glossary

refusal skills: a set of social strategies that enable people to competently resist the pressure by others to engage in dangerous or otherwise undesirable behaviors.

WORKSHEETS

Reproducible Study Outline and Reading Cloze worksheets for Chapter 3 are provided in the Teacher's Resource Box.

Reproducible Chapter Tests A and B are also provided in the Teacher's Resource Box.

Ask students to brainstorm qualities and characteristics that they think people have who listen to each music type. Then have students listen to selections from each of the different styles, identifying the music they would prefer to listen to.

Finally, ask students to review the qualities they listed for people who like that type of music. Would they like to be placed into a group with those characteristics, based solely on the type of musical choices they make? Ask students to think about whether they made their choice of music preference based on what they really enjoy or what their peer group thinks is the best music.

Review again the list of groups that students belong to. Ask students to consider whether they are in groups that are cultivating qualities they want.

A reproducible copy of the Life Choice Inventory is provided in the Teacher's Resource Box.

CLASS ACTIVITY

Ask students to think of an actual situation in which they went against their own values because of pressure from peers. Have them write answers to these questions: Why did I go against my value system even though I knew it was wrong for me? How big a part did "peer pressure" play in helping me "forget" my values? In the long run, did I gain, or lose, by going against my values?

Life Choice Inventory

How Sharp Are Your Refusal Skills?

These 20 skills have been determined to be important to refusing to give in to peer pressure. The more a person uses these skills, the stronger is that person's resistance. Answer each of the following questions. On a separate paper, list the number corresponding to how often you use this skill.

    5: Always   4: Almost always   3: Often
         2: Sometimes   1: Never

When dealing with peers, I: Score

1. Ask for help when I need it regarding a social interaction.
(For example, if someone suggests something dangerous or illegal, I ask for help from school authorities or parents.)   _____

2. Give instructions to others in my group.
(I think logically and break up tasks into parts that can be asked of others.)   _____

3. Convince others to do as I wish or to turn to my way of thinking.
(I use conflict resolution skills to understand both sides of the argument.)   _____

4. Identify my feelings accurately.
(I can usually tell whether butterflies in my stomach are from pleasant excitement, worry, or embarrassment.)   _____

5. Express my feelings appropriately.
(I make decisions about how, when, where, and to whom feelings should be expressed.)   _____

6. Effectively deal with other people's anger.
(I use the conflict resolution skills of Chapter 2, such as staying calm, not interrupting, and repeating what I've heard in my own words.)   _____

7. Handle my own fear when it arises.
(I decide on the spot how realistic fears are, and take appropriate action such as walking away.)   _____

8. Exhibit self-control under stress.
(I analyze my feelings and decide what to do to remain in control, such as count to ten, take a deep breath, etc.)   _____

9. Stand up for myself assertively.
(I recognize when I'm being mistreated, and I say assertively what's on my mind, while controlling my negative impulses.)   _____

10. Handle it when someone teases me.
(I can distinguish good-natured joking from mean-spirited teasing. I choose to ignore teasing, accept it, or use humor to make a real joke of it.)   _____

11. Identify and avoid trouble before it starts.
(I try to project into the future to decide whether the situation has the potential for trouble. If so, I come up with alternatives.)   _____

HEALTHY PEOPLE 2000

Increase to at least 20 percent the proportion of people aged 18 and older who seek help in coping with personal and emotional problems.

Most of the adult population reports experiencing personal or emotional problems in the course of a year. Half of these people say that they are unable to solve their problems, and approximately one-third report that they are unable to do anything to make their problems more bearable. Yet relatively few seek help, in part because they believe it better to handle problems alone, in part because helping resources are unknown, unaffordable, untimely, or believed to be inadequate to the problems. Those who do turn to others for support more often than not seek out family members and friends. Professional welfare or service organizations are usually contacted

12. Stay out of fights.
(I think about the long-term consequences of fighting, and take actions to avoid a fight, as described in Chapter 2.)   _____

13. Gracefully handle embarrassment.
(I know what makes me feel embarrassed and learn to accept embarrassment, change the cause of it, or distract others with humor.)   _____

14. Accept being left out.
(I decide if being left out is positive or negative. If it's negative, I accept it, tell the others how I feel, or ask to be included.)   _____

15. Consider the opinions of others.
(I do not immediately accept or reject the persuasion tactics of another. I judge each idea against my own beliefs.)   _____

16. Accept failure and respond appropriately.
(I decide what caused the failure, be it academic, social, or other. I make changes, when appropriate, to prevent a repeat.)   _____

17. Respond to accusations appropriately.
(I decide if the accusation is true, and I take appropriate action. If the accusation is false, I deny the charge and explain why it is false. If it is accurate, I apologize and offer to make amends.)   _____

18. Prepare effectively for a difficult conversation.
(I think about how I and the other person will both feel, and how my words might affect the other, before choosing an approach.)   _____

19. Handle group pressure.
(I listen to others, and understand what it is they want me to do. I then listen to my feelings and values to decide what to do.)   _____

20. Make decisions with intention, not impulse.
(I follow the steps to decision making presented earlier in this book when making difficult decisions.)   _____

SCORING:

On your separate score sheet, fill in how many times you answered the corresponding response.

5 (Always)   _____
4 (Almost Always)   _____
3 (Often)   _____
2 (Sometimes)   _____
1 (Never)   _____

If you answered at least 15 questions with either a 5 or 4, your refusal skills are serving you well. If you answered less than 15 questions with either a 5 or 4, reread the questions, and try to identify situations in which you can apply the new skills in your life. All of the skills are important, so if you scored 1 or 2 on any of them, this points to a skill that needs rehearsal and repetition to improve it. Imagine a situation to which the skill might apply. Think of how to apply it. Then rehearse your response until it becomes natural.

Source: The 20 skills presented here appeared originally in A. P. Goldstein, K. W. Reagles, and L. L. Amann, *Refusal Skills: Preventing Drug Use in Adolescents* (Champaign, Ill.: Research Press, 1990), pp. 33–52.

ON LINE WITH HEALTH

You may want to have your students visit the following URLs, where they will find information and additional Web site resources to enhance their study of this chapter. As with all Web sites, you should check these out first to be sure the information found there is appropriate for your students.

Life's Playbook Online **http://www.lifesplaybook.com**

National Association for Self-Esteem **http://www.self-esteem-nase.org/**

Life's Playbook Online provides a series of profiles of men and women who have distinguished themselves in business, community, school, and sports.

The National Association for Self-Esteem site has lots of information, too, as well as educational programs, research and references, and a chat room.

---

when assistance is not available within the network of family or friends or the emotional upset is particularly intense. Mental health professionals, physicians, and religious counselors are the most likely choices of those who seek professional help.

Given a high level of role strain, the activity level, intimacy, and dependability of the individual's social network have been found to reduce the level of distress. In addition, the dependability of one's network, more than its activity level or intimacy, buffers the effects of high levels of role strain on the individual. This buffering effect seems to be specific to situations in which emergency help, economic strain, or occupational problems are at issue. A confiding relationship with a spouse, a confidant outside of marriage, or membership in a mutual help group can be effective buffers.

ANSWERS TO CHAPTER 3 REVIEW VOCABULARY

1. **a.** adolescence, **b.** femininity, **c.** peer groups, **d.** gender roles, **e.** deviant, **f.** personality, **g.** positive self-talk, **h.** gender, **i.** self-esteem
2. **a.** Needs, **b.** Stereotypes, **c.** hierarchy
3. **a.** Self-image is the characteristic that a person sees in him or herself while body image is how a person thinks his or her body looks. **b.** Gangs usually tend to express aggression against laws and society. Members must obey the rules, which often include crimes, selling drugs, or other harmful activities. Cults are related to gangs, but are usually disguised as religious groups, healing centers, and addiction treatment centers. People are drawn in through guilt, brainwashing, threats, or legal action.

RECALL

SECTION 1

1. school age (6–12) (p. 54)
2. physiological, safety, love, esteem, and self-actualization (p. 55)
3. They feel a need to be important and appreciated. It also helps in the development of identity. (p. 56)

SECTION 2

4. age 12 or 13 (p. 57)
5. Girls develop more body fat, while boys develop more muscle tissue. (p. 57)

CHAPTER 3 Review

Summarizing the Chapter

Your ability to respond correctly to the following statements ensures your understanding of the main concepts in the chapter.

1. Describe the eight stages of life according to Erik Erikson.
2. Discuss the importance of developing an identity during the teen years.
3. Summarize Maslow's hierarchy of needs.
4. Describe how sexual maturation and gender identity affect personality.
5. Discuss how positive self-talk, positive body image, and self-acceptance help in the development of high self-esteem.
6. Identify the value of positive peer groups. Identify the dangers of deviant peer groups.

Learning the Vocabulary

personality	masculinity
self-image	stereotypes
psychology	sexual harassment
variables	self-esteem
hierarchy	positive self-talk
needs	body image
self-actualization	peer groups
adolescence	peer pressure
puberty	cliques
gender	gangs
gender roles	cults
gender identity	deviant
femininity	refusal skills

Answer the following questions on a separate sheet of paper.

1. **Matching**—*Match each of the following phrases with the appropriate vocabulary term.*
   a. the period of growth from the beginning of puberty to full maturity
   b. refers to biological, social, and physical

76

---

traits associated with being female
   c. groups of people who are similar in age and stage of life
   d. roles assigned by society to people of each gender
   e. outside the normal system
   f. the characteristics of a person that are apparent to others
   g. the practice of making affirmative statements about oneself to oneself
   h. classification of being male or female
   i. the value a person attaches to himself or herself

2. **a.** _____ are urgent wants for necessary things.
   b. _____ are fixed pictures.
   c. A _____ is a ranking system in which each thing is placed above or below others.

3. **a.** What is the difference between self-image and body image?
   b. What is the difference between a gang and a cult?

Recalling Important Facts and Ideas

Section 1

1. According to Erikson, during what age span should a person develop industriousness?
2. List Maslow's hierarchy of needs.
3. Why is it especially beneficial for teens to be helpful to those who really need help?

Section 2

4. When do adolescent boys usually begin a growth spurt?
5. What is the main difference between girls' and boys' body composition?
6. List three changes that have occurred in gender roles over the years.

Section 3

7. What are some qualities of a person with high self-esteem?
8. List five problems linked with poor self-esteem.
9. List four strategies for improving self-esteem.
10. What types of pressures are advertisers using to their advantage?
11. What is the danger in always comparing yourself to others?

Section 4

12. Give three examples of negative peer groups.
13. What are some benefits peer groups provide?
14. What are some common parental values that teens are likely to adopt?

---

6. Answers will vary; could include: acceptance of women in the ranks of the armed forces, men in the nursing profession, exclusive clubs opening to both genders, women becoming corporate executives, women building bridges, men enjoying cooking and other tasks in the home. (p. 60)

SECTION 3

7. They don't think they are perfect. They believe in and respect themselves and are emotionally healthy. (p. 62)
8. Answers will vary; could include: low self-esteem is linked to drug and alcohol abuse, crime, prostitution, gangs, teenage runaways, child and family abuse, and violence. (p. 62)

15. What common techniques do cults use to pressure people into doing what they want?

16. What tends to happen when people join groups that do not follow society's rules?

17. Give some suggestions for positive ways to find new interests and friends.

Critical Thinking

1. Think of some labels that were used to describe you as a young child. Were the labels positive or negative? Why do you think so?

2. Think of some labels that might describe you as a teenager. Are the labels positive or negative? How can you change the negatives to positives?

3. Analyze how each past and present label has influenced your self-esteem.

4. Many times people do not like the way others see them. Fortunately, you have the ability to change your personality and self-esteem if you so choose. List four labels you would like to have attached to you and describe how you could best achieve them.

Activities

1. Write a description of the person you think you will be ten years from now. What are you like? What is your lifestyle like?

2. Analyze an advertisement from a magazine in relation to the gender stereotypes that are used to sell that particular product. Write a brief report and include a copy of the advertisement.

3. Give yourself a boost! Write a letter to yourself convincing you of your worth as a person. Tell why you are special and include all your good points, talents, and skills.

4. Transfer your interpretation of Maslow's hierarchy of needs onto a poster by using pictures from magazines or your own original illustrations to portray each need.

5. Make a list of ten events that took place in one particular day. Evaluate each in relation to how it affected your self-esteem. Clearly state if the event raised, lowered, or had no effect on your esteem.

6. Identify a product being advertised in a magazine which you know to be a product that takes advantage of people's low self-esteem. Write a letter to the editor expressing your anger for running false advertising. Submit a copy of the advertisement and letter to your teacher before you mail it.

7. Look through some family photographs and find some pictures that represent different developing phases of your life. Coordinate these pictures with Erikson's theory. Create an album and label each photograph. Give your album a title and write a short script to tell the story of your life.

8. Watch television for two hours. List the commercials that appeal to gender identity and contain stereotypical gender roles. Write a one-sentence description of how each commercial used this theme.

9. Make three columns on a sheet of paper. Label the left column "Positive," label the center column "Stages," and label the right column "Negative." In the center column, list each of Erikson's eight stages: infancy, toddler stage, preschool age, school age, adolescence, young adulthood, adulthood, and older adulthood. In the left column, summarize the positive side of each stage. In the right column, summarize the negative side of each stage. For example, for the infancy stage, you would write in the left column something like: "To learn trust. The infant learns that needs will be met." In the right column you would write: "If neglected or abused, the person learns distrust that can last a lifetime." Rate your own development in the first five stages, on a scale from one to ten, with ten being the highest development. How did you rate your development? Share your answers with the class if you are comfortable doing so.

Making Decisions about Health

1. You have a friend who has been hanging out with a gang for quite a while, and who is beginning to feel uneasy about it. The gang members seem to be pressuring her into doing things that make her uncomfortable. She really would like to get out, but several questions keep running through her mind: Will my friends be angry with me if I quit? I don't really have many friends outside the gang—if I leave who will be my friends? How much longer can I keep my gang membership a secret from my parents?

She is becoming more and more confused each time she thinks about making a decision. How can you help your friend remedy this situation?

12. cliques, gangs, cults (p. 67)

13. By observing their peers, young teens learn valuable lessons and how to interact with others. Peer groups help bridge the gap between the dependent state of childhood and the independent state of adulthood. They see they are not alone in their problems. (pp. 67–68)

14. Answers will vary; could include: family, religion, work morals, standards. (p. 68)

15. They require people to pay large sums of money for "spiritual cleansing" or "clearing out internal evils;" use guilt, brainwashing, threats, and legal actions to take over. (p. 70)

16. They face rejection and punishment from the majority. (p. 71)

17. Answers will vary; could include: take a photography class, learn to work with pottery, try out for a school play, sign up for a nature course, learn a sport, enroll in a fitness class, volunteer, join a youth group, call someone you admire, attend a concert, join the ROTC. (p. 68)

9. Answers will vary; could include: write out positive statements, find activities related to goals, be grateful, practice positive self-talk, seek out books and movies with positive themes, support others, don't think negatively, celebrate your successes, give and receive affection. (p. 62)

10. A negative body image and intense pressure from society for a sexier appearance make teenagers easy prey for advertisers. (p. 63)

11. If you're an unhappy person, you rate yourself poorly. You should learn to see yourself as special and unique. Celebrate the strengths you see in others and those you know you possess. Believe in yourself. (p. 66)

KEY POINTS

Chapter 4 is 28 pages long and divided into five sections. Briefly, this chapter introduces students to the concept of stress, its effects on the body, and ways to reduce the stress. The chapter emphasizes the importance of the individual's need to deal with stress effectively to reduce harmful effects on the body systems. It also gives students some positive ideas for identifying stressors, developing time management skills, and using relaxation techniques to cope with everyday living.

ACTIVITY TO INTRODUCE THE CHAPTER

Have the students think of a time of day that is very stressful for them. Is it morning, a certain class at school, homework time? Have the students write all that they can about that stressful time. Who is involved? Why do they feel stressed? What are their feelings? Ask the students to decide what they could do to change the stress. List some changes that they would be willing to make to reduce the stress. List both the factors that they can and cannot control. Ask the students to describe how they feel when the stressful moment has ended.

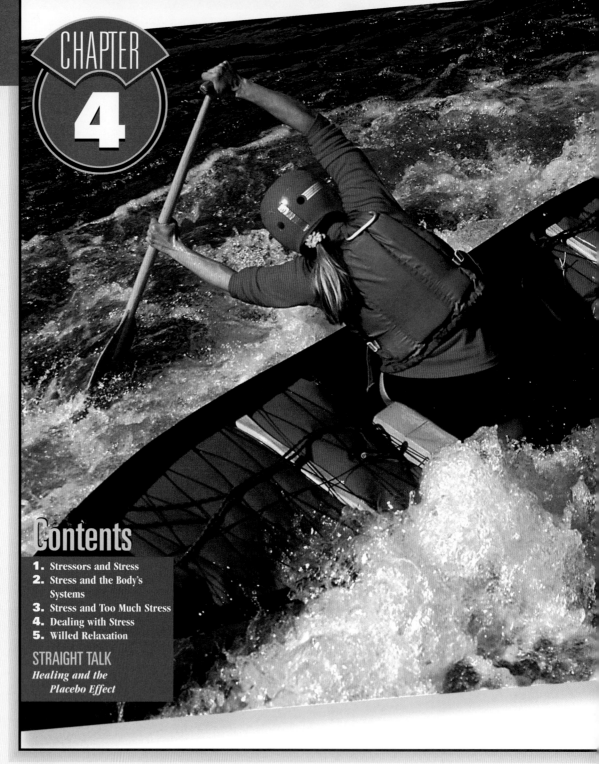

CHAPTER 4

Contents

NOT Enough Time?

Following are some suggestions to help you make sure that you cover the key topics in this chapter if you have limited time. (Refer to the daily lesson plans in your Teacher's Resource Box for additional suggestions.)

DAY 1 Assign students to read Sections 1, 2, and 3 ahead of time. Also, have the students study the "Psychological Stressors for High School Students" on page 82. During class have students do the Class Activity on page 82, the Group Activity on page 85, and the Class Activity on page 87. Conclude the class with a combination of quizzes listed under the Assess heading at the end of each section.

Stress and Stress Management

What do you think? Are the following statements true or false? If you think they are false, then say what is true.

1. Buying a new car and taking a final exam are more similar than different, as far as your body is concerned.
2. Prolonged stress can make a person likely to suffer diseases.
3. The fight-or-flight reaction only occurred in the days of our ancestors. People today do not experience it.
4. Whether an event is stressful depends more on the person experiencing it than on the event itself.
5. You cannot change the way you react to stress.
6. Machines can help you learn to relax.

(Answers on page 101)

Introduction

The word **stress** is widely used today. When a person says, "I am under stress," he may mean that he is ill, that his love life has gone off course, that he is under financial pressure, or any of a hundred other things.

In contrast, another person who says she is under stress may mean that things are going great—that she is thriving. Stress can be a threat to health, or it can be the fuel for progress and achievement. For some, it almost borders on inspiration. This kind of stress produces beneficial energy and alertness.

Stress tends to get out of hand in some people's lives. Life in today's urban world can be so demanding that people respond by constantly overloading themselves. They study on the way to school and eat on the run between classes. They drive cars and talk on their phones at the same time. Even when on vacation, people who are supposed to be at leisure sign up for tours that visit 15 countries in two weeks. For them, "hurry up" becomes a way of life. To make matters worse, people today report their stress to be greater than people reported 30 years ago.

This chapter describes the effects of stress on your body and mind. It also shows you ways of dealing with the stress in your own life.

BULLETIN BOARD IDEAS

Put together, or have students put together, a collage of magazine photos, advertisements, slogans, and so forth depicting stress, its effects, and products marketed to reduce stress. You might find it interesting to focus particularly on the marketing of stress relievers in our society. Use the collage as a springboard for discussing the prevalence of stress in our society, and the money-making aspects of this.

Answers to

1. **True.**
2. **True.**
3. **False.** We experience the fight-or-flight reaction today just as our ancestors did.
4. **True.**
5. **False.** You can change the way you perceive a stressor so that it will benefit you.
6. **True.**

FAST FACTS

Men who earn less than $10,000 per year suffer migraine headaches 60 percent more often than men who earn more than $30,000.

DAY 2 Assign students to read Sections 4 and 5 ahead of time. Also, have students read the Straight Talk feature, "Healing and the Placebo Effect," on pages 102–103. During class have students do the Class Activity on pages 91–92, or the Class Activity on page 95. Lead the students in the Discussion on page 96. Conclude the class with a combination of quizzes listed under the Assess heading at the end of each section. You may want to assign reteaching activities from the resource material for those students doing poorly on the quizzes.

DAY 3 Use class time for the Guest Speaker activity described on page 100.

SECTION 1

FOCUS

OUTCOMES

In this section students will learn:

1. What a stressor is.
2. How to differentiate between physical and psychological stressors.
3. To recognize some common stressors among teenagers during their high school years.

FOCUS ACTIVITY

Write the word *stressor* on the board and define the word for students. (anything that requires a person to cope with, or adapt to, a situation) Have students list stressors that exist in their lives. Compare how commonly the stressors given exist among teenagers. Now have students divide the stressors listed on the board into physical or psychological stressors. Discuss ways in which teenagers deal with these stressors. Have students list some more effective ways of dealing with the situations if their methods seem ineffective.

TEACH & APPLY

CLASS ACTIVITY

Do students think most people overload themselves? Ask students to make a list of ten adults and ten teenagers they know. Have them put a check next to the name of each person they think is living an overloaded lifestyle. Discuss the percentage of people who have this problem, if indeed it is a problem.

SECTION 1

Stressors and Stress

Never-ending, **chronic stress** is the kind that can damage body systems in a number of ways. The heart and blood vessels are especially responsive to stress and often suffer the brunt of its impact on the body. Tragically, some people have not learned how to deal with stress. Many seek relief in self-destructive habits such as using alcohol or other drugs. These substances cause stress themselves, and their effect is to worsen the toll being taken.

Figure 4–1 Signs of Stress

Physical Signs	Psychological Signs
Pounding of the heart	Irritability, tension, or depression
Rapid, shallow breathing	Impulsive behavior and emotional instability; the overpowering urge to cry or to run and hide
Dryness of the throat and mouth	Lowered self-esteem; thoughts related to failure
Raised body temperature	Excessive worry; insecurity; concern about other people's opinions; self-deprecation in conversation
Feelings of weakness, light-headedness, dizziness, or faintness	
Trembling; nervous tics; twitches; shaking hands and fingers	Reduced ability to communicate with others
Tendency to be easily startled (by small sounds and the like)	Increased awkwardness in social situations
High-pitched, nervous laughter	Excessive boredom; unexplained dissatisfaction with job or other normal conditions
Stuttering and other speech difficulties	Feelings of isolation
Insomnia—that is, difficulty in getting to sleep, or a tendency to wake up during the night	Avoidance of activities
	Irrational fears (phobias) about specific things
Grinding of the teeth during sleep	Irrational thoughts; forgetting things more often than usual; mental "blocks"; missing of planned events
Restlessness, an inability to keep still	
Sweating (not necessarily noticeably); clammy hands; cold hands and feet; cold chills	Guilt about neglecting family or friends; inner confusion about duties and roles
Blushing; hot face	Excessive work; omission of play
The need to urinate frequently	Inability to organize oneself, tendency to get distraught over minor matters
Diarrhea; indigestion; upset stomach; nausea	
Headaches; frequent earaches or toothaches	Inability to reach decisions; erratic, unpredictable decisions
Premenstrual tension or missed menstrual periods	
More body aches and pains than usual, such as pain in the neck or lower back; any localized muscle tension	Decreased ability to perform tasks
	Inability to concentrate
	General ("floating") anxiety; feelings of unreality
Loss of appetite; unintended weight loss; excessive appetite; sudden weight gain	A tendency to become fatigued; loss of energy; loss of spontaneous joy
Increased use of substances (tobacco, legally prescribed drugs such as tranquilizers or amphetamines, alcohol, other drugs)	Nightmares
	Feelings of powerlessness; mistrust of others
Accident proneness	
Frequent illnesses	

Pursuing wellness

A Stress-Free Life: Is It for You?

Ask students if they would really want to live a life that was absolutely and completely free of stress. Although they might think it sounds like a great life, in reality they would hate it. While it is true that continuously high levels of stress are undesirable and can be harmful, an absolutely stress-free life would not be desirable either. Such a life would most likely be dull and boring, with no challenges or excitement.

Most of us function best with stress levels that fluctuate around the midranges, between high and low. One example of these fluctuations is what results from an event such as a

You may have noticed some effects of another kind of stress, the short-term kind that arises when a problem suddenly demands to be solved—**acute stress**. This sort of stress may bring you new energy. You may be amazed at all you can accomplish. If the stress continues, though, it becomes chronic, energy gives way to exhaustion, and you may become sick. Students often push hard to study for tests and to complete assignments toward the end of the grading period, only to find that when they relax in the break that follows, they become ill.

Too many people wait for health problems to set in before they take steps to relieve their stress. You do not have to wait: you can take action as soon as you notice signs indicating too much stress. Cold hands and feet are among the first signs. Figure 4–1 on the opposite page lists others.

A **stressor** is anything that requires you to cope with, or **adapt** to, a situation. Physical stressors include all physical conditions, such as air temperature, intensity of lighting, bacteria, injuries, or radiation. Psychological stressors include life-changing events, both desirable and undesirable.

The Stressors of High School

The high school years are stressful, for they represent a period of change that requires teenagers to adapt. They are believed by many to be among the most stressful periods in life. Each person under stress responds to stressors in an individual way. Some researchers studied the effects of life changes on high school students and found that when students faced more than one change at a time, their grade point averages dropped. So did their scores on a test of self-esteem.

Those students who handled changes one at a time were least affected by stress. If you are experiencing many changes or stressors listed in Figure 4–2 on the next page, try focusing on them one at a time. You can then reduce your level of stress and protect your self-esteem.

 KEY POINTS   *A stressor is anything that requires you to cope with, or adapt to, a situation. High school students face many stressors.*

The Perception of a Stressor

Your reaction to an experience depends greatly on your **perception** of it. Your perception of something is not quite like anyone else's, because your life experiences that help determine your perceptions are unique to you.

Figure 4–3 on page 83 demonstrates how perceptions affect the way you respond to events. Suppose you see a snake at your feet. Your reaction may be any of the following, or something else entirely:

▶ "Snakes are poisonous"—fear.
▶ "Snakes are beautiful"—joy.
▶ "Snakes are my topic of study"—interest.

Obviously, whether or not the snake encounter was stressful depends upon your point of view about—your perception of—snakes. Likewise, a student who has prepared for a test experiences that test as much less stressful

"To be totally without stress is to be dead."

Hans Selye
(1907–1982)
Endocrinologist

MINI Glossary

stress: the effect of physical and psychological demands (stressors) on a person. Stress that provides a welcome challenge is *eustress* ("good" stress, pronounced YOU-stress); stress that is perceived as negative is *distress* ("bad" stress).

chronic stress: unrelieved stress that continues to tax a person's resources to the point of exhaustion; stress that is damaging to health.

acute stress: a temporary bout of stress that calls forth alertness or alarm to prompt the person to deal with an event.

stressor: a demand placed on the body to adapt.

adapt: to change or adjust in order to accommodate new conditions.

perception: a meaning given to an event or occurrence based on a person's previous experience or understanding.

COMPREHENSION CHECK

Acute means sharp, sudden, intense. This is in direct contrast to *chronic*, which is not so intense and lasts much longer.

BACKGROUND INFORMATION

If you want students to learn the terms *eustress* and *distress*, point out that the word *stress* is included in both terms. What they need to remember is that eu = "good," dis = "bad."

TEACHER SUPPORT

Key Passage

Ask students what strategy for handling stress is presented on this page. (deal with one stressor at a time) Ask students if they are currently feeling stressed from more than one source. If so, ask them to list those sources. Now, ask students if they are trying to deal with more than one of these stressors at once. Which one would they pick if they had to focus on just one stressor?

LEARNING WITH VISUALS

Have students do a personalized illustration of the stressors in their lives. Have them draw a picture of themselves (or paste in a school picture) and surround it with stress arrows (with the stressor written on the arrow). They can select the stressors that apply from Figure 4–2 on page 82, and add additional stressors as they feel appropriate to personalize the illustration.

big test. As the test gets closer and closer, your stress level goes up; when the test is over, your stress level goes down. Another example might be having a fight and breaking up with your boyfriend or girlfriend. During the breakup your stress level is high, but later if you find someone you like even better, your stress level goes back down.

Keep in mind that long-term exposure to

high levels of stress can be harmful to your health and should be avoided or properly handled. A moderate amount of stress in your life, however, is normal and to be expected. Use that stress as a motivating or driving force to enrich and improve the quality of your life.

CLASS ACTIVITY

Tell the students to list on a sheet of paper the stressors given in Figure 4–2 that apply to them. Have the students put a + next to all the psychological stressors on their lists over which they have control. Have them put a − next to the stressors over which they have no control. What does this tell them about the stress in their lives? Ask them if they are surprised with the results.

BACKGROUND INFORMATION

The rating scale in Figure 4–2 was adapted from the Social Readjustment Rating Scale (SRRS) developed by Dr. Thomas Holmes. What are simplified here for high school students as stress points, Dr. Holmes calls his *life change units (LCUs)*. The SRRS is not a foolproof way to rate stress, and it's necessary to remember that people differ greatly in their reactions to the same event. This means that the SRRS is, at best, a rough index for stress. Still, a high score should be taken seriously.

Other psychologists have examined the effect of minor, but more frequent, stressors. Psychologist Richard Lazarus refers to such daily frustrations as *hassles* or *microstressors*. According to one of his studies, frequent and severe hassles turned out to be better predictors of day-to-day emotional and physical health than major life events.

Vocabulary worksheets are provided in the Teacher's Resource Box.

Figure 4–2 Psychological Stressors for High School Students

People ranked these events according to how stressful they perceived them to be. Note that some "happy" events are included here. Individual people may score these events higher or lower than they are scored here and other individuals may be stressed by events not named here.

Life Event	Stress Points
• Death of parent	119
• Divorce of parents	98
• Death of a close family member (except parent)	92
• Breakup with boyfriend/girlfriend	79
• Expulsion from school	79
• Major personal injury or illness	77
• Death of a close friend	70
• Pregnancy	66
• Getting a job	62
• Money troubles	61
• Dating	57
• Gain of new family member	57
• Change in finances	56
• Major illness of family member or close friend	56
• Failing grades at school	54
• Change in number of arguments with peers	51
• Marriage	50
• Parent beginning or stopping work	46
• Peer difficulties	45
• Loss or death of loved pet	44
• Change in responsibilities at home or school	43
• Brother or sister leaving home	42
• Moving away	41
• School beginning or ending	38
• Trouble with parent	38
• Outstanding personal achievement	37
• Change in schools	35
• Christmas	30
• Change in recreation	29
• Trouble with teachers/principal	29
• Change in personal appearance	27
• Change in social activities (joining new group)	27
• Change in eating habits	27
• Change in sleeping habits	26
• Change in number of get-togethers	26
• Vacation	25
• Change in church activities	22
• Traffic tickets or other minor violations of the law	22

Check the list, and identify the events that have happened to you in the past year or that you expect within the next year. Use the number system to determine how many stress points you are experiencing in this period of your life. Then score yourself as follows:

Over 200: Urgent need of intelligent stress management.   100–149: Stressful life; keep tabs on your mental health.
150–199: Careful stress management indicated.   Under 100: No present cause for concern about stress.
Your answers are personal and private. Share them with others only if you are comfortable doing so.

Source: Events and stress points adapted from the work of M. A. Miller and R. H. Rahe, Life changes scaling for the 1990's, *Journal of Psychosomatic Research* 43 (1997): 279–292.

Chapter 4, Section 1

The following quiz will help you assess your students' understanding of the material covered in this section of the chapter. You might use the quiz as an oral exercise, which will lead into a class discussion of the topics covered. Or, you might use it as a paper/pencil quiz to evaluate your students individually.

Like the Quick Quiz, the Section Review can also be used as an assessment tool to spark class discussion or as an individual student evaluation. It can also be used as a review in preparation for this quiz.

1. Chronic stress is the kind of stress that produces beneficial energy. (False)
2. People appear to experience greater levels of stress today than they did 30 years ago. (True)

Threatening = Stress reaction.

Event.   Perception.

Threatening or not threatening?

Not threatening = No stress reaction.

Figure 4–3 Perceptions and Stressors. To produce stress, an event must be perceived as threatening.

than a classmate who forgot to study. Many things—family interactions, schoolwork, relationships, and more—have the potential to cause stress. The important thing is that an event must be labeled as a threat by you before it can produce stress in your body.

 KEY POINTS *To produce stress in your body, an event must first be labeled as threatening by your mind.*

SECTION 1 Review

Answer the following questions on a sheet of paper.

Learning the Vocabulary

The vocabulary terms in this section are *stress, chronic stress, acute stress, stressor, adapt,* and *perception.*

1. _____ is the effect of a physical or psychological demand on a person.
2. A _____ is anything that requires you to cope with, or _____ to, a situation.
3. What is the difference between chronic stress and acute stress?
4. The way you react to an experience depends on your _____ of it.

5. Name four physical and four psychological signs of stress.

Learning the Facts

6. What can happen when acute stress becomes chronic stress?
7. When you are dealing with many stressors at one time, what is the best way to handle things?

Making Life Choices

8. Add up your stress points as instructed in Figure 4–2 on the opposite page. What stressors are you currently facing that are not on the list? What stressors do you anticipate dealing with in the near future that are not on the list? Develop your own personal stress scale. List what you believe to be your top ten stressors in order of most to least stressful.

3. Alcohol and other drugs, while unhealthy in themselves, can help to reduce stress. (False)
4. Acute stress is beneficial on a short-term basis. (True)
5. A stressor is anything that requires your body to adapt to a situation, including air temperature. (True)
6. Psychological stressors always result from negative changes and events. (False)

7. The high school years are generally a time of low stress. (False)
8. When dealing with stress it is best to try to cope with everything at once. (False)
9. An individual's perception of an event determines his or her reaction to it. (True)
10. An event must be labeled as a threat by you before it can produce stress in your body. (True)

ASSESS

EVALUATE

 A reproducible quiz for Section 1 is provided in the Teacher's Resource Box.

 SECTION 1 Review Answers

1. Stress (p. 81)
2. stressor, adapt (p. 81)
3. Acute stress is a short-term stress, sometimes producing new energy; while chronic stress is unrelieved stress that can damage body systems. (pp. 80–81)
4. perception (p. 81)
5. Answers will vary. Refer to Figure 4–2. (p. 82)
6. Energy gives way to exhaustion and one may become sick. (p. 81)
7. It is best to focus on one change or stressor at a time. (p. 81)
8. Answers will vary.

CLOSE

Have the students describe as many physical and psychological stressors as possible that exist in the classroom. List them on the board. Ask the students to agree or disagree as a group with each item listed. Make some suggestions to reduce or eliminate the stressors within the classroom. Are the suggestions practical? If they are, try as a class to reduce or eliminate the stressors for one week. At the end of the week, decide if the environment in the classroom has improved.

SECTION
2

FOCUS

OUTCOMES

In this section students will learn:

1. That stress affects each of the body's systems.

2. How the various glands and the hormones they secrete react within the body during times of stress.

3. About effects that occur to the immune system as a result of prolonged stress.

FOCUS ACTIVITY

Create some major stressful situations within the classroom—using both positive and negative stressors. For example, bang on a desk, turn lights on and off, change the temperature of the room, have someone come into the room saying pizza is on the way for everyone, raise your voice, and end by announcing a pop quiz. Have students note what happened to their bodies physically and how they felt psychologically. Ask students to share and compare their responses.

TEACH & APPLY

COMPREHENSION CHECK

Have students explain the difference between the way the nervous system responds to a psychological stressor as compared to a physiological stressor. (There is no basic difference.) As a follow-up question ask, "What does the body always do in response to stress?" (It restores normal conditions inside the body.)

84

For Your Information

Anything that harms the immune system (such as the AIDS virus, which you'll read about in Chapter 16) threatens life. Anything that strengthens the system, such as exercise and a well-chosen diet, supports health.

People who live with psychological stress need to understand its effects on the body.

SECTION 2
Stress and the Body's Systems

Exercising, taking an exam, or buying a new car all affect your body in about the same way. Physically, your heart beats faster. You breathe faster than normal, signaling that your body is getting ready to act. All external changes stimulate you this way to some degree. They require you to change in some physical way—that is, to adapt. All environmental changes—changes in the temperature, the noise level around you, what is touching you, and countless others—require your body to adapt. So do all psychological events, both desirable and undesirable.

All of the body's systems, and especially the **nervous system**, the **hormonal system**, and the **immune system**, are affected by stress. Chapter 6 provides more information about the anatomy and workings of these three systems.

The Nervous System

A stressful event may be a mental challenge (such as an exam) or a physical challenge (such as cold weather). Whatever the challenge, the responses of the nervous system are always similar. That is, the nervous system always produces a set of reactions to restore normal conditions inside the body. As an example, let's look at the body's responses to cold weather.

When you go outside in cold weather, nerves in your skin act as a thermometer, sending "cold" messages to the spinal cord and brain. The central nervous system reacts to these messages and signals the smallest blood ves-

---

special needs

Linguistic

Each person deals with stress on some level almost on a daily basis. The strategies we choose determine the effect stress has on our lives. Thinking about alternative ways of dealing with stress will allow students to choose positive ways they can handle personal stressors when they arise.

Review the list of ways for dealing with stress as identified in this chapter: exercise, attitude control, time management, coping devices (displacement, ventilation), defense mechanisms (denial, fantasy, projection, rationalization, regression, selective forgetting, withdrawal), and changed perception.

Give students specific situations that can cause stress. For example: You walk into your toughest class and written on the board are the words—"Surprise Quiz Today!" Assign each of sels, closest to the skin's surface, to shut down. This action forces your blood to circulate deeper in your tissues, where its heat will be conserved. The system also signals the muscles just under the skin surface to contract, forming goose bumps. All muscle contractions, even goose bumps, produce heat as a by-product. If these measures do not raise your body temperature enough, the nerves signal your large muscle groups to shiver. The shivering (contractions) of these large muscles produces still more heat. All of this activity adds up to a set of adjustments that maintain a constant body temperature under conditions of an external extreme (in this case, cold).

Now let's say you come in and sit by a fire and drink hot cocoa. You are warm, and you no longer need the body's heat-producing activity. At this point, the nervous system signals the skin surface capillaries to open up again, the goose bumps to subside, and the muscles to relax. These responses show that the nervous system is helping to keep you from getting too warm. Your body has maintained its temperature throughout the cold time and the warm time.

This example described only the nervous system's role in managing a brief period of one type of stress. The nervous system plays many other roles, too, depending on the type and degree of stress.

 The nervous system responds to challenges by producing reactions that restore normal body conditions.

The Hormonal System

The hormonal system works together with the nervous system to maintain communication among body organs. The two systems complement each other in helping the body adapt to changes in the environment.

A **hormone** is a chemical messenger released by a **gland**. Glands receive information about body conditions. They then release hormones into the bloodstream to control those conditions. A hormone flows everywhere in the body. However, only the hormone's target organs respond to it, because only they possess the equipment to do so.

Like the nervous system, the hormonal system is busy during times of stress. It sends messages from one body part to another to maintain order. The hormones that control the stress response are called the **stress hormones**. Among the stress hormones, **epinephrine** and **norepinephrine** are well known. They regulate the body's activities during emergencies and between times.

 The hormonal system consists of glands that produce chemical messengers that communicate body conditions to target organs. Release of the stress hormones brings on the stress response.

The Immune System

Many tissues perform jobs in the immune system. The main cells of **immunity** are the white blood cells. These are made in the bone marrow and travel to other glands, where they mature. White blood cells make antibodies, the body's main ammunition against infections. All the body's tissues work together to provide immunity. All the body's fluids connect the parts of the immune system so that they act as a unit—one system.

MINI Glossary

nervous system: the body system of nervous tissues—organized into the brain, spinal cord, and nerves—that send and receive messages and integrate the body's activities.

hormonal system: the system of glands—organs that send and receive blood-borne chemical messages—that control body functions in cooperation with the nervous system.

immune system: the cells, tissues, and organs that protect the body from disease. The immune system is composed of the white blood cells, bone marrow, thymus gland, spleen, and other parts.

hormone: a chemical that serves as a messenger. Each hormone is secreted by a gland and travels to one or more target organs, where it brings about responses.

gland: an organ of the body that secretes one or more hormones.

stress hormones: epinephrine and norepinephrine, secreted as part of the reaction of the nervous system to stress.

epinephrine (EP-uh-NEFF-rin), **norepinephrine:** two of the stress hormones; also called *adrenaline* and *noradrenaline*.

immunity: the body's capacity for identifying, destroying, and disposing of disease-causing agents.

the ways of dealing with stress to a pair of students. Give them three minutes to discuss it, then ask them to present the reasons why that way is the best for dealing with the stressful situation. After all presentations have been made, have the class vote to decide which is actually the best way to handle that particular stress. Is there always one best way?

Other examples you may want to use:

1. Your best friend has a date for a big dance and you don't.
2. You fail your driving test.
3. The president has just announced that the United States is going to war.
4. A family member is diagnosed with a terminal illness.
5. Your best friend is supposed to drive you home after a party, but has been drinking.

ASSESS

EVALUATE

A reproducible quiz for Section 2 is provided in the Teacher's Resource Box.

SECTION 2 Review Answers

1. hormone, gland (p. 85)
2. nervous system (p. 84)
3. epinephrine, norepinephrine (p. 85)
4. nervous, hormonal, and immune systems (p. 84)
5. It sends messages from one body part to another to maintain order. (p. 85)
6. Long periods of stress weaken immunity and make a person more likely to suffer disease. (p. 86)
7. Answers will vary.

CLOSE

Discuss some career choices that your students have in mind for their futures. (See Appendix A for health-related careers.) Analyze the stress level of their career choices. Discuss the importance of the amount of stress involved in a job in their decision-making process for choosing a career.

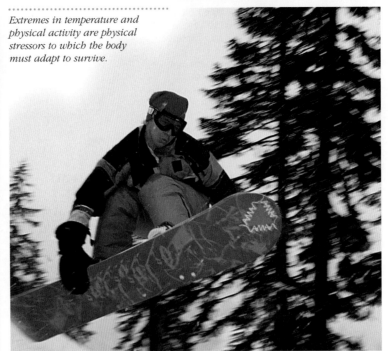

Extremes in temperature and physical activity are physical stressors to which the body must adapt to survive.

The activity of the immune system is lower than normal during the stress response. However, between times it recovers quickly. Short periods of stress, followed by periods of relief from stress, can strengthen the immune system. Long periods of unrelieved stress, however, can reduce the number of white blood cells or their effectiveness and so make a person likely to suffer diseases.

KEY POINTS *The immune system is the body's main defense against disease. Unrelieved stress can weaken the immune system.*

SECTION 2 Review

Answer the following questions on a sheet of paper.

Learning the Vocabulary

The vocabulary terms in this section are *nervous system, hormonal system, immune system, hormone, gland, stress hormones, epinephrine, norepinephrine,* and *immunity.*
Fill in the blank with the correct answer.

1. A _____ is a chemical messenger released by a _____.
2. The brain, spinal cord, and nerves make up the _____.
3. Two stress hormones are _____ and _____.

Learning the Facts

4. What are the three body systems most affected by stress?
5. How does the hormonal system react to stress?
6. What happens to the immune system when it is exposed to long periods of unrelieved stress?

Making Life Choices

7. List three things that upset you and cause you stress. Identify each stressful situation as acute or chronic. Have you or anyone you know ever experienced a chronic stress that in turn affected health in a negative way? Describe the situation and the outcome.

QUICK QUIZ

Chapter 4, Section 2

The following quiz will help you assess your students' understanding of the material covered in this section of the chapter. You might use the quiz as an oral exercise, which will lead into a class discussion of the topics covered. Or, you might use it as a paper/pencil quiz to evaluate your students individually.

Like the Quick Quiz, the Section Review can also be used as an assessment tool to spark class discussion or as an individual student evaluation. It can also be used as a review in preparation for this quiz.

1. The body adapts to both environmental and psychological changes. (True)
2. The immune system responds very little to stress. (False)
3. When under stress the nervous system

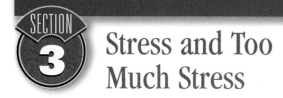

Stress and Too Much Stress

A little stress can be beneficial. However, too much stress, unrelieved, can be exhausting and harmful. Consider what causes stress, both physical and psychological, and what it does to you.

The Stages of the Stress Response

Whatever the stressor that triggers it, the **stress response** has three phases: alarm, resistance, and recovery or exhaustion.

Alarm   The first phase of the stress response is always **alarm**. Alarm occurs when you think that you are facing a challenge. The body releases the stress hormones, which activate the nerves and all systems.

Resistance   The second phase of the stress response is always **resistance**. Resistance is a state of speeded-up functioning. The stress hormones continue to flow, causing muscles to contract and other body functions to shut down. (We'll describe this *unbalanced state* in more detail shortly.)

During the resistance phase, your resources are mobilized just as an army mobilizes its equipment and supplies to fight a battle. In the case of your body, the resources are your attention, strength, and fuels. You can use your resources until they run out or wear out. Then you need to replace or repair them.

Recovery or Exhaustion   The third phase of the stress response may be either of two opposite states—**recovery** or **exhaustion**. Figure 4–4, on the next page, shows both. Recovery occurs when stress ceases to affect the body. It is hoped that before your resources run out, you deal with the source of stress or it goes away, and you recover. Then your stress hormone levels drop to normal, your body systems slow down, your muscles relax, blood flows to all body parts, needed repairs take place, fuel stores are refilled, and you become ready for the next round of excitement. It is because of the need for recovery between times of stress that the military provides "R and R" (Rest and Recreation) times for its personnel.

Stress can make you stronger. Each time you go through a period of stress and recover, you are better able to meet the next round of stress. Just as your muscles grow stronger with repeated use, so does your stress resistance—but you must have rest between times to build that strength.

If stress continues to affect you without a break and your body stays in overdrive for too long, your resistance finally breaks down. Then recovery is delayed or becomes impossible. This is exhaustion.

 KEY POINTS   *The stress response occurs in stages, and ends in recovery or exhaustion.*

Stress and the Fight-or-Flight Reaction

Although stress itself arises in the mind, the body's response is physical in nature. The stress response developed long ago to permit our Stone Age

MINI Glossary

stress response: the response to a demand or stressor. The stress response has three phases—*alarm, resistance,* and *recovery* or *exhaustion.*

alarm: the first phase of the stress response, in which the person faces a challenge and starts paying attention to it.

resistance: the second phase of the stress response, in which the body mobilizes its resources to withstand the effects of the stress.

recovery: a healthy third phase of the stress response, in which the body returns to normal.

exhaustion: a harmful third phase of the stress response, in which stress exceeds the body's ability to recover.

---

produces a set of reactions that restore normal conditions inside the body. (True)

4. Emotional stress takes a physical toll on the body. (True)

5. A hormone is a chemical messenger released by the nervous system. (False)

6. Both the hormonal and nervous system work to maintain communication among body organs. (True)

7. Stress hormones control the body's

response to stress. (True)

8. Among other hormones, the glands release epinephrine and norepinephrine. (True)

9. The main cells of immunity are the red blood cells. (False)

10. Stress increases the number of antibodies in the blood and, over long periods of time, strengthens the immune system. (False)

LEARNING WITH VISUALS

The transparency "Stress Ending in Recovery or Exhaustion" is provided in the Transparency Acetate Binder.

Use the transparency to help expand discussion of the stress response. To help students understand the illustration, ask them what the alarm represents. (first awareness of stress) What are they resisting? (the stress) Tell them that the straight line represents the normal level of resistance—it shows the body's behavior when no new stressors are encountered. Then, give students a sample situation such as a teacher asking a student to stay after class. This is alarm. Suppose that the teacher confronts the student with a failing grade. What sorts of resistance occur? Point out that if this happens only occasionally, the student recovers, goes on to the next class, and soon everything is back to normal. If it occurs regularly, the student will eventually become exhausted and could develop a serious health problem. Ask students to draw their own illustrations, identifying specific stressors and responses. Have them show recovery or exhaustion depending upon whether or not the type of stress is chronic.

DISCUSSION

Students should agree that today's stress situations rarely call for physical action. Have them brainstorm a list of stressors, then divide the list into those that do and those that do not call for physical action.

Figure 4–4 Stress Ending in Recovery or Exhaustion. Alarm briefly lowers resistance but is followed by a high level of resistance. Recovery restores the normal level. If resistance is required for too long, exhaustion sets in, and resistance temporarily falls below the level normally maintained.

The threats to your ancestors were physical, and the reaction was to fight or flee.

ancestors to react quickly to *physical* danger. While our ancestors had to cope with fierce tigers and spear-wielding foes, however, they were never faced with class speeches or final exams. Today, people facing class speeches or final exams feel fear, just as their ancestors did when facing tigers. Today's human body responds to the fear caused by these stressors in the same way as human bodies did long ago. The body still prepares to act physically. Unfortunately, while the stress response is perfectly suited to times when physical action is needed, today's crises rarely call for physical action.

The stress response is often called the **fight-or-flight reaction**, because when someone is faced with a physical threat, the two possible actions are to fight or run away. Every organ responds to the alarm:

▶ Heart rate speeds up.
▶ Pupils of the eyes widen (enhancing vision).
▶ Muscles tense (ready to jump, run, or struggle).
▶ Fuels, such as fat, are released from storage (for use by the muscles).
▶ Blood flow to skin is reduced (to protect against blood loss in case of injury).
▶ Blood flow to digestive organs is reduced (these can wait).
▶ Blood flow to muscles and brain increases (these need extra supplies right now).
▶ Immune system temporarily shuts down (to free up energy).

Earlier, we called the state of stress resistance an *unbalanced state.* Here's why. It is a state that favors muscular activity while it shuts down other necessary body functions, such as digestion and immune defenses. This unbalanced state is beneficial at times—it helps the body deal with an emergency. Later, when the danger has passed, the body functions become balanced once again—recovery. Digestive system activity and immune defenses can resume. Both states are important. You need normal functioning to keep you running smoothly during peaceful times, and stress resistance to get you through emergencies.

QUICK QUIZ

Chapter 4, Section 3

The following quiz will help you assess your students' understanding of the material covered in this section of the chapter. You might use the quiz as an oral exercise, which will lead into a class discussion of the topics covered. Or, you might use it as a paper/pencil quiz to evaluate your students individually.

Like the Quick Quiz, the Section Review can also be used as an assessment tool to spark class discussion or as an individual student evaluation. It can also be used as a review in preparation for this quiz.

1. Resistance is always the first phase of the stress response. (False)
2. During the alarm stage of the stress response, the body releases the stress hormones. (True)

Prolonged stress, however, can make diseases of the heart and arteries likely. The fat released into the bloodstream to serve as fuel for the muscles may not be used up if no physical action occurs. When this fat is left in the bloodstream, it tends to collect along artery walls, damaging them. You'll learn more about heart disease in Chapter 17. For now, you should realize that psychological stress is believed to contribute to the development of heart disease.

If a round of stress leads to recovery and to a greater ability to respond to the next round, then it has benefited you. On the other hand, if it leaves you drained and *less* able to respond the next time, it has harmed you. How can you make sure that your stressful experiences benefit you and do not harm you? The next section provides some insight.

 KEY POINTS *The stress response is an ancient, physical response to fear: the fight-or-flight reaction. The response occurs even if the stressor is a psychological one that does not demand physical action.*

SECTION 3 Review

Answer the following questions on a sheet of paper.

Learning the Vocabulary

The vocabulary terms in this section are *stress response, alarm, resistance, recovery, exhaustion,* and *fight-or-flight reaction.*
Fill in the blank with the correct answer.

1. _____ is the healthy third phase of the stress response, while _____ is the harmful third phase.
2. The stress response is often called the _____.
3. _____ is the first phase of the stress response, in which a person faces a challenge and begins paying attention to it.

Learning the Facts

4. What are the three phases of the stress response?

5. What occurs in the resistance phase of the stress response?
6. What parts of the body experience changes during the fight-or-flight reaction?
7. What diseases are associated with prolonged exposure to stress?

Making Life Choices

8. A little stress can be beneficial. Once it exceeds your limit, though, it can be both exhausting and harmful. Consider what stress, both physical and psychological, does to you. Describe a situation in which you experienced a stress response that followed the pattern of alarm, resistance, and recovery. Describe a situation in which the stress was chronic and resulted in a stress response of alarm, resistance, and exhaustion. Looking back on the second situation now, how might you have achieved a faster recovery?

MINI Glossary

fight-or-flight reaction: the body's response to immediate physical danger; the stress response. Energy is mobilized, either to mount an aggressive response against the danger, or to run away.

3. Resistance is an unbalanced state of increased bodily functioning. (True)
4. Recovery is always the third and last stage of the stress response. (False)
5. Successfully managed stress can make you stronger and better able to deal with future problems. (True)
6. Prolonged and unrelieved stress can result in exhaustion. (True)
7. Humans developed the fight-or-flight reaction during the Stone Age, as a response to the threat of physical danger. (True)
8. The fight-or-flight reaction is well-adapted to stressful situations in modern life. (False)
9. Every organ of the body is involved in the stress response. (True)
10. The digestive and immune systems continue to function normally during stressful situations. (False)

ASSESS

EVALUATE

A reproducible quiz for Section 3 is provided in the Teacher's Resource Box.

SECTION 3 Review Answers

1. Recovery, exhaustion (p. 87)
2. fight-or-flight reaction (p. 88)
3. Alarm (p. 87)
4. alarm, resistance, and recovery or exhaustion (p. 87)
5. There is a state of speeded-up functioning. Stress hormones continue to flow, causing muscles to contract and other body functions to shut down. (p. 87)
6. Every organ responds. The heart rate speeds up; the pupils of the eyes widen; the muscles tense; fat is released into the body; circulation to the skin, digestive system, and internal organs is reduced, and circulation to the muscles and brain is increased. The immune system temporarily shuts down. (p. 88)
7. diseases of the heart and arteries (p. 89)
8. Answers will vary.

CLOSE

For extra credit have the students tell stories that would follow along with Figure 4–4. The stories can be made up or something that really happened. The stories can be presented in written or oral form.

Dealing with Stress

SECTION 4

FOCUS

OUTCOMES

In this section students will learn:

1. The importance of managing stress while using physical strength, psychological strength, and knowledge.
2. The importance of time management in reducing stress.
3. Some coping devices that help people through difficult situations.

FOCUS ACTIVITY

Have students list some recognizable signs of stress and stressors that they have noticed among their peers. Now have each student think of a personally stressful time that occurred recently. Ask the students to recall the early warning signs that were present when this situation occurred (consult Figure 4–1). What did they do to relieve stress? Impress upon the students how important it is to be able to recognize their own personal signs of stress to be better able to deal with the situation. Depending upon the makeup of your class, you might also wish to have other students tell their classmates some signs that they have recognized in each other.

FAST FACTS

One study found that 15 percent of a group of 25-year-old doctors and lawyers who scored high on a hostility test were dead by age 50.

People who use stress management strategies are better able to cope with periods of stress than those who do not. Also, people who maintain strong programs of personal wellness are best able to cope with daily irritations and problems, common in the lives of teenagers. Figure 4–5 illustrates some of these stressors.

At the heart of such personal wellness programs is a strong sense of self-esteem. In addition to enhancing your wellness in general, high self-esteem can improve your ability to manage crises when they arise. People with high self-esteem learn to view challenges as positive, rather than

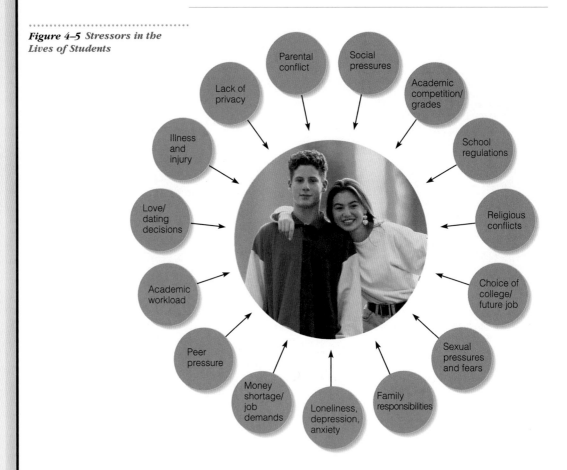

Figure 4–5 Stressors in the Lives of Students

COOPERATIVE LEARNING

Dealing with Stress

Explain to students that stress can be both positive and negative. Positive stress may help a person obtain a goal, whereas negative stress may prevent a person from obtaining a goal. Dealing with stress in a positive way may help a person make the winning free throw in basketball, give a speech to the stu-dent body, or ask someone special out on a date. Dealing with stress in a negative way may keep a person from even trying to make the basketball team, speak in front of other people, or ask for a date.

To give students practice in identifying positive stress and negative stress, divide the class into groups of three or four students. Have each group make a list of positive stress situations and a list of negative stress situations. Also have students list all the stressors that are

How Well Do You Resist Stress?

To determine how likely you are to be affected by stress, answer the following questions. Beside each question, fill in the number corresponding to how much of the time each statement applies to you. Your answers to the Life Choice Inventory are personal and private. Share them with others only if you are comfortable doing so.

4: Always   3: Almost always   2: Most of the time
      1: Some of the time   0: Never

During most of my life I: Score

1. Eat at least two full, balanced meals a day. ____
2. Get seven to eight hours' sleep. ____
3. Give and receive affection regularly. ____
4. Have at least one relative on whom I can rely. ____
5. Exercise to the point of perspiration at least twice a week. ____
6. Do not smoke, or smoke less than half a pack of cigarettes a day. ____
7. Do not drink alcohol or abuse drugs. ____
8. Am at an appropriate weight for my height. ____
9. Feel that my basic needs are being met. ____
10. Get strength from my values and beliefs. ____
11. Regularly attend club or social activities. ____
12. Have a network of friends and acquaintances. ____
13. Have one or more friends to talk to about personal matters. ____
14. Am in good physical health (including eyesight, hearing, and teeth). ____
15. Am able to speak openly about my feelings when angry or worried. ____
16. Have regular conversations with the people I live with about domestic issues (such as chores or money). ____
17. Have some fun each day. ____
18. Organize my time effectively. ____
19. Drink two or fewer cups of caffeinated beverages (coffee, tea, or cola drinks) a day. ____
20. Take quiet time for myself each day. ____

During stressful times I:

21. Organize my responsibilities and meet the most important ones first. ____
22. Refuse to take on too many responsibilities. ____
23. Express my feelings at intervals. ____
24. Use willed relaxation methods. ____
25. Seek outside help as needed. ____

                                Score ____

SCORING

81–100: Congratulations! Your defenses against daily stresses are strong.
61–80: You are well defended against stress, but you could still improve your defenses.
41–60: You are too vulnerable to stress. Try to improve.
0–40: You urgently need strategies for handling stress.

associated with each of the stress situations. Once students have made the list of situations and stressors have them make a list of all the positive ways they can think of to deal with that stress. Responses will vary but may include exercising, cleaning their room, helping an elderly person, reading, or watching a funny movie. Have students also make a list of all the negative ways they think people deal with stress. Responses again will vary but may include using alcohol or other drugs,

becoming violent towards others, taking frustrations out on others, or avoiding others or the situation.

Have groups then list all the benefits of handling stress in a positive way, and the detriments of handling stress in a negative way. How would the way(s) they handle stress affect their overall health? Follow up by having groups share their responses with each other.

Have students do the Life Choice Inventory, "How Well Do You Resist Stress?" (A reproducible copy is provided in the Teacher's Resource Box.) Discuss the ways in which the various scores indicate how well a person handles a stressful situation. Discuss students' scores with them. Have students decide whether or not they are happy with their scores. Now divide the class into groups of four and have the students share their answers within the groups. What did they discover that they had in common with their groups? What conclusion can the class make about how teenagers handle stress and what they all do to resist stress?

TEACH & APPLY

CLASS ACTIVITY

Not having enough time is often a major complaint among teenagers, as well as adults. Ask the students to repeat some clichés using the word *time*. "Time flies," "Time's up!" and so on. Write the phrases on the board or make them into signs that can be placed around the

(continued on next page)

(continued from previous page)

classroom. Have the students discuss what role time plays in their lives. Do they feel more time conscious with a digital watch or clock, or with a traditional (face) clock or watch? Does the school bell schedule affect their feelings about being ruled by time? What other parts of their lives are ruled by time?

Ask students to develop a time management chart. In the first column of the chart, have them list school, home, work, and social activities. In the second column they should record the amount of time spent in each of the four areas. In column three they should write what they can do, if anything, to reduce the amount of time spent on these activities. In the fourth column, have students include what they would do with the free time they have now created for themselves.

TEACHER SUPPORT

Key Passage

This probably happens to students frequently without their being aware of it. Ask them to think of three or four situations in which they were very tired, without knowing why. Can they think of stressful situations that might have preceded their periods of exhaustion?

---

negative, situations. Therefore, they react with less fear and experience less stress than people with low self-esteem. For example, a person with low self-esteem might fear meeting new people. This person would feel stress during these meetings. In contrast, a person with high self-esteem would feel at ease. This illustrates that whether an event is stressful or not depends more on the perception of the person experiencing it than on the event itself.

In addition to maintaining high self-esteem, the strategies of eating well, sleeping well, and being physically active can help equip you to withstand stress. Just as important are seeking out daily joy and laughter and acting in harmony with your values. These steps can help you move serenely through most of life.

To determine how well you protect yourself from stress during ordinary life, complete the first 20 questions of this chapter's Life Choice Inventory on page 91. Answer the last five questions to see how well you manage the stressful times.

The sections that follow present some key components of stress control. As you'll see, managing stress well takes all your capacities—physical strength, psychological strength, and knowledge. "Stress vitamins" do not help, though, as the Consumer Skills feature on page 94 explains.

Exercise

Physical activity is always important. It keeps your body strong and strengthens your immune system between times of stress. Then, during stress, physical activity plays a special role. Consider what happens if you experience alarm (anxiety, fear), but you *don't* fight or flee—that is, your body takes no physical action. The body gets *ready* to exercise, but it doesn't act.

Now your muscles are tense and can't relax. Your blood is rich with fuels that are building up and can damage your heart. You are in a state of high alert with no relief in sight. This state drains your reserves, exhausts you mentally, and lowers your resistance to diseases of all kinds. It's time to work out.

Physical activity works your muscles so they can relax again. It burns the fuels in your blood and prevents them from building up. It relieves your anxiety and brings temporary relief. When you've had a good workout, it helps you relax.

 KEY POINTS   *Between times of stress, physical activity strengthens stress resistance. During times of stress, physical activity can work off muscle tension, use up ready fuels, and help the body recover.*

Attitude Control

While physical activity works well to combat stress that has already set in, you can also change the way you react to events so that the events aren't so stressful. An example is performing on stage: the stress response can help you get "up for it." Some excitement ahead of the event will give you the physical energy to turn out a spectacular performance. You are most attractive when you are aroused and alert. Too much nervous energy, however, will hinder you. If you allow yourself to think about what a disaster it will be if you do less than a perfect job, you will be trembling visibly, your teeth

---

HEALTHY PEOPLE 2000

Reduce to less than 35 percent the proportion of people aged 18 and older who experienced adverse health effects from stress within the past year. (Baseline: 42.6 percent in 1985)

The effects of stress are most commonly described as nervousness, tension, anger, irri-

tation, depression, anxiety, and an inability to cope, as well as physical symptoms that include headache, muscleache or tension, stomachache or tension, and fatigue. It has been suggested that the effects of stress are related to a variety of clinically defined illnesses such as anxiety, eating disorders, depression, gastrointestinal and cardiovascular illnesses, and immune disorders, as well as suicide and other forms of aggression,

In Your Opinion, What Causes The Most Stress for Teens?

The most stress in teens, I think, is the pressure they get from school. The students that have goals in life and try to become something probably have the most stress because they are trying the hardest.
Aasima Afsar, 15,
Manzano High School, NM

I believe that it is peer pressure. Peer pressure is the thing that causes stress for so many other matters. For instance, with school, people try to fit in so they go to a party instead of doing their homework. That causes stress at school. Then at home, they try to be "cool" so they stay out all night, come home and then get smart with their parents. That causes stress in the home. So, peer pressure causes stress with students themselves, with students and school, and with students and their parents.
Danielia Williams, 17,
Wheeling Park High School, WV

The thing that causes the most stress in teens has to be juggling one's schedule. I find it very difficult to balance between spending time with my family and my friends as well as keeping up with my homework, my after-school activities, and my job. I sometimes miss out on some-

thing that is really fun to catch up on homework assignments that I did not have time to do on a busy night.
Matthew Himrod, 17,
Wheeling Park High School, WV

My home environment causes the most stress in my life. This involves my siblings, parents, and after-school activities. It seems the days get shorter and shorter. I never seem to have enough time to do everything. There is much pressure to be mature and responsible at home. When you're with your friends you can relax and be yourself, but at home there is a specific format you feel you must follow. Also, when you're home you have more time to think about your current problems, and they all come together at once.
Diane Lewis, 17,
Connellsville High School, PA

I think that school causes the most stress in my life. Starting high school was very stressful, and it still is. There are so many rules and so many things to worry about. You have to worry about your clothes, your hair, and fitting in; your grades, your future, and getting into college.
Karie Baker, 14,
Fargo South High School, ND

High school gives students the most stress. Today there are more and more AP and honor classes offered. Test grades play the biggest part in the stress problem. I personally have gone through four AP and honor classes. I tell myself I'm just human and doing the best I possibly can. I would recommend all high school students take one psychology course. Understanding psychology will solve many stress-related problems for students, and I am proof.
Andy Le, 18,
Woodrow Wilson High School, CA

I would have to pick violence. My family was raised under violence. We lived in and around the projects. There were drug sellers, drunks, fights, and shootings every week. I would worry where I was and who I was with.
Kenyana Greene, 14,
Somerville High School, MA

Following are some questions you may want to use to encourage discussion of the ideas expressed by the students in the Teen Views feature:

a. Do students' home lives create stress, or help relieve stress?

b. Do students have the feeling that there is not enough time to do all they want to do, or do they seem bored much of the time, with nothing to do?

c. Has divorce caused stress in their lives? Was there more stress before the divorce than during and after?

d. Many of the students in the feature say that school causes the most stress in their lives. Do your students agree? What aspect of school is most stressful? Is this stress a beneficial type of stress?

e. Are peers a source of stress? How?

CLASS ACTIVITY

Ask students to think of a very stressful time they have daily. (math class, getting home from school, and so on) What creates the stress? Why do they feel stressed out during this time? What can they do to prepare for this stressful time? Are they willing to do the preparation necessary to help reduce the stress? Have students write answers to these questions as an assignment.

substance abuse, and intentional and unintentional injuries.

Reports from both the medical and work sectors confirm the pervasiveness of perceived stress-related disability that emerges in epidemiologic self-report data. Worker compensation data confirm the magnitude of occupational stress problems in the United States. The economically disadvantaged—low income, poorly educated, nonprofessional—

and women seem to be at higher risk for both psychosocial and psychophysiologic stress reactions, with the unemployed and part-time employed, minorities, single parents, and adults under 30 also at higher risk for psychosocial distress. The older adults, older singles without children, those living alone, and those in poor general health or recently hospitalized are also at higher risk for psychophysiologic distress.

Consumer SKILLS

Answers to Critical Thinking Questions

1. Stress uses up protein from muscle and other lean tissue, calcium from the skeleton, and vitamins and minerals from every cell of the body. Stress vitamins seem to be a quick and easy way to provide the body with the vitamins it is lacking.

2. They can't provide all of the nutrients and substances that the body needs. They can't take the place of nourishing food. There are no quick fixes.

3. Eat well-balanced meals all the time so that your body is prepared when the crisis hits.

CLASS ACTIVITY

Use the time management chart developed by students earlier (Class Activity, pages 91–92) as a guide for developing a chart showing how weekend time is spent. Have students compare their two charts. What happens to their time on the weekends? If the weekends are as regulated as the weekday during the school year, what does this say about their levels of stress? What can be done to free up their time on weekends? Discuss answers to these questions with the class.

Claims Made about Stress Vitamins

People often wonder if any particular diet protects against the ill effects of stress. Stress does drain the body of its nutrients. It uses up protein from muscle and other lean tissue, calcium from the skeleton, and vitamins and minerals from every cell of the body. Yet most people cannot eat during crises or cannot digest their food, because the stress response shuts down digestive activity in favor of muscular activity. Going without food and nutrients further stresses the body.

To store the needed nutrients ahead of time, you need to eat foods that contain them. Proper nutrition, as described in Chapters 7 and 8 of this book, can build up your defenses.

As for the pills that advertise themselves as "stress vitamins," they are not the best choice. They simply cannot provide all of the nutrients and other substances that the body needs. If you cannot eat for a long time, you probably do need vitamins, but you need minerals as well. It may help a little to take a vitamin-mineral preparation that supplies a balanced assortment of nutrients, not in "megadoses" but in the amounts needed daily (see Chapter 7). Even the best pills can't take the place of nourishing food, though, so it's still important to eat as well as possible. There are no quick-fix pills that will make you strong in a crisis.

Critical Thinking

1. *In what ways can stress drain the body of its nutrients? Why are stress vitamins popular?*
2. *Why are stress vitamins not the best choice for supplying the needs of the body under stress?*
3. *How should a person prepare nutritionally for times of stress?*

will be chattering, and your knees will be knocking together. In such a state, you can hardly reach your audience at all. You will also suffer from exhaustion afterward. It is to your advantage to learn to react to the event as if it were not so stressful and to relax before and after it.

The stage performance example illustrates another stress control strategy: use the stress response to your advantage. Direct and control the energy it gives you. It is a magnificent response to challenges, after all. It's only when the energy is scattered and wasted that the stress response drains you without giving you anything in return. (In other words, it's OK to have butterflies in your stomach, as long as they're all flying in formation.)

 KEY POINTS *The energy of the stress response can be harnessed and used to a person's benefit. To do so, view events positively instead of negatively.*

Time Management

Efficient time management can also help you to minimize stress. Time is similar to a regular income: you receive certain amounts of it at regular intervals. In the case of time, you receive 24 hours of it each day. Time is like money, too, in that you have three ways in which to spend it:

COOPERATIVE LEARNING

Here are a few strategies that might make your cooperative learning groups work a little easier.

1. Assign students specific *roles* to play within the groups. (This role is in addition to the individual tasks assigned to the students.) Some easily implemented roles are *reader*, the person responsible for reading all materials to the group; *recorder*, a student who writes out the answers for any worksheets or questions the group must complete; and *materials handler*, the student responsible for getting and putting away any materials needed by the group.

▶ You can save ahead (do tasks now so you won't have to do them later).

▶ You can spend as you go.

▶ You can borrow from the future (have fun now and hope you will find the time later to do things you have to do).

The goal for managing time wisely is to ensure security for the future while enjoying the present. It takes skill to treat yourself to enough fun so that you enjoy your present life, and still save enough so that you will have time available when you need it. When your friends call on a Sunday to invite you out, you don't want to be caught with no money on hand, no clean clothes, and no studying done for the big exam on Monday. That is an avoidable stress. Planning ahead can prevent it.

Make a time budget. If this sounds boring, remember that you have to do it only once. Besides, an hour of time spent organizing buys many hours of time doing what you choose. One way is to make two records—one, a list of things to do, and the other, a weekly time schedule (see Figure 4–6 on the next page). To make the time schedule, set up a grid that lists the days of the week across the top, and lists blocks of time (such as each hour from waking to bedtime) down the left-hand side. Fill in your set appointments, such as class meetings, first. Then add study time, waking and travel time, and mealtimes. Allot a space each day to exercise. In the time left, decide when to take care of your regular weekly chores, such as laundry, yard work, or room cleaning. Then make time for your need to play and relax.

Now make a list of special things you have to do. Place tasks from this list in the empty spaces in your days. Decide how urgent each one is ("This I can do next week; this I have to do today"). Enter the most urgent items into today's schedule, carry it with you, and check off each item when you have completed it. Move uncompleted tasks to the next day's schedule.

To schedule a long-term assignment, such as a big report, first identify every task you must do to complete the project. Then, working backward from the due date, schedule the tasks. For example, if it will take you six hours to type a report, schedule those six hours on a grid that you have started for the due-date week. Back up and schedule time before that to write the final draft. Schedule time still earlier for the first drafts and the reading. If you have been realistic about the time each step will take, you will not be caught short at the end.

A part of wise time management is knowing your limits so you don't take on more tasks than you can handle. Spreading yourself too thin is a source of stress. After identifying your limits, learn to say no when others ask you to do more

Planning ahead can minimize stress.

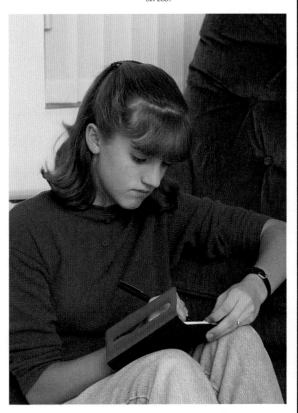

These roles should be rotated so that each student gets a chance to play each role during different class periods.

2. Another strategy that is easily implemented is that of *jigsawing* materials. To jigsaw a lesson, you must first distribute a set of materials to each group. The materials need to be divisible by the number of students in the group. Each group member

is assigned a different part of the material to learn and then teach to the other group members. Each student in the group is responsible for learning and teaching a section of the material.

DISCUSSION

Have students suggest positive ways that they can prevent stress. List them on the board. Ask the students for examples of appropriate coping devices. Then ask students to suggest negative examples of coping devices and list these beside the positive examples. Discuss how negative coping devices can create more stress.

COMPREHENSION CHECK

Ask students if they know the difference between treating the symptoms of an illness and dealing with the cause of an illness. Taking pain relievers to give relief to chronic headaches would be an example of treating symptoms. This is a distinction they should know since it applies to many different areas of health.

COMPREHENSION CHECK

Ask students to explain the main differences between coping devices and defense mechanisms. (Coping is nonharmful, defense mechanisms are self-destructive.) Ask students to study the list of defense mechanisms given in the text. (denial, fantasy, projection, rationalization, regression, selective forgetting, withdrawal) For their own consideration, not for class discussion, do they find themselves using any of these? What circumstances bring on these defense mechanisms? What steps can they take to relieve the stress?

BACKGROUND INFORMATION

The term *conscious* was used and discussed in earlier chapters. Tell students that *subconscious* refers to thoughts that are not immediately available to a

Figure 4–6 *Time Management (Example)*

Defense mechanisms: Forms of mental avoidance.

than you feel comfortable doing. (Assertiveness helps here, as was explained in Chapter 2.)

KEY POINTS *Wise time management helps control stress in life.*

Coping Devices and Defense Mechanisms

When major stressors strike, you may not be able to deal with them all at once. The human mind has some temporary measures it can use to get through the hardest times: **coping devices**. These are useful only for a while. They do nothing to solve problems permanently.

One coping device is **displacement**, the transferring of energy to a familiar, even pointless, activity for a while. Ignoring the pain caused by extreme stress, a person will clean house, rebuild a bicycle, play music, work at church, or manicure fingernails as if life depended on nothing else. Healthy people use displacement behaviors to handle tough times while giving themselves time to heal. Sooner or later, however, it is necessary to deal directly with problems, even painful ones.

Another way of coping is **ventilation**. To ventilate is to let off steam, by expressing feelings to another person. This helps to relieve pain. After ventilating, a person can often go on to work directly on solving a stressful problem.

Some coping devices have negative effects, especially when their use becomes habitual. They are useful only for short periods and only because

enrichment...

Tell students that more and more people in our society are being forced to adapt to dramatic changes in language, dress, values, and social customs as they grow up in cultures other than their native cultures. The difficulty that people encounter in these situations is sometimes referred to as *acculturative stress*, which is marked by confusion, anxiety, hostility, depression, alienation, and physical illness. Four common methods of adapting to this stress are: **a.** *integration*—maintaining old

A benefit of stress: the alertness that brings clear thinking.

they prevent a worse thing from happening: complete breakdown. These are sometimes known as **defense mechanisms**:

▶ Denial—the refusal to admit that something unpleasant or painful has occurred: "No, I don't believe it." Also called *repression*.

▶ Fantasy—imagining, in the face of a painful or unpleasant situation, that something positive has happened instead: "He hasn't really left me. He's gone to buy me a present."

▶ Projection—the belief, in the face of an unpleasant or painful situation you have caused, that it is the other person's fault: "The teacher asked the wrong questions on the exam."

▶ Rationalization—the justification of an unreasonable action or attitude by manufacturing reasons for it: "I couldn't prevent the accident, because I had to pay attention to something else."

▶ Regression—using inappropriate, childish ways of dealing with painful realities: chronic crying or whining.

▶ Selective forgetting—memory lapse concerning an experience or piece of news too painful to bear: not remembering it.

▶ Withdrawal—drawing away from people and activities to avoid pain: living in fantasy (daydreaming), refusing to talk with anyone, or sleeping excessively.

Coping devices, including defense mechanisms, help people survive bad periods of stress. They are especially useful when the stress is unexpected and severe, like the sudden death of a loved one. Often, though, you can see stress coming.

 KEY POINTS *Coping devices can help you deal with severe stress temporarily. Defense mechanisms are self-destructive, though, and are best used only for short periods, if at all.*

MINI Glossary

coping devices: nonharmful ways of dealing with stress, such as displacement or ventilation.

displacement: channeling the energy of suffering into something else—for example, using the emotional energy churned up by problems to do tasks or other familiar activities.

ventilation: the act of verbally venting one's feelings; letting off steam by talking, crying, swearing, or laughing.

defense mechanisms: self-destructive ways of dealing with stress; automatic, subconscious reactions to emotional injury, such as denial, fantasy, projection, rationalization, regression, selective forgetting, or withdrawal.

cultural identity, but participating in a new culture; **b.** *separation*—maintaining old identity and avoiding contact with new culture; **c.** *assimilation*—adapting to the new culture and having contact with its members; **d.** *marginalization*—rejecting the old culture, but

also suffering rejection by members of the new culture.

Ask students if they can guess which type of adaptation leads to the most stress. (Marginalization and separation cause high stress.)

person's consciousness. It refers to mental activities just below the threshold of consciousness.

BACKGROUND INFORMATION

Most students will have a general understanding of what *anxiety* is. You may want to elaborate somewhat, however, since it is such a key term. In context, anxiety is an emotional state in which a person feels tense, uneasy, apprehensive, worried, and vulnerable. Anxiety often leads to the defense mechanisms discussed in this section.

The handout *Stress Reducing Strategies*, which summarizes several of the additional strategies explained in this chapter, is provided in the Teacher's Resource Box.

COMPREHENSION CHECK

After the general strategy of maintaining overall wellness, physical activity is the first item on the list in the Health Strategies on page 98. Have students refer to the discussion on page 92 about the importance of exercise. Ask them why physical activity is important when under stress, and why it is important between times of stress. (during periods of stress: works muscles which were tensed by stress, burns the fuels released into the blood by stress, relieves anxiety; between times of stress: keeps body strong; strengthens immune system) Ask for a show of hands from students who feel they are stressed. Ask for a show of hands from students who exercise regularly. Encourage students to put this information into practice.

The handout "Interventions to Manage Stress" is provided in the Teacher's Resource Box.

BACKGROUND INFORMATION

Tell students that implementing a daily schedule is an effective method for combating depression. Students might check off each daily activity as they complete it. The advantage to this is that they begin to break the self-defeating cycle of feeling helpless and falling further behind. Some experts also say that depression is supported by self-critical or negative thoughts. They recommend writing down such thoughts as they occur. Students should then write a sound, logical answer to each of those thoughts. Another strategy is not to minimize or ignore positive results. When good things happen, take credit for them, note them, and use them as a sign that things will continue to get better.

ASSESS

EVALUATE

As a minimum, students should be able to answer these questions.

1. What are some signs of stress and what are some ways to reduce stress?
2. What is the importance of time management when dealing with everyday stressors?
3. What are some coping devices commonly used by teenagers to get them through a difficult situation?

Discuss the answers with the class.

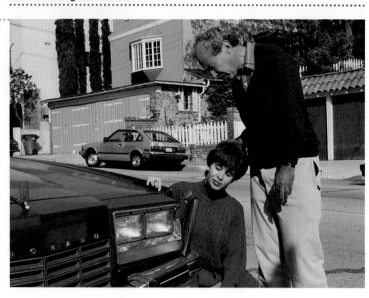

Short-circuit stress by focusing on the positive.

Health Strategies

Managing Stress

To manage stress:

1. During ordinary times, maintain a program of strong personal wellness.
2. Be sure to include regular physical activity.
3. Cultivate high self-esteem.
4. Maintain a positive attitude toward stressors—view them as opportunities for growth.
5. Manage time wisely.
6. Take on tasks only within your limits.
7. Practice assertiveness to maintain your limits.
8. Monitor your body for the early warning signs of too much stress.
9. Release tension by crying, laughing, talking with friends, or willing yourself to relax.
10. When stress becomes intense, identify which stressors you can control. Put the others out of your mind. Take action by focusing on the immediate task.
11. If stress becomes unmanageable, seek outside help.

Changed Perceptions

Stressors seem to appear from nowhere. They may seem out of your control. You may not be able to prevent an automobile accident, a losing streak in sports, or a period of strife in a relationship. You do, however, have control over your assessment of those events. As mentioned, it is your perception, more than the event itself, that causes the stress response in your body.

Armed with the knowledge that stress is a result of your own thinking, you can set about to reassess a situation in ways that reduce its power to cause you stress. Say you hit another car while driving, and your car is in bad shape. You might immediately begin listing all of your fears about potential consequences—your parents' anger, your lost transportation, your lost investment, and the threat of being unable to meet obligations. All of these fears are the result of a negative focus or appraisal. What if, though, you consciously directed your focus toward the positive—no one was hurt or killed, the other driver was at fault for the accident, your car is still repairable. Turning your focus to these more positive assessments short-circuits much of the unnecessary stress you might otherwise feel.

Daily hassles contribute greatly to most people's stress levels. Most people haven't learned to reassess these irritations positively. For example, getting stuck in traffic is not in itself stressful, but your thoughts can make it so. You can think, "This is horrible! I must get through this mess right now! My class has started . . . I'm missing information . . . I'll

QUICK QUIZ

Chapter 4, Section 4

The following quiz will help you assess your students' understanding of the material covered in this section of the chapter. You might use the quiz as an oral exercise, which will lead into a class discussion of the topics covered. Or, you might use it as a paper/pencil quiz to evaluate your students individually.

If students have difficulty with the concepts covered in the Quick Quiz and the Section Review, you might suggest they review the material using the Survey, Question, Read, Recite, Review (SQ3R) study method, which is described in detail in the introduction to this Teacher's Wraparound Edition.

1. High self-esteem cannot improve your ability to manage stress. (False)
2. Physical activity strengthens stress resis-

never catch up, and I'll fail my class!" It's not the traffic that is causing you stress, however. It's what you are saying to yourself about the traffic that is causing problems. In reality, your teacher will probably forgive a day or two of lateness, and you can catch up on your work with a little effort.

How can you reassess the daily hassles? One way is to focus on other things. While stopped in traffic, appreciate the "extra" time, and use it productively. Make a "to do" list, review your notes, or meditate until traffic starts moving again. You might try to analyze the situation to improve it: "I left 15 minutes before class time today and got stuck. Tomorrow, I'll leave 5 minutes sooner to miss the traffic." One woman defuses the stress from long grocery-store lines by taking the opportunity to page through magazines and books on the checkout counter racks.

Some experts in stress management recommend keeping a "stress log" to help you identify those situations and responses to them that cause you stress. Try keeping track of stressful moments and your thoughts at the time. If you see any unrealistic reactions causing stress consistently, you can work on changing negative attitudes or false beliefs.

The Health Strategies section on the opposite page, "Managing Stress," gives you some other suggestions for handling stress. If you find, however, that on most days you feel overwhelmed by stress and are unable to cope, it may be time to seek outside help.

KEY POINTS *Some situations may be out of your control, but your attitude is always within your control. When daily hassles occur, reduce their power to cause stress by reassessing them more positively.*

> 66 *To avoid sickness, eat less; to prolong life, worry less.* 99
>
> Chu Hui Weng
> Chinese philosopher

A reproducible quiz for Section 4 is provided in the Teacher's Resource Box.

SECTION 4 Review Answers

1. Coping devices (pp. 96–97)
2. Ventilation (p. 96)
3. defense mechanisms (p. 97)
4. Having high self-esteem improves one's ability to manage crises when they arise, and to view challenges as positive situations. (pp. 90, 92)
5. It can be directed into a performance or physical activity. (p. 92)
6. Answers will vary. Refer to the Health Strategies on page 98 for possible answers.
7. Answers will vary.
8. Answers will vary.

CLOSE

Ask the students to stand up and go to three people in the room they do not know very well. Have them introduce themselves to each one, exhibiting confidence, physical strength and stature, positive psychological attributes, and knowledge. Have the students say one complimentary thing to each of the other three students. After everyone is finished and seated again, discuss how acting positively helps one to be positive in dealing with stressful situations.

SECTION 4 Review

Answer the following questions on a sheet of paper.

Learning the Vocabulary

The vocabulary terms in this section are *coping devices, displacement, ventilation,* and *defense mechanisms.* Fill in the blank with the correct answer.

1. _____ are temporary, nonharmful, ways of dealing with stress.
2. _____ means venting one's feelings verbally.
3. Self-destructive stress outlets are _____.

Learning the Facts

4. How does a person's self-esteem affect the person's ability to manage stress?
5. How can the energy of stress be controlled and used to a person's benefit?
6. Give three suggestions for managing stress.

Making Life Choices

7. Describe an incident in which stress affected your judgment and caused you to behave in an unsafe way. If you could replay this situation, how would you behave differently?
8. Describe a situation in which stress worked to your advantage, enabling you to achieve more than you thought possible.

tance and can speed the body's recovery from stressful situations. (True)

3. It is possible to learn to use the stress response to your benefit. (True)
4. Time management is intended to reduce your free-time to a minimum. (False)
5. A coping device is often a good permanent solution to a problem. (False)
6. Displacement is a way to avoid directly confronting a problem by occupying yourself with something else. (True)

7. Ventilation is a special method of breathing designed to reduce stress. (False)
8. Coping devices that have negative effects are sometimes known as defense mechanisms. (True)
9. A stress log can help you to identify situations that cause you stress. (True)
10. You can alleviate your physical response to stress simply by changing your perception of the event. (True)

SECTION 5

FOCUS

OUTCOMES

In this section students will learn the:

1. Normal state of the body.
2. Ways in which the relaxation response and other techniques help return the body to a normal state.

FOCUS ACTIVITY

Produce a certain level of stress in the classroom, either by providing discordant background noise, reminding students of grades, exams, quizzes, perhaps even suggesting a pop quiz. Then tell them (order them) to relax. Give them a moment and inquire, in a non-relaxing voice, whether they are relaxed. Discuss why relaxation might be difficult. What factors made it difficult to relax? How easy do they find it to relax "on demand"?

TEACH & APPLY

GUEST SPEAKER

Contact your local hospital's wellness center. Ask them if they have an exercise specialist who could demonstrate exercises students can do to relax their necks, shoulders, arms, legs, and stomachs while sitting at their desks. These exercises are easy to do and can be done by the students at any time to help ease stress. Spend class time over a period of a week doing these exercises for five minutes at the beginning of each class session.

SECTION 5

Willed Relaxation

The exact opposite of the stress response is the **relaxation response**. This response reduces blood pressure, slows the pulse, quiets anxiety, and releases tension. Relaxation permits your body to recover from the effects of stress. You can will it to happen, even in the middle of a stressful situation. You can relax anywhere, at any time.

Willed relaxation always has these components:

▶ A comfortable position.
▶ A quiet, calm mind.
▶ A passive attitude toward mental thoughts.

The following paragraphs describe various methods of achieving this response.

"Relax!" When someone tells you this, can you do it? How do you know when you've succeeded? Many clinics use a **biofeedback** technique to teach people how to monitor their own physical condition. A machine (the electromyograph, or EMG) measures muscle tension and sounds a tone that changes in pitch as muscles tighten or relax. Harmless sensors are fastened to the forehead, neck, jaw, or anywhere muscles may be tense. The pitch drops lower and lower as the person relaxes. By listening and working to lower the tone, the person learns how to relax.

A way to relax without machines is **progressive muscle relaxation**. The technique involves lying flat and then locating and relaxing muscles all over the body, beginning at either the head or the feet. People who have never tried this are surprised to discover the tightness they may have in the muscles of the belly, the upper back and neck, and the face. Fifteen different sets of muscles in the face alone can become tense. Some people learn that the only thing prevent-

With practice, you can learn to relax whenever you need to.

Health Strategies

Steps to Relaxation

To relax at will:

1. Assume a comfortable sitting position.
2. When you are ready, close your eyes.
3. Become aware of your breathing. Breathe in deeply, hold the breath, then breathe out.
4. Allow each of your muscles to relax deeply, one after another. You may feel like you are floating, drifting, or gliding.
5. Maintain a passive attitude. Permit relaxation to occur at its own pace. Thoughts will pass through your mind. Allow them to come and go without resistance.
6. Continue for 20 minutes. You may open your eyes to check the time, but do not use an alarm. When you finish, sit quietly for several minutes. Open your eyes when you are ready.

COOPERATIVE LEARNING

Have students work in cooperative learning groups to analyze these case studies. The groups should formulate plans for the people to relieve stress. Allow groups to share their plans with the rest of the class.

CASE STUDY 1   Haley lives in a single-parent family with a mother who has lost her job. Haley has a ten-year-old sister who lives with them. Last week their utilities (gas, electricity, and telephone) were cut off in their apartment. Haley is failing her English class. She feels she has no friends. Lately she has suffered from stomachaches and headaches. She wants to sleep a lot.

CASE STUDY 2   James wants to become a physician. He thinks he must make all As to get into medical school. He also wants to get ing them from relaxing is that their shoulders are hunched up. Others find that they clench their jaws; others, that they are squinting or frowning without knowing it.

With practice, you can learn to relax your muscles whenever you think of it—not only when you have time to keep still for 30 minutes. Professional mountain climbers train themselves to do it while climbing—the so-called mountain rest step. Any time you take a step, you have to tense one leg—but why tense the other one? At each step, relax the unused leg. That way, you're resting throughout the climb, and you won't be exhausted when you get to the top. Students may not often have physical mountains to climb, but they do have mental ones. If your shoulders (for example) are tense while you are reading, what good does that do you? Relax them.

The Health Strategies section on the opposite page, "Steps to Relaxation," presents a summary of one method that might be used. Many variations are possible, and a complete set of instructions would provide many more details. If you practice the method as described here once or twice daily, then the relaxation response will come with little effort after a while.

To practice relaxation is to take control of the body's responses, and to enjoy a benefit beyond the simple pleasure it brings. Just as stress can lead to disease, stress management can help prevent it.

 KEY POINTS *People who learn to relax at will can enjoy the benefits of the relaxation response regardless of their circumstances and surroundings.*

SECTION 5 Review

Answer the following questions on a sheet of paper.

Learning the Vocabulary

The vocabulary terms in this section are *relaxation response, biofeedback,* and *progressive muscle relaxation.*

1. _____ is a clinical technique used to help a person learn to relax.
2. _____ is a technique of learning to relax by relaxing specific muscle groups.
3. The opposite of the stress response is the _____.

Learning the Facts

4. What occurs in the body during the relaxation response?

5. What does a machine that is used to teach biofeedback do?
6. What two relaxation methods can be practiced without the use of machines?

Making Life Choices

7. Refer to the Health Strategies section on the opposite page entitled "Steps to Relaxation." Take some time to try to relax at will. Then answer the following questions. How did you feel before, during, and after the exercise? Did you find this an effective stress reduction activity? Why or why not? Describe any variations in the activity you might incorporate.

MINI Glossary

relaxation response: the opposite of the stress response; the normal state of the body.

biofeedback: a clinical technique used to help a person learn to relax by monitoring muscle tension, heart rate, brainwave activity, or other body activities.

progressive muscle relaxation: a technique of learning to relax by focusing on relaxing each of the body's muscle groups in turn.

ASSESS

EVALUATE

 A reproducible quiz for Section 5 is provided in the Teacher's Resource Box.

 ### SECTION 5 Review Answers

1. Biofeedback (p. 100)
2. Progressive muscle relaxation (p. 100)
3. relaxation response (p. 100)
4. This reduces the blood pressure, slows the pulse, quiets anxiety, and releases tension. (p. 100)
5. It measures muscle tension and sounds a tone that changes in pitch as muscles tighten or relax. (p. 100)
6. progressive muscle relaxation and relaxation technique described in Health Strategies (p. 100)
7. Answers will vary.

CLOSE

Have students choose the method of willed relaxation from page 100 they feel would work best for them. Ask them to answer these questions about the technique: 1. Would you be willing to try the technique each day for one week? Why or why not? 2. If so, what benefits would you hope to achieve?

For extra credit, have the students try a technique and report on their results. Students should keep a diary to record the results and make notes of both physical and psychological benefits that the willed relaxation techniques have on the body.

---

an athletic scholarship, so he is working to be on the freshman basketball team. He likes to wear the latest clothing styles. Therefore, he has asked his parents to let him get a Saturday job to earn money to supplement his clothing allowance. Lately James has been in such a bad mood around his friends that he is not being invited to be a part of the group outings anymore. Also, he has a lot of neckaches and seesawing emotions.

CASE STUDY 3   Taketa was in a car wreck last month and broke both her legs. Recently she had the flu. Last week her face started breaking out more than ever. She is anxious to begin her piano lessons again. She also wants to go on the weekend camping trip with her church group.

DISCUSSION

DISCUSSION

Ask students to list the methods Mr. Cousins used to create a pleasant environment for his recovery. (hotel room rather than hospital room; watched comedy films, listened to funny stories) Have them think about the effects of laughter and why it helps. Is a good, hearty laugh a form of exercise? Does exercise help reduce stress? Is there a relationship between the two? Do students find that laughter also improves their outlook on life? Which produces more depression—a tragic story or a humorous one?

BACKGROUND INFORMATION

Medicine is beginning to study the importance of faith, particularly religious faith, in the healing process. Doctors are learning to encourage their patients to pray and seek comfort from religious services because studies have shown the benefits these provide in the healing process.

BACKGROUND INFORMATION

The term *placebo* can seem negative, yet students may want to consider that the *placebo effect* is verifiable healing which is unrelated to medication. It could be considered "natural medicine."

Healing and the Placebo Effect

An unusual story about surviving intense stress is that of Norman Cousins's bout with a crippling illness. Cousins, the editor of the famous *Saturday Review* magazine, took a stressful trip overseas and returned home exhausted. A week later, he found himself hardly able to stand up, and he had to go to the hospital. His story is one of an unexpected recovery.

What happened to Mr. Cousins?

At first, Cousins was told that the diagnosis was an ever-worsening disease of the connective tissue of the spine, almost always fatal. His physicians predicted that his spine would weaken until he was paralyzed. Stress and exhaustion had led to disease. The disease was expected to be totally disabling, the expectation caused further stress, and the end would be tragic.

Lying in his hospital bed, Cousins considered what he already knew about stress, diseases, and cures. It occurred to him that if negative emotional experiences could harm the body, then positive emotional experiences might restore health. To his way of thinking, the most positive emotional experiences would be "hope, faith, laughter, confidence, and the will to live."

Finding the hospital an unpleasant environment, Cousins checked out and moved, with his physician's approval, into a hotel room. There he could be equally well taken care of. Each day, he watched comedy films and had funny stories read to him. He had spent weeks with hardly any sleep and was in severe pain, but now he made a wonderful discovery. After a hearty laugh, he could relax and sleep soundly for an hour or two at a time.

The laughter, relaxation, and sleep brought about a healing that no medical attention could have achieved. The long of the story is in Cousins's article "Anatomy of an Illness," which was published in the *Saturday Review* and the *New England Journal of Medicine* as a landmark in medical history. The short of it is that Cousins recovered completely.

Well, how do you suppose he did it? What accounts for his recovery?

There has been much talk about that. Most people (including Cousins himself) agree that it was certainly due, at least in part, to the **placebo effect**. A placebo is an **inert**, or dummy, substance labeled "medicine" and used for its psychological effect. The placebo effect is the healing that occurs in people given such medication.

How common is the placebo effect?

It is not unusual for experiments using placebos to record a benefit in 30 to 60 percent of subjects. That is, people given only distilled water or sugar pills will recover about half the time, as completely as if they had received a powerful medication.

Placebos, given with encouragement ("This will make you better"), are sometimes so effective that physicians have on occasion prescribed them when they didn't know what else to prescribe. The curious thing is that people will recover, given placebos, when they would not recover without them. In other words, the placebo effect is valuable as a weapon against illness.

Are you telling me that my physician may give me fake medicine?

No, that would be against medical **ethics**. The point is that your response, even to the real drug, may be aided by your faith in the treatment, whether you or your physician knows it or not.

102

HEALTHY PEOPLE 2000

Decrease to no more than 5 percent the proportion of people aged 18 and older who report experiencing significant levels of stress who do not take steps to reduce or control their stress. (Baseline: 21 percent in 1985)

Baseline data source: Prevention Index, Rodale Press, Inc.

Most adult Americans report having a great deal of stress in their lives. More than a fourth of those who acknowledge a great deal of stress say they do not consciously take steps to control or reduce it. Among those who do take steps, emotional denial, physical exercise, and stress avoidance are the most popular measures. Yet the stress management literature describes an array of formal interventions, including relaxation, biofeedback, meditation, desensitization, development of

We want to warn you, though: **quacks** will sell you placebos every chance they get. Since 30 to 60 percent of people given anything will recover, there will be plenty of people around to praise the virtues of the quack's miracle cures.

 Are you saying I don't need to see a doctor when I get sick?

No, not at all. You *do* need to see a doctor. Pick the most competent, well-qualified physician that you can, so that your faith in him or her will help you get well.

How does the placebo effect work?

No one knows for sure. Part of the effect may come from the relaxation that brings relief from anxiety. The patient wonders what is wrong, feels helpless, and worries so much that symptoms become worse. Then the patient goes to a trusted expert. The expert names the disease. The patient feels reassured: the expert has the answer. The expert then prescribes a treatment, and the patient relaxes. Both stress and the symptoms begin to disappear.

The placebo effect can be measured. Blood pressure falls. Pulse rate slows. The patient gets well, whatever treatment has been prescribed. Faith heals.

 Do you suppose that witch doctors and other healers work their cures the same way?

Probably so. Don't forget that the body will often heal itself, given time. Frequently, all that healers have to do is to wait out the course of the illness. If they can offer reassurance and confidence, they will be providing support as important as any chemical or physical procedure might be. In fact, health-care providers in training are taught not only to manage their clients' medical care but also to dole out liberal doses of TLC, Tender Loving Care. Children given TLC recover faster than those deprived of it.

Does the placebo effect work for pain?

Yes. People in pain, given placebos, often experience relief of their pain. It is thought that placebo treatments stimulate the brain to produce natural chemicals that relieve pain even more powerfully than the drug morphine. People in pain who are given placebos along with a drug that blocks the brain's production of these natural painkillers experience no relief at all. This shows that placebos relieve pain by triggering the brain's production of painkillers.

 How powerful can the placebo effect be in relieving pain?

The natural chemicals of the brain don't necessarily produce a cure—you still need a surgeon to operate on a medical problem. However, mobilizing the body's natural resources speeds healing.

Some fascinating stories are told about healing in the hospital. Just physically touching people has been shown to hasten healing. Researchers now know it often works. They are experimenting to find out how and why.

 So faith really heals. I'm skeptical, though, about those faith-healing scenes we sometimes see on television.

Rightly so. Anything as dramatic as faith healing is bound to attract quacks. Fraud is most successful when it imitates amazing true events. A viewer should always watch such scenes skeptically and judge each one on its own merits. Just remember, though: the fact that a quack can try to rip off the public by faking "miracle cures" does not mean that the placebo effect is fake. It is real. Faith does heal—or at least it helps enormously—in any situation where stress has contributed to illness.

 I see what you mean. I think you've partially explained the healing effect of love, too.

You might be right. Anything that makes people feel cared for helps them to produce their own internal tranquilizers and strengthens their bodies. As Dr. Francis Weld Peabody of Harvard University put it, "The secret of the care of the patient is in caring for the patient."

Mini Glossary

placebo effect: the healing effect that faith in medicine, even inert medicine, often has.

inert: not active.

ethics: moral principles or values.

quacks: people pretending to have medical skills, and usually having products for sale.

WORKSHEETS Reproducible Study Outline and Reading Cloze worksheets for Chapter 4 are provided in the Teacher's Resource Box.

Reproducible Chapter Tests A and B are also provided in the Teacher's Resource Box.

ON LINE WITH HEALTH

You may want to have your students visit the following URLs, where they will find information and additional web site resources to enhance their study of this chapter. As with all web sites, you should check these out first to be sure the information found there is appropriate for your students.

On-line Stress Workshop **http://www.bbinst.org/home2.html**

This site is an interactive opportunity for self-assessment of stress and also offers ideas for coping with stress.

coping responses, assertiveness training, imagery, diet, exercise, and weight control. A service industry is evolving, although the efficacy of most of the techniques has not yet been rigorously evaluated.

Continual improvements in research methodology may permit more reliable identification of the sources of stress and the processes that mediate the transformation of stressful events into health and mental health problems, as well as evaluation of stress management and stress reduction techniques. As the results of these efforts are made available to primary care providers as well as to the public at large, the utility of stress management and stress reduction in general should become more apparent and the selection of techniques more informed and better differentiated. If the results of these efforts demonstrate the utility of stress management and stress reduction, then dissemination should be undertaken.

VOCABULARY

1. a. The stress response is the response to a demand or a stressor, and is the opposite of the relaxation response, which is the normal state of the body.
b. They are similar because both are the third phase of the stress response. They are different because the recovery phase goes into effect when the source of stress is dealt with. Exhaustion occurs when the stress continues to affect you without a break and your resistance finally breaks down. The body does not return to normal as quickly as it needs to during exhaustion.
2. a. immunity **b.** stress **c.** gland **d.** chronic stress **e.** inert **f.** hormone **g.** ethics **h.** immune system **i.** defense mechanisms **j.** biofeedback.
3. a. hormonal system **b.** norepinephrine, stress hormone **c.** displacement, coping devices **d.** resistance **e.** Quacks

RECALL

SECTION 1

1. Answers will vary; could include: physical—air temperature, intensity of lights, bacteria, injuries, or radiation. Psychological—refer to Figure 4–2 on page 82 for possible answers. (death of a parent, divorce of parents, breakup with

CHAPTER 4 Review

Summarizing the Chapter

Your ability to respond correctly to the following statements ensures your understanding of the main concepts in the chapter.

1. Identify signs of stress and common stressors experienced by high school students.
2. Describe how the nervous system, and immune system respond to stress.
3. Describe the three phases of the stress response.
4. Identify coping devices and defense mechanisms.
5. Explain how to prevent and manage stress.

Learning the Vocabulary

stress	resistance
chronic stress	recovery
acute stress	exhaustion
stressor	fight-or-flight reaction
adapt	coping devices
perception	displacement
nervous system	ventilation
hormonal system	defense mechanisms
immune system	relaxation response
hormone	biofeedback
gland	progressive muscle
stress hormones	relaxation
epinephrine	placebo effect
norepinephrine	inert
immunity	ethics
stress response	quacks
alarm	

Answer the following questions on a separate sheet of paper.

1. a. Explain the differences between the stress response and the relaxation response.
b. How are the recovery and exhaustion phases of the stress response similar? How are they different?

2. *Matching*—Match each of the following phrases with the appropriate vocabulary term from the list above:
a. the body's capacity for identifying, destroying, and disposing of disease-causing agents
b. the effect of stressors on a person
c. an organ of the body that secretes one or more hormones
d. prolonged, unrelieved, damaging stress
e. not active
f. a chemical messenger that travels to target organs
g. moral principles or values
h. the cells, tissues, and organs that protect the body from disease
i. fantasy, denial, and regression are examples.
j. a clinical technique that focuses on the brain waves and heart rate to teach relaxation

3. a. The _____ is made up of glands that control body functions in cooperation with the nervous system.
b. Epinephrine and _____ are each a _____ secreted as part of a reaction of the nervous system to stress.
c. Ventilation and _____ are non-harmful ways to deal with stress called _____.
d. The second phase of the stress response is called _____.
e. _____ are people pretending to have medical skills.

Recalling Important Facts and Ideas

Section 1

1. Identify three physical and three psychological stressors.
2. How do multiple stressors affect a high school student's self-esteem?

Section 2

3. Name two hormones that react to stressors.
4. How do short periods of stress followed by relief affect the immune system?

Section 3

5. How can stress make you stronger?
6. What causes the body to go into exhaustion rather than recovery?
7. What parts of the body experience reduced circulation and what parts experience increased circulation during a fight-or-flight reaction?

boyfriend/girlfriend, something bad happening to friend or family member, death of close family member other than parent, major personal injury or illness, marriage, falling grades at school, expulsion from school, dating, major illness of family member or close friend, pregnancy, peer difficulties, gain of new family member, money troubles, death of close friend, loss or death of pet, change in number of arguments with peers, change

in responsibilities at home or school, getting a job, brother or sister leaving home, trouble with parent, outstanding personal achievement, parent beginning or stopping work, school beginning or ending, change in personal appearance, trouble with teachers/principal, moving away, change in schools, change in recreation, change in church activities, change in social activities, change in sleeping habits, change in number of get-togethers,

8. Why is the phase of stress resistance called an unbalanced state?

Section 4

9. Why is physical activity considered an excellent stress management technique?

10. How can you change the way you react to stress so that events are less stressful?

11. What are three ways time can be spent?

12. What defense mechanism are you using when you blame someone else for your own problems?

13. What should you do if stress becomes so overwhelming that it affects your ability to function?

Section 5

14. What are the three essential components of willed relaxation?

Critical Thinking

1. What type of stressors did people living one hundred years ago have to deal with? Do you think life was more stressful then or is it more stressful now? Why? Would you want a life totally without stress? Why or why not?

2. Develop a personal plan for improved stress management. List three negative coping strategies that you tend to use. Describe how you can benefit from using a positive coping strategy in each situation.

3. Some people do not believe that stress has any effect on a person's mental health. Do you agree or disagree with this thought? Why do you feel the way you do?

Activities

1. Keep a diary for three consecutive days in which you record stressful situations you encounter. Each time you make an entry, include the following information:
   a. Describe the situation.
   b. Identify the stressor.
   c. Tell how you felt.
   d. Explain what you did to reduce the stress.
   e. Identify your coping strategy as beneficial or harmful.
   After you complete your diary, go over all your entries and describe any patterns that emerged.

2. Create some original cartoon illustrations that portray two defense mechanisms and two coping devices.

3. Create a collage on poster board. Divide the poster in half. On one side place pictures that depict teenage stressors and on the other side place pictures of positive stress outlets.

4. Develop a pictorial essay portraying the three phases of the stress response. You may use photographs, magazine pictures, or your own original illustrations.

5. Make a chart on which you keep track of the way you manage your time, hour by hour, for two full days. Do you think you managed your time well? How could you change the way you spend your time in order to reduce stress?

6. Cut out magazine and newspaper photos to create a collage of people experiencing stress. Mount the photos on poster board. On the poster board, identify the indicators (clenched jaw, tears, yelling, and so on) in the photos that make you think the people are experiencing stress. Now draw a stick figure that represents you. Draw in (or write in) the indicators that you display when you are under stress. If you can, ask a friend or family member to help you identify the indicators you display when you are under stress.

7. Have a partner trace your outline from the waist up onto a large sheet of paper. Draw in any significant items that will identify the drawing as you. On your head, write five things you are good at doing. On your heart, write five hopes or goals that you want to achieve in your lifetime. On your shoulders, list five things you are not good at doing. On your arms, list five coping skills that you use to handle stress. On your bellybutton, write five things that make you angry. On your stomach, write five things that worry or upset you.

Making Decisions about Health

1. Last year you found you experienced a tremendous amount of stress during final exam time. You don't want to find yourself in the same position this year. Final exams are one month away and already you are beginning to worry. Design a plan of effective stress management that you can follow to help you reduce your stress.

105

drive for too long, your resistance breaks down. This is exhaustion. (p. 87)

7. Circulation to the brain and muscles is increased, while circulation to the skin and digestive system is reduced. (p. 88)

8. It is a state that favors muscular activity while it shuts down other necessary body functions, such as digestion and immune defenses. (p. 88)

SECTION 4

9. Physical activity works your muscles so they can relax again. It burns the fuels in your blood and prevents them from building up. It relieves anxiety and brings temporary relief. (p. 92)

10. Learn to react to an event as if it were not so stressful and to relax before and after it. Also learn to direct and control the energy from a stressful situation. (pp. 92–94)

11. save ahead (do now so you won't have to do later), spend as you go, and borrow from the future (have fun now and hope to find time later) (p. 95)

12. projection (p. 97)

13. seek outside help (p. 98)

SECTION 5

14. a comfortable position; a quiet, calm mind; a passive attitude toward mental thoughts (p. 100)

change in eating habits, vacation, traffic tickets or other minor violations of the law)

2. grade point averages and scores on a test of self-esteem drop (p. 81)

SECTION 2

3. epinephrine, norepinephrine (p. 84)

4. It makes the immune system stronger. (p. 86)

SECTION 3

5. When a person goes through a period of stress and recovers, they are better able to meet the next round of stress. Just as muscles grow stronger with repeated use, so does stress resistance, but there must be rest between times of stress to build strength. (p. 87)

6. When stress continues to affect you without a break and your body stays in over-

KEY POINTS

Chapter 5 is 24 pages long and divided into four sections. This chapter identifies and describes several types of common emotional problems in a clear, straightforward manner and then identifies possible solutions. The chapter also focuses on the problem of teen suicide, warning signs to watch for, and means of preventing suicide.

ACTIVITY TO INTRODUCE THE CHAPTER

Have the class, all together or in small groups, brainstorm a list of words or phrases they think of when they hear the word *psychiatrist*. Write this list on the board and follow up with the questions listed under "Fact or Fiction." It is a good idea to bring the students' prejudices and ignorance out in the open, as well as to identify students with positive attitudes toward the mental health field before you begin the chapter.

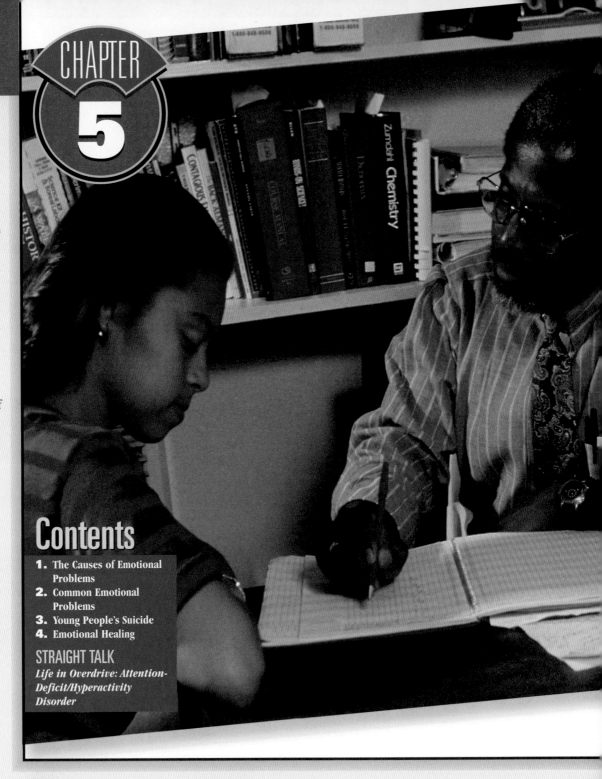

CHAPTER 5

Contents

NOT Enough Time?

Because it is likely that many of your students will have experienced some of the problems described in this chapter, it is important that you give the chapter as much time as possible. Students who identify with the problems in the chapter will be feeling many confusing emotions and may wish to discuss them if sufficient time is allowed.

DAY 1 Assign Section 1 to be read prior to class. Use the Activity to Introduce the Chapter on page 106. Do the Focus Activity on page 108. Discuss Section 1 and have students do the review. Do the Class Activity on page 109. Assign Section 2 and the review work as homework.

DAY 2 Correct the Section 2 review orally. During class do the Focus Activity on

Emotional Problems

What do you think? Are the following statements true or false? If you think they are false, then say what is true.

1. Emotionally healthy people handle life's problems without the help of counseling.
2. The people who most need professional help for emotional problems are often least likely to seek it.
3. People who engage in regular physical activity experience less depression than people who do not.
4. Anxiety can be beneficial.
5. Most people who survive a suicide attempt are glad they are alive.
6. An enabler is a person who assists people with problems in finding a good counselor or self-help group.

(Answers on page 124)

Introduction

Emotional problems are a normal part of everyone's life. Healthy people keep working to solve them much of the time, but sometimes problems become overwhelming and interfere with daily life. When that happens, the person may feel alone and ashamed. People can overcome problems or learn to deal with them, however, with the support of self-help groups, counselors, and others.

People are more aware of, and better informed about, emotional problems than they used to be. They also value psychological help more than in the past. Most people now realize that counseling is helpful for everyone.

Anyone who could use some help in coping with life's events should seek counseling. The hardest part of dealing with an emotional problem is facing it. From there on, things get easier.

The choice of exactly when to seek professional help is different for each person. Many people seek help right away. Others wait until problems begin to cause them distress and seem beyond their own control. Some people *never* obtain outside help, even for serious emotional problems. Some therapists claim that the people who most need professional help often are least likely to seek it.

BULLETIN BOARD IDEAS

Write the title of the various health care professionals discussed in the chapter (counselor, psychiatrist, psychoanalyst, psychologist, social worker) on large pieces of paper, one title per paper. Then, on five more pieces of paper, write the description of each professional. (See "Careers in Health," Appendix A.) On additional papers, write local agencies where such a professional might be found. Post the papers on the bulletin board and use five different colors of yarn, one per professional, to connect the professional title to the job description and to local agencies where he or she might be found.

Answers to

1. **False.** Emotionally healthy people often benefit from such help, and it is well worth seeking.
2. **True.**
3. **True.**
4. **True.**
5. **True.**
6. **False.** An enabler is a "misguided" helper who does harm by rescuing the person from the natural consequences of his or her behavior.

FAST FACTS

According to the National Institute of Mental Health, at any one time, 6 to 10 percent of the population is clinically depressed.

page 111 and lead the Discussion suggested on page 112. Assign the Class Activity on page 111 as homework.

DAY 3 Open class with a discussion of the homework. Do the Class Activity on page 113. Upon completion, do the Focus Activity on page 117 and assign Section 3 as homework.

DAY 4 Discuss homework. Lead the Discussion suggested on page 117 and the

Class Activity on page 118. Close class by assigning Section 4 for homework.

DAY 5 Open class with the Focus Activity on page 121. Follow this with the Class Activity on page 121. Use class time to begin the Group Project on page 122. The quiz can be given the next day or at the end of class. Have the class work on the chapter review.

SECTION 1

FOCUS

OUTCOMES

In this section students will learn:

1. The causes of emotional problems.
2. Traits of emotionally healthy and unhealthy people.

FOCUS ACTIVITY

Have each student choose two characters from television shows or movies, one character they think of as emotionally healthy and one they consider emotionally unhealthy. Then ask them to look at Figure 5–1, "Comparing Emotionally Healthy and Emotionally Unhealthy Traits." Have the students identify the healthy and unhealthy traits of the characters they selected. How correct was their initial thought on the emotional health of each character?

TEACH & APPLY

COMPREHENSION CHECK

The students' major question as they begin this chapter will probably be "What is an emotional problem?" Focus their attention on the definition given here—"*patterns of thinking or behavior that cause a person significant emotional pain or prevent normal functioning.*" The key words are *significant* and *prevent normal functioning.* Students need to be able to distinguish between the temporary, fleeting moments of emotional pain and the pains that don't go away.

SECTION 1

The Causes of Emotional Problems

This chapter uses the term **emotional problems** to describe patterns of thinking or behavior that cause a person significant emotional pain or prevent normal functioning. In truth, many such problems, such as hyperactivity and learning disorders (discussed in the Straight Talk section beginning on page 125), may be both physical and mental in origin. Emotional problems can affect any one or more of three important areas:

1. Social or family relations.
2. Performance of tasks (including schoolwork).
3. Leisure time activities.

Emotional problems range from common, mild, temporary depression or anxiety to severe long-term problems, such as a loss of the sense of reality. Some traits that are considered to be emotionally healthy are compared with those considered to be unhealthy in Figure 5–1 on the next page.

This chapter is devoted to the most common emotional problems. The emphasis is practical: how to recognize them, understand them, and deal with them.

 Even emotionally healthy people need help with emotional problems from time to time, especially when the problems interfere with social, occupational, or leisure activities.

No one but an expert can pinpoint the exact cause of an emotional problem. Sometimes even the experts can't do it. Many different causes can produce symptoms that, on the surface, may appear quite similar.

A student who feels too tired and unmotivated to study for a test may think the cause is psychological, but the tiredness could have a physical cause. The fumes given off by fresh paint, for example, could make a person feel sick. Alternatively, the cause might be a poor diet. Nutrient deficiencies can cause a long list of symptoms that resemble those of emotional problems. Lack of exercise can bring mental discomfort, as can lack of sleep.

For the reasons above, it is important to seek a professional diagnosis for an emotional problem. People should no more attempt to diagnose their own or their friends' emotional problems than they would their physical illnesses.

Some emotional problems run in families. These problems may be learned, inherited, or both. Children of families with problems, such as abuse or addiction, often grow up with emotional problems. Why some people who were abused as children grow up normally and others have long-term emotional problems is a mystery. Perhaps some people inherit a tendency to be emotionally healthy and so develop normally despite problems at home. Others may start life with a tendency to develop problems and do so even if they receive excellent parenting.

Some severe emotional problems are caused by brain damage from drugs; injuries; and diseases, such as syphilis and senility. Some emotional problems result from unbalanced body chemistry and can be worsened by stress. Regardless of cause, though, the majority of emotional problems can be treated and improved.

COOPERATIVE LEARNING

Emotional Disorders

Divide the class into ten different groups, assign each group one of the following emotional disorders to research and report on. Each report must contain a written portion and a visual aid, and must be presented orally to the class. Groups must cite their resources in their reports. Visual aids may include a video, poster, or overhead. Written reports should be turned in at the same time the oral report is due. The responsibility for, and the presentation of, the oral reports must be shared by all members of the groups.

Suggested report topics:

1. Schizophrenia
2. Insomnia
3. Neurosis
4. Psychosis

Emotionally Healthy People:	Emotionally Unhealthy People:
Have high self-esteem.	Have low self-esteem.
Are confident that their behavior is normal.	Guess at what normal behavior is.
Strive to be honest.	Often lie when it would be just as easy to tell the truth.
Accept themselves.	Judge themselves without mercy.
Can have fun.	Have difficulty having fun.
Don't take themselves seriously.	Are afraid to laugh at themselves.
Enjoy other people but do not make others the sole source of their happiness.	Are certain their happiness hinges on others.
Can have close relationships.	Find close relationships unusually difficult.
Accept the things they cannot control.	Try to change and control everything.
Find approval within themselves.	Constantly seek approval from others.
Are assertive and ask directly for what they want or need.	Manipulate others and try to get their way by underhanded means.
Usually feel they are similar to other people.	Usually feel they are different from other people.
Take responsibility appropriately, but do not take responsibility for others.	Are responsible or irresponsible to an extreme.
Give loyalty when it is appropriate and deserved.	Are extremely loyal (even when loyalty is undeserved) or are disloyal to those who have proved themselves worthy.
Consider consequences before acting.	Act on impulse.
Are not driven by compulsions (explained later in the chapter).	Are prone to addictions and compulsions.
Continue to mature emotionally throughout their lives.	Tend to remain immature.
Live with balance, not extremes.	Live lives that swing between extremes.
Accept and trust their observations, feelings, and reactions.	Deny and reject their observations, feelings, and reactions.
Attend to their physical and psychological needs.	Neglect their own needs.
Disclose family problems when appropriate.	Hide family or other secrets.
Refuse to tolerate inappropriate behavior.	Tend to tolerate inappropriate behavior.
Feel emotional pain; are able to grieve when they suffer losses.	Deny emotional pain; are unable to grieve losses.
Are not prone to stress-related illnesses.	Are prone to stress-related illnesses.

Figure 5–1 Comparing Emotionally Healthy and Emotionally Unhealthy Traits

An example of a serious mental illness that tends to run in families is **schizophrenia**. A person with schizophrenia gradually loses the ability to distinguish fantasy from reality, and becomes less and less able to function.

New technology, called *brain imaging*, has allowed researchers to look into the living brain itself. The brains of people with schizophrenia show signs of tissue shrinkage. Fluid-filled spaces exist in some areas where working brain tissue normally is found. New drug therapies, however, offer hope to some people with schizophrenia.

Other research looks at twins. If one identical twin develops schizophrenia, then the other twin is likely to develop it, too. Some think that this proves that schizophrenia is hereditary. However, many people with schizophrenia grew up in families with serious problems, including violence or sexual abuse. Possibly, an unsupportive upbringing also plays a role.

Whatever the role of heredity, some environmental factors clearly aggravate emotional problems. Among these factors are pressures from society. Each child arrives in this world with certain inborn traits. Some children

MINI Glossary

emotional problems: patterns of behavior or thinking that cause a person to feel significant emotional pain or to be unable to function in any one or more of three important areas—social or family relations, occupation (including school performance), or use of leisure time.

schizophrenia (SKITZ-oh-FREN-ee-uh): a mental illness, a condition of losing touch with reality accompanied by reduced ability to function.

5. Depression
6. Attention-deficit/hyperactivity disorder
7. Obsessive-compulsive disorder
8. Post-traumatic stress disorder
9. anorexia nervosa/bulimia
10. phobias

Allow groups to research their subject areas during class periods.

Each report should include a brief history of the disorder, a description of how the disorder affects an individual, and the available treatments for the disorder. Each group may also write up a quiz for their classmates to take after the presentation.

ASSESS

EVALUATE

A reproducible quiz for Section 1 is provided in the Teacher's Resource Box.

SECTION 1 Review Answers

1. eating disorder (p. 110)
2. schizophrenia (p. 109)
3. addiction (p. 110)
4. Only an expert can pinpoint the cause of an emotional problem. (p. 108)
5. Answers will vary; could include: brain damage from drugs; injuries; syphilis and senility; and unbalanced body chemistry. (p.108)
6. Answers will vary. Refer to Figure 5–1 on page 109 for possible answers.
7. Answers will vary.

CLOSE

Play or sing the song, "Rudolph the Red-Nosed Reindeer." Use the lyrics of the song as an example of how emotional problems can be increased by peer and family pressures, and decreased or eliminated by the realization of one's own value. Brainstorm ways people can come to realize their own worth. Be sure that seeking help from a qualified professional is on the list. You might encourage students to identify other song lyrics which promote self-esteem.

are physically strong, some artistic, some sensitive, and so forth. However, parents and society seem to want children to develop in specific ways. A parent who desperately wants a child to play sports is a familiar example. The child may not possess talent or interest in sports. Placed in a tug-of-war between the need to please the parent and the need to follow inner guidance, the child can develop emotional problems in a hurry.

Struggles such as the one just described may continue through life. People of all ages may try to please others at the cost of their own emotional growth. This damages self-esteem. If a chronic pattern develops, it can chip away at emotional health.

A young person who strives to meet, and falls short of, performance standards set by others may seek relief from the resulting stress in unhealthy ways, such as by using alcohol or other drugs. The person may develop an **addiction**. For some, it may be alcohol or drugs. For others, it may be gambling that consumes them. Other young people striving for an unreasonable ideal of slimness, may develop an **eating disorder** (discussed in the Straight Talk section in Chapter 8). These addictions and disorders require treatment, but they do not represent flaws within the person.

Part of the problems mentioned above may be caused by the society that puts such pressures on people. This situation shows one reason why it is so important to develop a working set of inner values to live by. With strong values, a person can act according to internal standards and not invite such harsh external judgment.

> **"** Your prayer must be for a sound mind in a sound body. **"**
>
> Juvenal
> (A.D. 55 to 60–ca 127)
> Roman poet and satirist

KEY POINTS *Emotional problems may be inherited or learned. Some people have tendencies toward emotional health, some toward emotional problems. Pressures from society can worsen problems.*

SECTION 1 Review

Answer the following questions on a sheet of paper.

Learning the Vocabulary

The vocabulary terms in this section are *emotional problems, schizophrenia, addiction,* and *eating disorder*. Fill in the blank with the correct answer.

1. An _____ is characterized by an abnormal intake of food stemming from emotional causes.
2. In _____, a person loses touch with reality.
3. A dependence on a substance, habit, or behavior is called an _____.

Learning the Facts

4. Why is it important to seek professional help for an emotional problem?
5. List four possible causes of emotional problems.
6. Name three emotionally healthy traits and three emotionally unhealthy traits.

Making Life Choices

7. Brainstorm a list of terms people use to describe people who suffer from emotional problems or mental illness. Circle all the terms that have a negative connotation. Why do you think people with mental illness continue to be feared and avoided? Suggest some ways that might help people to better understand it.

Chapter 5, Section 1

The following quiz will help you assess your students' understanding of the material covered in this section of the chapter. You might use the quiz as an oral exercise, which will lead into a class discussion of the topics covered. Or, you might use it as a paper/pencil

quiz to evaluate your students individually.

*If students have difficulty with the concepts covered in the Quick Quiz and the Section Review, you might suggest they review the material using the **S**urvey, **Q**uestion, **R**ead, **R**ecite, **R**eview (SQ3R) study method, which is described in detail in the introduction to this Teacher's Wraparound Edition.*

1. Emotional problems are normal but untreatable. (False)

SECTION 2
Common Emotional Problems

All people, from time to time, have negative feelings that require attention. Most common among these feelings are depression, anxiety, guilt, and shame.

Usually people can deal with, and get over, these feelings when they arise. Sometimes, though, intense feelings can overwhelm the ability and desire to solve a problem. The person may then need outside help to completely get over the negative feelings.

Problems vary in degree. Each can be mild or extreme, short-lived or long-lasting. The more severe the disorder, the more critical the need for professional help. Guilt and shame, while not strictly classified as emotional disorders themselves, are strong contributing factors to other emotional problems. These feelings can worsen and compound other emotional problems.

Sometimes problems become so overwhelming that they interfere with your daily routine. If this happens to you, seek support from parents, friends, or a counselor.

MINI Glossary

addiction: dependence on a substance, habit, or behavior.

eating disorder: abnormal food intake stemming from emotional causes and related to addiction. In *anorexia nervosa*, young people starve themselves to lose weight. In *bulimia*, they binge on food, then starve or vomit. (See the Straight Talk section at the end of Chapter 8 for details.)

2. Counseling is a legitimate and beneficial method of dealing with an emotional problem. (True)

3. Some "emotional" problems may actually have a physical cause. (True)

4. A person should instinctively understand his or her emotional problems. (False)

5. Emotional problems can be inherited. (True)

6. Brain imaging allows researchers to examine living brain tissue. (True)

7. Environmental factors play no part in the development of emotional problems. (False)

8. Emotional problems can result from conflicts between a child's inborn traits and his parents' desires. (True)

9. Addiction and eating disorders represent personal flaws. (False)

10. Strong inner values can decrease the negative impact of society's values and expectations. (True)

SECTION 2

FOCUS

OUTCOMES

In this section students will learn:

1. Common emotional problems.
2. Strategies for coping with emotional problems.
3. Effective communication of anger.

FOCUS ACTIVITY

Ask students to write descriptions of situations in which they have experienced each of the common negative feelings: anxiety, depression, guilt, shame, and resentment. Share your own experiences with these feelings to help students see how truly common these feelings are. Discuss how students have gotten over these feelings and how they can help others get over such feelings.

TEACH & APPLY

CLASS ACTIVITY

Assign the following homework. Each student must come to class the next day prepared with a joke or a comic strip to share. Be sure to set guidelines for jokes and comics. These guidelines should include: no sexual references, no racial heritage or gender slurs, no racial references, and no inappropriate language. Spend the next day sharing jokes and laughing. Discuss laughter's part in lifting depression.

COMPREHENSION CHECK

Ask students when, according to the text, a person needs outside help. (when intense feelings overwhelm a person's ability and desire to solve problems)

DISCUSSION

Have students study the Health Strategies. Ask them why it is important to study these strategies. Remind them that even if depression is not a problem they expect they will ever have, it strikes many people every year. They, or someone they care about, could develop it. Knowing now that there are strategies available for coping with mild depression may be helpful in the future.

TEACHER SUPPORT

Key Passage

Make sure students reread this important sentence: *"Physically active people feel less depressed and anxious than inactive people."* Remind students of a key strategy for combating stress—engage in regular physical activity. How does physical activity fight depression? (alters the body's chemistry; lifts mood and attitude; provides a benefit to those with heart disease, diabetes, alcoholism, and so on.)

Health Strategies

Coping with Mild Depression

To ease the passing of a mild depression:

1. Identify the cause by exploring your feelings.
2. Take action. Make a change in your life; change the terms of a negative relationship; stop wishing for something or someone you can't have; renew self-care activities you have been neglecting (bathe, exercise).
3. Force yourself to do something different, something fun (the first move in this direction is the hardest).
4. Do something physically active.
5. Eat a pick-me-up snack of fruit, yogurt, or other nutritious food.
6. If possible, avoid difficult or unpleasant tasks for a while.
7. Do not put pressure on yourself to achieve too much too soon (don't set the stage for failure).
8. Break large tasks into manageable parts. Set small, attainable goals.
9. Seek out other people.
10. Reject negative thinking. Replace it with positive thinking (see Chapter 2 for tips).
11. Find reasons to laugh. Time off from self-pity may end a depression.
12. Go outdoors. The green color of living plants in the sun has a known beneficial effect on the viewer.
13. If you feel stuck, get help.

Depression

If you have never felt "down," you are a most unusual person. Ten million U.S. citizens suffer from **depression** each year. Five of every 100 teenagers suffer its most severe form. Depression drives more people to seek counseling than does any other emotional problem.

Most likely, you know exactly what depression feels like. You have been there: taking no joy in life, looking forward to nothing, wanting to withdraw from people and activities. Being extremely tired can make you feel this way. In the case of depression, though, it doesn't go away, even after a night's sleep.

Depression can be difficult to diagnose, because it disguises itself as other illnesses—flu, chronic fatigue syndrome, or **insomnia**. A person in a long-term depression (more than two weeks) needs a skilled diagnosis. Learn to recognize the signs of serious depression listed in Figure 5–2 on the next page. Seek a diagnosis if any of these symptoms lasts for more than a week or two.

Sometimes a depression is the warning sign of a disease. Depressed mood is one of the early symptoms of certain kinds of cancer, for example. A major depression, at least sometimes, can be due to imbalances in the body's chemistry. The brain is extremely sensitive to chemical changes. Too much or too little of the normally present substances can greatly affect mood. It is important, therefore, to have a physical checkup if a depression sets in and refuses to go away. Blood tests can reveal imbalances that can be reversed by proper medication.

A mild depression may go away by itself. Often, though, you can hurry it on its way. Over a lifetime, most people learn what kinds of things depress them. Some people tend to become depressed at certain times of the day, month, or year. A loss of any kind, even of a cherished possession or pet, may bring depression as one of the stages of grief.

People can learn how to recognize the early signs of depression and how best to prevent or relieve it. The Health Strategies section on this page, "Coping with Mild Depression," reviews ways of dealing with these common feelings.

Physically active people often feel less depressed and anxious than inactive people. Running has been shown to be useful—even as useful as psychotherapy—to treat mild depression. Physical activity alters the body's chemistry; lifts mood and attitude; and provides a benefit to those with heart disease, diabetes, alcoholism, and other conditions. It makes people feel good, physically and emotionally.

Lasting serious depression, whatever the cause, can be terrifying. Some people who have experienced it say that they would rather endure any kind of physical pain than the mental torture of total hopelessness and helplessness. Serious depression affects not just the individual, but that person's family, co-workers, and others.

special needs

Musical

Music is often a daily part of teenage life. Some students listen to certain music because that is the music their peer group listens to. Others may make more independent musical choices. In either case, as young people listen repeatedly to a set of songs, they are being subjected to the messages conveyed by the music. They may or may not be aware of the types of messages they are receiving, but research has shown that many teens are deeply affected emotionally by the music they listen to.

Ask students to make a list of five songs they listen to most frequently. Next to each

Figure 5–2 Symptoms of Depression

Emotional:	Physical:
• Sad or down most of the time.	• Slowed down; always tired, with no drive.
• In depressed, downhearted mood.	• Restless, unable to sit still.
• The need to cry often.	• Unable to fall asleep, stay asleep, or get up.
• An unfillable "emptiness."	• Uninterested in food, without appetite.
• A feeling that the future holds no hope.	• Always tired, unexplainable fatigue.
• Worse in the mornings, better as the day progresses.	• A racing heartbeat.
• Feeling useless, like a fifth wheel, unimportant.	• Uninterested in dating.
• Unable to decide which option to take.	• Aches and pains (headache, backache).
• Unable to think clearly or to concentrate.	• Unable to care about your appearance (don't bathe, care for clothing, fix your hair).
• Difficulty making decisions.	• Digestive upsets (constipation, stomachache).
• Unable to remember things you should.	• A desire to drink alcohol or take drugs.
• No joy from things you once enjoyed (reading magazines, talking on the phone).	**Social:**
• Irritable, easily aggravated.	• Loss of affection or feelings for others.
• Thoughts of death come to mind.	• Problems in school and at home.
• Thoughts of suicide come to mind.	• A need to be alone much of the time.
	• A desire to stay away from classes, hobbies, or activities.

Source: Adapted from the pamphlet *Depression: Define it. Defeat it.* Available from D/ART, National Institute of Mental Health, Public Inquiries 15C–05, 5600 Fishers Lane, Rockville, MD 20857.

To the depressed person, it seems that all is lost, that help is unattainable, that only despair awaits in the future. Depressed people, by their very behavior, repel others as if they were saying, "Leave me alone." Too often, they get what they seem to be asking for. Also too often, they consider suicide as a means of bringing an end to their unbearable condition.

What the depressed person needs, however, is understanding, encouragement, and most of all, an accurate diagnosis. Depressed people need others to help them recover. They also need to realize that depression is treatable by proper medication. Too many people continue to suffer from depression, even though safe, effective and economical treatments are available for the asking. When help finally comes, depression can lift, and life can be restored to normal.

 KEY POINTS *Depression can be mild and short-lived or severe and long-lasting. Everyone should learn to recognize the signs of depression. People can often pull themselves out of mild depressions by changing their routines. Severe depression, however, requires competent diagnosis and treatment for its reversal.*

Anxiety

Like depression, **anxiety** is familiar to everyone. Also like depression, anxiety is a normal state, some of the time. However, while depression is a

 MINI **Glossary**

depression: the condition of feeling apathetic, hopeless, and withdrawn from others. A *major depression* is an emotionally crippling depressed state linked to physical causes; it may be, at the extreme, a suicidal state.

insomnia (in-SOM-nee-uh): sleep abnormalities, including difficulty in falling asleep and wakefulness through the night.

anxiety: an emotional state of high energy, with the stress response as the body's reaction to it.

song, ask them to indicate how listening to the song makes them feel. Finally, ask them to write a short summary of the lyrics of the songs. Do the words of the song make a difference in how the song makes them feel, or are they reacting solely to the music?

You may want to conclude this activity by selecting several of the songs students listen to most or several songs most-frequently

played on a popular radio station. Play the selections for the class, and discuss the mood expressed by the music as well as the lyrics of the songs. You might also make several selections of music to play for students that have particularly positive messages. Have students make a list of songs they can play to help them feel good emotionally, or to help them feel calm when they get stressed.

CLASS ACTIVITY

Since test taking is a common cause of anxiety among students, you may want to give them some general tips on how to deal with the stress they feel prior to an important test. Here are some tips:

1. *Preparation*—working hard to prepare for the test is by far the most effective way to combat test anxiety.
2. *Relaxation*—learning self-relaxation techniques can help; studying with a friend with whom you can share anxiety also helps you relax.
3. *Rehearsal*—imagine running out of time, feeling panic at ' not knowing an answer, or drawing a blank; try to simulate the test situation.
4. *Restructuring thoughts*—thinking before the test that you will fail can become a self-fulfilling prophecy; changing these negative thoughts to practical, positive thoughts will improve the performance.

CLASS ACTIVITY

Discuss with the class the emotional health benefits of physical exercise. Have students develop written exercise programs that fit their lifestyles. Encourage them to have a program that includes 20 minutes of aerobic exercise at least three days a week. Invite your physical education teacher as a guest speaker to address this issue.

DISCUSSION

Have students brainstorm times when anxiety can be beneficial in short spurts. Ideas generated may include: sports, tests, amusement park rides, performing, school dances. Have students apply the Health Strategies on this page.

114

CHAPTER 5: Emotional Problems

Too much anxiety can prevent a person from performing even the most routine tasks.

Health Strategies

Dealing with Anxiety

If you find yourself in an anxious state, it is wise to:

1. Identify the cause. What do you fear? State it in words.
2. Deal with the cause. Can you change it? How? Do it.
3. If you can't change the cause, let it go. Worry is not helpful, and it wastes energy. Replace worry with concentration, relaxation, or positive imaging.
4. Imagine a positive outcome. If you can, start working to bring it about. Live in the solution, not in the problem.
5. Use any extra energy in some physical way: be active.
6. Practice relaxation techniques.

low-energy state, anxiety is one of high energy and therefore can be beneficial in short spurts. A small dose of anxiety can spur a student to take a test with intense concentration. Too much test anxiety, though, can freeze the test taker's mind. Too much anxiety is disabling.

Anxiety can unexpectedly hit people who have been through stressful experiences such as bombings, wars, rape, floods, torture, kidnapping, or hurricanes. After such an experience, a person may have disturbed sleep and memory loss (especially memory of the stressful time). The individual is said to have a **post-traumatic stress disorder**. The person may repeatedly relive the experience and may be unable to focus on present tasks. Sometimes the person acts unresponsive to other people. At other times the person overreacts to minor disturbances.

Post-traumatic stress disorders may arise long after the stressful periods have ended. Many of the veterans who fought in Vietnam during the 1960s, for example, still had symptoms 15 to 20 years later. Not until the 1980s and 1990s did they begin to come to terms with their war experiences. Also, many women, after being raped or abused as children, show signs of distress months or years after the actual incident.

An **anxiety attack** is a sudden, extreme, and disabling attack of panic that often comes on for no apparent reason. You may have experienced an anxiety attack at some time in your life. You felt suddenly panicky and extremely stressed. Your heart started hammering, you felt dizzy, and you broke out in a sweat. It lasts only a few minutes, but an anxiety attack renders you helpless to cope with anything for as long as it is going on.

An occasional attack of anxiety can hit anyone. In fact, an overdose of caffeine (six to eight cola beverages in as many hours) can bring one on. The body's reaction to anxiety is the stress response. It includes rapid heartbeat and breathing, extreme alertness, and the other aspects of readiness to fight or flee, as discussed in Chapter 4. The Health Strategies section on this page, "Dealing with Anxiety," gives you some suggestions for dealing with ordinary anxiety.

For people who have severe anxiety attacks, self-help may not be enough. Some people have such attacks frequently and never know when to expect them. This makes them constantly fearful and handicaps them throughout life. These people can obtain outside help if they seek it. Qualified counselors have special skills in teaching people how to deal with anxiety attacks.

Focusing ON Self-Esteem

Self-esteem in teens is closely related to the way they see themselves and the amount of control they have over their lives. Eating disorders, especially anorexia nervosa and bulimia, are efforts to gain control and feel better about self.

Eating is not just about good nutrition to fuel our bodies. People attach many other meanings to the act of eating food.

Ask students to brainstorm all the reasons they eat. Suggestions to get them started are:

1. We eat to satisfy hunger or the basic physiological need.
2. Stress may cause some people to eat and others to be unable to eat.
3. Food can serve as protection. Eating gives us an excuse not to talk.

A special form of anxiety, a **phobia**, is a fear of some particular object or situation. People can develop phobias linked to all sorts of things:

- ▶ Acrophobia—fear of being in high places.
- ▶ Aerophobia—fear of flying.
- ▶ Agoraphobia—fear of being in large, open spaces, or of leaving home.
- ▶ Anthropophobia—fear of people.
- ▶ Aquaphobia—fear of water.
- ▶ Arachnophobia—fear of spiders.
- ▶ Astraphobia—fear of lightning.
- ▶ Brontophobia—fear of thunder.
- ▶ Claustrophobia—fear of being in small, closed spaces, such as elevators.
- ▶ Gephyrophobia—fear of bridges.
- ▶ Murophobia—fear of mice.
- ▶ Nyctophobia—fear of darkness.
- ▶ Thanatophobia—fear of death.
- ▶ Triskaidekaphobia—fear of the number 13.
- ▶ Xenophobia—fear of strangers.

Related to anxiety, **obsessive-compulsive disorder** is an uncontrollable need to perform an action, such as washing one's hands, over and over again. In extreme cases, the **compulsions** become so repetitive that the person cannot lead a normal life.

Long-term or intense anxiety out of line with any real danger or threat is a signal that the situation may be getting out of control. Signs of extreme anxiety are the same as those of extreme stress (listed in Figure 4–1 on page 80 in Chapter 4). If these symptoms persist, it is time to get help.

 Small doses of anxiety can energize a person to meet challenges, but too much anxiety is disabling. The emotionally healthy person uses slight anxiety to advantage and copes with extreme anxiety by finding relief for it.

Guilt and Shame

Ordinary **guilt**, like ordinary anxiety, is desirable up to a point. A guilty feeling means that you have crossed a line your values say you should not cross. The guilty feeling is a reminder from your conscience to act according to your values. Appropriate guilt can be useful to keep your values straight and your conscience functioning.

The extreme version of guilt is **shame**. While guilt begins within the self, shame originally comes from outside the self as a form of control. Shame is communicated with a look, with a tone of voice, or with words such as "Shame on you!" Shame is often used by well-meaning parents and other authorities to control behavior. In contrast to guilt, shame handicaps a person's functioning and destroys self-esteem.

While normal guilt separates the behavior from the person, shame bonds the behavior with the person. Guilt says, "What you did was bad, but you are OK, and you can decide not to do it again." Shame says, "What you did was bad, you are bad, and nothing you do will change that."

MINI Glossary

post-traumatic stress disorder: a reaction to stress such as wartime suffering or rape, arising after the event is over.

anxiety attack: a sudden, unexpected episode of severe anxiety with symptoms such as rapid heartbeat, sweating, dizziness, and nausea.

phobia (FOH-bee-uh): an extreme, irrational fear of an object or situation.

obsessive-compulsive disorder: the uncontrollable need to perform repetitive acts.

compulsions: irresistible impulses to perform senseless acts.

guilt: the normal feeling that arises from the conscience when a person acts against internal values ("I did a bad thing").

shame: the extreme feeling of guilt that arises when a person internalizes mistakes ("I am a bad person because I did it").

BACKGROUND INFORMATION

For enrichment, tell students that people suffering from *phobias* realize that their fears are unreasonable, irrational, and excessive, but they can't help it. Also tell students that a person is not suffering from a phobia unless the fear is strong enough to disrupt the person's daily life. Lots of people are afraid of spiders, but unless that fear is causing a problem every day, it would not be a phobia. One of the most destructive phobias is *agoraphobia*, which often begins after a stressful event. This leads to the fear of leaving the familiar settings of home.

DISCUSSION

Have students brainstorm a short list of physical ailments. (flu, cancer, measles) Ask students who they feel is at fault for these illnesses. Encourage a discussion that points out that disease is no one's *fault* and no one is to blame. (Lifestyle choices are important factors, but many people who make all healthy choices still contract lifestyle diseases.) Lead a discussion about the concept that all persons deserve compassion and understanding.

Introduce the idea that emotional problems also deserve compassion and understanding. Encourage students to realize that emotional problems are not the fault of the victim, nor are these problems a cause for shame by the victim or family members. Be sensitive to the possibility that some students may have a family member with emotional problems.

Ask students to think of times when they ate something even though they weren't really hungry. Ask them to describe the situations they were in at the time, and then tell why they think they were eating. List as many reasons as possible on the board.

Now ask students to consider the emotions attached to eating. Examples they might mention may include feeling happy, angry, frustrated, or frightened.

Are these pleasant or unpleasant emotions? Do students often associate these emotions with food?

Ask students to conclude this discussion by writing a paragraph about the connections they see between food and self-esteem.

Eating disorders are discussed in more depth in Chapter 7.

ASSESS

EVALUATE

Provide students with some role-play situations that allow them to practice effective communication of anger. Role plays may include: *Parent and child:* early curfew, too many chores, strict dating rules, strict dress code. *Friend and friend:* date competition, pressure to drink, broken trust/promise, exclusive activity.

SECTION 2 Review Answers

1. Guilt arises from your conscience while shame is the extreme version of guilt that arises when a person internalizes mistakes. Shame destroys self-esteem. (p. 115)
2. depression (p. 112)
3. anxiety (p. 113)
4. Ten million U.S. citizens suffer from depression and 5 of every 100 teenagers. (p. 112)
5. Answers will vary. Refer to the Health Strategies, "Dealing with Anxiety," on page 114 for possible answers. (p. 114)
6. keeps your values straight and your conscience functioning (p. 115)
7. Answers will vary

CLOSE

Discuss with students the differences between guilt and shame, and anxiety and depression.

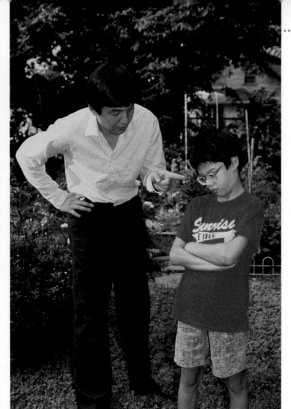

The parent who knows the difference between guilt and shame disciplines without damaging the child's emotional health.

To show the difference between guilt and shame, compare these two responses to a child who hits another:

Parent #1: *"Stop that, child. I don't ever want to see you hitting again. It's not right to hit."*

Parent #2: *"Stop that, child. Only bad boys hit. You are a bad boy."*

In the first case, the child learns appropriate guilt but knows he is still loved. In the second, the child learns that something about him (he hits) makes him bad. This chips away at his self-esteem.

Many adults have to work to reverse the effects of shame instilled in them from childhood. To regain self-esteem, they must reject shame, get in tune with appropriate guilt, and listen to its messages about their values. Someone who has lied to a friend, for example, may feel ashamed of doing so and take on the label of "liar." A more productive way of dealing with the situation is to allow the appropriate guilt ("I feel bad that I lied") to modify future behavior ("I'll tell the truth next time").

KEY POINTS *The emotionally healthy person tunes in to appropriate guilt to stay in touch with values. At the same time, the person rejects shame as destructive to self-esteem.*

SECTION 2 Review

Answer the following questions on a sheet of paper.

Learning the Vocabulary

The vocabulary terms in this section are *depression, insomnia, anxiety, post-traumatic stress disorder, anxiety attack, phobia, obsessive-compulsive disorder, compulsions, guilt,* and *shame.*

1. What is the difference between guilt and shame?

2. The condition of feeling discouraged and hopeless is known as _____.

3. _____ is an emotional state of high energy, with the stress response as the body's reaction to it.

Learning the Facts

4. How common is depression?
5. Give three recommendations for dealing with anxiety.
6. How can guilt be a useful emotion?

Making Life Choices

7. Why do you think depression is so common among teenagers?

Chapter 5, Section 2

The following quiz will help you assess your students' understanding of the material covered in this section of the chapter. You might use the quiz as an oral exercise, which will lead into a class discussion of the topics covered. Or, you might use it as a paper/pencil quiz to evaluate your students individually.

Like the Quick Quiz, the Section Review can also be used as an assessment tool to spark class discussion or as an individual student evaluation. It can also be used as a review in preparation for this quiz.

1. Depression, anxiety, guilt and shame are common problems. (True)

SECTION 3

Young People's Suicide

During one average day in the United States today, about 20 young people end their own lives—four times the number typical in 1950. On the same day, 1,000 attempt to do so but fail. Only accidents and homicides kill more teenagers than do suicides, and many accidents may be suicides in disguise. When a young person rides a bike into oncoming traffic on a superhighway, or climbs to a high rooftop and falls, experts suspect the incidents may be intentional.

Suicide may be the nation's number-one preventable cause of death among teens. The uncertainty of some victims' intentions is clear. Some have been found dead while still clutching the telephone, calling for help. Others have called the police to say they were planning to overdose. The majority of attempts are made in such a way that someone will be "sure" to save them.

Teenagers and Suicide

Most teens who commit suicide suffer from the deep gloom, loneliness, and hopelessness of depression—a fatal despair. Even without clinical symptoms of depression, teens may experience down moods and have repeated thoughts of death. This chapter stressed the urgency of learning to recognize the symptoms of depression. A reason to do so is that the symptoms of severe depression are the same ones that are associated with suicide.

Young people may attempt suicide because they think that life's bad feelings will last forever. In reality, of course, things almost always improve. A suffering teenager may see suicide as the only path out of the pain and hopelessness of the moment. Other reasons teens may attempt suicide include:

▶ Having an unrealistic, romantic view of death.
▶ Feeling like a failure.
▶ Inability to express anger or pain.
▶ Lacking firm values or rules on which to base life decisions.
▶ Suffering a loss and seeing no end to deep grief.
▶ Having a relative or friend commit suicide, making the act seem (falsely) reasonable.
▶ Trying to impress another person with the urgency of their feelings.

Researchers have studied the lives of teenaged suicide victims. The researchers found that two-thirds of those studied abused alcohol or other drugs on a regular basis. It appears that drugs and alcohol can cause or worsen symptoms of depression that lead to suicide and can interfere with rational thinking. Possibly the most important life feature that predicts suicide is a previous suicide attempt. Sadly, those who eventually succeed in suicide are often those who have sent the clearest of warnings of their intent beforehand.

Family issues often surround adolescent suicide. A suicidal teenager may live with an abusive family, or may have recently suffered losses such

2. Depression is very easy to diagnose (False)

3. Depression can result from a chemical imbalance in the body. (True)

4. Running and other forms of exercise can be effective in treating mild depression. (True)

5. Depression never requires professional treatment. (False)

6. Short-term anxiety can be beneficial. (True)

7. An anxiety attack is a disabling feeling of panic. (True)

8. A phobia is a general feeling of anxiety. (False)

9. Shame originates with the self. (False)

10. Shame is unnecessary and destructive to self-esteem. (True)

SECTION 3

FOCUS

OUTCOMES

In this section students will learn:

1. Reasons why some teens commit suicide or attempt suicide.
2. Facts and myths surrounding suicide prevention.
3. How to help prevent suicide.

FOCUS ACTIVITY

Begin the section by having the class brainstorm reasons why they think teens commit suicide. Write the reasons on the board as the students suggest them. Then have them read, either silently or as a class, the paragraphs under "Teenagers and Suicide." Have the students compare their class list with the list given in the text. Discuss those reasons on the class list which are mythical rather than real, as well as the solid reasons they suggested.

TEACH & APPLY

DISCUSSION

Teach the students the phrase, "Keep a secret, lose a friend." Tell students that often a suicidal teen will confide in a friend after asking the friend to promise not to tell. Have students brainstorm the feelings they might have if they keep the promise and their friend dies.

As a follow-up to this activity, assist the class in developing phrases that could be used in responding to a suicidal teen

(continued on next page)

(continued from previous page)

who elicits a promise of silence. Samples: "I care about you too much to keep this promise. Let's go talk to my mom (your mom, our teacher, and so on—any trustworthy adult) together. She'll help."

Direct students to use only adults as the choice of a person to go to for help. The adult may be named if desired. (i.e., a favorite teacher or school counselor)

CLASS ACTIVITY

Distribute two cards to each student. One card should be green and the other one red. Make the cards out of construction paper. Read a variety of responses one may make to a suicidal teen. Have students hold up the green cards for good responses (go) and the red cards for poor responses (stop). Students may enjoy making up their own responses for the class to evaluate. Use responses from the following list and/or make up your own. Sample responses:

"Okay, I promise to keep your secret."

"Yea, sure, like I really believe that you'd jump."

"I'm your friend and I'll stand by you."

"Let's go talk to (trusted adult). They can help."

"That's dumb. Don't worry about it."

"You're making too big a deal of this."

FAST FACTS

Approximately 1 person out of every 100 attempts suicide at some point in his or her life.

Trained volunteers stand by, ready to take calls. . .

as the divorce or death of a parent or other close family member. A family history of suicide or suicide attempts is also common among suicidal teens.

Other losses also often precede suicide. A teenager whose friend dies, especially if the friend dies of suicide, may be unprepared for the deep grief that follows. Sometimes a series of more modest losses produces the same reaction. Many a teenager who suffered seemingly ordinary and expected losses, such as rejection by peers, loss of a boyfriend or girlfriend, or suspension from school has committed suicide.

No one knows why, but some teenage suicides have occurred in clusters. This fact has led researchers to look for common links between the suicides. One finding is that clusters of teenage suicides have closely followed media reports of real suicides, or movies and television shows that tell stories of suicides. Some believe that the teenagers had mimicked the images they had seen in the media, or imitated one another.

 KEY POINTS *Although preventable, suicide claims the lives of teens every day. Characteristics associated with teenage suicide include alcohol and drug abuse, issues of family, parental and other losses, and depression.*

Preventing Suicides—Facts and Myths

The overwhelming majority of people who survive a suicide attempt are glad they are alive. The wish to die lasts only a few hours or days, not a lifetime. If victims can be helped through the crisis period, chances are good that life will go on normally, afterward. To help them, people must first obtain accurate information and forget any myths they might have heard about the potential for suicide.

"They Just Want Attention" A widely believed and dangerous myth is that a person who talks about suicide just wants attention, and is best ignored. This wrong idea can lull friends and family into complacency even while a person is plainly displaying suicidal intentions. It may even give victims added reasons to follow through—to prove the seriousness of the intent.

"Girls Are Not As Serious As Boys" A related false idea is that girls, because they survive more suicide attempts, are not as serious as boys in their threats. It's true that girls more often attempt suicide with drugs rather than firearms, increasing the chances for their discovery and rescue. It is also true, however, that a person who has tried suicide in the past will probably do so again—and may very possibly succeed.

HEALTHY PEOPLE 2000

Reduce by 15 percent the incidence of injurious suicide attempts among adolescents aged 14 through 17.

Attempted suicide is at once a morbid, potentially lethal health event, a risk factor for future completed suicide, and a potential indicator of other health problems such as substance abuse, depression, or adjustment and

stress reactions. Although much has been written about the increasing rates of youth suicide in the United States, little is known about patterns and trends in the occurrence of suicide attempts among the young. In several surveys of adolescents in the general population, as many as 10 percent of the respondents report having attempted suicide at least once. As a group, suicide attempters with serious medical injuries are at higher risk of repeated suicide attempts and completed

"They are Mentally Ill or Weak" Another myth is that people who commit suicide are mentally ill or weak in character. True, a few adolescents who kill themselves were suffering from a serious mental illness. The remaining great majority do not suffer mental illness at the time of death, but cannot see another way out of their problems.

"Don't Mention Suicide to Them" One of the more damaging myths concerns a fear of speaking openly about suicide for fear of "putting ideas in their heads." A suicidal person already has the idea, and if the person is not considering suicide, no harm is done through its mention. Talking openly with a clearheaded person about their intent can often act as a lifeline to people considering suicide. It opens the door to the possibility of help.

Warning Signs It is important to remember that suicide is a possibility. Otherwise you may miss the warning signs. Take any of the signs listed in Figure 5–3 on this page seriously. Notice that many are also the signs of depression.

"They Want to Die" Suicide attempts seem to mean that the victims want to die. However, except for a tiny percentage, those who attempt suicide truly want to live. As surprising as it may sound, a suicide attempt is really a call for help. People who attempt suicide usually believe that they are not loved or accepted. A suicide attempt says, "Look at me, help me, save me!" The person wants desperately to know that someone cares.

 Anyone talking about attempting suicide should be taken seriously—talk with them. People who attempt suicide usually want to live. Knowing the signs of depression can help you recognize when someone is reaching out for a helping hand.

> **If many of these signs are present and if they are long-lasting, the person may be at high risk for suicide.**
>
> - Abrupt changes in personality; aggressive, hostile behavior; impulsiveness; sudden mood swings.
> - Alcohol or drug abuse.
> - Anxiety at times of separation.
> - Ceasing to groom oneself or care for one's room, possessions, or clothes.
> - Ceasing to meet responsibilities (do homework or return calls).
> - Cessation of hobbies and activities.
> - Changes in eating or sleeping habits; weight loss or fatigue.
> - Feeling bad about oneself; feeling extremely sad, pessimistic, and helpless.
> - Giving away possessions; making a will or other final arrangements.
> - Inability to concentrate.
> - Not caring what happens; passive behavior.
> - Refusal to leave the room or the bed.
> - Slackening of interest in schoolwork and declining grades.
> - Thinking, talking, or writing about death; even outwardly lighthearted or vague references to death or dying.
> - Withdrawal from friends or family.
> - Sudden lifting of depression, signalling feelings of relief after deciding to commit "suicide" as a solution to problems.

Figure 5–3 Signs That May Warn of an Approaching Suicide

. . . from anyone who feels a need to talk about his or her problems.

DISCUSSION

Discuss the most common reasons teens commit suicide. Review the signs students can look for and the ways they can help. Help students understand that they are not responsible for the actions of a friend, but a friend is more likely to turn to them than to an adult. Learning the options now will help them respond more appropriately if this should ever occur.

ON LINE WITH HEALTH

You may want to have your students visit the following URLs, where they will find information and additional Web site resources to enhance their study of this chapter. As with all Web sites, you should check these out first to be sure the information found there is appropriate for your students.

Suicide Awareness/ Voices of Education **http://www.save.org/**

The Yellow Ribbon Project **http://www. geocities.com/Heartland/ Acres/8088**

These sites are devoted to education and awareness of signs of and alternatives to suicide. There is lots of good information on how to deal with emotions, rather than being overcome by them.

For reliable information on a variety of health topics try **http://www. healthfinder.gov**

suicide than are suicide attempters with minor injuries. This objective focuses on that part of the spectrum of suicidal behavior among high school students which results in injuries to the victim.

The overall suicide rate has changed relatively little since 1950. However, the rates vary substantially by gender, age, and race/ethnicity. Men are more likely to commit suicide. Although the rate for male adolescents is comparatively low, there has been a steady increase in suicide among all youth aged 15 to 19 since the 1950s. By 1986, suicide was the second leading cause of death in the 15- to 19-year-old group. Suicide rates among men (but not women) aged 20 through 34 increased dramatically in the last three decades and remained relatively high in the 1980s. Special goals have been set for these populations at unusual risk.

ASSESS

EVALUATE

A reproducible quiz for Section 3 is provided in the Teacher's Resource Box.

Review Answers

1. about 20 (1000 attempt but fail) (p. 117)

2. depression (p. 117)

3. alcohol and drugs (p. 117)

4. abusive family, recent loss of loved one by divorce or death, family history of suicide (pp. 117–118)

5. "They just want attention," "Girls are not as serious as boys," "They're mentally ill or weak," "Don't mention suicide to them," "They want to die." (pp. 118–119)

6. Answers will vary.

CLOSE

Review Figure 5–3 with students. Discuss each of the warning signs listed. Then review the important ways to help in the event of a student observing these warning signs in a friend.

How to Help

The first step in preventing suicide is to get involved or, if you cannot get involved, tell someone else who can help. Don't wait to see what develops, because tomorrow may be too late. Ask outright if the person is planning suicide. Be careful not to make light of your friend's feelings. If you imply that your friend doesn't mean it, you may unknowingly offer a dare. At the same time as you show your concern, try to offer reassurance that the crisis is temporary.

If the person seems on the verge of making a suicide attempt, the two most important things to do are these:

▶ Phone a suicide hotline or crisis intervention center immediately. Dial 911, the operator, or the police.

▶ Stay with the person until help arrives.

Stay aware that you may not succeed in preventing the suicide. Accepting that you were powerless to prevent a tragedy can be one of the hardest things in life to face. Still, you cannot change what has happened. Emotional support is available for survivors. Learning about the process of grief can also help.

In case you have thoughts about ending your life, you should know that most people feel like that, sometimes. Those thoughts and feelings come and go, just as others do. Things can seem very bad, but they always get better, given time. You can talk to someone during the bad times without their knowing who you are: call the helping hotline in your area. You can also ask someone you trust to listen to your thoughts. You'll both be glad you did.

For **Y**our **I**nformation

The grieving process is explained in the Straight Talk section in Chapter 21.

KEY POINTS *In preventing suicide, get involved by offering concern and reassurance to the person. Remember that suicide hotlines and 911 can provide assistance. Stay with the person until help arrives.*

SECTION 3 Review

Answer the following questions on a sheet of paper.

Learning the Facts

1. About how many young people end their own lives during an average day?

2. What do most teenagers who commit suicide suffer from?

3. What two things are often abused by suicide victims?

4. What kinds of family issues often surround young people's suicides?

5. List three myths about the potential for suicide.

Making Life Choices

6. Over the last six months your friend has stopped doing any homework and is getting poor grades. She doesn't go to dance class anymore and has given you a lot of her personal belongings. It seems like whenever you talk to her she brings up the topic of death. You're pretty certain she's been using alcohol a lot lately. Describe what you would do to try to help your friend.

Chapter 5, Section 3

The following quiz will help you assess your students' understanding of the material covered in this section of the chapter. You might use the quiz as an oral exercise, which will lead into a class discussion of the topics covered. Or, you might use it as a paper/pencil quiz to evaluate your students individually.

Like the Quick Quiz, the Section Review can also be used as an assessment tool to spark class discussion or as an individual student evaluation. It can also be used as a review in preparation for this quiz.

1. Suicide is a major cause of death among teenagers. (True)

2. Depression is not a common cause of suicide. (False)

SECTION 4

Emotional Healing

Y ou don't have to be sick to ask for help for an emotional problem. You just have to need or want help. The exact moment when a person decides to get help for an emotional problem is often the moment when that person starts to get better. Often, though, people hesitate to ask for help because they are afraid this will be an admission that they are "sick." Actually, emotionally healthy people often make this choice.

It's dangerous to go to the wrong person for therapy.

Types of Therapy

Any activity that has a healing or health-promoting effect is a form of **therapy**. For one person, going out for a softball team after work may serve as therapy. For another, it may be best to get away from noise and crowds, go home to a quiet kitchen, listen to music, and cut up fresh vegetables for a special dinner. Painting, writing, playing with children, walking on the beach—all these can serve as therapy.

Soothing activities can help relieve many emotional problems, but cannot, by themselves, solve severe problems. A person with a severe emotional problem may benefit from professional help. Professionals who can help may include any of the following:

▶ A *counselor*—a helping person. Be careful, though. Both qualified and unqualified people practice under this title. Many states require licensing for counselors to practice.

▶ A *psychiatrist*—a physician (M.D.) who, after completing medical school, received additional special training to treat emotional problems and is licensed to prescribe drugs.

Any activity that has a healing effect is therapy.

MINI Glossary

❙ **therapy:** treatment that heals.

3. The symptoms of severe depression are the same as those of suicide. (True)

4. Inability to express anger is a potential reason for suicide. (True)

5. Suicide victims do not have a high frequency of drug and alcohol abuse. (False)

6. Often people who talk about committing suicide are just looking for attention. (False)

7. People who commit suicide are usually

suffering from a serious mental illness. (False)

8. A suicide attempt is a call for help. (True)

9. It's better not to get involved with a person who seems suicidal. (False)

10. Suicide hotlines and 911 can assist you in coping with a suicide crisis. (True)

SECTION 4

FOCUS

OUTCOMES

In this section students will learn:

1. Various types of therapy for emotional problems.

2. Methods for seeking and finding help.

3. How to help friends with emotional problems.

FOCUS ACTIVITY

Have students brainstorm to compile a lengthy list of activities that may serve as therapy for mild emotional problems. This list should include any safe, nonviolent, legal activity that brings the participant enjoyment. Discuss the benefits of these activities as a class.

TEACH & APPLY

CLASS ACTIVITY

Write the titles of the emotional health and suicide prevention professionals listed in this section (counselor, psychiatrist, psychoanalyst, psychologist, social worker) on a set of index cards and their job descriptions on another set of cards. (See "Careers in Health," Appendix A.) Have the students play a matching game. This game can be played with the entire class or small groups. Students can even play this game on their own at a learning center in your classroom or as a free-time activity.

All the information from the cards can also be used to make a "Healing Sources" bulletin board in the classroom or guidance office. See the Health Strategies on page 122 for additional information.

121

▶ A *psychoanalyst*—a psychiatrist who specializes in seeking the root causes of emotional problems.
▶ A *psychologist*—a person with a graduate degree (M.S. or Ph.D.) in psychology from a university. Many states require licensing for psychologists to practice.
▶ A *social worker*—a person with a graduate degree in social work (M.S.W.). This degree includes training in counseling.

Other than these, people who claim to offer therapy may not be trustworthy. Effective therapy relationships always contain these three ingredients:

1. Respect and trust between the therapist and the client.
2. The exploration of the present problem's causes, effects, or both.
3. The search for new, more productive ways of dealing with the problem.

A way of dealing with some problems is through drug therapy. Especially for those suffering from depression, new medications can help relieve illness that was formerly unresponsive to therapy. The brain's chemistry is normally maintained with precision. When out of balance, the brain's chemistry affects a person's mood and thinking. Drugs, such as **Prozac**, can often restore the normal chemistry of the brain and so relieve depression.

Therapy need not be long or expensive to be effective. Many public health programs run therapy centers and counseling groups that charge on a sliding scale according to ability to pay. Some schools provide free counseling and may run groups of their own. In addition to formal therapies, many find help in the form of "Anonymous" self-help groups. Alcoholics Anonymous (AA) helps people recover from alcohol addiction. Overeaters Anonymous (OA) helps people recover from eating disorders. Alanon helps the family members of people with addictions. Alateen helps teens in dysfunctional families. The services of these groups are free, and members support them voluntarily.

KEY POINTS *Many activities can act as therapy, especially when they are soothing and bring relief from stress. An effective relationship between a professional therapist and client is based on respect, trust, exploration of the problem, and a search for ways of dealing with the problem. Effective therapy need not be expensive.*

Health Strategies

Finding Help

If you want some help working on an emotional problem:

1. Tell your parents you'd like to work out a problem. They may be able to help you themselves, or they may have a good idea regarding whom you should see.
2. Check with the teacher of your health or life management skills course. The teacher is likely to be well informed regarding local helping agencies.
3. Ask your family physician to suggest someone to help you.
4. Ask your school guidance counselor whom to see. You might also ask for the name of a helpful member of the clergy.
5. Look in your telephone book for a telephone counseling service. Call and ask what to do. You don't have to give your name if you don't want to.
6. Look up "Mental health," "Health," "Social services," "Drugs," "Alcohol," "Family services," "Suicide prevention," or "Counseling" in the telephone book. Call and ask what to do. Again, you can choose whether or not to give your name.

About Finding Help

If you have concluded that you might benefit from having psychological help, be selective. Not all "therapists" are well qualified. Some are even quacks. Try the possibilities listed in the Health Strategies section on this page, "Finding Help."

Stick with it. The first source of help you try may not work out well. However, there is someone out there for you to talk

decision making activity

Suicide Prevention

Suicide is recognized as one of the leading causes of death among young people in our country. Suicide prevention must involve learning to recognize the warning signs, developing good listening and communication skills, and knowing when to intervene and get the necessary professional assistance. Suicide

is a permanent solution to some temporary problems.

It must be stated that given the right set of circumstances, anyone could be a victim of suicide. At times, life and life's events become overwhelming. A caring person's responsibility is to recognize when a friend is going through a difficult time and act appropriately.

Some situations are clearly more threatening than others. For example, a person who to. You might start by seeing a counselor for anxiety but end up getting help learning how to deal with peers—which might solve the anxiety problem. Often a single, clearheaded discussion will lead to a simple solution.

People may hesitate to seek professional help for fear of what they may be forced to discover about themselves. Yet the most earthshaking discovery people are likely to make is that they are not alone—that other people have the same problem and that, with help, they can deal with it.

 Seeking professional help for an emotional problem is often the first step toward health. Choose therapists carefully, based on trusted advice and professional qualifications.

For a person who feels lonely or depressed, comfort may be just around the corner.

How to Help Another Person

It is sometimes possible to help another person who has an emotional problem. Simply caring and offering support is often enough. Listening is helpful, too. Often a person can work out problems, given enough chances to discuss them.

Helping skills are not inborn, however. The untrained person can do more harm than good by saying or suggesting the wrong things. For example, a person who hopes to help may become codependent, and weaken the other person. A **codependent** "helper" may allow the troubled person to avoid facing problems. This misguided attempt to help is termed **enabling**, because it supports the continuation of inappropriate behavior. Enablers, with the best intentions in the world, make it possible for other people to continue drinking, gambling, or other self-destructive behaviors by rescuing them from the natural consequences of their own actions (see Chapter 13). Without having to face consequences, troubled people have no reason to change.

In addition to enabling, a person may help another for the wrong reasons. Helping others may be a way of avoiding facing one's own problems. It provides an excuse: "I couldn't go to class because I was helping Jane." People who focus on other people's problems to this extent are often codependent and need help for themselves.

Helping people in crisis requires a special set of strategies. You sometimes have to break out of ordinary social behavior. If a person is clearly irrational and in danger, you may have to risk the friendship in order to help the person. To tell when to take this risk, ask yourself:

▶ Do I think that the person's life or health is in serious danger?
▶ Is the person threatening someone else's life or health?
▶ If I fail to help, will the situation become dangerous?

If the answer to any of these questions is yes, get involved. It is a risk, but the risk of not helping is worse. Your judgment may not be perfect, but it is the best you have available—so use it.

For **Y**our **I**nformation

The problems of a *codependent* relationship are discussed in Chapter 19.

MINI Glossary

Prozac: the brand name of one drug of a group of drugs used to restore normal brain chemistry in people with depression.

codependent: a person who is so focused on the needs of others that the person's own needs are neglected.

enabling: misguided "helping." An enabler is a person who actually does harm by supporting a troubled person's continued self-destructive attitude or behavior.

speaks generally of suicide should be taken seriously, but the presence of weapons, drugs, or the mention of them constitutes an emergency.

Example: "Do you have a plan?" "Not really, I just kind of thought about it," vs. "Well, my parents are out late tonight and my dad's pistol and ammunition are in the closet." Which response would be categorized an emergency?

In any case:

Listen, show interest and support (do not give advice).

Be non-judgmental (do not solve problems or give advice or glib* answers).

Get an adult involved (teacher, parent, counselor, youth director, or clergy member).

*Glib answers are simple answers to complex situations.

ASSESS

EVALUATE

Distribute three index cards to each student. Have each student write three questions and answers (one set on each card) from Section 4 that they feel should be included on a quiz over the section. Put the cards in a bag or box and choose ten or more of the questions to use as a quiz.

Review Answers

1. Answers will vary.
2. counselors, psychiatrists, psychoanalysts, psychologists, social workers (pp. 121–122)
3. Drugs can sometimes restore the brain's chemistry to normal. (p. 122)
4. Answers will vary. Refer to Health Strategies "Finding Help" on page 122 for possible answers.
5. You should know your own limits for your own emotional well-being. You can become emotionally drained. Continuing to listen may postpone a solution. Put the person in touch with an expert. (p. 124)
6. Answers will vary; could include: parents, friends, clergy, teacher, relatives.
7. Answers will vary.

CLOSE

Invite a school counselor to class and allow students to interview him or her.

Here are the answers to the questions at the start of the chapter.

1. **False.** Emotionally healthy people often benefit from such help, and it is well worth seeking.
2. **True.**
3. **True.**
4. **True.**
5. **True.**
6. **False.** An enabler is a "misguided" helper who does harm by rescuing the person from the natural consequences of his or her behavior.

When a crisis requires professional help, the person who needs help should be the one to call. Mental health agencies will not step in unless the person with the problem makes the request. If your friend is resistant, place the telephone call yourself. Then persuade your friend to talk to a helping person on the other end of the line. If that fails, or if your friend is very sick, weak, or debilitated, call the police or an ambulance. The move may be awkward, but the urgency of the situation justifies it.

Continue helping until you are satisfied that you have done what you can. Then let go. Should the outcome disappoint you, remember that you did your best.

Be sure to protect yourself. For your emotional well-being, it is important to be aware of the limits of your ability to give support. A depressed person can be a sort of emotional sink into which you pour your energy without getting anything back. Such a relationship drains you, to no useful purpose.

If such a situation drags on for very long, wisdom dictates that it is best for you and the other person if you remove yourself from it. Your continued listening may be postponing a solution. Put the person in touch with expert help, and bow out. Make it clear that you are taking this action to encourage truly effective help for your friend and peace of mind for yourself.

KEY POINTS *Offering emotional help to others is beneficial only if the help does not prevent their recovery. When a person becomes overly dependent, it is best to help the person form a link to professional help, and bow out.*

Answer the following questions on a sheet of paper.

Learning the Vocabulary

The vocabulary terms in this section are *therapy, Prozac, codependent,* and *enabling.*

1. Write a sentence using each vocabulary term.

Learning the Facts

2. List all the professionals who are trained to help people with emotional problems.
3. Why is drug therapy sometimes an effective treatment for depression?
4. Give three recommendations for finding help for an emotional problem.

5. Why is it important to know your limits when extending yourself to help someone with an emotional problem?

Making Life Choices

6. Many times personal problems are resolved through a discussion with someone in whom you have confidence. Develop a list of people you believe you could go to for help. List the reasons why you chose each particular person.
7. Why do you think people become enablers? Explain how you might discover that you were enabling a friend to keep up a drug problem. Discuss what you might do to stop enabling your friend.

Chapter 5, Section 4

The following quiz will help you assess your students' understanding of the material covered in this section of the chapter. You might use the quiz as an oral exercise, which will lead into a class discussion of the topics covered. Or, you might use it as a paper/pencil quiz to evaluate your students individually.

Like the Quick Quiz, the Section Review can also be used as an assessment tool to spark class discussion or as an individual student evaluation. It can also be used as a review in preparation for this quiz.

1. Only people with serious mental illnesses can benefit from professional assistance. (False)
2. Therapy can include any activity that has a healing or health-promoting effect. (True)

Straight Talk

Life in Overdrive: Attention-Deficit/ Hyperactivity Disorder*

Daniel, age eight, bounces into the living room, where his younger sister, Jackie is coloring. He snatches the crayon box from her hand, pulls out some crayons, and scrawls his name across the picture Jackie had been creating. Scattering crayons, he sprints for the television, pausing to stomp several of Jackie's favorite colors into the carpet. Next, Daniel climbs over the back of a chair, switches on the television, turns the volume up, and holds the channel button down as the programs flicker across the screen. The sounds of Daniel's stomping and his sister's sobbing remind their mother that she forgot to give Daniel his medication this morning.

Justine, a high school sophomore, cannot explain why she makes an F one day and an A the next, both in the same class. She studies her lessons, but she often gets distracted. Because she occasionally excels in her studies, her parents tell her she's lazy when she does poorly. She gets discouraged and feels disgusted with herself when she loses points for failing to follow directions and making careless mistakes.

 Daniel sounds like he's a hurricane. Is that what hyperactivity is like?

Yes, it is. Like millions of other U.S. schoolchildren, Daniel has **attention-deficit/hyperactivity disorder (ADHD)**. In an average classroom of 30 children, one or two, mostly boys, have this kind of **learning disorder**. ADHD differs from the "hyper" behavior, or excitability, that normal children fall into occasionally. Instead, it is as if Daniel lives all of his waking life in overdrive.

A collection of symptoms describes the child with ADHD:

- ▶ Having a short attention span, even while playing.
- ▶ Having trouble with tasks that require sustained mental effort.
- ▶ Having trouble learning, and failing to achieve in school.
- ▶ Having poor **impulse control**—acting out physically and verbally before thinking.
- ▶ Angering friends often by not waiting his or her turn or playing by the rules.
- ▶ Running instead of walking. Climbing instead of sitting still. Talking excessively.

These symptoms often act as clues to parents and teachers that a child might have ADHD. However, guessing is not helpful. A diagnosis by a knowledgeable clinician is needed so that much-needed treatment may begin.

 Do those kids have trouble in school? It sounds as if they might.

Children with ADHD find learning to be almost impossible, at least when they are placed in traditional classrooms. However, in a supportive learning environment, where distractions are few, where tasks are broken into manageable pieces, and where structure and routine are dependable, many can excel.

Children with ADHD often have some academic advantages, too. They are often extremely creative and inventive. They may be wild, funny, and bubbly children who love life and learning. Often, once they latch onto a topic that interests them, wild elephants cannot tear them away.

125

Straight Talk

Discussion
Have students compare the descriptions of Daniel and Justine. Which one has the more obvious difficulties? What are these difficulties? What are the standard discipline methods parents use to deal with behavior such as Daniel's? (time out, spanking, taking away privileges, and so on) How effective would these be? Why? Encourage students to refer to the list of symptoms of ADHD children in discussing these questions.

Now ask students to think about Justine. What would be standard discipline methods for dealing with her? (grounding, extra study requirements, encouragement to try harder, rewards for good grades, and so on) Why would these methods be ineffective?

---

3. A psychiatrist is not licensed to prescribe drugs. (False)

4. Respect is an important ingredient in a therapeutic relationship. (True)

5. Drug therapy can be an effective way of dealing with some emotional problems. (True)

6. There are many inexpensive therapy options available through self-help groups, schools, and public health programs. (True)

7. All therapists who advertise are well-qualified and trustworthy. (False)

8. Codependents unintentionally enable troubled people to continue their destructive behavior. (True)

9. Codependents rarely have emotional problems of their own. (False)

10. When attempting to help a depressed or troubled person, it is important to be aware of and to respect your own emotional limitations. (True)

WORKSHEETS

Reproducible Study Outline and Reading Cloze worksheets for Chapter 5 are provided in the Teacher's Resource Box.

Reproducible Chapter Tests A and B are also provided in the Teacher's Resource Box.

COMPREHENSION CHECK

Review with students the meaning of ADHD. (Attention Deficit Hyperactivity Disorder) Does Justine have ADHD? (No, since she does not have hyperactivity. She has Attention Deficit Disorder.) Ask students to look again at the list of symptoms for the child with ADHD and the information in Figure 5–4. Which symptoms apply to Daniel? Which to Justine? Which to both?

CLASS ACTIVITY

Assign students to read or reread the Straight Talk feature silently in class. While they are reading, provide a number of distractions in the classroom. (perhaps a dripping sound, a constant clanging, some music, a randomly scraping chair, writing on the chalkboard with squeaky chalk, and so on) After a few minutes, discuss with the class what difficulties they may have had in concentrating. How many students were able to completely tune out the noises? How many were at least partially distracted? How many were unable to concentrate at all? Discuss the fact that children with ADHD "seem to lack the ability to filter out distractions that other people can easily ignore." Talk about what distractions there are in the classroom that students automatically tune

Life in Overdrive: Attention-Deficit/ Hyperactivity Disorder* *(continued)*

The desirable side of ADHD also leads some adults with the condition to be highly successful at work because of their ability to make quick decisions. On the other hand, the same impulsiveness may make them prone to lose jobs or to leave jobs before they've made other plans for employment. The way ADHD affects someone's life can be highly individual. It may depend heavily on whether or not the person's self-esteem survived the misunderstandings of childhood.

 What causes ADHD?

No one knows for sure. It is likely that slight brain malfunctions change the way the brain uses energy, especially in areas of the brain that screen out distraction. Children with ADHD do seem to lack the ability to filter out distractions that other people can easily ignore. For example, to a child with ADHD, the sound of an air conditioner running or the sight of a passing car easily overpowers a teacher's words. Concentration and learning are both lost.

The condition runs in families. A child with one or both parents with ADHD is many times more likely to develop it than are other children.

What about Justine, the teenager in the second example? It sounds like that girl just needs to buckle down and study.

Justine suffers from a more subtle form of the same disorder: attention deficit without **hyperactivity**. Children with this form of the disorder often have normal intelligence, but they have trouble learning, they daydream, and they are easily distracted.

Because these children are quiet and do not disturb anyone with their behavior, their problems are easily overlooked by parents and teachers. It is thought that many more children have attention deficit than are diagnosed with it. These children can easily be mistakenly labeled unintelligent or lazy. Putting labels on people is never helpful, and it can be particularly destructive when it tears down the self-esteem of those with learning disorders.

Some children with attention deficit improve with age, but most continue having symptoms through life. Many reach the college years or even adulthood before they receive a diagnosis. When that day finally arrives, they breathe a sigh of relief to find out that their problem has a name, that it is not their fault, and that the possibility of treatment exists.

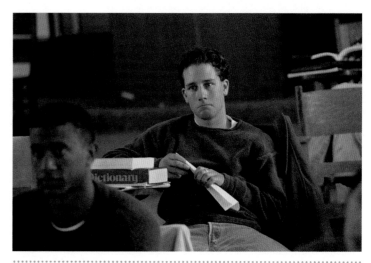

Students with ADHD need a classroom with few distractions to allow them to learn.

126

enrichment

Ask students to think about the development of self-esteem in children with ADHD. You may want to refer students back to the discussion in Chapter 3 of self-esteem development. Rereading this information in conjunction with

their study of this chapter should help students empathize more than they have previously with the concerns involved in the development of children with ADHD.

Have students consider the following questions:

1. How does a child's perception of self form?

Someone I know takes Ritalin every day. What is Ritalin, and how does it work?

Ritalin is a brand name for one of the stimulant drugs used in the treatment of ADHD. Ritalin helps many young people to control their behavior. It often works best when combined with counseling for the family.

It seems illogical that Ritalin, a stimulant that one would expect to pep people up, would calm down an already overpepped child. Ritalin works, though, because it "wakes up" areas of the brain that work to screen out distractions. Ritalin allows the child to calmly concentrate on one thing at a time without paying attention to random noises or distractions.

 I've heard that sugar and additives in children's food cause ADHD. Is that true?

No, it isn't true. Many parents resist the idea of treating their children with drugs. For them, the idea that a change in diet might improve their child's behavior sounds wonderful. Changing a child's diet may even seem to help for a while, but old behaviors return quickly once the placebo effect wears off. Proper nutrition is critical to mental and physical health, but eating sugar or other food doesn't cause hyperactivity. Using dietary "treatments" may only delay effective medical therapy.

 My little brother gets wild and "hyper" sometimes, but he doesn't have ADHD. How can we keep him calm?

No magic answers exist. However, a few ideas have sometimes helped to calm unruly, excitable children. Normal, everyday causes of such behavior seem to be:

▶ Desire for attention.
▶ Lack of sleep.
▶ Overstimulation.
▶ Too much television.
▶ Lack of exercise.

A child who often fills up on cookies, misses lunch, becomes too cranky to nap, misses out on outdoor play, and spends hours in front of a television can fall into a chronic pattern of crankiness and fatigue. This cycle of tension and fatigue often disappears when adults start insisting on regular hours of sleep, regular mealtimes of nutritious foods, and regular outdoor play.

 I wish that everyone with ADHD could get the help they need.

So do we. Without treatment, the problems faced by young people like Daniel and Justine can be overwhelming. They suffer intensely from the guilt and shame they feel, believing that they are somehow at fault for their problems. No matter how hard they try, though, they cannot get better by themselves. They are likely to become social outcasts, to develop emotional problems, to drop out of school, to have unsupportive social and family relationships, and even to commit crimes later on as adolescents and adults—unless they receive effective therapy.

Some parents resist seeking treatment for their ADHD child because they are embarrassed by the idea that their child is not perfect, or they may be too proud to seek help, or they believe the child will grow out of it if they just wait it out. Parents may also fear the expense of therapy. In truth, about a third of ADHD children do improve without help as they age, but they may carry the emotional scars of years of misunderstanding for life. Parents need to know that learning disorders are no one's fault. They should be proud to provide their children with the best available help. Low-cost, effective treatments are available, and the sooner they begin, the better. Their benefits can last a lifetime.

*Title "Life in Overdrive" borrowed from C. Wallis, Life in overdrive, *Time*, 18 July 1994, pp. 43–50.

MINI Glossary

attention-deficit/hyperactivity disorder (ADHD): an inability to pay attention, often with hyperactivity and poor impulse control. ADHD is most often diagnosed in children younger than age seven. It interferes with home life, schoolwork, or other functions.

learning disorder: any of a number of nerve or brain dysfunctions that interfere with normal learning, believed to affect 2 to 3 children in each class of 30. The disorders may affect attention, memory, language, organizational skills, problem solving, social awareness, and other aspects of learning.

impulse control: the ability to wait and think before acting or speaking.

hyperactivity: a condition of excessive activity. In children, hyperactivity is demonstrated by constant fidgeting, talking, moving, running, climbing, and so on. In adolescents and adults, hyperactivity takes the form of restless feelings and difficulty sitting still.

127

out. (heating or air conditioning system, noise outside, scraping feet, coughing, and so on) Encourage students to consider the difficulty they would have in focusing if those small distractions were as loud to them as the additional distractions you provided during their silent reading time.

COMPREHENSION CHECK

Ask students why Ritalin, a stimulant, is used for treating ADHD. (Ritalin "wakes up" areas of the brain that screen out distractions, allowing a child to concentrate without distractions.)

2. Do you think children with ADHD see themselves as abnormal?

3. What is the best way for siblings to interact with a child with ADHD?

4. What role do friends play in helping or hindering self-esteem?

5. What do you think happens to self-esteem when parents are very protective?

6. How do stereotypes of children with ADHD affect self-esteem?

Point out to students that when ADHD is viewed as a *fact of life*, the child will be better able to develop a high level of self-esteem.

VOCABULARY

1. a. anxiety attack;
b. insomnia; **c.** guilt;
d. eating disorder; **e.** post-traumatic stress disorder;
f. shame; **g.** emotional problems; **h.** schizophrenia

2. a. a habit or behavior;
b. Anxiety is a state of high energy, and can be beneficial in short spurts. Too much can be disabling. Phobias are a special form of anxiety that are an extreme, irrational fear of an object or situation.

3. Answers will vary.

RECALL

SECTION 1

1. social or family relations, performance of tasks, or leisure time activities (p. 108)

2. Society puts heavy pressure on people, and with strong values a person can act according to internal standards and not invite harsh external judgment. (p. 110)

SECTION 2

3. depression (p. 112)
4. Answers will vary; could include: identify the cause, take action, force yourself to do something different, do something physically active, eat a pick-me-up snack, avoid difficult or unpleasant tasks for a while, don't put pressure on yourself to achieve too much too soon, break large tasks into manageable goals, seek out other peo-

CHAPTER 5 Review

Summarizing the Chapter

Your ability to respond correctly to the following statements ensures your understanding of the main concepts in the chapter.

1. Describe the causes of emotional problems.
2. Identify common emotional problems.
3. Discuss the issue of teen suicide.
4. Identify professionals who can offer help for emotional problems. Explain how to find competent psychological services.
5. Discuss how to go about helping another person who has an emotional problem.

Learning the Vocabulary

emotional problems	compulsions
schizophrenia	guilt
addiction	shame
eating disorder	therapy
depression	Prozac
insomnia	codependent
anxiety	enabling
post-traumatic stress disorder	attention-deficit/hyperactivity disorder (ADHD)
anxiety attack	learning disorder
phobia	impulse control
obsessive-compulsive disorder	hyperactivity

Answer the following questions on a separate sheet of paper.

1. Matching—Match each of the following phrases with the appropriate vocabulary term from the list above:
a. a sudden, unexpected episode of severe anxiety with symptoms such as sweating and rapid heartbeat
b. a disorder that involves sleep abnormalities
c. a feeling a person gets when acting against internal values
d. anorexia nervosa is an example

e. a reaction to a stressful event such as rape, arising after the event is over
f. the extreme feeling of guilt that arises when a person internalizes blame for mistakes
g. patterns of behavior that impair a person's ability to function in social or family relations, occupation, or use of leisure time
h. a serious mental illness that tends to run in families
i. the ability to wait and think before acting or speaking

2. a. In an addiction, what sorts of things can people become dependent on, other than drugs?
b. How are anxiety and phobias similar and how are they different?

3. Create a story using as many of the vocabulary terms as you can. Underline each term you use from the vocabulary list.

Recalling Important Facts and Ideas

Section 1

1. What areas of your life can be affected by emotional problems?
2. Why is it so important to develop a working set of inner values by which to live?

Section 2

3. What is the most common emotional problem for which people seek counseling?
4. Give four recommendations for coping with mild depression.
5. How does physical activity affect the emotions?
6. Name three phobias.
7. Why is shame destructive to self-esteem?

Section 3

8. How common is teenage suicide?
9. What are some reasons why teenagers may attempt suicide?
10. How can you help a suicidal friend?

Section 4

11. What are the three ingredients necessary for an effective therapy relationship?
12. Name a few self-help groups.

Critical Thinking

1. Imagine that the community you live in has absolutely no mental health services. Design a comprehensive mental health services program to suit the needs of your community. Consider

128

ple, reject negative thinking, find reasons to laugh, go outdoors, and if you feel stuck, get help. (p. 112)

5. Physical activity alters the body's chemistry, lifts mood and attitude, and provides a benefit to those with heart disease, diabetes, alcoholism, and other conditions. (p. 112)

6. Answers will vary; could include: claustrophobia, agoraphobia, acrophobia, and any from the list of phobias on page 115.

7. When a person is made to feel shame, the person learns that he or she is bad. This chips away at self-esteem. (p. 115) the different age groups, cultures, and most common emotional problems within your community. What would you advise and why?

2. People who are feeling depressed or suicidal often see only one solution to their problems—taking their own life. List as many reasons as you can think of for teenage depression and for each reason listed develop a healthy way to deal with each problem. It is very important for people to realize there is more than one way to look at a problem. Name some people who could help teenagers in this way.

Activities

1. Contact a local hotline to find out some of the common problems people call in about. Find out what the staff training involves in order to work on the hotline.
2. Make a chart on poster board that lists the names of ten phobias on one side and their definitions on the other.
3. Find an article or watch a movie about an individual's struggle with an emotional problem. Describe the problem and how the person dealt with it. Include a copy of the article or the name of the movie.
4. Using your phone book, look up mental health facilities. Call five facilities to find out what services they provide. List each facility, address, phone number, and services provided.
5. Choose six traits of emotionally healthy people from Figure 5–1. Write a description of someone with those traits. Read the description aloud and allow classmates to guess the traits being described. Now, choose six traits of emotionally unhealthy people. Again, write a description of a person with those traits. Read the description aloud while classmates try to identify the traits being described.
6. Work in small groups of three or four people to complete this activity. Choose one of the following causes of mild depression:
   • death of a pet
   • poor sports performance
   • failed test
   • no partner for a dance
   • family fight
   • canceled plans
   • activity ruined by weather
   • break up with boyfriend or girlfriend
   • awkward injury

Work with your group to develop a plan to end the mild depression by choosing one or more activities from the Health Strategies section, "Coping with Mild Depression."

7. Working in the same groups you worked in for activity number 6, role play the mild depression your group chose and the strategies developed for coping with the mild depression.
8. Read the following saying, "If our problems were clothes and we hung them out on the line to dry, once we saw other people's problems we would be glad to take our own back." Do you agree or disagree with this saying. Explain why you feel the way you do.
9. Work in groups of four or five to develop puppet shows on child abuse, family violence, or divorce. Your target audience will be about eight years old. Use the local police department, newspapers, and magazines for your information. Perform the puppet show for your classmates, then find a class of eight year olds with whom you can share your puppet show.

Making Decisions about Health

1. Your friend's parents have not been getting along with each other for quite a while. They recently told your friend they are getting divorced. Lately, your friend has been having trouble eating, sleeping, and concentrating on school work. What steps can you share to help your friend?
2. What steps would you take to help a friend who is experiencing depression?
3. What steps would you take to help yourself out of a feeling of depression?

10. Answers will vary; could include: get involved; ask outright if the person is planning suicide; try to offer reassurance that the crisis is only temporary; phone a suicide hotline or crisis intervention center; dial 911, the operator, or the police; and stay with the person until help arrives. (p. 120)

SECTION 4

11. respect and trust between the therapist and client; the exploration of the present problem's causes, effects, or both; the search for new, more productive ways of dealing with the problem. (p. 122)
12. Answers will vary; could include: Alcoholics Anonymous, Overeaters Anonymous, Al-Anon, and Alateen. (p. 122)

129

SECTION 3

8. There are over 1,000 suicide attempts every day, with 20 young people succeeding at taking their own lives. (p. 117)
9. Answers will vary; could include: a way out of present circumstances; trying to impress others with the urgency of their feelings; having an unrealistic, romantic view of death; feeling like a failure; inability to express anger or pain; lacking firm values or rules on which to base life decisions; suffering a loss and seeing no end to deep grief; and having a relative or friend commit suicide. (p. 117)

	OUTCOMES	FEATURES
CHAPTER 6 **The Human Body and Its Systems**	• Differentiate among cells, tissues, organs, and systems. • Describe the importance of muscles and bones. • Identify the brain and spinal cord as the primary organs of the central nervous system. • Describe how the digestive system works. • Identify the cardiovascular system as the transportation system of the body. • Identify the male and female reproductive organs.	
CHAPTER 7 **Nutrition: The Nutrients**	• List the six Dietary Guidelines for Americans. • Discuss the impacts that overnutrition and undernutrition have on the body. • Identify the six classes of nutrients. • Design a balanced meal. • Describe the functions and food sources for carbohydrates, fats, and proteins. • Identify the essential vitamins, their functions and food sources. • Identify the essential minerals, their functions, and food sources.	*Health Strategies:* Dietary Guidelines for Americans (page 162); Getting the Fat Out of Your Diet (page 178) *Life Choice Inventory:* How Well Do You Eat? (page 168) *Consumer Skills:* Honey versus Sugar (page 176); How to Read a Food Label (page 181) *Straight Talk:* SOS: Selection of Supplements (page 196) *Teen Views:* Would you be healthier if you ate at fast food restaurants less often? (page 193)
CHAPTER 8 **Nutrition: Weight Control**	• Explain the problems associated with too little or too much body fat. • Explain the effects of an unbalanced energy budget. • Distinguish between loss of fat and loss of weight. • Identify unsound weight-loss programs. • Design a safe plan for weight loss and maintenance. • Design a healthful weight-gain program.	*Health Strategies:* Clues to Identifying Unsound Weight-Loss Programs (page 212) *Life Choice Inventory:* Eating Attitudes Test (page 224) *Consumer Skills:* Weight-Loss Schemes (page 213) *Straight Talk:* An Obsession with Thinness: Eating Disorders (page 225) *Teen Views:* Do teens diet too much or too little? (page 208)
CHAPTER 9 **Fitness**	• Discuss how fitness promotes all aspects of health. • Describe how you gain cardiovascular endurance, flexibility, muscle strength, and muscle endurance. • Recognize the dangers of using steroids and other drugs. • Describe preventive measures for sports injuries and accidents.	*Life Choice Inventory:* How Physically Active Are You? (page 236) *Consumer Skills:* Pills, Powders, and Potions for Fitness (page 250) *Straight Talk:* Food for Sports Competition (page 256)
CHAPTER 10 **Your Body: An Owner's Manual**	• Identify self-care practices to maintain healthy teeth, hair, nails, skin, and ears. • Explain the importance of correct posture to the health of the spine. • Determine when medical help is necessary.	*Life Choice Inventory:* Are Your Immunizations Up to Date? (page 282) *Consumer Skills:* Tricks, Traps, Quacks, and Gimmicks (page 294) *Straight Talk:* The Night Shift: Our Need for Sleep (page 284)

TEACHING SUPPORT

- *Vocabulary:* Learning Key Terms, Crossword Puzzle, Word Scramble
- *Study Outline; Reading Cloze*
- *Reteaching:* The Skeletal System, The Muscular System, The Nervous System, The Digestive System, The Cardiovascular System, The Urinary System, The Respiratory System, The Immune System, The Hormonal System, The Female Reproductive System, The Male

- Reproductive System
- *Tests:* Chapter 6 Test A, Chapter 6 Test B
- *Transparencies:* The Skeletal System; The Muscular System; The Nervous System; The Digestive System; The Cardiovascular System; The Urinary System; The Respiratory System; The Immune System; The Hormonal System; The Female Reproductive System; The Male Reproductive System

- *Vocabulary:* Learning Key Terms, Crossword Puzzle, The Scrambler
- *Study Outline; Reading Cloze*
- *Reteaching:* Nutrients, Vitamins and Minerals
- *Enrichment:* Calculations from Labels, Applying the Dietary Guidelines, Undernutrition vs. Overnutrition, Nutrient Advertisements, Analyzing Nutrient Labels, Vitamin Contracts
- *Career Briefs:* Dietitians and Nutritionists
- *Life Choice Inventory:* How Well Do You Eat?

- *Handouts:* Fast Foods Low in Fat and Calories, Selecting Nutritious Foods, Nutrients in Typical Lunches
- *Quizzes:* Sections 1–6
- *Tests:* Chapter 7 Test A, Chapter 7 Test B
- *Transparencies:* Daily Food Choices: Milk and Milk Products; Daily Food Choices: Breads and Cereals; Daily Food Choices: Vegetables; Daily Food Choices: Fruits; Daily Food Choices: Meat and Meat Alternatives; Daily Food Choices: Miscellaneous Group; The USDA Food Pyramid

- *Vocabulary:* Learning Key Terms, Crossword Puzzle, Weighty Matters
- *Study Outline; Reading Cloze*
- *Reteaching:* Basal Energy Needs
- *Enrichment:* Relate the Concepts, Fasting: A Fairy Tale, Calories and Qualities
- *Career Briefs:* Medical Assistants
- *Life Choice Inventory:* Eating Attitudes Test

- *Handouts:* Evaluating a Weight-Loss Diet, Tips for Reducing Sodium Intake, Seasoning without Your Salt Shaker
- *Teacher Information Sheets:* Basal Metabolic Rate, Poor Choices for Weight Loss
- *Tests:* Chapter 8 Test A, Chapter 8 Test B
- *Transparency:* What Happens Inside the Body During Overeating and Undereating

- *Vocabulary:* Learning Key Terms, Crossword Puzzle
- *Study Outline; Reading Cloze*
- *Reteaching:* Word Choice, Understanding Fitness, Stretches and Exercises Chart
- *Enrichment:* Exploring Fitness Centers, Designing a Personal Fitness Program

- *Career Briefs:* Physical Therapists
- *Life Choice Inventory:* How Physically Active Are You?
- *Handouts:* Fitness Objectives
- *Transparencies:* How to Take Your Pulse, Strength and Endurance Routines
- *Tests:* Chapter 9 Test A, Chapter 9 Test B

- *Vocabulary:* Learning Key Terms
- *Study Outline; Reading Cloze*
- *Reteaching:* Completion
- *Enrichment:* I Need a Doctor, Straighten Up!
- *Career Briefs:* Dental Hygienists
- *Handouts:* Terms Used on Cosmetic Labels

- *Tests:* Chapter 10 Test A, Chapter 10 Test B
- *Transparency:* Brushing and Flossing

MULTIMEDIA SUPPORT

- Health Video Library
- CNN Health and Fitness Update Videos
- Westest
- Student Review Software
- Diet Analysis Software
- Nutrition CD-ROM

LESSON PLANNING

You will find detailed daily lesson plans for both **traditional scheduling** and **block scheduling** in your Teacher's Resource Box.

INTRODUCING CHAPTER 6

KEY POINTS

Chapter 6 is 30 pages long and divided into the 12 sections listed below. The primary purpose of this chapter is to make students more aware of the miraculous workings of the human body and the fact that all the body systems work together, not independently. The chapter can also function as a review of the body systems. It begins with a short discussion of the structure of a system from the simplest cell to the collection of organs that perform a function. Although every system is responsible for a specific function, every system is dependent on all other systems for maintenance, protection, and life processes. It is this integration of all systems that maintains body homeostasis.

ACTIVITY TO INTRODUCE THE CHAPTER

Have students work in pairs to complete the following activity. Assign one member of each pair to perform a simple task, such as opening a book to a certain page and reading a paragraph, or doing a couple of jumping jacks. (All "performers" should do the same activity.) The second member of the pair should carefully observe the performance. The pair should then work together to generate a list of the individual movements that occurred during the performance. They should try to match movements to the body system(s) involved in making that movement. Have all pairs participate to help develop a class list on the board.

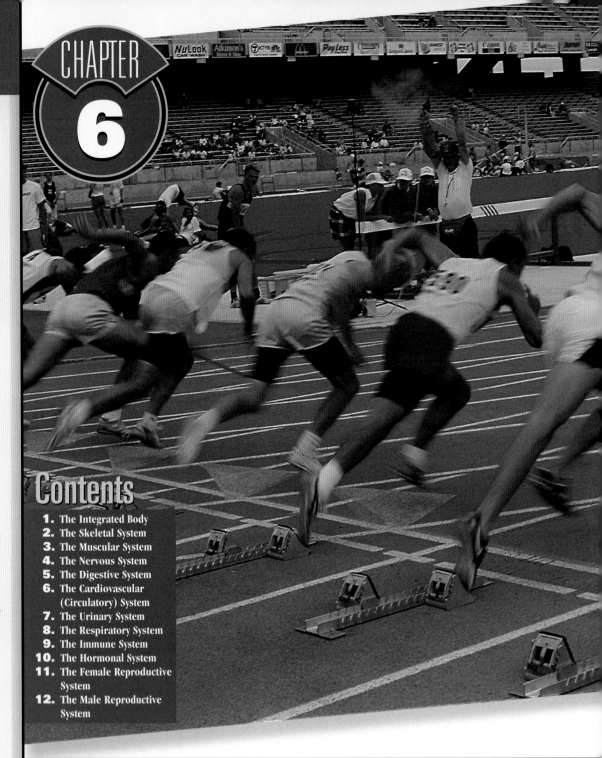

CHAPTER 6

Contents

NOT Enough Time?

You will probably want to use this chapter periodically throughout your course. If you teach the chapter in its entirety, as a review of the body systems, you may want to use the following plan.

DAY 1 Assign students to read Sections 1–6 prior to class. During class have students do the following activities: the Class Activity on page 136; the Focus Activity on page 138; the Focus Activity on page 140; the first Class Activity on page 143; and the Class Activity on page 144. If time permits, use some of the Evaluate activities for each section.

The Human Body and Its Systems

What do you think? Are the following statements true or false? If you think they are false, then say what is true.

1. Once bones have grown to adult size, they gain no more materials, although they may lose some.
2. Some muscle fibers are striped.
3. The brain is defenseless against the effects of alcohol.
4. If the digestive system did not protect itself, it would be digested by its juices.
5. Everyone's heart has a pacemaker.
6. The lungs are equipped with muscles in their walls that draw air in and out of the lungs' chambers.
7. Once a disease-causing organism enters the body, it is too late to prevent illness.
8. It is normal for men to produce female hormones in their bodies.

(Answers on page 135)

Introduction

How does your body do the things it does? For example, how can your legs "know" when your mind decides that it's time to walk to the VCR to change a video? What does it mean when you get the hiccups? How does food in your stomach nourish your toes?

To answer questions like these you need knowledge, not only of each of the **body systems** individually, but also of the ways the systems work together. The more you learn about the working of the integrated body, the more you will appreciate its miraculous everyday functions.

This chapter is unlike any other in this book. Its mission is to teach you just enough about the body to provide a basis for understanding the chapters that follow. Most sections of this chapter are written as questions and answers centered around figures showing each body system.

The figures present all of the structures discussed and named in the text. While reading about each system, look often at the related figure to see the body parts being discussed in the text. This way, learning how the parts work is easy. If you need to see definitions of any of the parts named in the figures, turn to the main glossary at the end of the book.

BULLETIN BOARD IDEAS

Write the names of the various systems of the body covered in this chapter (skeletal, muscular, nervous, digestive, cardiovascular, urinary, respiratory, immune, hormonal, and reproductive) on separate rectangles of construction paper. Then write a description of each system on additional rectangles of construction paper. Arrange the system rectangles down one side of the bulletin board, with the descriptions randomly placed down the other side. Use yarn to match the system to its description.

You might want to have students create and use the bulletin board as a study aid.

Answers to FACT or FICTION

1. **False.** Adult bones not only break down but also build up their structures throughout life.
2. **True.**
3. **True.**
4. **True.**
5. **True.**
6. **False.** The lungs lack muscles and, like balloons, fill passively with air only when the diaphragm contracts and creates a vacuum in the chest cavity.
7. **False.** Most often, when disease-causing organisms enter the body, the immune system destroys them and prevents illness.
8. **True.**

DAY 2 Assign students to read Sections 7–12 prior to class. During class, assign the following activities: Discussion on page 150; Group Project on page 152; the Focus Activity on page 154; and the Focus Activity on page 156. If time permits, use a variety of the Evaluate activities for each section.

SECTION 1

FOCUS

OUTCOMES

In this section students will learn that:

1. The body is made up of cells, tissues, organs, and systems.

2. All cells work in cooperation with other cells to support the whole by performing specific functions according to their genetic makeup.

3. All systems are dependent on each other and work together to maintain a state of homeostasis.

TEACHER SUPPORT

Key Passage
You will find another example of homeostasis in Chapter 4. The example in that chapter explains how the body reacts to the stress of cold weather.

FOCUS ACTIVITY

Obtain slides that show the different types of cells. Show them during a discussion of cell types.

TEACH & APPLY

COMPREHENSION CHECK

Remind students that all of the parts labeled in the illustrations and discussed in the various sections of this chapter are defined in the glossary.

The Integrated Body

No body system can function all alone, without help from the other systems. Each system depends on all the other systems to maintain the life of the whole person. Each adjusts to changing conditions to keep internal body conditions about the same at all times. This process of the body's striving to maintain constant internal conditions is called **homeostasis**, a word that means "staying the same."

As an example of homeostasis, the urinary system (see Figure 6–8 on page 146) is extremely sensitive to the composition of the blood in the cardiovascular system. When the body becomes flooded with too much water, the kidneys (in the urinary system) detect the extra water in the blood, draw it out, and release it from the body as urine. These steps bring the blood's water content back to normal. In the opposite case, when water becomes scarce and the blood's water content begins to diminish, the kidneys quickly step in to excrete less water in the urine.

The kidneys' management of the body's water balance is just one among thousands of examples of homeostasis. Each process goes on every minute of every day without your conscious awareness. The beauty of homeostasis is that the sum of its actions is expressed as wellness of the body.

Figure 6–1 The Organization of the Body

A **cell** is the basic unit of life within the body.

Tissues are formed by many cells together. They are the smallest working units of organs. All the cells of one tissue type work the same way.

Organs are collections of tissues and have many functions. Example: The pancreas.

Whole body systems are made up of organs all working together to meet the body's needs. Example: The digestive system.

The nucleus contains the genetic material of the cell.

Other structures support the cell's work and life.

In the pancreas two kinds of cells are mingled together in grapelike clusters. Some tissues of the pancreas make hormones, and some tissues make digestive juices.

The pancreas, along with many other organs, plays an important role in digestion.

COOPERATIVE LEARNING

The human body is made up of ten systems that work together to function as one system, although each system is unique and separate from the other systems they are still dependent on each other. It's important that we take care of all our body systems because when we neglect one system the other systems also

suffer. Explain to your students why it's important to keep your body systems healthy.

Divide the class into groups of three, allow one student in each group to have a text book open, one member has notebook paper and a pen or pencil, and one person takes the task of being the questioner. To make sure that all members of the group participate equally, have them switch roles in the group after they finish each section or body system in the chapter. Before the groups begin to work on

Cells

The body is made up of billions of microscopic **cells**. Each of the body's cells is a self-contained, living unit (Figure 6–1), although each depends on the rest of the body to supply its needs. Each cell keeps itself alive by taking up the substances it needs, such as oxygen, from the surrounding fluid and releasing the wastes it produces into that fluid.

In the human body every cell works in cooperation with every other to support the whole. The cell's **genes**, made of **DNA**, determine the nature of that work. Each gene is a blueprint that directs the cell in making a piece of machinery that helps to do the cell's work. For example, in a nerve cell, the genes guide the cell to make equipment needed to generate nerve impulses.

Each cell contains a complete set of genes inside its **nucleus**. The genes are lined up along slender bodies known as **chromosomes**. This means that all the information needed to make a whole human being is found in virtually every body cell. The reason why cells of different body parts are different from one another is that different genes are active in each kind of cell. For example, in some intestinal cells, the genes for making digestive enzymes are active. In the body's fat cells, the genes for storing fat are active.

Tissues and Organs

Groups of cells that perform similar functions form the **tissues**. Tissues perform tasks for the body. For example, some cells join together to form muscle tissue, which can contract. Tissues also are organized in sets to form whole **organs**. In the heart organ, for example, muscle tissues, nerve tissues, connective tissues, and other types all work together to pump blood.

Body Systems

Some jobs around the body require that several related organs cooperate to perform them. The organs that join together to work on a function are parts of a body system. For example, the heart and blood vessels work together to deliver blood to the body tissues as parts of the cardiovascular system (also called the circulatory system).

Figure 6–2 on the next page presents simple diagrams of all the body systems. Showing them together this way is intended to convey the meaning that no one system is completely independent of any of the others. All are responsible for functions that maintain homeostasis. Thus they work together to maintain the body's health:

▶ The *skeletal system* works with the muscular system to produce movement. Its bones release nutrients into the blood when they are needed by other body systems (Figure 6–3 on page 136).
▶ The *muscular system* responds to messages from the nervous system to move body parts. It works with the skeletal system to achieve movement (Figure 6–4 on page 138).
▶ The *nervous system* communicates with all other body systems. It directs activities of all the systems and receives information about the conditions in all other systems (Figure 6–5 on page 140).
▶ The *digestive system* breaks food down into nutrients. It delivers the nutrients to the cardiovascular system (Figure 6–6 on page 142).

MINI
Glossary

body systems: groups of related organs that work together to perform major body functions.

homeostasis (HOH-me-oh-STAY-sis): the maintenance of a stable body environment, achieved as body systems adapt to changing conditions.

cells: the smallest units in which independent life can exist. All living things are single cells or organisms made of cells.

genes (JEENZ): the units of a cell's inheritance, which direct the making of equipment to do the cell's work.

DNA (deoxyribonucleic acid): the genetic material of cells which serves as a blueprint for making all of the proteins a cell needs to make exact copies of itself.

nucleus: inside a cell, the structure that contains the genes.

chromosomes: slender bodies inside the cell's nucleus, which carry the genes.

tissues: systems of cells working together to perform special tasks.

organs: whole units, made of tissues, that perform specific jobs.

CLASS ACTIVITY

Have students brainstorm a list of body functions that they think are remarkable. If they had to list them in order, with the most remarkable listed first, how would they list them? Why?

BACKGROUND INFORMATION

As you discuss cells, students may ask about cancerous cells, which will be discussed fully in Chapter 17. For now, tell them that cancer is an abnormal growth of abnormal cells. Ask students what systems are not affected by cancers. (All systems are affected.)

DISCUSSION

In a class discussion, have your students define systems as being composed of organs; define organs as being composed of tissues; define tissues as being composed of cells, and, define cells as the basic, simplest form of life.

CLASS ACTIVITY

Divide the class into groups and have them try to think of machines, or mechanical or electrical systems that are designed to maintain a state of homeostasis. (Examples: cars, with such parts as oil and water gauges that light up; fuse boxes that blow out when overloaded; thermostats, which start furnaces.)

TRANSPARENCIES

The transparency "Delivery of Oxygen by the Heart and Lungs to the Muscles" is provided in the Transparency Acetate Binder.

the chapter share your class or group rules with them, such as working within their own group; giving only positive, cooperative comments to each other; and any others you find necessary.

To help groups study the body systems, have the person with the book read the information in the book about one of the body systems. The person with the paper and pen or pencil is to take notes and record any questions they or the questioner may have. The

questioner comes up with as many questions he or she can think of to help stir up debate on the body system for the group to discuss. The questioner may also facilitate questions that help the group understand how all the body systems relate to each other and work together. After the group has finished one body system, have them switch roles, and read and discuss the next body system. After all body systems have been covered, have the groups describe how the body systems work together.

ON LINE WITH HEALTH

You may want to have your students visit the following URL, where they will find information and additional web site resources to enhance their study of this chapter. As with all web sites, you should check this one out first to be sure the information found there is appropriate for your students.

BodyQuest
http://library.advanced. org/10348/

BodyQuest is specifically designed for students and includes lots of good activities. (Body systems are shown in computer-generated art.)

ASSESS

EVALUATE

Have students choose any body organ and list the many systems that require the function of that organ, or have them choose a system and list the ways in which that system is affected by or affects other systems. For both options, student points are determined by the number of relationships they can list.

Nervous system
Digestive system
Muscular system
Cardiovascular (circulatory) system
Skeletal system
Urinary system
Reproductive system
Respiratory system
Hormonal (endocrine) system
Immune system

Figure 6–2 The Integrated Body. While the systems can be studied separately, none can operate independently of the others.

QUICK QUIZ

Chapter 6, Section 1

The following quiz will help you assess your students' understanding of the material covered in this section of the chapter. You might use the quiz as an oral exercise, which will lead into a class discussion of the topics covered. Or, you might use it as a paper/pencil quiz to evaluate your students individually.

Like the Quick Quiz, the Section Review can also be used as an assessment tool to spark class discussion or as an individual student evaluation. It can also be used as a review in preparation for this quiz.

1. Each body system can function independently. (False)

2. Homeostasis is the bodily process of maintaining constant internal conditions.

▶ The *cardiovascular system* pumps blood and carries oxygen and nutrients to all other systems. It cleanses all systems of their wastes. It carries messages of the hormonal system. Its cells come from the bone marrow of the skeletal system (Figure 6–7 on page 144).

▶ The *urinary system* works with the cardiovascular system to maintain fluid and chemical balance in the body. It filters waste products out of the blood into the urine for removal (Figure 6–8 on page 146).

▶ The *respiratory system* delivers oxygen to, and removes wastes from, the cardiovascular system. It responds to the nervous and muscular systems to perform its tasks (Figure 6–9 on page 148).

▶ The *immune system* protects all other body systems from infection. Its cells travel through the cardiovascular system and through all body tissues (Figure 6–10 on page 150).

▶ The *hormonal system* communicates with many body systems to direct their activities. It monitors the blood for indicators of body conditions. It receives information and directions from the nervous system (Figure 6–11 on page 152).

▶ The *reproductive system* works with the nervous and hormonal systems to establish the gender of each human being. It responds to nerves, hormones, and muscles in creating new human beings (Figures 6–12 on page 154 and 6–13 on page 156).

For Your Information

Muscle cramps and muscle soreness are discussed in Chapter 9, which is about fitness.

SECTION 1 Review

Answer the following questions on a sheet of paper.

Learning The Vocabulary

The vocabulary terms in this section are *body systems, homeostasis, cells, genes, DNA (deoxyribonucleic acid), nucleus, chromosomes, tissues,* and *organs.*

1. Use each of the vocabulary terms listed above correctly in a sentence.

Learning the Facts

2. How do the kidneys manage the water balance in the body?

3. How do the cells in the body stay alive?

4. Which tissues in the cardiovascular system work together to pump blood?

5. List three body systems, and describe what they do.

Making Life Choices

6. The body systems can be affected by our behavior. Do you think that some healthy behaviors may benefit many of your body systems? List healthy behaviors that probably offer such benefits. Also list some unhealthy behaviors that you think may harm many systems.

Answers to FACT or FICTION
Here are the answers to the questions at the start of the chapter.

1. False. Adult bones not only break down but also build up their structures throughout life.
2. True.
3. True.
4. True.
5. True.
6. False. The lungs lack muscles and, like balloons, fill passively with air only when the diaphragm contracts and creates a vacuum in the chest cavity.
7. False. Most often, when disease-causing organisms enter the body, the immune system destroys them and prevents illness.
8. True.

A reproducible quiz for Section 1 is provided in the Teacher's Resource Box.

SECTION 1 Review Answers

1. Answers will vary.
2. When the body is flooded with too much water the kidneys detect the water, draw it out, and release it as urine. When water becomes scarce, the kidneys step in to excrete less water in the urine. (p. 132)
3. by taking up the substances needed, such as oxygen, from the surrounding fluid and releasing the wastes produced into that fluid (p. 133)
4. muscle tissues, nerve tissues, connective tissues and others (p. 133)
5. Answers will vary. Refer to the list in this section. (pp. 133–135)
6. Answers will vary.

CLOSE

Ask students to:

1. Tell what makes up a body system.
2. Discuss what makes each cell different and what cells need in order to function properly.
3. Give an example of a homeostatic process that occurs in the body.

(True)
3. Each of the body's cells is a self-contained, living unit. (True)
4. The nature of a cell is determined by its genes. (True)
5. Genes are made up of DNA. (True)
6. Sets of tissue join together to form genes. (False)
7. An organ is an organized set of tissues. (True)

8. The muscular system works with both the skeletal and the nervous system. (True)
9. The respiratory system is completely unconnected to the nervous system. (False)
10. All the body's organs work together to maintain homeostasis. (True)

135

FOCUS

OUTCOMES

In this section students will learn that:

1. Bones are living structures four times stronger than concrete.

2. Bones are equipped with both bone building cells and bone dismantling cells.

3. Bones give the body shape, protect vital organs, and help move the body.

FOCUS ACTIVITY

Bring in a couple of chicken or turkey bones and pass them around the room. Have students write down any noticeable characteristics about them. Discuss the properties of bones.

TEACH & APPLY

CLASS ACTIVITY

Using a replica or chart of the skeletal system, ask students to identify specific bones: the largest bone, smallest bone, long bones, flat bones, etc.

The transparency "The Skeletal System" (Figure 6–3) is provided in the Transparency Acetate Binder.

The Skeletal System

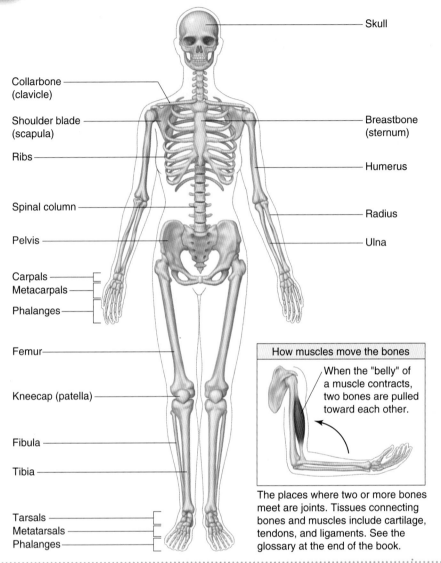

How muscles move the bones

When the "belly" of a muscle contracts, two bones are pulled toward each other.

The places where two or more bones meet are joints. Tissues connecting bones and muscles include cartilage, tendons, and ligaments. See the glossary at the end of the book.

Figure 6–3 The Skeletal System

Chapter 6, Section 2

The following quiz will help you assess your students' understanding of the material covered in this section of the chapter. You might use the quiz as an oral exercise, which will lead into a class discussion of the topics covered. Or, you might use it as a paper/pencil quiz to evaluate your students individually.

Like the Quick Quiz, the Section Review can also be used as an assessment tool to spark class discussion or as an individual student evaluation. It can also be used as a review in preparation for this quiz.

1. Bones allow movement and protect soft vital organs such as the kidneys and brain. (True)

2. Bones manufacture all of the body's

Without a skeleton, people would be made entirely of soft tissues. Like slugs, they would have few distinguishing features. They would be easily injured and would find movement difficult, at best. Bones determine the body's shape. Experts can reconstruct the facial likeness of a person who has died by working from the skull and jawbone alone.

Bones also protect soft vital organs, such as the brain and kidneys. They allow movement by acting as levers and anchors to which muscles attach. In addition, bones are warehouses that store many minerals and vitamins. Perhaps the most amazing feat performed by the bones is the manufacturing of all the body's blood cells—millions each day—without which life would come to an immediate halt.

Many people think of their bones as nonliving structures, sort of like the concrete girders that hold up a bridge. The true picture is far more spectacular. Bone tissue is more like solid aluminum or steel. It is four times stronger than reinforced concrete. Bones possess this remarkable strength thanks to a microscopic crystal structure similar to that of diamonds. Unlike concrete, bones are peppered with living bone cells that continuously maintain their solid parts, as well as their honeycombs of chambers and passageways. A rich network of blood vessels and nerves runs all through the bones, bringing nutrients and oxygen to bone cells and picking up stored nutrients to carry to body tissues.

How do bones grow?

Bones are equipped with both bone-dismantling cells and bone-building cells. Babies' bones are made mostly of connective tissue and are soft at first. Gradually, the bone-building cells add crystals of calcium and other minerals, making the bones more and more rigid. As the bones grow longer, they must also be reshaped. Bone-dismantling cells take apart the old structures while bone-building cells put the new ones together.

Once built, do bones ever change?

Throughout life, bone-dismantling cells are active. Whenever the blood needs more of the minerals stored in the bones, the bones give up those minerals. This reduces bone density.

Many older people suffer from a condition of weak bones—osteoporosis—because their bone-dismantling cells remain active while the bone-building

cells gradually slow down. If older people also fail to eat diets that provide enough calcium, or if they fail to exercise (along with other factors), their bones' calcium dwindles little by little, day after day over a lifetime.

It is now believed that the teen years are a once-in-a-lifetime opportunity for laying down bone material. Therefore, getting enough calcium in the diet is especially important for you right now. Physical activity is also a key.

How do the bones help the muscles to move the body?

Bones are connected to each other at flexible joints, as shown in Figure 6-3. A muscle connected to two bones across a joint can pull the two bones closer together. For example, the largest muscle of your arm (the biceps) is attached to the bone of your upper arm and to a bone of your forearm. The elbow joint separates the two bones. When you want to reach up to touch your shoulder, the muscle contracts. The whole structure works together like a pulley and lever.

Why does it hurt so much to hit your "funny bone"?

"Funny bone" is a nickname for the humerus—pronounced like the word *humorous*—but it hardly seems funny when you feel the intense pain and tingle caused by hitting your elbow against a corner. Actually, the sensation is not caused by the bone itself but by a nerve that nestles in a bony cradle of the humerus bone. When struck, the nerve compresses against the bony structures, sending a bolt of paralyzing pain and sensation from the fingernails through the neck and back—hardly a laughing matter.

Is it harmful to "crack" your knuckles?

The popping noise made when the joints of the fingers (and sometimes other joints) are bent slightly beyond their normal range is probably caused by the release of nitrogen gas that collects in microscopic bubbles inside the joint. The gap between the cartilage pads of each bone end is filled with a thick fluid that lubricates the joint. Physicians disagree whether cracking your knuckles can make them become larger than normal. Knuckle cracking does not seem to be related to arthritis. If practiced to extreme, however, it may cause slight impairment of hand function.

TRANSPARENCIES The transparency "The Spinal Column" is provided in the Transparency Acetate Binder. It may be useful in reinforcing the concept of bones protecting soft tissue.

COMPREHENSION CHECK

Emphasize that the bones in the skeletal system are alive. Bones are not lifeless objects, as students might think of them. The skeletal system grows, changes, and repairs itself. Ask students if they think of plants, flowers, and trees as being living things. Point out that the skeletal system is equally alive, constantly growing and changing. Ask students to consider what would happen to the body if it were not.

ASSESS

EVALUATE

WORKSHEETS A reproducible quiz for Section 2 is provided in the Teacher's Resource Box.

CLOSE

Ask students to:

1. Give an example of the bones that protect, give shape, allow movement, store vitamins, and produce blood cells.
2. Describe the changes that occur in the bones throughout life.

blood cells. (True)
3. Bone tissue is extremely fragile. (False)
4. Bones become softer as you grow older. (False)
5. Osteoporosis is a condition of weak bones which afflicts many elderly people. (True)
6. Teenagers should be especially careful to include adedquate amounts of calcium in their diets. (True)
7. The way bones and muscles move could be compared to a pulley and lever. (True)
8. Bone-building cells remain active while the bone-dismantling cells gradually slow down. (False)
9. The humerus is nicknamed the "funny bone." (True)
10. Knuckle-cracking has been linked to arthritis. (False)

SECTION 3

FOCUS

OUTCOMES

In this section students will learn that:

1. There are three main types of muscles.
2. The body relies on both fast twitch and slow twitch muscles to do most work.
3. Muscle tissues grow with work and shrink without work.

FOCUS ACTIVITY

Have students, at their desks, do a back push-up. To do this, they should hold onto the edge of their chairs with legs out straight and lower themselves down as far as they can and back to place. Have students list the muscles they worked.

TEACH & APPLY

CLASS ACTIVITY

Bring in several different cuts of meat—thigh, drumstick, heart; chicken parts work well. Have students, wearing gloves, look for how the part is attached to the bone. Examine the fat content around the muscle and identify any visible muscle fibers. Then have students identify the types of muscle.

The transparency "The Muscular System" (Figure 6–4) is provided in the Transparency Acetate Binder.

SECTION 3   The Muscular System

- neck
- upper back and neck (trapezius)
- shoulder (deltoid)
- chest (pectoralis)
- biceps
- triceps
- back (latissimus dorsi)
- side (oblique)
- abdominals
- buttocks (gluteus)
- inner thigh
- hamstrings
- quadriceps
- calf (gastrocnemius)
- (This tendon, the Achilles tendon, connects the calf muscle to the heel.)

Figure 6–4   The Muscular System

Chapter 6, Section 3

The following quiz will help you assess your students' understanding of the material covered in this section of the chapter. You might use the quiz as an oral exercise or, you might use it as a paper/pencil quiz to evaluate your students individually.

Like the Quick Quiz, the Section Review can also be used as an assessment tool to spark class discussion or as an individual student evaluation. It can also be used as a review in preparation for this quiz.

*If students have difficulty with the concepts covered in the Quick Quiz and the Section Review, you might suggest they review the material using the **S**urvey, **Q**uestion, **R**ead, **R**ecite, **R**eview (SQ3R) study method, which is described in detail in the introduction to this*

Movement of the body is possible thanks in part to the unique structure of muscle tissue. Layers upon layers of muscle tissue form strong sets of paired muscles that pull the bones back and forth in ways that make it possible to dance, ride a bike, and use sign language. Many muscles inside the body are not shown in Figure 6–4. Some inner muscles run the length of the digestive organs to move food through the digestive tract. Others surround and grasp the chambers of the heart and squeeze blood from them with each heartbeat.

Are all the muscles the same?

No, they vary. The ones that move your skeleton are under your control. They are called voluntary muscles. The ones that control your internal organs move automatically. They are called involuntary muscles. The voluntary ones appear striped under the microscope, and they are very strong. The involuntary ones appear smooth, and they are less strong.

One set of muscles appears mixed: the muscles of the heart. They are strong, like skeletal muscles, but under involuntary control. This mix allows the heart to beat without a rest, year after year.

Is it true that some people are born with the right muscles for running or swimming?

In a sense, it is. Some of the voluntary muscles are suited for fast action, like the jump of the basketball player. Some are suited for slow action, like the strokes of a long-distance swimmer. Everybody has some of both, but some people inherit more fast-action muscles, and some inherit more of the slow, sustained type.

How do muscles contract?

Muscle cells respond to signals from nerve cells. Nerves release powerful chemicals that create electrical impulses in the muscle cells. The electrical impulses travel along the cells' membranes, triggering the long, thin muscle cells to shorten and bunch up. When enough cells get the signal, the whole muscle contracts.

Why is it that the muscles of runners are long and slender, while the muscles of weight lifters are rounded and bulky?

Part of the answer lies in a person's genetic heritage. Some people are just born with bulky or slender muscles. Another part is in the work that each type of athlete does. Each type of work requires different characteristics in the muscle tissues. For the weight lifter, muscles must be extra strong. Thus each muscle cell builds up its membrane and contracting fibrils to be thick and bulky, providing strength. For the runner, strength is not as urgent as is the ability to contract repeatedly for prolonged times. Therefore, the body does not build bulky muscles in the runner, but packs the cells with the internal structures that sustain effort over a long time.

What does It mean to be "muscle bound"?

A person who trains incorrectly may lose the ability to use certain muscles normally. Muscles come in paired sets. The action of each muscle set opposes another. When one muscle set of the pair becomes greatly more developed than its mate, movement becomes difficult. A bodybuilder who becomes over-enthusiastic in developing biceps, for example, may neglect the opposing muscle, the triceps. As a result, the arms begin to hang abnormally when relaxed. Some movements can become almost impossible.

Is it true that to strengthen muscles, you must work them until they are sore?

Years ago the rule for gaining muscle was "no pain, no gain." People thought that injury was the trigger causing muscles to grow. This has been disproved. Scientists now know that muscle contractions themselves send messages to the genetic material of the muscles' cells. The genetic material receives messages about the work: how long it lasts and how intense it is. Based on this information, the cells build the equipment they need to perform the type of work that they are being called upon to do. Even without injury, muscles grow in size and gain in strength after working.

Which muscle is the strongest?

Strength in a muscle is directly related to its overall size, so it follows that the largest muscle is also the strongest. In the human body, the strongest muscle is the one that pushes the body from a squatting to a standing position—did you guess? It's the gluteus maximus, the major muscle of the buttocks (seat).

Teacher's Wraparound Edition.

1. Muscles are formed of many layers of muscle tissue. (True)
2. Muscles that move automatically are called voluntary muscles. (False)
3. Voluntary muscles are stronger than involuntary muscles. (True)
4. The muscles of the heart are voluntary but very weak. (False)
5. All voluntary muscles are best suited to fast action. (False)
6. Muscles respond to electrical impulses created by signals from the nerve cells. (True)
7. Over-developing particular muscles can actually impair body movement. (True)
8. All muscles are the same. (False)
9. Muscles help you to digest your food. (True)
10. The tongue is the strongest muscle in the human body. (False)

SECTION 4

FOCUS

OUTCOMES

In this section students will learn that:

1. The central nervous system is composed of the brain and the spinal cord.

2. The brain's many functions are divided among its many physical parts.

FOCUS ACTIVITY

Do some reaction tests for eye-hand coordination. Hold the zero edge of a ruler between a student's thumb and fingers. Drop the ruler and record how far the ruler fell before it was caught by the student. (The point at which the student grabs the ruler is the distance.) Now have the subject close his or her eyes and repeat the action when you say, "Now." Discuss which was faster—eye-hand or ear-hand coordination.

TEACH & APPLY

The transparency "The Nervous System" (Figure 6–5) is provided in the Transparency Acetate Binder.

SECTION 4 — The Nervous System

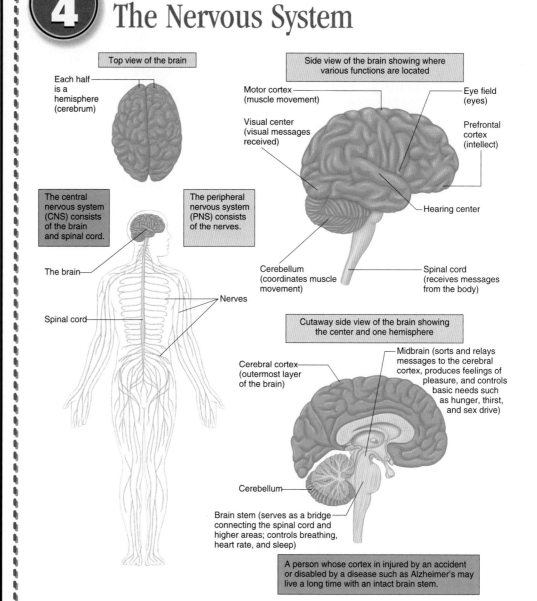

Top view of the brain

Each half is a hemisphere (cerebrum)

The central nervous system (CNS) consists of the brain and spinal cord.

The peripheral nervous system (PNS) consists of the nerves.

The brain

Spinal cord

Nerves

Side view of the brain showing where various functions are located

Motor cortex (muscle movement)

Visual center (visual messages received)

Eye field (eyes)

Prefrontal cortex (intellect)

Hearing center

Cerebellum (coordinates muscle movement)

Spinal cord (receives messages from the body)

Cutaway side view of the brain showing the center and one hemisphere

Cerebral cortex (outermost layer of the brain)

Midbrain (sorts and relays messages to the cerebral cortex, produces feelings of pleasure, and controls basic needs such as hunger, thirst, and sex drive)

Cerebellum

Brain stem (serves as a bridge connecting the spinal cord and higher areas; controls breathing, heart rate, and sleep)

A person whose cortex in injured by an accident or disabled by a disease such as Alzheimer's may live a long time with an intact brain stem.

Figure 6–5 *The Nervous System*

QUICK QUIZ

Chapter 6, Section 4

The following quiz will help you assess your students' understanding of the material covered in this section of the chapter. You might use the quiz as an oral exercise, which will lead into a class discussion of the topics covered. Or, you might use it as a paper/pencil quiz to evaluate your students individually.

*If students have difficulty with the concepts covered in the Quick Quiz and the Section Review, you might suggest they review the material using the **S**urvey, **Q**uestion, **R**ead, **R**ecite, **R**eview (SQ3R) study method, which is described in detail in the introduction to this Teacher's Wraparound Edition.*

1. The brain is the master organ of the body, and controls almost every physical

The brain, master organ of the body and the seat of the thinking mind, is a 3-pound mass of specialized nerve tissue. With its wrinkled, walnutty appearance, it lies motionless, armored within the skull, just a gray blob with no observable activity. One would never suspect the massive power of the brain, which lies not in physical movement but in its chemistry. Without so much as a quiver, the brain controls almost every physical body function, every thought, and every emotion.

To control things, the brain must obtain information about events and conditions around the body. It must also deliver instructions to tissues about what to do. The spinal cord consists of nerves that connect the brain to all the body parts. It lies safe within the bony spinal vertebrae and provides the body's main communication line. Nerves branch from the trunk of the spinal cord to carry messages back and forth between the tissues and the brain. The brain and spinal cord make up the central nervous system.

Do the different brain parts do different things?

In order to perform the fantastic number of tasks required of it, the brain must be organized. Indeed, its work is divided among its physical parts. In the outer layer (cortex) of the brain's two large hemispheres, conscious thought takes place. The small bulb lying at the base of the hemispheres, the cerebellum, maintains balance and directs muscle activities. The brain stem leading to the spinal cord controls breathing and other basic functions.

Within these large brain areas are smaller divisions, each with specific duties. The prefrontal cortex concerns itself with high intellectual tasks, such as reading a health textbook. When you chat with friends later, an area about the size of a quarter on the left side of your brain will control the muscles of your mouth and throat that produce speech. When you next hear your favorite song on the radio, the hearing center will become active. If the music sends a thrill through you, it has triggered tissues in your midbrain. These tissues create pleasure when stimulated—for example, by viewing a beautiful sight (received by the eye field); when savoring the flavor of a favorite food or the aroma of flowers (the smell center); and more perilously, from the direct stimulation produced by mind-altering drugs.

Many more functions are known. Some fascinating books have been written about them.

How does the brain protect its chemistry?

The brain maintains a barrier that excludes certain chemicals carried by the blood. The blood-brain barrier is a control system by which the brain's blood vessels control the environment inside the brain. It admits those chemicals the brain needs, but excludes those that could interrupt the brain's work. In this way, the brain's internal chemistry remains balanced, despite changes in the rest of the body's chemistry. The system fails to exclude some harmful chemicals, though, and these enter and affect the brain. Alcohol is a toxin against which the blood-brain barrier provides no defense. Other mind-altering drugs also pass freely into brain tissues.

What if nerve or brain tissues are injured? Do they heal?

Nerve cells, for the most part, cannot reproduce themselves to fully repair injury, as some other tissues do. However, they may be able to grow new parts in a limited way to reconnect with other nerves after being severed. Traditionally, it has been taught that brain cells are not able to reproduce at all. However, recent experiments have shown that at least some types of brain cells can be coaxed to reproduce in the laboratory. Still, many people suffer lifelong damage from injuries to the brain and nerves because regrowth of the tissue is limited.

How does tapping your knee make your whole leg jerk?

The jerk of the leg is an example of a reflex, a sort of intentional short circuit in the nervous system. The nerves that control reflexes form an arc—from tissue to spinal cord back to tissue—that can produce the needed response in a split second. Tapping the knee triggers a reflex that contracts the muscle at the front of the thigh. The thigh muscle jerks the leg.

Reflexes control situations that demand immediate action. They do not wait for judgments by the brain. Reflexes can prevent major damage. For example, when you touch something hot, your hand jerks away uncontrollably before you even feel your finger being burned.

body function. (True)

2. The brain delivers instructions to tissues about what to do. (True)

3. The spinal cord is the body's main communication line. (True)

4. Unconscious thought takes place in the brain's cortex. (False)

5. Each division of the brain performs a specific duty. (True)

6. Your brain tissues create emotion. (True)

7. The blood-brain barrier protects the brain from certain chemicals carried by the blood. (True)

8. The blood-brain barrier excludes all harmful chemicals from the brain. (False)

9. Regrowth of damaged brain tissue is very rapid. (False)

10. Reflex actions are not controlled by the brain. (True)

SECTION 5

FOCUS

OUTCOMES

In this section students will learn that the digestive system is:

1. Responsible for breaking down food into a form usable by cells.
2. Composed of acids and digestive juices that act on ingested substances.

FOCUS ACTIVITY

Give each student a soda cracker. Have students eat their crackers and describe the action of their digestive systems. (teeth, tongue, saliva, esophagus, and so on) Ask them to name all the digestive organs they can think of.

TEACH & APPLY

The transparency "The Digestive System" (Figure 6–6) is provided in the Transparency Acetate Binder.

COMPREHENSION CHECK

As students look at Figure 6-6, you may want to review with them the basic processes that occur during digestion. There are six basic steps:

1. Ingestion of food into the mouth;
2. movement of food along the digestive tract;
3. mechanical preparation of food for digestion;

CHAPTER 6: The Human Body and Its Systems

SECTION 5 The Digestive System

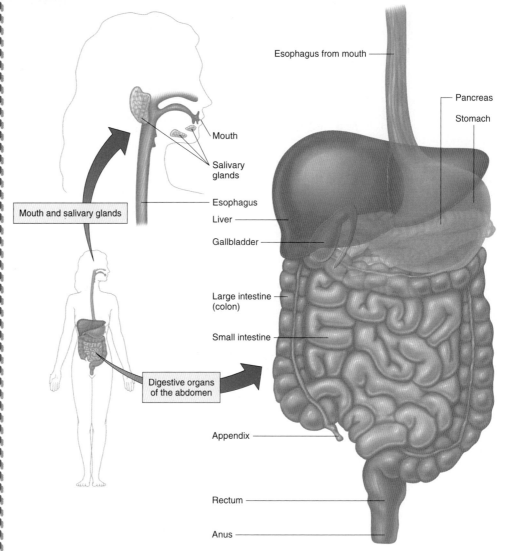

Figure 6–6 *The Digestive System*

Esophagus from mouth
Pancreas
Stomach
Mouth
Salivary glands
Esophagus
Liver
Gallbladder
Large intestine (colon)
Small intestine
Appendix
Rectum
Anus
Mouth and salivary glands
Digestive organs of the abdomen

Chapter 6, Section 5

The following quiz will help you assess your students' understanding of the material covered in this section of the chapter. You might use the quiz as an oral exercise, which will lead into a class discussion of the topics covered. Or, you might use it as a paper/pencil

quiz to evaluate your students individually.

*If students have difficulty with the concepts covered in the Quick Quiz and the Section Review, you might suggest they review the material using the **S**urvey, **Q**uestion, **R**ead, **R**ecite, **R**eview (SQ3R) study method, which is described in detail in the introduction to this Teacher's Wraparound Edition.*

1. An object can pass through the body without entering the tissues. (True)

The human body is shaped something like a doughnut, with the digestive tract running through the center to form the hole. If you were to accidentally swallow a small bead, the bead would pass right through your digestive tract and out of your body, never entering the tissues at all. Food in the digestive tract meets a different fate. Glands squirt digestive juices that contain powerful chemicals, called enzymes, into the tract to break the food molecules down into smaller pieces that can be absorbed into the tract's tissues. Only after a substance passes through the intestinal wall tissues is it truly inside the body.

Why doesn't the stomach digest itself?

The powerful acids and juices of the stomach, and of the whole digestive tract, would indeed digest the tract if it weren't for a protective layer of mucus that coats the tract's lining. The mucus coating forms a barrier between the system and its contents. If the layer of mucus is too thin to protect the tissue, ulcers can result. Alcohol also dissolves the layer. Ulcers are common in those with addictions to alcohol. Some infections can also cause ulcers.

What causes indigestion, and what is the best cure?

Indigestion is an aching pain in the digestive tract caused from the system's failing to cope with the stomach's contents in a normal way. It can occur when spice in food irritates the tract lining; when too much fat overwhelms the system's ability to digest it; or when too much air, food, or liquid is swallowed and expands the stomach and intestines, causing pain and pressure.

The best cure for indigestion is prevention. Avoid foods that have caused problems for you in the past. Eat mostly low-fat foods with only small portions of high-fat foods. Eat slowly; chew thoroughly; and eat only until you feel full. If you develop indigestion, you might obtain relief from over-the-counter remedies. It's best to ask a health-care provider, though, before turning to the use of medicines.

What is heartburn?

At the base of the esophagus, where it meets the stomach, circular muscles squeeze the opening shut to prevent the stomach contents from backing up in the esophagus. Sometimes the mixture of acid and food in the stomach splashes up through this opening into the esophagus. When this happens, the strong acid burns and irritates the sensitive esophagus lining—heartburn.

Heartburn has nothing to do with the heart. However, the esophagus lies near the heart, so people have been led to think that the pain they feel from heartburn is coming from the heart. The opposite can also happen. Some people have needlessly died from heart attacks because they attributed their chest pains to "indigestion" and failed to get help.

What does the appendix do, and why must some people have theirs removed?

The appendix is the little worm-shaped sac that hangs from the lower right side of the large intestine. It seems to have no purpose in digestion. It is notable only if undigested food particles and bacteria lodge in it and an infection gets started. Appendicitis is painful. It is also dangerous, because the sac can burst open. If this happens, digestive products and infected material flow into the normally sterile body cavity. This life-threatening condition can be prevented by surgically removing an inflamed appendix before it bursts. The operation carries little risk. If you have a pain in your lower right abdomen that doesn't go away, call a doctor.

Why does my stomach sometimes grumble?

As fluid and gas squeeze past the convoluted folds and turns of the digestive organ tissues, the bubbles produce a gurgling, grumbling sound. The sound may be inconvenient at times, but it is normal, especially when you are hungry.

Why do people "pass gas," and what causes its odor?

Technically, the gas is *flatus* (FLAY-tus). Everyone produces some gas all the time. Not much can be done to avoid it or to help control its release from the intestine. Gases are a normal waste product of digestion. Bacteria of the large intestine consume and thrive on fibers and food particles left in the tract after digestion and absorption. Most odors are from molecules that form when bacteria act on proteins. The nature of the odor depends on the food eaten, and on the type of bacteria in the system.

---

4. chemical digestion of food;
5. absorption of digested food into the blood and lymph for transport throughout the body;
6. elimination of indigestible substances and waste products from the body by defecation.

CLASS ACTIVITY

Have students research and compare the digestive systems of some animals with those of humans. (Possible animals might include: cow, owl, snake, and so on) Students should answer these questions: What animals' digestive systems have special characteristics? What are their advantages?

CLASS ACTIVITY

Put a few drops of hydrochloric acid on carbohydrates, proteins, and fats. (cracker, lean meat, and fat) Have students observe how long each takes to be acted upon. Discuss what this tells us about foods we ingest.

ASSESS

EVALUATE

A reproducible quiz for Section 5 is provided in the Teacher's Resource Box.

CLOSE

Ask students to:

1. Identify the organs involved in digestion.
2. Name some ways the digestive system protects itself from harmful substances.

---

2. Food molecules are broken down in the digestive tract by enzymes. (True)
3. The stomach is protected by a layer of mucus. (True)
4. The powerful acid found in the stomach can prevent ulcers. (False)
5. Indigestion is caused by the failure of the digestive system to cope with the stomach's contents. (True)
6. The best cure for indigestion is constant medication. (False)
7. Indigestion can usually be avoided by healthy eating habits. (True)
8. Heartburn is caused by stomach acid splashing onto the heart. (False)
9. The appendix plays a vital role in digestion. (False)
10. Gas is a normal waste product of digestion. (True)

SECTION 6

FOCUS

OUTCOMES

In this section students will learn that the:

1. Heart pumps continually to deliver nutrients to the cells and to pick up cellular wastes.
2. Blood can repair damage to the vessel system.

FOCUS ACTIVITY

Obtain an animal's heart from a local butcher. Describe and point out these characteristics: type of muscle, amount of fat, arteries surrounding it, valves and chambers visible.

TEACH & APPLY

BACKGROUND INFORMATION

You may want to tell students that blood consists of both the liquid component called *plasma* and a nonliquid portion whose structures are collectively called *formed elements*. Plasma is approximately 91% water. The portion of plasma that is not water consists of various dissolved materials. Formed elements include the red blood cells, various types of leukocytes (white blood cells), and cell fragments called platelets.

CLASS ACTIVITY

Using a diagram of the human heart, trace a drop of blood from the heart to the lungs and back to the heart.

CHAPTER 6: The Human Body and Its Systems

SECTION 6
The Cardiovascular (Circulatory) System

The lines in red represent arteries in the body, which carry oxygen-rich blood to the organs and muscles.

The lines in blue represent veins in the body, which bring oxygen-starved blood back to the heart

Cutaway view of the heart

Superior vena cava — Aorta — Pulmonary artery — Valve — Pulmonary veins — Right atrium — Left atrium — Valve — Valve — Valve — Left ventricle — Right ventricle — Septum — Inferior vena cava

Heart

Blood circulation

Head — Right lung — Left lung — Atria — Ventricles — Capillaries

From the heart, blood travels through arteries to the lungs to collect oxygen. Then it returns through veins to the heart. The heart then pumps the oxygen-rich blood through other arteries to every part of the body. Oxygen-starved blood returns to the heart through other veins.

Figure 6–7 The Cardiovascular System

Chapter 6, Section 6

The following quiz will help you assess your students' understanding of the material covered in this section of the chapter. You might use the quiz as an oral exercise, which will lead into a class discussion of the topics covered. Or, you might use it as a paper/pencil

quiz to evaluate your students individually.

*If students have difficulty with the concepts covered in the Quick Quiz and the Section Review, you might suggest they review the material using the **S**urvey, **Q**uestion, **R**ead, **R**ecite, **R**eview (SQ3R) study method, which is described in detail in the introduction to this Teacher's Wraparound Edition.*

1. The cardiovascular system transports the body's fluids and provides the cells with

With its vast network of arteries, veins, and capillaries, the cardiovascular system—also called the circulatory system—provides the transportation system for the body's fluids. Each cell in the body depends on this system's life-sustaining work. Cells dump their wastes into this system. They also pull from its rich abundance all the nutrients and other chemicals they need to live and function.

How does the heart know how fast to beat?

The heart responds to a small area of its upper right chamber (right atrium), its natural pacemaker. This area acts almost as a spark plug does. It sends an electrical impulse through the heart that causes both atria to contract immediately. Within less than a second, the ventricles also contract in response to the signal.

The pacemaker adjusts the heart rate in response to instructions carried by nerves from the brain. Also, when the heart itself detects the need, it can quicken the pace. The heart and blood vessel tissues monitor blood levels of carbon dioxide, the waste product of the tissues. When carbon dioxide reaches a high concentration, this indicates to the heart a need for faster delivery of oxygen from the lungs. The heart also quickens the heartbeat whenever the blood pressure falls, and whenever it receives any of several hormones from body organs.

Does the heart ever rest?

For as long as a person is alive, the heart never takes a break. In a sense, though, the heart rests continuously and efficiently in the moments of muscle relaxation between contractions. During these rest periods, the relaxed heart muscles allow blood to fill the heart's chambers.

When the blood picks up wastes from the cells, how does it get rid of them?

To try to answer this question in a paragraph or two is impossible, for many wastes are deposited in the blood, and they are removed by several systems. The urinary system, for example, is wondrously designed to scrub the blood of much of the cells' debris.

Carbon dioxide waste deposited in the blood trades places with oxygen during gas exchange in the lungs. Other wastes are pulled out of the blood by the liver. The liver processes these wastes and either tosses them out into the digestive tract to leave the body with the feces, or sends them to the kidneys for disposal in urine. Thus the cardiovascular system, the liver, the digestive system, the lungs, and the urinary system all work together on the task of cleansing the blood.

Blood is red, serum is yellow, and the veins look blue. Why?

Blood outside the body is red because of the enormous number of red blood cells it contains. Take away the red cells, and what's left is not red at all, but a clear, yellowish syrup (serum). The red cells contain hemoglobin, an iron-containing protein that turns red whenever it is in contact with oxygen.

As red cells move through the lungs, they pick up the oxygen of newly inhaled air and attach it to their hemoglobin. The oxygen gives the cells a red color. As they travel through the body, red cells give up their oxygen to the tissues and replace it with carbon dioxide. As they lose oxygen and gain carbon dioxide, the red cells take on a dark purple cast. You can see this blood on its way back to the lungs, because it is traveling through the colorless veins under the skin. If you were to accidentally cut a vein, though, the blood would flow bright red, because oxygen from the air would combine instantly with the hemoglobin.

What makes a wound stop bleeding?

Blood platelets in the blood form a net, which traps still more platelets and other blood cells. This forms a clot, which plugs the wound until it can heal.

What are blood types?

Human blood is classified into four types. The types are based on which, if any, of two proteins—antigen A and antigen B—are present in the red blood cells. The symbols used to identify the four types of blood—A, B, AB, and O—represent which of the proteins, or factors, are present. Type A contains antigen A, type B contains antigen B, type AB contains both, and type O contains neither.

The categories become important when people need transfusions, because some types of blood are hostile to others. Should blood of the wrong type be given, the native blood would attack the transfused blood as if it were an enemy invader. The blood would clump together within the vessels, with harmful or fatal results.

The transparency "Delivery of Oxygen by the Heart and Lungs to the Muscles" is provided in the Transparency Acetate Binder.

The transparency "An Overview of the Cardiovascular System," also provided in the Transparency Acetate Binder, will help you show students how this system is a transportation system.

ASSESS

EVALUATE

Have students use any five of the following terms in a sentence with either *heart* or *cardiovascular system*: aorta, carbon dioxide, cells, iron, left atrium, oxygen, right atrium, transportation system, urinary system. Give extra credit if they can correctly use *inferior vena cava*.

A reproducible quiz for Section 6 is provided in the Teacher's Resource Box.

CLOSE

Ask students to:

1. Describe the function of the cardiovascular system.
2. Explain how blood helps to eliminate cell waste.
3. List the four blood types.

needed nutrients. (True)

2. The left atrium of the heart acts as a pacemaker. (False)

3. The heart can quicken its pace independently, without a signal from the brain. (True)

4. The heart responds to the level of carbon dioxide in the blood. (True)

5. The heart does not help to regulate blood pressure. (False)

6. The heart frequently stops working while a person is living. (False)

7. The liver and lungs help to cleanse the body's blood. (True)

8. Hemoglobin combines with oxygen to give the blood its red color. (True)

9. Platelets form clots which plug a wound and prevent it from bleeding. (True)

10. Any type of blood can be given in a transfusion. (False)

SECTION 7

FOCUS

OUTCOMES

In this section students will learn:

1. That the urinary system monitors the composition of the blood and removes wastes.

2. How the urinary systems of men and women differ.

FOCUS ACTIVITY

Have students help you list the major organs of the urinary system.

TEACH & APPLY

The transparency "The Urinary System" (Figure 6–8) is provided in the Transparency Acetate Binder.

DISCUSSION

Have students compare how protected the kidneys and bladder are from injury and infection in relation to other organs. Discuss answers to these questions: Can one live without the kidneys? With one kidney? What problems might affect the bladder?

SECTION 7 — The Urinary System

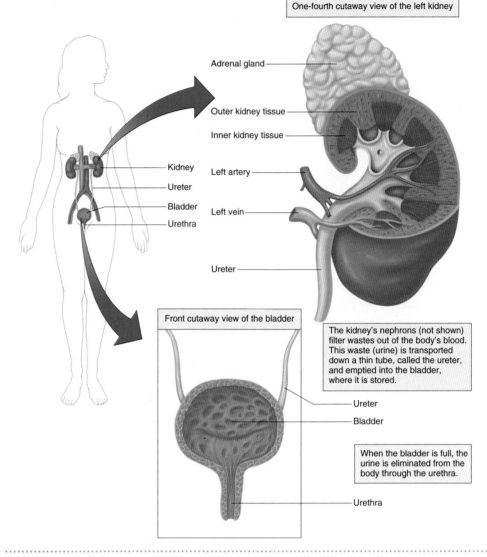

One-fourth cutaway view of the left kidney

Adrenal gland

Outer kidney tissue

Inner kidney tissue

Left artery

Left vein

Kidney

Ureter

Bladder

Urethra

Ureter

The kidney's nephrons (not shown) filter wastes out of the body's blood. This waste (urine) is transported down a thin tube, called the ureter, and emptied into the bladder, where it is stored.

Front cutaway view of the bladder

Ureter

Bladder

When the bladder is full, the urine is eliminated from the body through the urethra.

Urethra

Figure 6–8 *The Urinary System*

Chapter 6, Section 7

The following quiz will help you assess your students' understanding of the material covered in this section of the chapter. You might use the quiz as an oral exercise, which will lead into a class discussion of the topics covered. Or, you might use it as a paper/pencil quiz to evaluate your students individually.

Like the Quick Quiz, the Section Review can also be used as an assessment tool to spark class discussion or as an individual student evaluation. It can also be used as a review in preparation for this quiz.

1. The primary function of the urinary system is the task of waste removal from the blood. (True)

2. The kidneys are designed to monitor the

The task of waste removal from the blood is the specialty of the urinary system. Although this may seem unglamorous, it is absolutely essential to life. Without the careful monitoring of the blood's composition by the kidneys, toxic wastes would soon build up and interrupt functioning of all the body's tissues.

Among the first signs of kidney failure are confusion, inability to make judgments, and dizziness. Should the situation continue, the person would lose consciousness—pass out. These symptoms demonstrate the connection between the functions of the urinary system and the workings of the brain. The brain—and in fact all the body tissues—depends entirely on the correct composition of the blood, which the urinary system works to maintain.

How do the kidneys know what's inside the blood vessels?

The kidneys are designed perfectly for the job of monitoring the composition of the blood. They are made up of a million microscopic units, called nephrons. The nephrons draw fluid from the blood, but they leave the blood cells and large molecules inside the blood vessels. The fluid is then inside the kidneys' units, which detect and measure various substances. These measurements provide the kidneys with information about the condition of the blood.

Once informed of body conditions, the kidneys push some of the fluid—along with some minerals, blood sugar, and other useful substances—back into the blood. Some fluid, along with waste products, stays behind in the kidneys to become urine.

Of all the body's organs, second only to the brain, the kidneys are most like a master computer that controls conditions in the body. The number of measurements and fine adjustments they make, from moment to moment, is staggering.

How do the kidneys know how much water to put back into the blood, and how much to make into urine?

The water balance of the blood is important. If the kidneys take out too much water, this will dehydrate the body. If the kidneys put too much water back in, the tissues will swell. The kidneys have a partner that helps them to perform this balancing act—the

pituitary gland of the brain. This gland also monitors changes in the blood composition. When the water level begins to drop, the pituitary gland sends a hormone to the kidneys that tells them to conserve water.

The kidneys, on receiving this message, not only use less fluid to make urine but also respond with their own hormone that tells other tissues about the dehydration. One of the tissues that responds to this hormone is the brain, which then lets you know that you're thirsty. You then drink a glass of water to replenish the water in your blood.

Drinking too much fluid causes no problem to the body. The kidneys detect the excess and drain it out as urine. No matter how much water you drink in a day, your body water concentration stays the same, thanks to the skill of your kidneys.

How does the bladder know when to empty?

Urine formed in the kidneys carries the blood's waste products down the tubes, called ureters, that lead to the bladder. The bladder is the holding tank for urine.

The walls of the bladder are stretchy. They allow the bladder to expand as urine collects. When the bladder is full (this takes about 2 cups of urine), nerves in the bladder's walls, known as stretch receptors, inform the brain. The brain then arranges to urinate. On command from the brain, and under the person's control, a set of circular muscles at the opening of the urethra relaxes. Urine then flows through the urethra and out of the body.

Is the urinary system the same in men as in women?

Men and women have similar urinary systems, right up to the urethra. There, however, things change. The male urethra is three times as long as the female urethra. It conducts semen, as well as urine, out of the body. A special valve in the male urethra makes sure that the two functions never happen at the same time.

The female urethra is used for waste disposal only. Because of its short length, it is more prone to allow dangerous infectious bacteria to reach the bladder. Bladder infections thus are much more common among women than among men. Any infection of the urinary system should be treated immediately, before it has a chance to endanger the health of the kidneys.

acids in the stomach. (False)

3. Kidneys are made up of microscopic units called nephrons. (True)

4. Kidneys monitor the condition of the blood but do not collect harmful substances from the blood. (False)

5. The kidneys' functions are very simple. (False)

6. The kidneys work in harmony with the pituitary gland of the brain. (True)

7. Stretch receptors inform the brain of the need to urinate. (True)

8. The blood's waste products are known as ureters. (False)

9. The male urethra conducts semen as well as urine out of the body. (True)

10. Bladder infections are more common among men than among women. (False)

COMPREHENSION CHECK

Review with students the symptoms of kidney failure. These symptoms are probably very surprising to students. Ask them what they would have guessed to be symptoms of failure in the urinary system. Ask them what they would have guessed the symptoms given for kidney failure were associated with if they had been given the symptoms without being told what they indicated. How do these symptoms illustrate the connection between the functions of the urinary system and the workings of the brain? (The brain and all other body tissues depend on the urinary system to maintain the correct composition of the blood.) This should help them realize the importance of the urinary system. Ask students if they know anyone who has had a kidney transplant. What symptoms did they notice in this person prior to the transplant? Was the transplant successful?

ASSESS

EVALUATE

A reproducible quiz for Section 7 is provided in the Teacher's Resource Box.

CLOSE

Have students write a half-page essay that compares the kidneys to a filter or large net that monitors the composition of the blood.

The Respiratory System

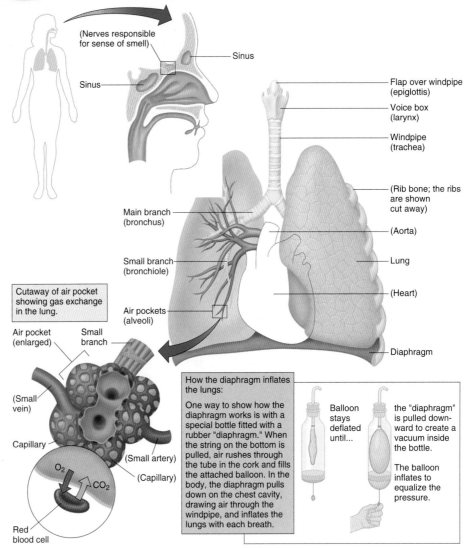

(Nerves responsible for sense of smell)

Sinus

Sinus

Flap over windpipe (epiglottis)

Voice box (larynx)

Windpipe (trachea)

(Rib bone; the ribs are shown cut away)

(Aorta)

Main branch (bronchus)

Lung

Small branch (bronchiole)

(Heart)

Air pockets (alveoli)

Diaphragm

Cutaway of air pocket showing gas exchange in the lung.

Air pocket (enlarged)   Small branch

(Small vein)

Capillary

(Small artery)

(Capillary)

O_2

CO_2

Red blood cell

How the diaphragm inflates the lungs:

One way to show how the diaphragm works is with a special bottle fitted with a rubber "diaphragm." When the string on the bottom is pulled, air rushes through the tube in the cork and fills the attached balloon. In the body, the diaphragm pulls down on the chest cavity, drawing air through the windpipe, and inflates the lungs with each breath.

Balloon stays deflated until...

the "diaphragm" is pulled downward to create a vacuum inside the bottle.

The balloon inflates to equalize the pressure.

Figure 6–9 *The Respiratory System*

SECTION 8

OUTCOMES

In this section students will learn:

1. That the respiratory system is responsible for delivering oxygen to all cells.

2. The functions and potential problems of the sinuses.

FOCUS ACTIVITY

Divide the class into groups. Have groups brainstorm all the organs involved in the respiratory system. The first group finished should write its list on the board. Other groups can then critique and correct this list.

TEACH & APPLY

TRANSPARENCIES

The transparency "The Respiratory System" (Figure 6–9) is provided in the Transparency Acetate Binder.

CLASS ACTIVITY

1. Have students sit upright and quiet for one minute. Have them count the number of breaths they take in one minute and compare the results with classmates.

2. Have them consciously breathe in and out and explain which muscles seem to be involved in inhalation and exhalation.

3. Discuss the benefits of breathing through the nose.

4. Explain what determines the rate of breathing.

148

QUICK QUIZ

Chapter 6, Section 8

The following quiz will help you assess your students' understanding of the material covered in this section of the chapter. You might use the quiz as an oral exercise, which will lead into a class discussion of the topics covered. Or, you might use it as a paper/pencil quiz to evaluate your students individually.

If students have difficulty with the concepts covered in the Quick Quiz and the Section Review, you might suggest they review the material using the **S***urvey,* **Q***uestion,* **R***ead,* **R***ecite,* **R***eview (SQ3R) study method, which is described in detail in the introduction to this Teacher's Wraparound Edition.*

1. Oxygen is a major waste product of the body. (False)

Every day, the lungs breathe in and out the amount of air in an average-size classroom. With each inhaled breath, the lungs pull from the surrounding atmosphere the oxygen that allows tissues to burn fuels for energy. On exhaling, the lungs return carbon dioxide to the air as the major waste product of the body's fuel use.

To say, as we just did, that the lungs breathe air in and out is not quite accurate. Lungs themselves possess no muscles to move air in and out of their chambers. Instead, the lungs rest like passive balloons within the chest cavity, inflating and deflating thanks to the work of the diaphragm and chest muscles.

When someone takes a breath, the curved diaphragm straightens and pulls downward, as shown in Figure 6–9. Muscles of the chest also pull the ribs outward. The combined effect is to enlarge the chest cavity. As a result, air rushes into the lungs through the only available opening—the windpipe: you inhale. When the diaphragm and chest muscles relax, air flows out of the lungs as the vacuum is released: you exhale. Thanks to this action, life-giving oxygen can be transferred from the surrounding air to the tissues that require it.

What determines how fast I breathe?

The same thing that determines how fast your heart beats—a brain center that measures your need for oxygen—also determines how fast you breathe. It can tell, from the amount of carbon dioxide in your blood, how fast you need to exchange that gas for oxygen in your lungs. Naturally, it is hard muscular work that creates this need, because muscles burn fuel as they work, and they need oxygen to do it.

Is it true that it is better to breathe through your nose than through your mouth?

The nose is superbly designed for breathing. While the mouth simply pulls air directly from the environment into the lungs, the nose acts as a filter and air conditioner. Nose hairs are the first line of defense against debris entering the lungs. The stiff hairs purify the air of most of the large particles it contains, such as dust or fibers. Any particles that get by this first barrier are likely to be forcefully expelled when they trigger the sneeze reflex. If tiny particles pass by these two defenses, they still must flow over the mucus-coated membranes lining the nasal passageway. Bacteria and other microscopic bits that fall into the mucus produced there are trapped, killed, and swept out into the throat by millions of tiny waving hairs that act as brooms. The mucus and its contents are swallowed. In the stomach, they are destroyed by acids and digestive enzymes.

In addition to filtering the air, the nasal passageways also warm it and add moisture. This protects the lungs from cold or dry air, which could injure the delicate lung tissue. While the mouth is superior for speaking and eating, the nose is indeed the organ of choice for breathing.

What are the sinuses, and why do they cause some people trouble?

Your skull contains eight air spaces—holes in your head, so to speak. The function of these sinuses is to lighten the weight of the skull. They also play a role in creating the sound of the voice as sound waves resonate inside them. The sinuses are located in the facial area—behind the nose, over the eyebrows, and in the cheek area.

The sinuses are lined with membranes that normally make a thick, cleansing liquid known as mucus, which drains into the throat. When infection or allergy causes the membranes to swell, though, the canals become blocked. Painful pressure can build up in the sinuses. This pressure can cause a severe headache. If infection from a cold settles into the sinuses, antibiotics may be needed to help the victim recover.

What is a hiccup?

A hiccup is an involuntary contraction of the diaphragm, caused by irritation. The sound is made when the sudden contraction of the diaphragm sucks air over the vocal cords. The cords then snap shut, cutting off the air flow and the sound.

How can you stop the hiccups?

Most people favor one or another hiccup remedy—drinking water, breathing into a paper bag, being startled. One cure backed by at least some scientific evidence calls for dissolving a teaspoon of sugar on the tongue and letting the sugar soothe the throat. If you cannot take the sugar cure for any reason, be assured that most bouts of hiccups resolve themselves in a few minutes. (Should your case last for a day or more, you may need a medical evaluation.)

2. The movement of the lungs draws oxygen into the body. (False)
3. Inhalation is the result of the action of the diaphragm and the muscles of the chest. (True)
4. Air enters the lungs through the windpipe. (True)
5. The lungs determine how fast you breathe. (False)
6. The nose's hair and mucus-coated membranes act as a filter which protects the lungs from foreign particles. (True)
7. The nasal passages cool air before it enters the lungs. (False)
8. The mouth is better adapted for breathing than the nose. (False)
9. Sinuses lighten the weight of the skull. (True)
10. A hiccup is an involuntary contraction of the sinuses. (False)

TRANSPARENCIES

The transparency "Delivery of Oxygen by the Heart and Lungs to the Muscles," provided in the Transparency Acetate Binder, will help your students better understand how oxygen is delivered to the body simultaneously with the removal of carbon dioxide.

ASSESS

EVALUATE

1. Have students give a short summary on the muscles involved in inhalation and exhalation. (The diaphragm goes down, the chest muscles pull the ribs out to create a vacuum. The diaphragm and chest muscles relax and force air out of the lungs.)
2. Have students give two important roles of the sinus cavities. (The sinus cavities help lighten the weight of the skull and create the sound of the voice.)

WORKSHEETS

A reproducible quiz for Section 8 is provided in the Teacher's Resource Box.

CLOSE

Ask students to:

1. Locate and describe the major parts of the respiratory system.
2. State the functions of the sinuses.

149

SECTION 9

FOCUS

OUTCOMES

In this section students will learn:

1. The functions of the lymphatic system.
2. How the lymphatic system provides immunity.

FOCUS ACTIVITY

Ask students to explain why their glands swell when they are experiencing an illness.

TEACH & APPLY

The transparency "The Immune System" (Figure 6–10) is provided in the Transparency Acetate Binder.

GROUP ACTIVITY

Divide the class into groups. Have each group prepare a chart showing the similarities and differences between the lymphatic system and the circulatory system.

DISCUSSION

Ask students to share experiences they have had to support the theory that one can "think oneself well."

You may want to continue this discussion by telling students that common observations suggest that the mind does have an effect on disease development. People under mental stress come down with colds

SECTION 9   The Immune System

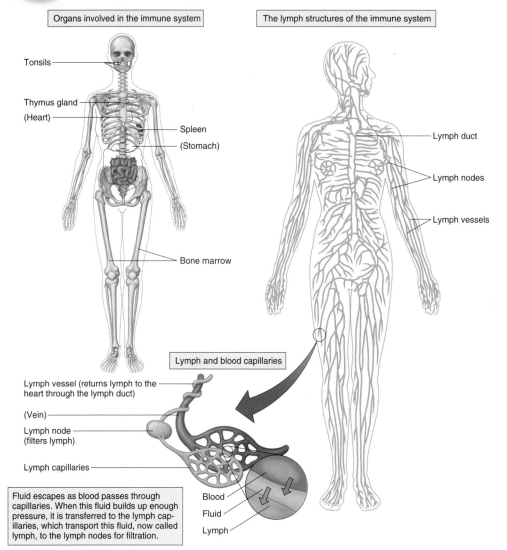

Figure 6–10 *The Immune System*

Chapter 6, Section 9

The following quiz will help you assess your students' understanding of the material covered in this section of the chapter. You might use the quiz as an oral exercise or, you might use it as a paper/pencil quiz to evaluate your students individually.

Like the Quick Quiz, the Section Review can also be used as an assessment tool to spark class discussion or as an individual student evaluation. It can also be used as a review in preparation for this quiz.

1. The immune system eliminates intruders in the body, including viruses, bacteria, and even diseased cells. (True)
2. The lymphatic system is similar to the cardiovascular system in that it moves

Each day, the immune system traps, kills, and eliminates many invaders in the body—bacteria, viruses, even cells that could start cancer. Immunity works because its special cells, described in Chapter 15, are busy everywhere in the body. Especially, they congregate in areas where invaders are likely to intrude, such as the throat, digestive tract, and reproductive organs. The lymphatic system is especially active in immunity.

What does the lymphatic system do?

The lymphatic system is similar to the cardiovascular system, in that it moves fluid around the body. This "second cardiovascular system" is important in many ways. It helps to clean the cells by carrying their wastes to the blood for removal by the kidneys. It helps to transport fats that have been absorbed from food in the digestive tract. Unlike blood, lymph does not always stay within its vessels. It can travel freely in the tissues.

An extremely important function of the lymphatic system concerns immunity. The lymph nodes—the structures resembling strung pearls in Figure 6–10—act as filters to remove bacteria from the body. Other lymph tissues also help to produce the body's fighting force of white blood cells that travel throughout the tissues, searching for invaders to destroy.

What good is the thymus gland?

The thymus gland is critical to immunity, especially in infancy, when it is responsible for the development of the immune system. As people age, the thymus shrinks in size. However, it still plays important roles in developing the white blood cells.

Certain white cells, the T cells, are named for the thymus, because they first become functional when they pass through there. White cells are first made by the bone marrow and released in an immature state. They fully develop when they are taken up by other tissues that give them their special functions.

What does the spleen do?

The spleen is a spongy organ that filters blood much as the lymph nodes do. In addition, the spleen destroys old, worn-out red cells. The spleen's spongy structure allows it to act as a sort of reserve for the blood supply. If the body needs more blood to carry oxygen to the tissues, the spleen contracts and squeezes blood from its chambers into the bloodstream. Still another talent of the spleen—if the bone marrow becomes unable to produce red blood cells, the spleen can take over this function.

Does the heart pump the lymph around the body?

The heart indirectly moves the lymph, through the action of the blood pressure. However, the heart doesn't pump lymph directly, as it pumps blood. Large lymph vessels have valves that keep lymph from flowing backward. The movement of body muscles helps to squeeze it on its way in the vessels.

Why do people with infections get "swollen glands"?

The swellings detectable at the juncture of the jaw and throat are really lymph nodes responding to infection. Nodes that are working extra hard cleaning up bacteria and fighting infection often become enlarged and painful to the touch. The swellings subside with the infection.

Can anything injure the immune system?

Yes, many things cause injury to the immune system. The virus that causes AIDS (see Chapter 16) is much feared because of its ability to completely disable the immune system of an infected person. Other illnesses can also injure the tissues of the system.

Nutrition also affects immune system tissues. The body's defenses are sensitive to nutrition status and are soon impaired when a person fails to eat a diet with adequate nutrients, even for a short time. This is why weight-loss dieting, poorly planned, can make a person sick. Another factor that depresses immune response is overexposure to ultraviolet radiation from the sun (sunburn).

Can your mental thoughts make the immune system work better?

A new field of psychology, psychoneuroimmunology, is dedicated to finding relationships between emotions, stress, depression, personality, and the physical immune response. Some people would like to believe that people can simply "think themselves well." However, the relationships between the mind's activity and diseases of the body are not clear.

more frequently than others. One study found that unhappy women had smaller numbers of certain immune cells than did women who reported themselves to be happy. The Chapter 4 Straight Talk, "Healing and the Placebo Effect," discusses the issue further.

ASSESS

EVALUATE

Write the following terms on the board and tell students to write the correct term as you read the sentences: lymphatic system, bacteria, disease, immunity, muscles, thymus, vessels, white.

1. The second circulatory system is the _____ _____. (lymphatic system)
2. Unlike blood, lymph does not need to travel in _____. (vessels)
3. Lymph nodes filter _____ out of the body. (bacteria)
4. The _____ gland is critical to immunity but gets smaller with age. (thymus)
5. _____ cells help fight disease. (White)
6. Lymph travels through the systems by the squeezing action of _____. (muscles)

A reproducible quiz for Section 9 is provided in the Teacher's Resource Box.

CLOSE

Ask students to:

1. Describe lymph.
2. Explain the actions of the white cells that attack bacteria and infections.
3. Name factors that negatively affect the immune system.

fluid around the body. (True)
3. Lymph, like blood, always remains within its vessels, and cannot travel freely about the tissues. (False)
4. Lymph nodes act as filters which remove bacteria from the body. (True)
5. The thymus gland is extremely important in the development of the immune system and in the development of certain white blood cells. (True)
6. The spleen's normal function is to produce red blood cells. (False)
7. The heart directly pumps the lymph around the body. (False)
8. "Swollen glands" are really lymph nodes that have become enlarged due to the effort of fighting infection. (True)
9. The immune system is vulnerable to numerous viruses and illnesses, and can be weakened by poor nutrition. (True)
10. Psychoneuroimmunology is a proven science. (False)

SECTION 10

FOCUS

OUTCOMES

In this section students will learn:

1. How the hormonal system, or endocrine system, operates as a communication system in the body.

2. That hormones can affect growth, basic metabolic rate, and an individual's mood.

FOCUS ACTIVITY

On a diagram of the human body, have students locate the major endocrine glands and discuss the function of each gland.

TEACH & APPLY

The transparency "The Hormonal System" (Figure 6–11) is provided in the Transparency Acetate Binder.

DISCUSSION

Discuss with students how the hormonal system differs from the nervous system even though both are communication systems.

GROUP PROJECT

Divide the class into seven groups. Assign each group a gland to research and report on. Students should be able to locate the gland, define its function, describe what would happen without the gland, and tell what systems of the body would be affected.

SECTION 10 The Hormonal System

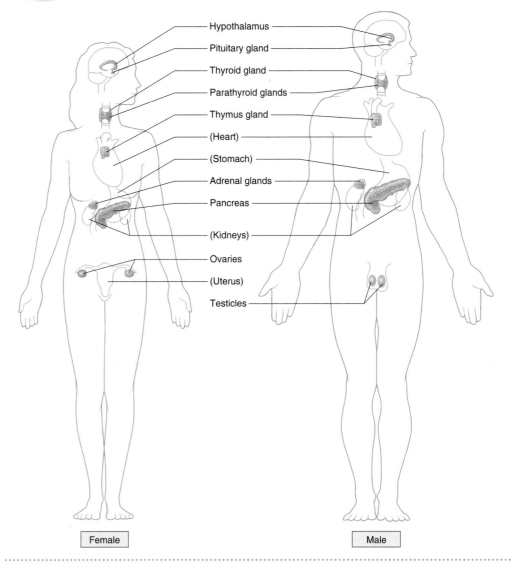

Figure 6–11 The Hormonal System

Chapter 6, Section 10

The following quiz will help you assess your students' understanding of the material covered in this section of the chapter. You might use the quiz as an oral exercise, which will lead into a class discussion of the topics covered. Or, you might use it as a paper/pencil quiz to evaluate your students individually.

Like the Quick Quiz, the Section Review can also be used as an assessment tool to spark class discussion or as an individual student evaluation. It can also be used as a review in preparation for this quiz.

1. The function of the hormonal system is to coordinate body functions by sending and receiving chemical messages. (True)

2. Only a hormone's target organ can

The body has yet another communication system—the hormonal, or endocrine, system. Like the nervous system, it coordinates body functions by sending and receiving messages. Instead of the impulses of the nervous system, which are electrical, the messages of the hormonal system are chemical—hormones released into the bloodstream. Over a hundred hormones are known.

When a gland of the hormonal system releases a hormone, it travels everywhere in the body. However, only the hormone's target organ can respond to it. The target organ is equipped with structures to receive the hormone, and to act in response to it. A message sent along a nerve is like a conversation that travels along a phone wire (the nerve fibers) through a central switchboard (the brain and spinal cord) to one listener. A hormonal message is like a radio talk show broadcast on the airways (the bloodstream). Any organ with the right receiver can pick it up.

What functions do hormones control?

Not all the functions of the many hormones are known. One well-known one is the growth-stimulating effect in children of human growth hormone (HGH). The brain's pituitary gland makes HGH. This hormone then stimulates other glands to make their own hormones. This second fleet of hormones acts on tissues such as the bones and muscles, rebuilding them into more and more adult forms. Later in life, after growth is complete, HGH remains an important regulator of the body's use of protein, as well as its use and storage of fat and carbohydrate.

Does HGH cause young teenagers to grow extra fast?

Growth hormone is produced at a more or less steady rate through the growing years. Another set of hormones, however, comes into play at about age 11 or 12—the sex hormones. During the teen years, these hormones act on the growing parts of the body and give growth an extra boost—the adolescent growth spurt. They are also responsible for the development of body hair, the maturation of the reproductive and genital organs, and many other characteristics associated with being male or female.

What would happen if a man or a woman started producing

the hormones of the opposite gender?

Years ago, the sex hormones were assumed to be exclusively male or female. However, now scientists know that men normally produce some "female" hormones, and normal women produce some "male" hormones. Male hormones in females are known to stimulate the normal growth of body hair. Female hormones in males help to maintain the appropriate percentage of body fat.

Do thyroid problems make people gain or lose body fat?

The thyroid gland, at the front of the throat, produces thyroxine, a hormone that regulates the use of fuel in the body. Thyroxine is essential both to feeling energetic and to the maintenance of normal body weight. Feelings of energy can reflect the body's basal metabolic rate (basal energy needs are discussed in Chapter 8). When the thyroid produces too little thyroxine, the person feels tired out most of the time. A person whose thyroxine level is just slightly above normal is more likely to feel nervous than extra energetic.

Theoretically, a person with low thyroxine could begin to gain weight if food intake were normal. However, most people with underactive thyroid glands have little appetite. They feel so sleepy and sluggish that they have no urge to prepare food or even to eat. The opposite condition, an overactive thyroid, causes an increased appetite, but an even greater increase in basal metabolic rate. The weight loss it causes is occasionally so extreme that the thyroid must be destroyed to save the person's life.

How do hormones affect mood?

Hormones may interact with the brain and affect how a person feels. When under stress, people feel hostile, irritable, or angry. These feelings may be related to the release of the stress hormones that make the body ready to fight. Experiments have shown that sex hormones also may partly determine a person's mood. For one thing, aggression is linked to male hormones in rats. For another, some researchers suspect that the ups and downs of female hormones within the menstrual cycle produce mood changes. Many women report feeling anxious or irritable a few days before menstruation, although a direct link to hormonal changes is yet to be proved.

respond to the hormone's message. (True)

3. Human growth hormone (HGH) causes teenagers to grow extra fast during puberty. (False)

4. Human growth hormone (HGH) becomes inactive during adulthood. (False)

5. The sex hormones are responsible for the development of secondary sexual characteristics. (True)

6. Males produce both "male" and "female" hormones. (True)

7. The thyroxine produced by the thyroid gland regulates the use of fuel in the body. (True)

8. A feeling of energy can indicate the body's basal metabolic rate (BMR). (True)

9. There is a proven, direct link between hormones and changes in mood. (False)

10. All the functions of hormones are known. (False).

FOCUS

OUTCOMES

In this section students will learn to:

1. Trace the path of an ovum.
2. Describe the functions of the female reproductive organ.

FOCUS ACTIVITY

Without the use of their books, have students generate a list of all the organs that make up the female reproductive system.

TEACH & APPLY

TRANSPARENCIES The transparency "The Female Reproductive System" (Figure 6–12) is provided in the Transparency Acetate Binder.

DISCUSSION

Discuss how the female reproductive system is protected as compared to the male reproductive system. Why is this important?

CLASS ACTIVITY

On a chart, trace the journey of an ovum from the ovaries to the vagina.

The Female Reproductive System

Front view of complete uterus side

This side has been cut away to show internal structures.

Fallopian tube

Uterus

Fallopian tube

Ovary

Fringe

Fringe

Ovary

Cervix

Vagina

Cutaway side view through the center of the body

Immature ova

Maturing ova

Fluid-filled pouch

Ruptured pouch with free ovum

Cutaway of ovary's internal structure

(Backbone)

Fallopian tube

Ovary

Uterus

Cervix

(Bladder, urinary)

Vagina

(Urethra)

Clitoris

Foreskin

The Menstrual Cycle

What's happening in the ovary

Immature ova | Ovum developing | Ovum released | Lining builds up | Bleeding or pregnancy

Days 1 2 3 4 5 6 7 8 9 10 11 12 13 14 15 16 17 18 19 20 21 22 23 24 25 26 27 28

Bleeding | Uterine wall starts to thicken

What's happening in the uterus

Figure 6–12 The Female Reproductive System

QUICK QUIZ

Chapter 6, Section 11

The following quiz will help you assess your students' understanding of the material covered in this section of the chapter. You might use the quiz as an oral exercise, which will lead into a class discussion of the topics covered. Or, you might use it as a paper/pencil

quiz to evaluate your students individually.

Like the Quick Quiz, the Section Review can also be used as an assessment tool to spark class discussion or as an individual student evaluation. It can also be used as a review in preparation for this quiz.

1. The female reproductive cell is called the ovum. (True)
2. The ovaries don't produce the female reproductive cell; they are present in the

The female reproductive system produces the female reproductive cells, the ova. It also supports each fertilized ovum from the beginning of pregnancy through birth. Starting from the ovaries, the ova travel by way of the fallopian tubes to the uterus and vagina.

Each month, one or the other of the ovaries releases one ovum. The monthly timing of this event is governed by the rise and fall in levels of the female sex hormones. This cyclic ebb and flow is described fully in Chapter 20, pages 551 to 552.

How do the ovaries produce ova?

Although the ovaries ripen and release the ova, they don't really make any new ones. All of the cells that will ever become ova are present in the ovaries at birth. A baby girl holds approximately one-half million of the immature ova in her ovaries. When she reaches age 12, only a quarter or so of those ova remain alive in her ovaries. At about the midpoint of each monthly cycle, through all her reproductive life, she releases one of the ova.

Each ovum starts out as an immature cell and is "ripened" by the ovary in a series of stages. The ovary houses the ovum in a small pouch of fluid that develops in stages and ruptures to release the ovum when it's ready. The beating fringe on the end of the ovary sweeps the ready ovum into the major tube of the female system, the fallopian tube.

What does an ovum look like?

An ovum is a large cell, about the size of the period at the end of this sentence. The ova pictured in Figure 6–12 have been greatly enlarged. Ova are like all cells, with one important exception: they possess only half the normal amount of genetic material. Male sperm cells also contain only half the regular amount of genetic material. When the ovum and sperm unite, they form a single cell that possesses a complete set of genetic material (both halves) and is unique in its makeup.

Where does an ovum become fertilized?

On being swept up by the gentle, beating fingers at the end of a fallopian tube, the ovum starts a journey. Once in the tube, the ovum may meet sperm that are swimming up from the vagina. The sperm may have been waiting there for a day or two for the ovum. Whether or not sperm are present, the ovum travels through the fallopian tube to the uterus. Unfertilized ova and some fertilized ones just keep on traveling through the cervix and out of the vagina, undetected. Frequently, though, a fertilized ovum will end its travels in the uterus, where it attaches to the wall lining and begins a pregnancy.

What is menstruation?

Each month, the uterus prepares itself to support a pregnancy. It does so by enriching its lining with tissue that can supply blood to a developing ovum that might implant there. If no ovum implants, the uterus sheds its lining by way of menstruation, a period of bleeding that lasts about four to seven days. The 28-day cycle shown in Figure 6–12 is typical. However, cycle lengths vary among individuals, and even in the same woman from time to time.

How does an infant fit through the vagina to be born?

The vagina is very elastic, from the point where it connects to the uterus at the cervix, to the outside of the body. At the time of childbirth, hormones make the vaginal walls especially able to stretch. As the baby's head passes through the cervix, the vagina expands to form a passageway large enough for an infant.

What is a hymen?

In many, but not all, young girls, the vaginal opening is partly or entirely covered by a thin membrane—the hymen. Later, through physical activity, tampon use, or sometimes by way of sexual intercourse, the membrane disintegrates.

What is a hysterectomy, and why might a woman need one?

Hysterectomy is the surgical removal of the uterus, and possibly the ovaries, which of course ends menstruation. As women age, they may develop tumors, severe menstrual problems, or other problems that require treatment by hysterectomy. So many women in this country undergo hysterectomy that some experts suspect that the procedure may be overused.

BACKGROUND INFORMATION

For enrichment, give students some information about the causes of infertility. The leading cause of female infertility is blocked fallopian tubes, resulting from such factors as pelvic inflammatory disease (PID), septic abortions, or abdominal surgery. The second leading cause is endometriosis. In this disease, uterine tissue grows outside the uterus, often appearing on the ovaries, fallopian tubes, and in the abdominal cavity. Why endometriosis causes infertility is not known. In addition to physical causes, there may be hormonal reasons why a woman is unable to conceive. As many as 20% of women with infertility problems have hormonal abnormalities. Finally, immunological causes may be present, the most significant of which is the production of sperm antibodies by the woman. Other factors are smoking and toxic chemicals.

ASSESS

EVALUATE

A reproducible quiz for Section 11 is provided in the Teacher's Resource Box.

CLOSE

Ask students to:

1. Describe the organs that transport the ova from the ovary to the vagina.
2. Relate menstruation to the cycle of time needed for the journey of the ova to the vagina.

ovaries at birth. (True)
3. The uterus is the major tube of the female reproductive system. (False)
4. Like all cells, an ovum possesses a normal amount of genetic material. (False)
5. The ovum travels through the fallopian tube to the uterus only if sperm are present. (False)
6. When an ovum becomes fertilized, it attaches itself to the lining of the uterus. (True)

7. After leaving the fallopian tube, unfertilized ova attach themselves to the uterus. (False)
8. Menstruation is the result of the uterus shedding a lining of tissue built up in preparation for pregnancy. (True)
9. The vaginal opening is always covered by a thin membrane called the hymen. (False)
10. Hysterectomy is the surgical removal of the uterus. (True)

SECTION
12

FOCUS

OUTCOMES

In this section students will learn to:

1. Identify the major organs of the male reproductive system and their functions.
2. Explain why the male reproductive organs are external to the body.
3. Describe the properties of semen and sperm.

FOCUS ACTIVITY

Without the use of their books, have students generate a list of all the organs that make up the male reproductive system.

TEACH & APPLY

The transparency "The Male Reproductive System" (Figure 6–13) is provided in the Teacher's Resource Box.

BACKGROUND INFORMATION

The primary causes of male infertility are low sperm count, a lack of sperm ability to move spontaneously, and blocked passageways. As with women, environmental factors may contribute to infertility. Increasing evidence suggests that toxic chemicals are responsible for decreased sperm counts in men and that smoking may reduce sperm counts.

SECTION **12** The Male Reproductive System

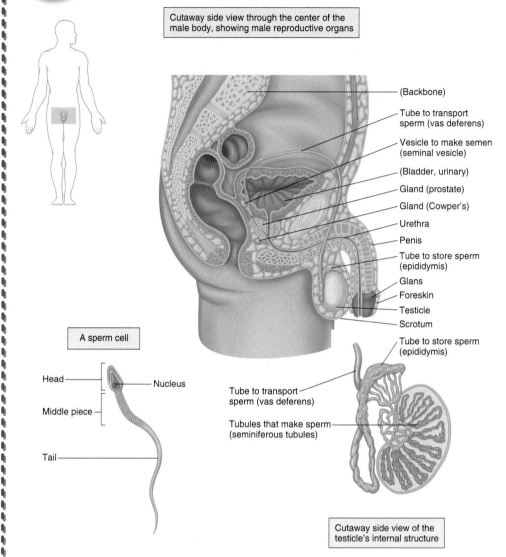

Cutaway side view through the center of the male body, showing male reproductive organs

(Backbone)
Tube to transport sperm (vas deferens)
Vesicle to make semen (seminal vesicle)
(Bladder, urinary)
Gland (prostate)
Gland (Cowper's)
Urethra
Penis
Tube to store sperm (epididymis)
Glans
Foreskin
Testicle
Scrotum
Tube to store sperm (epididymis)

A sperm cell
Head — Nucleus
Middle piece
Tail

Tube to transport sperm (vas deferens)
Tubules that make sperm (seminiferous tubules)

Cutaway side view of the testicle's internal structure

Figure 6–13 *The Male Reproductive System*

special needs

Spatial

This is a scientific vocabulary-intense chapter. To assist students in more fully comprehending the body so they can internalize the need to maintain physical health and fitness, this activity makes the anatomical terminology more concrete. It will especially help students with spatial or visual learning styles.

Have each student make a small (approximately 1" × 3") vocabulary card for the terms listed in the Chapter Review: aorta, appendix, artery, biceps, bladder, bone marrow, brain stem, cerebellum, cerebrum, cervix, cortex, diaphragm, endocrine gland, esophagus, femur, gastrocnemius, gluteus maximus, hamstrings, hypothalamus, kidney, large intestine, liver, lymph node, lymph vessels, mouth, ovaries, pancreas, pectorals, pelvis, phalanges, pituitary, pulmonary veins,

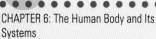

The male reproductive system is made up of a series of organs connected by tubes that lead out of the body through the penis. The entire unit is designed to continually produce, store, and deliver male reproductive cells to fertilize an ovum. In the male system, most organs, such as the penis and testicles, are external to the body. Most of the transportation route is within the abdominal cavity.

Why are the testicles outside the body?

The testicles are the only human organs able to produce male reproductive cells. Thus it seems surprising that they are located outside the protection of the abdominal cavity. Their location serves an important function, though—temperature regulation.

Sperm production requires a temperature 3 or 4 degrees Fahrenheit lower than normal body temperature. If the testicles were inside the abdomen, the heat of the internal body would bring sperm production to a halt. The scrotum, the tough sac of muscle and skin that contains the testicles, maintains the right temperature. When the testicles become too cool, the scrotum contracts by reflex action to bring them close to the body to warm them with body heat. When the temperature is right, the scrotum relaxes once again. This allows the testicles to drop away from the body.

Men should be aware that anything that holds the testicles too close to the body can interfere with sperm production. Even the wearing of tight pants is thought to interfere with the natural cooling of the testicles.

Where are the sperm produced, and how do they get to the penis?

The sperm are produced inside each testicle by thousands of tiny tubes that make millions of sperm cells each day. These tubes lead to another structure packed with yards of tubing whose function it is to store sperm until it is needed. Many other tubes, one leading to another, wind through the lower abdominal cavity and lead ultimately to the urethra, the passageway through which both sperm (in semen) and urine leave the body.

What is semen?

Semen is a thick mixture of fluids that carry the sperm from the male body. The fluids are produced by several glands. Semen helps to neutralize the normal acid from urine in the male urethra. This is important, because acid kills sperm. The vagina may also be slightly acidic, and seminal fluids neutralize this acid as well. Muscular contractions (ejaculation) propel semen out of the body.

Can sperm really swim?

Sperm are beautifully designed for movement in fluid. As you can see in Figure 6–13, their long, whipping tails make them look something like tadpoles when they are viewed under a microscope. Of course, sperm are as small as bacteria and so are much too small to be seen with the naked eye. Three or four million of them are present in each ejaculation. However, just one sperm fertilizes an ovum.

What is the prostate gland, and why does it cause trouble for older men?

The prostate is one of the glands of the male reproductive system. The urethra, which carries both semen and urine, runs through the prostate. Occasionally, disease of the prostate partly blocks off the urethra, making urination and sexual activity difficult. Around age 50, many men develop enlarged prostate glands. This may lead to bladder and kidney trouble unless the prostate is surgically reduced in size.

Prostate gland enlargement can indicate a risk of cancer. It is important for older men to have periodic checkups to make sure that their reproductive organs are healthy (see Chapter 17).

What is circumcision, and is it medically useful?

A covering of skin, the foreskin, folds over the glans of the penis at birth. Circumcision, the surgical removal of the foreskin, originated in ancient religions and is still meaningful for some. Most boys born in the United States are circumcised soon after birth.

An uncircumcised penis requires extra cleaning under the foreskin during bathing. It is thought that a buildup of bacteria and matter that can collect there may increase the risks of infections and cancer in older uncircumcised men. Some physicians recommend circumcision to reduce the risks of these conditions. Others say that the risks are small, that cleaning is easy, and that circumcision should be performed only if the parents request it—not as a routine procedure.

---

quadriceps, radius, rectum, right atrium, scrotum, sinus, small intestine, spleen, stomach, testicle, thymus gland, thyroid gland, tibia, triceps, ulna, ureter, urethra, uterus, vagina, vas deferens, vein, ventricle, voice box, windpipe

Then, using a 3–D model of the human body (you may need to borrow one from the science department), give each student an opportunity to place the cards on the corresponding location on the model. Have students keep track of terms they are not sure of,

as you may want to have them retry those terms later until mastery has been achieved.

An optional practice, or if a human-body model is not available, would be to have students work with a same-gender partner and tape the cards to the corresponding location of the body (except those pertaining to reproductive organs). For study at home, you may want to provide an illustration for students to identify and label.

DISCUSSION

Discuss the advantages and disadvantages of the location of the male reproductive system outside the body. Then have students write down the major organs of the male reproductive system and locate and describe each.

GROUP ACTIVITY

Have students describe the characteristics of a sperm cell. Then have them work in pairs to list some problems associated with the male reproductive system.

Reproducible Study Outline and Reading Cloze worksheets for Chapter 6 are provided in the Teacher's Resource Box.

Reproducible Chapter Tests A and B are also provided in the Teacher's Resource Box.

ASSESS

EVALUATE

A reproducible quiz for Section 12 is provided in the Teacher's Resource Box.

CLOSE

Ask students to:

1. Name and describe the organs of the male reproductive system.
2. Identify both differences and similarities between the male and female reproductive systems.

ANSWERS TO CHAPTER 6 REVIEW VOCABULARY

1. **a.** radius **b.** femur
   c. pelvis **d.** phalanges
   e. cerebrum **f.** right atrium
   g. aorta **h.** aorta **i.** kidneys
   j. rectum **k.** scrotum
2. **a.** triceps **b.** gastrocnemius
   c. pectorals **d.** gluteus
   maximus **e.** testicle **f.** pulmonary vein **g.** bladder
3. **a.** spleen **b.** veins
   c. lymph vessels **d.** thymus **e.** lymph nodes
   f. large intestines
   g. endocrine **h.** pituitary
   i. thyroid **j.** pancreas
   k. scrotum **l.** vas deferens

RECALL

SECTION 2

1. determine the body's shape, protect soft vital organs, store minerals and vitamins, manufacture all the body's blood cells (p. 137)

SECTION 3

2. voluntary, involuntary, and mixed, which are the muscles of the heart (p. 139)

SECTION 4

3. It consists of nerves that connect the brain to all parts of the body and provides the body's main communication line. (p. 141)
4. *cortex*—conscious thoughts take place; *cerebellum*—maintains balance and directs muscle activities; *brain stem*—controls breathing and basic functions (p. 141)
5. controls the environment inside the brain; admits those chemicals the brain needs, but excludes those that could interrupt the brain's work. (p. 141)

CHAPTER 6 Review

Summarizing the Chapter

Your ability to respond correctly to the following statements ensures your understanding of the main concepts in the chapter.

1. Differentiate among cells, tissues, organs, and systems.
2. Describe the importance of muscles and bones.
3. Identify the brain and spinal cord as the primary organs of the central nervous system.
4. Explain how the brain's numerous functions are divided among its many physical parts.
5. Describe how the digestive system breaks down food particles.
6. Identify the cardiovascular system as the transportation system of the body.
7. Compare the endocrine (hormonal) system to a communication system.
8. Identify the male and female reproductive organs responsible for uniting an ovum and a sperm.

Learning the Vocabulary

Use the illustrations, the information you learned in this chapter, and the glossary at the end of the book to complete the exercises below.

1. In each group one choice does not belong. List the one that doesn't belong and explain your answer.
   a. radius, hamstrings, triceps, quadriceps, biceps
   b. cerebrum, cerebellum, femur, cortex, brain stem
   c. pancreas, appendix, esophagus, pelvis, liver
   d. aorta, phalanges, ventricle, vein, artery
   e. ureter, bladder, kidney, cerebrum, urethra
   f. radius, ulna, phalanges, tibia, right atrium
   g. voice box, aorta, windpipe, sinus, diaphragm

h. aorta, lymph node, thymus gland, bone marrow, spleen
i. mouth, kidneys, esophagus, stomach, small intestine
j. ovaries, rectum, thyroid gland, hypothalamus, thymus gland
k. scrotum, cervix, uterus, vagina, ovary

2. Fill in the blank with one of the following terms: *pulmonary veins, pectorals, triceps, bladder, testicle, gluteus maximus, gastrocnemius.*
   a. The quadriceps muscle is opposite the hamstrings and the biceps muscle is opposite the _____.
   b. The gluteus maximus is the major muscle of the buttocks and the _____ is the major muscle of the calf of the lower leg.
   c. The trapezius is opposite the _____.
   d. The _____ is the biggest muscle in the body.
   e. The ovary serves the female as the _____ serves the male.
   f. The inferior and superior vena cava attach to the right atrium and the _____ attach to the left atrium.
   g. The rectum is the organ of elimination for the digestive system and the _____ is the organ of elimination for the urinary system.

3. *Matching*—Match each of the following phrases with one of the following terms: *lymph vessels, pituitary, pancreas, spleen, thymus, veins, large intestines, thyroid, endocrine, lymph nodes, scrotum, vas deferens.*
   a. filters blood to remove old blood cells
   b. vessels that carry used blood to the heart
   c. vessels that contain lymph nodes
   d. a gland at the base of the throat
   e. act as filters to remove bacteria from the body
   f. responsible for absorption of water and minerals
   g. another name for hormonal system
   h. the gland that makes HGH
   i. regulates the use of fuel in the body
   j. secretes insulin
   k. double pouch that contains testicles in males
   l. tube that transports sperm

6. A reflex is a sort of intentional short circuit. The nerves that control reflexes form an arc from tissue to spinal cord and back to tissue. (p. 141)

SECTION 5

7. *indigestion*—spicy foods irritate the lining, too much fat, or too much air, food or liquid is swallowed; *heartburn*—mixture of acid and food in the stomach irri-

tates the lining of the esophagus; *appendicitis*—particles lodge in the appendix and cause an infection (p. 143)

SECTION 6

8. The cardiovascular system, because each cell in the body depends on it. Cells dump their waste into it and pull all the nutrients and chemicals they need to live and function from it. (p. 145)

Recalling Important Facts and Ideas

Section 2
1. List some functions of the living structures we know as bones.

Section 3
2. Name three types of muscles present in the body.

Section 4
3. Describe the spinal cord and its part in the central nervous system.
4. Identify the physical parts of the brain and their functions.
5. What is the blood-brain barrier and why is it important?
6. How does a reflex action work?

Section 5
7. List three disorders of the digestive system and their causes.

Section 6
8. Which system is classified as the "transportation system" of the body and why?
9. When does the heart rest and what happens during these periods?
10. What is the function of the blood platelets?

Section 7
11. Name the organs and the systems that work together to cleanse the blood by removing wastes from the cells.
12. Describe how the kidneys act as a filter and tell what is filtered.
13. Which organs help monitor the amount of water in the blood?
14. Why are women more prone to urinary infections than men?

Section 8
15. Why is the nose the preferred organ of breathing?
16. List two functions of our sinuses.
17. List some remedies to stop hiccups.

Section 9
18. Why is the lymphatic system called the second circulatory system?
19. Why is damage to the spleen a serious injury?
20. What can you do to keep your immune system healthy?

Section 10
21. Explain how the hormonal system works as a communication system.
22. Name three hormones in the body and describe what they do.

Section 11
23. Trace the path of an egg from the ovary to the uterus.

Section 12
24. Why aren't the testicles located inside the body?

Critical Thinking

1. Many people who are hospitalized with heart complications or other infections die, not of heart failure, but of kidney failure. Why does this happen?
2. Even as a young girl, a female should maintain a healthy lifestyle to protect her future children. Why can her actions in her early life affect her children?

Activities

1. Take your pulse for 15 seconds and then multiply it by 4. This is your resting pulse rate. Then do two minutes of continuous exercise. Retake your pulse. Compare the two readings. What is the difference? Retake your pulse every minute until it returns to the resting rate. How long did it take to get back to normal? Compare your results with those of another person in your class. Whose pulse returned to resting rate more quickly?
2. Pick a partner in your class to check your lung capacity. Inhale as deeply as you can and then exhale into a balloon. Compare results with your partner. Which one of you has the larger lung capacity?
3. Read the following statement, "We cannot live life without taking some risks." Do you agree or disagree with this statement? Give reasons for your answer. What are some of the risks people take each day? What body systems are affected by these risks?

Making Decisions about Health

1. Discuss the subject of organ transplants as a method of prolonging life or curing disease. What organs are most likely to be needed?

---

9. between contractions; the relaxed heart muscles allow blood to fill the heart's chambers (p. 145)
10. They form a net which traps more platelets and other cells to form a clot so a wound can heal. (p. 145)

SECTION 7

11. cardiovascular system, the liver, digestive system, the lungs, and the urinary system (p. 147)
12. The nephrons in the kidney draw fluid from the blood. The kidney then detects and measures the substances in the fluid to obtain information about the blood. The kidneys push minerals, blood sugar, and useful substances back into the blood, while some fluids along with waste become urine. (p. 147)
13. kidneys (p. 147)
14. short length of the urethra allows bacteria to reach the bladder (p. 147)

SECTION 8

15. It acts as a filter and air conditioner. (p. 149)
16. lighten the weight of the skull, create the sound of the voice as sound waves resonate inside them (p. 149)
17. drinking water, breathing into a paper bag, being startled (p. 149)

SECTION 9

18. It moves the fluid around the body by cleansing cells, carrying wastes, and transporting fat. (p. 151)
19. The spleen filters blood, destroys all worn out red cells, and if bone marrow is unable to produce red blood cells, it can take over this job. (p. 151)
20. Eat a diet with adequate nutrients, avoid overexposure to ultraviolet radiation. (p. 151)

SECTION 10

21. It sends and receives messages—the messages are chemical hormones released into the bloodstream. (p. 153)
22. *HGH*—human growth; *sex hormones; thyroxine* (p. 153)

SECTION 11

23. egg travels through the fallopian tube to the uterus (p. 155)

SECTION 12

24. If the testicles were inside, the heat of the internal body would stop sperm production. (p. 157)

KEY POINTS

Chapter 7 is 40 pages long and divided into the 8 sections listed below. This chapter introduces students to the six nutrients the body requires and the ways in which the body uses food to produce energy. The chapter also provides knowledge to assist the students in daily food choices. Students will study carbohydrates, fats, proteins, vitamins, and minerals, and will analyze their existing eating patterns and compare what they eat to national guidelines. They will have the opportunity to make diet changes to meet the recommended amounts of each nutrient.

ACTIVITY TO INTRODUCE THE CHAPTER

Write the following statement on the board or an overhead transparency. "A body must be well nourished to be healthy and beautiful." Ask students to answer these questions: What kinds of foods do you eat that contribute to a healthy, beautiful body? What kinds of foods do you eat that do not contribute to a healthy, beautiful body?

BULLETIN BOARD IDEAS

Have students create a report on a diet tip to make a person's diet more healthy. The report should focus on something that people can do to improve the quality of foods they eat and persuasive arguments in favor of adopting this healthy eating habit. Take a vote in class on the four or five best tips to a better diet and put these up on the bulletin board under the title, "Fine Tune Your Diet."

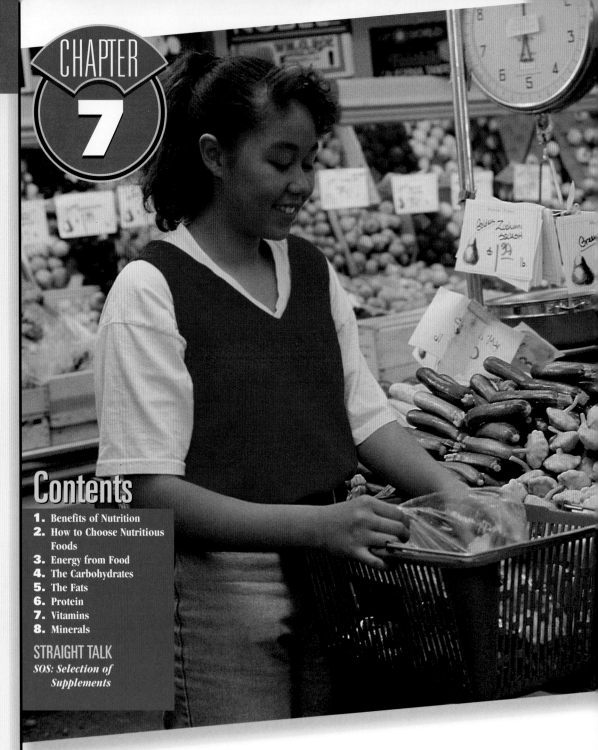

CHAPTER 7

Contents

STRAIGHT TALK
SOS: Selection of Supplements

NOT Enough Time?

Following are some suggestions to help you make sure that you cover the key topics in this chapter if you have limited time. (Refer to the daily lesson plans in your Teacher's Resource Box for additional suggestions.)

DAY 1   Assign students to read Sections 1 and 2 prior to class. Do the Activity to

Introduce the Chapter on page 160, followed by the Evaluate assessment on page 163 and the Focus Activity on page 164. If time allows, do the Class Activity on page 168. Assign Sections 3 and 4 for homework.

DAY 2   Discuss Section 3. Have students write down what they ate the day before. Then do the Focus Activity on page 171 and the Evaluate activity on page 173. Lead the

Nutrition: The Nutrients

What do you think? Are the following statements true or false? If you think they are false, then say what is true.

1. To be well nourished is simply a matter of eating foods with enough of the right nutrients.
2. Honey and sugar are the same, as far as the body is concerned.
3. Of all the things in foods that cause diseases, sugar is probably the biggest troublemaker.
4. A teaspoon of fat has more than twice the calories of a teaspoon of sugar.
5. To be sure to get enough protein, you must eat meat.
6. Vitamin supplements can be useful in treating many diseases.
7. As far as nutrients are concerned, the more, the better.
8. The best dietary measure against cancer is to take antioxidant vitamin pills each day.
9. Most people easily get enough calcium, because it is found in so many foods.
10. Electrolytes are dissolved minerals that carry electrical charges.

(Answers on page 192)

Introduction

You choose to eat a meal about 1,000 times a year. You will choose when to eat, what to eat, and how much to eat, about 65,000 times in your lifetime (if you live to be 65). You will consume about 50 tons of food. Each day's intake of **nutrients** may affect your body only slightly. Over a period of years, though, the effects of those intakes will build up. This is why it's important for you to learn now to make wise food choices.

Answers to FACT or FICTION

1. **False.** Eating foods with enough nutrients is important, but equally important is to keep from eating too much or too little food.
2. **True.**
3. **False.** Of all the things in foods that cause diseases, fat is by far the biggest culprit.
4. **True.**
5. **False.** You can easily get enough protein from grains, beans, vegetables, milk, and eggs without eating any meat.
6. **False.** The only disease that a vitamin supplement will cure is the one caused by a deficiency of that vitamin.
7. **False.** All of the vitamins and minerals can be toxic in large amounts.
8. **False.** The best dietary measure against cancer is to consume at least five servings of vitamin-rich fruits and vegetables each day.
9. **False.** Low intakes of calcium are common, because few foods contain it in large amounts.
10. **True.**

FAST FACTS

The average American consumes 130 pounds of fat per year. This amount of fat would be equal to eating more than one full stick of butter each day.

class in the Discussion suggested on page 175. Assign Sections 5 and 6 for homework.

DAY 3   Open the class period with the Focus Activity on page 178, followed by the Comprehension Check on page 179. Close with the Evaluate assessment on page 184. Assign Sections 7 and 8 for homework.

DAY 4   Open with the Focus Activity on page 185, followed by the Comprehension Check on the same page. Have students do the Group Activity on page 187 for both vitamins and minerals. Have students complete the Chapter Review on pages 198–199.

SECTION 1

FOCUS

OUTCOMES

In this section students will learn:

1. To identify the benefits of nutrition.
2. The six Dietary Guidelines for Americans.

FOCUS ACTIVITY

Have students study the Health Strategies "Dietary Guidelines for Americans" on this page. Have them think about the last three meals they have eaten. Now ask them to evaluate those meals based on these guidelines. Discuss their results.

TEACH & APPLY

COMPREHENSION CHECK

You may want to make sure that students understand the several different forms of the word *nutrition*. Write *nutrition, nutrients, well nourished,* and *nourishing* on the board. As a class, develop definitions for each word, then have students write sentences using each word.

Vocabulary worksheets are provided in the Teacher's Resource Box.

SECTION 1

> **❝** *Thou shouldst eat to live, not live to eat.* **❞**
>
> Cicero (1067–43 B.C.)
> Roman statesman,
> orator, and author

Health Strategies

Dietary Guidelines for Americans*

1. Eat a variety of foods.
2. Balance the food you eat with physical activity—maintain or improve your weight.
3. Choose a diet with plenty of grain products, vegetables, and fruits.
4. Choose a diet low in fat, saturated fat, and cholesterol.
5. Choose a diet moderate in sugars.
6. Choose a diet moderate in salt and sodium.

*The guidelines also make the recommendation that children and teenagers, among others, should not drink alcohol. Adults who do drink should limit their intake of alcohol to one or two drinks a day.

Benefits of Nutrition

Good nutrition helps make people's bodies strong, fit, and healthy—in short, beautiful. Bodies are beautiful in many different ways. Some people are tall, some short. Some have dark skin, some are fair. Some have curly hair, some have straight hair. Whatever your body is like, one thing is true: to be its most beautiful, it must be well nourished. Adequate intakes of all the nutrients underlie the health of your complexion, the straightness of your bones, the shape and strength of your muscles, and the gleam in your eye.

The Best Food for You   Your body is growing and renewing its parts all the time. Each day it adds a little to its tissues as you gain height and strength. It also replaces some old muscle, bone, skin, and blood with new tissues. In this way some of the food you eat today becomes part of "you" tomorrow. The best food for you, then, is the kind that supports normal growth and maintains strong muscles, sound bones, healthy skin, and enough blood to cleanse and nourish all the parts of your body.

The best food also reduces your risks of developing illnesses later in life. Your food choices weave together with other lifestyle choices you make to either raise or lower your chances of becoming ill. You will learn more about the connections between your food choices and diseases in Chapters 8 and 17.

To manage your nutrition in your own best interest, you have to learn what foods to eat, since not all foods are equally nutritious. The Health Strategies section on this page, "Dietary Guidelines for Americans," presents some general dietary guidelines put forth by the government. Although these guidelines are written for adults, they also apply to teens, with one exception—the recommendations about fat. A teen who has trouble eating enough food to grow at the expected rate should not cut fat from the diet, because energy from fat can help promote growth.

The Problems of Overnutrition and Undernutrition Some people do not obtain enough nutrients from their food. They may develop **nutrient deficiencies** or other forms of **malnutrition**. Pregnant women, especially pregnant teens, are very sensitive to nutrient deficiencies. These deficiencies can slow the growth of their infants, both before and after birth. Adolescents and teens are also sensitive to deficiencies, because they are growing at astonishing rates. A person who does not receive proper nutrition during the teen years may never reach full height, because all of the nutrients are needed for growth. After the person reaches adulthood, growth stops, even if the diet is then excellent. All the groups of people just mentioned are most likely to suffer from **undernutrition**—that is, too few nutrients for health and growth.

Focusing ON Self-Esteem

How are shopping, self-esteem and peer groups related to teens? If you ask teens why they do something, buy something, or wear particular clothes, they are likely to say, "Because everyone else does" or "Because it's the thing to do right now." Early in the teen years

self-esteem is tied to the group decision. Older teens become better able to make independent judgments and choices.

Much of this need to fit in and be like everyone else is tied to what teens wear and eat. Ask students to consider the last time they made a purchase decision based on peer choice. Examples might include

• blue jeans

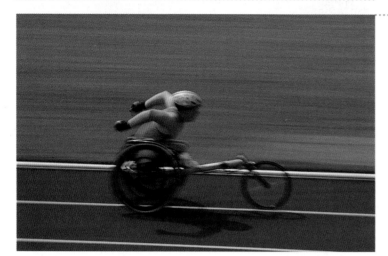

Sound nutrition helps make athletes strong and fit.

Another threat to people's health is **overnutrition**. Many people are overweight, or have daily intakes of salt, fat, cholesterol, and alcohol that may be too high for their hearts to remain healthy. Others eat too few vegetables and too much meat, choices linked to many diseases. Even vitamins and minerals can be poisonous if too many are taken in concentrated form. The key to good nutrition, then, is to eat foods that provide enough, but not too much, energy and nutrients.

 KEY POINTS *Good nutrition promotes growth and helps prevent diseases. Both undernutrition and overnutrition threaten health.*

SECTION 1 Review

Answer the following questions on a sheet of paper.

Learning the Vocabulary

The vocabulary terms in this section are *nutrients, nutrient deficiencies, malnutrition, undernutrition,* and *overnutrition.*

1. Write a sentence using each term.

2. Explain the difference between overnutrition and undernutrition.

Learning the Facts

3. List three benefits of good nutrition.

4. List the six Dietary Guidelines for Americans.

Making Life Choices

5. The food choices we make today influence our health in the future. Take a look at your diet, and guess what path your health may be likely to follow in the future.

MINI Glossary

nutrients: compounds in food that the body requires for proper growth, maintenance, and functioning.

nutrient deficiencies (dee-FISH-en-sees): too little of one or more nutrients in the diet; a form of malnutrition.

malnutrition: the results in the body of poor nutrition; undernutrition, overnutrition, or any nutrient deficiency.

undernutrition: too little food energy or too few nutrients to prevent disease or to promote growth; a form of malnutrition.

overnutrition: too much food energy or excess nutrients to the degree of causing disease or increasing risk of disease; a form of malnutrition.

ASSESS

EVALUATE

Quiz students on the glossary terms for this section. Read the terms and ask students to write definitions.

SECTION 1 Review Answers

1. Answers will vary.

2. *Undernutrition* occurs when the body receives too little food energy or too few nutrients for health and growth; *overnutrition* occurs when the body receives too much food energy or too many nutrients, causing or risking disease. (pp. 162–163)

3. helps make people's bodies strong, fit, and healthy (p. 162)

4. Refer to the Health Strategies Dietary Guidelines for Americans on page 162.

5. Answers will vary.

A reproducible quiz for Section 1 is provided in the Teacher's Resource Box.

CLOSE

Divide the class into six groups; assign each group one of the dietary guidelines. Have each group draw a simple picture or symbol to stand for its guideline. Have each group share and discuss its picture/symbol. Then have students close their books and name the dietary guidelines by using the pictures as a guide. Have students name them without the pictures.

- brand of soda or pop
- a new CD

Ask if they often buy items even though they know that a particular item is quite different from the "in" thing at the moment. Do they know anyone who often buys the unusual item? Does the person have high self-esteem? Then, ask students to consider when they last used comparison shopping techniques.

1. With what items are they more likely to compare?

2. Does price or parental influence have anything to do with these buying decisions?

3. Were they shopping with friends when they made the comparisons?

SECTION 2

FOCUS

OUTCOMES

In this section students will learn:

1. To identify healthier daily food choices.

2. To make sound choices about foods based on factual information.

FOCUS ACTIVITY

Before teaching about nutrients in foods, determine how much students already know. Write on the board: "What are nutrients? Name six classes of nutrients." Discuss their answers.

TEACH & APPLY

DISCUSSION

Explain that we sometimes eat foods that we do not want and should not eat just because they are readily available. Have students think of snacks that are waiting for them when they come home from school. Have them list the various snacks as you write them on the chalk board. Point out the foods that might be seen as junk foods and why. Circle all foods that are readily available (need little or no preparation). Have students discuss why it is important to think about food choices in advance. (so they will not make impulsive decisions to eat something just because it is available) Have students brainstorm a list of ways to have nutritious snacks readily available. What snacks would be good food choices? What snacks are high in fat? In salt? In sugar?

SECTION 2

How to Choose Nutritious Foods

The food you eat supplies nutrients, fiber, and other materials. The nutrients fall into six classes: **carbohydrate**, **fat**, **protein**, **vitamins**, **minerals**, and water. Altogether, people need about 40 vitamins and minerals and ample amounts of all the other nutrients. How can they meet their needs for all of these nutrients? Figure 7–1 on pages 166 to 167, which shows the Daily Food Guide diet-planning pattern, offers guidance.

Using the Daily Food Guide

Each nutrient has its own unique pattern among foods. It might seem a tricky business, then, to work them all into the meals you eat. Yet people all over the world meet their needs for these nutrients from an astonishing variety of diets.

Happily, eating wisely doesn't require giving up favorite foods and all the pleasures they provide, although it may require limiting yourself in choosing them. Most people's diets just need a little fine-tuning. Eat certain foods more often, and eat other foods less often. That's all.

The Food Guide Pyramid part of Figure 7–1 on page 167 helps you in choosing enough nutritious food of each kind to meet your nutrient needs. Note that the Food Guide Pyramid suggests choosing at least these servings daily:

► Six servings from the bread, cereal, rice, and pasta group.
► Three servings from the vegetable group.
► Two servings from the fruit group.

For **Y**our **I**nformation

Remember this pattern: six, three, two, two, and two.

Choose at least two servings of fruit each day.

•multicultural issues•

Ask the students to name their favorite, other than fast-food, local restaurants. (If students are unable to name restaurants other than fast-food restaurants, encourage them to ask their parents to take them to a local restaurant.) Based on their responses, ask the following questions about the restaurants that reflect either regional or national diversity.

1. Do you think the food served is nutritious?

2. What is your favorite food or foods served at the restaurant?

3. What does the type of food served tell you about the foods and seasonings available in that culture?

4. What does the type of food served tell

Your food can provide all the nutrients your body needs.

▶ Two servings from the milk, yogurt, and cheese group.
▶ Two servings from the meat, poultry, fish, dry beans, eggs, and nuts group.

These are the *minimum* numbers of servings. To find out how many servings you need, consult Figure 7–2 on page 170.

Controlling Calories   Now that you know how many servings of foods to eat to get enough nutrients, what about controlling calories? The Daily Food Guide can help here, too. Notice that the lists of foods in Figure 7–1 are color-coded with purple, red, or green dots. Foods with purple dots are lowest in calories. Those with red dots are intermediate. Those with green dots are highest in calories. A diet of the fewest recommended number of servings, all from the green-coded foods, provides the needed nutrients and only about 1,600 calories. Most people need more food energy than this to maintain a healthy body weight. More servings, and even a few of the items marked with yellow or red dots, can fill in extra energy.

The Daily Food Guide pattern is easy to learn. You can use it with great flexibility. (Example: replace milk with cheese, because both supply the same nutrients in about the same amounts.) You can choose dried beans and nuts to stand in for meats.

MINI Glossary

carbohydrate: a class of nutrients made of sugars; these nutrients include sugar, starch, and fiber. All but fiber provide energy. Often referred to in the plural, *carbohydrates*.

fat: a class of nutrients that does not mix with water. Fat is made mostly of fatty acids, which provide energy to the body. Technically referred to as *lipids*.

protein: a class of nutrients that builds body tissues and supplies energy. Protein is made of amino acids. Referred to only in the singular, *protein*.

vitamins: essential nutrients that do not yield energy, but that are required for growth and proper functioning of the body.

minerals: elements of the earth needed in the diet, which perform many functions in body tissues.

you about the food preparation and storage equipment used in that culture?
5. How would you describe the style of meal service?
6. Are any special manners or other customs expected?
7. How does the table setting compare to what you typically use at home?
8. Do the restaurant personnel wear any special type of clothing? If so, how does

the clothing contribute to the mood of the restaurant?
9. Is there any music? If so, describe it.
10. What appeals to you most about this restaurant?
11. Describe any insights into the people of that culture that you gain from this eating experience.

CLASS ACTIVITY

On a scratch piece of paper, have students list, in descending order, each of the six groups, included in Figure 7–1, "The Daily Food Guide." Their lists should begin with the group from which they need the most servings and end with the group from which they should have the least number of servings. Have them list the number of servings next to the group. Ask if they were surprised at which group is the most important in terms of number of servings. You may also want to ask them to make a second listing of the groups in the order in which students think they currently obtain the most servings. How do the lists compare?

COMPREHENSION CHECK

Make sure students notice and understand the key in Figure 7–1, which indicates the relative number of calories in the different foods.

CLASS ACTIVITY

Have students write a paper explaining at least two similarities between the food pyramid and the traditional concept of a square meal using the four food groups. Students should contrast at least two differences.

FAST FACTS

The average American consumes about 90 pounds of sugar every year.

Figure 7–1 The Daily Food Guide

Key:
- Foods generally lowest in calories
- Foods moderate in calories
- Foods generally highest in calories

Bread, Cereal, Rice, and Pasta Group

(For carbohydrate, fiber, and other nutrients.)
6 to 11 servings per day.
Serving = 1 slice bread; 1/2 cup cooked cereal, rice, or pasta; 1 ounce ready-to-eat cereal; 1/2 bun, bagel, or English muffin; 1 small roll, biscuit, or muffin; 3 to 4 small or 2 large crackers.

- Whole grains, enriched breads, rolls, tortillas, bagels, rice, pasta, air-popped corn.
- Pancakes, muffins, cornbread, crackers, biscuits, presweetened cereals, granola.
- Croissants, fried rice, doughnuts, pastries, sweet rolls.

Fruit Group

(For vitamin C, vitamin A, potassium, and other nutrients.)
2 to 4 servings per day.
Serving = 1/2 cup fresh or canned fruit or typical portion (1 medium apple, 1/2 grapefruit); 3/4 cup juice; 1/4 cup dried fruit.

- Apricots, cantaloupe, grapefruit, oranges, orange juice, peaches, strawberries, apples, bananas, pears.
- Canned or frozen fruit.
- Avocados, dried fruit.

Vegetable Group

(For vitamin A, folate, and other nutrients.)
3 to 5 servings per day.
Serving = 1/2 cup cooked or raw vegetables; 1 cup leafy raw vegetables; 3/4 vegetable juice.

- Bean sprouts, broccoli, brussels sprouts, cabbage, carrots, cauliflower, cucumbers, green beans, peas, leafy greens (spinach, collard), lettuce, legumes, mushrooms, tomatoes, summer and winter squash.
- Corn, potatoes, sweet potatoes, yams.
- French fries, olives, tempura vegetables.

Milk, Yogurt, and Cheese Group

(For calcium, riboflavin, protein, and other nutrients.)
2 servings per day for adults and children.
3 servings per day for teenagers, young adults, and pregnant and lactating women.
Serving = 1 cup milk or yogurt; 2 ounces processed cheese; 1 1/2 ounces natural cheese.

- Nonfat milk, 1% low-fat milk (and nonfat products such as yogurt, cottage cheese, cheese), fortified soy milk.
- 2% reduced-fat milk (and low-fat products such as yogurt, cheese, cottage cheese), sherbet, ice milk.
- Whole milk (and whole-milk products), custard, milk shakes, pudding, ice cream.

HEALTHY PEOPLE 2000

Nutrition is essential for sustenance, health, and well-being. But dietary factors also contribute substantially to the burden of preventable illness and premature death in the United States. Dietary factors are associated with 5 of the 10 leading causes of death: coronary heart disease, some types of cancer, stroke, noninsulin-dependent diabetes mellitus, and atherosclerosis. Three other major killers—cirrhosis of the liver, unintentional injuries, and suicides—have been associated with excessive alcohol intake. In general, once-prevalent nutrient deficiencies have been replaced by excesses and imbalances of some food components in the diet. However, undernutrition still occurs in some groups of people, including those who are isolated or

Figure 7–1 The Daily Food Guide, continued

Meat, Poultry, Fish, Dry Beans, Eggs, and Nuts Group

(For protein, iron, and other nutrients.)
2 to 3 servings per day.
Serving = 2 to 3 ounces lean, cooked meat, poultry, or fish; 1 egg, 1/2 cup legumes, or 2 tablespoons peanut butter equal to one ounce meat, or about 1/3 serving.

- Poultry, fish. lean meat (beef, lamb, pork), dried peas and beans, egg whites.
- Beef, lamb, pork, refried beans, whole eggs.
- Hot dogs, luncheon meats, peanut butter, nuts, sausage, bacon, fried fish or poultry.

Fats, Oils, and Sweets

(Not a food group, few nutrients.)

- Foods high in fat: margarine, salad dressings, oils mayonnaise, cream, cream cheese, butter, gravy, and sauces.
- Foods high in sugar: cakes, pies, cookies, doughnuts, candy, soft drinks, jelly, syrup, sugar, and honey.

Food Guide Pyramid

Fats, oils, and sweets **Use sparingly**

KEY
☐ Fat (naturally occurring and added)
☑ Sugars (added)

Milk, yogurt, and cheese group **2–3 servings**

Meat, poultry, fish, dry beans, eggs, and nuts group **2–3 servings**

Vegetable group **3–5 servings**

Fruit group **2–4 servings**

Bread, cereal, rice, and pasta group **6–11 servings**

economically deprived.

Many dietary components are involved in diet and health relationships. Chief among them is the disproportionate consumption of foods high in fats, often at the expense of foods high in complex carbohydrates and dietary fiber that may be more conducive to health. The *Dietary Guidelines for Americans* recommends that to stay healthy one should eat a variety of foods; maintain healthy weight; choose a diet low in fat, saturated fat, and cholesterol; choose a diet with plenty of vegetables, fruits, and grain products; use sugars only in moderation; use salt and sodium only in moderation; and if alcoholic beverages are consumed, do so in moderation.

A reproducible copy of the Life Choice Inventory, "How Well Do You Eat?" is provided in the Teacher's Resource Box.

CLASS ACTIVITY

Bring the following to school: one bag of chips, ten slices of bread, a jar of peanut butter, a small can of meat, a large soft drink, a box of cereal, measuring spoons, measuring cups, a small food scale, a variety of sizes of bowls and glasses, a butter knife, and a funnel.

- Have two students pour bowls of cereal like they would eat for breakfast.
- Have two more students pour snack-sized bowls of chips.
- Have two more students scoop out the amount of peanut butter that they would use for a sandwich.
- Have two more students pour themselves a soft drink.

Talk about serving sizes and how serving sizes are listed on most packages. (Of course, people do not always eat just one serving.) Hold up different items and ask students how many servings they think are in each container, then read the label. Show students how big servings really are, according to the package labels.

Measure each item either by weight on the scale or by cups

How Well Do You Eat?

How well do you eat? On another piece of paper, answer these questions to find out. Your answers to the Life Choice Inventory are personal and private. Share them with others only if you are comfortable doing so.

PART 1 Do you eat nutritious foods from all of these categories? Answer yes or no. For each yes answer, give yourself 2 points. Total possible points = 10. For serving sizes, see Figure 7–1, presented earlier.

                                Score

1. I have 2 or more cups of milk or 2 servings of milk products every day. _____
2. I have 2 or more servings of meat or meat alternates every day. _____
3. On some days I eat dried peas or beans instead of meat. _____
4. I generally have at least 6 servings of grain products (breads, cereals, rice, and the like) each day. _____
5. I have at least 2 servings of fruits and 3 servings of vegetables every day (total of at least 5). _____

Total for Part I _____

PART 2 Do you maintain appropriate weight? If yes, give yourself 20 points, skip Part 3, and go on to Part 4. If no, take no points, and complete Part 3 below.

6. I eat just enough food to stay within 5 to 10 pounds of the weight considered appropriate for my height (see Chapter 8). _____

PART 3 Do you choose a diet low in fat, saturated fat, and cholesterol? For each yes answer, give yourself 1 point. Total possible points = 10.

7. My milk and milk-product choices are mostly nonfat or low in fat (nonfat or low-fat milk rather than whole milk); and I eat ice cream or ice milk two or three times a week or less. _____
8. I seldom have more than about 3 teaspoons of margarine or butter per day. _____
9. My meat, fish, poultry, or egg choices usually amount to 2 servings a day or fewer. _____
10. In choosing meats, I eat chicken and fish more often than beef, ham, lamb, or pork. _____
11. I remove fat or ask that fat be trimmed from meat before eating. I avoid meats with fat ground in, such as sausages. _____
12. In choosing meat, I usually choose broiled, boiled, baked, or roasted; I usually don't choose fried. _____
13. On some days I eat dried peas or beans instead of meat. (This is the same as Question 3—it counts under both Part 1 and Part 3.) _____
14. In choosing or preparing vegetables, I use little or no fat. _____
15. The grain products I use have little or no fat added. _____
16. In buying foods, I read labels for fat content and choose mostly foods with less than 3 grams fat per 100 calories. _____

Total for Part 3 _____

CRITICAL THINKING

Have students develop a spreadsheet for recording foods they have eaten over a three-day period. They should include this information:

1. food eaten
2. amount eaten
3. time of day
4. location food was eaten
5. how they were feeling
6. who they ate with
7. number of calories eaten
8. fat content

PART 4 Do you get plenty of starch and fiber daily? For each yes answer, give yourself 2 points. Total possible points = 10.

17. When I am hungry, I choose starchy foods such as popcorn, cereals, pasta, potatoes, and breads rather than fatty foods such as fried snacks or chips. _____

18. The grain products I use are mostly whole grains (whole-wheat bread, whole-grain cereals, brown rice, and the like). _____

19. I eat abundant fruits and vegetables (this resembles Question 5 above; you get added points for these as high-fiber foods). _____

20. I eat salads or raw vegetables (such as carrots and celery) at least every other day. _____

21. I eat dried beans or peas at least once a week (again, you receive credit for these as high-fiber foods). _____

Total for Part 4 _____

PART 5 Do you eat reasonable quantities of sugar, honey, and other concentrated sweets? For each yes answer, give yourself 2 points. Total possible points = 6.

22. If I eat sweets (candy bars and the like), it is in addition to, not in place of, the nutritious foods I need, and only within the limits my weight allows. _____

23. If I drink cola beverages, it is in addition to, not in place of, the milk and fruit products I need, and only within the limits my weight and caffeine tolerance allow. _____

24. I don't let sweets and sugary drinks harm my dental health; I rinse or brush my teeth after eating and drinking them. _____

Total for Part 5 _____

PART 6 Do you use salt wisely? For each yes answer, give yourself 2 points. Total possible points = 4.

25. I generally choose foods salted lightly or not salted at all. _____

26. I add little or no salt to food after preparation. _____

Total for Part 6 _____

SCORING

50	Incredible.
40–49	Excellent.
30–39	Your diet has room for improvement.
20–29	Not so good. Work on your weakest areas.
Below 20	Poor. Make major efforts to improve.

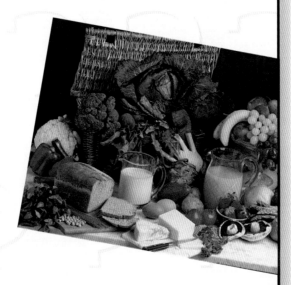

Have the students keep this three-day record as accurately as possible. You may need to supply calorie books and charts for students to use in completing the three-day records.

Have them exchange records with another student. Analyze and draw conclusions about:

1. daily caloric expenditure versus needs

2. snacks eaten (amount and kind)

3. fat content of diet

4. nutritional value

5. representation of food pyramid

6. overall assessment

7. changes needed for a healthier diet.

or tablespoons. Compare one serving from the package to what the student volunteers served themselves. How many servings of each item did they actually take as a serving?

Using the labels on the packages, calculate the amount of calories in each student's serving. Compare this to the amount of calories per suggested serving on the package.

You might have students tell you which nutrients are provided in each food.

You may want to distribute the handout "Nutrients in Typical Lunches," provided in the Teacher's Resource Box. This handout shows the amounts of vitamin A, vitamin C, calcium, and iron contained in three standard lunches.

The Teacher's Resource Box contains a handout entitled "Selecting Nutritious Foods." This handout pulls together ten strategies that are mentioned in this chapter.

The Teacher's Resource Box also contains a handout on U.S. Public Health Service Objectives, which gives the U.S. Department of Health and Human Services goals for nutrition.

The transparency "Nutrients in Whole-Grain, Enriched White, and Unenriched White Bread" is provided in the Transparency Acetate Binder.

ASSESS

EVALUATE

Have students bring in recipes or descriptions of dishes from other countries. Have them determine what servings from the food pyramid are represented, and ask them to suggest what other foods are still needed to fill in the rest of the day's requirements.

SECTION 2 Review Answers

1. Answers will vary.
2. Eat according to the pattern established in the Dietary Guidelines for Americans. (p. 164)
3. by selecting foods in Figure 7–1 that are color-coded with green dots. (p. 165)
4. bread, cereal, rice, and pasta (p. 164)
5. Answers will vary.

WORKSHEETS

A reproducible quiz for Section 2 is provided in the Teacher's Resource Box.

CLOSE

Ask students if modifying foods to get proper nutrition is a difficult or easy task. Ask students why the diet business is such a successful industry. Address the fact that poor nutrition choices are sometimes a result of a lack of knowledge, money, or time. Poor nutrition also results from behavioral problems. People need to figure out why they eat the less nutritious foods and what causes them to make poor choices. Discuss.

Figure 7–2 *How Many Servings?*

	Teenage Girls	Teenage Boys
Calories[a]	About 2,000	About 2,800
Bread, cereal, rice, and pasta group	9	11
Vegetable group	4	5
Fruit group	3	4
Milk, yogurt, and cheese group[b]	3	3
Meat, poultry, fish, dry beans, eggs, and nuts group	2 (6 ounces total)	3 (7 ounces total)
Total fat (grams)	73	93
Added sugar (teaspoons)	12	18

[a]Assumes mostly low-fat and low-calorie food choices.
[b]Pregnant or lactating teenagers need four servings.

Source: U.S. Department of Agriculture, *Home and Garden Bulletin* 252 (1992): 9.

Here's how the typical U.S. diet stacks up. What's wrong with this diet? (Hint: see the Food Guide Pyramid)

The food guide pattern can be applied to casseroles and other mixed dishes. It can also be applied to different national and cultural foods. A study of the Daily Food Guide and some thought about the questions asked in this chapter's Life Choice Inventory should help you develop a diet that meets your needs.

KEY POINTS *Diet-planning patterns, such as the Daily Food Guide pattern, help people meet their needs for vitamins and minerals, keep other nutrients in balance, and help with calorie control.*

SECTION 2 Review

Answer the following questions on a sheet of paper.

Learning the Vocabulary

The vocabulary terms in this section are *carbohydrate, fat, protein, vitamins,* and *minerals.*

1. Write a sentence using each term.

Learning the Facts

2. What is the best possible way to meet all of the body's nutrient needs?

3. How can you avoid consuming large amounts of calories and still meet the body's nutrient needs?
4. From which food group should you eat at least six servings daily?

Making Life Choices

5. Look at your scores on the Life Choice Inventory. List the areas in which you scored well. List the areas in which you were deficient. List three improvements you could make in your diet. What was your overall rating? Were you pleased with your scores? Why or why not?

Ability Levels

Remind students that practically all foods contain mixtures of the three energy-yielding nutrients. Foods are sometimes classified, however, by the predominant nutrient. It is incorrect to call meat a protein; it is a *protein-rich* food. Ask students why this is so. (Meats contain more than just protein. Beef, for example, contains fat as well as protein.) A *carbohydrate-rich* food such as corn also contains fat and protein. Ask students if they know of any single-nutrient foods. (Only a few refined foods are pure, single-nutrient foods; the most common ones being sugar,

SECTION 3

Energy from Food

Three nutrients—carbohydrates, fats, and protein—provide **energy** the body can use. The body uses energy from these nutrients to do its work and to create heat to maintain a steady temperature. Carbohydrates supply the body with one of its main fuels, the sugar **glucose**. The brain and nervous system can normally use only this fuel for energy to fuel their activities.

Fat supplies the body with another main fuel, **fatty acids**. The muscles, including the heart muscle, rely heavily on this fuel.

Protein is used mostly to build body tissues. It also can be broken down (into **amino acids**) and used for energy. In difficult conditions, such as starvation or severe stress, the body may burn much more protein for fuel than in normal times. In summary:

▶ Carbohydrate—provides energy as glucose.
▶ Fat—provides energy as fatty acids.
▶ Protein—builds working cell parts; is made from amino acids, which can also provide energy.

One other substance provides energy: the alcohol of alcoholic beverages. Alcohol is not a nutrient, because it does not promote growth, maintenance, or repair of the body. In fact, it is a **toxin**: the body can tolerate it in small quantities but in larger quantities is poisoned by it.

> **"** *Long meals make short lives.* **"**
>
> Sir John Lubbock
> (1834–1913)
> British financier and author

For perfect functioning, every nutrient is needed.

MINI Glossary

energy: the capacity to do work or produce heat.

glucose: the body's blood sugar; a simple form of carbohydrate.

fatty acids: simple forms of fat that supply energy fuel for most of the body's cells.

amino acids: simple forms of protein normally used to build tissues or, under some conditions, burned for energy.

toxin: a poison.

which is almost pure carbohydrate, and oil, which is almost pure fat.)

One way to think about the difference between glycogen molecules and glucose molecules (discussed on the next page) is to compare them to beads on a string. Strung together, the beads take on a new identity called a necklace. Similarly, glucose mole-

cules, when linked together, form glycogen. Just as a necklace can break and lose its beads one at a time, glycogen can break down, turning loose thousands of glucose molecules, one at a time.

FOCUS

OUTCOMES

In this section students will learn:

1. The role of carbohydrate, fat, and protein nutrients in providing energy.
2. What a calorie is, and how it is a measure of energy in food.
3. Why the body needs energy, and from where that energy is derived.
4. The advantages of a balanced meal.

FOCUS ACTIVITY

Write the following question on the chalkboard: What is meant by a balanced meal? Have students write their answers and give examples. Discuss student answers and explain the importance of eating a balanced meal to receive a variety of nutrients.

TEACH & APPLY

BACKGROUND INFORMATION

In this text, you'll find both the singular, scientific usage of *carbohydrate* and *fat*, and the more common, plural forms. *Carbohydrate* and *fat* are often referred to in the plural because individual members of their classes have specific effects on the body. This is not the case with *protein*. Since the body uses all members of the protein class in the same way as amino acids, this class is referred to only in the singular.

LEARNING WITH VISUALS

Have students draw a graphic representation of the role of glycogen, glucose, the hypothalamus, the liver, and blood in the body. Have them use arrows and labels with their drawings so that anyone can understand what process is going on and which parts of the body are included. They might use symbols to represent glucose and glycogen. They may want to refer to illustrations in other chapters of the text, especially Chapter 6.

COMPREHENSION CHECK

Students should be able to explain that the body changes fat from food very little; it is stored as is. On the other hand, the body changes glucose to glycogen and stores it in the liver. The liver also changes extra glucose into fat and releases the fat into the blood.

CLASS ACTIVITY

Assign each student one of the three nutrients discussed in this section (carbohydrate, fat, protein). Have students create a short radio or TV advertisement to advertise their nutrient and try to persuade others to try it. Encourage students to choose from a variety of advertising appeals to "sell" the nutrient such as: bandwagon—everyone uses this so you should, too; celebrity—a famous person endorses this product; sex appeal—a person might be more attractive or have attractive friends if they use that product, etc. Give students time in class to advertise. Have other students rate the advertisement and discuss its effectiveness.

***Figure 7–3** Energy Contributions of Carbohydrate, Fat, and Protein*

Fat =	9 calories per gram
Carbohydrate =	4 calories per gram
Protein =	4 calories per gram

The brain prefers using carbohydrates for fuel. The muscles use some carbohydrates, but they use much more fat.

Still, because people do drink alcohol, and because the body can turn it into fat, it has to be counted as an energy source.

Calories   The term **calories** is familiar to everyone as a measure of how "fattening" a food is. A more accurate definition of *calorie* is *a unit used to measure energy*. The calorie count of a food does reflect its fattening power. If you consume more carbohydrate, fat, and protein than you need, these nutrients will be stored in your body, mostly as fat. You should remember, though, that calories are more precisely units of energy, not units of body fat. Figure 7–3 shows the energy contributed by carbohydrate, fat, and protein.

Storing Glucose as Glycogen   The body stores extra energy in two fuels: glucose and fat. The glucose is stored in the liver and muscles as **glycogen**. The fat, as you know, is stored mostly under the skin as body fat.

The body's stores of glycogen are small, so you must eat regularly to maintain them. A regulatory center in the brain known as the **hypothalamus** sends out a hunger signal when blood glucose levels get too low. If you don't eat, the body starts to use its four or so hours' worth of glycogen (stored in your liver) to provide glucose.

The liver is generous with its glycogen. It releases it into the blood for use by the brain and other tissues. The muscles, on the other hand, keep their glycogen for their own use only. The Straight Talk in Chapter 9 tells more about the use of glycogen in muscles.

Storing Fuels as Body Fat   Within seconds after eating carbohydrates, your blood glucose level rises. Your liver and muscle cells store some extra glucose as glycogen. If still more glucose is available, the liver changes it, along with any excess protein, to fat. Then the fat cells in fat tissue store it.

Fat that comes from food isn't changed much in the body. It is stored in the fat cells as is. As a result of the body's storage of both glycogen and fat, you'll have two reserve fuel supplies to draw on the next time you have to postpone eating.

Energy from Food   When you get hungry, what should you eat? One obvious choice might seem to be a candy bar "for quick energy." It is true that the body can quickly raise its blood glucose level from the concentrated sugar in candy. The only trouble is that a dose of sugar by itself lasts only a short time in the blood. It is quickly used or stored. You'll soon be hungry again, and possibly shaky besides.

A better choice than candy is a **balanced meal**—that is, a meal that contains many kinds of food that offer carbohydrate, fat, and protein all together. Here's why a balanced meal is better:

▶ The carbohydrate in the meal provides a quick source of glucose energy.
▶ The fat in the meal slows down **digestion**, making the glucose last longer. The fat also provides most of the meal's food energy (calories).
▶ The protein in the meal slows down the body's use of carbohydrates, also making the glucose last longer.

An example of a balanced meal is shown in Figure 7–4.

KEY POINTS   *The body stores any extra energy from dietary carbohydrates, fats, or protein as glycogen or fat. The best source of energy for the body is a balanced meal.*

QUICK QUIZ

Chapter 7, Section 3

The following quiz will help you assess your students' understanding of the material covered in this section of the chapter. You might use the quiz as an oral exercise, which will lead into a class discussion of the topics covered. Or, you might use it as a paper/pencil

quiz to evaluate your students individually.

*If students have difficulty with the concepts covered in the Quick Quiz and the Section Review, you might suggest they review the material using the **S**urvey, **Q**uestion, **R**ead, **R**ecite, **R**eview (SQ3R) study method, which is described in detail in the introduction to this Teacher's Wraparound Edition.*

1. Carbohydrates, fats and proteins are the three nutrients that provide the body

Figure 7–4 A Balanced Meal. This meal presents a healthful balance of carbo-hydrate, fat, and protein. Less than 30 percent of its calories are from fat, and about 60 percent are from carbohydrate. The rest come from protein. Note the generous portions of vegetables and fruit. The bread is without butter, and the beverage is nonfat milk. Total calories: about 800. For fewer calories choose smaller por-tions, especially half the meat.

    A mistake people commonly make is to think that if fat should contribute 30 percent of the calories, then it should take up a third of the plate. On the contrary: a spoon of fat contains more than twice as many calories as a spoon of pure protein or of carbohydrate, and much of the fat in a meal is invisible. In this 800-calorie meal, the only visible fat is in the chicken skin and salad dressing, and yet fat contributes almost 30 percent of the calories.

SECTION 3 Review

Answer the following questions on a sheet of paper.

Learning the Vocabulary

The vocabulary terms in this section are *energy, glucose, fatty acids, amino acids, toxin, calories, glyco-gen, hypothalamus, balanced meal,* and *digestion.*
Fill in the blanks with the correct answer.

1. The units used to measure energy in food are ____.
2. The body's storage form of sugar is called ____.
3. The ____ sends out the hunger signal.
4. ____ is the body's blood sugar.
5. The capacity to produce heat or do work is ____.
6. ____ are simple forms of protein.

Learning the Facts

7. Explain how the number of calories in a food reflects its fattening power.
8. How does the body meet its glucose need if you have not eaten?
9. Why is a balanced meal consid-ered the best source of energy for the body?

Making Life Choices

10. Some people become obsessed with counting calories. Has anyone you know ever become obsessed with counting calo-ries? What was the result? Explain some of the dangers of such an obsession.

MINI Glossary

calories: units used to measure energy. Calories indicate how much energy in a food can be used by the body or stored in body fat.

glycogen: the form in which the liver and muscles store glucose.

hypothalamus (high-po-THALL-uh-mus): a brain regulatory center.

balanced meal: a meal with foods to provide the right amounts of carbo-hydrate, fat, and protein.

digestion: the breaking down of food into nutrients the body can use. The *digestive system* is a series of body organs that break foods down and absorb their nutrients. (See Chapter 6 for details of the system.)

with its main supply of energy. (True)
2. The brain and nervous system normally use only the sugar glucose as a source of energy. (True)
3. Fatty acids, which supply the muscles, are derived from carbohydrates. (False)
4. The body uses protein to build working tissues. (True)
5. Alcohol is a nutrient which provides energy to the body. (False)
6. A toxin, such as alcohol, is poisonous to the body in large quantities. (True)
7. A calorie is a unit of body fat. (False)
8. The hypothalamus sends out a hunger signal to the brain when the blood glu-cose level becomes too low. (True)
9. The body changes excess glucose into glycogen and body fat. (True)
10. "For quick energy" a candy bar can be better than a balanced meal. (False)

ASSESS

EVALUATE

Have students write three rea-sons to eat a balanced meal rather than a candy bar, when hungry.

SECTION 3 Review Answers

1. calories (p. 172)
2. glycogen (p. 172)
3. hypothalamus (p. 172)
4. glucose (p. 171)
5. energy (p. 171)
6. amino acids (p. 171)
7. If you consume more car-bohydrates, fat, and protein than you need, these nutri-ents will be stored in your body, mostly as fat. (p. 172)
8. The body uses the glyco-gen stored in the liver. (p. 172)
9. Answers to this question are contained in the three bulleted items at the end of this section. (p. 172)
10. Answers will vary.

A reproducible quiz for Section 3 is provided in the Teacher's Resource Box.

CLOSE

Have students write a definition of a calorie, explain how calo-ries are related to energy for the body, and tell what happens to extra calories.

SECTION 4

FOCUS

OUTCOMES

In this section students will learn:

1. The differences between the three types of carbohydrates and the role of each in the body.

2. How much fiber is recommended daily and what foods supply that fiber.

3. How to analyze their diets for the recommended amount of fiber.

FOCUS ACTIVITY

Bring a teaspoon, sugar, and a glass to class. Ask students how much sugar they put in coffee or tea. Start putting sugar in the glass and have the students tell you when to stop. Keep measuring until you have put in 10–15 teaspoons. Hold it up, and ask if they would drink something poured into the glass with that much sugar. Explain that this is the amount of sugar in one can of soda. Discuss.

TEACH & APPLY

LEARNING WITH VISUALS

Have students draw a diagram illustrating the characteristics that starch, fiber, and sugar have in common. Then have them illustrate the differences between starch, fiber, and sugar. Have students present these to the class, explaining the differences and similarities, and how they chose to represent these on paper.

The Carbohydrates

You have already read about two carbohydrates important in the *body*: (1) the sugar glucose in the blood and (2) the stored form of glucose, glycogen, in the liver and muscles. Carbohydrates important in the diet are **starch**, **fiber**, and **sugars**. The body converts the starch and sugars in food into blood glucose. Fiber passes unchanged through the digestive tract.

Starch

Starch, the main carbohydrate in grains and vegetables, is the chief energy source for people around the world. Starch serves the human body well. It provides glucose in a form the body uses best. And that's not all that starch does. If the starchy foods you eat are foods like whole-grain breads (not refined white bread), potatoes (not potato chips), or whole-grain cereals (not the sugary kind), then your body receives many of the *other* nutrients (vitamins and minerals) it needs, along with a steady supply of glucose. Most people would do well to boost their intakes of starchy foods.

The brain needs glucose to perform at its best. Studies of schoolchildren show that those who do not eat breakfast cannot concentrate on school work or pay attention as long as their well-fed peers can. Without breakfast, their bodies run out of glucose. Starchy breakfast foods like cereal, or even just toast, may be enough to keep them going.

College students are unable to pay attention when their blood glucose runs low in the late afternoon. Students who eat a carbohydrate-rich snack in the afternoon perform better on tasks of thinking and memory than students without snacks. The carbohydrates in foods

Everyone needs carbohydrate to be at their best.

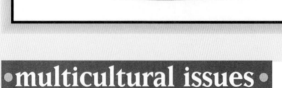

•multicultural issues•

Have students pick out a country they would like to represent. Ask them to bring to class a small food sample of a nutritious dish from the country they chose to represent. Have them make a replica of the flag of the country that dish represents and lay the dish near its flag. Tell students to write on an index card such as grains, breads, cereals, pasta, potatoes, and beans, as well as the sugars of fruits and vegetables, provide the brain with the glucose it needs to perform at its best.

 Starch is the main source of energy for the world's people. Starchy foods provide the body with glucose and many other nutrients.

Fiber—Not an Energy Source

Another form of carbohydrate in foods—fiber—is not digestible by human beings and so provides no calories. However, it helps to maintain the health of the digestive tract. Most people need to obtain more fiber. The body should have about 25 grams of fiber each day to remain healthy. Each serving of any food listed here provides about 2 grams of fiber:

▶ Fruits in the natural state with skins, 1 piece; ¾ cup berries; ½ cantaloupe; 2 prunes.

▶ Whole grains, including 1 slice whole-wheat bread or 2 slices cracked-wheat (light brown) bread; 2 Rye Crisp, Triscuit, or other whole-wheat crackers; ½ shredded wheat biscuit; ⅓ cup any bran cereal; 1 teaspoon wheat bran or 1 tablespoon All-bran cereal; 1½ cup puffed wheat cereal; 2 cups popped popcorn.

▶ Vegetables, lightly cooked, ½ cup most types; 1 cup raw celery; 2 cups lettuce; ½ cup most cooked dried beans; 1 large tomato; 1 small potato (in jacket); ⅓ cup corn.

▶ Other sources: 2½ teaspoons peanut butter; ¼ cup most nuts; 1 large pickle; 1 tablespoon strawberry jam.

Most types of fiber in foods move through the digestive tract almost unchanged—in one end and out the other. They aid in digestion by making the digestive tract contents (stools) soft and bulky and keep it moving through the tract. This subject may not be a glamorous one, but it is of interest to anyone who suffers from a lack of fiber. Fiber lack leads to **constipation** (hard, sluggish stools), **hemorrhoids** (swollen, painful veins in the **rectum** that bulge out from straining to pass hard stools), and many other painful intestinal ills.

Also, fiber binds with cholesterol and carries it out of the body in the stools. Thus it reduces the risk of heart disease. Fiber also helps to balance the blood glucose and so helps to control the most common form of the disease diabetes. Some fibers bind cancer-causing agents in the digestive tract, reducing the risk of cancer. In all of these ways, fiber helps fight diseases.

Fiber may also help to prevent the accumulation of too much body fat. The person who eats fiber-rich foods chews longer and fills up sooner on fewer calories than the person who eats too little fiber. It is hard to eat a diet high in fiber and also gain weight.

Clearly, fiber benefits the body, but is there such a thing as too much fiber? There certainly is. Some years ago, many college students overdid a high-fiber diet, much to their digestive distress. They suffered dangerously severe diarrhea. Also, a man wolfed down a half dozen oat bran muffins. He required emergency surgery to remove a blockage of bran lodged in his intestine. Too much of anything, especially in nutrition, is as harmful as too little.

MINI Glossary

starch: a carbohydrate, the main food energy source for human beings.

fiber: indigestible substances in foods, made mostly of carbohydrate.

sugars: carbohydrates found both in food and in the body.

constipation: hard, slow stools that are difficult to eliminate; often a result of too little fiber in the diet.

hemorrhoids: swollen, painful rectal veins; often a result of constipation.

rectum: the last part of the digestive tract, through which stools are eliminated (see Chapter 6).

what makes the dish nutritious. Students will go to each display and take a spoonful to taste. Have students vote on the top ten dishes. Ask those students to bring the recipes to class and pass them out to students. Or, the top ten recipes of each class can be put into a recipe book, which could be printed and sold to raise money for programs at the school.

Consumer SKILLS

Answers to Critical Thinking

1. Fruit is one possible answer. Encourage students to brainstorm other answers and to defend those answers.

2. Fruit also contains fiber, and larger amounts of vitamins and minerals.

COMPREHENSION CHECK

Ask students to give examples of empty-calorie foods and explain why they are called that. (Examples include soda pop, "sports drinks," candies, sugar, honey, candy bars, candy coated nuts and fruits, doughnuts, tortilla chips, butter, margarine, oils, salad dressings, and gravies.) They are considered empty-calorie foods because they are high in calories without other nutrients. Encourage students to look at the nutritional information on their snack foods.

ASSESS

EVALUATE

Have students analyze a friend's diet for sources of fiber. They should calculate the grams of fiber found in food items and suggest foods to add to the diet until the recommended daily intake of fiber is achieved.

Review Answers

1. Fiber benefits the digestive tract because it softens stools. Lack of fiber leads to constipation. (p. 175)

176

Honey versus Sugar

Some salespeople market honey as the ideal substitute for sugar. They say it offers nutrients, so it is not empty calories.

It's true that honey contains tiny bits of a few vitamins and minerals. Compared with a person's daily need, however, these nutrients don't add up to much. A tablespoon of honey (65 calories) offers ⅒ milligram of iron, for example. An adult's daily need for iron may be 15 milligrams. To meet the need for iron, then, the adult would need 150 tablespoons of honey in a day—almost 10,000 calories of honey! (Most people can eat only 2,000 to 3,000 total calories a day without getting fat.)

The nutrients in honey just do not add up as fast as the calories do. Therefore honey, like sugar, is a relatively empty-calorie food.

Critical Thinking

1. *If honey has too many calories and too few nutrients for health, what sorts of sweet foods do you suppose might better provide for the body's needs?*
2. *Why do you think so?*

Plant foods are high in fiber, animal foods have none. Plants with their skins and seeds intact are especially rich in fiber. Fiber can be destroyed when foods are refined or cooked. Apples have more fiber than applesauce. Apple juice has none. Baked potatoes with the skins have more fiber than mashed potatoes. Potato chips have almost none. If you want to choose foods with enough fiber for your health, choose whole grains, whole fruits, and whole vegetables most of the time. Eat some of these foods cooked lightly, and eat some raw.

KEY POINTS *Fiber is a plant form of carbohydrate that is not digestible by human beings. Fiber helps maintain the health of the digestive tract.*

Sugars

The last type of dietary carbohydrate is the sugars. All sugars are chemically similar to glucose and can be converted into glucose in the body. The four sugars most important in human nutrition are:

▶ Glucose (the body's fuel).
▶ Fructose (the sweet sugar of fruits and honey).
▶ Sucrose (table sugar).
▶ Lactose (milk sugar).

In foods, the four sugars just named come in diluted form mostly from fruits, vegetables, and milk. They also come in concentrated form as sugar, honey, and other sweets (see the Consumer Skills feature above).

QUICK QUIZ

Chapter 7, Section 4

The following quiz will help you assess your students' understanding of the material covered in this section of the chapter. You might use the quiz as an oral exercise, which will lead into a class discussion of the topics covered. Or, you might use it as a paper/pencil

quiz to evaluate your students individually.

Like the Quick Quiz, the Section Review can also be used as an assessment tool to spark class discussion or as an individual student evaluation. It can also be used as a review in preparation for this quiz.

1. Starch, fiber and sugars are carbohydrates that the body can convert into glucose. (True)
2. Fiber is the main energy source for peo-

Nutritionists recommend that you consume large quantities of fruits and vegetables that contain sugars, but they urge you in the same breath to "avoid consuming too much sugar." What's the difference?

The answer lies in the phrase **empty calories**. When you eat an apple, you receive about 100 calories from the sugars in it, together with a few of the vitamins, a moderate dose of fiber, and some minerals. By contrast, a 12-ounce regular cola beverage gives you about 150 calories from sugar without any other nutrients. The calories you receive from the cola are empty calories. Another reason experts say to avoid sugar: the bacteria that cause dental caries (cavities) thrive on sticky sugar.

 KEY POINTS *Sugars may benefit health when they are consumed in fruits or milk. Sugars may harm health when eaten in the form of concentrated sweets.*

A spoonful of honey has twice as many calories as the same amount of sugar, but in terms of nutrients they are equally poor.

SECTION 4 Review

Answer the following questions on a sheet of paper.

Learning the Vocabulary

The vocabulary terms in this section are *starch, fiber, sugars, constipation, hemorrhoids, rectum,* and *empty calories.*

1. Explain the relationship between fiber and constipation.
2. What does fiber have to do with hemorrhoids?
3. Foods that contribute a lot of calories but insufficient nutrients contain _____.

Learning the Facts

4. Explain the effect of starchy foods on brain functioning.
5. Why is it beneficial to obtain adequate amounts of fiber in your diet?
6. What danger is there in consuming a large amount of sugar?
7. Give two examples for each: foods high in carbohydrates, foods high in fiber, foods high in sugar.

Making Life Choices

8. Make a list of your ten favorite foods. Which ones on your list do you suspect are empty-calorie foods? Which ones do you think are the most nutritious?

MINI Glossary

empty calories: a popular term referring to foods that contribute much energy (calories) but too little of the nutrients.

2. Hemorrhoids develop as a result of straining to pass hard stools. Fiber helps soften stools. (p. 175)
3. empty calories (p. 177)
4. Starchy foods provide the body with glucose, which the brain needs to function properly. (p. 174)
5. Answers will vary; could include: lack of fiber leads to constipation, hemorrhoids, and other intestinal ills; fiber helps to prevent appendicitis, reduces risk of heart disease, balances blood glucose, helps control the most common form of diabetes, keeps cancer-causing agents from touching intestinal walls, and assists in maintaining balanced weight. (p. 175)
6. Large amounts of sugar equal empty calories. Dental cavities thrive on sticky sugar. (p. 177)
7. Answers will vary; could include: carbohydrates— grains, breads, cereals, pasta, potatoes, and beans; foods high in fiber—broccoli, apples, and pears with skin; foods high in sugar—regular colas and concentrated sweets. (pp. 174–177)
8. Answers will vary.

WORKSHEETS

A reproducible quiz for Section 4 is provided in the Teacher's Resource Box.

CLOSE

Have students review the benefits of carbohydrates, fiber, and sugar in a person's diet. Ask for any negative effects associated with having too much or too little of any of these in your diet.

---

ple all around the world. (False)
3. Fiber is a good source of calories. (False)
4. Most people need to include more fiber in their diet. (True)
5. Constipation and hemorrhoids are the potential results of a lack of fiber in the diet. (True)
6. Fiber increases the risk of heart disease. (False)
7. Too much fiber, like anything else, can be harmful to the body. (True)
8. Glucose, fructose, sucrose, and lactose are the four sugars that are most important to human nutrition. (True)
9. Foods containing sugars may be beneficial or harmful. (True)
10. Empty calories come from food with few nutrients. (True)

FOCUS

OUTCOMES

In this section students will learn:

1. Ways in which too much fat in a person's diet can have a negative effect on health.
2. How to estimate their daily fat gram allowances.
3. Strategies to lower the amount of fat in their diets.

FOCUS ACTIVITY

(This activity is to help students increase their awareness of the emotional as well as the medical aspects of being overweight. The hope is that students will become more sensitive and empathetic toward overweight people. You should consider whether there are overweight students in your class who might be sensitive about their weight before you assign this activity.) Ask students to name health risks related to being overweight. Ask students to describe feelings that a person might have who is noticeably overweight. Have students read their answers and discuss. Tell them that weight can often be managed by proper nutrition and exercise. Tell them that it is not easy, but it might be the price someone would pay not to go through life being over-weight and at an increased risk of health problems.

The Fats

Fat supplies most of the fuel for the body. Nearly all the body's tissues (all but the brain and nervous system) rely on fat to provide most of the energy they need.

The body has small stores of carbohydrate (glycogen) and not much protein to spare, but it can store fat in almost unlimited amounts. Fat is stored in a layer of cells beneath the skin and also in many pads in the chest and abdomen. As well as providing energy, fat layers help to insulate the body from cold and from quick changes in temperature. Pads of fat also cushion the body, protecting it from bruises, strains, and breaks.

Forms of Fat

The fats you eat come in two forms—**saturated** and **unsaturated** (unsaturated fat includes **polyunsaturated** fat). For people who are developing heart and artery disease, the most important preventive dietary step to take is to reduce their *total* fat intakes. At the same time they should switch from saturated fat to mostly unsaturated fat in foods.

Saturated fats come mainly from animal sources, including meats, butter, and cream. They tend to be solid at room temperature. Unsaturated fats come primarily from vegetable oils, including olive oil, corn oil, and canola oil. These tend to be liquid at room temperature. Some foods high in *unsaturated* fats, including the *polyunsaturated* type, are listed in the margin on page 180. Some foods high in *saturated* fats are listed below them.

Another form of fat is **cholesterol**. Some cholesterol is made from other fats in the body. Cholesterol is essential for the health of each cell. Too much cholesterol, though, is linked with heart and artery disease. Cholesterol forms deposits that build up along arteries and increase the risk of heart attacks and strokes.

People trying to lower blood cholesterol cannot do so by limiting only their cholesterol intakes. They must limit their total fat intakes, and especially limit their saturated fat intakes. Details about dietary fats and blood cholesterol are provided in Chapter 17.

 Fat is the major source of fuel for the body. Food fat comes in saturated and unsaturated forms. Saturated fats come mainly from animal sources. Unsaturated fats come mainly from plant sources (vegetable oils).

Health Strategies

Getting the Fat Out of Your Diet

To get the fat out of your diet:

1. Choose foods that have been grilled, roasted, broiled, boiled, baked, or microwaved. Don't choose fried.
2. Tell the food server, "No gravy," or cut your portion of gravy by half.
3. Pizza can be high in fat. Order it with thick crust and more vegetables than meat. Never ask for double cheese.
4. Choose lean meats with no visible fat. Don't eat meats with fat ground in, such as sausages and cold cuts.
5. Reduce meat servings by half. Load up on grains, beans, and vegetables.
6. Use canned tuna or chicken packed in water, not in oil.
7. Trim all the fat you can see from the meat on your plate.
8. Remove skin from chicken or turkey before eating.
9. Use oil-free salad dressings, reduced-calorie mayonnaise, and diet margarine. Use butter-flavored sprinkles instead of butter.
10. If you must fry something, use cooking spray instead of oil or butter.
11. Choose low-fat or nonfat dairy products. Use nonfat yogurt or nonfat sour cream substitute in place of regular sour cream.

COOPERATIVE LEARNING

Making Sense of Food Labels

Using the information in the text on pp. 180–182, guide students in reading food labels. Have students bring foods and beverages, or just their labels, to class. Have the class break into teams of two or more students. Have teams choose one or two labels, and answer the following about each item:

1. What constitutes a serving, according to the label?
2. How many servings are in a container?
3. How many calories are in one serving?
4. How many grams of fat are in one serving?
5. What vitamins and minerals does the item supply? (The answer may be "none," if no vitamins or minerals are listed on the label.)

Benefits of Reducing Fat Intake

More than any other diet factor, a high fat intake contributes to disease. Especially, saturated fat is damaging to the heart. Many forms of cancer are linked to high total fat intakes. Many other diseases may be, too, including arthritis, gallbladder disease, diabetes, and others. The most important dietary step you can take to prevent these diseases is to limit your total fat intake. When your fat intake falls lower, saturated fat falls with it. One more diet-related step is also critical to preventing diseases: keep your weight within a healthy range. The Health Strategies section, "Getting the Fat Out of Your Diet," on the opposite page describes some choices you can make to cut down on fat.

Reducing fat intake offers another benefit to people who wish to cut calories. A spoon of fat contains more than twice as many calories as a spoon of sugar or pure protein. By removing the fat from a food, you can drastically cut its calorie count. Figure 7–5 on the next page shows that the single most effective step you can take to reduce the calorie count of a food is to eat it with less fat.

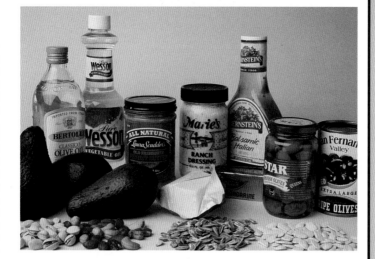

Unsaturated fats come primarily from vegetable oils.

 KEY POINTS *A high-fat diet is linked to many diseases. When you remove the fat from a food, you drastically cut its calorie count.*

How Much Fat Is Enough?

Recommendations for a healthy diet include holding fat to 30 percent of total calories. Carbohydrates should supply about 60 percent of calories, with protein filling in about 10 percent. Eating this way doesn't have to be complicated. A simple plan of low-fat foods can easily meet these recommendations.

Most important, the nutrient percentages just recommended are intended to be averages of a day's or week's worth of food. The percentages mean nothing when applied food by food. For example, foods (like peanut butter) may be very high in fat but also high in nutrients. Include these foods by balancing their fat with low-fat foods in the same meal or in the day's total foods. Peanut butter alone is over 70 percent fat, but when a little peanut butter is spread on two thick slices of bread and is eaten with a banana and a glass of nonfat milk, the fat content of the *meal* is well within recommendations. Figure 7–6 on page 182 shows how to get a rough estimate of how many **grams (g)** of fat you are allowed each day based on recommendations.

MINI Glossary

saturated: concerning fats and health, those fats associated strongly with heart and artery disease; mainly fats from animal sources.

unsaturated: concerning fats and health, fats less associated with heart and artery disease; mainly fats from plant sources.

polyunsaturated: a type of unsaturated fat especially useful as a replacement for saturated fat in a heart-healthy diet.

cholesterol: a type of fat made by the body from saturated fat; a minor part of fat in foods.

grams (abbreviated **g**): units of weight in which many nutrients are measured; 28 grams equals 1 ounce.

TEACH & APPLY

CLASS ACTIVITY

Have students research the role of fats in arctic animals and migratory animals. Discuss how animals prepare themselves for the cold or for migration by eating extra foods, which convert to fat. (They do not necessarily eat extra fat, but extra foods.) These fats insulate them from the cold temperatures and provide energy for their bodies when food is scarce, either in winter, or during a migration when they need extra energy to make the trip.

COMPREHENSION CHECK

Try the following exercise to help students remember which type of fat they should choose and which type they should avoid. Put the following eight words on the board in random order: *animal, solid, saturated, avoid, plants, liquid, unsaturated, choose.* On a sheet of paper, have each student separate the eight words into two separate columns with the four related words in each column. (The first four words listed should be in one column, the second four words in another column.) Have one student come to the front of the class and write the words in the proper columns. Then ask students to brainstorm ways to remember which fats they should choose and which they should avoid.

Then, ask the teams to discuss the following questions, and present their ideas to the class:

1. Did the serving size on the label surprise you? In what way?

2. What serving size do you typically consume?

3. Are calories in a serving too high, too low, or just right?

4. How many calories do you need in a day? (See Appendix B, Figure B–2 at the back of the text for this information.)

5. Is the product high or low in fat? (Read the right-hand column of the label—% of Daily Value—to find the percentage of a typical day's fat allowance provided in a serving.)

6. Is the item a rich source of any vitamin or mineral? (Again, consult the % Daily Value column.)

The handout, "Analyzing Nutrient Labels" is provided in the Teacher's Resource Box. You may want to use it to help students learn to read labels more critically and thereby help them make wiser food choices for their own health as well as for the health of our environment.

COMPREHENSION CHECK

Ask students to study Figure 7–5, "Fat and Calories," on this page. Have them look at the pairs of pictures and consider whether it would be difficult to choose the foods with less fat in any of the three situations. What choice would be the most difficult for them to make? Have they ever tried that choice? Suggest that they give it a try if they haven't. They could find that they like the choices with less fat just as well.

DEBATE

Divide the chairs in your room into three sections. Two groups of chairs face each other—these will be the pro and con sides. The other group will be against a wall facing the other two groups. The persons who will sit against the wall are the undecided individuals.

Make a statement about a controversial issue dealing with nutrition, such as, "There is enough stress in our lives without having to worry about what we eat." Students who agree with the statement sit in the pro section; those who disagree sit in the con section; those who are undecided sit in the section against the wall and listen to arguments from each side until they are persuaded by their classmates' arguments to take a

Figure 7–5 Fat and Calories

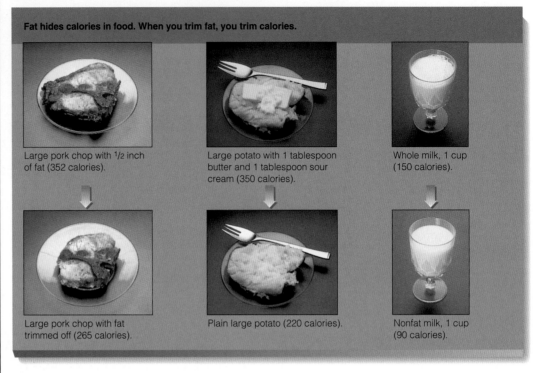

Fat hides calories in food. When you trim fat, you trim calories.

Large pork chop with ½ inch of fat (352 calories).

Large potato with 1 tablespoon butter and 1 tablespoon sour cream (350 calories).

Whole milk, 1 cup (150 calories).

Large pork chop with fat trimmed off (265 calories).

Plain large potato (220 calories).

Nonfat milk, 1 cup (90 calories).

For **Y**our **I**nformation

Unsaturated fat sources:

► Avocados, nuts, seeds, olives, peanut butter.
► Margarine, mayonnaise, salad dressing, oils (liquid types).

Saturated fat sources:

► Bacon, sausage, cold cuts, lunchmeats, hot dogs, hamburgers, chitterlings.
► Butter, lard, coconut and coconut oil, cream (sour or sweet), cheeses, palm oil.

 KEY POINTS *A diet that supports health provides about 30 percent of its calories from fat, 60 percent of its calories from carbohydrate, and 10 percent of its calories from protein.*

Reading Food Labels

One of the most helpful tools for tracking fat intake is the food label. Label-readers can glean all sorts of interesting details about the nutrients in foods. The Consumer Skills feature on the opposite page shows a typical cereal box label. Notice that the Nutrition Facts panel lists some percentages down the right-hand side, including some pertaining to fat. Those percentages reflect how much of a day's total allowance for a nutrient is contributed by 1 serving of the food inside the container.

The Daily Values were developed for use on food labels. They act as a sort of general average of people's needs for nutrients. They assume that everyone needs to consume either 2,000 or 2,500 calories of food in a day. They also assume everyone is adult, not pregnant, not lactating, not aged, and other assumptions. The Daily Values are therefore limited, but they are useful enough for their purpose in allowing nutrient comparisons among food labels. The Daily Values are listed in full in Appendix B at the back of the book.

special needs

Logical-mathematical

To give students an opportunity for real-life practice in making nutritious food choices after reading the Consumer Skills feature, ask each student to bring in samples of food labels from five different foods. Divide the class into small cooperative learning groups

so that each group has at least fifteen different food labels to work with. Ask students to use the labels to develop two different menus of approximately 2000 calories each. Each menu must contain at least seven different food items. The first menu should be as nutritious as possible, considering calories as well as total fat, sodium, carbohydrates, and the % daily value of protein, vitamins, and minerals. The second menu, while still containing at

How to Read a Food Label

Consumer SKILLS

Food labels on everything from a package of potato chips to a box of cereal provide consumers with meaningful nutrition facts. Knowing the proper way to read food labels can put you many steps ahead of the average buyer. Here's an example to show you what's on a food label.

Critical Thinking

1. *Why would a product package need to have the name and address of the manufacturer?*
2. *Why do you think the percentages of daily values are based on a 2,000 calorie diet?*
3. *What does it mean when the ingredients are listed in "descending order of predominance"?*

side. Anyone has the right to change his or her stand on the statement at any time, providing they move only when a speaker is finished speaking. Speakers from the two sides alternate speaking.

The undecided students can ask a question at any time by raising their hands and being recognized by you. If an undecided person wants to make a statement, he or she needs to move to either the pro or con side and wait his or her turn. You act as the facilitator and fact checker.

What's on a Label

The package must always state the product name, the name and address of the manufacturer, and the weight or measure.

The label may state information about sodium, calories, fat, or other constituents.

Approved health claims may be made, but only in terms of total diet.

West's ACTION CEREAL

Low in Fat, Good Source of Fiber

NET WT. 11 OZ. (311g)

Development of heart disease depends on many factors. A healthful diet low in saturated fat may reduce heart disease risks.

West's ACTION CEREAL

Nutrition Facts
Serving size ¾ cup (55g)
Servings per Box 10

Amount Per Serving	
Calories 167	Calories from Fat 27

	% Daily Value*
Total Fat 3g	5%
Saturated Fat 4g	20%
Cholesterol 0mg	0%
Sodium 250mg	10%
Total Carbohydrate 32g	11%
Dietary Fiber 4g	16%
Sugars 11g	
Protein 3g	

Vitamin A 25%	•	**Vitamin C** 25%	
Calcium 2%	•	**Iron** 25%	

* Percent Daily values are based on a 2,000 calorie diet. Your daily values may be higher or lower depending on your calorie needs:

	Calories:	2,000	2,500
Total Fat	Less than	65g	80g
Sat Fat	Less than	20g	25g
Cholesterol	Less than	300mg	300mg
Sodium	Less than	2,400mg	2,400mg
Total Carbohydrate		300g	375g
Dietary Fiber		25g	30g

Calories per gram
Fat 9 • Carbohydrate 4 • Protein 4

Ingredients: Whole oats, Milled corn, Enriched wheat flour (contains Niacin, Reduced iron, Thiamin mononitrate, Riboflavin), Dextrose, Maltose, High-fructose corn syrup, Brown sugar, Partially hydrogenated cottonseed oil, Coconut oil, Walnuts, Salt, and Natural flavors. Vitamins and minerals: Vitamin C (sodium ascorbate), Vitamin A (palmitate), Iron.

Serving size, number of servings per container, and calorie information

Percentages of Daily Values for nutrients based on a 2,000-calorie diet

Daily Values for selected nutrients for a 2,000- and a 2,500-calorie diet.

Calorie/gram reminder

Ingredients in descending order of predominance

Consumer SKILLS

Answers to Critical Thinking

1. Buyers might want to contact the manufacturer to make comments or complaints about the product. Therefore, it is necessary for the consumer to know where to locate the manufacturer.

2. 2,000 calories is probably a good average intake for most of the population.

3. The ingredients are listed in order of the amounts used in the product. An ingredient used most would be listed first, an ingredient used least would be listed last.

least seven different food items totaling around 2000 calories, should *not* be nutritious, so that students can see the difference between nutritious calories and empty calories.

You may want students to use a chart or table as a guide in their planning. It should contain information in the following categories for both Menu 1 and Menu 2: List of foods with number and size of servings, calo-

ries, total fat, sodium, total carbohydrates, and % daily values of protein, vitamins, and minerals.

When completed, have groups share their menus with each other by presenting an oral report and their charted findings. Ask the students to determine the most nutritious menu, the least nutritious menu, the menu they would most like to follow, and the menu they would be the least likely to follow.

ASSESS

EVALUATE

Have students describe how being overweight can have a negative impact on a person's health. Have them describe activities that have a positive impact on their health.

SECTION 5
Review Answers

1. Saturated fat comes from animal sources and is usually solid at room temperature. Unsaturated fat comes from vegetable sources and is liquid at room temperature. (p. 178)

2. cholesterol (p. 178)

3. grams (p. 179)

4. major source of fuel (p. 178)

5. reduces diseases, including heart disease, many forms of cancer, arthritis, gallbladder disease, diabetes, and diseases made worse by overweight; it also reduces calorie count of a food (p. 179)

6. Answers will vary. Refer to the Health Strategies "Getting the Fat Out of Your Diet" on page 178.

7. Foods high in fat can be balanced in the diet with low-fat or nonfat foods. (p. 179)

8. They give a sort of general average of people's needs for nutrients. (p. 180)

9–11. Answers will vary.

WORKSHEETS A reproducible quiz for Section 5 is provided in the Teacher's Resource Box.

CLOSE

Have students name as many reasons as they can think of to monitor the amount of fats in their diets.

Figure 7–6 How to Estimate Your Daily Value for Fat

1. Determine your daily calorie intake (see Recommended Energy Intakes in Appendix B in the back of the book). Example: 1,800.
2. Divide your total calories by10. Example: 1,800 ÷ 10 = 180.
3. Divide the answer to Step 2 by 3. Example: 180 ÷ 3 = 60.
4. In this example, the total daily fat intake should not exceed 60 grams.

The label shown in the Consumer Skills feature on the previous page "How to Read a Food Label" lists fat information as follows:

Amount per Serving	% Daily Value
Total fat 3 g	*5%*

Assuming a diet of 2,000 calories, this means that a serving of the cereal in the box shown contributes just 5 percent of the entire day's allowance for fat. It would take 20 servings of foods like this one to reach the day's fat limits.

$$\frac{3g}{\text{(total fat per serving of cereal)}} \div \frac{65g}{\text{(total fat Daily Value)}} \times 100 = 5\% \text{ of Daily Value for fat}$$

A label coming instead from a can of chili or other meaty item can easily list closer to 21 grams of total fat. In that case, a single serving of that one food contributes about a third of the total fat allowance for the whole day. Such foods are not necessarily off limits to a person watching fat intakes, but they are best used sparingly. A day's meals that include such a food should be finished off with low-fat grains, vegetables, fruits, and nonfat milk to keep fat from exceeding the recommended limits.

There is much more information to be learned from reading food labels. It is well worth the time and effort spent in learning about them.

KEY POINTS *Food labels provide a wealth of information to the knowledgeable consumer.*

SECTION 5 Review

Answer the following questions on a sheet of paper.

Learning the Vocabulary

The vocabulary terms in this section are *saturated, unsaturated, polyunsaturated, cholesterol,* and *grams.*

1. What is the difference between saturated and unsaturated fat?
2. A type of fat made by the body from saturated fat is called _____.
3. Many nutrients are measured in _____.

Learning the Facts

4. What is the main function of fat in the body?
5. List two benefits of limiting the amount of fat in your diet.

6. List three steps you can take to control the amount of fat in your diet.
7. Why should nutrient percentages be averaged over a day or week, rather than applied food by food?
8. What information is given by the Daily Values on food labels?

Making Life Choices

9. Give a few suggestions on how you might best keep your blood cholesterol level down through your dietary choices.
10. Generally speaking, most of the foods from fast-food restaurants are high in fat and lacking in other essential nutrients. Do you find yourself eating at this type of restaurant often? Why or why not?
11. Do you know of any low-fat foods that fast-food restaurants serve? What are they?

QUICK QUIZ

Chapter 7, Section 5

The following quiz will help you assess your students' understanding of the material covered in this section of the chapter. You might use the quiz as an oral exercise, which will lead into a class discussion of the topics covered. Or, you might use it as a paper/pencil

quiz to evaluate your students individually.

Like the Quick Quiz, the Section Review can also be used as an assessment tool to spark class discussion or as an individual student evaluation. It can also be used as a review in preparation for this quiz.

1. Fat supplies very little of the body's fuel. (False)
2. Fat insulates the body and cushions it from bruises, strains, and breaks. (True)

SECTION 6

Protein

SECTION 6

Protein is well known as the bodybuilding nutrient, the material of strong muscles—and rightly so. No new living tissue can be built without it, for protein is part of every cell, every bone, the blood, and every other tissue. Proteins are the body's machinery—they do the cells' work. The energy to fuel that work comes mainly from carbohydrate and fat. As mentioned earlier, protein donates a little energy as well.

Proteins are made of building blocks, the amino acids. A set of 20 different amino acids form proteins (much as letters of the alphabet form words and sentences). Your body can make some of the amino acids for itself. The other amino acids, which the body cannot make, are the **essential amino acids**. You must eat foods that contain them.

Your body loses protein every day. Digestive tract cells wear out and exit the body in the stools. Skin cells flake off or are rubbed off. Hair and nails (made of protein) grow longer daily and are shed or trimmed away. An adult loses about one-quarter cup of pure protein a day. People need to eat protein-containing foods every day to replace the protein they lose.

You know you are eating protein when you eat meats, fish, poultry, eggs, cheese, and milk. Protein also is contained in plant foods such as grains and beans (chili beans, lima beans, and the like). Other vegetables eaten in quantity also provide protein. In fact, a teenager receives more than a day's protein from one egg, two cups of milk, and an assortment of grains and vegetables—without a single serving of meat. Yet many teens choose two or three eggs for breakfast, a couple of hamburgers for lunch, and a big portion of roast for dinner.

Meats, eggs, and cheese are often high in fat and calories, and all are low in fiber. Too much of these foods can cause weight gain and threaten health. Vegetables, beans, grains, and low-fat milk are better choices for providing most of the day's protein.

Well-informed **vegetarians** can easily get enough protein from plant foods alone. Figure 7–7 on the next page lists some high-protein vegetarian food combinations.

Animal proteins supply all of the essential amino acids in the right amounts for building human tissues. Most plant proteins, in contrast, contain limited amounts of certain of the essential amino acids. To build muscles, make new cell parts, and grow, the body needs all of the essential amino acids. Therefore, single plant proteins alone usually won't serve the need. People who eat only plant foods must eat combinations of them each day to receive the full range of needed amino acids. The foods need not be eaten together in one meal, but may be spread among several of the day's meals. The food combinations suggested in Figure 7–7 and others like them provide the full range of essential amino acids, beneficial starch and fiber, and many more nutrients besides.

A person who fails to consume enough protein is taking a grave risk. The body wastes away its lean tissues and is left defenseless against diseases (the immune cells are made of protein). This often happens in remote places

Milk provides protein as well as many other nutrients.

MINI Glossary

essential amino acids: amino acids that are needed, but cannot be made by the body; they must be eaten in foods.

vegetarians: people who omit meat, fish, and poultry from their diets. Some vegetarians also omit milk products and eggs.

3. Unsaturated fats come mainly from animal sources. (False)

4. Cholesterol is a form of fat which is linked with heart and artery disease. (True)

5. Saturated fat is especially damaging to the heart. (True)

6. Limiting your fat intake is the most important dietary step you can take. (True)

7. Removing fat from a food does not sig-nificantly reduce the food's calorie count. (False)

8. To prevent diseases, it is critical to keep your body weight within a healthy range. (True)

9. Calories from fat should make up about 50 percent of a healthy diet. (False)

10. Food labels provide valuable information about the nutritional content of food. (True)

CLASS ACTIVITY

Using Figure 7–7, have students put together a vegetarian diet for a week. Remind them to make sure the necessary amino acids are included. Have students underline sources of protein, circle sources of fiber, and put a check mark beside those the provide carbohydrates. They should put a dot by those that are high in fat.

ASSESS

EVALUATE

Have students answer in essay form, Why is protein necessary in the diet?

Review Answers

1. Answers will vary.
2. the body's machinery, does the cells' work (p. 183)
3. meats, fish, poultry, eggs, cheese, milk, grains, beans, and other vegetables (p. 183)
4. The body wastes away its lean tissues and is left defenseless against disease. Hair loss and changes in skin occur. (p. 183)
5. Answers will vary.
6. Answers will vary.

CLOSE

Divide the class into two teams. Give each side five seconds to think of a food that is protein-rich. Have students go back and forth until one of the sides is stumped and cannot think of a protein source in time. The other team wins.

Figure 7–7 Vegetarian Protein Combinations

Choose foods from two or more of these columns in a day to obtain the needed amino acids:			
Grains	**Legumes**	**Seeds and Nuts**	**Vegetables**
Barley	Dried beans	Cashews	Broccoli
Bulgur	Dried lentils	Nut butters	Leafy greens
Cornmeal	Dried peas	Other nuts	Other vegetables
Oats	Peanuts	Sesame seeds	
Pasta	Soy products	Sunflower seeds	
Rice		Walnuts	
Whole-grain breads and other grain products.			

of the world. However, it also happens here among neglected and homeless children, sick people in hospitals, substance abusers, and others. Dieters who starve themselves may notice that, within a few months of dieting, their hair begins to fall out or their skin starts to change. These are signs of protein deficiency. For most people who eat a normal diet, though, protein deficiency is almost never a problem.

 KEY POINTS   *Protein is made of amino acids and serves as the building material for many body structures. The essential amino acids must be obtained from food each day. The consequences of protein deficiency are severe, but most people consume enough protein.*

 Review

Answer the following questions on a sheet of paper.

Learning the Vocabulary

The vocabulary terms in this section are *essential amino acids* and *vegetarians.*

1. Write a sentence using each vocabulary term.

Learning the Facts

2. What is the function of protein in the body?

3. What foods are the best sources of protein?
4. What are some signs of protein deficiency?

Making Life Choices

5. How can vegetarians best meet the body's protein needs without consuming animal proteins? Develop your own vegetarian protein combinations.
6. Most teenagers seem to get more than enough protein to meet their bodies' needs. Do you think the protein-rich foods you eat are the best ones for your health? Why or why not?

QUICK QUIZ

Chapter 7, Section 6

The following quiz will help you assess your students' understanding of the material covered in this section of the chapter. You might use the quiz as an oral exercise, which will lead into a class discussion of the topics covered. Or, you might use it as a paper/pencil

quiz to evaluate your students individually.

*If students have difficulty with the concepts covered in the Quick Quiz and the Section Review, you might suggest they review the material using the **S**urvey, **Q**uestion, **R**ead, **R**ecite, **R**eview (SQ3R) study method, which is described in detail in the introduction to this Teacher's Wraparound Edition.*

1. The body can substitute for protein in building cells. (False)

SECTION 7
Vitamins

The discovery of the vitamins thrilled people around the globe. Whole groups of people had been unable to walk, or to see, or to stop bleeding. Then, like a miracle, they recovered when one vitamin was added to their diets. On reading stories like these, people came to believe that vitamins could cure almost anything. Today we see a stream of advertisements for "miracle vitamins." The quacks say, "Are you nearsighted? Do you have pimples? The right vitamin pill will cure what ails you!" As a result, the **supplement** business is a multi*billion*-dollar industry.

The truth is, a vitamin can cure only the disease caused by a **deficiency** of that vitamin. Also, an overdose of any vitamin can make people as sick as a deficiency. It can even cause death (see Figure 7–8). While vitamins are dangerous in high doses, minerals (discussed later in this chapter) are even more dangerous. They can cause illness when taken in amounts not far above the recommended levels of intake. A balanced diet of ordinary foods supplies enough, but not too much, of each of the vitamins and minerals.

Vitamins themselves provide no energy to the body. Instead, many help to release energy from carbohydrate, fat, and protein. Other vitamins serve as helpers of other body processes.

The vitamins fall naturally into two classes—the **fat-soluble** ones and the **water-soluble** ones. The fat-soluble vitamins dissolve in the body's fats and tend to remain in the body. For this reason, the fat-soluble vitamins can build up to dangerous levels if a person takes supplements of them.

The water-soluble vitamins travel in the body's watery fluids and leave the body readily in the urine. This means that you must be sure to eat foods that provide water-soluble vitamins regularly to replace those that you have lost.

This section discusses a few of the vitamins and the importance of meeting your body's needs for them. A later section does the same for some of the minerals. The next section provides some current information about the vitamins called antioxidants.

 KEY POINTS *Too little or too much of any vitamin or mineral is harmful to health. Vitamins serve as helpers in body processes. Fat-soluble vitamins dissolve in fat. Water-soluble vitamins dissolve in water.*

Figure 7–8 Vitamin and Mineral Safety. Most people think, wrongly, that vitamins and minerals are safe in any amount. The truth is that too much can be as dangerous as too little.

Mini Glossary

supplement: a pill, powder, liquid, or the like containing only nutrients; not a food.

deficiency (dee-FISH-en-see): too little of a nutrient in the body. Severe deficiencies cause diseases.

fat-soluble (SOL-you-bul): a chemist's term meaning "able to dissolve in fat."

water-soluble: able to dissolve in water.

2. Energy to fuel the work performed by proteins comes mainly from carbohydrates and fat. (True)
3. Proteins are made of building blocks called fatty acids. (False)
4. The body produces essential amino acids. (False)
5. The body loses a significant amount of protein every day. (True)
6. The body's protein can be replaced only by protein-containing foods. (True)
7. Protein is contained in plant foods as well as meat, eggs and poultry. (True)
8. Vegetarians cannot get enough proteins from plant foods alone. (False)
9. Vegetarians must be careful to eat specific combinations of plant food each day in order to receive the full range of needed amino acids. (True)
10. Protein deficiency is a common problem. (False)

SECTION 7
FOCUS
OUTCOMES
In this section students will learn:
1. The functions of different vitamins in the human body.
2. How to analyze their diets for vitamin content.
3. The effects of various vitamin deficiencies and overdoses.

FOCUS ACTIVITY
Write the word *deficiency* on the board or overhead. Ask students to define the word in their own terms and to give examples of deficiencies: (Students learned the term *nutrient deficiency* in previous sections; you may want to refer them to the Mini Glossary definition.) Discuss student examples and compare these with the federal deficit. (Most students are probably familiar with this term.) Have students tell you what it would mean to have a vitamin or mineral deficiency.

TEACH & APPLY
COMPREHENSION CHECK
Ask students to read the definition of supplement, then ask them to explain what a supplement is in their own words. Ask them why a variety of pills, powders, and liquids are called *supplements*. (People use them to *supplement*, add to, the nutrients they get from foods they eat.)

COMPREHENSION CHECK

Ask students if it is better to eat too many vitamins or too few. (neither—both can be harmful)

TEACHER SUPPORT

Key Passage

The medical term for permanent blindness is *xerophthalmia*. Children deprived of vitamin A do become blind from this preventable condition. If the deficiency is discovered early, it can be reversed by two or three capsules of vitamin A daily. Vitamin A deficiency is the major cause of childhood blindness in the world. More than five million of the world's children suffer from less obvious signs of vitamin A deficiency—stunted growth, poor appetite, and impaired immunity resulting in infections. In Asia, vitamin A deficiency is charged with destroying the vision of 250,000 preschool children each year.

CLASS ACTIVITY

Ask students to list how often in the past week they have eaten dark green vegetables, deep orange and yellow fruits and vegetables, and milk. How many think they might be deficient in vitamin A intake? Ask them what problems this can cause in addition to night blindness. (Infections occur more readily, the skin becomes dry, and growth slows.)

Figure 7–9 Night Blindness

Night blindness is one of the earliest signs of vitamin A deficiency. A person who takes in too little vitamin A might experience this change in vision. Figure 7–10, on page 188, lists food sources of vitamin A.

A. In dim light, you can make out the details in this room.

B. A flash of bright light momentarily blinds you.

C. You quickly recover and can see the details again in a few seconds.

D. With too little vitamin A, you do not recover but remain blinded for many seconds; this is night blindness.

Vitamin A

Vitamin A deficiency is the major cause of childhood blindness in the world. More than half a million young children lose their sight each year because of vitamin A deficiency. One of the earliest signs of vitamin A deficiency is **night blindness**, which is illustrated in Figure 7–9 above. As vitamin A deficiency grows worse, it leads to permanent blindness.

Vitamin A also helps the body fight infections. It maintains normal, healthy skin and promotes growth. The symptoms of vitamin A deficiency therefore make themselves known not only in the eyes, but throughout the body. Infections occur readily, the skin becomes dry, and growth slows. In short, vitamin A deficiency interferes with many body processes.

Vitamin A deficiency often occurs along with protein deficiency. In countries where food is scarce, then, protein and vitamin A deficiencies are major nutrition problems.

In developed nations such as ours, people who take supplements of vitamin A should beware. Vitamin A dissolves into body fat, and can build up to toxic levels. Food sources of vitamin A are chemically different from the vitamin A in supplements. Vitamin A from foods does not cause dangerous buildups to occur. Only vitamin A from supplements does.

The best food sources of vitamin A are dark green vegetables, deep yellow and orange fruits and vegetables, and milk. Fast foods such as burgers and fries are poor sources of vitamin A. It is not surprising that many teenagers' diets tend to be low in vitamin A.

 KEY POINTS *Night blindness can be an early sign of vitamin A deficiency. Vitamin A is important to many body processes. Teens must make special efforts to eat enough vitamin A–rich foods.*

Pursuing wellness

Vitamins are nutrients that help control growth and help your body release energy to do work. Vitamin C is a water-soluble vitamin that needs to be consumed on a regular basis. In the early 1700s, the British navy found that sailors could not take voyages longer than about three months because the crew would develop the vitamin C deficiency called scurvy.

While vitamin C is an important vitamin and critical to good health, it has not been shown to be a miracle vitamin. A deficiency of vitamin C can result in disease; however, the presence of vitamin C or extremely large

Thiamin

Thiamin is typical of the water-soluble vitamins. It helps the body use energy from other nutrients, such as carbohydrates. Your body cannot feel its presence, but its absence makes itself known by causing symptoms.

The victim of a serious thiamin deficiency suffers severe symptoms: paralyzed limbs, loss of muscle tissue, swellings, enlargement of the heart, irregular heartbeat, and ultimately death from heart failure. Luckily, such extreme deficiencies almost never occur, but a mild lack of thiamin also produces symptoms. These include stomachaches, headaches, fatigue, restlessness, problems sleeping, chest pains, fevers, feelings of anger and aggression, and a whole string of symptoms often mistaken for mental illness. It takes a professional diagnosis based on chemical tests to determine the true causes of such common symptoms.

Mild thiamin deficiencies are likely to be seen in people who eat "junk" diets—that is, diets low in nutrients and high in calories, sugar, fat, and salt.

What foods in particular supply thiamin, then? Almost no one food you can eat will supply your daily need in a single serving. In fact, a teenager must eat *sixteen or more servings of nutritious foods each day* to get enough thiamin. The Daily Food Guide advises this number of servings (see Figure 7–1, earlier in this chapter).

Vitamins fall into two classes—fat soluble and water soluble.

 KEY POINTS *Thiamin is essential for health. To get enough thiamin and other nutrients, a teenager must eat sixteen or more servings of nutritious foods each day.*

Vitamin B$_6$

Vitamin B$_6$ is a classic example of a nutrient that can be toxic in excess. Whenever people start overusing a nutrient, no matter how harmless the nutrient may seem at first, it is only a matter of time before toxic effects appear. A few years ago, people were "diagnosing" themselves as having vitamin B$_6$ deficiencies, and then "prescribing" large doses for themselves.

The first major report of toxic effects of high doses of vitamin B$_6$ described people who had numb feet, then lost sensation in their hands, and then became unable to work. Later, their mouths became numb. Since then, other reports have shown nervous system damage from overdosing with vitamin B$_6$.

Not everyone suffers toxicity symptoms with high doses of vitamin B$_6$. Compared with fat-soluble vitamins, vitamin B$_6$ is relatively nontoxic. However, people vary in how much is too much for them. We cannot say that supplements are "safe" for anyone. This fact holds true for every vitamin. Food sources are safe, though. Figure 7–10 on the next page presents the best food sources of vitamin B$_6$ and the other vitamins. The figure also lists the jobs the vitamins do in the body.

 KEY POINTS *Vitamin B$_6$ is needed to maintain health. Too much vitamin B$_6$, like too much of any nutrient, is harmful.*

Antioxidant Vitamins

Many people are excited about new studies linking heart disease and cancer with low intakes of **antioxidant** vitamins. Their first reaction was to

MINI Glossary

night blindness: slow recovery of vision after flashes of bright light at night; an early symptom of vitamin A deficiency.

antioxidant (AN-tee-OX-ih-dant): a chemical that can stop the destructive chain reactions of free radicals. Among the nutrients, vitamins C and E, beta-carotene, and the mineral selenium are examples.

amounts of the vitamin do not enhance your health or guarantee freedom from disease. In fact, very large doses of vitamin C can cause health problems such as diarrhea, kidney stones, damage to growing bone, gout, and a burning sensation during urination. A healthy and balanced diet should provide all the vitamin C needed for most people. If you take vitamin supplements, be careful not to exceed the established dietary allowances established by the Food and Nutrition Board of the National Academy of Sciences and National Research Council.

BACKGROUND INFORMATION

You may want to tell your students that scientists studied some people who snack heavily on empty-calorie foods and found that these people had below normal thiamin activity in their blood. They also had the mental and physical symptoms of a mild thiamin deficiency. The scientists gave these people thiamin supplements for a month or so. The symptoms disappeared as the thiamin measures in the blood returned to normal. If you give students this information, also caution them against relying on supplements. It is better to obtain vitamins and minerals from foods than from supplements.

GROUP ACTIVITY

Assign groups of students different vitamins and have them create a skit showing how that vitamin functions in the body. You might also want them to show what happens if too much or too little of the vitamin is consumed. Tell students to be creative and make these funny, but to make sure the information portrayed in the skit is accurate. You may want to have them use visual aids.

FAST FACTS

57 percent of youngsters surveyed in a Gallup Poll said they had skipped breakfast.

188

CLASS ACTIVITY

Have students list ten foods that they eat on a regular basis. Have them list the vitamins contained in these food sources, then list the vitamins they need to include in their diets and what foods they will eat to include those vitamins. Have them use this list to make a vitamin contract so they will know which foods to add to their existing diets in order to get a variety of vitamins.

GROUP PROJECTS

Divide the class into small groups and have each group research a vitamin deficiency (which you assign to the group) and good sources of foods to supply those vitamins related to the deficiency. After listening to the research reports, other students should be able to list the vitamins in which people can easily become deficient and foods that supply those vitamins.

LEARNING WITH VISUALS

Have students draw a picture depicting the lack of a certain vitamin in the body. The picture should make an obvious connection between the vitamin and the related symptoms of the deficiency. It should contain the name of the vitamin and perhaps some depiction of food sources from which the vitamin is derived. You may want to have the students present their pictures to the rest of the class. They should be able to answer any questions about their vitamins and the related deficiencies.

Figure 7–10 *Major Roles and Sources of the Vitamins*

Vitamin	What It Does In the Body	Major Sources
Fat-soluble		
Vitamin A	Maintains normal vision and healthy bones, skin, internal linings, and reproductive system; strengthens resistance to infection	Vitamin A–fortified milk and dairy products; margarine; liver
Beta-carotene	A form of vitamin A and an antioxidant	Dark green vegetables (broccoli, spinach, greens); deep orange fruits and vegetables (cantaloupe, apricots, sweet potatoes, carrots)
Vitamin D	Promotes growth and health of bones	Vitamin D–fortified milk; eggs; liver; sardines; sunlight on the skin
Vitamin E	Protects the body cells from attack by oxygen: an antioxidant	Vegetable oils and shortening; green, leafy vegetables; whole grains; nuts and seeds
Vitamin K	Helps with blood clotting and bone growth	Normal bacteria in the digestive tract; liver; dark green, leafy vegetables; milk
Water-soluble		
Vitamin C	Acts as the "glue" that holds cells together; strengthens blood vessel walls; helps wounds heal; helps bones grow; strengthens resistance to infection but does not cure colds; an antioxidant	Citrus fruits; dark green vegetables; cabbage-like vegetables; strawberries; peppers; potatoes
Thiamin	Helps the body use nutrients for energy	Small amounts in all nutritious foods
Riboflavin	Helps the body use nutrients for energy; supports normal vision; helps keep skin healthy	Milk; yogurt; cottage cheese; dark green vegetables; whole-grain products
Niacin	Helps the body use nutrients for energy; supports normal nervous system functions	Milk; eggs; poultry; fish; whole-grain products; all protein-containing foods
Vitamin B_6	Helps the body use protein and form red blood cells	Green, leafy vegetables; meats; fish; poultry; whole-grain products; beans
Vitamin B_{12}	Helps form new cells	Meats; fish; poultry; shellfish; eggs; milk; cheese
Folate	Helps form new cells	Dark green, leafy vegetables; beans; liver
Biotin and pantothenic acid	Helps the body use nutrients for energy	Widespread in foods

Note: The names given here are the official names. Other names still commonly used and seen on labels are *alphatocopherol* for vitamin E, *vitamin B_1* for thiamin, *vitamin B_2* for riboflavin, *pyridoxine* for vitamin B_6, *folic acid* and *folacin* for folate, and *ascorbic acid* for vitamin C.

purchase supplements containing these vitamins. Two examples, however, help to show that people considering taking supplements of these vitamins should approach them with caution.

People who suffer from certain types of cancer often report eating few fruits and vegetables that contain a form of vitamin A, an antioxidant called **beta-carotene**. When these findings first became known, some people made the mistake of equating food with pills. They rushed out to buy beta-carotene

Pursuing wellness

Health Foods, Natural Foods, and Organic Foods

Health food is a term often used to imply that a food is special and can benefit people's health. This term, however, is inherently misleading due to the fact that almost all foods are healthy when eaten in moderation and can be unhealthy when eaten in excess. Any food that has caloric value (a measurement of energy) would contribute to your health. By this definition, snack cakes, ice cream bars, and soft drinks would all fit into the category of health foods!

Free radical   Molecules in the body

Cancer
Heart disease
Other diseases
Aging

1. Free radicals destroy molecules in the body.
2. This causes a chain reaction, destroying more molecules

3. The chain reaction injures tissues and causes disease and aging.

Vitamin E

4. Vitamin E and other antioxidants stop the chain reaction of the free radicals.

Figure 7–11 Free Radicals in the Body. Free radicals are formed in the body with normal body function. They are also formed during disease and aging.

supplements. Then, when research determined that beta-carotene pills have no protective effect, they flocked to the next vitamin fad.

No one yet knows why foods rich in beta-carotene might be protective, when the substance itself clearly is not. Perhaps some other beneficial chemical travels with beta-carotene in foods. Perhaps a number of such chemicals work in harmony to lower disease risks.

In any case, smart consumers look for beta-carotene-rich foods to include in the diet, such as those listed in the margin. Foods that contain beta-carotene typically appear deep orange or a deep, dark green.

Another antioxidant, vitamin E, seems masterful at defending the heart and arteries against diseases. Vitamin E has the knack of stopping the destructive activities of **free radicals**, which would otherwise damage body tissues. Given the chance, these dangerous free radicals start chemical chain reactions in the cells of the lungs, blood, heart—and, in fact, all of the tissues of the body. The chain reactions are believed to trigger or worsen cancer and diseases of the heart and arteries. Vitamin E stops the chain reaction, and so prevents the diseases, as shown in Figure 7–11 above.

People who eat diets rich in Vitamin E—either from foods or supplements—have fewer heart attacks than those whose diets lack the vitamin. Supplement makers are therefore proclaiming vitamin E pills as the new magic bullet against aging, diseases, and even death itself. However, some nutritionists warn that taking vitamin E supplements is not risk-free.

In amounts common in supplements, vitamin E in the body acts as a drug, not as a nutrient. For example, vitamin E supplements slow the clotting of blood, which can cause excessive bleeding should the person undergo surgery or be injured. Vitamin E supplements are also linked with an increased risk of bleeding in the brain (stroke), as well as with diseases such as asthma and one form of arthritis.

For **Y**our **I**nformation

Foods high in beta-carotene: apricots, broccoli, brussels sprouts, cantaloupe, carrots, leafy greens (collards, turnip, or mustard greens), orange juice, oranges, pumpkin, spinach, winter squash).

MINI Glossary

beta-carotene (Bay-tah CARE-oh-teen): an orange vegetable pigment that the body can change into the active form of vitamin A; one of the antioxidant nutrients.

free radicals: chemicals that harm the body's tissues by starting destructive chain reactions in the molecules of the body's cells. Such reactions are believed to trigger or worsen some diseases.

Natural foods are promoted as those foods produced and marketed with a minimum of processing and without the use of additives or artificial ingredients. This really applies only to meat and poultry. There is no legal meaning for the term *natural* when used with baked goods, processed foods, or beverages.

Organic foods are said to be foods grown without pesticides or synthetic fertilizers. In scientific usage, "organic" refers to compounds that contain carbon, which virtually all foods contain. Like the word *natural*, organic still lacks a legal meaning, though lawmakers are currently working to define it.

ASSESS

EVALUATE

Create a meal that is unbalanced as far as vitamin content. Have students circle foods that provide the same vitamins in abundance and add foods for vitamins that are not provided by the meal. Have students write the vitamins that are supplied in abundance and those that they have attempted to add.

Review Answers

1. fat-soluble, water-soluble (p. 185)
2. supplement (p. 185)
3. deficiency (p. 185)
4. Fat-soluble vitamins dissolve in fat and remain in the body longer. Water-soluble vitamins travel in the body's fluids and pass through the body quickly. (p. 185)
5. childhood blindness and slow growth (p. 186)
6. thiamin (p. 187)
7. Answers will vary.

A reproducible quiz for Section 7 is provided in the Teacher's Resource Box.

CLOSE

Have students define the word *vitamin* and name as many vitamins as they can with their books closed. Write the vitamins on the board and have students call out food sources that supply those vitamins. Write these on the board next to the appropriate vitamins.

Beta-carotene is found abundantly in foods like these.

One more antioxidant vitamin is worth mentioning: vitamin C. Like vitamin E, vitamin C protects body tissues from free radical destruction. Unlike vitamin E, however, vitamin C is found in abundance in fruits and vegetables. Pills of vitamin C are not necessary, even for people who have colds. Studies show that the effects of large doses of vitamin C are small or nonexistent on colds for most people. Extra large doses of vitamin C can be toxic.

In truth, the final word about antioxidants remains to be written. Most scientists agree that it is too early to recommend that people start taking antioxidant supplements. It's better to wait, they say, until all the risks are known.

Foods, however, deliver antioxidant vitamins safely. Foods also contain thousands of other chemicals that may benefit health in ways we are only beginning to appreciate. (Read more about them in Chapter 17.) For now, choose at least five generous servings of fruits and vegetables each day for their antioxidant vitamins, other nutrients, and all their health-promoting secrets still awaiting discovery.

 KEY POINTS *People who eat foods rich in the antioxidant vitamins beta carotene, vitamin E, and vitamin C, may lower their risks of disease. Foods deliver antioxidant vitamins safely. Antioxidant vitamin supplements can be toxic.*

 Review

Answer the following questions on a sheet of paper.

Learning the Vocabulary

The vocabulary terms in this section are *supplement, deficiency, fat-soluble, water-soluble, night blindness, antioxidant, beta-carotene,* and *free radical.*

1. The two classes of vitamins are _____ and _____.
2. A powder or pill that contains only nutrients is called a _____.
3. A _____ is a condition in which the body lacks an essential nutrient.

Learning the Facts

4. What is the difference between a fat-soluble and a water-soluble vitamin?
5. What is one result of a vitamin A deficiency?
6. Which vitamin helps the body use energy from other nutrients?

Making Life Choices

7. Why is it better to obtain the nutrients you need from foods, rather than supplements? Have you ever taken supplements? If so, what were your reasons for doing this?

QUICK QUIZ

Chapter 7, Section 7

The following quiz will help you assess your students' understanding of the material covered in this section of the chapter. You might use the quiz as an oral exercise, which will lead into a class discussion of the topics covered. Or, you might use it as a paper/pencil

quiz to evaluate your students individually.

Like the Quick Quiz, the Section Review can also be used as an assessment tool to spark class discussion or as an individual student evaluation. It can also be used as a review in preparation for this quiz.

1. Vitamin deficiencies cause illnesses that can usually be cured by a supplement of the vitamin. (True)
2. Vitamins are harmless, even in high

SECTION 8

Minerals

If you could extract all of the minerals from a single human body, they would easily fit into a box about the size of a cracker box and would weigh just a few pounds. Then, if you could remove all of the calcium and phosphorus from the box, only a small handful of dust would remain. Were you then to separate out of the handful each of the 16 or so remaining minerals, you'd want to close the window before you did so. Most are present in amounts so small that the slightest breeze might blow them away.

All minerals, even those present in just tiny amounts, are essential for proper body functioning. A tiny trace of a mineral contains billions of molecules that play vital roles in the body.

Teenagers need three servings of calcium-rich foods like these each day.

Calcium

Calcium is the most abundant mineral in the human body. Most of the body's calcium is stored in the bones and teeth. Milk and milk products are the best food sources of calcium. Everyone knows that children and teens need milk daily to support the growth of their bones. Calcium is not found in many other kinds of foods, however, and low intakes of milk are common.

A deficiency of calcium during childhood, and especially in the teen years, threatens the strength of the bones for the rest of the person's life. It sets the stage for loss of bone tissue, **osteoporosis**, which can totally cripple a person in later years. Chapter 21 tells more about who is at risk for osteoporosis and what is known about its prevention and treatment.

The obvious way to meet the need for calcium is to drink milk or eat milk products daily, because they are almost the only foods that contain much calcium per serving. Figure 7–12 on the next page shows the amounts of milk that will meet the calcium intake recommendations. A few other foods contain calcium, too: almonds, canned sardines (with the bones), leafy greens, broccoli, and beans. Orange juice sometimes has calcium added to it. This can be valuable for people who are allergic to milk. The photo above shows some calcium-rich food choices.

 KEY POINTS *Calcium is the body's most abundant mineral and is needed to form and maintain strong bones. Milk and milk products are its primary food sources.*

For Your Information

Teens, especially girls, should make sure they get enough calcium every day to build bones while bones are being made. The only time to strengthen the bones is before the mid-twenties. After about age 25, bones stop growing stronger and gradually lose their calcium over the remaining years of life.

MINI Glossary

osteoporosis (OS-tee-oh-por-OH-sis): a disease of gradual bone loss, which can cripple people in later life.

FOCUS

OUTCOMES

In this section students will learn:

1. What functions minerals perform in the human body.
2. The role of minerals as electrolytes.
3. The food sources of minerals and how students can analyze their diets for mineral content.

FOCUS ACTIVITY

Discuss with students the idea that young people who drink milk grow up to be big and strong. Ask students if this is accurate. Why or why not?

TEACH & APPLY

BACKGROUND INFORMATION

The major minerals are calcium, chloride, magnesium, phosphorus, potassium, sodium, and sulfur. The trace minerals are arsenic, boron, chromium, cobalt, copper, fluoride, iodine, iron, manganese, molybdenum, nickel, selenium, silicone, and zinc.

---

doses. (False)

3. Vitamins provide energy to the body. (False)
4. Vitamins fall into two classes: fat-soluble and water-soluble. (True)
5. Water-soluble vitamins need to be replaced regularly, because they are not retained long in the body. (True)
6. Night blindness is an early sign of Vitamin B$_6$ deficiency. (False)
7. Thiamin deficiency can cause symptoms

ranging from headache to death from heart failure. (True)

8. Vitamin B$_6$ is not essential to maintaining health. (False)
9. The antioxidant called beta-carotene has been proven to prevent certain kinds of cancer. (False)
10. Vitamin E stops the destructive activities of free radicals. (True)

COMPREHENSION CHECK

Ask students to close their books and give you the different symptoms listed for iron deficiency. Ask if any of them feel that they have these symptoms or know someone who does. Do they think there is a chance the symptoms are caused by a lack of iron? Figure 7–13 on page 194 lists foods that supply iron.

Key Passage

You may want to tell students about an additional cause of iron deficiency. Iron deficiency can sometimes be caused by poor absorption of the iron that is in the food. Factors that impair iron availability are tea, coffee, soy protein, wheat bran, calcium supplements, and fiber. Even without these influences, however, a normal, healthy person absorbs only about 10 percent of the iron from a mixed diet.

BACKGROUND INFORMATION

You may want to tell students that certain researchers, such as Randall Lauffer at Harvard Medical School, believe that many people have a disorder known as iron overload, which may lead to heart disease and cancer. Their suggestion is to skip the iron-enriched vitamins and foods and cut down on meat.

Answers to FACT or FICTION

Here are the answers to the questions at the start of the chapter.

1. **False.** Eating foods with enough nutrients is important, but equally important is to keep from eating too much or too little food.
2. **True.**
3. **False.** Of all the things in foods that cause diseases, fat is by far the biggest culprit.
4. **True.**
5. **False.** You can easily get enough protein from grains, beans, vegetables, milk, and eggs without eating any meat.
6. **False.** The only disease that a vitamin supplement will cure is the one caused by a deficiency of that vitamin.
7. **False.** All of the vitamins and minerals can be toxic in large amounts.
8. **False.** The best dietary measure against cancer is to consume at least five servings of vitamin-rich fruits and vegetables each day.
9. **False.** Low intakes of calcium are common, because few foods contain it in large amounts.
10. **True.**

Figure 7–12 *Amounts of Milk Needed to Meet Calcium Recommendations*

Age	Recommended Daily Intake
Children	2 cups
Teenagers	3 cups
Adults[a]	2 cups
Pregnant women	3+ cups
Pregnant teens	4+ cups
Older women	3 to 5 cups

[a]Nonfat or low-fat milk is recommended for adults.

Iron

Iron is present in every living cell and is the body's oxygen carrier. In the red blood cells, iron carries oxygen from the lungs to the tissues. Tissues must have oxygen to produce the energy they need to do their work. Too little iron causes **anemia**, with symptoms of weakness, tiredness, apathy, and headaches. A paleness develops that reflects a reduction in the number and size of the red blood cells. (In dark-skinned people, this paleness can be seen in the corner of the eye.) With too few or too small red blood cells, the person with this anemia grows weak and tires quickly. Energy will return, though, after a few weeks of eating the needed iron-rich foods.

Iron is one of the **trace minerals**, so called because only tiny amounts are needed in the diet. Even so, as many as half of all people—especially children, teens, and women—suffer from iron deficiency. Children and teens are prone to iron deficiency because of their rapid growth. Women in their reproductive years also tend to become iron deficient for two reasons: they lose iron in the blood of menstruation each month, and pregnancy brings extra demands for iron to support the growth of the developing infant.

People who are low on iron begin to feel tired long before they are diagnosed with iron-deficiency anemia. With no obvious disease, they seem lazy and careless. They cannot work or play with zest, and they become unfit physically. Schoolchildren and teens who lack iron even slightly perform poorly on tests of concentration and memory. If this one worldwide malnutrition problem could be solved, millions of people's lives would brighten. A person who feels bad day after day should suspect that something is wrong. That something might turn out to be poor nutrition. The cause of iron deficiency is usually poor nutrition. Two reasons people may receive too little iron are a sheer lack of food (starvation) or a steady diet of iron-poor foods. Other reasons are medical—blood loss or infection with parasites, for example.

Meats, fish, poultry, and beans are rich in iron. An easy way to obtain the needed iron is to eat these foods regularly. Foods that are rich in iron, however, are low in calcium, and vice versa. Any plan for a balanced diet must provide enough of both. Figure 7–13 on page 194 presents the minerals important in the diet, what they do in the body, and food sources of each one.

 KEY POINTS *Iron carries oxygen in the red blood cells. Too little iron in the diet causes anemia. Meats, fish, poultry, and beans are rich sources of iron and should be included in the diet each day.*

HEALTHY PEOPLE 2000

Increase calcium intake so at least 50 percent of youth aged 12 through 24 and 50 percent of pregnant and lactating women consume 3 or more servings daily of foods rich in calcium, and at least 50 percent of people aged 25 and older consume 2 or more servings daily. (Baseline: 7 percent of women and 14 percent of men aged 19 through 24 and 24 percent of pregnant and lactating women consumed 3 or more servings, and 15 percent of women and 23 percent of men aged 25 through 50 consumed 2 or more servings in 1985–86)

Note: The number of servings of foods rich in calcium is based on milk and milk products. A serving is considered to be 1 cup of skim milk or its equivalent in calcium (302 mg).

Would You Be Healthier if You Ate at Fast Food Restaurants Less Often?

It was once said by a wise scholar that, "Knowledge is the food of the soul." But what of our bodies? Today, in order to keep up with the rigorous pace of modern industry and business, personal sacrifices must be made. Time is a most valuable commodity as any business will tell you, and in an effort to utilize time spent during business hours, the masses of the employed are swept up in a daily sprint to feed themselves. This is where fast food comes in to the picture. Feeding the face is the main concern while health takes the back seat. My point is simply this, healthy eating comes as naturally to Americans these days as adjusting national debt comes to congress. The temptation is that much greater when you consider the convenience, cost, and that little thing called self-control, which according to recent magazine polls, few people have. To change our unhealthy eating habits we must change how we perceive our diet. I don't think I have to remind everyone that fast food is chock full to the brim with high sodium, even higher calories, and retains little, if any, nutrition, which your body requires. Essentially the group is aptly named "junk food" because that's exactly what it is, junk. In conclusion, fast food is a treat and should be treated as such. Remember, "an apple a day keeps your coroner at bay."
Christopher Diamond, 19,
Billings West High School, MT

I would not necessarily be healthier if I ate at fast food places less often, but on a road to better health. There are many different aspects to health. If I ate at fast food restaurants less often, I still might do something that could set me back. I would have to avoid other risky behaviors to achieve better health.
Emilee Owen, 15,
Manzano High School, NM

I wouldn't be healthier if I ate at fast food restaurants less often. I only eat fast food on weekends in the first place, not even every weekend. When I do eat fast food, I usually steer clear of the overly greasy food.
Katye Blackwell, 14,
Northeastern High School, NC

Mini Glossary

anemia: reduced number or size of the red blood cells; a symptom of any of many different diseases, including some nutrient deficiencies.

trace minerals: minerals essential in nutrition, needed in small quantities (traces) daily. Iron and zinc are examples.

electrolytes (ee-LECK-tro-lites): minerals that carry electrical charges that help maintain the body's fluid balance.

salt: a compound made of minerals that, in water, dissolve and form electrolytes.

Electrolytes

Three minerals—sodium, chloride, and potassium—serve as **electrolytes**, minerals that dissolve in body fluids and carry electrical charges. Electrolytes help maintain the proper balance of fluids in the body. Fluid is the environment in which the cells' work takes place—work such as nerve-to-nerve communication, heartbeats, contraction of muscles, and so forth. When people lose fluid—whether it is in sweat, blood, or urine—they also lose electrolytes. Sometimes too many body fluids and electrolytes are lost, as in heat stroke, diarrhea, or injury. This constitutes a medical emergency and requires expert medical assistance.

Sodium is best known as part of sodium chloride, the most common **salt** in foods. Sodium chloride is ordinary table salt, a much-loved food seasoning. Because salt is so widespread in foods, people easily meet their need for

Following are some questions you may want to use to encourage discussion of the ideas expressed by students in the Teen Views feature:

a. What are some healthy meal options within fast food restaurants?

b. Are there other options for meals that are just as quick and perhaps healthier?

LEARNING WITH VISUALS

Have students research the role of electrolytes in the body and draw a graphic representation of how they affect the balance of bodily fluids with their electrical charges. Students should research what events might cause a person's electrolytes to become unbalanced and what would happen as a result.

INTERDISCIPLINARY ACTIVITY: CREATIVE WRITING/ART

Instruct students to use poetry or artwork to link proper nutrition or poor nutrition to mental wellness.

Calcium is essential for the formation and maintenance of bones and teeth. The level of bone mass achieved at skeletal maturity (peak bone mass) is a factor modifying the risk for developing osteoporosis. Peak bone mass appears to be related to intake of calcium during the years of bone mineralization. Opinion is divided as to the age at which peak bone mass is achieved. Most of the accumulation of bone minerals occurs in humans by about 20 years of age. However, after the linear growth phase, there is a period of consolidation of bone density that continues until approximately 30 to 35. A high peak bone mass is thought to be protective against fractures in later life.

CLASS ACTIVITY

Bring various items to school such as meats, grains, vegetables, nuts, and candy. Ask students to list all the minerals contained in each food item using Figure 7–13. This will accustom students to using the figure.

CLASS ACTIVITY

Have students research common mineral deficiencies and report their findings to the class. Also have the students include in their reports foods that supply the mineral.

CLASS ACTIVITY

Assign students to develop an oral report on a mineral. They should bring in food items when they give their reports. They should report on deficiencies as well as overdoses of the mineral and what the results of each might be.

COMPREHENSION CHECK

Define *hypertension.* (high blood pressure) Ask students what mineral is related to hypertension (sodium) and how this mineral can worsen the problem.

Reproducible Study Outline and Reading Cloze worksheets for Chapter 7 are provided in the Teacher's Resource Box.

Reproducible Chapter Tests A and B are also provided in the Teacher's Resource Box.

Figure 7–13 Major Roles and Sources of the Minerals

Mineral	What It Does In the Body	Major Food Sources
Calcium	Structural material of bones and teeth; helps muscles contract and relax; helps nerves communicate; helps blood to clot	Milk and milk products; small fish with bones; dark green vegetables; beans
Phosphorus	Structural material of bones and teeth; supports energy processes; part of cells' genetic material	All foods that come from animals
Magnesium	Helps build bones and teeth; helps build protein; helps muscles contract and relax; helps nerves communicate	Nuts; beans; dark green vegetables; seafood; whole grains; chocolate
Sodium	Maintains cell fluids; helps nerves communicate	Salt; soy sauce; processed foods; celery; milk
Potassium	Helps build protein; maintains fluids; helps nerves communicate; helps muscles contract	All nutritious foods; meats; milk and milk products; vegetables; whole grains; beans
Iron	Helps red blood cells carry oxygen; helps tissues use oxygen to release energy; supports normal immunity	Red meats; fish; poultry; shellfish; eggs; beans; dried fruits
Zinc	Helps build genetic material and protein; supports normal immunity; supports growth; helps make sperm; helps wounds heal	Protein-rich foods; meats; fish; poultry; whole grains
Iodine	Part of thyroid hormone needed for growth	Iodized salt; seafood
Selenium	An antioxidant; works with vitamin E	Seafood; meats; vegetables
Copper	Helps make red blood cells; helps build protein; helps the body use iron	Organ meats such as liver; seafood; nuts
Chromium	Helps the body use carbohydrates and fats	Liver; nuts; whole grains; cheese
Fluoride	Helps strengthen bones and teeth	Water; seafood
Manganese	Helps with many processes	Whole grains; fruits; vegetables
Molybdenum	Helps with many processes	Milk; beans

sodium. For this same reason, however, some people must try consciously to reduce salt intakes to avoid making high blood pressure (**hypertension**) worse. Details about hypertension and cutting down on salt are presented in Chapter 17.

For **Y**our **I**nformation

Later chapters on fitness and first aid make clear the importance of drinking enough water, especially during hot, humid weather.

KEY POINTS *Electrolytes are dissolved minerals that carry electrical charges and help maintain the proper balance of fluids in the body. Sodium is an electrolyte. Some people must limit salt intakes to control their blood pressure.*

Water

Water is mentioned last in this chapter, but it is first in importance to the body. Water is the major substance of which bodies are made. About 60 percent of your body's weight is water. It is the most vital of nutrients: you

QUICK QUIZ

Chapter 7, Section 8

The following quiz will help you assess your students' understanding of the material covered in this section of the chapter. You might use the quiz as an oral exercise, which will lead into a class discussion of the topics covered. Or, you might use it as a paper/pencil

quiz to evaluate your students individually.

If students have difficulty with the concepts covered in the Quick Quiz and the Section Review, you might suggest they review the material using the **S**urvey, **Q**uestion, **R**ead, **R**ecite, **R**eview *(SQ3R) study method, which is described in detail in the introduction to this Teacher's Wraparound Edition.*

1. Calcium is the mineral contained in the largest quantity in the body. (True) can live for many days, weeks, or even months without consuming many other nutrients, but you can live only a few days without water.

Water carries oxygen, nutrients, wastes, and other materials from place to place in the body. It also provides the environment that human tissues require to live. Your body loses about 6 to 8 cups of water daily in **urine** and sweat, and in exhaled breath. You must replace all the water you lose, so you need to drink between 6 and 8 glasses of water and other beverages each day.

 KEY POINTS *Water is vital to life. It carries materials in the body and provides the needed environment in which human tissues must live.*

Conclusion

Your body is unique. It responds to foods and the nutrients contained in those foods in its own characteristic ways based on its genetic inheritance and its current needs. No doubt you already know your body's tendencies. For example, one person may tend to gain weight and may need to take steps to reduce fat intake. Another person may stay thin and may be best advised to ignore at least some fat-reduction suggestions. The overweight person needs to avoid storing excess calories as fat. The thin one needs many calories to help build up body weight.

The point is to think carefully about your own body and its needs before changing your diet. The Straight Talk feature that follows helps you to decide whether you need a vitamin or mineral supplement, and if so, which one. The next chapter is about weight control for those who need to gain, lose, or just maintain their body weight.

Water is the most vital nutrient of all.

SECTION 8 Review

Answer the following questions on a sheet of paper.

Learning the Vocabulary

The vocabulary terms in this section are *osteoporosis, anemia, trace minerals, electrolytes, salt, hypertension,* and *urine.*

1. Write a sentence using each term.

2. _____ is a disease of gradual bone loss.

3. _____ is a condition in which a reduction in the number and size of red blood cells is seen.

Learning the Facts

4. Where is most of the body's calcium stored?

5. List four foods that provide calcium.

6. Give an example of a trace mineral and a food source for that mineral.

7. What is an important function of electrolytes?

Making Life Choices

8. List all the ingredients and nutrition information that appear on the label of a popular sports drink. List any other label information you feel might encourage you to buy this product. Are you convinced this drink is the best fluid replacement? Explain.

MINI Glossary

hypertension: high blood pressure.

urine: fluid wastes removed from the body by the kidneys.

ASSESS

EVALUATE

Have students create a collage with pictures depicting sources of minerals and sketches or words associated with the deficiency of those minerals. Have them group all items related to one mineral together. Tell students that you will be grading their work on accuracy of information, proper labeling, good organization, and presentation to the class.

SECTION 8 Review Answers

1. Answers will vary.
2. Osteoporosis (p. 191)
3. Anemia (p. 192)
4. bones and teeth (p. 191)
5. Answers will vary; could include: milk and milk products, almonds, small fish with bones, leafy green vegetables, broccoli, and beans. (p. 191)
6. iron (red meats, fish, poultry, shellfish, eggs, beans, dried fruits) (p. 192)
7. help maintain proper levels of fluids in the body (p. 193)
8. Answers will vary.

 A reproducible quiz for Section 8 is provided in the Teacher's Resource Box.

CLOSE

Have students close their books and name minerals as you write them on the board. Have students tell you any information they remember about each mineral, which you might write on the board as well.

Straight Talk

SOS: Selection of Supplements

Each year, people spend billions of dollars on vitamin pills. You may be among the almost two-thirds of the population who take some sort of nutrient supplement. You may be wondering, after studying nutrition, whether supplements can really help clear up the skin, make glossy hair and strong nails, or build broad chests and strong muscles, as many advertisers claim. Read on.

I've read advertisements making fabulous claims for supplements. Are there any supplements that can improve my appearance or physique?

Claims that supplements can do these things are based on a tiny kernel of truth. Nutrients do support human growth and are absolutely necessary for clear skin, glossy hair, strong muscles, and all the rest. The trickery comes in when sellers imply that supplements of nutrients, given to people who are already well nourished, will produce even better results. The truth is that supplements do not improve the physical features of a person who eats well.

Can people get the nutrients they need from food alone?

People who haven't learned enough about nutrition think they need supplements as insurance against their own poor food choices. Indeed, their food choices may be poor, but taking supplements is no guarantee that they will get the particular nutrients they need. It's more likely that they'll get a duplication of the nutrients their food is supplying and still lack the ones they need. The only way to be sure to get the needed assortment of nutrients is to construct a balanced diet from a variety of foods.

Are you saying that no supplement supplies all the nutrients you can get from food?

Yes, that's right. Even if you could get all your vitamins and trace minerals from a supplement, there is no way you can package the bulk of protein, fiber, carbohydrate, calcium, and others you need into a pill. No one knows enough, yet, to construct a synthetic substitute for food. Even hospital formulas that are called "complete" do not equal food. The most these formulas can do is to enable sick people to survive. They won't thrive until they are back on food.

In the chapter I read that fat-soluble vitamins can build up to dangerous levels in the body. How dangerous is this?

Dangerous indeed. Excess vitamin A, for example, can damage the same body systems that are damaged by vitamin A deficiency. Symptoms such as blurred vision, blood abnormalities, organ damage, bone pain, pressure inside the skull, and fatigue can occur with vitamin A excess. Water-soluble vitamins can be toxic as well, but are less likely to cause such severe symptoms. Minerals, too, can be extremely dangerous and even deadly in high doses.

Do people ever have unusually high nutrient needs that require that they take supplements?

No two people have exactly the same nutrient needs. However, people's requirements differ, at the most, only by two or three times. An ordinary diet of mixed foods can easily meet the highest of those needs.

In rare instances, genetic defects may alter nutrient needs considerably. However, only 1 person in 10,000 has such a defect. That person needs a diagnosis and treatment by a qualified health-care provider.

196

HEALTHY PEOPLE 2000

Increase to at least 50 percent the proportion of overweight people aged 12 and older who have adopted sound dietary practices combined with regular physical activity to attain an appropriate body weight. (Baseline: 30 percent of overweight women and 25 percent of overweight men for people aged 18 and older in 1985)

Overweight occurs when too few calories are expended and too many consumed for individual metabolic requirements. The results of weight loss programs focused on dietary restrictions alone have not been encouraging. Physical activity burns calories, increases the proportion of lean to fat body mass, and raises the metabolic rate. Therefore, a combi-

What about high nutrient needs caused by different lifestyles? I've seen vitamins for stress, for cigarette smokers, for athletes—things like that.

Stresses, including smoking, do deplete people's nutrient stores somewhat. However, which supplements to give stressed people is just guesswork on the part of the manufacturers. The way to supply lost nutrients is still to eat well, not to take supplements. Another way is to learn to control stress. People who smoke should give up smoking, not take supplements. As for athletes, they need supplements *less* than other people, because their bodies require more food to replace the energy they burn off in physical activity. Larger food intakes mean higher nutrient intakes.

 Would there ever be a time when I should be taking a vitamin pill?

Yes, when a health-care provider recommends it, and yes, in at least two other instances:

► When your energy intake is below about 1,500 calories and you can't eat enough food to meet your vitamin needs. (People who can't exercise have this problem.)
► When, for whatever reason, you are going to be eating irregularly for a limited time.

Remember that if vitamins are needed, minerals are needed, too. A vitamin pill is not enough. A vitamin-mineral supplement is called for.

 When I do need a supplement, what kind should I take? I've heard the organic, natural ones are best.

Organic and *natural* are terms that only mean that the product will be expensive. Don't let them fool you. Read the ingredient lists, and buy the one that contains the nutrients you are looking for at the lowest price.

When selecting a supplement, look for one that contains no more than the RDA for nutrients. (Look up your RDA in Appendix B.)

 Can taking supplements prevent heart disease or cancer?

Good nutrition certainly helps protect you. People who eat diets low in nutrients do develop more cancer and many other ills than do well-nourished people. However, to say that a nutrient pill will protect you is to overstate the case drastically. The chapter's section on antioxidant vitamins made the point that even supplements of antioxidant vitamins are not as helpful as food in preventing diseases. You need every nutrient contained in foods, with all the other compounds foods contain, if you really want protection.

 Suppose I just want to take a supplement to be sure I get enough nutrients. There's no harm in that, is there?

Perhaps not—if you keep the dose low, and if you do not fall into a sense of false security. Pills can never make up for a poorly chosen diet. The right mix of foods is simply indispensable to the health of the body.

197

ON LINE WITH HEALTH

You may want to have your students visit the following URLs, where they will find information and additional Web site resources to enhance their study of this chapter. As with all Web sites, you should check these out first to be sure the information found there is appropriate for your students.

Food and Nutrition Information Center
http://www.nal.usda.gov/fnic/

Nutrition and Your Health: Dietary Guidelines for Americans
http://www.nalusda.gov/fnic/dga/dguide95.html

Healthy Eating Index
http://www.nal.usda.gov/fnic/HEI/HEI.html

Hot Topics—The American Dietetic Association
http://www.eatright.org/nufactsheet.html

All of these sites are packed with current resource information on many aspects of nutrition.

nation of both caloric control and increased physical activity is important for attaining a healthy body weight.

Neither frequent fluctuations in body weight nor extreme restrictions in food intake are desirable. Overweight people should increase their physical activity and should avoid calorie-dense foods, especially those high in fat. Diets that are lower in fat and higher in vegetables, fruits, and grains can facilitate weight reduction. Extremely low-calorie diets, cyclic weight reduction, and fad weight-loss regimes of unscientific merit should be avoided. Practices should be adopted that are safe and that lead to long-term maintenance of appropriate weight. Extreme behaviors as exhibited in bulimia or anorexia nervosa should be medically treated.

ANSWERS TO CHAPTER 7 REVIEW

VOCABULARY

1. **a.** salt; **b.** vitamins; **c.** trace minerals; **d.** electrolytes; **e.** carbohydrate; **f.** digestion; **g.** sugar; **h.** malnutrition; **i.** fiber
2. Answers will vary.
3. **a.** Calories are units that measure energy to be used by the body, while empty calorie refers to foods that supply much energy, but few nutrients. **b.** Glucose is the body's blood sugar, while glycogen is how glucose is stored in the liver and muscles.
4. A supplement is given if a person has a deficiency or too little of a particular vitamin in his or her body.
5. **a.** Cholesterol; **b.** vegetarians; **c.** rectum; **d.** vitamins; **e.** minerals

RECALL

SECTION 1

1. Choosing a wide variety helps assure that you receive all the necessary nutrients. Adequate intake of nutrients has an effect over a period of years. The best foods support normal growth, maintain strong muscles, and nourish all parts of the body. Good nutrition promotes health and growth and prevents disease. (p. 162)
2. pregnant women—slows down the growth of their infants; teenagers—may not reach full height (p. 162)

SECTION 2

3. Answers will vary.

CHAPTER 7: Nutrition: The Nutrients

CHAPTER 7 Review

Summarizing the Chapter

Your ability to respond correctly to the following statements ensures your understanding of the main concepts in the chapter.

1. List the six Dietary Guidelines for Americans.
2. Discuss the impacts that overnutrition and undernutrition have on the body.
3. Identify the six classes of nutrients.
4. List the types and quantities of nutritious foods suggested for teenagers in the Daily Good Guide.
5. Design a balanced meal.
6. Describe the functions and food sources for carbohydrates, fats, and proteins.
7. Estimate your daily fat gram allowance, and describe some strategies to control the amont of fat in your diet.
8. Explain why some amino acids are called essential amino acids.
9. Describe the difference between fat-soluble and water-soluble vitamins.
10. Identify the essential vitamins, their functions and food sources.
11. Explain the dangers of consuming high doses of vitamins and minerals.
12. Identify the vitamins that act as antioxidants in the body, and describe their role in disease prevention.
13. Identify the essential minerals, their functions, and food sources.
14. Discuss the problems associated with a vitamin or mineral deficiency.

Learning the Vocabulary

nutrients	protein
nutrient deficiencies	vitamins
malnutrition	minerals
undernutrition	energy
overnutrition	glucose
carbohydrate	fatty acids
fat	amino acids

toxin	essential amino acids
calories	vegetarians
glycogen	supplement
hypothalamus	deficiency
balanced meal	fat-soluble
digestion	water-soluble
starch	night blindness
fiber	antioxidant
sugars	beta-carotene
constipation	free radicals
hemorrhoids	osteoporosis
rectum	anemia
empty calories	trace minerals
saturated	electrolytes
unsaturated	salt
polyunsaturated	hypertension
cholesterol	urine
grams	

Answer the following questions on a separate sheet of paper.

1. *Matching*—*Match each of the following phrases with the appropriate vocabulary term from the list above:*
   a. the common one contains the mineral sodium
   b. essential nutrients that help release energy from foods
   c. minerals needed only in small amounts daily
   d. minerals that carry electrical charges
   e. sugar, starch, and fiber
   f. breaking down food into nutrients the body can use
   g. fructose
   h. underweight or overweight
   i. not digestible by human beings
2. Write a paragraph or create a story using at least ten vocabulary terms. Underline each term that you use.
3. Explain the difference between the following terms:
   a. calorie and empty calorie
   b. glucose and glycogen
4. Explain the relationship between a supplement and a deficiency.
5. a. _____ is a type of fat made from saturated fats by the body.
   b. People known as _____ basically eliminate meat, poultry, and fish from their diets.
   c. The last part of the digestive tract is called the _____.
   d. Riboflavin, niacin, and thiamin are examples of _____.

198

SECTION 3

4. It does not promote growth, maintenance, or repair of the body. (p. 171)

SECTION 4

5. Starchy foods supply the body with glucose, which is what the brain needs to function at its best. (p. 174)

6. Fiber keeps the stools softer and bulkier and easy to pass, so that constipation does not occur and hemorrhoids are less likely. (p. 175)
7. glucose, sucrose, lactose, fructose (p. 176)

SECTION 5

8. Answers will vary; could include: heart disease, many forms of cancer, arthritis,

e. Calcium, fluoride, and phosphorus are examples of _____.

Recalling Important Facts and Ideas

Section 1

1. Why do you need to include a wide variety of foods in your diet?

2. Name two groups of people that are prone to nutrient deficiencies and discuss the resulting problems.

Section 2

3. Plan a meal using the Food Guide Pyramid. The foods you choose should help you meet your body's needs and at the same time keep your calorie count down.

Section 3

4. Explain why alcohol is not a nutrient.

Section 4

5. Explain how starchy foods improve the efficiency of the body.

6. Explain how fiber aids the digestive process.

7. What are the four sugars that are important in nutrition?

Section 5

8. List three dangers of a high-fat diet.

9. What are the recommended percentages of carbohydrate, fat and protein for a healthy diet?

10. List three types of information found on a food label.

Section 6

11. What is the difference between amino acids and essential amino acids?

12. List four foods that are high in protein but low in fat and calories.

Section 7

13. Explain why excess amounts of fat-soluble vitamins are more dangerous than excess amounts of water-soluble vitamins.

14. Why do teenagers' diets tend to be deficient in vitamin A?

15. Name the diseases antioxidants are supposed to protect against.

Section 8

16. What is the most abundant mineral found in the body?

17. How much milk do teenagers need to drink to meet daily calcium recommendations?

18. What is the major function of iron in the body?

19. Give two reasons why a person might be iron deficient.

20. What is the connection between salt and hypertension?

Critical Thinking

1. Can you think of any guidelines you would add to the list of Dietary Guidelines for Americans? What are they?

2. According to research, many Americans do not have healthy diets. Discuss some of the barriers people might face in making nutritious food choices. What barriers do you find yourself facing?

3. What influence does advertising exert on our food choices? Do you see this as having a positive or negative impact on your diet? Explain why and give some examples.

4. Food product labels are sources of nutrition information. Do you generally read food labels? Why or why not?

Activities

1. Find a recent article from a newspaper or magazine on the topic of nutrition and write a summary. Be sure to include the date, source, and a copy of the article.

2. Analyze the food selections on your favorite restaurant's menu. Does the menu provide a variety of foods, including low-fat foods? What changes would you make in the menu in order to make the choices more nutritious?

3. Watch television for two hours. List all the foods you see advertised. Categorize the foods into various groups, such as high-calorie, low-calorie; high-fat, low-fat; healthy, etc. Write a report on your findings and discuss in class.

4. Create a set of healthy meal plans for yourself for a full day. Include breakfast, lunch, dinner, and two snacks. Use the Daily Food Guide on pages 166–167 as a guide. Be sure to use only foods that you like when making diet selections. Avoid empty-calorie foods and be conscious of calorie content, especially if you are trying to lose or gain weight.

Making Decisions about Health

1. You have noticed that your friend has a habit of skipping breakfast. Your friend is not at all worried because she has been taking a multivitamin every morning. What would you say to her to let her know your concern? Describe a more effective meal planning strategy for her to follow.

12. vegetables, beans, and low-fat milk (p. 183)

SECTION 7

13. Fat-soluble vitamins dissolve in the body's fat and remain in the body. If excess amounts are taken in supplements, they can build up to dangerous levels. Water-soluble vitamins travel in the body's fluids and leave the body in urine. (p. 185)

14. Teenagers' diets often consist of fast foods, such as burgers and fries, which have little vitamin A. (p. 186)

15. heart disease and cancer (p. 187)

SECTION 8

16. calcium (p. 191)

17. three cups of milk (p. 192)

18. It is the body's oxygen carrier. (p. 192)

19. Answers will vary; could include: children and teens because of their rapid growth; women in their reproductive years because of loss of blood during menstruation and extra demands for iron from infants during pregnancy; starvation; eating too many iron-poor foods; blood loss; and infection with parasites. (p. 192)

20. Too much sodium, found in salt, makes hypertension worse. (pp. 193–194)

gallbladder disease, diabetes, and all the diseases made worse by overweight. (p. 179)

9. fat—30 percent of total calories, carbohydrates—60 percent of total calories, protein—10 percent of total calories. (p. 179)

10. Answers will vary; could include: serving size, number of servings per container, calorie information, percentages of Daily Values for nutrients based on a 2,000-calorie diet, Daily Values for selected nutrients, for a 2000- and a 2500-calorie diet, calorie/gram reminder, and ingredients in descending order of predominance. (pp. 180–182)

SECTION 6

11. The body can make amino acids for itself, but must receive essential amino acids from foods (p. 183).

KEY POINTS

Chapter 8 is 30 pages long and divided into 6 sections. This chapter deals with maintaining ideal weight and having realistic expectations about body size. It gives students valuable information that will help them to make good decisions when considering a weight-loss or weight-gain program. It also gives students behavior modification tips and the knowledge to evaluate diet plans.

ACTIVITY TO INTRODUCE THE CHAPTER

Students as well as adults are often made to believe false or exaggerated claims for weight-loss diets and products. Billions of dollars are spent on dieting products each year.

To help students evaluate the reliability of advertisers' claims, try this activity. Ask the class if they think the following diet claim could be true: ***Lose 25 pounds in one week!*** Take a vote to see how many believe it is possible and how many don't. Then give the class the following information:

1. To lose 1 pound of body fat a person must go without 3,500 calories.
2. The imaginary person going on this diet has an energy requirement of 2,500 calories per day.

Ask students to figure out if it would be possible for this person to lose 25 pounds in one week using the following formula: 7 (days in a week) × 2,500 (daily calorie requirement) = 17,500 calories normally eaten in one week. 25 pounds × 3,500

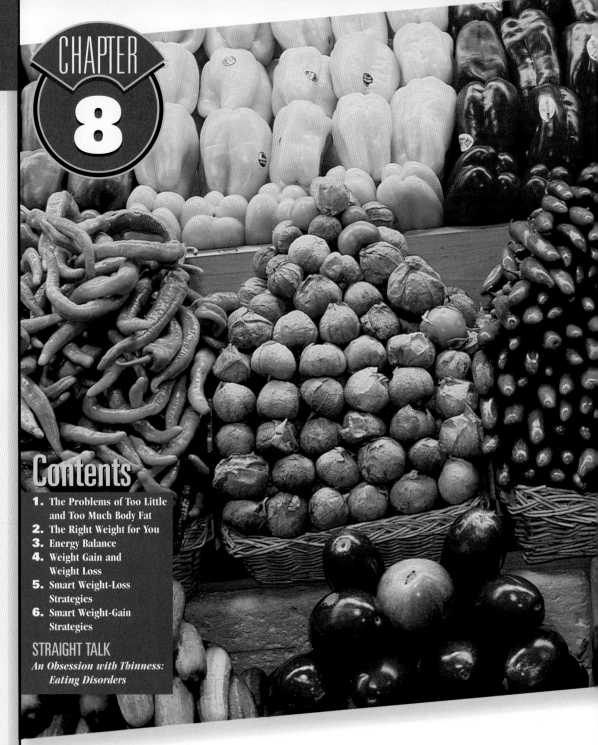

CHAPTER **8**

Contents

NOT Enough Time?

Following are some suggestions to help you make sure that you cover the key topics in this chapter if you have limited time. (Refer to the daily lesson plans in your Teacher's Resource Box for additional suggestions.)

DAY 1 Have the students do "Fact or Fiction" on page 201 on their own and give their answers in class. Do the Activity to Introduce the Chapter on page 200, the Evaluate assessment on page 202, and the Focus Activity on page 204.

Nutrition: Weight Control

What do you think? Are the following statements true or false? If you think they are false, then say what is true.

1. Being underweight presents a risk to health.
2. The dieter who sees a large weight loss on the scale can take this as a sign of success.
3. The way to lose body fat most rapidly is to stop eating altogether.
4. To succeed in losing weight, you have to stop eating carbohydrates.
5. You can eat any food on a weight-loss diet, as long as you don't eat too much of it.
6. A person who exercises daily spends more calories all day, even during sleep.
7. It is harder to lose a pound than to gain one.

(Answers on page 223)

Introduction

Are you pleased with your body weight? If you answered yes, you are a rare person. Nearly all people in our society think they should weigh more or less (mostly less) than they do. Usually, their main reason is that they want to look good by society's standards. They may know, too, that weight is related to physical health.

People also think they should control their weight. Two false ideas make their task difficult. The first is to focus on *weight*; the second is to focus on *controlling* weight. To put it simply, it isn't your weight you need to control. You need to control the amount of fat in your body in proportion to the lean. Furthermore, it isn't possible to control either one, directly. It is possible only to control your *behavior*.

calories (calories to lose 1 pound) = 87,500 calories. (must be burned to lose 25 pounds) Ask students for their answers.

Even if a person ate nothing all week, which would not be advised, the person would still have 70,000 calories to burn to lose the 25 pounds. What about exercise? To burn 70,000 calories in one week a person would have to run at a fast rate of speed, 24 hours a day, for all seven days.

This exercise will help students to see through some of the outrageous claims diet advertisers make.

BULLETIN BOARD IDEAS

Make a collage of diet advertisements, including both written and photographic claims. You could also include fashion photographs of tall, thin models.

Answers to **FACT or FICTION**

1. **True.**
2. **False.** A weight loss may reflect loss of water or lean tissue rather than loss of fat.
3. **False.** Fasting promotes rapid weight loss, but a balanced low-calorie diet can promote more rapid fat loss.
4. **False.** Carbohydrate is a necessary part of a healthy, balanced weight-loss diet.
5. **True.**
6. **True.**
7. **False.** It is as hard for a person who tends to be thin to gain a pound as it is for a person who tends to be fat to lose one.

DAY 2 On Day 2 do the Class Activity on page 207, the Section 3 Quick Quiz on page 208, and the Comprehension Check on page 211.

DAY 3 On Day 3 complete either the Class Activity on page 216 or the one on page 219. Use the Close activity on page 223. Discuss the Straight Talk feature on page 225. If time allows, use some of the reviews for the Evaluate sections.

SECTION 1

FOCUS

OUTCOME

In this section students will:

1. Examine the physical, social, and economic factors associated with being underweight or overweight.

FOCUS ACTIVITY

Ask students what they feel is the most important reason ideal weight should be maintained. Write the different responses on the board. Discuss.

TEACH & APPLY

COMPREHENSION CHECK

Ask students to write a sentence stating what it is that a person should be doing if that person is concerned about his or her weight. The sentence should begin, "If I want to weigh more or less than I do now, I should learn to . . ." Have them complete this sentence, then discuss their sentences in class.

ASSESS

EVALUATE

Have students close their books and take out a piece of paper. Tell the class to write down four problems associated with being underweight, four with being overweight, and four benefits of maintaining ideal weight.

The Problems of Too Little and Too Much Body Fat

Both too little and too much body fat carry health risks. Thin people usually die first during a famine or any time food is in short supply. A fact not always recognized, even by health-care providers, is that overly thin people are also at risk in the hospital. They may have to go for days without food so that they can undergo tests or surgery. In fact, people with cancer and other diseases lose their appetites, and so may die from starvation rather than from the disease itself. Women need a certain minimum amount of body fat to menstruate normally. If they become **underweight**, with too little body fat, their cycles are disrupted. Underweight people are urged to gain body fat as an energy reserve and to eat foods that provide all the nutrients.

Consequences of Obesity   As for too much body fat, for one thing, it makes hypertension (high blood pressure) worse. For another thing, weight gain can bring on diabetes in some people. If hypertension or diabetes runs in your family, you urgently need a sensible program to keep from getting too fat.

Excess body fatness also increases the risk of heart disease. Oversized fat pads crowd the heart muscle within the body cavity. Excess fat demands to be fed by miles of extra capillaries, overworking the heart to the point of damaging it. Meanwhile, fat clogs up the very arteries that bring energy and oxygen to the heart's muscles, starving these muscles.

Many other conditions are brought on or made worse by overfatness. These include breast cancer, diseases of the gallbladder, arthritis, breathing problems, problems in pregnancy, and even a high accident rate. The health risks of overfatness are so many that it has been declared a disease: **obesity**.

Underweight and overweight both present hazards to health.

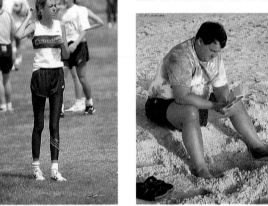

If you are obese, you are urged to reduce your fat intake. You can expect your health risks to lessen as you do this.

Some obese people can escape these health problems, but no one who is fat in our society quite escapes the social and economic handicaps. Excess body fatness often makes it difficult to be physically active, and so limits people's success in sports. Overweight people may find it difficult to meet dating partners. They also find it hard to purchase good-looking clothes that fit well. Overweight people pay high insurance premiums, they pay high prices for clothes, and they may be passed over at hiring time when looking

Chapter 8, Section 1

The following quiz will help you assess your students' understanding of the material covered in this section of the chapter. You might use the quiz as an oral exercise, which will lead into a class discussion of the topics covered. Or, you might use it as a paper/pencil quiz to evaluate your students individually.

Like the Quick Quiz, the Section Review can also be used as an assessment tool to spark class discussion or as an individual student evaluation. It can also be used as a review in preparation for this quiz.

1. Underweight people have few calorie and nutritional reserves to fall back on in cases of emergency, such as famine or hospitalization. (True)

for work. Psychologically, too, a body size that embarrasses a person reduces self-esteem. With lowered self-esteem, the person may say, "What's the use in trying to lose weight?" In this way, obesity and low self-esteem worsen each other.

Chronic Dieting How thin, then, is too thin—and how fat is too fat? The next section helps to draw the lines. In any case, many teenagers believe that no one can ever be too thin. They become **chronic dieters** who diet recklessly because everyone is doing it. They worry that their healthy bodies are not as thin as some unrealistically thin ideal. One study found almost half of high school girls to be on a diet, even though many were not overweight. About a quarter of the boys were dieting, too.

Even worse, teens often use harmful methods, such as taking diet pills, vomiting, misusing laxatives or other drugs, or fasting. Even children as young as nine or ten, and who are healthy and of normal weight, have taken on these unhealthy behaviors. Some have stunted their own growth and may never attain their full adult height—others develop eating disorders—all in the name of dieting.

This situation has been called a national crisis. Some blame movies and magazines for the constant pressure aimed at young people, and especially at girls, to be thin to the bone. Meanwhile, more and more teenagers are becoming obese. A mission of this chapter is to paint a more honest picture of body weight and to provide ways of deciding whether weight loss is needed. It also helps distinguish between healthy and harmful weight-control strategies. The next section helps to define overweight, healthy weight, and underweight.

 KEY POINTS *Both too much and too little body fat carry health risks. Overfatness carries social and economic handicaps as well.*

 SECTION 1 Review

Answer the following questions on a sheet of paper.

Learning the Vocabulary

The vocabulary terms in this section are *underweight, obesity,* and *chronic dieters.*

1. What is the difference between being underweight and being obese?
2. Write a sentence using each vocabulary word.

Learning the Facts

3. Why might being extremely thin pose a health risk?

4. List four health problems associated with excess body fatness.
5. Give one economic and one social handicap of obesity.
6. What do some people blame for the national crisis of chronic dieting?

Making Life Choices

7. Many people in our country look down on obese people. How can you help to lessen the social handicaps that obese people experience? Have you ever been in a situation where you or someone you know discriminated against an overweight person? Explain the situation, and describe how it could have been handled more sensitively.

 MINI Glossary

underweight: weight too low for health. Underweight is often defined as weight 10 percent or more below the appropriate weight for height.

obesity: overfatness to the point of injuring health. Obesity is often defined as 20 percent or more above the appropriate weight for height.

chronic dieters: people who frequently diet in unhealthy ways in an attempt to lose weight.

 For Your Information

The Straight Talk section explains how dieting and eating disorders are related.

SECTION 1 Review Answers

1. Underweight is weighing 10 percent below the appropriate weight for height; obesity is weighing 20 percent above the appropriate weight for height. (p. 203)
2. Answers will vary.
3. die first in a famine, at risk during hospitalization, and women do not menstruate normally (p. 202)
4. Answers will vary; could include: hypertension, diabetes, heart disease, breast cancer, diseases of the gallbladder, arthritis, breathing problems, problems in pregnancy, and high accident rate. (p. 202)
5. Answers will vary; could include: economic—pay high price for insurance premiums and clothes, and may be passed over at hiring time; social—difficult to be physically active and successful in sports, difficult to meet dating partners. (p. 202)
6. Some blame movies and magazines for the constant pressure aimed at young people to be thin. (p. 203)
7. Answers will vary.

 WORKSHEETS

A reproducible quiz for Section 1 is provided in the Teacher's Resource Box.

CLOSE

Lead a class discussion on problems students have had with weight control.

2. Obesity is considered a disease because of the many health risks associated with being overweight. (True)
3. Obesity minimizes the risk of hypertension/high blood pressure. (False)
4. Obesity can speed the onset of diabetes in people who are predisposed to it. (True)
5. Excess body fat has not been related to heart disease. (False)
6. There is no social stigma attached to being overweight. (False)
7. Obesity can increase the cost of insurance premiums and even make finding work more difficult. (True)
8. Chronic dieters feel the need to diet constantly in order to meet an unrealistic body ideal. (True)
9. Diet pills, laxatives, and fasting are effective dieting techniques. (False)
10. The obsessive dieting of young adults has been called a national crisis. (True)

203

FOCUS

OUTCOMES

In this section students will learn:

1. There is no way to determine ideal weight for adolescents.

2. There is no perfect way to determine the ideal weight for adults.

FOCUS ACTIVITY

Have students write on a piece of paper how they determine if their own weights are at a healthy level. They should fold the papers to insure privacy and not put their names on them. Collect the papers in a small box, then read the students' responses and discuss. Also discuss the answers to the following questions: Do these responses refer to appearance, energy, or health? How much should we be concerned with appearance, if we have energy and are healthy? Why is a scale not necessarily an accurate measure of how much one should weigh?

TEACH & APPLY

CLASS ACTIVITY

Have students approximate their ideal weights by using some of the examples listed in Figures 8–2 and 8–3. Ask students how many feel these methods are realistic for their weights. If they think they are not realistic, ask why. Discuss their responses.

The Right Weight for You

Your body's weight reflects its composition—the total mass of its bones, muscles, fat, fluids, and other tissues. The more of any of these you have, the more you weigh. Each type of tissue can vary in quantity and quality. The bones can be solid or brittle; the muscles can be well developed or underdeveloped; fat can be abundant or scarce; and so on. One tissue, though, stands out as varying the most: your body fat. Fat is the material in which the body can store the most food energy. It is fat that responds most to changes in food intake and exercise. Finally, it is fat that is usually the target of efforts at weight control.

Measuring Body Fatness

Health-care professionals would like to measure body fatness, rather than weight. However, body fatness is hard to measure directly. A **fatfold test** uses a **fatfold caliper**—a pinching device that measures the thickness of a fold of fat on the back of the arm, below the shoulder blade, on the side of the waist, or elsewhere (see Figure 8–1). When taken by a skilled professional, fatfold measures reflect total body fat fairly well, because about half of the body's fat lies beneath the skin.

However, not everyone's body fat is distributed in the same way, and the distribution itself turns out to be meaningful to health. Excess fat around the waist represents a greater risk to the health of the heart than excess fat on the hips, chest, or legs. Some quick but not-too-accurate ways of guessing at body fatness are provided in Figure 8–2 below.

KEY POINTS *Body fatness can be measured with a fatfold caliper.*

Figure 8–2 *Quick Ways to Estimate Body Fatness*

> **Just for fun, try the following methods for estimating body fatness.**
>
> • A crude measurement of body fatness is the **pinch test**. (This is a fatfold measure without the equipment to make it accurate.) Pick up the skin and fat at the back of either arm with the thumb and forefinger of the other hand. Keep your fingers still, so as not to lose the "measurement" when you pull them away from your arm. Measure the space between your fingers on the ruler. A fatfold over an inch thick reflects too much body fat.
>
> • Another shortcut method is to measure your waist compared to your chest (not bust). Every inch by which your waist measurement exceeds your chest measurement is said to take two years off your life.
>
> • Another crude measure: lie down, relax, and place a ruler across your abdomen from one hipbone to the other. If the ruler doesn't easily touch both bones while you're relaxing, you may be carrying too much body fat.

Figure 8–1 *Fatfold Test. In a fatfold test, a skilled professional lifts a fold of skin from the back of the arm or other area and measures its thickness. The caliper applies a fixed amount of pressure gently (it doesn't hurt).*

For Your Information

The standards for measuring triceps fatfolds are presented in Figure B–3 of Appendix B at the back of this book.

Pursuing wellness

There are a number a health concerns that are associated with obesity. Heart disease, high blood pressure, atherosclerosis, and stroke are more common in obese persons. Liver disorders, gallbladder disease, respiratory problems, and diabetes are also seen in a higher incidence.

The burden of extra fat puts a strain on the skeletal system. Arthritis is more common, particularly in the hips, knees, and lower spine. The more weight a person carries, the greater the wear and tear on the joints. This wear and tear can cause pain that results in

Height (in Inches)	Females Weight Range (in Pounds)					
	12	**13**	**14**	**15**	**16**	**17**
53–54.9	58–78	—	—	—	—	—
55–56.9	76–101	74–98	—	—	—	—
57–58.9	79–106	84–112	84–112	95–127	104–139	86–115
59–60.9	87–116	88–118	95–127	99–132	103–137	99–132
61–62.9	96–128	99–132	102–136	103–137	105–140	109–145
63–64.9	105–140	105–140	108–144	113–151	114–152	114–152
65–66.9	109–145	115–154	116–155	121–161	122–163	121–161
67–68.9	126–168	115–154	128–170	130–173	126–168	123–164
69–70.9	—	—	121–162	126–168	144–192	130–174

Height (in Inches)	Males Weight Range (in Pounds)					
	12	**13**	**14**	**15**	**16**	**17**
53–54.9	65–86	65–86	—	—	—	—
55–56.9	68–91	73–97	—	—	—	—
57–58.9	78–104	77–103	80–107	—	—	—
59–60.9	85–114	85–113	91–121	—	—	—
61–62.9	94–125	94–125	94–126	104–139	99–132	108–144
63–64.9	101–134	105–140	103–138	105–140	105–140	114–152
65–66.9	111–148	111–148	115–154	114–152	118–157	124–166
67–68.9	124–166	123–164	124–166	125–167	124–166	133–178
69–70.9	—	135–180	130–173	130–174	133–178	136–181
71–72.9	—	—	144–192	143–191	144–192	146–194
73–74.9	—	—	—	148–197	161–215	151–202
75–76.9	—	—	—	166–221	—	162–216

Notice that some older teens weigh less than some younger teens the same height, because gains in weight often don't keep up with gains in height. *Note:* The lower number in each weight range was derived by calculating 10 percent *below*, and the higher number was derived by calculating 20 percent *above*, the expected weight for height and age of youths 12 to 17 years old.

Figure 8–3 *Expected Weight Ranges for Teenagers (Based on Height and Age)*

Scale Weight

Body *weight*, by itself, says little about body *fatness*. A person with strong muscles and bones may not be overweight, but may seem overweight on the scale. Also, a person who doesn't seem overweight on the scale may have too much body fat for health. Even though scale weight is a poor measure of body fatness, it is still the measure people use to get an idea of whether they need to lose weight. People compare their weights to those listed on height-weight tables to find out what they "should" weigh.

The height-weight tables show the weights of adults who lived long and healthy lives. No one under age 25 is ever included on the tables. Thus, for *adults*, using the height-weight tables is reasonable.

For children and teenagers who want to know how much they should weigh, however, the height-weight tables for adults are useless. Children and teenagers are still growing. Weights and heights change rapidly during the teen years. These facts make any guess at what they "should" weigh at a given age or height just that—a guess.

MINI Glossary

fatfold test: a test of body fatness done with a *fatfold caliper*.

fatfold caliper: a pinching device that measures body fat under the skin.

pinch test: an informal way of measuring body fatness.

even less physical activity and the risk of additional weight gain. Low-back pain is also more common in people who are obese.

Surgical procedures on obese persons involve an increased risk, and postsurgical complications such as infection are also increased. In addition, anesthetic risk is increased due to obesity.

Overweight mothers tend to have a higher infant and maternal mortality rate.

Finally, cancer is more prevalent in obese persons. Men who are obese tend to have a higher incidence of cancer in the colon, rectum, and prostate. In women who are obese, there is a higher incidence of cancer of the ovaries, uterus, cervix, and breasts.

BACKGROUND INFORMATION

Appendix B contains instructions and charts that will enable you to obtain fairly accurate measurements of your students' body fatness using fatfold calipers.

ASSESS

EVALUATE

Have students give three reasons why it is difficult to determine ideal weight. Students should also be able to name three methods that can help estimate ideal weight.

Review Answers

1. caliper (p. 204)
2. pinch test (p. 204)
3. fatfold test using calipers; refer to Figure 8–2 on page 204 for answers. Some informal methods include: the pinch test, measuring the waist in comparison to the chest, lying down and placing a ruler from hip bone to hip bone.
4. Teens are still growing. (p. 205)
5. Answers are personal.

A reproducible quiz for Section 2 is provided in the Teacher's Resource Box.

CLOSE

Ask students to write a paragraph on what criteria they use in determining their ideal weights.

Figure 8–4 *Rule-of-Thumb Method for Estimating Appropriate Weight*

- A quick way to estimate a female's appropriate weight is to give the height of 5 feet (barefooted) a weight of 100 pounds. For every inch above 5 feet, add 5 pounds.

  Example: A female who is 5 feet 4 inches tall would add 20 pounds (4 inches times 5 pounds per inch) to 100 pounds, making her appropriate weight 120 pounds.

- For males, use the same method, but start at 110 pounds for 5 feet tall.

  Example: A male, 6 feet tall, adds 60 pounds (12 inches times 5 pounds per inch) to 110 pounds. This makes his average appropriate weight 170 pounds.

The tables of expected weight ranges for teenagers shown in Figure 8–3 on the previous page are no exception. They simply reflect the measures of many adolescents across the nation. You can use these tables, together with the rule-of-thumb method of Figure 8–4 above, to get a rough idea of how your weight compares with standards. Don't take the results too seriously if you don't fit in. The best indicators for you are these two: if you are growing normally, and if your fatfold is average, your weight is probably just right.

KEY POINTS *Height-weight tables used for adults are useless for children and teenagers. If children and teenagers are growing normally and their fatfolds are about average, their weights are probably fine.*

SECTION 2 Review

Answer the following questions on a sheet of paper.

Learning the Vocabulary

The vocabulary terms in the section are *fatfold test*, *fatfold caliper*, and *pinch test*.
Fill in the blank with the correct answer.

1. A _____ is a device that measures the thickness of the body fat under the skin.
2. A _____ is a fatfold measurement taken without the use of any equipment.

Learning the Facts

3. What methods can be used to measure body fatness?
4. Why are height-weight tables considered inaccurate for teenagers?

Making Life Choices

5. For your own information, use the rule-of-thumb method in Figure 8–4 above to estimate your "appropriate" weight. Are you satisfied with your current weight? Use some of the methods described in this section to estimate your body fat. Are you satisfied with your body fat test results? What changes, if any, do you feel need to be made in your weight and/or amount of body fat?

QUICK QUIZ

Chapter 8, Section 2

The following quiz will help you assess your students' understanding of the material covered in this section of the chapter. You might use the quiz as an oral exercise, which will lead into a class discussion of the topics covered. Or, you might use it as a paper/pencil quiz to evaluate your students individually.

Like the Quick Quiz, the Section Review can also be used as an assessment tool to spark class discussion or as an individual student evaluation. It can also be used as a review in preparation for this quiz.

1. Body weight is the total mass of bones, muscles, fat, fluids and other tissues of the body. (True)
2. Everyone's bones and tissues have the same density and weight. (False)

SECTION 3

Energy Balance

Suppose you are told by a health-care provider that you are too fat or too thin. How did you get that way? By having an unbalanced energy budget—that is, by eating either more or less food energy than you used up. In other words, your body fat reflects your energy income and expenses in much the same way as your savings account reflects your money income and expenses. In the case of body fat, though, more is not better.

A day's energy budget (in calories) looks like this:

*Food energy taken in (calories) minus
Energy spent by the body (calories) equals
Change in fat stores (calories).*

More simply:

Energy in – Energy out = Change in fat.

Energy In   You know about the "energy in" side of this equation. An apple brings in 100 calories; a candy bar, 425 calories. Perhaps you also know that for each 3,500 calories you eat over the amount you spend, you store a pound of body fat. The reverse is also true: for every 3,500 calories you spend beyond those you eat, you will use up a pound of body tissue as fuel.

Energy Out: Basal Energy   As for the "energy out" side, the body spends energy in two major ways: to fuel its **basal energy** needs and to fuel its **voluntary activities**. You can change both of these to spend more or less energy in a day, as you will see in a moment.

The basal energy supports the work that goes on all the time, without your awareness. The basal processes include:

▶ Beating of the heart.
▶ Inhaling and exhaling of air.
▶ Maintenance of body temperature.
▶ Working of the nerves and glands.

These basal processes support life.

Basal energy needs are surprisingly large. A person whose total energy needs are 2,000 calories a day spends 1,200 to 1,400 of them to support basal activities. This means that you use up 1,200 to 1,400 calories a day even if you just sit still and do nothing.

Energy Out: Voluntary Activity   The number of calories a person spends on a voluntary activity depends on four factors:

1. *The number and size of the muscles that are working.* The larger the active muscle mass, the more energy needed. This means that using the large muscle groups of the legs and buttocks to walk upstairs takes more energy than lifting books to a shelf with your arms and shoulders.
2. *The total weight of the body parts being moved.* The heavier the body parts, the more energy required to move them. This explains why a 200-pound person uses more energy than a 100-pound person does

Vigorous physical activity helps you to spend energy and burn fat.

MINI Glossary

▯ **basal energy:** the sum total of all
▯ the energy needed to support the
▯ chemical activities of the cells and to
▯ sustain life, exclusive of voluntary
▯ activities; the largest component of a
▯ person's daily energy expenditure.

▯ **voluntary activities:** movements
▯ of the body under the command of the
▯ conscious mind; one component of a
▯ person's daily energy expenditure.

FOCUS

OUTCOMES

In this section students will learn:

1. That calories fuel the basal energy needs and the voluntary activities.
2. How the number of calories taken in versus those burned off are balanced.

FOCUS ACTIVITY

Over time, small changes in diet may result in large gains or losses in weight. To maintain ideal weight, exercise more and make good food choices. For instance, if a person left total calories in the diet exactly the same, but increased exercise by walking an additional ten minutes a day, five pounds would be lost in a year. Drinking two less cans of pop per week is equivalent to about four pounds lost in a year. A knowledge of calories in foods can lead to making better food choices. Ask students to describe for the class similar calorie comparisons they know about.

TEACH & APPLY

CLASS ACTIVITY

Give students the Calorie Quiz from the Teacher's Resource Box with these directions: "Number your paper 1 through 15. I will name two

(continued on next page)

---

3. Fat is the body tissue that responds least to changes in food intake and exercise. (False)
4. A fatfold caliper measures fatness by pinching folds of fat on various parts of the body. (True)
5. The distribution of body fat has important health consequences. (True)
6. Fatness can be calculated from body weight. (False)
7. Scale weight is the measure most people

use to decide whether or not to diet. (True)
8. Excess fat around the abdomen is less dangerous than excess fat around the arms and legs. (False)
9. National height-weight tables give a reasonable indication of what children and teenagers should weigh. (False)
10. If a teenager is growing normally and has approximately average fatfolds, his or her weight is probably fine. (True)

(continued from previous page)

foods. By the number, write the food that you think has the most calories, or if you believe they are the same, write *same.*" After the quiz, give the students the correct answers and discuss students' reactions to the calories.

Following are some questions you may want to use to encourage discussion of the ideas expressed by the students in the feature.

a. Do students know of anyone who has taken diet pills? Were they effective? Did anyone regret taking them because of complications?

b. Do students agree that today's society makes everyone feel they have to be thin and beautiful?

ASSESS

EVALUATE

A reproducible quiz for Section 3 is provided in the Teacher's Resource Box.

Do Teens Diet Too Much Or Too Little?

Teens diet too much because in society, you are not considered pretty unless you are thin. We all know that teens want to look perfect and they will do anything to make them that way.

Aasima Afsar, 15,
Manzano High School, NM

I believe that the word *diet* is understood incorrectly by most teens. Most teens think of *diets* as short-term ways to lose weight. Really you should make your diet a long-term, lifelong commitment, not a way to fit into a dress for a dance in two weeks. Teens should try to eat foods filled with nutrients and low in fat and calories. Two candy bars and a can of soda just don't do it.

Joseph Brooks, 15,
Connellsville Senior High School, PA

I think teens diet too much by far. Today's society makes everyone feel like they have to be thin and beautiful to be accepted. I'm really tired of seeing what today's society does to today's youth. We are all a bunch of robots trying to be accepted by anyone and everyone who's popular. Who really cares more about your image, you or them? Learn to like yourself the way you are.

Andrea Bright, 16, East High School, MN

You can't just throw all teens in a pot and say "they do this" or "they don't do that." Teens are always changing. One day we're up; the next we're down. One day we're dieting; the next we're not. I think the problem, instead of dieting, is more how we eat in the first place. Yes, teens diet too much, but it's the result of our own stupidity. We eat ourselves to giddy heights on the scale, then crash diet ourselves back to near nonexistence. It's not just teens, though. All of America diets too much.

Kimberly Secora, 15,
Great Falls High School, MT

I think this question cannot be answered about teenagers as a whole. I believe some teens diet too much, some too little, and some just right. The teens who diet too much may become obsessive about exercise and eating, and therefore worry about it constantly. They tend to be thin or regular sized females. Compulsive dieters can eventually develop anorexia, bulimia, or both. The second type of teen, who diets too little, usually does not care what goes into his body (drugs, alcohol, food, etc.). He eats what and when he pleases and does not exercise regularly. Lastly, there are teens who diet just right. These people eat healthy foods and exercise regu-

larly. They maintain a constant, healthy body weight by living a healthy lifestyle. I think that the opinion of whether teens diet too much or too little depends on the person's point of view and the individual being judged.

Joy Womack, 15, West High School, MT

I think it depends on the teen. It's mostly in girls who diet. I think they diet because they're not happy with their bodies mentally and physically so they try to make themselves look like toothpicks and they feel better about themselves! I think a lot of the dieting is caused by stress. For example, there could be this really skinny popular girl and they'll try to be like her so the guys will like them. So they go on a diet to be as skinny or skinnier than that popular girl.

Jennifer Lusk, 15,
Manzano High School, NM

Most teens diet too much because of society's standards and ways of thinking, which make everyone so self-conscious that they have low self-esteem. I think it happens with more females than males because of the way society pictures them.

Hannah Gleason, 15,
Manzano High School, NM

Chapter 8, Section 3

The following quiz will help you assess your students' understanding of the material covered in this section of the chapter. You might use the quiz as an oral exercise, which will lead into a class discussion of the topics covered. Or, you might use it as a paper/pencil

quiz to evaluate your students individually.
Like the Quick Quiz, the Section Review can also be used as an assessment tool to spark class discussion or as an individual student evaluation. It can also be used as a review in preparation for this quiz.

1. An energy budget refers to the balance between calorie intake and the number of calories expended. (True)

2. An imbalance in the energy in/energy

when both are doing the same activity with equal effort.

3. *The length of time of exercise.* The longer the activity lasts, the more calories are spent.

4. *The amount of effort put into the movement—the exercise intensity.* Hard work takes more fuel.

Total Energy Expenditure A typical breakdown of the total energy spent by a moderately active person (for example, a student who walks from class to class) might look like this:

Energy for basal activities:	*1,400 calories*
Energy for voluntary activities:	*500 calories*
Total energy needs:	*1,900 calories*

The basal energy is the larger part. You can't change it much, today. You can, however, change the second part—voluntary activities—and so spend more calories today. In addition, you can, if you want to, increase your basal energy output over the long term by making physical activity a daily habit. As you develop lean tissue and drop fat, your basal energy output will pick up the pace as well. The end of this chapter shows how to alter energy spent on both basal and voluntary activities—with diet and physical activity—to regulate body weight.

 KEY POINTS *The balance between food energy taken in and energy spent determines how much fat a person's body stores in its fat tissues or how much it uses from storage. Two major ways in which the body spends energy are for basal processes and voluntary activities.*

> *"One man eats very little and is always full, but another man constantly eats and is always hungry. Why is that?"*
>
> Zen Riddle

SECTION 3 Review

Answer the following questions on a sheet of paper.

Learning the Vocabulary

The vocabulary terms in this section are *basal energy* and *voluntary activities*.

Fill in the blank with the correct answer.

1. _____ is the sum total of all the energy needed to support the chemical activities of the cells.

2. Movements of the body under the command of the conscious mind are _____.

Learning the Facts

3. What happens to the calories you eat in excess of those your body expends?

4. What are the two major ways the body spends energy?

5. Name three factors that determine the number of calories spent on a voluntary activity.

Making Life Choices

6. Is your body's energy budget balanced, or do you generally eat more or less food energy than you spend? Give specific reasons for your answer. Are you satisfied with your body's energy budget? Why or why not? What changes, if any, would you make?

SECTION 3 Review Answers

1. Basal energy (p. 207)
2. voluntary activities (p. 207)
3. The body stores them as fat. (p. 207)
4. basal energy, voluntary activities (p. 207)
5. Answers will vary; could include: the number and size of the muscles that are working, the total weight of the body parts being moved, the length of time of exercise, and the amount of effort put into the movement. (pp. 207–208)
6. Answers will vary.

CLOSE

Ask students to imagine they have gained ten pounds of unnecessary weight due to a broken leg. The cast has now been removed, and the doctor has said it is all right to resume normal activities. Ask students how they would try to lose this weight. What would be the healthiest and most sensible approach to take?

out equation results in a change in the amount of fat stored in the body. (True)

3. 3,500 excess calories result in one pound of stored body fat. (True)

4. Basal processes include voluntary activities such as walking. (False)

5. Inhaling and exhaling air are basal processes. (True)

6. The amount of energy required for basal processes is surprisingly small. (False)

7. The larger the active muscles mass, the

more energy is expended to perform movement. (True)

8. A two-hundred pound person expends the same amount of energy as a one-hundred pound person performing exactly the same activity. (False)

9. The greater the effort put into an action, the greater the amount of energy expended. (True)

10. You can control the amount of energy expended on basal activities. (False)

SECTION 4

FOCUS

OUTCOMES

In this section students will learn:

1. Body composition and the storage of energy nutrients.

2. The right and wrong ways to lose weight.

FOCUS ACTIVITY

Ask students to read the first four paragraphs of Section 4. Then give students the following information:

If dieting is done with exercise, 95 percent of the weight lost will be fat, and 5 percent will be lean tissue. If dieting is done without exercise, 75 percent of the weight lost will be fat, and 25 percent will be lean tissue.

Ask students to explain the significance of exercise as it relates to dieting. Discuss.

TEACH & APPLY

CLASS ACTIVITY

Request that students bring in advertisements for weight-reduction diets, pills, exercise gadgets, and clothes that are supposed to melt away fat. Have students evaluate the ads' claims. Have volunteers come to the front of the class, show their ads, and tell whether or not they think the products would work and why.

SECTION 4 — Weight Gain and Weight Loss

The cautious consumer distinguishes between loss of fat and loss of weight.

For **Y**our **I**nformation

A teenager 5 feet tall who weighs 100 pounds has only 20 pounds of lean.

You step on the scale and note that you weigh a pound more or less than you did the last time you weighed. This doesn't mean you have gained or lost body fat. Changes in body weight reflect shifts in many different materials—not only fat, but also water, bone minerals, and lean tissues such as muscles. It is important for people concerned with weight control to realize this.

Fat Tissue, Lean Tissue, and Body Water

A healthy 18-year-old teenager, who is about 5 feet 10 inches tall and who weighs 150 pounds, carries about 90 of those pounds as water and 30 as fat. The other 30 pounds are the lean tissues: muscles; organs such as the heart, brain, and liver; and the bones of the skeleton. Stripped of water and fat, then, the person weighs only 30 pounds!

The body's lean tissue is vital to health. When a person who is too fat seeks to lose weight, it should be fat, not this precious lean tissue, that is lost. For someone who wants to gain weight, it is best to gain both lean *and* fat, not just fat.

The type of tissue gained or lost depends on how the person goes about gaining or losing weight. Some of the most dramatic weight changes people achieve reflect losses and gains in the body's fluid content, which ideally shouldn't change much at all. Yet people seek to bring about such weight changes because they like to see the quick results. They fail to realize how useless such changes are in changing what really matters—the body's lean and fat tissue.

One dangerous way to lose fluid is to take a "water pill" (**diuretic**). These pills cause the kidneys to draw extra water from the blood into the urine. Another quick-weight-loss trick is to exercise heavily in the heat, losing large amounts of fluid in sweat. This practice is dangerous, too, and is not being recommended here.

Most quick-weight-loss diets cause large fluid losses that look like dramatic changes on the scale but are really temporary. Such diets cause little loss of body fat. Later sections of this chapter come back to how *not* to lose weight.

KEY POINTS *To lose weight safely and permanently, a person must lose fat tissue, not lean tissue or water.*

Feasting: Weight Gain

When you eat more food than you need, where does it go in your body? An excess of any energy nutrient—carbohydrate, fat, or protein—can be stored as follows:

▶ Carbohydrate is broken down, absorbed, and changed into glucose. Inside the body, glucose may be stored as glycogen or body fat.

enrichment

Tell students that what has been considered a fashionable amount for people to weigh has varied throughout the centuries, and from country to country. Also tell them that empha-

sizing different parts of the body has been popular with clothes designers. Then have students brainstorm examples of how people have been slaves to fashion, sometimes at the expense of health. (Examples: foot binding; having the lower ribs removed to have a smaller waist; eating arsenic to make the

▶ Fat is broken down mostly to fatty acids and absorbed. Then these may be stored as body fat.

▶ Protein, too, is broken down to its basic units (amino acids) and absorbed. Inside the body, these may be used to replace lost body protein. Any extra amino acids are changed into body fat and stored.

Notice that although three kinds of energy nutrients enter the body, they are stored there in only two forms: glycogen and fat. No matter whether you are eating steak, brownies, or baked beans, then, if you eat enough of them, the excess will be stored as fat within hours.

 The energy from any food can build up in body fat if a person eats more calories than are spent.

Fasting: A Wrong Way to Lose Weight

When the tables are turned and you stop eating altogether, your body has to draw on its fuel stores to keep going. Nothing is wrong with this. In fact, it is a great advantage to us that we can eat a meal, store fuel, and then use it until the next meal. (Some animals, such as cattle, have to spend almost all their waking hours eating—leaving them little time for daydreaming.)

People can store fat and glycogen, but their stores are not unlimited. A person with just average fat stores has enough fat to provide the body with energy for weeks, even when no food at all is eaten (fasting).

On the other hand, the body's supply of carbohydrate, stored as glycogen, is small by comparison. When too little carbohydrate is taken in, such as when the eater consumes a diet too low in carbohydrates or fails to eat at all, the glycogen stores last for less than a day. While glycogen runs out, the body's demand for the carbohydrate fuel glucose is as strong as ever.

So how does the fasting body get the needed glucose? It begins to convert protein to carbohydrate. In fasting, the body has no external source of protein, and so it takes apart the protein in its own muscles and organs to keep up the supply of glucose needed to feed the brain and nerves.

For this reason, dieters should avoid both fasting and diets too low in carbohydrates. People who follow weight-loss schemes that employ fasting or low-carbohydrate diets drop weight quickly, especially at first. This is because they are using up protein from muscles and organs as fuel. Protein contains only half as many calories per pound as fat, so it disappears twice as fast. Furthermore, with each pound of body protein used for fuel, 3 or 4 pounds of water are also lost from the body. Because of this, the person who stops eating altogether sees a great change in weight on the scales.

The body is thrown into a crisis. If it were to continue to feed on itself at this rate, death would occur in about ten days. Instead, the fasting body changes gears to an emergency route of energy use that allows it to wring every possible calorie from its stored fuel. In addition, vital functions slow down to reduce the need for basal fuel. The person slows down mentally, too, and feels too tired to exercise.

For the person who wants to lose weight, fasting has drawbacks and is not the best way. A balanced low-calorie, adequate-carbohydrate diet has in fact been proved to promote the same rate of *weight* loss and a faster rate of

For Your Information

Chapter 7 explained that the body stores its carbohydrate fuel, glucose, as the substance called glycogen. The relationship of glucose to glycogen can be compared with the relationship of beads to a necklace. The individual beads (glucose molecules), when strung together, become something else: a necklace (glycogen).

Glossary

◖ **diuretic** (die-yoo-RETT-ick): a drug
◖ that causes the body to lose fluids; not
◖ effective for loss of body fat.

COMPREHENSION CHECK

There are many poor weight-loss programs, and some that are actually dangerous. Have students look at the Health Strategies, "Clues to Identifying Unsound Weight-Loss Programs," on page 212. Then have the students analyze the following diet:

The Stewardess Diet
Day 1—Eat seven boiled eggs
Day 2—Eat seven wieners
Day 3—Eat seven bananas
Drink only water, tea, coffee, or diet soda. Repeat until the desired amount of weight is lost.

Write student responses on the board. If students don't bring it up, have them calculate each day's total calories to see whether the days have at least 1,000 calories. (seven eggs = 560 calories; seven hot dogs = 875 calories, seven medium bananas = 560 calories) Students also might not mention the high cholesterol content of the eggs or the high fat content of the hot dogs.

Discuss the importance of evaluating the healthiness of a diet before trying it.

complexion white; binding the bosom to appear flatter for the flapper look in 1920s; wearing very tight corsets to have a small waist, though it interfered with breathing and women would swoon or faint.) Being overweight was fashionable several hundred years

ago because it was considered a sign of wealth and affluence.

Have students discuss why people are willing to risk health for whims of "here today, gone tomorrow" styles.

The transparencies "Percent Nutrients in Food Versus the Human Body," and "What Happens Inside the Body During Overeating and Undereating," is provided in the Transparency Acetate Binder.

FAST FACTS

Approximately 50 million Americans went on diets in 1992. Only 5 percent will keep off any weight that they lost.

GROUP ACTIVITY

Put students into groups of four. Each group must have a reporter. Give groups five minutes to write down all of the things Section 4 mentioned that people should *not* do when dieting. Come back together as a large group. Ask each reporter to read an item from his or her list. After each has contributed, any reporter may add another. Discuss the answers.

fat loss than a total fast. A rule of thumb: to lose weight safely and effectively, do not go below 10 calories per pound of *present* body weight per day.

 When no food or too little carbohydrate is eaten, the body uses up its glycogen and then breaks down its own protein tissues to supply the brain with glucose. Then the body slows its rate of energy use. Fasting and low-carbohydrate diets are not healthy ways to lose weight.

Other Wrong Ways to Lose Weight

You can judge a good weight-loss diet not by the speed of weight loss but by how well those who use it maintain their new weight. By this standard, fad diets and fasting are not smart ways to lose weight. True nutrition experts never recommend them.

Health Strategies

Clues to Identifying Unsound Weight-Loss Programs

Don't trust any weight-loss programs that:

▶ Promise rapid weight loss (that is, more than 1 percent of total body weight per week).
▶ Use diets that are extremely low in calories (below 1,000 calories per day).
▶ Use diets that are too low in carbohydrates (providing less than 6 servings of cereals, breads, pasta, or rice in a day).
▶ Make people dependent upon special products rather than on regular foods.
▶ Do not teach permanent, realistic lifestyle changes, including regular physical activity and behavior modification.
▶ Misrepresent salespeople as "counselors" supposedly qualified to give guidance in nutrition or general health.
▶ Require large sums of money at the start or require that clients sign contracts for expensive, long-term programs. Programs should be on a pay-as-you-go basis.
▶ Fail to inform clients about the risks associated with weight loss in general or with the specific program being promoted.
▶ Claim that "cellulite" exists in the body. (Cellulite is supposed to be a hard-to-lose form of fat, but in reality, there is no such thing as cellulite. All fat is hard to lose.)

Source: Adapted with permission from *National Council Against Health Fraud Newsletter*, March/April 1987.

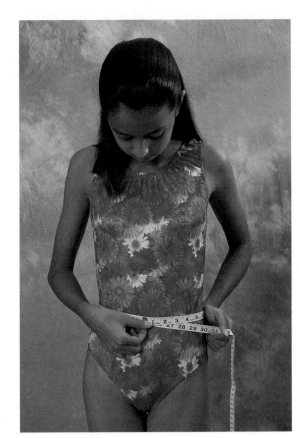

It's hard for some young girls to know how thin is too thin.

COOPERATIVE LEARNING

Losing and Gaining Weight

Explain to students that there are safe and unsafe ways of losing and gaining weight. Not all diet programs are safe, even if they lead to weight loss or gain. A number of diet programs offer quick results that can lead to a rapid return of the weight when the dieter quits the program. A diet that doesn't change a person's long term behavior usually will not be successful. Diets that have quick results may also be hazardous, whether they are designed to help a person lose or gain weight.

Divide your class into groups of three or four. Instruct students to bring advertisements for diet programs to class. In their groups,

Weight-Loss Schemes

Consumer SKILLS

One survey of 29,000 weight-loss schemes found fewer than 6 percent of them effective—and 13 percent dangerous. People may respond to this fact with the question, "Can't the government do something about that?" The government tries to find and crack down on diet swindles. Watchdog agencies, however, have too few staff members and too little money to handle the huge number of reported cases. They can't stop books from being published no matter how untrue. They can stop only the most dangerous products at best. This results in a free market for others who can rake in billions of dollars on products that are only slightly less dangerous than the worst ones.

It is easy for a swindler to get a product on the market and hard for the government or other groups to get it off. That puts the burden of identifying and avoiding frauds on you. To keep from being taken in, remember: if it sounds too good to be true, it probably is. The Health Strategies feature on the opposite page, "Clues to Identifying Unsound Weight-Loss Programs," offers clues to help you recognize bad weight-loss ideas.

Critical Thinking

1. *Do you think it might be worth it to some people to take a risk trying a new diet scheme for weight loss? If so, why? If not, why not?*
2. *Under what circumstances might you try one?*
3. *What might be a better plan?*

Other ways *not* to lose weight are water pills, diet pills, health spa regimens, muscle stimulators, passive exercise machines, hormones, and surgery. Water pills (diuretics, mentioned earlier) do nothing to solve a fat problem. They only bring about the loss of a few pounds on the scale for half a day. As for over-the-counter **diet pills**, they reduce appetite by triggering the stress response. One ingredient in such pills, ephedrine, has been declared hazardous, because thousands of people using it fell ill, and hundreds are believed to have died from its effects. Other pills leave the dieter with another problem: how to get off the pills without gaining more weight back.

Health spas may be a nice place to exercise, but you cannot "jiggle" or "melt" pounds away on their special machines. Muscle stimulators reduce body measurements by making muscles tighter, not by reducing their fat content—and only for an hour or so.

Hormones are powerful body chemicals, but most have proved useless and often hazardous as weight-loss aids. Researchers do see hope on the horizon, though, in a newly discovered hormone. In the photo on the next page, the mouse on the right lacks the ability to produce the hormone, leptin, that helps to control eating. The mouse on the left also lacks the hormone, but it remains thin because researchers inject it with the missing hormone. Research like this promises hope for future obesity treatments.

MINI Glossary

diet pills: medications that reduce the appetite or otherwise promote weight loss. Pills available over the counter usually contain caffeine and other drugs that cause more nervousness than weight loss. Prescription pills include amphetamines.

have students analyze at least two advertisements by answering the following questions about each one. **1.** Does the advertisement promise quick results? **2.** How much weight loss or gain is promised per week? **3.** Does the advertisement warn of any health risks? **4.** What is the total cost of the program?

Have students share their findings with the class. Remind the class that successful programs are those that include exercise and loss or gain of only 1 or 2 pounds per week. In order to lose weight, people need to burn more calories than they take in and to gain weight they need to take in more calories than they burn.

ASSESS

EVALUATE

Without using their books, have students write down five key points they remember from Section 4. Go around the room and have students give an item from their lists. Write the items on the board.

SECTION 4 Review Answers

1. Answers will vary.
2. The body's lean tissues and fluid levels are vital to health. (p. 210)
3. takes apart the protein in its own muscles and organs (p. 211)
4. Answers will vary; could include: fasting, fad diets, water pills, diet pills, health spa regiments, muscle stimulators, passive exercise machines, hormones, and surgery. (pp. 212–214)
5. Answers will vary.

A reproducible quiz for Section 4 is provided in the Teacher's Resource Box.

CLOSE

Have students write, without using their books, five of the eight clues to identifying unsound weight-loss programs. They are listed in the Health Strategies box entitled "Clues to Identifying Unsound Weight-Loss Programs" on page 212.

What's the difference between the lean mouse and her obese sister? The mouse on the left was treated with the hormone leptin.

For Your Information

Ineffective or dangerous weight-loss gimmicks:

▶ Chromium picolinate
▶ Diet pills
▶ Ephedrine or ephedra-containing products
▶ Expanding pills
▶ Glucomannan, bee pollen, spirulina
▶ Herbal products and teas, including aloe, buckthorn, cascara, castor oil, ma huang, rhubarb, and senna
▶ Hormones (most types)
▶ Laxatives
▶ Lipectomy and suctioning
▶ Massages, muscle stimulators
▶ Spa belts, rollers, saunas, whirlpools
▶ Stomach stapling, surgery, balloons

Surgery (such as stomach stapling) sometimes succeeds in treating severe weight problems, but it has dangerous side effects. Most types lead to digestive tract damage, diarrhea, and malnutrition.

Risks of these and other procedures outweigh the benefits for all except those whose obesity threatens their lives. Success, as measured by long-term weight maintenance, is seldom achieved by these methods. As the Consumer Skills feature on the previous page points out, however, bringing out new diet books and products is a profitable business.

 The best form of weight loss is one that is safe and that promotes the maintenance of the person's new weight. Pills, spas, muscle stimulators, and other gimmicks fail by this standard.

SECTION 4 Review

Answer the following questions on a sheet of paper.

Learning the Vocabulary

The vocabulary terms in this section are *diuretic* and *diet pills*.

1. Write a sentence using each vocabulary term.

Learning the Facts

2. Why is it important to lose mostly fat tissue and not water or lean tissue when you diet?

3. Where does the body get the glucose it needs when a person has not eaten in a while?

4. List four methods that you should not use in attempting to lose weight.

Making Life Choices

5. List as many dangerous methods of weight loss as you can think of. Why do so many people try these strategies and invest money thinking they will solve their weight problems? Do you know of anyone who has ever tried any of these methods? What was the end result?

Chapter 8, Section 4

The following quiz will help you assess your students' understanding of the material covered in this section of the chapter. You might use the quiz as an oral exercise, which will lead into a class discussion of the topics covered. Or, you might use it as a paper/pencil

quiz to evaluate your students individually.

Like the Quick Quiz, the Section Review can also be used as an assessment tool to spark class discussion or as an individual student evaluation. It can also be used as a review in preparation for this quiz.

1. Changes in body weight reflect shifts in water, bone minerals, and lean tissues as well as fat. (True)
2. Lean tissues, such as bones, muscles, and

SECTION 5

Smart Weight-Loss Strategies

With so many weight-loss schemes guaranteed to fail, what works? How can a person lose weight safely and permanently? The secret is a sensible approach (we didn't say *easy*) that uses diet, exercise, and behavior changes. It takes a great deal of effort, at first, for a person whose habits have all led to overfatness to adopt the hundred or so new habits that bring about thinness. When people succeed, they do so because they have used the methods described here.

Before embarking on such a plan, you must learn to distinguish between **hunger** and **appetite**. Most people would name hunger as the reason for eating, and often this is true. The physical need for food is not the only reason people eat, though. Another reason is appetite, the psychological desire for food. Appetite may arise in response to the sight, smell, or thought of food even when you are full. An example of this occurs when a server offers dessert after you've finished eating, and suddenly you desire a piece of cake.

Other factors influence eating, too. Some people react to stress by losing their appetites, while others indulge in **stress eating**. Some eat in response to all sorts of complex human feelings other than hunger or appetite. Sensations such as boredom, depression, or anger can sometimes be lessened for a while by eating. All your reasons for choosing foods contribute to the nature of your diet. All must be recognized, honored, and sometimes, controlled, as you develop your weight control plan. In weight control, eating becomes a deliberate process, rather than an automatic one.

The following sections are written as advice to "you." This is to give you the feeling that you are listening in on a counseling session in which an overfat person is being given advice about the methods known to be effective.

Diet Planning

No plan is magical. You needn't include or avoid any particular food. You are the one who will have to live with the plan, so you had better be the one who designs it. Don't think of it as a "diet" you are going "on"— because then you may be tempted to go "off." Think of it as an eating plan that you will adopt for life. It must consist of foods that you like or can learn to like, and foods that are available to you. You can see from Figure 8–5 on the next page that even fast foods can undermine weight-loss efforts or support them.

Calories and Nutrients   Choose a calorie level you can live with. A shortage of 500 calories a day for seven days is a 3,500-calorie weekly shortage—enough to lose a pound of body fat. There is no point in rushing. If you adopt an eating plan rather than a "diet," you can be practicing positive behaviors all the time you are losing weight. You will be ready to succeed for the rest of your life, once you arrive at your goal weight.

Make your meals meet your nutrient needs. This is a way of putting yourself first. "I like me, and I'm going to take good care of me" is the right

> **❝** *A little with quiet is the only diet.* **❞**
>
> Proverb

MINI Glossary

hunger: the physiological need to eat, experienced as a drive for obtaining food, an unpleasant sensation that demands relief.

appetite: the psychological desire to eat, a learned motivation and a positive sensation that accompanies the sight, smell, or thought of food.

stress eating: eating in response to stress, an inappropriate activity.

---

organs supply a very large proportion of total body weight. (False)

3. Dramatic weight changes often reflect only changes in the body's fluid content. (True)

4. Diuretics are a harmless and effective way to achieve rapid weight loss. (False)

5. Excess energy from carbohydrate, fat and protein is stored in the body as fat. (True)

6. The body can store only limited amounts of fat and glycogen. (False)

7. A fasting body must rely on the protein stored in its muscles and organs to provide glucose. (True)

8. Crash diets are a quick way to lose fat. (False)

9. The best way to lose weight is through a balanced low-calorie, adequate-carbohydrate diet. (True)

10. Diet pills, muscle stimulators, surgery and water pills can be healthy, effective ways to solve a fat problem. (False)

SECTION 5

FOCUS

OUTCOMES

In this section students will learn:

1. How to lose weight sensibly.
2. Strategies that help people keep weight off.

FOCUS ACTIVITY

Have students write down several reasons why a weight-loss diet must be approached seriously. Discuss the students' answers.

TEACH & APPLY

INTERDISCIPLINARY ACTIVITY: MATH

Bring to class a tape measure and male and female 11½-inch fashion dolls. Discuss how children learn from toys and the media what their bodies are "supposed" to look like. Ask students if the images shown in many advertisements are realistic. What about toys? Could real people have bodies like fashion dolls? Show the dolls and tell the students they will do an exercise to find the answer to that question.

You can do this activity yourself or it can be done by groups of students using many dolls and tape measures. Measure the dolls' heights, hips, waists, chests, hands, and feet. Have students multiply each measurement by six. Ask the students for their answers. Doll sizes may vary but the female will be about 5'9" tall with a 34½" chest,

(continued on next page)

215

(continued from previous page)

21½" waist, 30" hips, and 4½" hands and feet. The male will be about 6' tall, 36" chest, 27" waist, 34½" hips, 20¼" across the shoulders, 8¼" feet and 6¾" hands. Discuss the findings. Some students will want tape measures to compare their measurements to determine realism.

Discuss the fact that a leading toy company introduced a new fashion doll with more normal proportions due to consumer pressure. Do students think the more "normal" doll will be more or less popular?

CLASS ACTIVITY

Discuss Figure 8–5 with the students. Have students study the two choices for each of the meals (taco, burger, breakfast, and pizza). Which choices do they believe most students would make? Do any of the students already choose the meals with less fat? You could have the students calculate the actual calorie differences and calories-from-fat differences between the choices. This will help them realize the benefit of the trimmed-down choices. For example, choosing the trimmed meal under tacos would cut the calorie intake by 408 calories. It would cut the fat calorie consumption by 338 calories. As an additional activity for the students who complain that the trimmed meal is too sparse and not appetizing, have them develop a compromise meal.

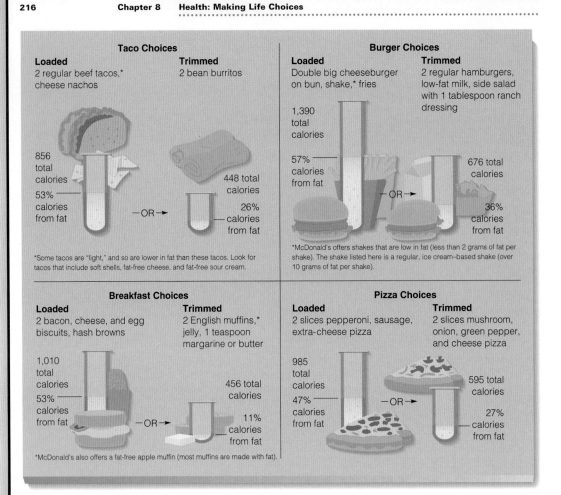

Figure 8–5 Fast-Food Choices. *Depending on the foods chosen, fast foods can be high or low in calories and fat.*

attitude. A good pattern to follow is the Daily Food Guide of Chapter 7, pages 166 and 167.

Most people could lose weight at a reasonable rate following such a plan and meet their nutrient needs, too. If you resolve to include a certain number of servings of food from each group each day, you may be so busy making sure you get what you need that you will have little time or appetite left for high-calorie or empty-calorie foods. Foods such as fruits, vegetables, and whole grains take a lot more eating, too. Crunchy, wholesome foods offer bulk and a feeling of fullness for far fewer calories than smooth, refined high-calorie foods. Limit your portions of meats: an ounce of ham contains more calories than an ounce of bread, and many of them are from fat.

Timing of Meals   Three meals a day is standard for our society, but no law says you shouldn't have four or five meals—only be sure they are

special needs

Intra-personal

This chapter opens with this, "Are you pleased with your body weight? If you answered yes, you are a rare person." Most students will indeed, answer no. After studying the information in this chapter, they will

be better able to attain or maintain a healthy body weight. This activity can add a more personal awareness of diet and exercise habits so that any needed changes can be made. As they work on this activity, stress the importance of lifestyle changes and help students focus on the fact that a healthy body weight may not be achieved instantaneously.

smaller, of course. What is important is to eat regularly and, if at all possible, to eat before you are very hungry. When you do decide to eat, eat the entire meal you have planned for yourself. Then don't eat again until the next meal. Save "free" (lowest-calorie) or favorite foods or beverages for a snack at the end of the day, if you need insurance against late-evening hunger. Also, remember to drink plenty of water.

Eating sensibly is the best way to control weight.

Other Helpful Hints   At first it may seem as if you have to spend all your waking hours planning and eating your meals. Such a huge effort is always needed when a new skill is being learned. (You spent hours practicing writing the alphabet when you were in the first grade.) After about three weeks, though, it will be much easier. Reward yourself often, but never with food. Imagine yourself as a person who "eats thin." Visualize your future self as fit and trim. Your new eating pattern will become a habit.

Do not weigh yourself more than every week or two. Gains or losses of a pound or more in a matter of days disappear as quickly. The smoothed-out average is what is real. Don't expect to continue to lose as fast as you do at first. A sizable water loss is common in the first week, but the loss slows down dramatically soon after. If you have been working out lately, your scale weight may show no loss or even a gain. This may reflect a welcome development: the gain of lean body mass—just what you want, if you want to be healthy.

If you slip, don't punish yourself. If you ate an extra 1,000 calories yesterday, don't try to eat 1,000 fewer calories today. Just go back to your plan.

 KEY POINTS   *To design a successful weight-loss diet, design it to last a lifetime. Be realistic and make it adequate.*

Behavior Modification

Behavior modification also offers ideas that make sticking with your plan easier. Figure 8–6 on the next page offers some of these ideas.

You may have to get tough with yourself if you stop losing weight or start gaining. Ask yourself honestly (no one is listening in), "What am I doing wrong?" A period of weight gain can usually be explained by a person's own choices. Be aware that you may be choosing that course. Your food behaviors are under your control. Rather than feeling ashamed or guilty, hold your head high and take the attitude, "This is me, and this is the way I am choosing to be right now."

Have students keep a health diary for at least a 24-hour period; an entire week would give a more realistic picture. Ask them to keep track of what they eat and drink (water, too!), including quantities, and where and when they eat. They should also include physical exercise, including walking to and from school, and so on.

To make this activity meaningful, help students analyze their own health habits. Each

student's profile will be different. Students must first have an honest picture of where they are in relation to having a healthy goal. Ask them to look for patterns in their diets and exercise habits. They probably have some good patterns as well as some that have a negative effect on their overall health. To conclude, help students find places where they can make any needed changes in their eating and exercising habits.

MINI Glossary

behavior modification: changing one's choices or actions by manipulating the cues that trigger the actions, the actions themselves, or the consequences of the actions.

DISCUSSION

Ask students where, other than the kitchen, they eat. Do they consume more calories in these other locations than in the kitchen or dining room? More empty calories?

CLASS ACTIVITY

Before class, fill several 1-gallon plastic jugs with water or sand. Ask for student volunteers to come forward and hold the jugs in their hands. Each jug represents approximately 8½ pounds. You may want the students to walk back and forth on the side of the room. Meanwhile, explain to the class the relationship between being overweight, exhaustion from carrying the extra weight, and not having the energy to exercise. Ask the students who have been holding the jugs if they would feel like doing a lot of physical exercise if they had to carry the weights with them wherever they went.

DISCUSSION

Have students think of one behavior modification strategy that was not listed in Figure 8–6. Go around the room and ask each student to give his or her answer. Make a master list on the board, and discuss the suggestions.

Figure 8–6 Using Behavior Modification for Weight Control

Using Behavior Modification for Weight Control

1. *To eliminate inappropriate eating cues:*
   - Let other family members buy, store, and serve their own sweets. When the television shows food commercials, change channels or look away.
   - Stay away from convenience stores.
   - Carry appropriate snacks from home.
   - Avoid vending machines.

2. *To reduce the cues you cannot eliminate:*
   - Eat only in one place, in one room.
   - Clear plates directly into the garbage.
   - Create obstacles to the eating of problem foods (for example, make it necessary to unwrap, cook, and serve each one separately).
   - Minimize contact with excessive food (serve individual plates, don't put serving dishes on the table, and leave the table when you are finished).
   - Make small portions of food look large (spread food out, and serve it on small plates).
   - Don't deprive yourself (eat regular meals, and don't skip meals).

3. *To strengthen the cues to appropriate eating and exercise:*
   - Encourage others to eat appropriate food and exercise.
   - Keep your favorite appropriate foods in the front of the refrigerator.
   - Learn appropriate portion sizes.
   - Save foods from meals for snacks (and make these your only snacks).
   - Prepare foods attractively.
   - Keep your roller blades (hiking boots, tennis racket) by the door.

4. *To practice the desired eating and exercise behaviors:*
   - Slow down (pause for two to three minutes, put down utensils, chew slowly, swallow before reloading the fork, and always use utensils).
   - Leave some food on the plate.
   - Join in and exercise with a group of active people.

5. *To arrange negative consequences of inappropriate eating:*
   - Eat your meals with other people.
   - Ask that others respond neutrally to your deviations (make no comment). This is a negative consequence, because it withholds attention.

6. *To arrange positive consequences of appropriate eating and exercise behaviors:*
   - Keep records of food intake, physical activity, and weight change.
   - Arrange for rewards (not food) for each behavior change or weight loss.
   - Ask for encouragement from your friends and family.

KEY POINTS *Reward yourself for following your weight-loss diet.*

Physical Activity

Some people who want to lose weight hate the very idea of physical activity. A word to them: weight loss, at least to a point, is possible without exercise. Even if you choose not to be physically active at first, however, let

HEALTHY PEOPLE 2000

Overweight acquired during childhood or adolescence may persist into adulthood and increase the risk for some chronic diseases later in life. Obese children also experience psychological stress. Concern has been expressed that the prevalence of obesity in adolescents may be increasing, but definitive data are lacking. There is also concern that overemphasis on thinness during adolescence may contribute to eating disorders such as anorexia nervosa and bulimia. Therefore, the target for this objective for adolescents is set at no more than 15 percent to prevent an increase in overweight above the baseline. The objective should be achieved through emphasis on physical activity accompanied by properly balanced dietary intake so that growth is not impaired. For adults who are overweight, achieving this objective will your mind be open to the idea. As the pounds come off, moving your body becomes a pleasure. You may want to take up an activity later on.

The next chapter gives many details about developing fitness, but a few points are important here. Physical activity contributes to weight control physically. It develops the body's lean tissue. It raises the rate of basal energy use. Physical activity also helps mentally. Looking and feeling healthy boosts self-esteem. High self-esteem helps a person to stay with a weight-control effort—a beneficial cycle.

Weight loss without activity can have a negative effect. A person who diets without exercising loses both lean and fat tissue. If the person then gains weight without exercising, the gain is mostly fat. Compared with lean tissue, fat tissue burns fewer calories to maintain itself. The person who slides back into eating the same amount as before the diet gains body fat, but not lean. This cycle of gaining, losing, and gaining again can leave people fatter than if they had not dieted at all.

On the other hand, the more lean tissue you develop, and the more calories you spend, the more you can afford to eat. This brings you both pleasure and nutrients. It must be clear by now that physical activity speeds up your body's energy use *permanently*—that is, for as long as you keep your body fit.

Physical activity, of course, also spends energy while you are doing it. Figure 8–7 on the next page lists energy costs of activities.

Whether you are trying to gain or lose weight, physical activity is essential for health.

require a combination of calorie restriction—particularly calories from dietary fat—accompanied by increased physical activity to achieve weight reduction.

Overweight affects a large proportion of the U.S. population and the prevalence of overweight has not declined among adults for two decades. Given the trend and the fact that weight management is difficult for most people, the target set for adults is very ambitious. Nonetheless, the potential benefits from

reduction in the prevalence of overweight are of considerable public health importance and deserve particular emphasis and attention. Achieving this objective and its special population targets will require a concerted public effort to prevent the development of overweight and to encourage and facilitate weight reduction among the overweight. All efforts should be culturally relevant to the population target groups.

COMPREHENSION CHECK

Figure 8–7 gives students the exact amount of calories burned in 15 different activities and for different intensities for three of those activities (bicycling, running, and swimming). For example, a person weighing 110 pounds who bicycles at 13 m.p.h. will burn 5 calories per minute. Using the column that most closely matches their weights, students can find approximately how many calories they will burn for each of these activities. To find an exact amount for their exact weights, they can use the number factor under the heading Cal/Lb/Min. Directions at the bottom of the figure explain the equation the students need to use to find the number of calories spent for their exact weights. Give them the following problem to make sure they understand how to use the equation:

Assume a person weighing 98 pounds plays basketball vigorously for 2 hours. How many calories would be spent? The equation would be 0.097 × 98 = 9.506 × 120 (the 2 hours must be changed to 120 minutes). The answer would be 1,140.72 calories.

ASSESS

EVALUATE

Ask students to summarize, in a written paragraph, what they have learned in Section 5. Emphasize that students should interpret what they have read in their own words. Have them write down what they think were the most important things to remember about safe dieting.

Figure 8–7 Energy Demands of Activities

This figure shows how many calories per minute are spent in activities for people at five different body weights. The calories per pound per minute (cal/lb/min) number makes it possible for you to calculate the number of calories for your own body weight, if it is not exactly one of the five weights listed here.

Activity	Cal/Lb/Min[a]	Calories Spent per Minute (for 5 Body Weights, in Pounds)				
		110	125	150	175	200
Aerobic dance (vigorous)	0.062	6.8	7.8	9.3	10.9	12.4
Basketball (vigorous, full court)	0.097	10.7	12.1	14.6	17.0	19.4
Bicycling						
13 miles per hour	0.045	5.0	5.6	6.8	7.9	9.0
19 miles per hour	0.076	8.4	9.5	11.4	13.3	15.2
Canoeing (flat water, moderate pace)	0.045	5.0	5.6	6.8	7.9	9.0
Cross-country skiing (8 miles per hour)	0.104	11.4	13.0	15.6	18.2	20.8
Golf (carrying clubs)	0.045	5.0	5.6	6.8	7.9	9.0
Handball	0.078	8.6	9.8	11.7	13.7	15.6
Horseback riding (trot)	0.052	5.7	6.5	7.8	9.1	10.4
Rowing (vigorous)	0.097	10.7	12.1	14.6	17.0	19.4
Running						
5 miles per hour	0.061	6.7	7.6	9.2	10.7	12.2
7.5 miles per hour	0.094	10.3	11.8	14.1	16.4	18.8
10 miles per hour	0.114	12.5	14.3	17.1	20.0	22.9
Soccer (vigorous)	0.097	10.7	12.1	14.6	17.0	19.4
Studying	0.011	1.2	1.4	1.7	1.9	2.2
Swimming						
20 yards per minute	0.032	3.5	4.0	4.8	5.6	6.4
45 yards per minute	0.058	6.4	7.3	8.7	10.2	11.6
Tennis (beginner)	0.032	3.5	4.0	4.8	5.6	6.4
Walking (brisk pace)						
3.5 miles per hour	0.035	3.9	4.4	5.2	6.1	7.0

[a]*Cal/lb/min* is an abbreviation for *calories* (cal) per *pound* (lb) of body weight per *minute* (min). You can use it to calculate the number of calories you use at your body weight for a minute of activity. To calculate the total number of calories you spend for a longer time, multiply the cal/lb/min factor by your exact weight. Then multiply your answer by the number of minutes you spend on the activity. For example, if you weigh 142 pounds, and you want to know how many calories you spend doing 30 minutes of vigorous aerobic dance: 0.062 cal/lb/min × 142 lb = 8.8 calories per minute. 8.8 cal/min × 30 minutes = 264 total calories spent.

If an activity is to help with weight loss, it must be active. Being moved passively, as by a machine or a massage, does not help. The more muscles you move and the longer and more vigorously you move them, the more calories you spend.

Weight loss is not the only reward to be won from working out. If you incorporate the right kinds of workouts into your schedule, your heart and lungs, as well as your muscles, will become and stay fit. The "right kinds" of workouts are described in the next chapter.

KEY POINTS *Physical activity is helpful in weight loss because it increases lean tissue, expends energy, and boosts self-esteem.*

QUICK QUIZ

Chapter 8, Section 5

The following quiz will help you assess your students' understanding of the material covered in this section of the chapter. You might use the quiz as an oral exercise, which will lead into a class discussion of the topics covered. Or, you might use it as a paper/pencil

quiz to evaluate your students individually.

Like the Quick Quiz, the Section Review can also be used as an assessment tool to spark class discussion or as an individual student evaluation. It can also be used as a review in preparation for this quiz.

1. Successful weight loss involves changes in diet, exercise and behavior patterns. (True)

2. Appetite results from a psychological

Weight Maintenance

Finally, be aware that it can be much harder to maintain weight loss than to lose weight. An appropriate calorie intake for maintenance is higher than the level of intake to promote loss, but it still may take effort not to overeat. (Appendix B at the back of the book includes suggested calorie intakes for people of various ages.) Those who succeed in maintaining appropriate weight have some key traits in common:

▶ They take responsibility for their weight. They do not place the responsibility on programs, professionals, pills, or potions.
▶ They have confidence that they can maintain weight—they believe in themselves.
▶ They expect to have **lapses**, times when they fall back into the old patterns.

A word about lapses—people who maintain weight have learned to cope with them. They identify the triggers that lead to lapses and keep learning to avoid them. For example, a person who unexpectedly overate at a party would forgive the lapse, and then get tough. One action might be to promise to eat a balanced meal before attending the next party (to defend against hunger) and to stay away from the buffet (to reduce temptation). When normal lapses occur, cope by saying, "I'm doing it again, but I do it less often now. I'm making progress."

 KEY POINTS *People who maintain weight take responsibility for their weight. They have confidence in themselves. They do not let normal lapses bother them.*

> ❝*The one way to get thin is to reestablish a purpose in life.* ❞
>
> Cyril Connolly
> (1903–1974)
> English author and editor

SECTION 5 Review

Answer the following questions on a sheet of paper.

Learning the Vocabulary

The vocabulary terms in this section are *hunger, appetite, stress eating, behavior modification,* and *lapses.*

1. Write a sentence using each vocabulary term.

Learning the Facts

2. List four recommendations for developing a successful weight-loss program.

3. Give three strategies for using behavior modification for weight control.

4. What are some advantages of including physical activity in a weight-loss and weight-maintenance program?

Making Life Choices

5. A sound exercise program is important in losing and maintaining weight and overall health. Look over Figure 8–7 on the opposite page. Choose several activities on the list that you enjoy. Make up a schedule for a week that includes at least one activity for each day. Calculate the number of calories you'll spend on each activity.

MINI Glossary

lapses: times of falling back into former habits, a normal part of both weight change and weight maintenance.

desire for food. (True)

3. Anger, boredom, depression, and stress do not significantly affect appetite. (False)

4. A diet should be approached as a short-term change in eating habits. (False)

5. When dieting you should eat only when you are really hungry. (False)

6. When dieting you should weigh yourself every day in order to keep track of your progress. (False)

7. The first three weeks of a diet are especially difficult, because they are spent learning new eating skills. (True)

8. Long-term increase in physical activity raises the rate of basal energy use and therefore contributes to weight control. (True)

9. Dieting without exercise can result in a loss of lean tissue. (True)

10. Low body weight, once achieved, is easy to maintain. (False)

SECTION 6

FOCUS

OUTCOME

In this section students will learn:

1. How to gain weight wisely.

FOCUS ACTIVITY

Explain to the class that because so many people have difficulties with being overweight, it is sometimes hard to relate to the problems associated with being underweight. Have students take out a piece of paper. Give them five minutes to write down drawbacks that would come from being underweight. Tell them not to forget social and economic factors, as well as physical ones. Discuss students' answers.

TEACH & APPLY

GUEST SPEAKER

Invite a registered dietitian to class. Have the dietitian discuss why an underweight person trying to gain pounds has as difficult a task as an overweight person trying to lose pounds. This will also give students a chance to ask questions from throughout the chapter.

Smart Weight-Gain Strategies

It is as hard for a person who tends to be underweight to gain a pound as it is for a person who tends to be overweight to lose one. Like the weight loser, the person who wants to gain must learn new habits and learn to like new foods.

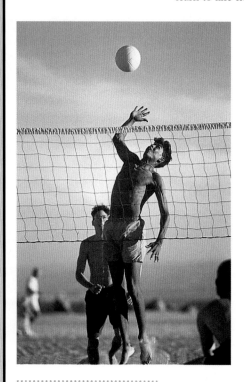

Active exercise helps people achieve and maintain healthy weights.

An underweight person must decide whether gaining weight is best for health. If the person is healthy, it may be that weighing less than average is an advantage. Thin people are unlikely to suffer from heart disease, for example. For teens who are still growing, it could be that they will "fill out" naturally in a year or two—the low weight is temporary. However, if an underweight person is unwell and eats poorly, then learning to eat well in ways that support the body's healthy weight is the best course. Some people may want to gain just for the sake of their appearance. This is a personal choice.

Physical Activity   Although physical activity costs calories, it is essential for health. Thus it should continue unless body weight is so low as to be life-threatening. The healthy way to gain weight is to build it up by patient and consistent physical training and, at the same time, to eat enough calories to support the weight gain. If you are not dangerously underweight, adopt an activity program designed to build lean body tissue. (For more details, see the next chapter.)

Selecting High-Calorie Foods   In addition to exercising appropriately, you must eat enough calories to support weight gain. If you add 700 to 800 extra calories of nutritious foods a day, you can achieve a healthful weight gain of 1 to 1½ pounds per week.

A person who wants to gain weight often has to learn to eat new foods. No matter how many helpings of boiled carrots you eat, you won't gain weight very fast. Carrots simply don't offer enough calories. The person who can't eat much volume should select high-calorie foods (the very ones the dieter is trying to stay away from). To gain weight, then:

▶ Eat an extra 700 to 800 calories per day.
▶ Use more high-calorie foods—those items marked in green in Figure 7–1 of Chapter 7 (pages 166–167).

Also, take an independent view of the low-fat diet plan that is recommended for the general U.S. population. Most people are too fat. For you, if you need to gain weight, a diet very low in fat might do more harm than good. Ignore recommendations about fat and calories made to overweight people.

enrichment

Ask students to consider the following scenario. Imagine there are two identical twins, one regularly eats 2,600 calories, 50 percent of it coming from fat. The other also eats 2,600 calories daily, with only 30 percent of it coming from fat. All other aspects of their lives—exercise, metabolism, and so on—are the same. Ask the class if the twins would have the same body composition (the same amount of fat and lean). Take a class vote. The answer is that the twin with the higher fat content in

To increase calorie intake:

▶ Choose milkshakes instead of milk, whole milk instead of nonfat milk, peanut butter instead of lean meat, avocados instead of cucumbers, whole-wheat muffins instead of whole-wheat bread.
▶ Add margarine to cooked vegetables. Use creamy dressings on salads, whipped cream on fruit, sour cream on potatoes, and so forth. (Because fat contains twice as many calories per teaspoon as sugar, it adds calories without adding much bulk.)

Additional Strategies   Since you need many more calories in a day, you will also need to:

▶ Eat more often. Make three sandwiches in the morning to eat as snacks between the day's three regular meals.

Most people who are underweight have simply been too busy (sometimes for months) to eat enough to gain or maintain weight. In this case:

▶ Plan ahead what to eat at your mealtimes and snack times.
▶ Plan time for eating each meal. If you fill up fast, eat the highest-calorie items first. Don't start with soup or salad. Eat meaty appetizers or the main course first.

Expect to feel full, sometimes even uncomfortably so. Most underweight people usually eat small quantities of food. When they begin eating significantly more food, they complain of being too full. This is normal, and it passes when the stomach adapts.

For the person who tends to be underweight, maintenance of the new weight is a final challenge. The weight-maintenance methods described on page 221 for the person who tends to gain weight work equally well in this case. Just swap strategies—for example, stand *near* the buffet at a party.

KEY POINTS   *Healthful weight gain can be achieved by a program of exercise and increased intake of calories.*

Answer the following questions on a sheet of paper.

Learning the Facts

1. What is the healthiest way to gain weight?
2. How many extra calories of nutritious food must be added daily to gain 1 to 1½ pounds per week?

3. Give three recommendations for increasing calorie intake.

Making Life Choices

4. Have you or anyone you know ever had difficulty gaining weight? Explain some of the frustrations involved. How are these problems similar to those of a person who is trying to lose weight? How are they different? Why is it that there are not as many fad programs or gimmicks on the market targeted at weight gain as there are for weight loss?

Here are the answers to the questions at the start of the chapter.

1. **True.**
2. **False.** A weight loss may reflect loss of water or lean tissue rather than loss of fat.
3. **False.** Fasting promotes rapid weight loss, but a balanced low-calorie diet can promote more rapid fat loss.
4. **False.** Carbohydrate is a necessary part of a healthy, balanced weight-loss diet.
5. **True.**
6. **True.**
7. **False.** It is as hard for a person who tends to be thin to gain a pound as it is for a person who tends to be fat to lose one.

ASSESS

EVALUATE

A reproducible quiz for Section 6 is provided in the Teacher's Resource Box.

Review Answers

1. build up weight by patient and consistent physical training and eat enough calories to support the weight gain (p. 222)
2. 700–800 calories a day (p. 222)
3. Answers will vary; could include: choose milk shakes instead of milk, whole milk instead of non-fat milk, peanut butter instead of lean meat, avocados instead of cucumbers, whole-wheat muffins instead of whole-wheat bread; add margarine to vegetables; use creamy dressing on salads, whipped cream on fruit, sour cream on potatoes; eat more often; plan ahead what to eat at your mealtimes; and plan time for eating each meal. (p. 223)
4. Answers will vary.

CLOSE

Have students design a list of behavior modification strategies for underweight people. Give students 15 minutes and then discuss their findings.

---

the diet would have a higher percentage of body fatness. Why? Our bodies use the energy nutrients differently. Dietary fat is changed to body fat with little effort. Carbohydrates, on the other hand, require a larger energy expenditure to be changed to body fat.

To give an example of this, Japanese people eat 20 percent more calories than Americans, but 33 percent less fat. The Japanese as a group of people are generally leaner than Americans. However, as Japanese people adopt Western eating habits, their body fatness usually increases.

A repro-ducible copy of the Life Choice Inven-tory is provided in the Teacher's Resource Box.

BACKGROUND INFORMATION

We have learned that weight loss or gain happens when the number of calories we eat does not equal the number of calories we burn. One method of deter-mining calorie requirements for the day is to use the following formula: Multiply your ideal healthy weight by the number below that best describes your activity level. The answer you get will represent your calorie needs for the day:

13—very sedentary person, inactive.

14—sedentary, does light house-work, moves slowly.

15—average, activities such as doing errands and light yard work, moves at a normal pace.

16—above average, does hard work involving heavy lifting and moving at a brisk pace, exer-cises regularly for fun.

17—strenuous, has a demand-ing exercise program and works hard physically, moving at a fast pace the major portion of the day.

If weight is above desired level, try exercising more. About five calories are burned for every minute walked. Remind students that small changes in behavior add up.

Eating Attitudes Test

Answer these questions on a separate piece of paper using the following responses:

A = Always   U = Usually   O = Often
S = Sometimes   R = Rarely   N = Never

1. I am terrified about being overweight.
2. I avoid eating when I am hungry.
3. I am preoccupied with food.
4. I have gone on eating binges where I feel that I may not be able to stop.
5. I cut my food into tiny pieces.
6. I know the calorie and fat content of every food I eat.
7. I avoid foods with a high carbohydrate content or a high fat content.
8. I feel that others would prefer if I ate more.
9. I vomit after I have eaten.
10. I feel extremely guilty after eating.
11. I am preoccupied with a desire to be thinner.
12. I think about burning up calories when I am physically active.
13. Other people think I am too thin.
14. I am preoccupied with the thought of having fat on my body.

15. I take longer than other people to eat my meals.
16. I avoid foods with sugar in them.
17. I eat only diet foods.
18. I feel that food controls my life.
19. I display self-control around food.
20. I feel that others pressure me to eat.
21. I give too much time and thought to food.
22. I feel uncomfortable after eating sweets.
23. I engage in dieting behavior most of the time.
24. I like my stomach to be empty.
25. I enjoy trying new, rich foods.
26. I have the impulse to vomit after meals.

SCORING

Now calculate your score, counting 3 for never; 2 for rarely; 1 for sometimes; 0 for always, usually and often. Total scores under 20 points indicate abnor-mal eating behavior.

Your answers to the Life Choice Inventory are per-sonal and private. Share them with others only if you are comfortable doing so.

Source: Adapted from J. A. McSherry, Progress in the diagnosis of anorexia nervosa, *Journal of the Royal Society of Health* 106 (1986): 8–9. (Eating Attitudes Test developed by Dr. Paul Garfinkel.)

CRITICAL THINKING

Have the students bring in:

1. some type of diet plan (from a magazine, book, or computer search; or one that a friend or someone in their family has used), and
2. an advertisement for some type of weight

loss plan (the more unusual the better).

First, discuss diet plans in general, using good plans and poor plans to make key points. Students need to be able to examine any diet plan critically, as statistics show that the majority of Americans will diet during their lifetimes.

Have each student take two of the diet plans submitted by the class and summarize

An Obsession with Thinness: Eating Disorders

Our society and others like it favor thinness, especially in women. Magazines, newspapers, and television screens display camera-ready women, flaws hidden, unrealistically thin. The message is clear—the way you are isn't good enough. It is as if they are saying, "You should become like the cover girl who doesn't sweat; doesn't grow hair on her slender legs; has a flat stomach, a perfect face, and small feet; and is always perfectly happy. If you, young woman, are not perfectly happy, it is because your body is not perfect by these standards." Acceptance of such unreasonable standards has driven many young women in our society to be obsessed with thinness.

 I thought being thin was healthy. Isn't it OK to want to be thin?

Being fit is healthy. Being thin may not be. Wanting a healthy body weight is safe and wise. The extreme desire for thinness is linked with three eating disorders: **anorexia nervosa, bulimia,** and **binge eating disorder (BED)**.

The Life Choice Inventory on the opposite page measures some attitudes related to eating disorders. Tests like this one give a general idea of a person's tendencies, but they cannot diagnose eating disorders. It takes a professional evaluation to do that.

 What happens to someone who has anorexia nervosa?

The story of Julie is typical. Julie is 18 years old. She is a superachiever in school and a fine dancer. She watches her diet with great care, and she exercises and practices ballet daily. She is thin, but she is not satisfied with her weight and is determined to lose more. She is 5 feet 6 inches tall and weighs 85 pounds, but she's still trying to get thinner.

 How could she possibly think she's too fat, weighing only 85 pounds?

Her self-image is false. Against her will, Julie's family took her to see a psychiatrist, who tested her. When given a self-image test, she drew a picture of herself that was grossly oversized. When asked to draw her best friend, Julie drew a fair likeness.

 Can't she see that she's starving herself?

Julie is unaware that she is undernourished, and she sees no need for treatment. She stopped menstruating several months ago and has become very moody. Her eyes lie in deep hollows in her face. She is close to physical exhaustion, but she claims never to be tired.

 How can someone get so thin and continue to diet?

Julie controls her food intake with great discipline even

MINI Glossary

anorexia (an-or-EX-ee-uh) **nervosa:** a disorder of self-starvation to the extreme.

bulimia (byoo-LEEM-ee-uh): repeated binge eating, usually followed by vomiting (also spelled *bulemia*).

binge eating disorder (BED): repeated binge eating, but not followed by vomiting.

Discussion

Help students make the association between eating disorders and other addictive or obsessive behaviors. Ask students to name things that people become obsessed with or addicted to. (drugs, cigarettes, food, gambling, sex, thinness, money, and so on) List their ideas on the board.

Ask students if they think people with these different addictions have something in common. The answer is that they are all looking for something outside of themselves to make them feel good. Ask students why this doesn't work, or only works temporarily. Explain that people have to be happy with themselves inside. If a person is hurting on the inside, the pain is not relieved by engaging in destructive behaviors even if at first it seems the pain is temporarily gone. Usually people need counseling to solve problems related to addictions, whatever they are. Once they can deal with the inner problems they have been hiding, they may be able to kick their addictions because they are happier with who they are.

---

positive and negative benefits of each plan in relation to proper nutrients, food pyramid, caloric intake compared to caloric needs of individuals, and so on.

Second, have students analyze the advertisements presented in class according to:

1. claims made
2. common denominators in the advertisements
3. positive benefits
4. negative aspects (especially if a drug is involved)
5. nutritional value
6. whether exercise is recommended as part of the plan

though she is starving. If she feels that she has slipped and eaten too much, she runs or jumps rope until she is sure she has exercised it off. Her fierce self-control, not lack of hunger, prevents her from eating.

 What could have caused her to behave this way?

Certain attitudes among coaches, trainers, and especially parents contribute to eating disorders. For example, the family may value achievement and outward appearances more than an inner sense of self-worth. For Julie, rejecting food is a way of gaining control. While some of her behaviors appear out of control, they are part of her plan.

Young women often look to their male parents for important feedback on their self-worth. If they don't receive it, they may tend to become too sensitive to society's messages. In Julie's case, her father's alcoholism makes him an ineffective parent.

 What is happening to her physically, and how serious is this condition?

Julie is suffering the physical effects of starvation in all of her body's organs. Her hormone output has become abnormal. Her blood pressure has dropped. Her heart pumps inefficiently. Its muscle has become weak, thin, and small in size. Her heart's rhythms have changed, with a characteristic abnormality appearing on the heart monitor. Sudden stopping of the heart, due to lean tissue loss or mineral deficiencies, causes many sudden deaths among victims of anorexia nervosa.

In bulimia, a binge episode ends with shame or self-loathing.

 Can a person with anorexia be cured?

Julie, like others, is proud of her dieting. She has, after all, made progress toward achieving society's goal for her—to be thin. Treatment is therefore an uphill battle for everyone.

Treatment centers use more effective methods today than they used to. Many people are helped to a degree, although two thirds fail to eat normally after leaving the centers. About 6 percent die, 1 percent by suicide.

 What happens to someone with bulimia?

The case of Sophie is typical of the person with bulimia. Sophie is female, single, Caucasian, in her early 20s, well educated, and close to her ideal body weight. Sophie is a charming, intelligent woman who thinks constantly about food. She sometimes starves herself, and sometimes she engages in **binge eating**. When she has eaten too much, she makes herself vomit.

Sophie's periodic binges take place in secret, usually at night. They last an hour or more. She usually starts the binge after having gone through a period of strict dieting, so that she eats with haste from hunger. Each time, she eats thousands of calories of cookies, cake, ice cream, or bread. The binge is not like normal eating. It is a compulsion and occurs in stages: planning, anxiety, urgency to begin, rapid and uncontrollable eating, relief and relaxation, disappointment, and finally shame or disgust.

226

HEALTHY PEOPLE 2000

Increase to at least 50 percent the proportion of overweight people aged 12 and older who have adopted sound dietary practices combined with regular physical activity to attain an appropriate body weight. (Baseline: 30 percent of overweight women and 25 percent of overweight men for people aged 18 and older in 1985)

Baseline data source: National Health Interview Survey, CDC.

Overweight occurs when too few calories are expended and too many consumed for individual metabolic requirements. The results of weight loss programs focused on dietary restrictions alone have not been encouraging. Physical activity burns calories, increases the

What are the physical effects of bulimia?

Swollen hands and feet, bloating, fatigue, headache, nausea, and pain are common. More serious are fluid and electrolyte imbalances caused by vomiting, abnormal heartbeat, and injury to the kidneys. Vomiting causes irritation and infection of the throat, esophagus, and salivary glands; erosion of the teeth; and dental caries (cavities). The esophagus may rupture or tear, as may the stomach. The eyes become red from the pressure of vomiting.

Some people with bulimia use strong laxatives or **emetics**, which can injure the intestinal tract. Emetics are poisons. Their overuse brings a very real threat of death.

 What makes a person become bulimic?

We don't know, but family structure and personality factors may be partly to blame. Much like Julie, who has anorexia nervosa, Sophie has been a high achiever, but dependent on her parents. The family of a person with bulimia may be emotionally, physically, or sexually abusive.

Sophie feels anxious in social settings and has difficulty in making friends and in dating. She is sometimes depressed. Feelings of failure make Sophie passive with men, to whom she looks for a sense of self-worth. When she is rejected, either in reality or in her imagination, her bulimia becomes worse. In fact, many women point to feelings of male rejection as the event that led to their first binge.

Some people with bulimia become antisocial. They may abuse drugs, steal, or become sexually uninhibited.

 How common are eating disorders?

Eating disorders occur only in wealthy nations and are increasing steadily. Women are the most likely victims (although men are not immune).

Many people have symptoms of eating disorders. For example, in one California study, researchers found that more than 80 percent of girls (age 17 to 18) feared body fatness, restrained their eating, and occasionally binged. These attitudes and actions are all symptoms of eating disorders. Boys also report such symptoms, but in greatly reduced numbers.

 What can be done about this situation?

One school of thought labels eating disorders as social problems. Perhaps they begin when young people develop low self-esteem and adopt the ideal of some false, "perfect" image as portrayed in the media.

Slowly, society is changing. Women are finding honor and esteem in such traditionally male fields as athletics, science, law, and politics. This has raised all women's self-esteem. Perhaps anorexia nervosa, bulimia, and binge eating disorders will disappear as human roles and ideals change. Prevention may be possible if, early in children's lives, they are nurtured to respect themselves. The simple concept—to respect and value your own uniqueness—may be lifesaving for a future generation.

 If bulimia involves binge eating, why is there also a condition called binge eating disorder?

Binge eating disorder (BED) has only recently been identified and named, although people have always suffered its effects. People with BED secretly and destructively binge, just as people with bulimia do, but they do not vomit. Over the years, this behavior leads to severe overweight, a condition that brings many of them to the doorstep of a health professional. People with BED suffer all of the physical and emotional ills of obesity, as described in the chapter, and the guilt and shame of those with bulimia, too. The circumstances leading to BED are thought to be the same as those that cause bulimia.

MINI Glossary

binge eating: overeating to an extreme degree.

emetics (em-ETT-ics): drugs that cause vomiting.

ON LINE WITH HEALTH

You may want to have your students visit the following URLs, where they will find information and additional Web site resources to enhance their study of this chapter. As with all Web sites, you should check these out first to be sure the information found there is appropriate for your students.

Healthy Weight, Healthy You
http://www.eatright. org/nfs12.html

Shape Up, America
http://www.shapeup. org/sua

These sites deal with understanding weight control and offer strategies for diet and exercise for a healthy balance.

FAST FACTS

An estimated 2 million people in the United States, primarily girls and young women, have been diagnosed with some form of eating disorder.

proportion of lean to fat body mass, and raises the metabolic rate. Therefore, a combination of both caloric control and increased physical activity is important for attaining a healthy body weight.

Neither frequent fluctuations in body weight nor extreme restrictions in food intake are desirable. Overweight people should increase their physical activity and should avoid calorie-dense foods, especially those high in fat. Diets that are lower in fat and higher in vegetables, fruits, and grains can facilitate weight reduction. Extremely low-calorie diets, cyclic weight reduction, and fad weight-loss regimes of unscientific merit should be avoided. Practices should be adopted that are safe and that lead to long-term maintenance of appropriate weight. Extreme behaviors as exhibited in bulimia or anorexia nervosa should be medically treated.

ANSWERS TO
CHAPTER 8 REVIEW

VOCABULARY

1. **a.** pinch test **b.** diet pills
   c. bulimia **d.** underweight
   e. anorexia nervosa
   f. diuretic **g.** fatfold test
2. **a.** Basal energy **b.** Emetics

RECALL

SECTION 1

1. Answers will vary; could
   include: they die first in a
   famine, they are at risk
   during hospitalization, and
   women do not menstruate
   normally. (p. 202)

SECTION 2

2. bones, muscles, fat, fluids,
   and other tissues (p. 204)
3. A person with strong muscles and bones may not be
   overweight, but may seem
   overweight on the scale.
   Also, a person who doesn't
   seem overweight on the
   scale may have too much
   body fat for health. (p. 205)
4. Teenagers are still growing;
   weights and heights
   change rapidly. (p. 205)

SECTION 3

5. They gain a pound of fat.
   (p. 207)
6. beating of the heart, inhaling and exhaling of air,
   maintenance of body temperature, working of the
   nerves and glands (p. 207)
7. The heavier the body parts,
   the more energy required
   to move them. (p. 207)
8. by making physical activity
   a daily activity (p. 209)

CHAPTER 8 Review

Summarizing the Chapter

Your ability to respond correctly to the following statements ensures your understanding of the main concepts in the chapter.

1. Explain the problems associated with too little or too much body fat.
2. Describe a method used to measure body fat and a method used to estimate appropriate weight.
3. Explain the effects of an unblanced energy budget.
4. Distinguish between loss of fat and loss of weight.
5. Identify unsound weight-loss programs.
6. Design a safe plan for weight loss and maintenance.
7. Design a healthful weight-gain program.

Learning the Vocabulary

underweight	hunger
obesity	appetite
chronic dieters	stress eating
fatfold test	behavior modification
fatfold caliper	lapses
pinch test	anorexia nervosa
basal energy	bulimia
voluntary activities	binge eating disorder
diuretic	binge eating
diet pills	emetics

Answer the following questions on a separate sheet of paper.

1. **Matching**—*Match each of the following phrases with the appropriate vocabulary term from the list above:*
   a. a fatfold measurement taken without the use of equipment
   b. over-the-counter medications that reduce appetite
   c. repeated binging sometimes followed by vomiting
   d. weight 10 percent or more below the appropriate weight for height
   e. a disorder of self-starvation to the extreme
   f. a drug that causes the body to lose fluids
   g. measurement of body fatness using a fatfold caliper
2. **a.** _____ makes up the largest component of a person's daily energy expenditure.
   b. _____ are drugs that cause vomiting.

Recalling Important Facts and Ideas

Section 1
1. List two problems associated with too little body fat.

Section 2
2. What components make up the sum total of your body weight?
3. Explain why body weight by itself is not an indicator of body fatness.
4. Why are the traditional height-weight charts considered reasonable for adults but useless for teenagers?

Section 3
5. What happens when a person consumes 3,500 calories more than he or she spends?
6. What are the basal processes that support life?
7. Why does a 200-pound person expend more energy than a 100-pound person does, doing the same activity with equal effort?
8. How can you increase your basal energy output over the long term?

Section 4
9. Why is the use of a diuretic considered a dangerous weight-loss method?
10. What happens to excess carbohydrates, fats, and protein a person consumes?
11. In order to lose weight safely and permanently, what must a person lose? What must the person retain?
12. Why is fasting a dangerous way to lose weight?
13. Identify three dangerous and three sound weight-loss strategies.

Section 5
14. How is physical activity helpful in weight loss?

Section 6
15. Give two recommendations for a successful and healthy weight-gain program.

228

SECTION 4

9. causes the kidneys to draw extra water from the blood into the urine (p. 210)
10. They are stored as either glycogen or fat. (p. 210)
11. lose fat tissues; retain lean tissue or water (p. 210)
12. The body uses up its glycogen and then breaks apart its own muscles and organs to keep the needed supply of glucose. (p. 211)

13. Answers will vary; could include: danger-ous—fasting, fad diets, diuretics, diet pills, health spa regimens, muscle stimulators, passive exercise machines, hormones, surgery; sound—diet, exercise, behavior changes. (pp. 211–215)

SECTION 5

14. It increases lean tissue, expends energy, and boosts self-esteem. (p. 219)

16. What are two common characteristics of a person with anorexia nervosa?

17. List four health problems that can result from bulimic behavior.

Critical Thinking

1. The diet industry makes billions of dollars off the American public. Choose one popular marketed diet plan and evaluate it using the information presented in Chapter 7, Nutrition, and Chapter 8, Weight Control. Answer the following questions: Do you feel this diet could be effective? Will it meet the body's nutrient needs? Could health problems arise from using this diet? Does this diet include a program for maintaining weight after goal weight is achieved?

2. After reading the Straight Talk section about eating disorders, answer the following questions: If you were Julie's friend, how would you deal with her anorexic behavior? What do you feel could have been done to prevent Sophie's bulimic behavior prior to her teenage years? What personality traits do Julie and Sophie have in common? Why do you think anorexia nervosa and bulimia appear more often in girls than boys? Why do you think the incidence of eating disorders in our country is steadily increasing?

3. Take a close look at your own personal program of diet and exercise. List four positive and four negative dietary habits you have. List four positive and four negative exercise habits you have.

Activities

1. Find some advertisements for weight-loss methods or programs. Analyze each weight-loss method using the Health Strategies section on page 212 entitled "Clues to Identifying Unsound Weight-Loss Programs."

2. Watch television for one hour before dinner. List all the food products that you see advertised during that time. Discuss the possible reasons for airing these commercials at that time.

3. Find three advertisements that seem to encourage teenagers to be thin. Analyze the techniques used in advertising the products that encourage thinness.

4. Visit a local diet center such as Weight Watchers, Jenny Craig, Nutri-System or the like. Write a one-page report discussing your findings.

5. List as many diets and weight-loss devices as you can think of and label each one as either safe or unsound. Explain why you judged them as you did.

6. Work together as a class to develop a survey on dieting and its problems. First, work in small groups to brainstorm questions to be used on the questionnaire for the survey. Then compile a list of all the questions generated by the groups and as a class, vote on the questions to be used on the questionnaire. Survey twenty females and twenty males. Make sure the questionnaires are filled out anonymously. Ensure those filling out the questionnaires that their privacy will be protected. Work together as a class to compile the data from the questionnaires. Then try to draw conclusions from the results.

7. Imagine that you have just gotten the cast off your leg after you broke it some time ago. While you had the cast on, you were very limited as to how much exercise you could do. Unfortunately, you gained ten pounds. The doctor has said you can resume normal activities. What will you do to lose the weight? Write out a step-by-step plan that describes how you will go about losing the extra ten pounds. Be sure to include exercise and sensible eating in your plan.

Making Decisions about Health

1. Your friend gets up on a Monday morning determined to start a weight-loss diet. She skips breakfast, and for lunch she has a modest, healthful meal of soup and salad. By midafternoon she is famished, but holds off, exerting her strongest will power. At dinner, the smell of food being served is overwhelming. She eats much more than she had intended, and later that evening, still hungry, she indulges in a sweet dessert.

    a. What errors in planning did your friend make?

    b. What could she have done to make it easier to practice moderation at dinnertime?

    c. Describe a more effective meal-planning strategy to help her lose weight.

229

SECTION 6

15. physical activity, eating enough calories to support the weight gain (p. 222)

STRAIGHT TALK

16. Answers will vary; could include: certain attitudes among coaches, trainers, and parents; family values achievement and outward appearances more than an inner sense of self-worth. (p. 226)

17. Answers will vary; could include: swollen hands and feet; bloating; fatigue; headache; nausea; pain; abnormal heartbeat and injury to kidneys; irritation and infection of the throat, esophagus, and salivary glands; erosion of the teeth; dental cavities; red eyes from pressure of vomiting; hands bruised and cut from scraping on the teeth while inducing vomiting. (p. 227)

KEY POINTS

Chapter 9 is 34 pages long and divided into six sections. Briefly, this chapter introduces the physical aspect of health. It stresses the importance of fitness and provides students with factual information about fitness. Students will discover the psychological and physical benefits of fitness. Many practical ideas for becoming fit and staying fit are also covered. At the conclusion of the chapter, the students should be able to properly set up an individual fitness program.

ACTIVITY TO INTRODUCE THE CHAPTER

Give the Presidential Fitness Test before teaching this chapter so that students will have a comparative personal learning experience. Allow them time to discover their personal fitness levels and set goals for themselves. You may invite local college physical education majors to help test.

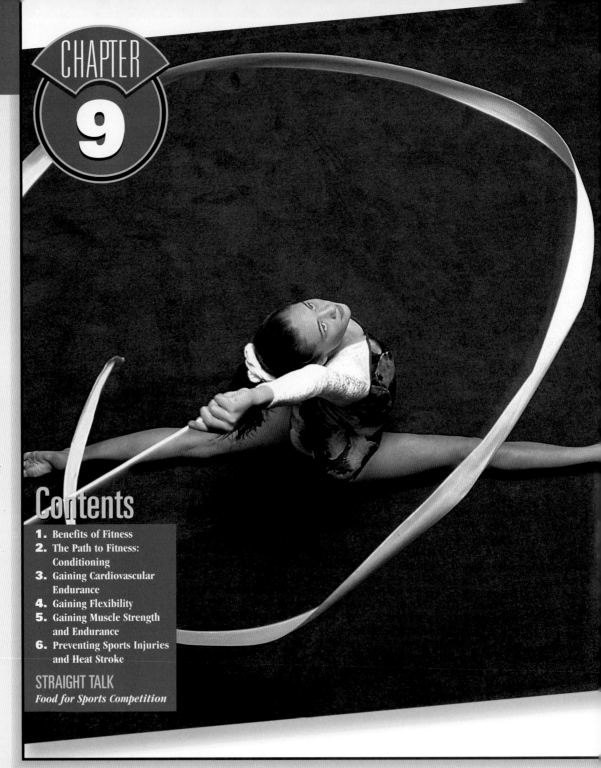

CHAPTER
9

Contents

NOT Enough Time?

Following are some suggestions to help you make sure that you cover the key topics in this chapter if you have limited time. (Refer to the daily lesson plans in your Teacher's Resource Box for additional suggestions.)

DAY 1   Assign Sections 1 and 2 ahead of time. During class do the Focus Activity on page 232, followed by the Group Activity on the same page. Do the Cooperative Learning activity on pages 236. Assign the Focus Activity on page 234. Have students read Sections 3 and 4 before the next class.

Fitness

BULLETIN BOARD IDEAS

Reproduce Figure 9–1, "Fitness Contributes to All Aspects of Health and Wellness" page 232, on a bulletin board. Show the three areas interlocking or overlapping. You could border the bulletin board with pictures of people involved in physical activity found in magazines or drawn by hand.

What do you think? Are the following statements true or false? If you think they are false, then say what is true.

1. In gaining fitness, striving to meet goals set by others is not as useful as striving to meet your own internal goals.
2. You should never overload your body, because overload can cause damage.
3. When performing stretching exercises, you should feel tightness but no pain.
4. Weight training is useful mainly to males who wish to build big, bulky muscles.
5. If you feel minor pain in your feet or legs while running, it is best to keep going and try to work through it.
6. You should not stop exercising to satisfy your thirst.
7. On a hot day, if you tend to perspire freely when you exercise, you should take a salt tablet.

(Answers on page 255)

Introduction

If you are a physically fit person, the following description applies to you.

You are graceful and move with ease. You are strong. Your weight is appropriate for your height, and your body's contours appear pleasing. You have endurance; your energy lasts for hours. You meet normal physical challenges with ease and have energy left over to handle emergencies.

In addition, you are well able to meet mental and emotional challenges. Physical fitness supports not only physical work but also mental and emotional endurance. Your confidence is high in all areas of life: social, academic, work, and athletic—you name it.

If these statements do *not* describe you today, take heart. You can gain fitness through practice. Activities that help you gain fitness are themselves enjoyable, and they quickly lead to improvement.

Answers to FACT or FICTION

1. **True.**
2. **False.** Although an extreme and sudden exertion can damage the body, a gradual increase in overload will produce a strengthened body.
3. **True.**
4. **False.** People of both genders use weight training for trimming and firming the body. Bodybuilders, whether male or female, follow special weight-training programs to gain muscle size and bulk.
5. **False.** You should stop to avoid serious injury.
6. **False.** It's best to rehydrate as you go.
7. **False.** You need water, not salt.

DAY 2   On Day 2 have the students begin the Group Projects on page 241. Do the suggested Guest Speaker activity on page 245 and close with the Evaluate assessment on page 246. Assign the Interdisciplinary Activity: Creative Writing on page 242. Have students read Sections 5 and 6 prior to the next class.

DAY 3   On Day 3 do the Role Playing activity on page 250, followed by the Group Activity on page 251. Close with the Close activities on page 255.

SECTION 1

FOCUS

OUTCOMES

In this section students will learn:

1. The difference between fitness and sedentary behavior.

2. The benefits of fitness.

FOCUS ACTIVITY

Give small groups of students markers and poster paper. Have them list the characteristics of a person they consider to be physically fit. Then have them create a list of characteristics of a person with a sedentary lifestyle. Compare the two lists. Students may want to illustrate their posters.

TEACH & APPLY

WORKSHEETS

Reproducible vocabulary worksheets for Chapter 9 are provided in the Teacher's Resource Box.

GROUP ACTIVITY

Follow up the Focus Activity by having the class as a whole compare the lists developed in the small groups. After each group has presented its poster, students will brainstorm to determine the numbers of hours they are sedentary compared to the amount of time they are physically active.

Figure 9–1 Fitness Contributes to All Aspects of Health and Wellness

Physical Health

Fitness:
Makes physical activity easy to perform.
Promotes rest, relaxation, sleep, and healing.
Aids weight control.
Contributes to nutritional health.
Enhances disease resistance (see Figure 9–2).
Strengthens accident resistance.

Mental, Emotional, and Spiritual Health

Fitness:
Strengthens resistance to depression and anxiety.
Strengthens defenses against stress.
Allows freedom from drug abuse.
Enhances self-esteem.
Enhances ability to learn.
Raises self-confidence.
Instills joy in life.
Inspires courage to face challenges.

Social Health

Fitness:
Provides social opportunities.
Enhances intimate relationships.
Strengthens family ties.
Opens the way for social support.
Encourages citizenship.
Enhances energy for productive work.

SECTION 1

Benefits of Fitness

itness is the reward of a person who leads a physically active life. The opposite of such a life is a **sedentary** life, which means, literally, "sitting down a lot." Today's world permits many people to lead sedentary lives, and even rewards them for doing so. It provides elevators, cars, automatic garage openers, even electric can openers, so that people can exert a minimum of physical effort.

Unfortunately, too many people in our country lead sedentary lives. According to the 1996 surgeon general's report on physical activity, 60 percent of Americans do not exercise regularly, and 25 percent do not exercise at all. The report is clear on this point: people need physical activity, even just moderate activity, to reduce their risks of diseases such as heart disease and high blood pressure.

Everyone's capacity to develop fitness differs. Some people are born with great potential; others are not. Whoever you are, though, you have the ability to improve. This is an important concept in fitness: strive to achieve improvements based on your current fitness level and potential. Do not compare yourself with others or with written sets of standards, at least not right away. Your first goal should be to develop and maintain fitness to support your health. Then later you can go further if you wish: you can set higher goals.

The term **fitness** means *the characteristics of the body that enable it to perform physical activity.* These characteristics include the flexibility of your joints; the strength and endurance of your muscles, including your heart muscle; and a healthy body composition. Add to that definition *the ability to meet routine physical demands, with enough reserve energy to rise to sudden challenges.* This shows even better how fitness relates to everyday life. Ordinary tasks such as carrying heavy suitcases, opening a stuck window, or climbing four flights of stairs might strain an unfit person. However, such tasks are easy for one who is fit. Add still one more detail to the definition of fitness: *the body's ability to withstand stress,* including psychological stresses. Now the definition is finished. It expresses all the aspects of the wonderful condition of the fit body. You can achieve all of these characteristics through regular physical activity.

A fit person benefits in all areas of life (see Figure 9–1 to the left). The most obvious of the benefits are the physical ones. Someone who is physically active, who sleeps soundly, and who eats adequately is one who has every chance for superb health, both physical and mental. Internally, those who are fit have all the advantages—they feel good. Figure 9–2, on the next page, shows that physical activity helps defend against physical disorders and also helps promote psychological well-being. If only half of the rewards listed in Figures 9–1 and 9–2 were yours for the asking, wouldn't you step up to claim them?

Imagine for a moment that the benefits in Figure 9–2 are associated not with regular physical activity, but with a newly discovered "miracle pill." A stampede of people would try to buy it. In fact, miracle products claim to offer many of these benefits. People spend billions of dollars each year in

QUICK QUIZ

Chapter 9, Section 1

The following quiz will help you assess your students' understanding of the material covered in this section of the chapter. You might use the quiz as an oral exercise, which will lead into a class discussion of the topics covered. Or, you might use it as a paper/pencil quiz to evaluate your students individually.

Like the Quick Quiz, the Section Review can also be used as an assessment tool to spark class discussion or as an individual student evaluation. It can also be used as a review in preparation for this quiz.

1. Physical fitness increases mental and emotional endurance. (True)

2. Confidence, endurance, weight and grace of movement are all a part of fitness. (True)

Figure 9–2 *Benefits of Physical Activity*

Regular Physical Activity Helps Protect against These Conditions:		
Physical		**Psychological**
• Acne • Backaches • Cancer (colon cancer, breast cancer, and others) • Diabetes • Digestive disorders (ulcers, constipation, diarrhea, and others) • Headaches • Heart and blood vessel disease (heart attacks and strokes)	• High blood cholesterol and triglycerides, high blood pressure • Infections (colds, flu, and many others) • Insomnia (sleep disorders) • Kidney disease • Menstrual irregularities, menstrual cramps, and mood swings, associated with the menstrual cycle • Obesity • Osteoporosis (adult bone loss)	• Physically active people experience less anxiety and depression than do sedentary people. • Fit people deal better with emotionally stressful events than do sedentary people. • Depressed people who adopt a routine of regular running become as well and stay as well as others who obtain psychotherapy.

hopes of obtaining them, yet they won't spend effort on physical activity. Why is money so much easier to spend than effort?

Sadly, regular physical activity requires more effort than pill taking, and more time. The choice is personal, but this chapter will, of course, try to influence your decision.

 KEY POINTS *Fitness enables the body to perform physical activity, to meet routine physical demands, to meet sudden challenges, and to withstand stress. Fitness is the product of a physically active life. Physical activity promotes fitness. Fitness promotes all aspects of health.*

 SECTION 1 Review

Answer the following questions on a sheet of paper.

Learning the Vocabulary

The vocabulary terms in the introduction are *sedentary* and *fitness*.

1. _____ enables the body to perform physical activities.
2. A person who is basically inactive is considered _____.

Learning the Facts

3. Describe a physically fit person.
4. List four benefits of physical activity.

Making Life Choices

5. What do you think has caused the interest in fitness in our country? Has the interest in fitness influenced your attitudes and behavior in any way? Why or why not? What do you have to gain by becoming more physically active?

 MINI Glossary

sedentary: physically inactive (literally, "sitting down a lot").

fitness: the characteristics of the body that enable it to perform physical activity, to meet routine physical demands with enough reserve energy to rise to sudden challenges, and to withstand stresses of all kinds.

3. A person with a sedentary lifestyle engages in a lot of physical activities. (False)
4. The majority of people in this country lead physically active lives. (False)
5. Physical activity is essential to good health. (True)
6. Fitness refers to the characteristics of the body that enable it to perform physical activity, such as flexibility, strength, and endurance. (True)
7. The ability to withstand stress is not a characteristic of fitness. (False)
8. The ability to meet routine physical demands without difficulty is a characteristic of fitness. (True)
9. Physical fitness has little impact on emotional health. (False)
10. People are born with different capacities to develop fitness, but everyone has the ability to improve his/her physical health. (True)

ASSESS

EVALUATE

 A reproducible quiz for Section 1 is provided in the Teacher's Resource Box.

 SECTION 1 Review Answers

1. Fitness (p. 232)
2. sedentary (p. 232)
3. Answers will vary; could include: graceful and moves with ease; strong; weight is appropriate for height; body's contours appear pleasing; has endurance, energy lasts for hours; meets normal physical challenges with ease, has energy left over to handle emergencies; able to meet mental and emotional challenges; and confidence is high in all areas (social, academic, work, and athletic). (pp. 231–232)
4. Answers will vary. Refer to Figures 9–1 and 9–2 for possible answers. (pp. 232–233)
5. Answers will vary.

CLOSE

Students should be able to list the benefits of fitness. Tell the students they have 30 seconds to list as many benefits of fitness as possible. Time them. When time is up, ask them to turn in their lists. Give credit for correct responses.

SECTION
2

FOCUS

OUTCOMES

In this section students will learn to:

1. Identify the four components of fitness and to name the benefits of these components.

2. Explain the overload principle and tell how to apply it.

3. List strategies for warm-ups and cool-downs.

FOCUS ACTIVITY

Have students keep a diary of all their physical activities for one week. Have them label their activities according to the four components of fitness. Share the lists in class (while providing student anonymity) to give and show examples of the types of exercises needed to establish these components.

TEACH & APPLY

BACKGROUND INFORMATION

One study found that adults who exercised regularly did better on cognitive tests than those who did not. The exercisers scored higher in memory, reaction time, and reasoning ability.

The Path to Fitness: Conditioning

The path to fitness is physical conditioning, which you can achieve through practice or training. **Conditioning** is the microscopic nuts and bolts of fitness: the hundreds of small changes that cells make so that the body can do the work that training demands.

Even routine daily activities can help condition the body. Small choices you make each day can either add to your fitness or take away from it. The person who chooses to walk upstairs gains more fitness than the one riding an elevator, for example. Parking the car a mile from your destination, or getting off the bus several stops early and walking the rest of the way, is a fitness-promoting strategy. Many other such strategies are listed later in the chapter. All can help you become more fit.

Components of Fitness

Fitness expresses itself differently in different body systems. With respect to the heart and lungs, endurance is important. This type of endurance is **cardiovascular endurance**. With respect to the joints, **flexibility** is important. With respect to the muscles, **muscle strength** and **muscle endurance** are important. Fitness also expresses itself in **body composition**—the proportions of muscle, fat, bone, and other tissue that make up a person's body weight. As you become physically fit—improving your cardiovascular endurance, flexibility, muscle strength and endurance, and body composition—you improve the health of your entire body.

Physical activity leads to fitness. You can get an estimate of how physically active you are by answering the questions in this chapter's Life Choice Inventory on page 236. The way to get a truly accurate measure of your own fitness is to visit an **exercise physiology** laboratory and have measurements taken by a professional.

The sections that follow give general principles that govern training and show how to train for a fit body. Before actually starting an activity, though, make sure it is safe to begin. Ordinary physical activity is not hazardous to any healthy person, especially to a young person. However, if you answer yes to any of the questions in the margin, you should proceed with caution. A fitness professional can test you to make sure you start your program at a level high enough to bring about the desired changes but not so high as to be dangerous. The key questions for a young person are listed in the margin.

If, during activity, you become uncomfortable, have trouble breathing, or feel any pain, stop exercising. Consult your health-care provider before continuing. The rest of this chapter assumes your fitness program will go well.

KEY POINTS *The components of fitness are cardiovascular endurance, flexibility, muscle strength, muscle endurance, and body composition. Before beginning a fitness program, check your health.*

For Your Information

Before beginning a fitness program, ask yourself these questions:

▶ Have you been sedentary for a long time?

▶ Are you more than 20 pounds heavier than you should be?

▶ Do you have any chronic illness?

▶ Has a health-care provider ever said you had heart trouble?

▶ Did you ever have, or do you now have, a heart murmur?

▶ Have you ever had a diagnosed or suspected heart attack?

▶ Do you have chest pains at any time?

enrichment

Figure 9–1 on page 232 lists 20 ways that physical fitness contributes to wellness. To reinforce these ideas, divide the students into three groups. Assign each group one of the three health categories (physical health; mental, emotional, and spiritual health; social health). Ask each group to choose two of the fitness benefits in their assigned category that seem the least obvious to them. Each group

Physical fitness brings many rewards.

The Overload Principle

Every day your body works. The stronger and more fit you are, the less you must strain to do that work. If your body is weak, you can't trade it in as you might trade in a run-down car. Fortunately, though, you don't have to. Unlike a run-down car, which will break down when overloaded, your body responds to **overload** in a positive way. It gets itself into better shape to meet the demand next time.

You can apply overload by using the **progressive overload principle** in several different ways. You can do the activity more often—that is, increase its **frequency**. You can do the activity more strenuously—that is, increase its **intensity**. You can do it for longer periods of time—that is, increase its **duration**.

All three strategies work well. You can pick one or a combination, depending on your preferences. For example, if you love your workout, do it more often. If you run out of time, shorten your workout time, but increase its intensity. If you hate hard work, take it easy and go longer. Any way you apply it, the progressive overload principle improves fitness.

Progress Slowly   Don't try to do too much too soon. It's better to progress slowly than to risk serious injury by pushing yourself too hard. To safely increase the frequency, intensity, or duration of your workout, exercise to a point that is only *slightly* beyond what is comfortable.

You've probably heard the expression "No pain, no gain." However, pain won't help you gain fitness; sustained effort will. It doesn't make sense to start with activities so demanding that pain stops you within two days. Learn to enjoy the small steps along the way, because fitness builds slowly. A worthwhile goal is to develop a fitness program that you can stick with, year in and year out.

MINI Glossary

conditioning: the hundreds of small changes that cells make in response to physical activity that make the body more able to do the work at hand.

cardiovascular endurance: a component of fitness; the ability of the heart and lungs to sustain effort over a long time.

flexibility: a component of fitness; the ability to bend the joints without injury.

muscle strength: a component of fitness; the ability of muscles to work against resistance.

muscle endurance: a component of fitness; the ability of muscles to sustain an effort for a long time.

body composition: a component of fitness; the proportions of lean tissue as compared with fat tissue in the body.

exercise physiology: the study of how the body works and changes in response to exercise. An exercise physiology laboratory has equipment to measure the components of fitness and to take other measurements.

overload: an extra physical demand placed on the body.

progressive overload principle: the training principle that a body system, in order to improve, must be worked at frequencies, intensities, or durations that increase over time.

frequency: the number of activity units per unit of time (for example, the number of exercise sessions per week).

intensity: the degree of exertion while exercising (for example, jogging takes more exertion than walking and so is more intense).

duration: the length of time spent in each exercise session.

will then pass its choices to another group. Now each group will develop examples of ways in which the two benefits chosen by their classmates *do* contribute to health. Groups may need to do library research or interview friends in order to have "proof" that

the two benefits of fitness thought to be most questionable are real. Finally, ask all the students whether or not they agree that "a fit person benefits in all areas of life."

Discussion

Athletes may feel these examples are limited—that fitness includes much more than what is listed here. They may want to mention components of fitness related to skill, which are more properly referred to as performance characteristics, such as agility, balance, coordination, power, speed, and reaction time. The focus of the discussion in the textbook, however, is on the health-related aspects of fitness: flexibility, muscle strength and endurance, and cardiovascular endurance.

Comprehension Check

Tell students about the Use-Disuse Principle, which says that fitness develops in response to demand and decreases when demand stops. This may help motivate those students who scored in the inactive range. Muscles enlarge after being called upon repeatedly to do a certain type of work. This muscle growth is called hypertrophy. When the activity is stopped for a few days and the muscles shrink and lose strength, it is called atrophy. Unused muscles do not "turn to fat," as many people believe.

How Physically Active Are You?

On a separate piece of paper, answer the following questions with either yes or no. For each question answered yes, give yourself the number of points indicated. Your answers to the Life Choice Inventory are personal and private. Share them with others only if you are comfortable doing so.

Occupation and Daily Activities

1. I usually walk to and from school and work (at least 1/2 mile each way). 1 point.
2. I usually take the stairs rather than use elevators or escalators. 1 point.
3. My typical daily physical activity is best described by the following statement:
   a. Most of my day is spent walking to class, sitting in class or at home, or in light activity. 0 points.
   b. Most of my day is spent in moderate activity such as fast walking. 4 points.
   c. My typical day includes several hours of heavy physical activity (football, volleyball, basketball, gym workout, or the like). 9 points.

Leisure Activities

4. I spend a few hours in light leisure activity each week (such as slow canoeing or slow cycling). 1 point.

5. I hike or bike (at a moderate pace) once a week or more on the average. 1 point.
6. At least once a week, I participate for an hour or more in vigorous dancing, such as aerobic or folk dancing. 1 point.
7. I play racquetball or tennis at least once a week. 2 points.
8. I often walk for exercise or recreation. 1 point.
9. When I feel bothered by pressures at school, work, or home, I use physical activity as a way to relax. 1 point.
10. Two or more times a week, I perform calisthenic exercises (sit-ups, push-ups, etc.) for at least ten minutes per session. 3 points.
11. I regularly participate in yoga or perform stretching exercises. 2 points.
12. Twice a week or more, I engage in weight training for at least 30 minutes. 4 points.
13. I participate in active recreational sports such as volleyball, baseball, or softball:
    a. About once a week. 2 points.
    b. About twice a week. 4 points.
    c. Three times a week or more. 7 points.
14. At least once a week, I participate in vigorous fitness activities like jogging or swimming (at least 20 continuous minutes per session):
    a. About once a week. 3 points.
    b. About twice a week. 5 points.
    c. Three times a week or more. 10 points.

Total points earned _____

SCORING

0 to 5 points—inactive. This amount of physical activity leads to a steady decline in fitness.

6 to 11 points—moderately active. This amount of physical activity slows fitness loss but will not maintain fitness.

12 to 20 points—active. This amount of physical activity will build or maintain an acceptable level of physical fitness.

21 points or over—very active. This amount of physical activity will maintain a high level of physical fitness.

Source: Adapted with the permission of Russell Pate (University of South Carolina, Dept. of Exercise Science).

COOPERATIVE LEARNING

Place the students into five small groups. Give each group a piece of poster paper and a marker. Give each group a component of fitness as its topic (cardiovascular endurance, flexibility, muscle strength, muscle endurance, and body composition). Each group needs a recorder. Give the groups one minute to write as many exercises as possible that fit that component. At the end of one minute, have the groups trade papers, but keep the same color markers. (The markers are their identi-

You have to overwork just a little. Pushing your body a little beyond its normal level of demand releases hormones that stimulate muscle and bone growth. In a day or two, nature repairs any slight injuries to the muscles, although injury is not required or desirable. It also remodels and strengthens the muscles and bones so that next time, the body will meet the more vigorous challenge more easily.

Proceed with Caution   The following are some other pointers about applying overload:

▶ Use proper equipment and attire.
▶ Exercise regularly.
▶ Train hard only once or twice a week, not every time you work out. Between times, do light workouts.
▶ Listen to your body and cooperate. If you feel energetic, work hard. If you are tired or in pain, go lightly or stop, even if that was not in your original plan.
▶ Perform approved activities with proper form.

Also, keep in mind that work that develops one component of fitness usually does little to improve other components. For example, stretching develops flexibility, but has no effect on cardiovascular endurance. Strive for balance in your fitness program. Include activities of different kinds, so as to develop all the components of fitness.

 Overload is extra physical demand that improves fitness. The progressive overload principle states that to improve, one must increase the frequency, intensity, or duration of physical activity over time.

Principles of Warm-Up and Cool-Down

The body needs to prepare for activity in two ways. It needs to get its fuels ready. It also needs to warm up its muscles and connective tissues, so that they

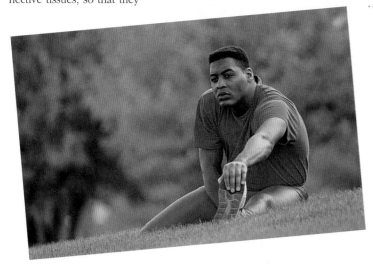

After physical activity, spend a few minutes cooling down and stretching the muscles.

ties.) For the next minute have the groups write injuries that could occur if the exercise technique is not done correctly. Again have the students trade papers so that each group has a new component. For the next minute, have students list as many results as possible from not meeting this component. Trade again for the last time. In the last minute, have groups list positive results for that component. Have the recorders bring the posters to the front for discussion.

SECTION 2 Review Answers

1. Muscle strength is the muscle's ability to work against resistance, while muscle endurance is the muscle's ability to sustain that effort for a long time. (pp. 234–235)

2. Cardiovascular endurance (p. 234)

3. progressive overload principle, frequency, intensity, duration (p. 235)

4. cardiovascular endurance, flexibility, muscle strength, muscle endurance, and body composition. (p. 234)

5. Answers will vary; could include: if you love your workout, do it more often; if you run out of time, shorten it but increase intensity; if you hate hard work, take it easy and go longer. (p. 235)

6. to get the body's fuels ready and warm up the muscles and connective tissues, so that they will stretch without tearing (pp. 237–238)

7. Answers will vary.

CLOSE

Have students set and write a goal to exercise for one week. The goal must describe the types of exercise, number of repetitions, when and if each will be increased, and time of day they will be completed. Help students include exercises for each muscle group. At the end of the week, have students orally present their goals. Students may then comment on how the program actually went, if their goals were set too high or too low, and what health improvements they have seen.

> 66 *Those who think they have no time for bodily exercise will sooner or later have to find time for illness.* 99
>
> Edward Stanley, Earl of Derby
> (1799–1869)
> English statesman

will stretch without tearing. A warm-up activity helps to do both. It frees the needed fuels from storage, and it sends extra blood through the tissues, warming them.

To warm up, take a brisk walk, take a light jog, or do some easy cycling or other light activity followed by a stretching routine. Another way to warm up is to do a light version of what you plan to do intensively later. A runner may start out walking; break into a jog; and finally, when it feels right, pick up the pace to an outright run. A person who bodybuilds may start with light weight repetitions; a tennis player, with a few lobs. This strategy is thought to best prepare the muscle groups that will be needed to perform the task ahead.

After activity, the body also needs to cool down so it can begin to relax again. A few minutes of light activity after a workout helps relax tight muscles and allows blood to circulate freely, cooling the body. This is also a good time to stretch the muscles. Stretching helps to prevent muscle cramps and soreness that might otherwise occur. Cool-down activities can also help to prevent symptoms—dizziness, for example—that people sometimes feel when they suddenly stop exercising.

Now that you know what fitness is and have learned some general principles about conditioning, you are ready to start some physical activities. The next few sections provide pointers on how, exactly, one goes about getting fit.

KEY POINTS *Warm-up activities help the body get ready for physical activity. Cool-down activities help muscles to relax and cool off.*

SECTION 2 Review

Answer the following questions on a sheet of paper.

Learning the Vocabulary

The vocabulary terms in this section are *conditioning, cardiovascular endurance, flexibility, muscle strength, muscle endurance, body composition, exercise physiology, overload, progressive overload principle, frequency, intensity,* and *duration.*

1. What is the difference between muscle strength and muscle endurance?

2. _____ is the ability of the heart and lungs to sustain effort over a long time.

3. The _____ states that to improve fitness, one must increase the _____, _____, or _____ of an activity over time.

Learning the Facts

4. What are the five components of fitness?

5. Give some pointers about applying overload in a fitness program.

6. What is the purpose of warming up before you begin an activity?

Making Life Choices

7. Determine how physically active you are by taking the Life Choice Inventory on page 236. Then answer the following questions: What was your score? Are you satisfied with your score? Why or why not? Discuss any changes you feel need to be made in your physical activity level.

QUICK QUIZ

Chapter 9, Section 2

The following quiz will help you assess your students' understanding of the material covered in this section of the chapter. You might use the quiz as an oral exercise, or, you might use it as a paper/pencil quiz to evaluate your students individually.

Like the Quick Quiz, the Section Review can *also be used as an assessment tool to spark class discussion or as an individual student evaluation. It can also be used as a review in preparation for this quiz.*

1. Conditioning is the process of becoming physically fit. (True)

2. Cardiovascular endurance refers to the capacity of the heart and lungs. (True)

3. Flexibility is not a component of fitness. (False)

SECTION 3

Gaining Cardiovascular Endurance

You're exercising. Your heart beats faster, your blood quickens through your arteries, your breathing delivers great lungfuls of air. How long can your heart and lungs keep going? How developed is your cardiovascular endurance?

Aerobic Activity

Cardiovascular endurance training demands that the heart and lungs work extra hard to deliver oxygen to the muscles for as long as the activity lasts. Cardiovascular endurance training is therefore **aerobic**—it demands oxygen. The more a person performs cardiovascular endurance activities, the better the heart and lungs become at delivering oxygen.

Not all physical activities are aerobic. Activity that lasts just a short time, but that is very intense, doesn't require as much oxygen as aerobic activity does. This type of activity is called **anaerobic** activity.

Aerobic versus Anaerobic Work A way to think of the difference between the two types of activity is to imagine two athletes. The first is a distance runner on an endless stretch of beach. The runner strides steadily across miles of sand. Now imagine a track meet. A sprinter bursts across the starting line in an explosion of energy. The burst lasts only a few seconds, followed by exhaustion at the finish line.

Split-second surges of power involve anaerobic work.

Sustained muscular efforts involve aerobic work.

MINI Glossary

aerobic (air-ROE-bic): refers to energy-producing processes that use oxygen (aero = air).

anaerobic (AN-air-ROE-bic): refers to energy-producing processes that do not use oxygen (an = without).

SECTION 3

FOCUS

OUTCOMES

In this section students will learn to:

1. Identify the differences between aerobic and anaerobic exercise.

2. Take their pulses.

3. Name several activities that benefit cardiovascular endurance.

FOCUS ACTIVITY

Have students develop a list of physical activities in which they participate. Then have them classify the activities as primarily aerobic or anaerobic. Question individual students about which type they tend to do more or less of. If they tend to favor one or the other, why do they think this is?

TEACH & APPLY

CLASS ACTIVITY

Hang two posters on the board, one labeled Aerobic and one labeled Anaerobic. Have an index card for each student and a piece of tape. On each index card list an activity such as walking, basketball, tennis, and so on. Have students tape their index cards under the appropriate sign. Have the student explain the reasons for the placement. When all have placed their cards, discuss them thoroughly.

---

4. Body composition refers to the proportion of muscle, fat, bone, and other tissues that make up a person's body weight. (True)

5. You shouldn't stop exercising if you experience some pain or some difficulty breathing. (False)

6. The body responds to physical overload by breaking down. (False)

7. The progressive overload principle includes increasing the frequency, intensity, or duration of exercise in order to become physically fit. (True)

8. When starting a fitness program it is best to exercise for as long and as strenuously as possible. (False)

9. Fitness requires listening to and cooperating with your body. (True)

10. Warm-up and cool-down exercises prepare the body for exercise and help to prevent symptoms such as cramps and dizziness. (True)

BACKGROUND INFORMATION

This illustration shows how the cardiovascular system delivers oxygen to the muscles. For a review of the cardiovascular system as a whole, refer students back to Chapter 6, pages 144–145. Tell students that the person with more fit muscles extracts more oxygen from the inhaled air than a person with less fit muscles. The cardiovascular system responds to the demand for oxygen by building up its capacity to deliver oxygen. Researchers can measure cardiovascular fitness by measuring the maximum amount of oxygen a person consumes per minute while working out—a measure called VO_2max.

The transparency "Delivery of Oxygen by the Heart and Lungs to the Muscles" is provided in the Teacher's Resource Box.

BACKGROUND INFORMATION

Muscles are made up largely of two different types of contracting cells called muscle fibers. The two types are slow-twitch muscle fibers, best suited to aerobic work, and fast-twitch muscle fibers, best suited to anaerobic work. Aerobic work develops the slow-twitch fibers; anaerobic work develops the fast-twitch fibers. Athletic talent is inborn, partly because of an inherent maximum capacity to develop each type of fiber. In a sense, an individual is born to be either a sprinter or a long-distance runner.

Figure 9–3 Delivery of Oxygen by the Heart and Lungs to the Muscles. The more fit a muscle is, the more oxygen it draws from the blood. That oxygen is provided to the blood by the lungs. Chapter 6 presented details of the cardiovascular system. Here, an oval-shaped diagram represents the body's blood vessels.

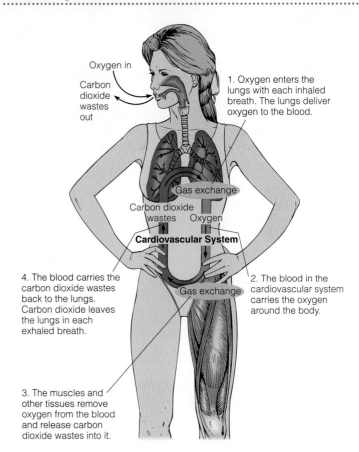

Oxygen in

Carbon dioxide wastes out

1. Oxygen enters the lungs with each inhaled breath. The lungs deliver oxygen to the blood.

Gas exchange

Carbon dioxide wastes   Oxygen

Cardiovascular System

4. The blood carries the carbon dioxide wastes back to the lungs. Carbon dioxide leaves the lungs in each exhaled breath.

Gas exchange

2. The blood in the cardiovascular system carries the oxygen around the body.

3. The muscles and other tissues remove oxygen from the blood and release carbon dioxide wastes into it.

The distance runner is performing mostly aerobic work, the kind that requires endurance. The ability to continue swimming until you reach the far bank, to continue hiking until you are at camp, or to continue pedaling until you are home reflects aerobic fitness.

The sprinter is performing mostly anaerobic work, which requires strength, agility, and split-second surges of power. The jump of the basketball player, the slam of the tennis serve, the weight lifter's heave at the barbells, and the fullback's blast through the opposing line are all anaerobic work.

Aerobic Work Brings Cardiovascular Benefits   At the start of this chapter, Figures 9–1 and 9–2 listed some of the health benefits of physical activity. All of the benefits listed there can be credited to cardiovascular endurance training. Some of the benefits, such as sound sleep, building of lean body tissue, and improved self-image, can also be gained by way of flexibility and strength training. However, cardiovascular endurance training promotes each and every one.

HEALTHY PEOPLE 2000

Increase to at least 30 percent the proportion of people aged 6 and older who engage regularly, preferably daily, in light to moderate physical activity for at least 30 minutes per day.

Note: Light to moderate physical activity requires sustained, rhythmic muscular movements, is at least equivalent to sustained walking, and is performed at less than 60 percent of maximum heart rate for age. Maximum heart rate equals roughly 220 beats per minute minus age. Examples may include walking, swimming, cycling, dancing, gardening and yardwork, various domestic and occupational activities, and games and other childhood pursuits.

A poorly conditioned cardiovascular system limits a person's ability to perform daily activities more than a lack of flexibility or muscle strength does. For this reason, cardiovascular endurance is the part of fitness most important to health and life. However, stretching to keep the joints flexible and strength training to build stronger muscles are important to total fitness, too, as later sections show.

 KEY POINTS *Cardiovascular endurance training demands oxygen—it is aerobic. With cardiovascular endurance training, the heart and lungs become better at delivering oxygen to the body.*

Principles of Cardiovascular Endurance Training

With cardiovascular endurance training, the blood increases in volume and can carry more oxygen. The heart muscle gains size and strength. The larger, stronger heart pumps more blood with each beat, so fewer beats are necessary to support a given task. The heartbeat (**pulse rate**) slows. The muscles that work the lungs gain strength and endurance, and breathing becomes more efficient. Blood moves easily through the body's arteries and veins, and the blood pressure falls. Muscles throughout the body become firmer. Figure 9–3 on the opposite page shows how the heart, cardiovascular system, and lungs all work together to deliver oxygen to the tissues and carry away the waste product carbon dioxide.

A slow resting pulse rate means the cardiovascular system is healthy. You may want to check your pulse right now. As a rule of thumb, the average resting pulse rate for teenagers and young adults is around 70 beats per minute. However, the rate can be higher or lower. Active people can have resting pulse rates of 50 or even lower. Instructions for taking your pulse are given in Figure 9–4.

Professional athletes may use stopwatches, graphs and charts to measure improvements in their pulse rates. The next section discusses the details of such measurements for those who want them. However, you need not get tangled up in all this. To improve your pulse rate, just get up and run, dance, or do any physical activity you'd like. Do it again every other day forever. A guideline for those who wish to gain fitness but who do not aspire to compete in the Olympics is to walk, jog, or run for 20 minutes or more at a rate at which you can talk but not sing. If you can't talk, you're going too fast—slow down. If you can sing, your pace is too slow to build fitness—speed up.

Figure 9–4 How to Take Your Pulse. Get a watch or clock with a second hand. Rest a few minutes for a resting pulse. Place your hand over your heart or your finger firmly over an artery in any pulse location (shown by the yellow circles) that gives a clear rhythm. Start counting your pulse at a convenient second, and continue counting for ten seconds. If a heartbeat occurs exactly on the tenth second, count it as one-half beat. Multiply by 6 to obtain the beats per minute. To ensure a true count:

▶ *Use only fingers, not your thumb, on the pulse point (the thumb has a pulse of its own).*

▶ *Press just firmly enough to feel the pulse. Too much pressure can interfere with the pulse rhythm.*

MINI Glossary

- **pulse rate:** the number of heartbeats per minute.

Physical activity is defined as any bodily movement produced by skeletal muscles that results in caloric (energy) expenditure. Energy use enhances weight loss or control, and maintaining health through physical activity prevents coronary heart disease. Engaging in light to moderate physical activity for at least 30 minutes per day, five or more days per week, will confer health benefits. A sustained walk for 30 minutes per day would result in an energy expenditure of about 1050 calories per week. A consistent weekly caloric deficit of 1,000 calories would translate into a weight loss of roughly one-third pound per week. Furthermore, epidemiologic studies suggest that a weekly expenditure of 1000 calories could have significant individual and public health benefit for coronary heart disease prevention, especially for those who are originally sedentary. (For calorie costs of activities, see Figure 8–7 on page 220.)

DISCUSSION

Lead the class in a short discussion on the differences in cardiovascular endurance and muscular strength. Have them give examples of each.

GUEST SPEAKER

Invite someone to speak about body image. Ask the speaker to include discussions about self-esteem, our perceptions of ourselves, advertising, and stereotypes in the presentation.

INTERDISCIPLINARY ACTIVITY: CREATIVE WRITING

Have the students write a paragraph expressing what life would be like for someone who was perfectly fit, or as fit as possible. Also describe what a normal day would include. In a second paragraph, have students write what life would be like for a person with no cardiovascular endurance. For the last paragraph, have students compare the two lives and decide which is the smarter life to live.

INTERDISCIPLINARY ACTIVITY: RESEARCH

Plan a research trip to the library. Assign a fitness topic to each student. (Fitness Crazes, Walking vs. Running, Effects of Exercise, Effects of Not Exercising, and so on) Help the students find recent articles and books on the topics. Allow the students enough time to begin their research. Give the students one week to accomplish the research and writing of their fitness papers. Allow time in class for students to share their findings.

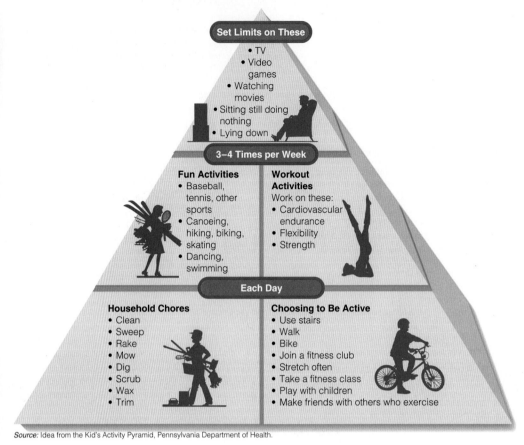

Source: Idea from the Kid's Activity Pyramid, Pennsylvania Department of Health.

Teens' Activity Pyramid

 KEY POINTS *Cardiovascular endurance increases the blood volume, improves the heart muscle's size and strength, slows the pulse rate, makes breathing more efficient, lowers the blood pressure, and firms muscles throughout the body.*

Activities for Cardiovascular Endurance

To improve cardiovascular endurance, you must work up to a point where you can perform aerobic activity for 20 minutes or more at a session. This means you must raise your heart rate (pulse) for that long. You should shoot for a heart rate that is quite a bit faster than your resting rate to "push"

CRITICAL THINKING

Have students interview people of different ages who are currently involved in an exercise program. They should ask questions similar to the following:

• What kind of exercise do you do?
• For how long do you do the exercise?

• When did you start your exercise program?
• What physiological and psychological benefits have you noticed?
• How does the program fit with your lifestyle and schedule?
• What motivates you to stick with the exercise program?

Then have students interview people of different ages who are not exercising on a the heart, but not one so fast as to strain it. Athletes call this the **target heart rate**. You can calculate yours from your age.

To calculate your target heart rate, first subtract your age from 220. The resulting number is close to the absolute *maximum heart rate* for a person your age. You should never exercise at this rate, of course. Now multiply your maximum heart rate number by 0.75 to get your target heart rate. For example, to calculate the target heart rate for a 16-year-old person:

▶ Maximum heart rate = 220 − 16 = 204.
▶ Target heart rate = 204 × 0.75 = 153 beats per minute.

When you first work out at this rate, you may find that even mild activity will push your heart to the target rate. As your cardiovascular fitness improves, you will have to work harder to push your heart to beat this fast. When you can work out at the target heart rate for 20 to 30 minutes, you know that you have arrived at your fitness goal.

Which Activities?   You can develop cardiovascular fitness only if you choose aerobic activity. This activity must:

▶ Be steady and constant.
▶ Use large muscle groups, such as legs, buttocks, and abdomen.
▶ Be uninterrupted and last for more than 20 minutes.

The activities listed in the margin all fit this description. You probably know something about these activities already. However, a few more facts about them might help.

Walking   Walking is good exercise, but the walker must put some "oomph" in the pace to achieve an aerobic workout. Strolling along at a pace of 1 or 2 miles per hour might help you to warm up. Striding along at 3.5 to 5 miles per hour, however, is the way to get a workout for your heart. Walking practically never injures people (so long as they wear supportive walking shoes and watch for traffic), because walking is easy on the joints.

Aerobic Dance and Step Aerobics   Aerobic dance and **step aerobics** can provide balanced, full-body workouts, as well as cardiovascular workouts. In dance and step, a good pair of shoes is a must for the safety of the feet and legs. Equally important is the choice of fitness center. Check the flooring to make sure that it is made of materials that absorb shock, such as wood platforms. (Cement, even when under carpeting, shocks the lower back.) Flooring becomes less critical in **low-impact aerobic dance**, in which one foot always remains in contact with the floor.

In dance, move around the room and change directions freely, take long strides, and lift your legs high. These movements, performed with control and vigor, provide the work your heart needs.

Running   Running is a passion for some. The challenge, simplicity, freedom, and mental and physical well-being that come with running keep many people returning to the road, day after day. However, with the joys come risks. Running injuries are common.

The right shoes are essential, of course. A runner hits the ground with a force of about two to three times the weight of the body, hundreds of times per mile. Running shoes stabilize the feet and cushion the enormous impact of each stride. Most injuries in running result from pushing too hard and too fast, trying to get fit too quickly. To begin a program, start slowly. Do not rush your progress. Watch and listen for traffic (don't wear a headset). If you

For Your Information

Some activities to help you gain cardiovascular endurance:

▶ Aerobic dancing
▶ Basketball
▶ Bicycling
▶ Fast walking
▶ Hockey
▶ In-line skating
▶ Jogging
▶ Lacrossse
▶ Rope jumping
▶ Rugby
▶ Soccer
▶ Stair climbing
▶ Step aerobics
▶ Swimming laps
▶ Water polo

MINI Glossary

target heart rate: the heartbeat rate that will condition a person's cardiovascular system—fast enough to push the heart, but not so fast as to strain it.

step aerobics: aerobic activity in which each participant steps up and down on a stable platform called a step bench ranging from about 6 inches to 12 inches high.

low-impact aerobic dance: aerobic dance in which one foot remains on the floor to prevent shock to the lower body.

regular basis. They should ask questions similar to the following:

• Why aren't you involved in an exercise program?
• Do you feel you have adequate knowledge about exercise and diet? Why or why not?
• Describe your past attempts at developing an exercise program.

• Describe your current lifestyle (work, leisure-time activities, risk factors).

After the interviews are complete, have students analyze the information they collected and draw conclusions. Encourage them to find similarities in the people of both groups.

ASSESS

A reproducible quiz for Section 3 is provided in the Teacher's Resource Box.

SECTION 3 Review Answers

1. pulse rate (p. 241)
2. target heart rate (p. 243)
3. aerobic activity demands oxygen—anaerobic activity is less intense and doesn't require as much oxygen (p. 239)
4. Answers will vary.
5. Answers will vary; could include: aerobic—swimming, bicycling, long-distance running, aerobic dancing; anaerobic—requires surges of power, weight lifting, sprinting, and tennis serve. (pp. 239–240)
6. Answers will vary; see the first paragraph under "Principles of Cardiovascular Endurance Training" on page 241 for possible answers.
7. be steady and constant, use large muscle groups (legs, buttocks, and abdomen), be uninterrupted and last for more than 20 minutes (p. 243)
8. Answers will vary.

CLOSE

Collect videos of athletic activities. Collect as many as possible, representing a wide variety of activities. Use these videos for a quiz. Play a 30-second spot of each video. The students must write whether the activity is aerobic or anaerobic.

---

are a female, run or walk with a partner. Heed the advice on rape prevention in the Straight Talk section of Chapter 18.

Swimming and Cycling As for swimming and cycling, these, too, provide work that strengthens the heart. These activities are almost stress-free for joints and connective tissues. Swimming not only develops cardiovascular endurance, but also develops strength and endurance in the upper body. However, swimming may not improve body composition as much as some other aerobic activities do. Cycling, on the other hand, superbly develops the lower body while it improves cardiovascular endurance. It also promotes a lean body composition effectively. Taken together, the two activities make a nice conditioning package—swimming for upper body and heart, and cycling for lower body, heart, and body composition.

The activities just described are only a few of many that people enjoy while gaining cardiovascular endurance. Don't limit yourself. Just use your imagination and go for it. For a lifestyle that encourages general fitness, the "Teens' Activity Pyramid" on page 242 offers some novel ideas.

KEY POINTS *Activities that promote cardiovascular endurance are those that raise the heart rate, are sustained for 20 or more minutes, and are performed every other day or more often. Many activities fit this description.*

SECTION 3 Review

Answer the following questions on a sheet of paper.

Learning the Vocabulary

The vocabulary terms in this section are *aerobic, anaerobic, pulse rate, target heart rate, step aerobics,* and *low-impact aerobic dance.*

1. Your _____ is the number of times your heart beats per minute.
2. Your _____ is fast enough to push the heart, but not so fast as to strain it.
3. What is the difference between aerobic and anaerobic activity?
4. Write a sentence using each vocabulary term.

Learning the Facts

5. Name two aerobic and two anaerobic activities.
6. List three effects of cardiovascular endurance training.
7. List three characteristics of activities that promote cardiovascular fitness.

Making Life Choices

8. After taking your resting pulse rate (Figure 9–4), answer the following question: Is your pulse below average, average, or above average? Now calculate your target heart rate (see page 243). Do you generally reach your target heart rate when you exercise? Why or why not? What activities do you regularly participate in to improve your cardiovascular endurance? Identify any changes you feel need to be made in your program.

QUICK QUIZ

Chapter 9, Section 3

The following quiz will help you assess your students' understanding of the material covered in this section of the chapter. You might use the quiz as an oral exercise, which will lead into a class discussion of the topics covered. Or, you might use it as a paper/pencil

quiz to evaluate your students individually.

If students have difficulty with the concepts covered in the Quick Quiz and the Section Review, you might suggest they review the material using the **S***urvey,* **Q***uestion,* **R***ead,* **R***ecite,* **R***eview (SQ3R) study method, which is described in detail in the introduction to this Teacher's Wraparound Edition.*

1. Cardiovascular endurance is improved through aerobic exercise. (True)

SECTION 4

Gaining Flexibility

Figure 9–5 Range of Motion of the Hip Joint

Full range of motion

Have you noticed that some people find reaching movements to be difficult? For a person who lacks flexibility, it is uncomfortable even to reach to the feet to tie the shoes. Contrast this person with a dancer of the same age taking a graceful bow after a performance, hands almost brushing the floor. These people represent both ends of the flexibility spectrum. The first person is stiff from years of limited movement. The second person has worked for years to maintain flexibility.

If the body is flexible, it can move as it was designed to move and will bend instead of tearing or breaking in response to sudden stresses. Flexibility depends on **elasticity** of muscles and **connective tissues** and on the health of the joints.

Range of Motion   Each body joint has its own limits on how far it can move—its **range of motion** (see Figure 9–5). A joint's range of motion is determined by the shape of its bones, and the placement and condition of its connective tissues. The bones and connective tissues of knees and elbows, for example, limit their movements to two directions only. The design of the shoulder joint, on the other hand, permits movements in many directions. A flexible joint moves smoothly through its entire range of motion.

Stretching Techniques   Stretching improves flexibility. When you stretch, remember that your goal is to get limber, not to push your joints beyond their range of motion. (Observe a cat stretching, and notice the technique. The stretch is long and lazy, a few moments of pure pleasure.)

Choose easy stretches, and stretch only to the point where you feel tightness but not pain. As you hold the stretch, even the feeling of tightness should gradually ease. If the tightness does not ease, or the stretch becomes painful as you hold it, you are overstretching.

Stretch in smooth motions—do not bounce. Bouncing can easily overstretch or tear a ligament until it can no longer support its joint, making the joint prone to injury. Nerves can overstretch painfully, too, if you are only slightly too enthusiastic. Figure 9–6 on the next page lists some dangerous stretches.

Never stretch a cold muscle. Warm up first with five minutes of light activity or with a hot shower. Then, to get a full stretch, relax the muscles, allow each body part to move slowly through its full range of motion, and hold each stretch position for 10 seconds. Breathe normally. Repeat each stretch once or twice. To improve, add 2 seconds to the time you hold each stretch until you are holding it for 30 seconds. Choose stretches that work all body areas: neck, shoulders, back, pelvis, thighs, calf muscles, and ankles. Figure 9–7 on page 247 illustrates some recommended stretches.

 KEY POINTS   *Flexibility depends on the elasticity of the muscles and connective tissues and on the condition of the joints. A joint's range of motion sets limits on its movements. Stretching improves flexibility.*

MINI Glossary

elasticity: the characteristic of a tissue's being easily stretched or bent and able to return to its original size and shape.

connective tissues: fluid, gelatin-like, fibrous, or strap-like materials that bind, support, or protect other body tissues; tendons, cartilage, and ligaments are connective tissue.

range of motion: the mobility of a joint; the direction and the extent to which it bends.

SECTION 4

FOCUS

OUTCOME

In this section students will learn:

1. The fundamentals of proper stretching.

GUEST SPEAKER

Have an athletic trainer take the class through some stretching exercises. Ask the trainer to discuss each exercise and its importance as it is being done by the students. Ask the trainer to share updated information on any changes in traditional exercises.

TEACH & APPLY

DISCUSSION

Have students, as a class, prepare a questionnaire of five to ten questions. Students will interview ten people (not students in the same class) using the questionnaire.

Following are some samples of questions:

1. Do you exercise? If so, how often? If not, is there a reason?

2. Do you think exercise is important? Why or why not?

3. Do you know the difference between aerobic and anaerobic exercise?

4. Why is flexibility important?

5. How much exercise do you get in a typical week?

Have students assure the participants that they will remain anonymous.

(continued on next page)

2. All physical activities are aerobic. (False)

3. Aerobic activities require good endurance. (True)

4. Sprinting is considered an anaerobic activity. (True)

5. Flexibility and muscle strength are more important to health than cardiovascular endurance. (False)

6. Cardiovascular endurance training increases the volume of the blood and the amount of oxygen the blood can carry. (True)

7. Cardiovascular endurance training increases the pulse rate. (False)

8. The heart's muscle size and strength improves with cardiovascular activity. (True)

9. Aerobic activity must be steady and constant, and must continue uninterrupted for at least twenty minutes. (True)

10. Weight lifting is an aerobic exercise. (False)

(continued from previous page)

Students should share their findings with the class. Discuss the results of the questionnaires. Were students surprised by their findings? Were people exercising more or less than they had anticipated?

DISCUSSION

Ask students if they have done any of the stretches and exercises in Figure 9–6. Has doing these exercises resulted in any injuries?

The transparencies "Recommended Stretches" are provided in the Transparency Acetate Binder. You may want to use them in your classroom presentation of this lesson.

ASSESS

EVALUATE

Divide the class into five teams. Give each team all the Mini Glossary definitions in Sections 1 through 4. Without using books, have the groups write the correct word for each definition. The first team with all the definitions matched with the correct words, wins. You may also write the words to choose from on the board. A more challenging variation of the activity is to give the words and ask for the definitions.

***Figure 9–6** Stretches and Exercises to Avoid*

Stretches and Exercises to Avoid	Why Avoid Them?
Unsupervised yoga	May cause many types of knee injury
Hurdler's stretch (sit with one leg bent under at the knee, reach for toe of outstretched leg)	May cause knee injury
Toe touching with straight knees	May overstretch tendons and damage major nerves and vertebrae
Deep knee bend; duckwalk (thighs touch heels)	May cause knee injury
Straight-leg lift (lie on back and lift both legs)	Aggravates lower back problems
Hyperextension of the back (arch the back and then let it sag, performed to extremes)	May injure lower back
Toe standing	May damage the foot arch
Straight-leg sit-up	Aggravates lower back problems
Ballet stretch (designed for dancers)	May cause many types of injuries

SECTION 4 Review

Answer the following questions on a sheet of paper.

Learning the Vocabulary

The vocabulary terms in this section are *elasticity*, *connective tissues*, and *range of motion*.

1. Write a sentence using each vocabulary term.

Learning the Facts

2. Give three recommendations for safe stretching.

3. Name one stretching exercise to avoid and one safe stretching exercise.

Making Life Choices

4. Try each of the recommended stretches in Figure 9–7 on the opposite page. Be sure to follow the guidelines for stretching listed in this section. Which exercises did you find the easiest, and which did you find the hardest? What parts of your body seem to need the most work in terms of improving flexibility? Why? Do you stretch on a regular basis? Why or why not? How might you safely measure improvements in your flexibility?

Ability Levels

Basic

Have student volunteers stand beside their desks. Take them through a range of motion exercises for their arms and hips (arm circles and bending over). After taking the students through the motions, use a rubber band to show how it stretches in the same way as

Figure 9–7 Recommended Stretches. These stretches can help you meet flexibility goals safely. The muscles being stretched are highlighted.

Whole-body stretch

Neck stretches

Lower back stretch

Lower back stretches

Calf muscle stretch

Buttocks stretch

Hamstring stretch

Inner thigh stretch

Upper body

Upper back and side stretch

SECTION 4 — Review Answers

1. Answers will vary.
2. do not push joints beyond their ranges, choose easy stretches, stretch in smooth motions, never stretch a cold muscle (p. 245)
3. Avoid—Answers will vary. Refer to Figure 9–6 on page 246 for possible answers. Safe—Answers will vary. Refer to Figure 9–7 on this page for possible answers. (pp. 246–247)
4. Answers will vary. (p. 245)

WORKSHEETS

A reproducible quiz for Section 4 is provided in the Teacher's Resource Box.

CLOSE

Be sensitive to students who may not wish to perform the following activity in front of the class.

Have a student sit on the floor with legs extended in front of him or her, knees slightly bent. Place the zero end of a yardstick against one heel so that it extends out in front of the student. Keeping hands together, student should stretch as far as is comfortable toward the yardstick. Have another student record the number of inches the student stretches. Repeat for each student who wishes to participate.

Have students set flexibility goals for themselves and develop plans to reach their goals. Give the students a chance to retest themselves in two weeks to see if their flexibility has improved.

muscles do. Show the proper technique with the rubber band—a smooth, not jerky, pull. Explain that this is how to stretch. People should not bounce. While you are discussing bouncing, continually jerk on the rubber band. As you discuss the proper, smooth, one-motion stretch, pull the rubber band slowly.

FOCUS

OUTCOME

In this section students will:

1. Determine proper ways to gain muscle strength and endurance.

FOCUS ACTIVITY

On the board write the words *females* and *males*. Have students brainstorm physical characteristics related to fitness activities for both males and females. Write them under the proper heading. Include words such as weight lifting, strong, powerful, and aerobics. Review the lists and discuss any stereotypical responses that were made. Discuss the fact that everyone has different body frames and muscular ability, and how, in trying to achieve personal best, stereotypes can be inhibiting.

TEACH & APPLY

BACKGROUND INFORMATION

Caution students against reading this section and then running off to a gym to work with weights or weight machines without first obtaining instruction from a knowledgeable coach/trainer or weight specialist. Emphasize the possibility of serious injury in working with weights improperly.

Gaining Muscle Strength and Endurance

Strength is a familiar concept. It is the ability of the muscles to work against **resistance**: to pull weeds from the ground, to push a stalled car, or to open a jar of jam. Strong muscles, tendons, ligaments, and bones also best protect the body's internal organs from injury. Many of today's mechanical helpers spare us effort but also rob us of opportunities to develop strength. For example, a thermostat makes it easy to turn up the heat without chopping firewood.

Muscle endurance is closely related to strength. Muscle endurance is the ability of a muscle to hold a contraction for long periods of time or to contract repeatedly.

Strength Conditioning

Two ways people gain muscle strength and endurance are through **weight training** and **calisthenics**. Weight training is the most efficient way. It uses weights or machines to provide resistance against which the muscles can work. Calisthenics are exercises that develop muscle strength and endurance by using the body's parts as weights pulled or pushed against gravity. Familiar examples are sit-ups, push-ups, and pull-ups.

Setting Goals Weight training can be an ideal workout for both males and females, and it need not produce big, bulky muscles. Bodybuilders can follow programs designed to do just that, but you can tailor your weight routine to meet other goals. To gain strength without bulk, you can use light weights and more repetitions. Rumor has it that weight training will lead to muscle-bound inflexibility; it does not. Inflexible joints do not result from weight training, but from unbalanced training and from leaving stretching exercises out of any fitness routine.

Weight-Training Tips To develop maximum strength from the smallest number of repetitions, lower the weight especially slowly. A group of ten repetitions of a particular exercise should take about a minute. Such a group of repetitions is called a **set**. Performing many sets with lighter weights mostly increases endurance. Doing fewer sets with heavier weights favors bulk and strength.

Figure 9–8 on the next page shows exercises that build strength and endurance. Some use small weights, called dumbbells, to provide resistance. Others use parts of the body working against gravity for resistance (calisthenics). One repetition of any of these exercises is easy to do. Thus the exerciser must apply overload by repeating the exercise many times in a set. Another way is to perform many sets in an exercise session. Remember, overload just a little—not so much as to injure yourself.

Whether your goal is strength, endurance, or improved body composition, weight training every other day or so seems to produce the best results.

MINI Glossary

resistance: a force that opposes another; in fitness, the weight or other opposing force against which muscles must work.

weight training: exercise routines for strength conditioning that use weights or machines to provide resistance against which the muscles can work.

calisthenics: exercise routines for strength conditioning that use the parts of the body as weights.

set: a specific number of times to repeat a weight-training exercise.

enrichment

There are three basic categories of muscular exercises: isometric, isotonic, and isokinetic. Isometric exercises are carried out by pushing or pulling against a fixed or immovable object. Each muscle contraction should be held for five–ten seconds. These exercises are easy to do and require no special equipment or machines.

Isotonic exercises occur when a muscle moves a moderate load several times, such as in weight lifting. Flexibility, coordination, and endurance can best be achieved with low resistance and high repetitions, while muscu-

Figure 9–8 Muscle Strength and Endurance Routines. *Some of the exercises show people using dumbbells. Should you wish to use other equipment to achieve the same effects, consult a qualified trainer. The muscles worked by each exercise are highlighted.*

lar strength can best be achieved with high resistance and low repetitions. Examples of isotonic exercises would be using free weights, such as barbells and dumbbells, or Nautilus or Universal equipment.

Isokinetic exercises are carried out with special machines that provide resistance to overload muscles throughout the entire range of motion. These exercises can be very effective at isolating and strengthening specific muscle groups, but the equipment is usually very expensive and available only at commercial fitness centers.

Consumer SKILLS

Background Information

Emphasize to students that no product has any special beneficial effects on either muscles or athletic performance. People must learn to defend themselves against the lies told by some sellers of fitness products. Students must be knowledgeable and think critically.

Answers to Critical Thinking

1. The herbs may contain toxins and can have unexpected side effects. Tell students not to make the mistake of equating "natural" with "harmless."

2. Answers will vary, but students should realize that many people want the benefits of fitness without doing the work. Advertisers realize this and develop their ads around the idea of quick and easy fitness and performance.

3. Making a profit.

ROLE PLAYING

Have the students read the Consumer Skills feature on this page. Have them assume roles as advertising agents. The students must advertise one of the pills or powders. Encourage students to create their ads using selling points that companies use in selling products. Display the advertisements and discuss why they are effective.

Pills, Powders, and Potions for Fitness

Athletes and other active people can be easy targets for quacks who sell an endless river of products—herbal steroid-drug substitutes, protein or amino acid supplements, vitamin or mineral supplements, "complete" drinks, "muscle-building" powders, electrolyte pills, and many other so-called **ergogenic** aids. The term *ergogenic* claims to mean that such products have special work-enhancing powers. Actually, no food or supplement is ergogenic.

Advertisements for commercial products may read as these do: "SWINDLE amino acids deposit slabs of muscle bulk"; "HOODWINK enzymes ram the body into turbo charge"; "Ultrapotent TECHNO-HYPE vitamins and minerals blast carbs through your system." Many ads like these are easy to see through. They are trying to pick readers' pockets. Others are harder to see through, though just as false.*

If potions do seem to work, they probably work by the power of suggestion. Don't discount that power, because it is awesome. In fact, use it instead of the potions. Imagine yourself as a winner. Visualize yourself as capable in your sport. You don't have to rely on magic for an extra edge. You already have a real advantage—your mind.

Critical Thinking

1. Taking pills and other supplements may seem like a scientific approach to athletics, but experts recommend against it. Especially with regard to the herbal steroids, why do you think experts say to avoid supplements?
2. Why is it so easy for some people to believe false advertising claims for improved athletic performance?
3. What motivates the sellers of such fake products?

*If you have questions about a fitness product, book, or program, write to the American College of Sports Medicine, P.O. Box 1440, Indianapolis, IN 46204.

Rest is as important as work. Muscles use the time between workouts to repair small injuries, to replenish their fuel supplies, and to build themselves up. If you like to work out every day, just be sure to work different muscle groups today from those you worked yesterday. Give each muscle group a day off.

Remember to breathe when you work with weights. Holding your breath puts pressure on the heart and lungs and can damage them. Exhale as you raise or push the weight away. (A way to remember this is to "blow the weight away from you.") Inhale as you lower the weight. Also, raise and lower the weight smoothly using your full range of motion. Jerking it up or letting gravity pull it down fails to improve strength and threatens to injure your joints. Also, heavy weights can be dangerous.

Work Muscles Equally Small muscles fatigue quickly, and this can stop your workout. Therefore, strengthen the larger muscle groups first, then the smaller ones. Make sure to distribute the weight work equally over the arms and legs, both sides—all the muscles. Overdeveloped muscles in one part of the body that work in opposition to weak muscles in another part, can cause damage. For example, strong back muscles and weak stomach

Pursuing wellness

If a person takes steroids, the reason is usually to get bigger, stronger, or faster. However, steroid use during adolescence can result in permanent stunting of growth due to the premature closure of the epiphyseal plates of the bones.

Steroid use in competitive sports is banned and drug testing is carried out to enforce this ban. In 1988 Ben Johnson, a Canadian sprinter, was stripped of his Olympic medal and world record for the 100-meter sprint after traces of the anabolic steroid stanolozol were detected in his system.

But losing a medal or being disqualified

muscles can pull the back out of line, injuring the spine. An overdeveloped muscle that opposes a weak one can also interfere with movement—the person becomes muscle bound. The discussion of the muscular system in Chapter 6 shows all the major muscles of the body.

Seek Expert Advice A wise beginning exerciser seeks guidance from a seasoned, professional trainer who has a reputation for getting results safely. (New employees of spas and gyms may be long on enthusiasm but short on knowledge and experience.)

Some false "short cuts" to strength, such as taking nutrient drinks, pills, and powders without hard work always fail, as the Consumer Skills feature on the opposite page points out. Muscles grow in response to work. Muscles do not helplessly build tissue whenever extra nutrients float by. Hard work itself triggers the muscles to grab what they need from the bloodstream to build themselves up. Muscle building is an active process, started by activity itself. A few hormones can also signal muscles to build tissue, but the price to health of taking them is high.

KEYPOINTS *Strength develops when muscles work against resistance.*

Strength Sought from Steroids and Growth Hormones

It is unwise to use hormones or other drugs to improve strength. Hormones and drugs that athletes take to gain strength or improve endurance have many dangerous side effects. Despite the hazards, these products often tempt those who want to gain a competitive advantage over others.

The Effects of Steroid Hormones Men generally develop bulkier muscles than do women, in response to exercise. This is because men produce larger amounts of certain hormones known as **steroids** in their bodies. These hormones are also available as drugs, which were developed to treat children born lacking in the ability to produce the hormones.

Like all drugs, steroids can be abused. Some athletes, both men and women, take steroid drugs in the attempt to develop bulky muscles. Many studies of these practices show that steroid drugs can indeed increase body weight (especially lean body weight). The drugs can increase muscle strength in some highly conditioned athletes who also exercise intensely.

Athletes struggling to be the best are tempted by the promise of muscles bigger and stronger than those that training alone can produce. Athletes who are not born superstars, and who normally would not be able to compete at high levels, can suddenly compete with born champions. This tempts other athletes to abuse the drugs, too. Especially among professionals for whom enormous salaries reward excellent performances, illegal steroid abuse is common.

The Hidden Price of Steroids Steroid abuse comes at a very high price, however. For one thing, all steroid abusers experience a sharp change in their blood fats that reflects an increased risk of heart disease. In addition, steroids are known to interrupt the normal work of the liver; cause cancerous liver tumors, liver rupture, and hemorrhage (bleeding); produce permanent changes in the reproductive system; and alter the structure of the face.

Men generally develop bulkier muscles than women do, in response to exercise.

Glossary

ergogenic (ER-go-JEN-ick): a term that claims to mean "work-enhancing." In fact, no products enhance the ability to do work.

steroids: hormones of a certain chemical type that occur naturally in the body, some of which promote muscle growth. Available as drugs, they are abused by athletes seeking a shortcut to large muscles.

DISCUSSION

Discuss how steroids are a short-term method of self-esteem building. Include in this discussion the reasons people want quick methods instead of long-term gains. Also discuss how steroids can be dangerous. You can approach this from the standpoint of side effects, as well as the deadly effect of AIDS (from the use of infected needles for the injection of steroids).

Your supplementary material contains an information sheet on steroids entitled "More on the Effects of Steroid Hormones on the Body."

GROUP ACTIVITY

Have the students write a pro and con list for the use of steroids. After completing their lists, have students cut their lists so that each pro and con is on a separate slip of paper. They should then cut off the pro and con headings. In small groups have the students paste their lists on poster board under the proper headings. This activity will reinforce knowledge as well as encourage small-group discussion. Their lists should contain many more cons than pros. Emphasize that even if they think there are some pros, steroids are dangerous—they should not use them.

from competition is a small penalty compared to the health risks involved. Some of the side effects and adverse reactions of anabolic steroid use include liver and other forms of cancer, heart disease, high blood pressure, high cholesterol, depression, hostility, mood swings, suicidal tendencies, baldness, acne, testicular atrophy, impotence, breast enlargement in males, and masculinizing effects in females. The former actor and NFL lineman Lyle Alzado blamed his brain cancer, from which he died in 1992, on his steroid abuse. If injectable steroids are abused, there is the additional risk of HIV infection and AIDS from the sharing of needles.

ASSESS

EVALUATE

 Review Answers

1. Weight training uses weights or machines to increase strength, calisthenics use the body's parts as weights pulled or pushed against gravity. (p. 248)
2. steroids (p. 251)
3. human growth hormone, acromegaly (p. 252)
4. resistance (p. 248)
5. weight training and calisthenics (p. 248)
6. every other day or so (p. 248)
7. Answers will vary. See pages 251–252 for possible answers.
8. Answers will vary. See the Consumer Skills on page 250 for possible answers.
9. Answers will vary.

A reproducible quiz for Section 5 is provided in the Teacher's Resource Box.

CLOSE

Have students bring to class one article from a magazine or newspaper that pertains to the information presented in this section Have the students present the article orally to the class.

In males, steroids cause the testicles to shrink. In females, they cause mustaches and other body hair to grow, and the breasts to shrink.

Steroids stunt growth in those who haven't yet reached full height. They also may cause acne. Steroids also affect the mind, bringing on mood swings, aggressive behavior, and changes in the sex drive. Some steroid users suffer deadly effects right away. Others may live longer. The effects on the body of years of abuse are unknown.

For now, serious athletes are forced to make a hard choice. They can use no steroids and face a field full of artificially gifted opponents, or use the drugs and risk death or disease. Many athletes choose steroids, but they fail to realize that the risks from the drugs far outweigh any consequences of losing a competition.

Human Growth Hormone   Steroids are illegal in competition and can be detected in urine tests. Therefore, some athletes have switched to other unsafe hormones that are not detectable—**human growth hormone**, for example. Then they develop symptoms of the disease **acromegaly**— huge body size, widened jawline, widened nose, protruding brow and teeth, and an increased likelihood of death before age 50. The American Academy of Pediatrics and the American College of Sports Medicine speak out against the use of all hormones by athletes.

> **" A feeble body weakens the mind. "**
>
> Jean-Jacques Rousseau
> (1712–1778)
> French philosopher
> and writer

KEY POINTS *Hormones promote muscle growth, but the taking of hormone drugs to improve strength and endurance for athletic competition is illegal and dangerous to health. There is no quick road to fitness.*

 Review

Answer the following questions on a sheet of paper.

Learning the Vocabulary

The vocabulary terms in this section are *resistance, weight training, calisthenics, set, ergogenic, steroids, human growth hormone,* and *acromegaly.*

1. What is the difference between weight training and calisthenics?
2. Drugs that are abused by some athletes seeking a shortcut to large muscles are called _____.
3. High doses of _____ can cause a disease known as _____.
4. Strength develops when muscles work against _____.

Learning the Facts

5. What are the two ways people gain muscle strength and endurance?
6. How frequently should weight training be done?
7. What are four dangerous physical side effects of steroid use?
8. Name some products that are marketed as ergogenic aids.

Making Life Choices

9. Has anyone you know ever used steroids or any pills, powders, or potions for fitness? What were the results, both positive and negative?
10. Set up a personal strength-conditioning program for one week that you would enjoy following. Don't make it too demanding—assume you will add to it as time goes on.

QUICK QUIZ

Chapter 9, Section 5

The following quiz will help you assess your students' understanding of the material covered in this section of the chapter. You might use the quiz as an oral exercise, which will lead into a class discussion of the topics covered. Or, you might use it as a paper/pencil quiz to evaluate your students individually.

Like the Quick Quiz, the Section Review can also be used as an assessment tool to spark class discussion or as an individual student evaluation. It can also be used as a review in preparation for this quiz.

1. Strength is measured by the ability of the muscles to work against resistance. (True)

SECTION 6
Preventing Sports Injuries and Heat Stroke

Fitness-minded people talk a lot about **shin splints**, **stress fractures**, **tennis elbow**, and other athletic injuries. These and other injuries can be avoided by exercising properly and by building fitness slowly (see Figure 9–9 on the next page).

You can become a marathon runner in time. However, you can do it without joint damage only if you build slowly. Another obvious measure is to use proper equipment, such as supportive shoes designed specifically for your sport.

Be consistent, too. An "occasional athlete," one who is inactive for days and then suddenly plays hard, invites injury. Vigorous and sudden demands on out-of-condition muscles, ligaments, and tendons lead to sprains. Take on a regular program of fitness to develop the strength that safe play demands.

Pain during activity is a signal that something is wrong. For example, if a jogger feels leg pain, a change of posture may be needed. If the pain continues or gets worse, stop jogging until the pain goes away. Then try again slowly, increasing just a little at a time.

To prevent dehydration and the fatigue that accompanies it, drink plenty of liquids before, during, and after physical activity.

MINI Glossary

human growth hormone: a non-steroid hormone produced in the body that promotes growth; taken as a drug by athletes to enhance muscle growth; also called *somatotropin*.

acromegaly (ack-ro-MEG-a-lee): a disease caused by above-normal levels of human growth hormone.

shin splints: damage to the muscles and connective tissues of the lower front leg from stress. Such damage usually heals with rest.

stress fractures: bone damage from repeated physical force that strains the place where ligament is attached to bone.

tennis elbow: a painful condition of the arm and joint, usually caused by strain, as from poor form in playing tennis.

SECTION 6
FOCUS

OUTCOME
In this section students will learn:

1. Ways of preventing heat stroke and sport injuries.

FOCUS ACTIVITY
Without using their books, ask the students to describe as best they can shin splints, stress fractures, and tennis elbow. Ask for other examples of injuries they have heard about. List them on the board as they are mentioned. Have students select one of the listed injuries to report on the next day. Each presentation should not take more than three minutes. If there are not enough injuries listed for each student to report on one, have them report in pairs.

TEACH & APPLY

DISCUSSION
With permission from the coach, have students watch a school wrestling team during its workout. Afterwards, have students talk to the wrestlers to find out the importance of making weight. Ask about wrestlers losing water weight and any other stories they may have heard. After watching and discussing, have your students bring their findings back to class for further discussion on the negative and positive aspects of wrestling.

2. Muscle endurance is not closely related to strength. (False)

3. Strong muscles can effectively protect the body's internal organs from injury. (True)

4. Weight training and calisthenics improve muscle strength and endurance. (True)

5. Calisthenics is more effective than weight training in increasing muscle strength. (False)

6. Push-ups are a form of calisthenics. (True)

7. Performing many weight-lifting sets with lighter weights promotes bulk and strength rather than endurance. (False)

8. In any weight-training program, rest is as important as work. (True)

9. Steroid hormones are a safe way to increase body weight and improve muscle strength. (False)

10. Human growth hormone is an unsafe and illegal alternative to conventional steroids. (True)

In your Teacher's Resource Box you will find a handout for students, "Strategies for Overcoming Fitness Obstacles," which lists barriers to obtaining fitness and suggested solutions for each of the barriers. Or you may use the Enrichment Activity "Honoring Your Commitment to Exercise," on which students are to provide solutions to the excuses given for not exercising.

DISCUSSION

Ask students for examples of athletic injuries they have incurred. Have the injuries been temporary or nagging? How severe were they? What do they think caused the injuries? What could have been done to prevent the injuries?

ASSESS

EVALUATE

Divide students into groups of four or five. Have each group design a poster teaching ways to avoid heat stroke. Display the posters around the room, gym, and school.

Review Answers

1. Heat exhaustion is a serious stage of overheating. The loss of water (dehydration) and the buildup of body heat can be fatal. (p. 255)
2. shin splints (p. 253)
3. Vigorous and sudden demands on out-of-condition muscles, ligaments, and

For **Y**our **I**nformation

To avoid heat stroke:

▶ Rest during times of high humidity, high temperature, or both.
▶ Limit exposure to any source of heat.
▶ Wear lightweight, loose-fitting clothing.
▶ Drink several extra glasses of water in the hours before you exercise heavily. Drink enough to cause you to urinate (this means your tissues are full to the maximum with water).
▶ Replace water lost during the activity with about a half cup of a dilute, cool beverage every 15 to 20 minutes. Cold, plain or lightly flavored water is recommended.
▶ Listen for your body's distress signals, and if you have to, stop exercising. Take a rest in the shade.

Figure 9–9 Common Injuries and Their Prevention

Injury	Prevention
Achilles tendon[a] pain	Stretch the ankles and calves frequently and gently. When running, avoid or go easy on steep hills. Wear running shoes with a slightly elevated heel.
Ankle/knees: inflammation on outer side of joint	Exercise on flat surface, or change sides often on a sloping surface.
Blisters	Wear socks and shoes that do not rub and slip on the feet.
Cramps	Drink plenty of fluids, eat a balanced diet, increase workload gradually, and stretch often.
Foot pain	Perform calf stretches. Run, dance, or play on firm, springy surfaces. Wear proper shoes.
Lower back pain	Increase the back's workload gradually. Stretch the lower back. Strengthen abdominal muscles.
Pain around or under knee	Build lower body gradually. Use proper equipment and form. If untrained, do not sprint. Slow your pace when cycling or running on hills. Stop at first sensation of pain.
Shin pain	Slow down, and work out on proper surfaces.
Shoulder: inflammation of soft tissues	Build upper body gradually. Don't overtrain.

[a]The Achilles tendon is shown in Figure 6–4 of Chapter 6, page 138.

Dehydration Be alert to the dangers of overheating and **dehydration**. Muscles heat up during exercise because they are burning fuel. To help control the body's temperature, blood flows through the muscles and carries heat to the skin. There the surrounding air and the evaporation of sweat can carry the heat away. (Ordinarily, a bead of sweat the size of a pearl can cool a liter of blood by 1 degree Fahrenheit.) On humid days, though, sweat does not evaporate well. Heat builds up. Then the body sweats even more heavily in an attempt to cool itself. This heavy sweating can be extremely dangerous, because fluid and electrolyte losses beyond a certain point cause cells to stop functioning. It can even be fatal.

Dehydration interferes with the body's ability to exercise. Muscle weakness and unusual fatigue on a hot day may mean you need more fluids. You

COOPERATIVE LEARNING

Developing A Fitness Program

Physical fitness is best achieved not only when people understand the benefits and meaning of fitness, but also when they understand the best means of becoming fit. The following activity will help students understand the meaning of cardiovascular endurance, flexibility, muscular strength, and muscular endurance, as well as give them an understanding of what exercises improve those components. You may alter this activity to also include power, speed, agility, coordination, balance, and body composition.

Divide the class into groups of four. Assign each member of the group a letter (A, B, C or D). After each member of all the groups has been assigned a letter instruct the class to separate into jigsaw groups. All the A's form one group, the B's form one group, the C's form do not need salt tablets or other forms of salt. These may make dehydration worse, because they pull water from the tissues into the digestive tract. Some people like commercial sports drinks, but these are usually unnecessary. (In the case of endurance athletes, though, who work out for more than an hour without stopping, the sugar in sports drinks may be of some benefit.) You do not need supplemental vitamins and minerals, either. Ordinary foods and beverages replace losses naturally.

Dangers of Overheating Overheating progresses through several stages. Early symptoms may be just swelling of the hands and feet or cramps in the legs or other muscles. Then comes **heat exhaustion**, and finally **heat stroke**.

The symptoms of heat exhaustion are signals of distress, such as headaches, nausea, chest pains, or diarrhea. They warn that heat stroke may be threatening. Extreme fatigue, intense dizziness, and fading-out consciousness are signs of heat stroke.

The most important preventive steps are to stop the activity immediately, seek out shade and a cool place, rest, and drink water. See the margin on the opposite page for more tips to avoid heat stroke.

It is unwise to exercise in a plastic or rubber suit in hopes of losing pounds. The waterproof material stops evaporation, causing the body to sweat heavily. This can lead to heat stroke. Similarly, too long a stay in a hot whirlpool bath, hot tub, or sauna can cause heat stroke.

 Most sports injuries are preventable. The most important preventive measures are to follow proper form; stop working if you feel pain; and take precautions against dehydration, heat exhaustion, and heat stroke.

Answers to FACT or FICTION Here are the answers to the questions at the start of the chapter.

1. **True.**
2. **False.** Although an extreme and sudden exertion can damage the body, a gradual increase in overload will produce a strengthened body.
3. **True.**
4. **False.** People of both genders use weight training for trimming and firming the body. Bodybuilders follow special weight-training programs to gain muscle size and bulk.
5. **False.** You should stop to avoid serious injury.
6. **False.** It's best to rehydrate as you go.
7. **False.** You need water, not salt.

SECTION 6 Review

Answer the following questions on a sheet of paper.

Learning the Vocabulary

The vocabulary terms in this section are *shin splints, stress fractures, tennis elbow, dehydration, heat exhaustion,* and *heat stroke.*

1. How are dehydration and heat exhaustion related?
2. _____ involve damage to the muscles and connective tissues of the lower front leg due to stress.

Learning the Facts

3. What is the problem with being an "occasional athlete"?
4. How can heat stroke be avoided?
5. List three steps you can take to prevent injury.

Making Life Choices

6. Your friend has begun a fitness program that includes running. While running, he experiences back and leg pain. Use your knowledge gained from studying this section to develop a checklist of things for your friend to consider as causes for his pain.

MINI Glossary

dehydration: loss of water. The symptoms progress rapidly from thirst to weakness to exhaustion, confusion, and even death.

heat exhaustion: a serious stage of overheating which can lead to heat stroke.

heat stroke: a life-threatening condition that results from a buildup of body heat; can be fatal.

tendons lead to sprains. (p. 253)

4. Answers will vary; could include: rest during times of high humidity or high temperature; limit exposure to any source of heat; wear lightweight, loose-fitting clothing; drink several extra glasses of water in the hours before you exercise heavily; replace water lost during the activity, and listen to your body's distress signals and stop exercising. (p. 255)

5. Follow proper form, stop working if you feel pain, take precautions against heat exhaustion; also refer to Figure 9–9. (pp. 254–255)

6. Answers will vary.

A reproducible quiz for Section 6 is provided in the Teacher's Resource Box.

CLOSE

As a class, compile a resource list of local places to call for preventive methods or treatments for athletic injuries. For example: fitness club, fitness director of a company, nurse, doctor, athletic trainer.

Reproducible Study Outline and Reading Cloze worksheets for Chapter 9 are provided in the Teacher's Resource Box.

Reproducible Chapter Tests A and B are also provided in the Teacher's Resource Box.

one group, and the D's form one group. Assign each group one of the four fitness components (cardiovascular endurance, flexibility, muscle strength, or muscle endurance).

Have the jigsaw groups define the components they are given, give examples of what types of exercises relate to the component, and explain how would they apply the overload principle (exercise frequency, intensity, and duration). Instruct students to explain what type of warm-up and cool-down activi-

ties should be used before and after the exercises.

After the jigsaw groups have completed their fitness concepts, have students return to their original groups and share their findings. By doing this, groups will quickly learn about the components of fitness. If time allows, have the groups practice the exercises.

Straight
Talk

Food for Sports Competition

You may wonder if athletes need special foods or nutrients to help them perform. Right away, you should know that no supplement or nutrient product has ever proved helpful in this way. On the other hand, the foods athletes choose at every meal matter greatly. The meals they eat can help or hinder their performance.

 I work out each day, and I'd like to go out for the track team. Can my diet help me make the team?

While the right diet can help you in your efforts, it would be an exaggeration to say that diet alone can help you make the team. Rather, a balanced diet that provides adequate nutrients and fuels can support your efforts. Once these things are in place, dedication and hard work can win your spot on the team. Without the needed raw materials, though, your efforts will be an uphill battle.

 What fuels are best to support my activity? I've heard that carbohydrates are the best.

Yes, carbohydrate-rich foods are best.

 Why?

The way your body handles fuels during exercise plays a major role. At rest, your body uses a fuel mix of about equal parts of fat and carbohydrate. However, when you begin to work physically, the fuel mix changes. The type of work you choose—aerobic or anaerobic—determines the fuel mix your body uses. Fat "goes with" aerobic exercise. Activities such as jogging or distance running use mostly fat for fuel.

Glucose "goes with" anaerobic activities. Sprinting, tennis, and football use much more glucose for fuel.

If you are a jogger or distance runner, you'll use mostly fat to provide your energy (but you'll still use some carbohydrate). On the other hand, sprinters and weight lifters use mostly carbohydrate (although they still use some fat). Athletes of both kinds depend on their storage form of glucose, glycogen, to provide the carbohydrate they need.

 How does glycogen in the working body relate to carbohydrate in the diet?

To see the relationship, try to imagine the body packing away into storage some of the nutrients it receives from foods. It will draw on these stored nutrients later, during activity. Your body can store unlimited amounts of fat, and fat is abundant in the diet. Thus you needn't worry about obtaining enough fat.

Carbohydrate is a different story. The body's glycogen stores are very small. Also, they run out quickly, after only an hour or so of intense activity. You must fill your glycogen stores from food daily. Most people rarely include enough carbohydrate-containing foods in their days' meals to keep their glycogen stores full. They must make special efforts to eat enough carbohydrate-containing foods.

 What would happen if I ran out of glycogen?

Most times, when glycogen runs out, a person just feels tired and hungry. During physical activity, though, to run out of glycogen is to "hit the wall." Continuing activity beyond this point is possible only through great effort, and the quality of performance is lowered. Figure 9–10 shows that a high-carbohydrate diet can triple an athlete's endurance.

256

special needs

Bodily-kinesthetic

Personal fitness, functional health, and a physically active lifestyle can be limited by a physical disability. Many disabled students exhibit limited aerobic fitness. If you have students who are restricted in their ability to be physically active because of a disability, encourage them to strive for personal fitness, functional

health, and an active lifestyle, within their limitations.

A topic for discussion might include how the meaning of fitness varies with the nature and severity of the disability. The physical educator might find information the doctor can share about the student's ability helpful in assisting the student in designing a personal fitness program. It's important to have as much information as possible about students prone to cardiopulmonary problems. Oxygen

Fat and protein diet

Normal mixed diet

High-carbohydrate diet

Maximum endurance time

57 min

114 min

167 min

For people who exercise lightly for an hour or less, such as casual joggers, glycogen stores rarely matter much. These people simply do not go long or hard enough to run out of glycogen. For distance runners, others who exercise for more than an hour at a stretch, and for people who work anaerobically, such as weight lifters and sprinters, glycogen is important.

 I've heard of a method called glycogen loading to improve performance. What is glycogen loading?

Athletes who compete in long-distance endurance events want to have as much stored energy in their muscles as they can. Glycogen loading tricks the muscles into storing more glycogen than normal. Old ways of doing this were dangerous, but the plan described here is safe.

Exercise physiologists recommend this glycogen-loading plan. First, about two or three weeks before competition, the athlete increases exercise intensity while eating a normal, high-carbohydrate diet. Then, during the last week before competition, the athlete does two things. With respect to exercise, the athlete gradually cuts back and, on the day before competition, rests completely. Meanwhile, with respect to foods, the athlete eats carbohydrate as usual until three days before competition, and then eats a very-high-carbohydrate diet. Endurance athletes who follow this plan can keep going longer than their competitors.

In hot weather, extra glycogen has one more advantage—it holds water. As glycogen breaks down, it releases its water, which helps to meet the athlete's fluid needs.

 I'm sold. What's the best high-carbohydrate food? Candy bars have sugar, and sugar is a form of carbohydrate, right?

From the standpoint that candy provides carbohydrate, candy bars might seem, at first glance, to be useful. Candy is available, needs no preparation, and tastes delicious. Before you load up on candy, though, you should know that most candy also contains a lot of fat. In fact, most types contain many more calories of fat than of carbohydrate.

Another thing about candy—while it provides concentrated sugar and fat for energy, it provides almost no other nutrients with them. Vitamins and minerals are just as important to performance as is carbohydrate. So consider candy, always, as a treat, not as a food to support health and performance. Bread, baked beans, potatoes, and pasta provide carbohydrate as starch, plus many other nutrients along with it.

 Are you telling me I should eat more bread, beans, potatoes, and pasta to provide carbohydrate?

Yes, those are the foods to choose, along with fruits (almost pure carbohydrate), low-fat milk products, cereals, grains, and vegetables. Olympic training tables are laden with such choices.

257

---

intake differs greatly depending on the disability. The greater the damage to the central nervous system, the less efficient oxygen transport can be. A 55 percent to 70 percent threshold level of the maximum heart rate (MHR) is appropriate for the health impaired (i.e. 55 percent to 200 is 110). Some medically disabled students who have limited large muscle use may be unable to maintain their MHR for a time period long enough to improve cardiorespiratory endurance. Students who are diagnosed with asthma should only begin an exercise program with direct input from a physician.

Possible teacher resources: *Fitness for Special Populations,* Roy J. Shephard, Human Kinetics Books, Champaign, IL, 1990; *Fitness for the Handicapped: An Instructional Approach,* James V. Sullivan, Charles C. Thomas, Publisher, Springfield, IL, 1984.

With the increased interest in sports medicine, exercise physiology, physical fitness, and conditioning, more men and women are entering these professions. Men and women are doing research on how the human body reacts during exercise, what helps people improve their cardiovascular condition, and what roles certain nutrients play in physical fitness. While some individuals are doing research, many are specializing in sports medicine, others are working in fitness centers, and still others are working as dietitians. Have the students prepare a report, either oral or written, on a career in this field. Encourage the students to talk with their science teacher, librarian, sports medicine professionals, registered dietitians, and vocational guidance counselors as they work on the assignment. Have students share their reports with the class.

Straight Talk

Food for Sports Competition (continued)

 Are there special foods I should be sure to include?

It's a mistake to think in terms of special foods. No one food must be either included or avoided. Try to adopt an athlete's diet as part of your lifestyle. Make it something you do every day—all three meals and all snacks eaten every day of every week. Instead of "special foods," try to think in terms of "special diet."

 Is there anything I can do before competition to help me perform my best?

On the day of competition, carefully plan your pregame meal. Eat it three to four hours before the event. The meal should be light (300 to 1,000 calories) and easy to digest. The meal should provide carbohydrate-rich foods such as potatoes, beans and lentils; refined pastas and breads; and fruit juices. Not only do these foods supply glucose, but they are quickly absorbed.

The juice provides fluids to help guard against dehydration and heat stroke.

Stay away from foods high in fat (such as meat) or foods high in fiber (such as raw vegetables). These require long times for digestion and can cause nausea during exercise. Tradition may call for a steak-and-salad dinner before a big game, but the needs of the players are better served by a new tradition—pasta or other high-carbohydrate meal to support performance. (See Figure 9–11 on the opposite page.)

 Speaking of steaks, you haven't mentioned protein. Don't athletes need more protein than other people do?

Athletes need just slightly more protein than other people do. They use much of the extra to build muscles, and a little of it for fuel. While exercising, the muscles use more of certain amino acids for fuel, because these can provide energy in much the same way as glucose.

This does not mean, though, that athletes need to take amino acid pills or powders or eat more meat. A diet of regular high-carbohydrate foods provides all of the protein and amino acids that athletes need, and in just the right amounts. Vegetarian athletes don't need amino acid pills either. They do need to be careful to include generous servings of protein-rich foods such as beans, seeds, whole-grain bread, pasta, and cereals, as well as low-fat milk and milk products in their diets.

 Almost every athlete I know takes vitamin C pills. Do athletes need more vitamin C than the amount in their diets?

Your question is part of a large issue: whether athletes need more of *any* vitamin. It goes without saying that athletes need *enough* vitamins and minerals to do what they do. However, they do not need *more* than the RDA (Recommended Dietary

258

enrichment....

Since 1962, when President Kennedy sent the first consumer protection message to Congress, legislation has been passed that is directed at product safety and protection against fraud.

Nutrition is a big consumer concern and, therefore, big business. Have students brainstorm a list of items that have been advertised as nutritional aids or healthy choices. Identify the topics that are of the most concern or interest to the students.

Then, assign groups to find out the number of different products there are within a topic,

Some Good Ideas for a Pregame Meal:	Not Recommended:
Angel food cake	Biscuits
Apricot nectar	Butter
Baked beans	Cheeses
Baked white or sweet potatoes	Creams
Black beans	Croissants
Black-eyed peas	French fries
Dried fruit	Frosted cakes
Frozen yogurt	Gravy
Graham crackers	Ice cream
Grape juice	Margarine
Jell-O	Meats
Lentils	Mayonnaise
Pancakes	Meats
Pasta	Muffins
Pineapple juice	Nuts
Popsicles	Onion rings
Sherbet	Pies
Sponge cake	Potato chips
Tortillas	Salad dressings
	Stuffing

Figure 9–11 Pregame Meal *Tips*

Allowance) amount of any of them (Appendix B at the back of the book lists the RDA). Much research supports this statement, and virtually no true scientific evidence exists to oppose it.

As for vitamin C, it follows the same rule as for all the other vitamins (although faddists say otherwise). Studies show that more is not better. Athletes who take vitamins in addition to an ample diet do not perform any better than those who get enough from food.

Besides, for vitamin C, anyone eating a reasonable diet would find it almost impossible *not* to receive two or three times the RDA. A person who drinks a small glass of orange juice and eats a baked potato and a serving of broccoli in a day receives about five times the RDA for vitamin C from these foods alone. When they learn this fact, athletes have been known to throw away their pills and learn to cook broccoli.

 Are you saying that no supplements have any effects on performance at all?

No, that's not quite true. Some concentrated nutrients may hurt an athlete's performance. For exam-

ple, niacin supplements interfere with the body's release of fat. Without enough fat to use as fuel, the muscles are forced to use extra glycogen in place of fat. This may make the body run out of glycogen sooner. It also makes the work seem more difficult to the exerciser.

 Can I relax my diet and rely on the drinks and candy-like bars that claim to provide "complete" nutrition to supply the nutrients I need?

Such bars and drinks usually taste good and provide extra food energy. However, they do not come close to providing "complete" nutrition, as they claim. They lack fiber, many nutrients, and other important constituents of real food.

In one case, though, a liquid meal may be useful. An athlete who gets nervous and so cannot eat before a game might try such a drink to supply some of the needed fluid and carbohydrate. However, a homemade milkshake of nonfat milk, ice cream, and a banana blended with flavorings can do the same thing, and less expensively.

259

their availability, cost range, merits, negative qualities, and how they compare to competitive products. Groups might choose to develop charts that report their research and consumer recommendations in a clear and informative way. The information provided should assist classmates in making rational choices.

Encourage the class to evaluate the reports and determine if the data provided would make them better consumers or if there is additional information they would need to make an informed decision. As a class, recommend helpful consumer resources.

CLASS ACTIVITY

Have students bring into class or bring in yourself, a selection of nutritional bars and powdered health drinks. Have the students compare the nutritional value of these products. What would they be missing if they depended on these products for their daily nutrition? Do these products give any recommendations for additional foods or meals to go with the product? Have students evaluate which of the products would be the best for someone as a supplement to a balanced nutritional day.

COMPREHENSION CHECK

Make sure that students are aware of both the positive and negative effects of caffeine on the body. If possible, have a health care provider come into class and lead a talk on the ways that caffeine affects the body. Have the students prepare questions ahead of time.

CLASS ACTIVITY

Have the students study the list of foods in Figure 9–11 and the meal modifications from Figure 9–12 on page 261. Have students plan an entire week's worth of meals for an athlete who has a competition on the Saturday at the end of the week. Compare students' meal choices and discuss possible alternatives.

ON LINE WITH HEALTH

You may want to have your students visit the following URL, where they will find information and additional Web site resources to enhance their study of this chapter. As with all Web sites, you should check this out first to be sure the information found there is appropriate for your students.

FitnessLink
http://www.fitnesslink.com

FitnessLink is a comprehensive site, full of information, resources, and real-life suggestions.

Straight Talk

Food for Sports Competition (continued)

Can the athlete find any other help in the diet?

Yes, there are two more things to be aware of. One is the use of caffeine. A moderate dose of this mild stimulant (the amount of one or two cola beverages or glasses of iced tea) one hour prior to exercise seems to help some people's performance. Caffeine stimulates the body's release of fat. Exercise does, too, but caffeine taken before exercise gets the fuel flowing before the exercise begins.

Remember, though, that a warm-up activity stimulates fuel release, too. Also, caffeine has adverse effects—upset stomach, nervousness, sleeplessness, irritability, headaches, breast disease, and diarrhea, among others. It also has a diuretic (water loss) effect that is potentially hazardous. Finally, caffeine in amounts greater than in five or six cups of coffee is illegal in competition and can disqualify a competitor. Use caffeine-containing beverages, if at all, with extreme care, as you would use any medical drug. Also, use them in *addition* to other fluids, not as substitutes.

You said there were two things concerning diet and exercise to be aware of. What's the other?

The other help that comes from diet is a real advantage in sports for the athlete who eats right. A diet that is low in fat, high in complex carbohydrates, and adequate in protein and other nutrients serves all the needs of human beings. Such a diet meets the needs of those who place physical demands on their bodies especially well.

Figure 9-12 on the opposite page shows how a normal, high-carbohydrate diet can be boosted with nourishing foods to meet an athlete's energy needs while providing abundant nutrients. Athletes need extra helpings of cereals, rice, beans, and bread; more milk and fruit; and even some sweet snacks, such as angel food cake or puddings. Meats provide important nutrients, but athletes need only the same amounts as do other people.

Training and genetics being equal, who would win a competition—the person who habitually consumes too few nutrients or the one who arrives at the event with a long history of full nutrient stores and well-met needs? Be sure you give your active body the food it needs if you expect it to perform its best.

260

Ability Levels

Advanced

Have students investigate, through articles and interviews at health clubs, how our society idolizes professional athletes, their performances, the products they endorse, and their salaries. Students should also investigate how society's view of these athletes affects the use of steroids. Divide the class into two groups in preparation for a class debate. One group will

Figure 9–12 Normal Diet and an Athlete's Diet—How to Modify a Regular Day's Meals to Meet an Athlete's Needs

Regular Meal Choices ➤ **To Modify** ➤ **Athlete's Meal Choices**

The regular breakfast plus:
2 pieces whole-wheat toast
4 teaspoons jelly
1/2 cup orange juice
2 teaspoons brown sugar on the oatmeal
2-percent-fat milk instead of nonfat milk

Both enjoy the same snack

The regular lunch plus:
1 more beef and bean burrito
1 banana
Plus an afternoon snack:
1 cup 2-percent-fat milk
1 piece angel food cake

The regular dinner plus:
1 dinner roll
2 teaspoons butter
1/4 cup more noodles
1/2 cup more sherbet
2-percent-fat milk instead of nonfat milk

Total calories 1,759
57 percent calories from carbohydrate
24 percent calories from fat
19 percent calories from protein

Total calories 3,119
61 percent calories from carbohydrate
24 percent calories from fat
15 percent calories from protein

261

argue that professional athletes must live up to a higher standard than the average citizen because they are emulated and adored by so many people. The other group should argue that professional athletes are just like everybody else. They just happen to make millions of dollars for their athletic talent. The average citizen should be able to discern how to act—it is not the athlete's job to be a role model for everyone.

VOCABULARY

1. **a.** frequency **b.** anaerobic **c.** fitness **d.** heat exhaustion **e.** flexibility **f.** set **g.** overload **h.** stress **i.** elasticity **j.** tennis elbow
2. **a.** Exercise duration is how long an exercise is performed—exercise intensity is the degree of exertion with which an exercise is performed. **b.** Target heart rate is the heartbeat rate that will condition a person's cardiovascular system, and thus develop cardiovascular endurance.
3. **a.** Cardiovascular endurance, flexibility, muscle strength, endurance, and body composition **b.** Low-impact aerobic dance

RECALL

SECTION 1

1. Answers will vary; could include: protection against: acne; backaches; cancer; diabetes; digestive disorders; headaches; heart and blood vessel disease; high blood cholesterol and triglycerides; infections; infertility; insomnia; kidney disease; menstrual irregularities, menstrual cramps, menstrual mood swings; obesity; and osteoporosis. (p. 233)

SECTION 2

2. If you love your workout, do it more often. If you run out of time, shorten your workout time, but increase intensity. If you hate hard

CHAPTER 9 Review

Summarizing the Chapter

Your ability to respond correctly to the following statements ensures your understanding of the main concepts in the chapter.

1. Discuss how fitness promotes all aspects of health.
2. Identify the five components of fitness.
3. Describe how you gain cardiovascular endurance, flexibility, muscle strength, and muscle endurance. Describe the benefits of each.
4. Recognize the dangers of using steroids and other drugs.
5. Describe preventive measures for sports injuries and accidents.

Learning the Vocabulary

sedentary	elasticity
fitness	connective tissues
conditioning	range of motion
cardiovascular endurance	resistance
flexibility	weight training
muscle strength	calisthenics
muscle endurance	set
body composition	ergogenic
exercise physiology	steroids
overload	human growth hormone
progressive overload principle	acromegaly
frequency	shin splints
intensity	stress fractures
duration	tennis elbow
aerobic	dehydration
anaerobic	heat exhaustion
pulse rate	heat stroke
target heart rate	
step aerobics	*Answer the following*
low-impact aerobic dance	*questions on a separate sheet of paper.*

1. ***Matching***—*Match each of the following phrases with the appropriate vocabulary term from the list above:*
   a. the number of weight training sessions per week
   b. energy-producing processes that do not use oxygen
   c. the characteristics that enable the body to perform physical activity
   d. a serious stage of overheating which can lead to heat stroke
   e. ability to bend the joints without injury
   f. a specific number of times to repeat a weight-training exercise
   g. an extra physical demand placed on the body
   h. bone injuries caused by repeated physical shocks at the point of ligament and bone attachment
   i. the ability to be stretched or bent and then return to the original size and shape
   j. painful condition of the arm joint usually caused by strain
2. **a.** What is the difference between exercise duration and exercise intensity?
   b. What is the relationship between target heart rate and cardiovascular endurance?
3. **a.** ____, ____, ____, and ____ are all components of fitness.
   b. ____ is a dance activity in which one foot always remains on the floor to prevent shock to the lower body.

Recalling Important Facts and Ideas

Section 1
1. List four physical benefits of fitness.

Section 2
2. Offer some pointers for applying the overload principle.
3. Explain the principles of warm-up and cool-down.

Section 3
4. Why must cardiovascular endurance training involve aerobic activities?
5. How does cardiovascular endurance affect the heart?
6. How long must aerobic activity last to improve cardiovascular endurance?
7. How do you determine your target heart rate?

262

work, take it easy and go longer, increasing duration. Exercise regularly, train hard only once or twice a week, and listen to your body. (p. 235)
3. A warm-up helps the body to get needed fuels ready and warms up muscles and connective tissues, so that they will stretch without tearing. A cool-down helps relax tight muscles and allows blood to circulate freely, cooling the body. (pp. 237–238)

SECTION 3

4. It demands that the heart and lungs work extra hard to deliver oxygen to the muscles for as long as the exercise lasts. Cardiovascular endurance training is aerobic. (p. 239)
5. The heart muscle gains size and strength and pumps more blood with each beat. (p. 241)

8. Give three strategies for including daily physical activity in your schedule.

Section 4

9. What are some signs and symptoms of overstretching?

10. Why is gentle stretching recommended over bouncing?

Section 5

11. How can you best increase muscle firmness and endurance when weight training?

12. Why do men generally develop larger muscles than women when they exercise?

13. What are some psychological side effects of steroid use?

14. How can steroid use be detected?

Section 6

15. What are the signs of heat stroke?

16. Why is exercising in a plastic or rubber suit dangerous?

17. How can injury best be prevented when you exercise?

Critical Thinking

1. List some of the reasons why being physically fit is especially important in today's world. Do you need to join a fitness center in order to keep in shape? Why or why not? What are some of the advantages and disadvantages of belonging to a fitness center? List some ways to become physically fit at a minimal expense. In your community, what sports activities can you participate in without paying any fees?

2. List your personal fitness goals. Make a list of all the physical activities you participate in within a one-week period. Identify which fitness component is promoted by each activity and which activities are anaerobic and aerobic. Will these activities help you to develop all your fitness goals? Now that you have read this chapter, what changes do you think you need to make in your program?

Activities

1. Interview a podiatrist or a doctor whose specialty is sports medicine and write a one-page report on your findings.

2. Investigate a particular type of exercise equipment: for example, Stairmaster, Nordic Track, stationary bike, or the like. Discuss which fitness components the machine is designed to improve. Explain the different features of the equipment and state the approximate cost.

3. Write a letter to the President's Council on Physical Fitness to obtain literature about fitness. The address is: President's Council on Physical Fitness and Sports, Suite 250, 701 Pennsylvania Ave. NW, Washington, DC 20004.

4. Investigate the different types of steroids that are commonly abused and write a one-page report.

5. Visit a local fitness center. Find out about the types of equipment, programs, classes, and instructors the center offers. What is the fee for joining? Overall, would you consider joining this center? Would it be a worthwhile investment? Why or why not?

6. Make a poster of newspaper and magazine advertisements for physical fitness products. Label one half of the poster "Safe and Effective Products" and the other half "Dangerous and Suspicious Products." Place each advertisement under the appropriate title, forming a collage.

7. Write a one-page story about a person who is completely unfit. What would this person be able to do? What wouldn't this person be able to do? What would his or her lifestyle be like? Describe in detail a day in the life of a totally unfit person.

8. Read the following statement: "A sound mind in a sound body, is a short but full description of a happy state in this world." (John Lock, 1632–1704, from *Some Thoughts Concerning Education*, 1693) What do you think the author meant by this statement? Do you agree with the statement? Why or why not? Discuss your answers with the rest of your class.

Making Decisions about Health

1. Your classmate considers himself to be in "perfect health." He rarely gets sick, eats right, and is not overweight. His blood cholesterol and blood pressure are within the acceptable range. He insists there is no need for him to participate in any type of exercise program. Do you agree with your classmate? Why or why not?

263

12. They produce larger amounts of certain hormones known as steroids in their bodies. (p. 251)

13. Answers will vary; could include mood swings, aggressive behavior, and changes in sexual drive. (pp. 251–252)

14. urine test (p. 252)

SECTION 6

15. extreme fatigue, intense dizziness, and fading-out consciousness (p. 255)

16. It stops evaporation, causing the body to sweat heavily, which can lead to heat stroke. (p. 255)

17. exercise properly, build fitness slowly, and use proper equipment (pp. 253–254)

6. at least 20 minutes (p. 243)

7. Subtract your age from 220 and multiply that number by .75. (p. 243)

8. Answers will vary; refer to the Teens' Activity Pyramid on page 242.

SECTION 4

9. tightness does not ease, stretch becomes painful (p. 245)

10. Bouncing can easily overstretch or tear alignment until it can no longer support its joint. Nerves can also overstretch with bouncing. (p. 245)

SECTION 5

11. Use small weights to provide resistance, repeat exercises many times in a set, perform many sets in a session, and train every other day. (p. 248)

KEY POINTS

Chapter 10 is 24 pages long and divided into four sections. This chapter is designed to acquaint the students with the knowledge and skill for proper care of the body, through good hygiene, self-exams, and proper posture.

ACTIVITY TO INTRODUCE THE CHAPTER

Divide the class into groups of four or five students each and give them ten minutes to list all the strategies that they use to maintain healthy bodies. Have them record these on chart paper. Allow each group to share and discuss their lists with the entire class. Then post their charts around the room.

BULLETIN BOARD IDEAS

Divide the bulletin board into two sides. On the left-hand side post advertisements for products (or the actual products) truly needed for personal hygiene. (examples: toothbrush, toothpaste, comb, soap, deodorant, shampoo) On the right-hand side, post advertisements, labels, or actual products of the great number of items people use in their hygiene routine. (examples: tooth whiteners, lotions, make-up, hair styling products, special hair brushes, colognes and perfumes, and so on) As a possible activity, students could bring in the advertisements of the products they use.

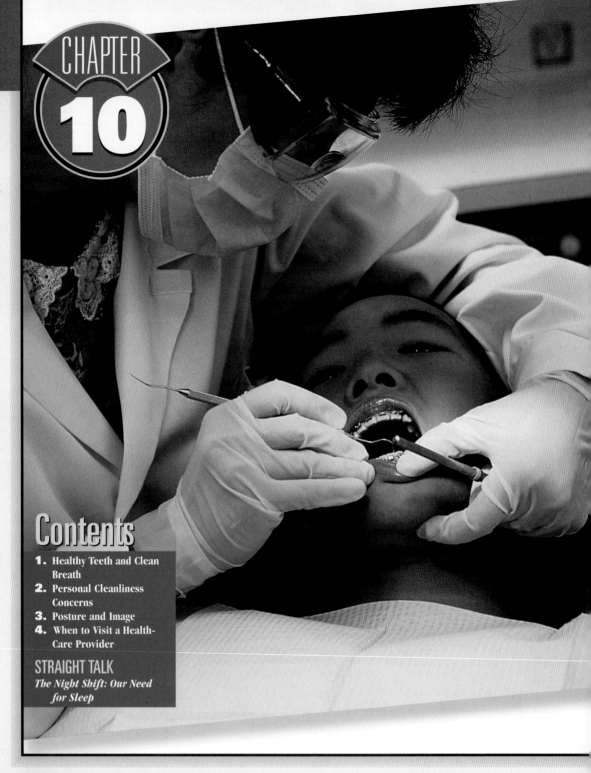

CHAPTER 10

Contents

1. **Healthy Teeth and Clean Breath**
2. **Personal Cleanliness Concerns**
3. **Posture and Image**
4. **When to Visit a Health-Care Provider**

STRAIGHT TALK
The Night Shift: Our Need for Sleep

NOT Enough Time?

Following are some suggestions to help you make sure that you cover the key topics in this chapter if you have limited time. (Refer to the daily lesson plans in your Teacher's Resource Box for additional suggestions.)

DAY 1 Assign students to read Sections 1 and 2 prior to class. In class do the Group Activity on page 267 and the Comprehension

Your Body: An Owner's Manual

What do you think? Are the following statements true or false? If you think they are false, then say what is true.

1. A dental plaque is an award given to students of dentistry at graduation.
2. Flossing is more important to the fight against gum disease than is brushing tooth surfaces.
3. People who get acne simply need to keep their faces cleaner.
4. Acne often clears up during summer vacations.
5. Douching is not necessary.
6. For every one product people truly need, a hundred other unneeded ones are for sale.
7. The advertising tricks used to sell unneeded products are easy to see through.

(Answers on page 281)

Introduction

A dvice about health care usually has more to say about curing illnesses than it does about staying healthy. Such advice emphasizes other people—health-care providers, who help cure illnesses. Usually, though, the most important aspect of health care is *self*-care. Doing a few simple things for your body can enable you to maintain it at least as lovingly as you would maintain a fine car.

This chapter starts by going over the body head-to-toe and instructs you in some simple self-care techniques. If you faithfully follow its advice, you can spend less time trying to cure illnesses and more time doing the things you like doing. There are times, though, when you must seek out help from a health-care provider. The last section tells when you should do so. The Straight Talk section points out the importance of sleep.

Answers to FACT or FICTION

1. **False.** Dental plaque is a sticky substance that builds up on teeth, damaging them.
2. **True.**
3. **False.** Although cleanliness is important, there are no simple answers to preventing or curing acne.
4. **True.**
5. **True.**
6. **True.**
7. **False.** False advertisements sound convincing, but many people fail to see through them.

FAST FACTS

Research by the Academy of General Dentistry in England indicates that eating cheese at the end of the meal helps prevent tooth decay. If you eat or drink anything else with the cheese, however, you weaken the protective effect. The best cheeses to eat are Edam, Gouda, mild cheddar, and Danish blue.

Check on page 272. Also do a variety of Evaluate activities if time permits. Assign students to read Sections 3 and 4 prior to the next class.

DAY 2   In class do the Background Information activity on page 280 and the Section 3 Review on page 281. Conclude with the Evaluate assessment on page 283.

FOCUS

OUTCOMES

In this section students will learn:

1. The benefits of proper dental care.

2. The consequences of improper dental care.

3. To identify dental diseases, procedures, and terminology.

FOCUS ACTIVITY

Ask the class to respond to the following questions before you have them read this section or do any of the activities:

1. Why would brushing back and forth be better than brushing up and down?

2. Why should the upper teeth be brushed first?

3. What difference does it make how you hold a toothbrush?

4. Why should we not "saw" with dental floss? What could be some of the consequences of sawing?

5. Why is it important to use a long section of floss?

Allow time for students to explain their answers; let others make additional comments. Discuss each question thoroughly.

TEACH & APPLY

DISCUSSION

Ask students to name the teeth and gum products that they buy and use regularly. Do they use a particular brand of toothpaste? Why?

SECTION 1
Healthy Teeth and Clean Breath

A bright smile says something about its owner—that the person has high enough self-esteem to tend daily to tooth care. You probably already know how to brush your teeth. However, you may not know that tooth decay can lead to major illness of the whole body. Even without decay, teeth that collect food particles and **dental plaque** create unpleasant mouth odor.

Cavities and Gum Disease The bacteria that live in plaque break down food particles and create acid. The plaque holds this acid like a sponge. This acid dissolves away the tooth's outer layer, its **enamel**. The person may not feel a **cavity** forming in its early stages. However, as the decay advances into the tooth's middle layer, its **dentin**, it eats into nerves. The pain at this stage can be shocking. Should the decay infect the tooth's deepest layer, its **pulp cavity**, it might kill the tooth. If a cavity is discovered in the early stages, a dentist can drill away the damaged part of the tooth surface and replace it with a substance that seals and saves the tooth.

Today, dentists often fill and seal healthy teeth to prevent decay from getting started. Figure 10–1 shows how cavities form and how sealants work.

As for **gum disease**, it causes mouth odor. It also causes more tooth loss than tooth decay does. Fifty percent of all adults will develop gum disease. An early

Red, swollen areas on the gums are telltale signs of serious gum disease.

Figure 10–1 How Cavities Form in Teeth

Healthy teeth have deep crevices and pits where decay can get started.

Sealants (shown here in blue) fill the tooth's normal crevices, protecting them from decay.

Cavities begin when acid dissolves away the tooth's enamel (A), its outer layer. At this stage, a cavity is easily treated. As the decay advances through the dentin (B) to the pulp cavity (C), hope for saving the tooth diminishes.

HEALTHY PEOPLE 2000

Reduce untreated dental caries so that the proportion of children with untreated caries (in permanent or primary teeth) is no more than 20 percent among children aged 6 through 8 and no more than 15 percent among adolescents aged 15.

Early diagnosis and timely treatment of caries can halt tooth destruction and prevent tooth loss. Yet in 1986–1987 the proportions of children aged 6, 7, and 8 with untreated decay in primary teeth were 32, 27, and 25 percent, respectively; in permanent teeth 39, 32, and 24 percent of children had decay that had not been treated.

Surveys have shown that, because of inad-

Brush your teeth after each meal and choose a toothbrush that bears the American Dental Association seal of approval.

symptom is gums that bleed easily. Treatment of advanced gum disease often involves the dentist's cutting away diseased gum tissue and scraping the teeth below the gum line. Even then, however, gum disease often returns, especially if the person fails to floss. Happily, gum disease is a problem that everyone can avoid by brushing and flossing.

Brushing and Flossing Brushing the teeth after each meal and flossing once each day can remove particles and plaque—that is, if brushing and flossing are done correctly. Some people brush and floss wrong, every day, all their lives, and suffer tooth and gum disease despite their efforts. Figure 10–2 on the next page shows how to get rid of plaque that takes hold at the gum line and beneath it.

Choose any soft- to medium-bristled inexpensive toothbrush approved by the American Dental Association (ADA). The angled head, flexible handles, pretty colors, and national advertising of fancy brushes do nothing extra for teeth, but they drive up the prices. Since any toothbrush should be replaced every three to four months to prevent bacterial buildup, the less expensive, the better. Electric toothbrushes, though expensive, do a better job of removing plaque for older people, children, or others who lack the skill or strength to brush properly.

To ensure that your flossing is effective, use the floss to pull plaque up from below the gum line, between the teeth. If you do this only once a day,

MINI Glossary

dental plaque (PLAK): a buildup of sticky material on the surfaces of the teeth; a forerunner of tooth damage.

enamel: a tooth's tough outer layer.

cavity: a hole in a tooth caused by decay. (Tooth decay is also called dental *caries*.)

dentin: a tooth's softer, middle layer.

pulp cavity: a tooth's deepest chamber, which houses its blood vessels and nerves.

gum disease: inflammation and degeneration of the pink tissue (gums) that is attached to the teeth and helps to hold them in place.

equate receipt of routine dental care, certain populations experience higher rates of untreated caries. For example, the prevalence of untreated decay may be higher among the children of migrant workers than the total population; migrant workers' use of dental services is well below the national average.

Dental caries is a unique microbial infection. Once established, it is progressive, does not heal without treatment, and leaves visible evidence of past infection. Because early diagnosis and prompt treatment of caries can halt tooth destruction and prevent tooth loss, low prevalence of untreated caries should be attainable. Financial, cultural, psychological, social, and geographic barriers contribute to lack of treatment.

COMPREHENSION CHECK

Use an oversized model of teeth and a toothbrush and the steps illustrated on this page to demonstrate the steps to cleaning teeth properly. Ask two or three volunteers to demonstrate the brushing techniques. Have the other students critique the volunteers' techniques.

DISCUSSION

Make sure students read the sentence "Years ago, people expected to lose their teeth in old age." (This sentence is on page 269.) Ask them if any of their older relatives or friends have false teeth. Then have them read the next sentence. Why do they think this change has occurred? (more knowledge and more preventive health care)

ASSESS

EVALUATE

Prepare a set of cards, each with a question, vocabulary word, or dental problem. Have students draw a card, prepare a quick answer or response, and then recite that to the class. The class should evaluate whether or not the statement given by the student is correct. The student giving the responses may intentionally give an incorrect response to challenge the class. Use all the terms covered in the Group Activity for this section. You may want to give extra credit for knowledge of terms in addition to the glossary terms.

Angle the brush at the gum line. Brush tooth surfaces back and forth, not up and down, so as not to push food particles below the gum line.

Brush the gums, especially beneath the gum line (gently), to dislodge plaque there.

Use floss to pull plaque up from below the gum line between the teeth.

Use a toothpick or brush to dislodge plaque from below the gum line along the teeth.

Figure 10–2 Brushing and Flossing the Teeth and Gums

you will be doing more to protect your teeth and gums than you can do by any amount of brushing of your tooth surfaces.

By the way, you need not buy expensive toothpastes and mouthwashes for a clean mouth. They do taste good and freshen the breath for a few minutes. Some even provide a little of the mineral fluoride, which helps protect teeth against decay. However, the fluoride in a mouthwash is not nearly as effective as the treatments given by dentists.

It is wise to avoid teeth-whitening products such as the kits sold in drugstores. Products sold as teeth whiteners contain bleaching substances and acids that may damage the teeth, gums, and tongue. Some toothpaste makers claim that their brands whiten teeth better than others. Unfortunately, these pastes do not make a measurable difference in tooth color, and they are not worth their substantial price.

For everyday cleaning, a toothbrush, clean water, and baking soda or toothpaste are all you need. Tablets or solutions that temporarily color existing plaque may be useful to show you where to concentrate your cleaning efforts.

Other Hints for Healthy Teeth To support your daily efforts, you should visit a dentist. A professional cleaning about once every six months and a full examination about once a year can go a long way toward helping you keep your teeth for life. Of course, you should also follow your dentist's advice about fluoride rinses or supplements.

One more thing about tooth care: choose snacks with care. The delicious snacks listed in the left column of Figure 10–3 do not promote dental decay. The sticky, sweet foods and other snacks listed in the right column cling to the teeth and are used by the bacteria in plaque to make acid.

QUICK QUIZ

Chapter 10, Section 1

The following quiz will help you assess your students' understanding of the material covered in this section of the chapter. You might use the quiz as an oral exercise, which will lead into a class discussion of the topics covered. Or, you might use it as a paper/pencil

quiz to evaluate your students individually.

*If students have difficulty with the concepts covered in the Quick Quiz and the Section Review, you might suggest they review the material using the **S**urvey, **Q**uestion, **R**ead, **R**ecite, **R**eview (SQ3R) study method, which is described in detail in the introduction to this Teacher's Wraparound Edition.*

1. Tooth decay can lead to major illness in all parts of the body. (True)

Some foods are more likely to cause tooth decay than are others. Sugar is one factor, but it's not just the sugar in foods that makes the difference. Other factors, such as fat, fiber, and stickiness matter as well.

These Foods Do Not Contribute to Tooth Decay

- Milk, cheese, plain yogurt
- Popcorn, toast, hard rolls, pretzels, corn chips, pizza
- Fresh fruits, fruits canned in water, salad greens, cauliflower, cucumbers, radishes, carrots, celery, diet soft drinks
- Lean meats, fish, poultry, eggs, beans
- Water, sugarless gum

These Foods Do Contribute to Tooth Decay; Brush Your Teeth after Finishing Them

- Chocolate milk, ice cream, milkshakes, sweetened yogurt
- Cookies, sweet rolls, pies, cakes, cereals, potato chips, crackers
- Dried fruits, fruit canned in syrup or juice, jams, jellies, fruit juices, regular soft drinks
- Peanut butter with added sugar, most luncheon meats (with added sugar), glazed meats, hot dogs
- Candies, sugar-sweetened gum, fudge

Figure 10–3 *How to Choose Snacks for Dental Health*

Years ago, people expected to lose their teeth in old age. Today, teens who care for their teeth have every reason to expect to be chewing with them at age 90.

 KEY POINTS *Brushing and flossing teeth and gums properly are needed to prevent tooth decay and gum disease. Some snacks help to support dental health, while others damage it.*

 SECTION 1 Review

Answer the following questions on a sheet of paper.

Learning the Vocabulary

The vocabulary terms in this section are *dental plaque, enamel, cavity, dentin, pulp cavity,* and *gum disease.*

1. The _____ is the deepest chamber of a tooth, which has blood vessels and nerves in it.
2. The tough outer layer of a tooth is called the _____.
3. Another name for dental caries is a _____.

Learning the Facts

4. How do cavities form?
5. How can gum disease be avoided?
6. How often should you schedule dental visits?

Making Life Choices

7. Why do you think some people avoid going to the dentist? What could you tell such people to convince them to go? How might a person's dental health affect the person's physical, mental, and social health?

2. Cavities are caused by acid contained in plaque. (True)
3. Cavity-forming bacteria first attack the tooth's enamel, then its pulp cavity, then its dentin. (False)
4. Gum diseases can be avoided by careful brushing and flossing. (True)
5. A toothbrush should be replaced every one to two years. (False)
6. Electric toothbrushes can be effective for people who lack the skill or strength to brush properly. (True)
7. All soft- to medium-bristled toothbrushes approved by the ADA are equally effective. (True)
8. Brushing is more effective in protecting teeth and gums than flossing once a day. (False)
9. Tooth whitening kits and toothpastes are inexpensive and effective. (False)
10. Sticky, sweet foods damage teeth. (True)

FOCUS

OUTCOMES

In this section students will learn:

1. The structure of hair and proper care procedures.

2. The structure of skin and proper care.

3. Routine cleanliness techniques for all-around body maintenance.

4. To identify cosmetic quackery and unneeded or fake health products.

FOCUS ACTIVITY

Divide the class into four groups. Assign each group one of the following topics: hair, skin, special care areas, quackery. Distribute instruction sheets for each topic, and tell students their assignment is to create a way to present their topics to the class. Choices may be an oral report, skit, center display, charts, posters, panel discussions, and so on. Give a set time to prepare and present. Instruction sheets might require that the group deal with the following aspects of its topic: natural body maintenance, personal care procedures, problems, diseases, professional help resources, drugs used, consequences of improper care, hereditary factors, and applicable statistics. Encourage the use of visual aids in presentations.

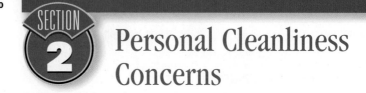

Personal Cleanliness Concerns

Along with tooth care, the care of your hair, nails, skin, ears, and eyes is important for both appearance and health. Some things such as daily bathing are too obvious to mention. Others, however, may not be learned during childhood and are important.

Care of Hair and Nails

For many, hair makes a personal statement—from dramatic shaved heads to long, glossy curls. People often choose hairstyles that reflect their personalities and lifestyles. During the identity-seeking teenage years, hairstyles can become almost an obsession. This is normal, but sellers of hair-care products may take advantage of the interest placed on hair. Learning something about hair and hair products can save you many wasted dollars.

The Nature of Hair Each hair strand is a fiber made of long, parallel strands of protein. Hair is a product made in the skin's **follicles**, vessel-like structures that contain the oil glands, the muscles that control hair movement (and also goose bumps), and the roots of hairs (see Figure 10–4). In cross-section, a strand of hair may be round (straight hair), oval (curly), or flat

Figure 10–4 Skin and Hair Structures

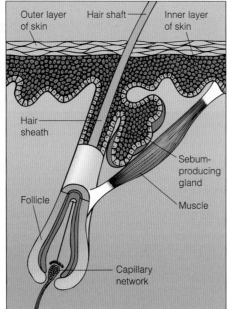

(wavy). Hair is a product of living tissue but is not alive itself. Therefore, it has no real needs of its own. It contains cells, but they are dead cells, woven into strands of protein.

Products that claim to "nourish" the hair are using the term *nourish* loosely. At best, most product ingredients sit atop the hair strands, and their effects are usually temporary. The exceptions are permanent coloring, hair straighteners, and permanent waves. These enter hair strands to change the chemical nature of the treated parts of hair.

Hair Products To keep normal hair looking healthy, simple cleansing is all that is needed. Soap would do the job, but it tends to make hair sticky. Shampoos are mild detergents that leave the hair cleaner. Shampoos vary in their effects because of their chemistry. Some are more acid, and this smoothes hair down. Some are more alkaline, and tend to fluff hair up. Choose an inexpensive one that works for you.

Shampoos for oily hair have more or stronger detergents. Those with protein additives that supposedly "repair damage" can do no such thing. Protein can be added to hair only during its creation within the hair follicles. The protein in shampoos just rinses down the drain, along with "herbal ingredients," "botanicals," and the extra money the user spent to buy them. Conditioning products may be useful, however, because they coat the hairs, mak-

COOPERATIVE LEARNING

Personal Hygiene Videos

This is a great activity that reminds students of the importance and benefits of good hygiene. Many students believe learning how to wash their hair, brush their teeth, or just cleaning themselves is boring or a waste of time.

Divide your class into groups of three or four students. Make arrangements with the audio and/or visual department in the school to supply video cameras and other audio and/or video aids. You may also need to make arrangements with the art department for poster paper and art supplies.

Have your students produce advertisements about health care products that promote good personal hygiene; these products may be ing them slide freely against one another rather than tangling. If hair becomes split or roughened from hot hair dryers, rough brushes, curling irons, or harsh chemicals (such as permanent waves, colorings, or the chlorine in swimming pools), the only cure is to trim off the damaged parts.

Controlling Dandruff Some people worry about dandruff—do they need to use dandruff-fighting shampoos? The scalp is like other skin in that it sheds bits of its thin outer layer each day. When these bits of skin are washed away daily or almost daily, they are unnoticeable. When they are allowed to build up and mix with the scalp's oils, they cling together into flakes (dandruff) and become an embarrassing social problem. By the way, no harm comes from washing your hair each day, and this alone often prevents or clears up a dandruff buildup. If regular washings with ordinary shampoo fail to control flaking, ask a pharmacist for an effective treatment.

The Nature of Nails As for nails, they are much like hair in composition. Like hair, nails grow from a root structure. Under the **cuticles** (see Figure 10–5), nail-forming cells bind together the protein **keratin** into sheets that form the nails. Once formed, nails can no longer accept protein. People who use polishes, hoping to strengthen their nails, may actually weaken them, because the solvents in polish and removers can disrupt normal nail protein structures.

Biting the free part of the nails isn't really harmful. Biting or clipping below the line of attachment, however, may start an infection that is difficult to treat and may linger for years. To stay healthy, nails need only be kept clean and trimmed.

Artificial Nails Artificial nails look nice, but they can cause problems. Nails applied incorrectly or touched up infrequently may gape away from the natural nail, leaving areas open to infection from bacteria, fungi, or wart viruses. Some infections are easily treatable. Others, however, can last for years or cause permanent nail loss. People with artificial nails should see a doctor if they notice pain, itching, redness or other discoloration, or discharge in the nail area.

To help keep your hair looking healthy, find an inexpensive shampoo that works for you.

Figure 10–5 How Fingernails Grow. *Underneath the cuticle, in the nail root, nail-forming cells collect the protein keratin. The cells then flatten and die to form the nail body.*

Nail body
Cuticle
Nail root

Glossary

follicles: vessel-like structures in the skin that contain the oil glands, the muscles that control hair movement (and also goose bumps), and the roots of hairs.

cuticles: the borders of hardened skin at the bases of the fingernails.

keratin: the normal protein of hair and nails.

made up or may be real. Have students tell their viewers about the benefits of using this product (health benefits, emotional benefits, social benefits, and so on), as well as the consequences of not using the product. Why is this product better than other products and why should people buy it over other products?

Students are to make a one-minute video advertising their product and at least one

poster. Both the video and the poster must explain how the use of the product will improve one's personal hygiene and health. Make sure that all members of the group are in the video and share somewhat equal roles.

At the conclusion, have all the groups watch the other videos and have the class vote on best advertisement, actor, and so on. This brings some fun to the class, and still offers a valuable learning experience.

GUEST SPEAKER

Invite a cosmetologist to your classroom or visit a cosmetology classroom or salon. Have the cosmetologist wash and fix a volunteer's hair, explaining proper hair care procedures as the class observes. Have the cosmetologist perform a facial. Ask him or her to speak on proper skin care as the class observes. Hold a question-and-answer session following the demonstration. Ask the class to share what they observed and learned from the demonstration. Ask the class to share some ideas for better hair and skin care, which they can include in their daily hygiene routines.

COMPREHENSION CHECK

Have students compile a class collage of advertisements that gives inaccurate or deceiving information about a product. Have them highlight the inaccurate parts of the advertisement.

GROUP PROJECT

Divide the class into six groups. On the board or overhead list the topic for each group: 1. skin; 2. special care areas—feet, hands, nails and ears; 3. hair; 4. teeth; 5. diet; 6. fitness. Give each group some plain white paper. Instruct them to design their own pamphlets about their assigned area of hygiene. They should use content, color, creative design for attractiveness and readability, cartoons, pictures, or charts to make the pamphlet one that will teach others proper care of the assigned hygiene area and be interesting and easy to read and use. Display the finished products on a classroom bulletin board.

A nail technician is licensed upon learning how to apply artificial nails safely, and clients should ask to see licenses that are not displayed. Sterilized equipment, antimicrobial hand washes, and clean work surfaces are all essential to stop the spread of infection. The work area should also be well ventilated to carry away potentially harmful fumes. Thinking safety, and not just beauty, can often help prevent problems.

Nourishing the Hair and Nails   While products do little to enhance hair and nails, proper diet helps a great deal. No nutrient supplement, not even gelatin, improves hair or nails so long as the person receives an adequate diet. However, too few nutrients from food can exert dramatic effects on nails. The body conserves nutrients when they run low. It meets essential functions, such as making immune system cells, before it spends resources making "optional" products such as hair or fingernails. Young people who go on "crash" weight-loss diets often begin losing their hair after a few weeks or months. Their fingernails may also become cracked or odd-shaped.

Hair loss and changes in fingernails are two early signs of malnutrition. Dietitians in a hospital are trained to watch for these signs. The most effective way to ensure that hair and nails look their best is to nourish the whole body. If the cells that make hair and nails are in top condition, and are given plenty of materials with which to build, the healthiest possible hair and nails are assured.

Some over-the-counter acne treatments are worth a try.

 KEY POINTS   *Hair and nails grow from root structures and are made mostly of protein. Once formed, they do not have the same needs as living tissues do. Cleanliness of hair and nails is important, but cosmetic products are unnecessary. During their formation, both hair and nails are sensitive to malnutrition.*

Help for Acne

No one knows why some people get **acne** and others do not. However, it is known to run in families. If both your parents had acne, the odds are high of your having it, too. The hormones of adolescence also play a role by making the glands in the skin more active.

How Pimples Form   Acne is related to the skin's natural oil, **sebum**. Sebum is made all the time in deep glands and is supposed to flow out of the glands to the skin's surface through the tiny ducts around the hairs. In acne, the oil is not brought to the surface of the skin.

Each of the ducts is lined with a skinlike tissue that normally sheds by scaling and flaking. The oil carries these scales and flakes to the surface of the skin. At times, the scales stick together and form a plug, halting the flow of oil and allowing bacteria to migrate down into the duct. As the plug grows bigger, it weak-

Focusing ON Self-Esteem

Feeling satisfied with one's appearance is a major factor in positive self-esteem for teens. Practical information and specific details for taking care of the body are important. You might want to contact a local cosmetologist to demonstrate proper hair and nail care for your students. If the cosmotologist cannot come personally, perhaps she or he might send visual aids such as posters, brochures, or product samples for you to share with your class.

Be sure that students understand that there is much they can do to enhance the appearance of their hair and nails without buying lots of expensive products.

ens the duct, allowing oil and bacteria to leak into the surrounding skin. The oil and bacteria irritate the skin and cause redness, swelling, and **pus** formation—the beginning of a **whitehead**, or pimple. A **cyst** may be formed—a sort of enlarged, deep pimple. The skin may open above the plug, revealing an accumulation of dark skin pigments just below the surface—a **blackhead**.

Many people think skin bacteria cause acne, but they do not. Bacteria make it worse, once the process has begun. Also, the color of a blackhead is caused by pigments, not by dirt, so cleanliness alone isn't the answer. Squeezing or picking at pimples to try to remove their contents does not help. In fact, it can cause more scars than the acne itself does.

Treating Acne   How, then, can you treat acne? Most young people with acne are willing to go to considerable trouble and expense to find a remedy. Many remedies have been suggested: washing constantly, sunbathing, taking antibiotics, spreading prescription acne medicines on the skin, avoiding certain foods and beverages, avoiding **comedogenic** cosmetics, or obtaining relief from stress. Each of these has helped some people. However, everyone responds differently to them. Nothing works for everyone.

Some products are worth a try. Among the over-the-counter treatments for mild acne are those that contain one of the following effective ingredients:

- ▶ Benzoyl peroxide.
- ▶ Salicylic acid.
- ▶ Resorcinol.
- ▶ Sulfur.

These ingredients have been proved safe and effective. However, they may have side effects such as drying or irritating the skin. Careful washing twice daily with mild soap helps remove skin-surface bacteria and oil and helps to keep the oil ducts open.

People who fail to find relief from their acne will try almost anything. Before trying unproved "therapies," read this chapter's Consumer Skills feature (on the next page) for hints about detecting the tricks used by quacks. The price of valid medical help is small when compared with the dangers that may lurk in a fraud's potions.

If nonprescription methods fail to clear up acne, see a **dermatologist** for a prescription medication. Antibiotics may be either applied on the skin's surface or taken internally. Retin-A cream works because it contains an acid that loosens the plugs that form in the ducts. The oil is then able to flow again so that the ducts will not burst. A new prescription gel is called Differin. So far, Differin seems as effective as Retin-A, but may be less irritating to the skin.

Skin clearing may begin within a month or so of using the prescribed products. Both drugs make the skin more easily damaged by sunlight and may cause drying or peeling. These side effects may make the acne look worse at first.

Accutane is an internal medicine reserved for severe acne that scars the skin. Its effectiveness for reversing severe acne is so high that for some people the drug is hailed as a miracle.

The miracle can involve risks, though. Side effects range from irritation and drying of the nose, mouth, and skin to miscarriage in pregnant women. Birth defects in infants of women who take Accutane during pregnancy are also possible.

Glossary

acne: a continuing condition of inflamed skin ducts and glands, with a buildup of oils under the skin, forming pimples.

sebum (SEE-bum): the skin's natural oil—actually a mixture of oils and waxes—that helps keep the skin and hair moist.

pus: a mixture of fluids and white blood cells that collects around infected areas.

whitehead: a pimple filled with pus, caused by the plugging of oil-gland ducts with shed material from the duct lining.

cyst (SIST): an enlarged, deep pimple.

blackhead: an open pimple with dark skin pigments (not dirt) in its opening.

comedogenic (coh-MEE-doh-JEN-ick): causing acne.

dermatologist: a physician (M.D.) who specializes in treating conditions of the skin.

BACKGROUND INFORMATION

Distribute the "Personal Care Products Shopping Analysis" handout from the Teacher's Resource Box. Instruct the students to go shopping for personal care products. They must choose one for skin, hair, eyes, ears, and one cosmetic/make-up type item. Have them complete the worksheet on their own. Labels will have to be read and information recorded at the store. Products do not have to be purchased. Encourage the students to choose items they do not usually use or have at home.

DISCUSSION

How many students have tried the different acne remedies mentioned here? What additional remedies have students tried? Which products seem to be most effective?

BACKGROUND INFORMATION

You may want to tell students that women who require accutane should make sure they are not pregnant before starting use of the drug. Accutane has been associated with miscarriage and birth defects.

Remind students that a well-balanced diet is a first step toward healthy hair and nails. Shampooing hair often to keep it oil and dirt free is important. For nail care, you might share the following list with students.

- Wear gloves for work during which your hands will be in water for long periods of time.

- Wear gloves for rough work like weeding flowerbeds or mowing the lawn.
- Use oil on your nails to discourage brittle nails.
- Keep nails manicured.
- Never bite your nails.
- Don't use your finger nails as tools.

Tricks, Traps, Quacks, and Gimmicks

Consumer SKILLS

Many advertisements twist the truth to dream up problems for us, or to make small problems seem large. Then they twist the truth again to make us think that they have just the solutions we need for these problems. Suppose you have a few freckles (or a thousand). A television commercial might start there, and take these steps:

- ► You have freckles. (So far, that's true.)
- ► Freckles make you look younger than you are. (This is, at most, only partly true, and it's not a problem.)
- ► That's a problem. (The commercial wants you to think freckles are a problem, so that it can go on to say . . .)
- ► You need Product X to hide those freckles.

People buy many Product Xs they don't need because they believe the twisted advertisements.

A common case of created problems is premenstrual syndrome (PMS), which has been said to "disable" women before their menstrual periods each month. PMS is not a made-up problem. It does seriously affect some women (see page 278). Advertisers make it out to be more common than it is, though, and claim that it needs treatment when it does not. Women are led to think that anyone who menstruates needs to buy PMS remedies. Only an informed critical thinker can recognize the difference between a real need and a created one.

Other gimmicks to get your attention include personal reports, opinions, exaggerations, vague statements that hide the facts, and glowing reports from people who have tried products and saw improvement

from the placebo effect. Other claims familiar to television watchers are:

- ► Our product is better than theirs (brand loyalty appeal).
- ► Everyone uses our product (peer pressure appeal).
- ► Rich and famous people use our product (snob appeal).
- ► You'll receive bonuses and free items if you buy our product (bribery).
- ► Our product is new and improved (newness appeal).
- ► Ordinary people use our product (just-plain-folks appeal).
- ► Funny, happy people use our product (smile appeal).
- ► Beautiful people use our product (beauty appeal).
- ► Scientific people approve our product (appeal to reason).

Quacks also offer special machines (special technology), secret formulas (mysterious chemistry), and medical "breakthroughs" (miracles and magic for the child in everyone). These selling techniques work. Otherwise, they would not be used.

Critical Thinking

1. *Do you think such advertisements have ever worked with you or someone you know?*
2. *Have you ever bought useless products because of an advertisement?*
3. *With so many grasping fingers reaching for your wallet, how can you protect yourself?*

Acne Prevention Many people think that certain foods and drinks worsen their acne. Chocolate, cola beverages, fatty or greasy foods, nuts, sugar, and foods or salt containing iodine have all been blamed for worsening acne. It's not proved that these foods do worsen acne. If they do seem to affect your skin, however, there's no harm in avoiding them.

Some cosmetics do cause acne flare-ups in susceptible people, so a change of products may be worth a try. Stress clearly worsens acne by way of the hormones that are secreted in response to it. Vacations from school or other pressures slow secretion of stress hormones and so help to bring relief. The sun, the beach, and swimming also seem to help. The sun's rays kill bacteria. Swimming can help cleanse the skin. Avoid excessive sun exposure, though; it can cause skin cancer.

One remedy always works: time. Acne is most common among teenagers and young adults. While waiting for acne to clear up, keep the symptoms under control with treatments that work for you.

 Acne results from a buildup of sebum and flakes of skin that get trapped in the skin's ducts. Cleanliness and relief from stress may help control it. Nothing but time is a permanent cure.

Ear Piercing, Body Piercing, and Tattooing

Recently, fashion has promoted the piercing of not just earlobes, but of upper ears, lips, noses, and, in fact, just about any other body part. Tattooing, an ancient art of decorating the skin by injecting permanent dyes into it, recently became popular again. Both these practices require making puncture wounds to the skin, so both present the danger of infection.

Some body parts are prone to infections. The upper ear is mostly cartilage, with little blood flowing through it. If bacteria enter the upper ear when pierced, they can grow with little opposition from the white blood cells and antibodies that normally would destroy them. Such infections are difficult to treat, and have left some teenagers with scarred, malformed ears. Moist body areas, such as the nose or mouth, also make easy targets for infections.

Diseases such as hepatitis or AIDS can be spread by the use of unsanitary equipment. Viruses survive in the tiniest traces of blood left on piercing and tattooing needles. A practitioner who sterilizes equipment between clients, wears latex gloves, and never reuses needles minimizes this danger.

Many people discover, too late, that tattoos are much more easily acquired than removed. Techniques such as laser surgeries, scraping away the skin with wire brushes, or burning the skin away with acids often remove tattoos. However, they leave visible scars. Anyone considering a tattoo might try a temporary one first. Advantage: You don't need surgery to get rid of it.

 Fashion that demands puncturing the body brings risks of local infections and infectious diseases. Sanitation measures reduce these risks.

Eyes and Ears

Sight and hearing are easy to take for granted, especially when they are working perfectly. Your eyes and ears are designed to serve you throughout life and will do so with just a little careful treatment and common sense.

Eyes   The eyes have imperfect defenses against the sun's ultraviolet rays. When out-of-doors in bright sun, or for long times, wear sunglasses that screen such rays out. Never look directly into the sun.

For Your Information

Eye Cosmetics—Safety Tips

▶ Remove eye makeup before sleeping. Mascara can flake into the eye during sleep to cause infection or injury.
▶ Keep makeup containers closed when not in use to keep bacteria out.
▶ Store makeup in a dark, cool place to protect its preservatives.
▶ If you develop an eye infection, don't use makeup. Throw away any makeup you were using when you discovered the infection.
▶ Throw away any makeup if the color or consistency changes, or an off-odor develops. These may be signs that the product has spoiled.
▶ Don't keep any eye makeup for longer than six months.
▶ Never share eye makeup.

hygiene. Review each section of the chapter as needed to make sure all areas are included. Discuss with students the cycle that can develop when people have serious difficulties. For example: A man is out of work. The family struggles to maintain their usual lifestyle for as long as possible, but ends up losing their home. The money or facilities for good daily hygiene are not available, and as a result it is embarrassing to go for job interviews.

Without work, the family can't reestablish those good hygiene habits. . . and the cycle continues.

If possible, have students make a list and bring items from home to put into kits to be donated to those who need them. You may want to have a fund-raising event to earn money for the purchase of the items to be donated.

***Figure 10–6** Healthy and Damaged Ears.*

A. *This inner ear had healthy nerve cells and the person had normal hearing.*

B. *This ear was exposed to loud noise, which damaged the nerve cells and caused permanent hearing loss. Notice that the hairlike nerve structures are missing along the bottom of the ear canal.*

***Figure 10–7** A Noise Thermometer. This shows the time required to damage hearing at various noise levels. The scale on the thermometer is marked off in decibels, the unit of measure for sound.*

Source: Adapted from Noise Thermometer, *Know* Noise, Copyright 1993, Sight and Hearing Association, St. Paul, MN. All rights reserved.

On the other hand, the eyes are well defended against infection and injury by the brows, lids, lashes, and tears. If something does get into the eye and tears don't wash it out, hold the eye open and gently drop plain, clean water or a commercial eyewash into the lower or upper lid.

Contact lenses, because they are applied directly to the eye, require careful handling. They must be cleaned thoroughly each day, as directed by the prescribing physician. If left in overnight, contacts are very likely to cause an eye infection, even if the lenses are the kind recommended for extended wearing. Girls who use eye makeup, and especially those who also wear contacts, should take note of the tips in the margin of the previous page.

Some vision problems can be corrected by surgery. Surgery to correct nearsightedness requires that small cuts be made in the eye's clear outer layer, the cornea, to reshape it. Once healed, the eye's new shape allows clearer distance vision, often without glasses. Some people must have repeat surgeries to make small adjustments. Some may require reading glasses at an earlier age than normal. However, most also find the surgery helpful.

Noise and Hearing   The ears cannot shut out loud noises, which can injure their delicate inner structures and impair hearing (see Figure 10–6). Many people, even young children, have hearing loss and are not even aware of it. Hearing loss caused by noise gets worse with repeated exposures, and damage to the inner ear lasts for life. Figure 10–7 points out some dangerous noise levels.

After the ears have been exposed to loud sound, words may sound muffled, or the ears may ring. These are two ways that your ears can tell you that the sound was harmful. Some hearing is destroyed every day at rock concerts, on hunting trips, at construction sites, and even at loud pep rallies.

The best way to prevent such damage is to stay away from loud sound. If that is impossible, wear commercially made earmuffs or earplugs. As soon as possible, move away from the loud sound to give the ears a rest.

Pursuing **wellness**

Tell students that it is important to check the health of the eyes, ears, nose, and throat before beginning an exercise program. Students may wonder why this is so. Tell students that their eyes help them to be able to see dangers and hazards that they may encounter during an exercise program. If they have difficulty seeing uneven ground or some object in the path while jogging, they may become injured.

Their ears allow students to be aware of

To protect vision, shield the eyes from the sun's ultraviolet rays and gently remove any foreign objects that get into the eyes. To protect hearing, avoid loud noises.

Avoiding Body Odor

Everyone knows to bathe daily to remove the collected sweat and grime of the day. Some may wonder, though, whether they need products to help them stay clean: underarm antiperspirants or deodorants, vaginal sprays, douches, scented powders, or cologne. The truth is that none of these products are needed for *health*. Most simply mask odors for a while.

Body odor is caused by the action of normal skin bacteria on sweat and skin debris. Soap makes bacteria slippery enough to be washed away. While no threat to health, unpleasant odors may make others withdraw and damage a person's self-esteem. People who perspire heavily may want to use antiperspirants to reduce the sweat that feeds the bacteria that cause body odor. Also, a deodorant may help a little to mask any odor that may form during the day. Antiperspirants and deodorants are not substitutes for cleanliness, though. Even the most aromatic ones cannot mask an unclean odor.

Both male and female external reproductive organs require a careful daily washing to keep them free of infections and odors. An unpleasant discharge or bad odor may indicate an infection and should be checked out by a physician.

 Cleanliness is the key to freedom from body odors. Some people may want to use antiperspirants or deodorants, but most other products are unneeded.

Menstrual Concerns

A healthy vagina cleans itself. Even during **menstruation**, gentle external cleaning is all that is needed. "Personal deodorant" sprays are not needed, and **douches** can be downright dangerous. Douching interrupts the normal cleaning cycle and may wash bacteria up into the normally bacteria-free areas of the reproductive tract. (Douching has been linked with reproductive tract cancer, but it is uncertain whether douching can *cause* cancer.) Women should know that the vagina can easily become infected with the normal bacteria from the digestive tract. Soiled toilet paper should be kept away from the vaginal area.

Many women use tampons to absorb menstrual flow internally. They should be aware that while using tampons is convenient, the user stands a risk of developing **toxic shock syndrome (TSS)**. TSS develops when bacteria begin to break down the menstrual blood trapped inside the vagina. These bacteria release dangerous poisons that are absorbed into the blood, causing high fever and a sunburn-like rash. The way to avoid TSS from tampons is to not use tampons, of course. However, some women choose to use tampons anyway. They can reduce TSS risk by using the lowest absorbency needed to control menstrual flow, changing the tampons every four to eight hours, and alternating their use with pads.

Pads or sanitary napkins are used to collect menstrual flow externally. Pads should be changed every four to eight hours (depending on menstrual

> ❝ *Henry IV's feet and armpits enjoyed an international reputation.* ❞
>
> Aldous Huxley
> (1864–1963)
> English novelist and critic

menstruation: the monthly shedding of the uterine lining in nonpregnant females.

douches (DOOSH-es): preparations sold to cleanse the vagina. Actually, vaginas clean themselves constantly with no help. Douches can wash dangerous bacteria into the reproductive tract.

toxic shock syndrome (TSS): a type of poisoning that can occur when bacteria break down menstrual blood; often associated with use of super-absorbent tampons.

unseen dangers such as traffic, dogs, running water, or machinery. The ears also need to function well for communication during team sports and for verbal warnings in activities such as racquetball or snow skiing.

The nose may alert them to a potential hazard such as fire or a chemical leak. It is also important for the nose to function well for air exchange during endurance-type exercise. The throat needs to function well in order to transport sufficient air to the lungs.

INTERDISCIPLINARY ACTIVITY: HISTORICAL RESEARCH

In coordination with the history/social science department, have the students research the ways in which people in the past have dealt with the personal hygiene issues that have been presented in this section (acne, fingernails, body odor, and so on). Have the students write a short report and present it to the class. Evaluate the report in terms of historical accuracy and presentation style. You may want to have a representative of the social science department come into class to assist you in the evaluation.

ASSESS

EVALUATE

Provide a cross-section diagram, or have the students draw their own, of a hair follicle and skin structure. Have them label the parts: blood vessels, oil gland, hair follicle, sweat gland, and skin layers. Have a class discussion about the effect these glands and parts play in the cleanliness of the body.

SECTION 2 Review Answers

1. dermatologist (p. 273)
2. cyst (p. 273)
3. Keratin (p. 271)
4. Sebum is the skin's natural oil that can cause acne. (p. 272)
5. premenstrual syndrome (p. 278)
6. because the only time protein can be added to hair is during its creation (p. 270)
7. It may cause a loss of hair. (p. 272)
8. Answers will vary; could include: those that contain benzoyl peroxide, resorcinol, salicyclic acid, or sulfur. (p. 273)
9. Answers will vary. Refer to Consumer Skills on page 274 for possible answers.
10. to prevent bacterial growth, which leads to toxic shock syndrome (p. 277)
11. Answers will vary.

A reproducible quiz for Section 2 is provided in the Teacher's Resource Box.

CLOSE

Utilize the students' displays, reports, collages, and analyses to review. If you have kept cooperative groups the same throughout the series of assignments, assign each group a specific personal care area (hair, skin, and so on) to report on. The group will compile its resources on that area. Each group will give an oral presentation of its findings.

flow) to prevent bacterial growth. Bacteria cause odor when they break down menstrual blood externally.

Girls and women who menstruate may experience normal contractions of the muscular uterus—**menstrual cramps**. Some find relief from the over-the-counter drug ibuprofen. Should cramping become severe, a health-care provider should check for problems.

Some symptoms, such as nervousness, cramping, moodiness, and fatigue, may announce the menstrual period several days in advance of bleeding. Called **premenstrual syndrome (PMS)**, such symptoms can be a problem for some women. PMS often responds to simple remedies such as getting enough rest, exercise, relaxation, and nourishing food. No vitamin pills of any sort are effective against PMS. However, reducing intakes of colas, iced tea, and other caffeine sources may help.

Many other products are on store shelves, sold for many reasons. Don't be misled by sellers trying to force unneeded products on you.

 KEY POINTS *For health, bodies need only routine cleansing. Feminine sprays, powders, and perfumes may be enjoyable, but are not essential.*

SECTION 2 Review

Answer the following questions on a sheet of paper.

Learning the Vocabulary

The vocabulary terms in this section are *follicles, cuticles, keratin, acne, sebum, pus, whitehead, cyst, blackhead, comedogenic, dermatologist, menstruation, douches, toxic shock syndrome (TSS), menstrual cramps,* and *premenstrual syndrome (PMS).*

1. A _____ is a physician who specializes in treating conditions of the skin.
2. An enlarged, deep pimple is a _____.
3. _____ is the protein of hair and nails.
4. How are acne and sebum related?
5. Physical discomfort, moodiness, and nervousness can be signs of _____.

Learning the Facts

6. Why are protein additives in shampoos ineffective in repairing damaged hair?
7. How does malnutrition affect hair?
8. Name two over-the-counter treatment ingredients that are effective for acne.
9. List three gimmicks that are commonly used to sell health products.
10. Why is it important to change tampons at least every four to eight hours?

Making Life Choices

11. Look at advertisements for skin-care products on television or in magazines. What tactics or gimmicks are used in the ads to try to get you to use their products? If you have used any of the products, do you think they are as effective as the ads claim? Why or why not?

Chapter 10, Section 2

The following quiz will help you assess your students' understanding of the material covered in this section of the chapter. You might use the quiz as an oral exercise, which will lead into a class discussion of the topics covered. Or, you might use it as a paper/pencil

quiz to evaluate your students individually.

*If students have difficulty with the concepts covered in the Quick Quiz and the Section Review, you might suggest they review the material using the **S**urvey, **Q**uestion, **R**ead, **R**ecite, **R**eview (SQ3R) study method, which is described in detail in the introduction to this Teacher's Wraparound Edition.*

1. Hair is made of strands of protein and is

Posture and Image

Why is it that some people seem to radiate energy, have a bounce in their step, and seem to be a picture of high self-esteem. They have good posture. One of the best things proper posture does is give a person that energetic, positive look.

The Health of the Spine   The way you walk, sit, and sleep greatly affects your skeleton over the years. The bones and cartilage disks of your **spine** are sensitive, as those who have had even a twinge of back pain are aware. Think of your spine as a set of 33 delicate, hollow bones **(vertebrae)** stacked up on one another like doughnuts with pads between them (the cartilage disks). Think of your spinal cord running right up through the holes in the doughnuts. (A difference from doughnuts is that the holes in the vertebrae are near their edges, not at the center.)

Major nerves exit and enter the spaces between vertebrae. If the bones or cartilage disks are damaged, they can bulge out and pinch those nerves (see Figure 10–8). The result is stabbing pain, like an electric shock, torturing the muscles of the neck, shoulders, back, or legs.

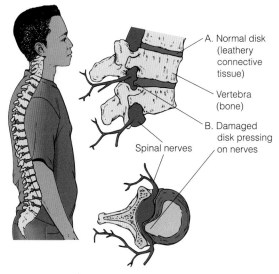

A. Normal disk (leathery connective tissue)

Vertebra (bone)

B. Damaged disk pressing on nerves

Spinal nerves

Normal curve of the spine. When the bones are stacked this way, the disks bear the weight evenly, and the nerves feel the least pressure.

Figure 10–8 The Spinal Column

MINI
Glossary

menstrual cramps: contractions of the uterus, during and a few days before menstruation, that may cause pain.

premenstrual syndrome (PMS): symptoms such as physical discomfort, moodiness, and nervousness that occur in some women each month before menstruation.

spine: the stack of 33 vertebrae that form the backbone and hold the spinal cord, whose nerves enter and exit through spaces between the bones.

vertebrae (VERT-eh-bray; singular, **vertebra**): the delicate, hollow bones of the spine.

FOCUS

OUTCOME

In this section students will learn:

1. The importance of good posture and a healthy spine.

FOCUS ACTIVITY

Have the students design a questionnaire to interview someone about common back ailments. Have the students do research on the ailment(s) they learned about. Also suggest they research treatment and preventative measures for this ailment.

TEACH & APPLY

TEACHER SUPPORT

Key Passage
Tell students that at birth spinal columns consist of 33 vertebrae separated into 5 different types: 7 cervical, 12 thoracic, 5 lumbar, 5 sacral, and 4 coccygeal. In adults, the sacral vertebrae will fuse into a single sacrum and the coccygeal vertebrae will fuse to form a coccyx. The result is an adult spinal column of 26 separate bones.

produced in the skin's follicles. (True)

2. Hair is living tissue. (False)

3. Acne is caused by the skin's natural oil sebum. (True)

4. Blackheads are caused by skin bacteria. (False)

5. Certain medicines, stress-reduction, skin-cleansing, time, and sunshine can all help to reduce acne. (True)

6. Tattoos and body piercing bring risks of

infection. (True)

7. The eyes are naturally protected from the sun's ultraviolet rays. (False)

8. Loud noise can cause permanent damage to the ear. (True)

9. Deodorants are an effective substitute for daily cleansing. (False)

10. Tampons increase the risk of toxic shock syndrome (TSS). (True)

GROUP ACTIVITY

Divide the students into groups of four or five. Assign each group to construct a model of a human spine using household materials (blocks, toothpicks, pieces of wood, bottle caps, popsicle sticks, and so on). Instruct them to simulate a head on top of the 7 cervical, 12 thoracic, and 5 lumbar vertebrae, plus the sacrum and coccyx to show the normal curve and weight-bearing construction of the back.

CLASS ACTIVITY

Four different areas in which students can evaluate and possibly correct improper posture are shown in this illustration. Have students write the four areas (sleeping, sitting, standing, and walking) down the left side of a sheet of paper leaving several lines of space between each heading. For each heading have them pick the illustration that most closely matches their most typical posture. They should then describe whether or not they are satisfied with their posture in that area, whether or not they have had any trouble with their backs, and what they will try to do if they are not satisfied with their posture or have experienced back pain.

BACKGROUND INFORMATION

Use a model of the back to teach the structure of the vertebrae, names of its parts, and the weight-bearing responsibility of the back. Instruct students on which muscles surround the back area and the physiology of these. Point out the relationship of these to the abdominal muscles, as well.

Figure 10–9 *Care of the Spine*

enrichment....

Share with students the following information about low-back pain.

Most low-back pain is caused by mechanical factors such as poor posture, excess body weight, and generally poor physical fitness.

To combat low-back pain, proper standing, lying-down, and sitting postures are important. (Refer students to Figure 10–9.) Have students work in pairs to check their standing posture. When a student is standing properly, the partner should be able to draw an imagi-

Preventing Spinal Damage Eight out of ten adults have at least one episode of back pain bad enough to send them to a doctor. People who don't get enough exercise are the most likely victims. As their back and abdominal muscles become weak, their spines tend to become less well supported and slip out of shape. Happily, most such back problems are preventable with proper posture and exercise. Posture do's and don'ts are shown in Figure 10–9. Chapter 9 provided guidance about how to safely strengthen the abdomen and back.

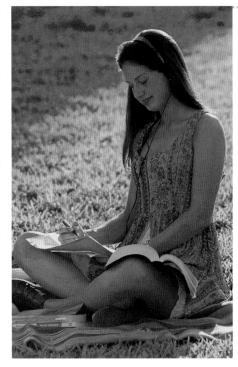

People with good posture seem to radiate energy and high self-esteem.

 Correct posture improves the way a person looks and helps protect the health of the spine.

Review

Answer the following questions on a sheet of paper.

Learning the Vocabulary

The vocabulary terms in this section are *spine* and *vertebrae*.

1. The _____ is made up of the _____, which are hollow bones.

Learning the Facts

2. What three things affect your skeleton over the years?

3. Which people are most at risk for developing back pain?

4. Why is sleeping on your back not recommended?

5. Besides improving the health of the spine, why is good posture important?

Making Life Choices

6. Spend a few minutes observing the posture of people as they walk, sit, or stand. What does their posture say about them? Think about your own posture. What does it say about you? Does it need to be improved? If so, how can you go about improving it?

Answers to FACT or FICTION

Here are the answers to the questions at the start of the chapter.

1. False. Dental plaque is a sticky substance that builds up on teeth, damaging them.
2. True.
3. False. Although cleanliness is important, there are no simple answers to preventing or curing acne.
4. True.
5. True.
6. True.
7. False. False advertisements sound convincing, and many people fail to see through them.

nary straight line from the ear lobe to the outside of the ankle bone. Students should stand against a wall with their backs pressed against it for this activity.

Exercises to develop low-back and abdominal muscles will help prevent low-back pain. Exercises to develop physical endurance will not only help a person lose weight, but will also give increased energy. In turn, this will help with good posture because physically fit people are less inclined to slouch.

SECTION 4

FOCUS

OUTCOMES

In this section students will learn:

1. When a person needs to see a doctor.

2. When a person does not need to consult a professional physician

FOCUS ACTIVITY

Ask students to name and describe the duties of as many health-care providers as possible.

TEACH & APPLY

BACKGROUND INFORMATION

Have students choose one of the health-care providers identified in the Focus Activity and research that occupation. Students should report back to class on the educational requirements, the duties, and any other interesting facts they can find about the particular health-care provider.

DISCUSSION

Ask students why it is just as important to know when NOT to go to the doctor as to know when to go. (excessive, unnecessary costs)

Are Your Immunizations Up to Date?

On separate paper, answer yes (Y) if you've been immunized for all that apply to you. If you answered no (N) and the description applies to you, ask a parent or school nurse about it. Your answers to the Life Choice Inventory are personal and private. Share them with others only if you are comfortable doing so.

Age:	Vaccine:	Response:	
Birth	Hepatitis B (Hep B)	Y	N
2 months	DTP (diphtheria, tetanus, pertussis) HIB (haemophilus influenza, type b), oral polio, Hep B	Y	N
4 months	DTP, HIB, oral polio	Y	N
6 months	DTP, HIB	Y	N
12 months	Tuberculin test, Hep B		
15 months	MMR (measles, mumps, rubella), HIB, DTP, oral polio, chicken pox (varicella zoster virus, or VZV)[a]	Y	N
4 to 6 years	DTP, oral polio, MMR	Y	N
11 to 12 years	MMR (if not given at age 4 to 6), VZV (if not given at 15 months), Hep B (if not given during infancy)	Y	N
14 to 16 years	Tetanus-diphtheria toxoid, adult type; booster every ten years or after a contaminated wound if more than five years have passed since the previous injection.	Y	N

[a]Chicken pox (varicella zoster virus, or VZV): a relatively new vaccine for children 12 to 18 months old who have not had chicken pox. Older children who have not had the disease can receive the vaccine at any time, preferably before age 13. Recommended, but not yet a required vaccine.

CRITICAL THINKING

Tell students that only about 33 percent of all doctors today are family physicians, general internists, and pediatricians. Only 17 percent of all medical school graduates are choosing to become generalists. In comparison, in England 73 percent of physicians are generalists. Is the trend toward specialists (surgeons, oncologists, dermatologists, and so on) good or bad for the students as patients?

Divide the class into two groups: One group that says there should be more general

SECTION 4

When to Visit a Health-Care Provider

Part of caring for yourself involves seeking help from a health-care provider when needed. For one thing, growing children and teens need to be checked to make sure they are growing as expected and to receive their **immunizations** on time. This chapter's Life Choice Inventory challenges you to think about your own immunization history.

Almost as important as knowing when to go see a health-care provider is knowing when *not* to go. One time not to go is when you have an ordinary cold. You also need *not* go if you have:

- ► A mild rash without other symptoms.
- ► A single episode of vomiting or diarrhea without abdominal pain.
- ► A temperature of 102 degrees Fahrenheit (39 degrees centigrade) or less.
- ► Other mild self-limiting ailments, such as a mild headache.
- ► A condition treatable with self-care and over-the-counter medications (see the next chapter).

As for when *to* see a health-care provider, Figure 10–10 provides some guidelines.

See a health-care provider for:

1. Temperature above 102 degrees Fahrenheit.
2. Any serious accident or injury.
3. Any fall with possible injury.
4. Sudden severe pain in the abdomen.
5. Breathing difficulty.
6. Loss of consciousness, even if brief.
7. Severe headache for more than two hours.
8. Intense itch.
9. Bleeding with unknown cause. (Blood in vomit or stools may appear dark; blood in urine may appear pink.)
10. Faintness; dizziness; abnormal pulse; abnormal breathing; cold or clammy skin; bluish cast to lips or fingernails.
11. Sudden loss of mental ability, vision (especially a halo effect), hearing, touch, or ability to move.
12. Any symptoms after taking medication.
13. Diarrhea or vomiting for a day or more.
14. Any symptom, even if mild, lasting longer than a week or two, or one that recurs.

Figure 10–10 *When to Ask for Medical Help*

KEY POINTS *Knowing when to get medical help is an important part of maintaining your body.*

SECTION 4 Review

Answer the following questions on a sheet of paper.

Learning the Vocabulary

The vocabulary term in this section is *immunizations*.

1. Write a sentence using this term.

Learning the Facts

2. List some symptoms of illnesses or injuries that indicate the need to seek medical help.

Making Life Choices

3. Check with your parents to find out if your immunizations are up to date. If there are any that are not current, discuss how and when they should be updated.

MINI Glossary

immunizations: injected or oral doses of medicine that stimulate the immune system to develop the long-term ability to quickly fight off infectious diseases; also called *vaccinations*.

physicians, and one that says more general physicians aren't necessary. Arguments of the first group could include: Most people don't need specialized care; if general physicians had fewer patients they could be more involved, thus helping prevent the need to go to a specialist. Arguments for the second group could include: People with complicated conditions need doctors in that specialty for better care; research into new techniques might slow down if more doctors were only general physicians.

Background Information

For enrichment, tell students that people appear to be somewhat alert even while asleep. Studies have shown that people are more likely to wake up if their own names are spoken; sleeping mothers seem to be more responsive to soft noises from their children than other loud noises; and some subjects in studies have even learned to touch a switch to avoid electric shocks, while still asleep.

Background Information

You may want to expand upon this discussion of sleeping pills. Tell students drugs create a dependence, as well as interfere with normal sleep patterns. This combination can leave a person exhausted and hooked. Better than taking drugs is to find the cause of the insomnia, with a health care provider if necessary. The most common cause is pain or discomfort. Other causes are anxiety, change of surroundings, change in schedule, caffeine, alcohol, and nicotine. Possible cures are changing bedding, relaxation exercises, "white" noise (air conditioner or fan), maintaining a regular daily schedule, exercise, and bedtime rituals (snacks, boring books, counting, and so on).

Straight Talk

The Night Shift: Our Need for Sleep

During sleep, people recover from physical and emotional stresses and injuries. They also dream. Chapter 1 said that people who had regular, adequate sleep were physically younger for their years than people who did not. This Straight Talk explores the importance of sleep and tells what is known about its effects on the health of the body.

What exactly does sleep do for me?

This question is difficult to answer. Even though people spend a third of their lives sleeping, no one seems to know for sure what goes on during all that time. However, we know some of the things that happen physically: the blood pressure falls, breathing and heartbeat slow down, the muscles relax, and the body temperature falls. Perhaps most important, growth hormone is released at almost no time other than during sleep. Growth hormone provides for growth and renewal of body cells. It is probably growth hormone that brings about the physical recovery that sleep brings.

What happens if a person doesn't get enough sleep?

All body systems work less and less well. People become irritable, can't concentrate, think and learn more slowly, and lose coordination. If deprived of sleep long enough, people may start feeling confused, begin seeing imaginary things, or even feel that they are going insane. Irregular sleep or chronic lack of sleep over years can shorten life. Other problems with too little sleep include fatigue, reduced ability to work, reduced infection-fighting immunity, and

increased risks of heart disease and digestive disorders. A few reports suggest that going without sleep for many months may even prove fatal, although such reports are extremely rare.

People who do not sleep enough at night tend to nod off during the day. This can be dangerous if they are driving. Drivers who fall asleep at the wheel cause 6,000 auto-related deaths a year.

Does everybody need eight hours of sleep a night?

People's sleep needs vary. About 2 percent of adults habitually sleep ten hours a night, and some even more. Children need more than eight hours a night. Babies sleep 16 hours or even more; most adults, about six to seven hours. Teenagers may need as much as nine and a half hours to feel fully rested. These differences seem to reflect the rate of cell growth, which is fastest in the young and which slows throughout life. Amazingly, though, by the age of 60, you will have slept for about 20 years of your life.

I've heard that an hour of sleep before midnight is worth two afterward, but I rarely get to bed before 11 o'clock.

There's nothing special about the hour of midnight. Teenagers often get sleepy later than young children, and may naturally want to sleep later in the morning. It is true, however, that early hours of sleep are "deeper" than others, and therefore more restful.

You go through several stages during sleep. First, after you start to sleep, your body temperature falls, and your brain slows its activity. At this point, you may suddenly jerk half awake—the sign of a sudden burst of brain activity that signals the start of the first stage of sleep. During the first stage of sleep, your

284

Pursuing wellness

Ask students if they routinely do anything for the purpose of maintaining good health and preventing disease. List all of the behaviors

they mention on the board. Many of the students may overlook some basic things such as sleep and hygiene procedures (bathing, brushing their teeth, and so on).

Ask if any students have ever had a severe toothache. Can they describe the pain to muscles relax, and your heartbeat slows down.

Minutes later, you enter the second stage of sleep. Brain activity slows still more. Your eyes roll from side to side, but if they were to open, they would not see. This lasts for about half an hour.

The third and fourth stages of sleep bring very slow brain activity, relaxed muscles, and even breathing. This is the deepest sleep of all. It occurs mostly in the early hours of a night's sleep.

It is during the deepest stage that **REM sleep** occurs. (REM stands for "rapid eye movements.") The rapid eye movements seem to reflect dreaming, as if the person's eyes were following the actions of the dreams. You cycle several times a night through REM, into other stages of sleep, and back into REM.

 That's amazing. I had no idea so much was going on while I was asleep. What do you suppose it's all for?

We don't know. But we do know that REM sleep seems to be essential to a person's well-being. People deprived of REM sleep become hostile, irritable, and anxious. When sound sleep is again possible, people who have been deprived of REM sleep will experience longer periods of REM to "make up" for what they've missed. This is one reason why sleeping pills may actually harm people. Many of them interfere with this important phase of sleep.

People who drink alcohol, consume caffeine, or smoke cigarettes may also be interrupting their normal sleep patterns without knowing it. Even a single alcoholic drink before bedtime has caused abnormal stoppage of breathing in sleep experiments. Caffeine and nicotine, the drug of tobacco, are both stimulants and can change the brain's activity to prevent normal sleep.

 I like to remember my dreams. Do dreams have any functions?

There have been many theories about what purpose dreaming may serve. The emerging view seems to be that dreams are tied to the workings of the unconscious mind. Some researchers who earlier dismissed dreaming as meaningless or random now believe that dreams may have some significance.

Should I try to remember my dreams?

Dreams may be useful. It is thought that dreaming helps the brain to make sense of events that occur in awake life. The theory holds that the subconscious mind "learns" the day's events during REM sleep. Even if people don't become aware of their dreams, says the theory, dreaming still affects their minds.

Some people try to remember their dreams and write them down. They say this provides valuable insights into their waking lives.

ON LINE WITH HEALTH

You may want to have your students visit the following URL, where they will find information and additional Web site resources to enhance their study of this chapter. As with all Web sites, you should check this out first to be sure the information found there is appropriate for your students.

Choosing a Doctor
http://www.ohiohealth. com/fsdoc.htm

This site offers some helpful guidelines to keep in mind when choosing a doctor.

Glossary

REM (rapid eye movement pronounced as the syllable *rem*) **sleep:** the periods of sleep in which a person is dreaming.

other students?

Do any of the students know anyone who has had serious gum problems? While keeping the anonymity of the person being discussed, ask the students what problems, expenses, and/or painful procedures have been the result of gum disease. Try to elicit enough stories to help impress the students with the importance of preventative care now and throughout their lives.

VOCABULARY

1. **a.** dermatologist **b.** follicles
   c. cuticle **d.** douches
   e. dental plaque **f.** pus
   g. sebum **h.** dentin
   i. immunizations **j.** toxic
   shock syndrome
2. **a.** A cavity is a hole in a
   tooth caused by decay. A
   pulp cavity is a tooth's deepest chamber, which houses
   its blood vessels and nerves.
   b. The vertebrae are the delicate, hollow bones of the
   spine. The spine is the stack
   of 33 vertebrae that form the
   backbone and hold the
   spinal cord.

RECALL

SECTION 1

1. Angle the brush at the gum
   line; brush tooth surfaces
   back and forth, not up and
   down; brush the gums,
   especially beneath the gum
   line; use floss to pull
   plaque up from below the
   gum line between the
   teeth; use a toothpick or
   brush to dislodge plaque
   from below the gum line
   along the teeth. (p. 268)
2. They contain bleaching
   substances and acids that
   may damage the teeth,
   gums, and tongue. (p. 268)
3. Promote tooth decay—
   Answers will vary; could
   include: chocolate milk, ice
   cream, milkshakes, sweetened yogurt, cookies,
   sweet rolls, pies, cakes,
   presweetened cereals,
   potato chips, crackers,
   dried fruits, fruits canned in
   syrup or juice, jams and jellies, peanut butter with

CHAPTER 10 Review

Summarizing the Chapter

*Your ability to respond correctly to the following
statements ensures your understanding of the main
concepts in the chapter.*

1. Identify self-care practices to maintain healthy
   teeth, hair, nails, skin, and ears.
2. Identify sales gimmicks and quackery.
3. Explain the importance of correct posture to
   the health of the spine.
4. Identify immunizations you have received and
   those you still need.
5. Determine when medical help is necessary.

Learning the Vocabulary

dental plaque	comedogenic
enamel	dermatologist
cavity	menstruation
dentin	douches
pulp cavity	toxic shock syndrome
gum disease	(TSS)
follicles	menstrual cramps
cuticle	premenstrual syndrome
keratin	(PMS)
acne	spine
sebum	vertebrae
pus	immunizations
whitehead	REM (rapid eye
cyst	movement)
blackhead	

*Answer the following questions on a separate sheet of
paper.*

1. **Matching**—*Match each of the following phrases
   with the appropriate vocabulary term from the
   list above:*
   a. a skin doctor
   b. the structures that contain the roots of hairs
   c. the borders of hardened skin along the
   bases of the fingernails

d. preparations used to clean the vagina
e. material that builds up on the tooth
f. a mixture of fluid and white blood cells
around an infected area
g. acne-causing
h. a tooth's soft middle layer
i. also called vaccinations
j. dangerous poisoning that can occur when
bacteria break down menstrual blood

2. **a.** What is the difference between a cavity
   and a pulp cavity?
   b. What is the relationship between the spine
   and the vertebrae?

Recalling Important Facts and Ideas

Section 1

1. Describe correct flossing and brushing
   techniques.
2. Why should teeth-whitening products be
   avoided?
3. Identify two foods that promote tooth decay
   and two foods that do not promote tooth
   decay.

Section 2

4. What is the only cure for damaged hair?
5. What happens when oil and bacteria irritate
   the skin?
6. Why is the upper ear prone to infections?
7. How can foreign particles best be removed
   from your eye when tears fail to remove them?
8. What precautions should be taken by a practitioner who does body piercing or tattooing?
9. What are some techniques used to remove
   tattoos?

Section 3

10. List one thing correct posture can do for you.
11. How can strong abdominal muscles help you
    avoid back pain?

Section 4

12. Why do children and teenagers need to have
    regular medical check-ups?
13. List four situations that would require a visit to
    the doctor.

Critical Thinking

1. What are the benefits to the medical profession
   when people become more involved in self-
   care? What are some of the specific benefits of

286

added sugar, glazed meats, hot dogs, candies, sugar-sweetened gum, and fudge.
(p. 269)

SECTION 2

4. trim off the damaged parts (p. 271)
5. redness, swelling and pus form, the beginning of a whitehead or pimple (p. 273)
6. It is mostly cartilage with little blood flowing through it. If bacteria enter a puncture
   there, they grow with little opposition

from the white blood cells and antibodies
that would normally destroy them.
(p. 275)
7. Hold the eye open and gently drop plain,
   clean water or a commercial eyewash into
   the lower or upper lid. (p. 276)
8. The practitioner should sterilize equipment
   between clients, wear latex gloves, and
   never reuse needles. (p. 275)
9. laser surgery, scraping away the skin with
   wire brushes, or burning the skin away
   with acids (p. 275)

practicing self-care? Are there any risks involved in self-care?

2. Compare and contrast personal health care today with personal health care in the nineteenth century. Give specific examples.

3. Why is quackery such a profitable business? Why do so many people fall victim to deceptive practices? List some examples of products quacks might sell based on fear. How can you avoid spending your money on worthless products?

Activities

1. Submit a copy of an advertisement and analyze the gimmicks used based on the Consumer Skills feature on page 274.

2. Interview a dental hygienist or a dentist about the dental care practices they recommend. Hand in a short report or a tape recording of the interview.

3. Make a list of various activities that damage hair and some precautions that will help minimize the risk of damage.

4. Produce an original video commercial. Pretend to be a quack and use some of the deceptive practices listed on page 274 in the Consumer Skills feature.

5. Submit a copy of a newspaper or magazine advertisement for a health-care product you suspect is making a false claim. Attach a one-page report explaining the reasons for your suspicions.

6. Contact some local community health agencies and make a list of educational programs they have available on self-care.

7. Call your water district and find out if the water in your community is fluoridated, the cost of fluoridation, and when this practice began.

8. Make a poster of the do's and don'ts of personal health care by either collaging pictures you cut out from magazines or creating original drawings.

9. List all the ways to protect eyes to keep them healthy. Identify what occupations and sports commonly use protective eyewear.

10. Write a report on how your life would be different if you could not hear or see.

11. Develop a file on personal appearance tips for teenagers. Create the file so that it can be used by younger students or by the next group of students to take this course. The file should include tips on the following:

- Skin care
- Teeth care
- Hair care
- Nail care
- Grooming tips
- Acne
- Health problems

An example of tips for nail care would be: eat a well-balanced diet, wear gloves for rough work, never bite your nails, don't use your nails as tools, and so on. Add any topics that you feel are important. Color code the file so the different types of tips are easy to find.

12. Work with three or four other students to design a bulletin board of strategies for maintaining a healthy body. Use creative ideas. Include drawings, photos from magazines or newspapers, and interesting type to make the bulletin board visually appealing.

13. Talk with an optometrist or ophthalmologist about the types of eye problems they see in teenagers. What are the most common problems? How do they treat them? What strategies do they have for keeping the eyes in good health? Make a poster with the information you collect from the person interviewed.

Making Decisions about Health

1. You have the nagging feeling that something is wrong with your body. There's pain here, discomfort there, and a feeling of nausea that's almost overwhelming sometimes. These symptoms seem to come and go and you wonder if you should see a physician. What course of action should you follow?

2. Josh is the drummer for a band that plays rock music. The music is played very loudly. (Josh says, "The louder, the better.") Lately, Josh has been asking people to repeat what they say to him. His grades in class are going down because he misses important points during the discussions and lectures. He does assignments wrong because he doesn't get the instructions right. What do you think is Josh's problem? How can you help him understand that he has a problem? What would you advise Josh to do?

287

SECTION 3

10. Answers will vary; could include: give a person a positive energetic look; keep a person free from back pain. (p. 279)

11. Strong abdominal muscles support the back and help keep it from slipping out of place. (p. 281)

SECTION 4

12. to make sure they are growing as expected and to receive immunizations on time (p. 283)

13. Answers will vary. Refer to Figure 10–10 on page 283 for possible answers.

	OUTCOMES	FEATURES
CHAPTER 11 **Drugs as Medicines**	• List five ways medicines benefit people. • Describe the factors that alter or influence the effects of drugs. • Explain the procedures the FDA must follow in order to approve a drug. • Describe the differences between over-the-counter drugs and prescription drugs. • Explain how advertising affects the sales of over-the-counter drugs. • Describe the purpose of over-the-counter drugs. • Discuss the purposes of prescription drugs. • Describe the effects of caffeine on the body.	*Health Strategies:* Taking Medicines Safely (page 302) *Life Choice Inventory:* How Wisely Do You Choose OTC Medicines? (page 299) *Consumer Skills:* OTC Medicine Advertising (page 298) *Straight Talk:* Caffeine (page 304)
CHAPTER 12 **Drugs of Abuse**	• Define and differentiate among drug use, drug misuse, and drug abuse. • Describe the three factors that lead people to drug abuse. • Explain the problems associated with physical and psychological addiction. • Identify the effects of marijuana and related drugs. • Define and discuss the abuse of stimulants, narcotics, and depressants. • Describe the effects of inhalants, look-alike drugs, and designer drugs. • List the signs of drug abuse.	*Health Strategies:* Enjoy Life (page 333) *Life Choice Inventory:* Is Any Drug or Medicine a Problem for You? (page 334) *Consumer Skills:* Look-alikes (page 328) *Straight Talk:* How to Refuse Drugs without losing Friends (page 338) *Teen Views:* How Has Drug Abuse Affected Your School or Community (page 332)?
CHAPTER 13 **Alcohol: Use and Abuse**	• List three reasons why young people start to drink alcohol. • Explain what alcohol is and how it affects the body. • Identify the immediate effects of intoxication. • Discuss what is meant by fetal alcohol syndrome. • Describe the effects of drinking on driving. • Explain why alcoholism is a family disease. • Identify how an enabler's behavior affects the person with an alcohol problem. • List what kinds of help are available to the alcohol-dependent person.	*Health Strategies:* How Not to Enable (page 360) *Health Strategies:* How to Give a Great Party without Alcohol (page 363) *Life Choice Inventory:* Does Someone You Know Have a Drinking Problem? (page 348) *Consumer Skills:* Advertisements for Alcohol (page 347) *Straight Talk:* Alcoholism, the Disease (page 365)
CHAPTER 14 **Tobacco**	• Describe the immediate effects of nicotine on the body. • Describe the effects of smoking on the respiratory and cardiovascular systems. • List negative aspects of tobacco use other than health hazards. • Identify ways in which other people's tobacco smoke harms nonsmokers who are exposed to it. • Identify the health problems associated with the use of smokeless tobacco. • Describe the withdrawal symptoms that follow quitting smoking and the pleasures of doing so.	*Health Strategies:* Giving Up Smoking (page 388) *Life Choice Inventory:* What Motivates a Smoker? (page 390) *Consumer Skills:* Tobacco as a Gateway Drug (page 376) *Straight Talk:* The New Tobacco Rules: Will They Stop Teenagers from Smoking? (page 394) *Teen Views:* Why Do So Many Teens Think Smoking Is Cool? (page 374)

TEACHING SUPPORT

Vocabulary: Learning Key Terms, Crossword Puzzle, Fill in the Blank
Study Outline
Reading Cloze
Reteaching: Effects of Medicines, What Are Medicines?, Word Choice
Enrichment: Reading a Label, Over-the-Counter Medicine
Career Briefs: Pharmacists
Life Choice Inventory: How Wisely Do You Choose OTC Medicines?

Handouts: How New Drugs Are Discovered, Attitudes about Over-the-Counter Drugs, Analyzing Medicine Use, Caffeine Content of Beverages, Foods, and OTC Drugs
Teacher Information Sheet: Food/Drug Interactions
Quizzes: Sections 1–4
Tests: Chapter 11 Test A, Chapter 11 Test B
Transparencies: The FDA, Risk/Benefit Ratio

Vocabulary: Learning Key Terms, Crossword Puzzle, Fill-In Puzzle
Study Outline
Reading Cloze
Reteaching: All about Marijuana, All about Cocaine
Enrichment: Kinds of drugs, Making Healthy Decisions, Party Situation, Strengthen Your Refusal Skills
Career Briefs: Human Services Workers
Life Choice Inventory: Is Any Drug or Medicine a Problem for You?

Handouts: Attitudes about Drug Abuse, Mini Glossary of Drug Abuse Terms
Teacher Information Sheet: Stopping Drug Addiction
Quizzes: Sections 1–7
Tests: Chapter 12 Test A, Chapter 12 Test B
Transparencies: The Downward Spiral of Physiological Addiction, The Cycle of Psychological Addiction, Stimulation to Depression

---

Vocabulary: Learning Key Terms, Crossword Puzzle, Fill in the Missing Term
Study Outline
Reading Cloze
Reteaching: The Facts about Alcohol, Alcohol and the Human Body
Enrichment: Alcohol Awareness Designs, Alcoholism and the Family, You Be the Judge and Jury
Career Briefs: Social Workers
Life Choice Inventory: Does Someone You Know Have a Drinking Problem?
Handouts: Thinking about Drinking, Test Your Knowledge, Classify Your Drinking Behavior,

Blood Alcohol Concentration by Number of Drinks and Body Weight, The Disguises of Alcoholism, Characteristics of Alcoholism, Attitudes about Drunk Driving, The Progression of Alcoholism, Myths about Alcoholism
Teacher Information Sheets: Withdrawal from Alcohol, The Family Dynamics of Alcohol Abuse
Quizzes: Sections 1–5
Tests: Chapter 13 Test A, Chapter 13 Test B
Transparencies: Alcohol's Effects on the Brain, The Liver, The Hangover, The Fates of Two Drinkers, Comparing Excessive vs. Moderate Drinking

---

Vocabulary: Learning Key Terms, Crossword Puzzle, Find a Clue
Study Outline
Reading Cloze
Reteaching: Tobacco and Disease, True or False
Enrichment: Fact and Fantasy, Keep Them Going in Circles, Concerned Students
Career Briefs: Respiratory Therapists
Life Choice Inventory: What Motivates a Smoker?
Handouts: Smokers and Their Smoking Habits, Smoking Facts, Analyzing Advertising for Tobacco, International Smoking, Public Health Objectives

Teacher Information Sheet: Set-up for Demonstration
Quizzes: Sections 1–5
Tests: Chapter 14 Test A, Chapter 14 Test B
Transparencies: Normal Lung, Lung with Emphysema, Carbon Monoxide Sources Compared

---

MULTIMEDIA SUPPORT

- Health Video Library
- CNN Health and Fitness Update Videos
- Westest
- Student Review Software
- Diet Analysis Software
- Nutrition CD-ROM

LESSON PLANNING

You will find detailed daily lesson plans for both **traditional scheduling** and **block scheduling** in your Teacher's Resource Box.

287b

KEY POINTS

Chapter 11 is 20 pages long and divided into four sections. Briefly, this chapter describes the effects of medicines on the body and the regulatory role of the FDA. It stresses the importance of the proper selection and use of medicines. It also gives students guidelines to follow for taking medicines.

ACTIVITY TO INTRODUCE THE CHAPTER

Have students inventory sections of a local drug store. This inventory should include: names of medicines, purpose, active and inactive ingredients, classification (generic or brand name, over-the-counter or prescription), costs, and expiration dates.

BULLETIN BOARD IDEAS

Use the Health Strategies feature, "Taking Medicines Safely," on page 302, as the basis for your bulletin board. Condense some of the longer tips so that each one can be made large enough to be seen easily.

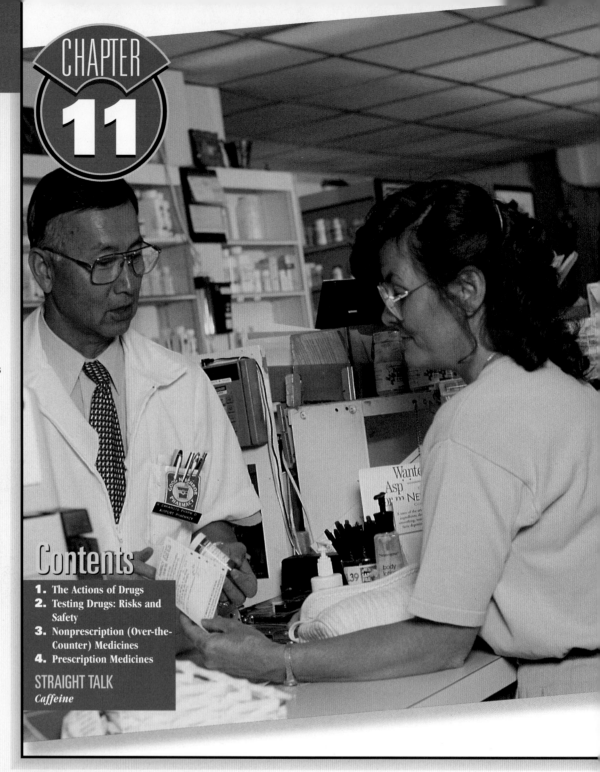

CHAPTER 11

Contents

1. The Actions of Drugs
2. Testing Drugs: Risks and Safety
3. Nonprescription (Over-the-Counter) Medicines
4. Prescription Medicines

STRAIGHT TALK
Caffeine

NOT Enough Time?

Following are some suggestions to help you make sure that you cover the key topics in this chapter if you have limited time. (Refer to the daily lesson plans in your Teacher's Resource Box for additional suggestions.)

DAY 1 Assign students to read Sections 1 and 2 prior to class. During class have students do the Focus Activity on page 290 and

Drugs as Medicines

FACT or FICTION

What do you think? Are the following statements true or false? If you think they are false, then say what is true.

1. Prescription medications can be dangerous, but over-the-counter medicines are safe.
2. The effect aspirin has on the body depends on why a person takes it.
3. The action of a drug can depend on whether or not it is taken with meals.
4. People who drink alcohol often need higher doses of certain drugs than other people.
5. Generic drugs are exactly the same as their brand-name equivalents, only cheaper.

(Answers on page 303)

Introduction

Within this century, remarkable discoveries of **drugs** that help prevent, cure, or relieve symptoms of disease have spared much suffering and saved countless lives. Today, people use thousands of different drugs as **medicines** to treat hundreds of different illnesses or symptoms of illnesses. The health effects of such widespread use of medicines, however, are not always those that people expect.

This chapter presents drugs used as medicines. The Straight Talk section discusses one of the most common of all drugs—caffeine. The next chapter focuses on drug abuse.

Answers to FACT or FICTION

Here are the answers to the questions at the start of the chapter.

1. **False.** All drug use involves risk.
2. **False.** Everyone who takes aspirin receives *all* of its effects.
3. **True.**
4. **False.** People who drink alcohol may experience enhanced effects from certain drugs, and alcohol consumption may make larger amounts of some drugs dangerous.
5. **False.** Generic drugs contain the same active ingredients, but may contain different inactive ingredients.

FAST FACTS

Americans consume ten billion aspirin annually, or one every three seconds.

---

the Group Project on page 291. Conclude the class with the Quick Quiz on pages 294–295.

DAY 2 Before Day 2 have students read Sections 2 and 3. During class have students do the Focus Activities on pages 295 and 297.

Conclude with the Quick Quiz on page 301. Assign Section 4.

DAY 3 During class have students do the Group Activity on page 302 and the Close Activity on page 303.

FOCUS

OUTCOMES

In this section students will learn the:

1. Actions of drugs.
2. Side effects of commonly used medicines.
3. Factors that change medicines' effects.

TEACHER SUPPORT

Key Passage

Discuss the text statement, "Drugs do not cure diseases by themselves." Have students describe how drugs help the body cure diseases.

FOCUS ACTIVITY

Write the word *medicine* on the chalkboard. Have students list all the medicines they can. Write the students' responses under the word *medicine*. To encourage class participation in this brainstorming activity, reserve comments until all students are satisfied with the list. Discuss. Suggest medicines that may have been omitted. (penicillin, cortisone, polio vaccine, and so on) Divide the class into teams of four. Have each team examine the list of medicines and incorporate each medicine into one of the five categories: prevents disease, cures disease, makes the disease less severe, relieves symptoms, or brings about other desired effects. Discuss.

The Actions of Drugs

People often believe that drugs can cure diseases, but this is not entirely true. Only the body can actually cure diseases. Drugs can only help the body in its efforts. Medicines benefit people in these ways:

▶ They may help *prevent* disease (example: vaccines are used to convey immunity to diseases).
▶ They may help in the *cure* of disease (example: penicillin kills the bacteria that cause some forms of pneumonia).
▶ They may make diseases less severe without helping cure them (example: steroid hormones reinforce the body's defense against incurable arthritis).
▶ They may relieve symptoms (example: aspirin relieves inflammation, aches, and pains).
▶ They may bring about other desired effects (example: minoxidil, rubbed on a balding scalp, helps promote hair growth).

All drugs, including aspirin, have far-reaching chemical effects on the body.

All drugs work by changing the body's own processes. One familiar drug, **aspirin**, illustrates this concept.

Most people think they understand aspirin. Their reasoning goes something like this: "Aspirin is cheap and familiar. Many people take it for headache or fever. It's not addictive, and it certainly can't be as powerful as the drugs physicians prescribe. It must be safe." If this is how you think about aspirin, then you may be surprised by its far-reaching chemical effects on the body. All drugs (whether drugs used medically or abused drugs) affect users physically. Their use always involves risks.

Aspirin works by blocking the actions of powerful body chemicals. These chemicals exist in

Pursuing wellness

Tell students that at some time in life most people are likely to suffer some type of flexibility-related injury such as muscle pull, muscle strain, or low back pain. There are a number of over-the-counter drugs and medicines that are considered analgesics, or pain relievers. However, for flexibility-related injuries it is beneficial to select a medicine that has an anti-inflammatory action. While all body tissues. They produce fevers, cause **inflammation**, cause the blood to clot, and make nerves sensitive to pain. Aspirin changes all these body responses through its actions on body chemistry. Thus aspirin reduces fever and inflammation, prevents the blood from clotting, and is still the best drug available to relieve certain kinds of pain.

You cannot use aspirin for any one purpose without bringing on all its other effects. A person might take aspirin to prevent blood clotting, but this same effect also occurs in people who take aspirin to treat pain. For people who do not expect it, the anticlotting effect may be dangerous, since it can prolong bleeding. A single two-tablet dose of aspirin doubles the bleeding time of wounds, an effect that lasts from four to seven days. For this reason, it is important not to take aspirin before any kind of surgery or in the weeks before childbirth.

Another thing you should know about aspirin is that its use is associated with a rare, but often fatal, disease: Reye's (pronounced "RISE") syndrome, which damages the liver and brain. The most likely victims of Reye's syndrome are children under 15 years of age who are given aspirin to relieve symptoms of chicken pox or flu. The lives of victims who are promptly treated can sometimes be saved. However, they may be left mentally retarded or with disorders of voice and speech.

Warning signs of Reye's syndrome are listed in Figure 11–1 above. In a child recovering from chicken pox, any of those signs means that a medical emergency is developing. See a health-care provider right away.

Almost all cases of Reye's syndrome can be prevented by treating children's symptoms of flu or chicken pox with pain relievers other than aspirin. For example, **acetaminophen** (sold under brand names such as Tylenol or Datril), **ibuprofen** (whose brand names are Advil, Motrin, and others) **naproxen sodium** (brand name Aleve), or **ketoprofen** (brand names Actron and Orudis KT) can reduce fever and relieve pain. Those medicines are not associated with Reye's syndrome.

Aspirin is typical of all drugs: they all have **side effects**. Some are harmful (see Figure 11–2 on the next page). For example, many drugs impair driving ability. Cold medicines and **antihistamines** can cause drowsiness. Other drugs can slow down a driver's reaction time. If there is any question about a drug's effect on driving, talk with a pharmacist or other health-care provider. All drugs have many effects. All of them occur when you take the drugs, whether you expect them and want them to occur or not.

 KEY POINTS   *Medicines help prevent disease, help cure disease, make disease less severe, relieve symptoms, or produce other desired effects. Drugs act by altering body processes. All drugs have side effects.*

Figure 11–1   Warning Signs of Reye's Syndrome

A child may seem to be recovering from flu or chicken pox when these symptoms appear:

- Nausea with severe vomiting.
- Fever.
- Inactivity.
- Loss of consciousness.
- Uncontrollable behavior while unconscious.

 MINI Glossary

drugs: substances taken into the body that change one or more of the body's functions.

medicines: drugs used to help cure disease, lessen disease severity, relieve symptoms, prevent disease, help with diagnosis, or produce other desired effects.

aspirin: a drug that relieves fever, pain, and inflammation.

inflammation: pain and swelling caused by irritation.

acetaminophen (ah-SEET-ah-MIN-o-fen): a drug that relieves fever and pain.

ibuprofen (EYE-byoo-PRO-fen): a drug that relieves fever, pain, and inflammation.

naproxen sodium (na-PROX-en): a drug that relieves fever, pain, and inflammation. It provides longer relief from a single dose than other common pain relievers.

ketoprofen (KEE-toe-PRO-fen): a drug that relieves fever, pain, and inflammation. Its small pill size eases swallowing for those who have trouble swallowing regular pills.

side effects: effects of drugs other than the desired medical effects.

antihistamines: drugs that counteract inflammation caused by histamine, one of the chemicals involved in allergic reactions.

acetaminophen may be fine for headache or fever, it does not have an anti-inflammatory property. A better choice would be plain aspirin (acetylsalicylic acid), ibuprofen, naproxen, or ketoprofen.

For a stronger drug, a doctor's prescription

would be required. In any case, for concerns regarding the proper treatment for a flexibility-related injury, see the family doctor.

TEACHING WITH VISUALS

Refer students to Figure 11–2. Tell students that they should not be frightened of the list of possible hazards associated with each of these drugs. In almost all cases, the drugs are perfectly safe. They were tested extensively before the government permitted their sale. These are potential problems and reactions that take place, which people should be aware of. Following are some additional side effects that you might want to tell students about.

a. acetaminophen—difficulty in diagnosing overdose because reaction may be delayed for up to a week after taking medication

b. antacids—possible concealment of ulcer, prevention of certain antibiotics' functioning (for example, antacids that contain aluminum)

c. aspirin—excessive bleeding during surgery or childbirth

d. diet pills—nervousness and crabbiness

DISCUSSION

Have students tell of times when they suffered the side effects of a drug. Were any of the situations frightening or life-threatening? Do students feel that they take the warnings that accompany medicines and drugs seriously enough? Would someone who drove under the effects of an antihistamine be acting as irresponsibly as someone who drove while intoxicated?

Figure 11–2   Side Effects of Commonly Used Medicines

Medicine	Possible Hazard
Acetaminophen	Bloody urine; painful urination; skin rash; yellowing of the eyes or skin (even at normal doses); severe liver damage and death from overdose or chronic low-level excesses
Acid reducers	Fever; diarrhea; headache; anxiety; confusion; depression; dizziness; hallucinations; sleepiness; rarely, severe allergic reactions, heart and liver abnormalities
Antacids (such as Tums)	Reduced mineral absorption from food; reduction of effectiveness of other medications; possible worsening of high blood pressure; aggravation of kidney problems
Aspirin	Stomach bleeding; vomiting; worsening of ulcers; enhancement of the action of anticlotting medications; severe allergic reactions in some people; association with Reye's syndrome in children and teenagers; prolonged bleeding time
Cold medications	Loss of consciousness (if taken with prescription tranquilizers)
Diet pills	Organ damage or death from bleeding of the brain
Ibuprofen	Allergic reactions in some people with aspirin allergy; fluid retention; liver damage similar to that from acetaminophen; enhancement of action of anticlotting medications
Ketoprofen	Stomach ulcers with bleeding
Laxatives	Reduced absorption of minerals from food; creation of dependency
Naproxen sodium	Stomach ulcers with bleeding; kidney damage in the elderly, in people with liver disease, or in those taking other drugs
Toothache medications	Destruction of the still-healthy part of a damaged tooth (for medications that contain clove oil)

Factors That Change Medicines' Effects

When you take a drug, many factors work together to determine its effects on you. One is the nature of the drug itself—the substance. Another factor is the form in which you take the drug. Liquid drugs, for example, may be absorbed faster than capsules or tablets, so liquids tend to go to work faster.

Another factor is the route by which the drug is taken. Drugs taken by mouth must travel through the digestive tract to be absorbed. Those injected into the bloodstream or absorbed through the skin (**transdermal** delivery) go to work right away.

Ability Levels

Advanced

Have students discuss the following statement: "News of 'new' medicines often hits the media years before the drugs are ready for use. This raises false hopes in those who urgently need drugs for medical problems, such as cancer and AIDS."

Have the students work in teams of four. Each team represents a different TV station's editorial staff, responsible for what news goes on the air and what is omitted. After discussing the above statement, the teams are to decide whether to release news of a new drug

When you take the drug is another factor. For example, whether or not the drug is taken at mealtimes affects how fast it can act on the body. Food in the digestive tract can slow down the absorption of medicines. Still another factor is you—your body and mind. Your age, your weight, and what you expect the drug to do modify its effects.

Probably the strongest factor affecting the actions of medicines is the use of other drugs, such as alcohol, nicotine (the drug of tobacco), drugs of abuse, medicines, and others. Two or more drugs taken at the same time can strongly affect one another's actions. They may slow down one another's absorption. They may work against one another in the tissues. One drug may get in the way of the other's breakdown and removal from the body. A person's history of drug use also affects a medicine's action. This is so important that the next section tells of its effects on the body. Figure 11–3 above sums up factors that affect the action of medicines.

This person might have an unexpected reaction to medicine.

Figure 11–3 *Factors That Change Medicines' Effects*

1. The nature of the drug
2. The form in which it is taken
3. The route by which it is taken
4. When it is taken (with or without food, for example)
5. You (your age, weight, expectations, etc.)
6. Other drugs taken with it
7. The taker's history of drug use

KEY POINTS *Factors that alter a drug's effects on you include the drug itself, the form in which it is taken, the route by which it is taken, whether or not it is taken with food, your age, your weight, your expectations, and what other drugs you may take with it.*

Previous Drug Use, Other Drug Use

A drug may produce one set of effects when used for just a few days but produce an entirely different set of effects when used over weeks, months, or years. Often, after taking a drug over a long time, a person will need higher doses to get the desired effect. This is because the body has developed **tolerance** to the drug.

How Tolerance Works   Tolerance means the body has grown used to being exposed to the drug. The longer the exposure, the better the body becomes at breaking the drug down, and the faster it gets rid of it. Many organs work together on this. The liver breaks down the drug faster. The kidneys throw it out in the urine faster. Other tissues begin to ignore the drug—they no longer respond to it.

Tolerance varies from person to person. One person may come to tolerate a certain drug well, but another may hardly adjust to it at all. When you understand the body's tolerance to a drug, you begin to catch a glimpse of how drug **addiction** can set in.

Drug Synergy   Drugs also interact, sometimes to the benefit of the users, and sometimes to their peril. Two drugs taken together may produce a new or stronger effect, called **drug synergy**, than either drug can produce alone. Sometimes this is beneficial, as when medicines are intended to work

MINI Glossary

transdermal: literally, "across the skin." In a drug delivery system, a drug is placed in contact with the skin by way of an adhesive patch. The drug is absorbed across the skin and into the bloodstream.

tolerance: a state that develops in users of certain drugs that makes larger and larger amounts of the drugs necessary to produce the same effect.

addiction: a physical or psychological craving for higher and higher doses of a drug that leads to bodily harm, social maladjustment, or economic hardship.

drug synergy: the combined action of two drugs that is greater than or different from the action of either drug alone.

In the Teacher's Resource Box you will find an information sheet entitled "Food/Drug Interactions." This sheet will give you more in-depth information about some of the ways that foods can affect the actions of drugs in the body.

DISCUSSION

Ask students if any of them or their family members have had to take a particular drug long enough to build up a tolerance to it. What has been the result? Has the physician prescribed heavier doses, changed drugs, or attempted some other strategy?

COMPREHENSION CHECK

Because students are so used to hearing the word *drugs* used to mean the drugs of abuse, you should emphasize the actual meaning of the term, which is any substance taken into the body that changes one or more of the body's functions. Have students write sentences using the word *drug* or *drugs*, without referring to drugs of abuse. Ask students to volunteer their sentences to be read aloud.

Vocabulary worksheets are provided in the Teacher's Resource Box.

not yet approved by the FDA, or to wait for FDA approval of the drug. Tell them that the maker of the drug claims that this drug will cure any form of cancer, with absolutely no side effects. Have each team report its decision and reasons to the class.

Ask the students if they think that people who suffer from a terminal or incurable illness should be allowed to take experimental drugs, even if the side effects could kill them. If these people know they will die soon, should they be allowed any chance, no matter how small, for a cure?

ASSESS

SECTION 1

Review Answers

1. a. aspirin **b.** side effects
   c. drugs **d.** addiction
   e. medicines
2. when they are used to help prevent, cure, or relieve symptoms of disease (p. 290)
3. reduces fever and inflammation, relieves pain, prevents blood from clotting, and doubles the bleeding time of a wound; four to seven days (p. 291)
4. drowsiness, loss of consciousness (if taken with prescription tranquilizers) (pp. 291–292)
5. Answers will vary.

A reproducible quiz for Section 1 is provided in the Teacher's Resource Box.

CLOSE

COMPREHENSION CHECK

Students should be able to complete the following:

1. List five ways medicines benefit people.
2. Describe the advantages and disadvantages of aspirin.
3. Describe the factors that influence the effects of drugs.

together to help cure an illness. Other times, the interactions are dangerous, as when sleeping pills and alcohol are combined. The body breaks down both of these drugs in the same way. Taken by itself, the dose of the sleeping medicine is broken down little by little as it enters the body. The presence of alcohol changes things, though, because the body gives highest priority to breaking down alcohol. Meanwhile, the body ignores the sleeping medication, which could build up in the blood to high, or even deadly, levels. Many accidental deaths occur in this way. Many drugs, taken with alcohol, cause dangerous reactions.

Antagonist Drugs   One drug can also prevent the action of another, acting as an **antagonist**. Such drugs are often useful in the treatment of accidental overdoses or poisonings. Drugs that block the action of snake venoms are examples of antagonists. Some forms of addiction therapy use antagonist drugs to oppose the effects of the addictive drug.

KEY POINTS   *Tolerance to a drug develops when the body gets used to exposure to the drug. Tolerance sets the stage for the development of addiction. Synergy can lead to accidental overdoses. Alcohol and medicine can be a dangerous combination.*

SECTION 1 Review

Answer the following questions on a sheet of paper.

Learning the Vocabulary

The vocabulary terms in this section are *drugs, medicines, aspirin, inflammation, acetaminophen, ibuprofen, naproxen sodium, ketoprofen, side effects, antihistamines, transdermal, tolerance, addiction, drug synergy,* and *antagonist.*

1. Match each of the following phrases with the appropriate term:
   a. a drug that relieves fever, pain, and inflammation that should not be given to children
   b. effects of a drug other than the desired medical effect
   c. substances taken into the body that change one or more body functions
   d. a physical or psychological craving for higher and higher doses of a drug
   e. drugs used to help cure diseases, lessen disease severity, and relieve symptoms

Learning the Facts

2. When do drugs become medicines?
3. What are the effects of a single, two-tablet dose of aspirin? How long do the effects of this dose last?
4. List a side effect of cold medicines and antihistamines.

Making Life Choices

5. Your friend's father is a smoker and has a beer every night. He has a bad cold with a fever. He decides to treat his cold with over-the-counter antihistamines. With his smoking and drinking, what do you now know about the dose he takes? Why is it dangerous to take drugs when you drink or smoke?

QUICK QUIZ

Chapter 11, Section 1

The following quiz will help you assess your students' understanding of the material covered in this section of the chapter. You might use the quiz as an oral exercise, which will lead into a class discussion of the topics covered. Or, you might use it as a paper/pencil

quiz to evaluate your students individually.

If students have difficulty with the concepts covered in the Quick Quiz and the Section Review, you might suggest they review the material using the **S**urvey, **Q**uestion, **R**ead, **R**ecite, **R**eview (SQ3R) *study method, which is described in detail in the introduction to this Teacher's Wraparound Edition.*

1. Medicines cannot help prevent diseases. (False)

SECTION 2

Testing Drugs: Risks and Safety

Ingredients in medicines must be proved both safe and effective before the Food and Drug Administration (FDA), a watchdog agency of the federal government, allows the medicines on the market. The term **safe** means that an ingredient will not hurt you. The term **effective** means that the ingredient will do what the maker claims it will do. The FDA keeps tabs on drug companies as they develop new drugs and bring them to market. Then, after the drug is on the market, the FDA continues to check for side effects. Procedures for bringing new medicines to market, especially for medicines to treat AIDS, have been "streamlined," but can still take years.

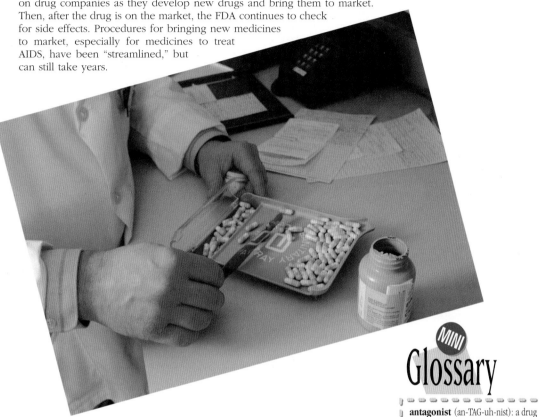

There is a fine line between correct and incorrect use of drugs. They must be effective, but they must also be safe.

MINI Glossary

antagonist (an-TAG-uh-nist): a drug that opposes the action of another drug.

safe: causing no undue harm; part of the legal requirement for a drug.

effective: having the medically intended effect; part of the legal requirement for a drug.

SECTION 2

FOCUS

OUTCOMES

In this section students will learn:

1. The role of the FDA.
2. How antibiotics work.
3. The importance of correct dosage of any drug.

FOCUS ACTIVITY

Write the following statements on the board: "Miracle drug discovered. It has been claimed that this drug will raise the IQ of those who take it by 20 points. The FDA stands in the way, refusing distribution to the public." Have students list the pros and cons of the FDA being able to regulate the release of drugs to the general public. Provide a forum for debate.

TEACH & APPLY

WORKSHEETS

For enrichment your Teacher's Resource Box contains a handout entitled "How New Drugs Are Discovered."

TRANSPARENCIES

You may also want to use a transparency entitled "The FDA," which can be found in your Transparency Acetate Binder. The overhead gives an overview of the FDA's process for checking and approving drugs.

---

2. Medicines may help cure or relieve the symptoms of an illness. (True)
3. Drugs cure diseases without the body's assistance. (False)
4. Drugs work by changing the body's chemical processes. (True)
5. Aspirin is a drug that has little effect on the body's chemical processes. (False)
6. Reye's syndrome is a dangerous disease associated with aspirin use. (True)
7. Only prescription drugs have side effects. (False)
8. There are many factors that can alter a drug's effect on you. (True)
9. Developing tolerance to a drug decreases the chance of addiction. (False)
10. When two drugs taken together produce a stronger or unexpected effect, it is called drug synergy. (True)

ASSESS

CLOSE

No drug is totally safe for all people at all times at any dose. The saying "the dose makes the poison" means that the safety of any substance depends on how much of it a person consumes. Part of the evaluation of a drug's safety compares the dose that presents risks to health with the dose needed for the medical effect.

Drugs that are safe to use in the amounts that work are the best ones for treating diseases. Among the safest drugs are many **antibiotics**. Antibiotic drugs stop all living cells from dividing. Antibiotic drugs can be used to work against bacteria in the body, because bacteria normally divide more rapidly than most body cells. Because they divide faster, the bacteria die off faster than the body's own cells do when exposed to an antibiotic. Once the drug is out of the system, the body's own cells soon recover. This is why antibiotics are relatively safe for human beings, but deadly to bacteria. As you can see, the dose and length of treatment have to be just right to wipe out the bacteria and leave the person able to recover.

Some drugs are less safe. An example is the drug alcohol, which was used to kill pain during wartime, in surgery, and in childbirth before the development of safer **anesthetics**. A little alcohol dulls pain. More alcohol produces unconsciousness. Only a little more stops the heartbeat and breathing. The amount of alcohol needed for the anesthetic affect is dangerously close to a **lethal dose** (one that causes death)—making alcohol unsafe to use in this way. Today, better, safer drugs are used for pain management instead.

KEY POINTS   *Companies must prove that ingredients in medicines are safe and effective before the Food and Drug Administration (FDA) allows their sale. Scientists study the risks of each drug compared with its benefits. Drugs that carry low risks to health in comparison to their benefits are most desirable in the treatment of disease.*

SECTION 2 Review

Answer the following questions on a sheet of paper.

Learning the Vocabulary

The vocabulary terms in this section are *safe, effective, antibiotics, anesthetics,* and *lethal dose.*
Fill in the blank with the correct answer.

1. A _____ is the amount of a drug necessary to produce death.
2. Drugs that kill pain, with or without producing loss of consciousness, are called _____.
3. An _____ drug is one that has the medically intended effect.

Learning the Facts

4. How do antibiotic drugs work to fight infection?
5. What are the medical problems associated with the use of alcohol as an anesthetic?

Making Life Choices

6. You are going to a party to celebrate your friend's 16th birthday. He is planning to drink 16 shots of alcohol. What do you think could happen to him? How are you going to react? Will you try to stop him? How would you argue your opinions?

HEALTHY PEOPLE 2000

Reduce nonfatal poisoning to no more than 88 emergency department treatments per 100,000 people.

While death from poisoning of children less than 5 years old has declined and is quite low, incidence of nonfatal poisoning is still alarmingly high. In 1987, there were over 107,000 children under 5 years of age treated in hospital emergency departments for poisoning. Approximately 700,000 poison exposures involving children in this age group were reported to poison control centers during the same year.

Past actions such as the Poison Prevention Packaging Act (PPPA), the annual poison prevention week, the shift to less toxic fuels (natural gas and LP gas) for cooking and heating, and safety standards for products that release

SECTION 3

Nonprescription (Over-the-Counter) Medicines

The FDA divides medicines into two classes: **over-the-counter (OTC) drugs**, sold freely; and **prescription drugs** (which you will read about in the next section), sold only with a physician's prescription.

Use of OTC Drugs

People buy over-the-counter (OTC) medicines in the belief that they will bring relief from medical problems. Fortunately, buyers often choose correctly and obtain relief from minor and **chronic** medical problems at reasonable costs. Many ailments respond to the OTC treatments people choose for themselves. Sometimes, though, people buy medicines that are not necessary and may be quite costly. Net sales for OTC medicines are in the many billions of dollars every year.

Unlike prescription drugs, which need a physician's prescription, OTC drugs are freely available. This is because they are relatively safe. Also, most people require about the same doses, so OTC drugs can be used without individualized guidance. The instructions are easily understood. Finally, OTC drugs are not abused in the usual sense. That is, although they may be misused, they do not produce sensations that drug abusers seek. All of these

When using OTC medicines, follow safety guidelines.

MINI Glossary

antibiotics: drugs used to fight bacterial infection.

anesthetics (an-us-THET-icks): drugs that kill pain, with or without producing loss of consciousness.

lethal dose: the amount of a drug necessary to produce death.

over-the-counter (OTC) drugs: drugs legally available without a prescription.

prescription drugs: drugs legally available only with a physician's order.

chronic: in relation to illness, this term refers to a disease or condition that develops slowly, shows little change, and lasts a long time.

SECTION 3

FOCUS

OUTCOMES

In this section students will learn the:

1. Difference between active ingredients and inactive ingredients.
2. Difference between over-the-counter and prescription drugs.
3. Difference between brand-name and generic drugs.
4. That some illnesses are best treated with rest and good nutrition, rather than the overuse of over-the-counter drugs.

FOCUS ACTIVITY

Display the packages of a variety of generic and brand-name medicines. If possible, include packages from over-the-counter and prescription medicines. Ask students which drugs they think are most effective and which they would prefer to use. Have students compare the ingredients and prices. Have students examine their motives for selection. Does packaging influence their selections? What role does product identification play in their choices? Is someone more likely to buy a medicine advertised on TV, on the radio, or in a magazine? Ask students to examine which is more important when buying medicine: the cost or the fact that it has been advertised.

---

combustion byproducts have all helped to reduce the risk of poisoning.

Prescription drugs and some other hazardous materials are sold primarily in child resistant containers as required by the PPPA. Improvements in child resistant containers should be sought so they can be more readily used by older people than current containers.

People aged 65 and older have the second highest death rate from poisoning. Drug inter-

actions, inadvertent overdoses, and deliberate overdoses may cause lethal ingestion. Better knowledge of details about this cause of injury will allow communities to develop targeted interventions.

The public needs to be informed of the potential for household poisoning, especially when children visit households where poisons have not been adequately secured. (These topics are addressed in Chapter 22.)

Consumer SKILLS

Answers to Critical Thinking

1. to protect everyone's right to freedom of the press
2. Answers will vary; students may think that a large segment of the population would be in favor of such laws. They should realize, however, that it would be difficult to write laws in such a way that they would eliminate the "information" that needs to be eliminated while still allowing accurate information to be published.
3. Again, answers will vary, but students should realize that they are responsible for their own protection. The government can do a great deal to make advertising honest, but as students have seen, there are limits to what the government can do. Finally, each individual must make wise decisions and read information critically.

TEACHER SUPPORT

Key Passage

This is a key sentence: "Pain or discomfort is a signal from your body that something is out of balance." Students should not be in the habit of taking medicine the second they experience discomfort. They should think about what's causing the discomfort.

OTC Medicine Advertising

Consumer SKILLS

Although the law states that labels *on* products must be truthful, dishonest companies may place "information" sheets or cards of *mis*information *near* the display shelf where products are being sold. This trick is especially common in places that sell "health" products or dietary supplements and herbs. However, such sheets can appear in regular drugstores and grocery stores, too. Be suspicious of claims of cures or benefits displayed near products for sale.

A similar trick is used in some magazines. You might open a magazine and start reading a scientific-looking article written by Dr. Rip Off, M.D., who boasts that vitamin X pills clear up acne. Already you think this is strange—*the claim seems too good to be true*. As you read on to the next page, an advertisement jumps out at you: "BALLYHOO vitamin X tablets—only $6.95 per bottle." The advertisement says only that the company sells vitamin X tablets, a legal claim. However, if you were to search for the origins of the article on the previous page, chances are you would find that the BALLYHOO Company sent it, as well as the advertisement, to be published.

The article is full of lies, but it is legal to print it. The FDA prevents companies from printing lies in advertisements, but no law forbids lies in other writing. Lies on labels are illegal, but "information" sheets can say anything and claim the constitutional right to freedom of the press. Your first clue to the hoax is the claims in the article. Your second is the advertisement for the product nearby.

Critical Thinking

1. *Why do you think the government allows these tricks of publishing?*
2. *What would happen if the government tried to stop people from using these publishing tricks?*
3. *Who protects consumers from falling for such tricks?*

factors make them safe to use, and easy to use correctly, without a physician's help.

Overusing OTCs   Many people, however, use too many OTC medicines, too often. Advertisers seeking to sell their products suggest that people pay attention to feelings in their bodies, label them as "problems," and then seek cures through pills. For example, a person who has a headache may quickly take a dose of aspirin rather than trying to identify the cause of the headache. Maybe the person's headache is from hunger or tension. Maybe the person needs to rest more, to eat better, to exercise more, or to learn and use stress-reduction techniques. This chapter's Consumer Skills feature warns you of other tricks advertisers use to sell pills.

Pain or discomfort is a signal from your body that something is out of balance. Before heading for the medicine cabinet for every minor ailment, stop and listen to your body. Try to find and relieve the *cause* of the pain. Instead of taking a tablet for indigestion, try eating more slowly or eating smaller portions. See if that relieves your discomfort.

Misusing OTCs   Many people misuse OTC diet pills in an effort to lose weight. As Chapter 8 discussed, the way to lose weight safely and permanently is to eat an adequate, balanced diet and be physically active. Diet

Ability Levels

Basic

1. Have students work in teams of four to list as many of the guidelines for taking medicines safely as they can. Each student in turn describes a guideline to his or her teammates. Allow 15 minutes for this review activity, then have one representative from each team report to the class. Compile a class list. Discuss which team offered the most comprehensive list, and if any guidelines were omitted.

Life Choice Inventory

How Wisely Do You Choose OTC Medications?

On your own paper, answer yes or no to these questions to find out how smart an OTC drug shopper you are.

1. When I have an ailment, I do not go straight to the drugstore. First, I ask myself honestly if there's a lifestyle change I need to make, such as getting more sleep, eating better, or exercising more. If so, I make the change. 4 points

2. If I have an ailment that I think would respond to an OTC medicine, I first consult a medical book or a pharmacist to confirm my suspicions. 3 points

3. I buy only the medicines I need to relieve my symptoms. (Example: a cough suppressant, not an inflammation reliever, for a cough). 3 points

4. I read drug labels and buy by chemical names, not by brand names. 3 points

5. In taking medicines, I read their labels and follow directions as to dose, timing, and duration. 3 points

6. I do not overbuy, and I throw away drugs after their expiration dates have passed. 2 points

7. Before taking two or more drugs, I check with my health-care provider or pharmacist to be sure there is no cross-reaction. 3 points

8. If my symptoms persist, I see a health-care professional. 2 points

SCORING

For each yes answer, give yourself the number of points indicated. Your answers to the Life Choice Inventory are personal and private. Share them with others only if you are comfortable doing so.

23: Perfect score! You are a wise user of OTC medicines.

18–22: Very good. Identify the questions you missed, and raise your score to 23.

13–17: Not so good. You could be harming your health or wasting money by using OTC drugs unwisely or unnecessarily.

12 or under: Improvement needed. Think, revise your behaviors, and take this quiz again.

---

pills contain stimulants that raise the heart rate and blood pressure. Misuse of diet pills has been linked to seizures and death from heart failure or stroke.

KEY POINTS *Medicines are divided into two classes: over-the-counter (OTC) drugs and prescription drugs. OTC drugs are safe if used correctly and according to the directions. OTC drugs can be overused, however.*

Choosing OTCs Wisely

Sometimes, though, medicines are truly needed. When they are, how can you tell which medicines to buy? You need to know how to read their labels to find what's in them.

---

2. Ask students if they are careful to take their prescription medicines safely. Do they read the instructions on the bottle? Do they read any accompanying literature? Do they ask their parents for guidance in taking their medicines?

3. Tell students that some experts recommend eating yogurt while taking antibiotics. Antibiotics kill good bacteria as well as bad ones. The acidophilus in yogurt may introduce beneficial bacteria back into your system.

A reproducible copy of the Life Choice Inventory is provided in the Teacher's Resource Box.

TEACH & APPLY

BACKGROUND INFORMATION

In your Teacher's Resource Box you will find a handout entitled "Attitudes About Over-the-Counter Drugs." The handout provides students with an opportunity to explore their own attitudes about OTC drugs.

DISCUSSION

Ask students to estimate how much money their families spend on OTC drugs in a year. They'll need to talk to their parents and make some guesses. Have them report back to the class and compare the averages.

BACKGROUND INFORMATION

Among many suggestions for selecting OTC medicines are:

a. Consult a home medical guide to determine the condition you're trying to treat.

b. Ask a pharmacist to help you decide what is needed.

c. Do not buy a decongestant spray for a runny nose.

d. Be careful about using two different medications at the same time.

GROUP ACTIVITY

Have students work in teams of four. Allow students two minutes to list the medicines they have taken in the past year. When the lists are complete, have the teams categorize the medicines as prescription or over-the-counter. After teams have categorized their lists, have a class discussion. Make a class chart. What medicine is taken most often?

DISCUSSION

Ask students what they can do when they have a headache, other than grab a pain reliever. (eat a solid meal, take a short nap, massage their neck) What can they do to relieve a stuffy nose that would not involve medicine? (take a hot bath, breathe steam from a bowl of hot water or from a vaporizer, use saline nasal drops) Why does our society seem to go for the "quick fix," even though it may not be the best one?

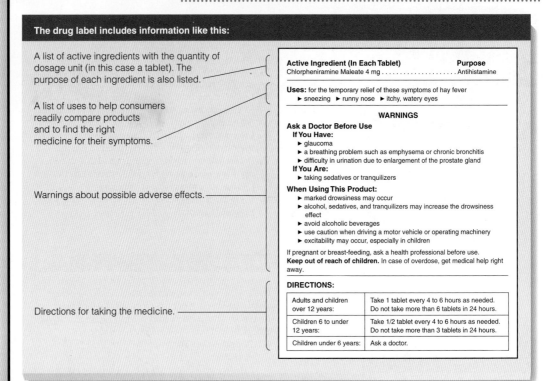

The drug label includes information like this:

A list of active ingredients with the quantity of dosage unit (in this case a tablet). The purpose of each ingredient is also listed.

Active Ingredient (In Each Tablet)	Purpose
Chlorpheniramine Maleate 4 mg	Antihistamine

A list of uses to help consumers readily compare products and to find the right medicine for their symptoms.

Uses: for the temporary relief of these symptoms of hay fever
► sneezing ► runny nose ► itchy, watery eyes

WARNINGS

Ask a Doctor Before Use
If You Have:
► glaucoma
► a breathing problem such as emphysema or chronic bronchitis
► difficulty in urination due to enlargement of the prostate gland

If You Are:
► taking sedatives or tranquilizers

When Using This Product:
► marked drowsiness may occur
► alcohol, sedatives, and tranquilizers may increase the drowsiness effect
► avoid alcoholic beverages
► use caution when driving a motor vehicle or operating machinery
► excitability may occur, especially in children

If pregnant or breast-feeding, ask a health professional before use.
Keep out of reach of children. In case of overdose, get medical help right away.

Warnings about possible adverse effects.

DIRECTIONS:

Adults and children over 12 years:	Take 1 tablet every 4 to 6 hours as needed. Do not take more than 6 tablets in 24 hours.
Children 6 to under 12 years:	Take 1/2 tablet every 4 to 6 hours as needed. Do not take more than 3 tablets in 24 hours.
Children under 6 years:	Ask a doctor.

Directions for taking the medicine.

Figure 11–4   How To Read an OTC Medicine Label
Labels provide consumers with information such as you see in this sample label.

Reading Labels   By reading labels of OTC drugs, you can protect yourself against ingredients that may harm you. If you are allergic to the yellow dye tartrazine, for example, you can choose drugs not colored with it. The FDA makes sure that medicine companies tell the truth on labels. A drug label must list approved uses for drugs—that is, conditions against which the drugs have been proved effective. If products have other, unproved claims on their labels, they can be removed from store shelves.

While you're reading the label, check the expiration date. Medicines change with time into other substances that are not effective in treating illnesses. Do not buy medicines if they've passed the date stamped on the label. Throw away medicines you bought earlier, if they've passed their expiration dates. Figure 11–4 above shows what else you might find on a medicine label.

Generic and Brand Names   Both OTC drugs and prescription drugs are referred to by two terms. First, **generic names** are the chemical names of drugs. These generic names never begin with capital letters. Second, **brand names** are the names given to drugs by the companies that make them. They are always capitalized. (They also have a circled *R* by their

QUICK QUIZ

Chapter 11, Section 3

The following quiz will help you assess your students' understanding of the material covered in this section of the chapter. You might use the quiz as an oral exercise, which will lead into a class discussion of the topics covered. Or, you might use it as a paper/pencil

quiz to evaluate your students individually.

Like the Quick Quiz, the Section Review can also be used as an assessment tool to spark class discussion or as an individual student evaluation. It can also be used as a review in preparation for this quiz.

1. You need a physician's prescription in order to buy over-the-counter (OTC) drugs. (False)

2. OTC drugs can offer relief from many

names, meaning "registered trademark.") One generic drug may have several brand names.

You can often save money by using a generic drug rather than the same drug sold with a brand name. Ask your physician or pharmacist first, though. A generic drug contains the same **active ingredients** as the brand-name drug. However, it may have different **inactive ingredients**—which may affect its use in the body.

Evaluating Your OTC Drug Choices While OTC drugs can help relieve symptoms, they often do nothing to treat the underlying illness. Sick people who take OTC drugs can be tempted to carry on with their regular routines instead of resting in bed until they are well. This makes it likely that they'll be sick longer. They may even suffer **relapses**.

If OTC medicines don't bring you the relief you seek, it's time to visit your health-care provider. Any health-care provider can advise you on what actions to take. If you need prescription medicine, you'll need to consult a physician. To see how well you choose OTC medicines, try this chapter's Life Choice Inventory on page 299.

 KEY POINTS *Both OTC and prescription drugs are given two names: generic names and brand names. Drugs have both active and inactive ingredients.*

SECTION 3 Review

Answer the following questions on a sheet of paper.

Learning the Vocabulary

The vocabulary terms in this section are *over-the-counter (OTC) drugs, prescription drugs, chronic, generic names, brand names, active ingredients, inactive ingredients,* and *relapses.*

1. Explain the differences between the following terms:
   a. active ingredients and inactive ingredients
   b. over-the-counter drugs and prescription drugs

Learning the Facts

2. What are the benefits of buying generic drugs?

3. What makes over-the-counter drugs relatively safe?
4. Describe the problems associated with the misuse of diet pills.
5. List at least five things you find on a medicine label.
6. Who gives brand names to drugs?

Making Life Choices

7. Angela has a cold and sore throat. At the drug store she buys a nighttime cold medicine so she can sleep, something else to take during the day so she won't be drowsy, a cough medicine, nasal spray, and throat gargle. Should she be taking all these together? What advice would you give Angela?

MINI Glossary

generic (jeh-NEHR-ick) **names:** the chemical names for drugs, as opposed to the brand names; the names everyone can use.

brand names: the names companies give to drugs; the names by which they are sold.

active ingredients: ingredients in a medicine that produce physical effects on the body.

inactive ingredients: ingredients that give a medicine qualities other than medical effects. For example, oils and waxes may be mixed with a medication to be used on the skin; water, colorants, and flavors may be added to liquid medicines taken by mouth.

relapses: illnesses that return after being treated and almost cured. Relapses are often more severe than the original illnesses.

minor and chronic medical problems at reasonable costs. (True)
3. OTC drugs are relatively safe, and so can be used without individualized medical guidance. (True)
4. OTC medications are rarely overused or used unnecessarily. (False)
5. Misuse of OTC diet pills has been linked to severe serious health problems. (True)
6. Only health professionals can understand the labels of OTC drugs. (False)
7. The labels of OTC medications sometimes contain false claims or other forms of misinformation. (False)
8. You should always discard medicines whose expiration dates have expired. (True)
9. Generic drugs contain the same active and inactive ingredients as the name brands. (False)
10. OTC drugs often treat only the symptoms of an illness. (True)

FOCUS

OUTCOMES

Simpsons

In this section students will learn:

1. Why prescription drugs are not freely available.
2. What to ask the physician before taking a prescribed drug.
3. How to take medicines safely.

FOCUS ACTIVITY

Have students call out illnesses and disorders that are treated with prescription drugs. Compile the list on the board. Discuss what life would be like without prescription drugs.

TEACH & APPLY

GROUP ACTIVITY

In teams of four, have each student in turn give one reason prescribed drugs can be obtained only by a physician's order. Have students check this page to ensure that they listed all the reasons.

WORKSHEETS

As you conclude the chapter, you may want to use the handout, "Analyzing Medicine Use," which presents students with two different scenarios involving medicines and asks students to analyze the situation.

Health Strategies

Taking Medicines Safely

To take medicine safely, follow these guidelines:

1. Check with your physician or pharmacist before substituting generic for brand-name prescription medicine.
2. Read and follow instructions on labels or on package inserts.
3. Do not share prescription medicine with other people who seem to have the same illness that you did. Their illnesses could be different. Furthermore, a drug or dose that is safe for you may be dangerous for someone else.
4. Do not mix drugs (including OTC and other drugs) without checking first with your physician or pharmacist.
5. Avoid alcohol when using medicine.
6. Throw away any unused prescription medicine or an OTC drug that has expired. Drugs break down into unknown, untested chemicals as they age.
7. Store drugs in a cool, dark place. Be especially careful in the summertime—medicines left in a hot car can turn into who-knows-what. Some drugs must be refrigerated and others protected from light.
8. Call your physician if the drug isn't doing what you expect it to.
9. Call your physician if you develop side effects.
10. Keep the drug in its original container.
11. When taking medicine at night, turn on the light to see the label and your dose.
12. Take the entire prescription of medicine, even if you feel better right away. After the symptoms are gone, the underlying cause remains, and the drug must wipe it out completely.
13. Keep all medicines where young children cannot get them.

Prescription Medicines

Prescription drugs are drugs that are not freely available. You can't buy them over the counter. They can be obtained only if prescribed (ordered) by physicians, because:

- They may be dangerous. They can easily be misused.
- The doses must be adjusted to body weight, age, drug use, or other factors.
- They require guidance to use them correctly. They may have complicated directions.
- They can be abused. They can cause addiction or have other serious side effects.

Prescription drugs are true miracles of our time, when they are used correctly. As an example, for a person whose cells cannot properly use the sugar glucose in the blood, insulin is a life-saving medicine. Another miracle: a person whose heart can no longer use calcium may take a calcium channel blocker, so that the life-giving heartbeat can go on.

Prescription medicines can be misused, though. A physician may prescribe these drugs, but the taker has a part to play, too, in using them correctly.

Suppose your cold symptoms do not go away, but instead grow worse after two weeks of rest and OTC medication. You begin to wonder if your illness is more serious than a cold. You wisely decide to see a health-care professional, who prescribes a medicine for you. Before leaving the physician's office with your prescription, be sure that you know:

- The name of your condition.
- The name of the prescribed medicine.
- Whether the physician recommends using a generic version of the drug, if available.
- How often, how long, and in what doses you should take the medicine.
- Whether to take the medicine with meals or between them.
- What side effects you should look for and report.
- What you should do if you forget to take a dose on time—double the next one, take it late, or leave it out entirely.

Also, be sure that your physician knows about other medicines you are taking. Other strategies for taking med-

special needs

narios to allow students to practice the other guidelines.

Linguistic

Give students an opportunity to practice identifying good health strategies in taking medicines safely. (Refer to the Health Strategies on this page for a list of 13 guidelines.) Have students present short scenarios, and then decide which of the 13 guidelines applies to each situation. You may want to write additional sce-

Scenario 1:

Matthew's little sister Baylee has an ear infection for which her pediatrician prescribed a liquid antibiotic that must be kept refrigerated. She takes it three times a day. As Matt's family prepares to drive to his grandparent's in a town three hours away, they need to . . .
(Answer: Health Strategies #7)

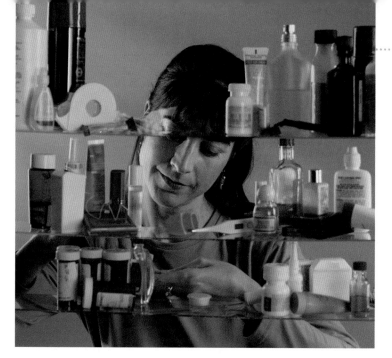

Take care to store medicines properly. Too much heat or light can turn them into who-knows-what.

ications, both OTC and prescription, are summed up in the Health Strategies section on the opposite page, "Taking Medicines Safely."

 KEY POINTS *Taking prescription medication safely requires that you understand the diagnosis, know what medicine is being prescribed, and follow instructions. Follow recommended guidelines for use, storage, disposal, and replacement of medicines, too.*

SECTION 4 Review

Learning the Facts

1. List four reasons why prescription drugs can only be obtained with a physician's order or prescription.
2. Prescription drugs are true miracles of our time, when they are used correctly. What are the two examples discussed in this section?

3. The Health Strategies feature "Taking Medicines Safely" offers 13 guidelines for taking medicines. List five of them.

Making Life Choices

4. After taking the Life Choice Inventory on page 299, are you satisfied with your results? What will you do to improve your results? What guidelines can you offer to your family and friends who use over-the-counter drugs to help ensure that they do so safely and effectively?

Answers to FACT or FICTION Here are the answers to the questions at the start of the chapter.
1. **False.** All drug use involves risk.
2. **False.** Everyone who takes aspirin receives *all* of its effects.
3. **True.**
4. **False.** People who drink alcohol may experience enhanced effects from certain drugs, and alcohol consumption may make larger amounts of some drugs dangerous.
5. **False.** Generic drugs contain the same active ingredients, but may contain different inactive ingredients.

Scenario 2:
Taylor went to a football game and yelled and cheered until she lost her voice. Three days later she still could barely whisper and her throat really hurt. Her doctor gave her a prescription, which she took faithfully. The next day she had a horrible stomach ache and stayed home from school. Because her stomach still hurt after two days, she should . . . (Answer: Health Strategies #9)

Scenario 3:
Damon was practicing for basketball tryouts while Ashley watched. To impress her, he did his famous lay-up shot, jumping higher than he ever had. When he came down, he landed on the side of his foot, and twisted his ankle. Ashley said she had some pain pills left from the time she had broken her wrist. Damon should . . . (Answer: Health Strategies #3)

Straight Talk

Caffeine

In our society, people start using **caffeine** during youth with their first cola drink, chocolate bar, or glass of iced tea. Caffeine in coffee and medications comes later, as adults look for a wake-up effect. Lately, though, some people have been cutting back on their caffeine use because they fear that caffeine may cause harm.

What exactly does caffeine do?

Caffeine is a **stimulant** drug, so it peps up the activity of the central nervous system (the brain and spinal cord). Some of its effects feel like a pick-me-up, with reduced drowsiness and fatigue and a sharpened focus on tasks at hand. The effect on you depends on how much you take in and how much you're used to, as well as your individual makeup. Most people notice a speeded-up heart rate and feel their muscles tense when they take in the amount contained in two to five cups of brewed coffee. More than this can cause abnormal symptoms.

What symptoms does caffeine produce?

It produces signs of stress. Prolonged stress can weaken the body. Caffeine also acts as a diuretic— a drug that makes the body lose water through frequent urination. Caffeine also stimulates stomach acid secretion, so it irritates the stomach, especially in a person with ulcers.

The most severe effect of caffeine is fatal poisoning, but that occurs only with huge doses. For example, if a child accidentally ate 30 or so caffeine wake-up pills, emergency treatment would be required to save the child's life.

Scientists are studying links between caffeine and high blood pressure, adult bone loss, and a painful breast condition called fibrocystic breast disease.

How can I tell if I'm getting too much caffeine?

If you take more caffeine than the amount in about five cups of coffee in about an hour's time, your heartbeat may become irregular, and you may feel your heart pounding. You may have trouble sleeping. You may have headaches, trembling, nervousness, and other symptoms of anxiety.

A physician who is unaware of a person's caffeine use may mistakenly prescribe calming tranquilizers or recommend a psychiatrist for symptoms brought on by caffeine. All the person really needs is to cut down on caffeine intake.

All of caffeine's symptoms seem to hit children the hardest. Children love colas and chocolate, but these must be strictly limited. As people age, they once again become sensitive to caffeine and must restrict intakes.

I've heard a friend say, as a joke, "I'm addicted to cola!" Is caffeine addictive?

Your friend may have built up a tolerance to caffeine by taking in large amounts daily. If your friend were to suddenly stop using caffeine, withdrawal symptoms might start: anxiety, muscle tension, and a headache that no painkiller can relieve. A dose or two of caffeine can reverse withdrawal symptoms.

Is that why they put caffeine in headache medicines, then?

Yes. Someone with a caffeine-withdrawal headache may try plain pain relievers, but these fail to cure the headache. When the person tries an "extra-strength" kind that includes caffeine, the headache

304

COOPERATIVE LEARNING

Snowball Fight

Divide the class into pairs. Give each pair a list of vocabulary words and/or categories (such as factors that change medicines' effects). Have one person in each pair write down a vocabulary word or category on a half sheet of paper and the other partner write the definition or answer on a half sheet of paper. Divide all the vocabulary words and categories up throughout the class so that all of them have been used. After the students have written all of the vocabulary words and definitions ask them to put their desks in one large circle. Instruct them to wad each half sheet of paper up and throw it at someone across the disappears. The pills increase the person's caffeine intakes even more.

If caffeine is addictive, as you say, is my friend engaging in drug abuse?

You may want to read the next chapter and then ask yourself that question. Certainly, if your friend takes caffeine *pills* to avoid withdrawal, then yes, your friend is abusing drugs. However, if your friend drinks only colas, then the caffeine is a food component, not officially a drug. That is why caffeine can be added to soft drinks—it occurs naturally in the kola nut and is an expected part of the product. Figure 11–5 lists the caffeine amounts in some products.

Do you think we should all do without caffeine?

Not necessarily. The equivalent of one or two cola beverages or a cup or two of coffee a day is almost certainly safe for any teenager or adult. Pregnant women and young children might be wise to do without it, though, just because some questions about caffeine are still unanswered.

What are some alternatives to beverages that contain caffeine?

Many sodas are caffeine-free these days. Decaffeinated coffee is an old standby. (By the way, there is no truth in the rumor that decaffeinated coffee or tea contains dangerous chemicals.) Decaffeinated tea and teas made from mint or other herbs are delicious. Don't forget the best thirst quencher—a glass of ice-cold water. Also, juice and milk are "natural" drinks with a health bonus—nutrients your body needs.

Beverage or Food	Average Milligrams
Coffee, 5-ounce cup, brewed	110
Coffee, 5-ounce cup, decaffeinated	3
Tea, 5-ounce cup, steeped	50
Iced tea, 10-ounce glass	70
Soft drinks (12 ounces):	
Colas (diet, regular), Mellow Yellow, Mountain Dew, Surge	50–55
Big Red, Dr. Pepper, Sunkist Orange	40
Jolt (extra caffeine)	90
Caffeinated water drinks (17 ounce or half-liter)	
Aqua Java	50–60
Java Water	125
Krank$_2$O	100
Water Joe	60
Hot cocoa (5 ounces), chocolate milk (8 ounces)	5
Milk chocolate candy (1 ounce)	6
Dark chocolate candy (1 ounce)	20
Starbucks coffee ice cream (1 cup)	40–60
Dannon coffee yogurt (1 cup)	45

OTC Medicines	Average Milligrams
Diuretics	
Aqua Ban	200
Pre-Mens Forte	100
Pain relievers	
Anacin, Midol (2 tablets)	64
Excedrin, extra strength (2 tablets)	130
Stimulants	
No Doz, Vivarin (1 tablet)	200
Weight control aids	
Dexatrim, Dietac	200
Prolamine	280

Figure 11–5   Caffeine in Beverages, Foods, and Medicines

305

Glossary

caffeine: a mild stimulant of the central nervous system (brain and spinal cord) found in common foods, beverages, and medicines.

stimulant: any of a wide variety of drugs, including amphetamines, caffeine, and others, that speed up the central nervous system.

classroom presentations, see the *Classroom Guide to the CNN Health and Fitness Updates*. The **CNN Health and Fitness Updates** are available with West Educational Publishing's *Health: Making Life Choices*.

FAST FACTS

Caffeine raises body temperature because it stimulates metabolism. When running a fever avoid fluids with caffeine in them.

ON LINE WITH HEALTH

You may want to have your students visit the following URLs, where they will find information and additional Web site resources to enhance their study of this chapter. As with all Web sites, you should check these out first to be sure the information found there is appropriate for your students.

Nonprescription Medicines—What's Right for You?
http://www.pueblo.gsa. gov/press/nfcpubs/ nonmeds.txt

Problem-Free Prescriptions
http://www.cigna.com/ upbeat/prescrip.html

These sites have information for making informed decisions regarding medication. The CIGNA site also has links to other related sites.

room. (Make sure they don't get carried away with this part but, allow them to enjoy the activity.) When all the vocabulary words and definitions have been thrown, have the pairs hunt for matches, matching the vocabulary word with its definition or the category with the proper answers.

You can make a contest out of the activity, offering extra credit for the group that finds the most matches, and so on. You may also give extra credit for the number of matches a group gets. This allows for all groups to earn extra credit and to be successful. Groups may also bargain with other groups to exchange sheets that they have in their possession. This encourages classmates to cooperate with each other.

VOCABULARY

1. Answers will vary.
2. Generic names are the chemical names of drugs and never begin with capital letters. Brand names are the name given to the drugs by the company that makes them and are always capitalized.
3. **a.** caffeine **b.** antagonist **c.** prescription drugs **d.** relapses **e.** active ingredients **f.** stimulant **g.** addiction
4. **a.** antibiotics **b.** aspirin, acetaminophen, ibuprofen, naproxen sodium, and ketoprofen **c.** safe **d.** Over-the-counter drugs

RECALL

SECTION 1

1. Answers will vary; could include: prevent disease, help in the cure of disease, make diseases less severe, relieve symptoms, and bring about other desired effects. (p. 290)
2. reduces fever, reduces inflammation, relieves pain, prevents the blood from clotting (p. 291)
3. nausea with severe vomiting, fever, inactivity, loss of consciousness, uncontrollable behavior while unconscious (p. 291)
4. Answers will vary. Refer to Figure 11–2 on page 292 for possible answers.
5. Answers will vary; could include: nature of the drug; form in which it is taken; route by which it is taken; whether or not it is taken with food; age; weight;

CHAPTER 11 Review

Summarizing the Chapter

Your ability to respond correctly to the following statements ensures your understanding of the main concepts in the chapter.

1. List five ways medicines benefit people.
2. Describe the factors that alter or influence the effects of drugs.
3. Explain the procedures the FDA must follow in order to approve a drug.
4. Describe the differences between over-the-counter drugs and prescription drugs.
5. Explain how advertising affects the sales of over-the-counter drugs.
6. Discuss the purpose of over-the-counter drugs.
7. Discuss the purposes of prescription drugs.
8. Describe the effects of caffeine on the body.

Learning the Vocabulary

drugs	effective
medicines	antibiotics
aspirin	anesthetics
inflammation	lethal dose
acetaminophen	over-the-counter (OTC)
ibuprofen	drugs
naproxen sodium	prescription drugs
ketoprofen	chronic
side effects	generic
antihistamines	brand names
transdermal	active ingredients
tolerance	inactive ingredients
addiction	relapses
drug synergy	caffeine
antagonist	stimulant
safe	

Answer the following questions on a separate sheet of paper.

1. Write a paragraph using at least ten vocabulary terms. Underline each term used.

306

2. Explain the differences between a drug's generic name and its brand name.
3. **Matching**—Match each of the following phrases with the appropriate vocabulary term from the list above:
   a. a stimulant drug
   b. a drug that opposes the action of another drug
   c. drugs available only with a physician's order
   d. illnesses that return after being treated and almost cured
   e. substances in medicines that produce physical effects on the body
   f. any of a variety of drugs that speed up the central nervous system
   g. physical or psychological craving for higher doses of drugs
4. **a.** _____ are drugs used to fight bacterial infections.
   b. There are five different drugs that are used to relieve fever, pain, and inflammation. They are _____, _____, _____, _____, and _____.
   c. A drug that is _____ causes no undue harm.
   d. _____ are legally available without a prescription.

Recalling Important Facts and Ideas

Section 1

1. List three ways in which medicines benefit people.
2. List four things aspirin does to the body.
3. List the five warning signs of Reye's syndrome.
4. Refer to Figure 11–2, "Side Effects of Commonly Used Medicines." Name one hazard from each type of medicine.
5. Describe the factors that alter a drug's effects on the body.
6. Define *tolerance* (to a drug). What body organs are affected by an increase in drug tolerance?
7. Many accidental deaths occur when two particular drugs are taken together. What are the two drugs?
8. What is the purpose of a drug that acts as an antagonist?

Section 2

9. List two things the FDA must do in order to approve a new drug.

expectations; other drugs taken; and taker's history of drug use. (pp. 292–293)
6. a state that develops in users of certain drugs that makes larger and larger amounts necessary to produce the same effect; liver, kidneys (p. 293)
7. sleeping pills and alcohol (p. 294)
8. to prevent the action of another drug, in cases such as an overdose, poisoning, or snake bite (p. 294)

SECTION 2

9. They must evaluate drug safety and effectiveness. (p. 295)
10. Because they divide faster, the bacteria die off sooner than the body's own cells do when exposed to an antibiotic. Once an antibiotic is out of the system, the body's own cells soon recover after the bacteria has been killed. (p. 296)

10. Why are antibiotics among the safest drugs?

Section 3

11. What is the difference between generic drugs and brand name drugs?

12. How much money is spent yearly on over-the-counter drugs?

13. What is the legal difference between information sheets and printing on drug labels?

Section 4

14. What information should you know before leaving the physician's office with your prescription?

Straight Talk

15. What effects does caffeine have on the central nervous system?

16. List three side effects of caffeine.

17. Describe the withdrawal symptoms of caffeine addiction.

Critical Thinking

1. Discuss some of the problems people may face from taking aspirin regularly. How can healthier alternatives to aspirin be promoted? How could you publicize this information in your school?

2. Other countries put drugs on the market faster than the United States. Many people go out of the United States to obtain these drugs. Do you think it is safe for many Americans to use drugs from other countries? What possible problems could occur?

3. On Friday night, Kyle suffered a painful swollen shoulder during the football game. To relieve the pain he took a friend's prescription drug containing codeine. Soon Kyle experienced nausea. What should he do? What should he have done after the injury?

Activities

1. Watch TV for one hour and write down all the advertisements that relate to drugs. How many advertisements are for over-the-counter drugs? What does that tell you about our society and the use of drugs? Take an advertisement that promotes the use of a drug to relieve a health problem and change it to an advertisement that promotes healthful activities instead of drugs, for relief.

2. Bring in one article from a newspaper or magazine about the problem(s) of over-the-counter drug use. Highlight information the class has discussed. Read aloud parts of the article the class has not discussed.

3. Make a video for local elementary schools and high schools showing the effects caffeine has on the body.

4. Work with a partner to develop a list of the side effects of aspirin. Your partner should name all the side effects he or she can think of while you write them down. Then you should name any additional side effects while your partner adds them to the list. Work with another pair to combine your list with their list. Then work with the entire class to compile one list. Check the final list against information given in this chapter.

5. Compile a list of home remedies that are commonly used. Information can be gathered by asking friends, family, or by doing some research in the library. Try to determine if cultural differences contribute to the types and uses of home remedies.

Making Decisions about Health

1. Your friend has been feeling tired and run-down lately. Her hectic schedule, which includes school full-time, work part-time, and participation on a softball team, leaves no time for adequate rest or proper nutrition. She decides to make a trip to the health food store to see if she can buy something to give her more energy. She spots a bottle that looks interesting. An information sheet nearby promises that the product will give her renewed energy, stamina, and mental alertness. It also promises the product will clean toxins out of her blood. Are such remedies more effective or safer than non-prescription, over-the-counter drugs? Why or why not? What can you say about the reliability of the information presented on the information sheet next to the remedy?

307

STRAIGHT TALK

15. It peps up the activity of the central nervous system. (p. 304)

16. Answers will vary; could include: produces stress, acts as a diuretic, stimulates stomach acid, and fatal poisoning when taken in huge doses. (p. 304)

17. anxiety, muscle tensions, and a headache that no painkiller can relieve (p. 304)

SECTION 3

11. The generic name is the chemical name of a drug, while the brand name is the name given to a drug by the company that makes it. (p. 300)

12. many billions of dollars (p. 297)

13. The FDA regulates what is printed on the labels, but not what is printed on information sheets. This allows for lies to be printed on information sheets. (p. 298)

SECTION 4

14. name of our condition; name of the prescribed medicine; whether the physician recommends using a generic version of the drug, if available; how often, how long, what doses; whether to take the medicine with meals or between them; what side effects you should look for and report; what you should do if you forget to take a dose on time (p. 302)

KEY POINTS

Chapter 12 is 34 pages long and is divided into seven sections. The chapter explains the difference between drug use, misuse, and abuse. It introduces students to all the personal problems associated with these national problems, and explains why people still use drugs. The chapter then gives students effective tools to use to help kick the habit of drug abuse and to replace it with their own drug-free highs. This chapter includes opportunities for students to acknowledge how drug abuse might affect their future goals. It provides them opportunities to practice refusing drugs, tobacco, or alcohol, and to protect others from drug, alcohol, and tobacco use.

ACTIVITY TO INTRODUCE THE CHAPTER

To emphasize to students just how big a problem drug abuse is in our society, invite a judge or lawyer to visit your class and explain how drug abuse affects all aspects of our society. This should introduce the chapter as well as establish why students should learn how they can help on an individual level. Also have students brainstorm a list of why students take drugs. Follow up by reading current event articles related to crime or death as a result of drug abuse.

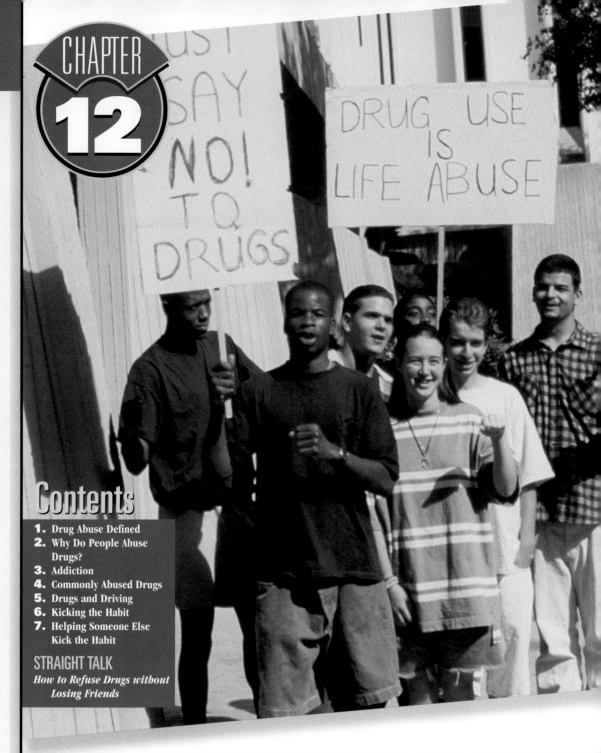

CHAPTER 12

Contents

NOT Enough Time?

Following are some suggestions to help you make sure that you cover the key topics in this chapter if you have limited time. (Refer to the daily lesson plans in your Teacher's Resource Box for additional suggestions.)

DAY 1   Have students read Sections 1 and 2 prior to class. Do the Discussion activity on page 310. Have students practice their refusal skills by doing the Evaluate assessment on page 314. Assign students to read Section 3 before the next class.

DAY 2   On Day 2, have students do the Comprehension Check on page 316. Spend any remaining time doing the Group Activity on page 317. Assign students to read Section 4 for homework for the Day 3 lesson.

Drugs of Abuse

FACT or FICTION

What do you think? Are the following statements true or false? If you think they are false, then say what is true.

1. People with low self-esteem are more likely to abuse drugs than people with high self-esteem.
2. People who abuse drugs are unaware of the hazards the drugs present.
3. When people become addicted to drugs, the primary reason they continue to use them is to experience pleasure.
4. A physical addiction is more powerful than a psychological addiction.
5. Smoking marijuana provides a harmless high.
6. Smoking marijuana is more damaging to the lungs than smoking tobacco cigarettes.
7. Amphetamines improve people's driving because they speed up the nervous system.
8. People usually recover from drug dependency on their own.

(Answers on page 337)

Introduction

A concerned mother tells her husband that she is upset about her son's smoking marijuana—his drug abuse. She is so upset that she takes a double dose of prescribed sleeping pills to calm her nerves.

A young man comes home from a stressful day at his high-pressure job and drinks a six-pack of beer to relax. On the 11 o'clock news, he hears a report of a local cocaine drug bust. He thinks to himself, "Those people who abuse drugs are such a problem to our society."

You've probably guessed that in the two scenes just described, the people concerned about drug abuse were also engaging in it. A discussion of drug abuse with these people could lead to heated debate. People trying to define drug abuse often disagree and end up in emotional discussions. What is drug abuse? Let's try to define it in an objective, nonemotional way.

BULLETIN BOARD IDEAS

Using Figure 12–5 on page 339 for ideas, create a bulletin board with creative ideas for "just saying 'no' to drugs." Use pictures of students in your classes or pictures of people in advertisements. Use cartoon balloons for each statement of drug refusal, and make it look like each person has a different way of saying "no" to drugs. Make some of the statements humorous and others more serious. Ask students' permission before putting their pictures on the bulletin board.

Answers to FACT or FICTION

1. **True.**
2. **False.** Even people who are fully aware of the hazards abuse drugs.
3. **False.** People continue abusing drugs to avoid the pain of withdrawal symptoms.
4. **False.** Psychological addictions can be as powerful as physical ones.
5. **False.** Smoking marijuana is associated with harmful health effects.
6. **True.**
7. **False.** Amphetamines impair driving ability.
8. **False.** People rarely recover from drug dependency on their own.

DAY 3 On Day 3, have students develop a drug-free plan for their futures (Comprehension Check, page 325). Discuss the drug categories and the effects of drugs, using Figure 12–2 and the Discussion activity on page 320. Assign Section 5 as reading homework for the Day 4 lesson.

DAY 4 On Day 4, take a few minutes for the Focus Activity on page 331. Assign students to answer the Section 5 review questions on page 331. Go over answers, then have students complete the Close activity on page 332. Ask students to read Sections 6 and 7 for the Day 5 lesson.

DAY 5 Have students answer the essay question in the Evaluate assessment on page 337. Have students explore the issue of protecting their friends from drug abuse by using the Role Play activity on page 336 or the Close activity on page 337.

SECTION 1

FOCUS

OUTCOMES

In this section students will:

1. Define drug use, abuse, and misuse.
2. Explore society's views of drug use and abuse.

FOCUS ACTIVITY

List some drug use, abuse, and misuse situations on the board. An example of each would be taking aspirin for a headache, snorting cocaine at a party, and taking sleeping pills each night. Ask students to add to each list.

TEACH & APPLY

DISCUSSION

Have students brainstorm a list of positive and negative consequences that can result from drug use, abuse, misuse, and even recreational or social use. If any positive consequences are listed, discuss them with the class and decide under what circumstances they might be positive.

As students begin this chapter, you may want to use the handout in your Teacher's Resource Box entitled "Attitudes About Drug Abuse" to help students evaluate their present attitudes about drugs, before they begin the chapter. Be sure they realize there are no right or wrong answers.

SECTION 1

Drug Abuse Defined

Definitions of drug abuse vary. Medical experts and the Food and Drug Administration (FDA) have created one set of formal definitions. Society has created another set of definitions. Individual people have created still others, based on their own drug histories and attitudes.

The FDA's definitions are these. **Drug use** is the taking of a drug, as medicine, correctly—that is, for its proper medical purpose and in the right amount, frequency, strength, and manner. In contrast, **drug abuse** is the tak-

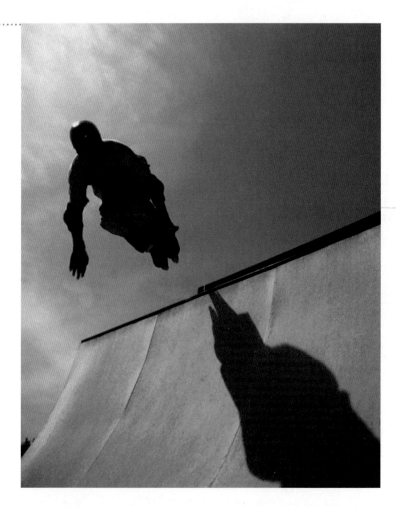

Life is full of natural pleasures, but drug abuse prevents their enjoyment.

Pursuing wellness

It could be argued that wellness is a strictly personal matter. It is, however, important for students to consider that everything in their lives has an effect on them.

Ask students what influence *family* can have on wellness. To prompt discussion, have students consider:

1. The methods family members use to deal with stress.
2. The use of tobacco, alcohol, and drugs in their families.

ing of a drug for a nonmedical purpose, and in a manner that can damage a person's health or ability to function. All drugs can be abused, even those prescribed by physicians. The FDA also defines **drug misuse** (of medical drugs only) as the taking of a drug for its correct medical purpose, but not in the right amount, frequency, strength, or manner. These definitions classify any use of drugs for nonmedical reasons as drug abuse. There is no such thing as mere "use"—for example, to socialize with friends—of a nonmedical drug.

Some individuals try to define drug abuse differently. Many people who take mind-altering drugs call themselves drug users, not abusers. They use the label **recreational drug use**. They claim to suffer no harmful health effects and no problems on the job, in the family, or in society. (People who call themselves *social drinkers* make these same claims.) The term *recreational drug use* does not hold much meaning, because abusers of drugs are not able to judge themselves fairly—their opinions are slanted.

Society's view of drug abuse can be seen in its laws. Society clearly displays its disapproval of mind-altering drugs—except for alcohol for adults—by making it illegal to possess, use, or sell them. By making these laws, society has defined the use of mind-altering drugs, except alcohol, as abuse.

 Drug abuse is the taking of a drug for a nonmedical purpose and in a manner that can damage a person's health or ability to function. Both legal and illegal drugs can be abused.

Review

Answer the following questions on a sheet of paper.

Learning the Vocabulary

The vocabulary terms in this section are *drug use, drug abuse, drug misuse,* and *recreational drug use.* Match each of the following phrases with the appropriate term.

1. Taking a drug for its medically intended purpose but not in the proper dose.
2. A term made up by people who claim their drug taking produces no harmful social or health effects.
3. Deliberate taking of a drug for other than medical purposes.
4. Taking of a drug for its medically intended purpose.

Learning the Facts

5. What two groups have gotten together to define drug abuse?
6. Why doesn't the term recreational drug use hold much meaning?
7. Describe how society's views of drug abuse are reflected in its laws.

Making Life Choices

8. The neighbors are growing marijuana in their backyard. They have told your parents that they use marijuana as a recreational drug. You have just learned in school that this drug is illegal and can harm health. How do you feel about confronting the neighbors? What will you do about the neighbors, if anything? Why?

Glossary

drug use: the taking of a drug for its medically intended purpose, and in the appropriate amount, frequency, strength, and manner.

drug abuse: the deliberate taking of a drug for other than a medical purpose and in a manner that can result in damage to a person's health or ability to function.

drug misuse: the taking of a drug for its medically intended purpose, but not in the appropriate amount, frequency, strength, or manner.

recreational drug use: a term made up, to describe their drug use, by people who claim their drug taking produces no harmful social or health effects; a term not defined by the FDA.

3. Methods used by their families to have fun.
4. The use of, or failure to use, devices such as seat belts as an indication of practicing safe living.

The *community* also influences personal wellness. Have students think of specific examples of the following:

1. Hotline availability for drugs or teen pregnancy.
2. Community commitment to chemical-free teen activities.
3. Recreation programs for teens.
4. Active community involvement in DARE or similar programs.

ASSESS

EVALUATE

Have students finish the following sentences without using the book:

1. A drug abuser is . . .
2. A drug misuser is . . .
3. A drug user is . . .

Students should be able to give descriptions that help define these classifications.

SECTION 1 Review Answers

1. drug misuse (p. 311)
2. recreational drug use (p. 311)
3. drug abuse (pp. 310–311)
4. drug use (p. 310)
5. medical experts and the FDA (p. 310)
6. because the abusers of drugs are not able to judge themselves fairly—their opinions are slanted (p. 311)
7. clear disapproval of mind-altering drugs—except for alcohol—by making it illegal to possess, use or sell them (p. 311)
8. Answers will vary.

A reproducible quiz for Section 1 is provided in the Teacher's Resource Box.

CLOSE

Have students describe, in a few short paragraphs, the different ways in which drugs are abused in our society.

SECTION 2

FOCUS

OUTCOMES

In this section students will:

1. Practice refusal skills in situations involving drug and alcohol abuse.
2. Learn why people take drugs.
3. Learn the consequences of drug abuse.

FOCUS ACTIVITY

Ask students why people abuse drugs. List their reasons on the board. Emphasize euphoria as a reason people continue to abuse drugs.

TEACH & APPLY

DISCUSSION

Three reasons for abusing drugs are given on this page. (a person's physical or genetic nature; personality traits; peer pressure) Ask students to identify these reasons and then state what they believe is the most common reason of these three and why. Discuss.

SECTION 2

Why Do People Abuse Drugs?

Different factors lead different people to abuse drugs. Among them are the nature of the person, the nature of the drug, and the possible consequences that await the abuser from both the family and the larger society.

The Nature of the Person

A person's physical or genetic nature affects the way that person relates to drugs. Scientists are studying people's genetic makeups in hopes of finding clues as to what makes some people abuse drugs.

Personality traits, too, may play a role in a person's tendency toward or away from drug abuse. For example, some people are naturally curious, and curiosity can be a strong motivator. Many people try drugs to see what they are like. Most of these people don't, however, become chronic drug abusers. A few do continue trying drugs, and some become unable to stop.

A strong factor that motivates people to abuse drugs is peer pressure, already discussed in the Straight Talk section of Chapter 3. In some crowds, drugs are often a part of social events, and the desire to fit in socially is strong. The need to belong to a group is normal throughout life. The problem comes when drug taking provides all or part of the reason that a group gets together. The drive to belong is also responsible for other dangerous decisions, such as gang membership.

Some teenagers are easily impressed by how much money people spend and which possessions they own. They lack strong internal values such as the values of good grades, high moral standards, and legitimate work. Such a youngster can make easy prey for an adult **drug trafficker**, who promises the youth big money fast in exchange for carrying or selling drugs for the adult. The teenager is led to believe, falsely, that a **juvenile** caught trafficking drugs is punished only lightly, if at all. The scheme may even work for a few weeks or months. Eventually, though, the drug dealer, who ends up with the cash, betrays the young person, who ends up out of school, in a detention facility, or even being killed in a drug deal. Meanwhile, the trafficker goes free and lures another teenager to carry and sell the drugs.

While it is important to have friends and status, it is more important to resist the pressure to take or sell drugs. Often, when one or two key people stand up for their own rights, the behavior of a whole group can change.

Are you wondering how you can stand up for yourself among friends who are taking drugs? A place to start is to ask why your friends take them.

People who focus their attention on themselves rather than on other people or activities are likely to abuse drugs. People may also abuse drugs because they pride themselves on their "differentness" from the rest of society. Drugs fit their image of themselves as different. Others may lack excitement or fun and look to drugs to fill this void. Still others may lack money or friends or parental love, and they look to drugs as a substitute for these things. Drug abuse may temporarily distract the person—feel like an

For **Y**our **I**nformation
Chapter 2 made clear that a person's values play a role in the choices that person makes.

CRITICAL THINKING

Ask students to give examples of proper drug use. (Two examples are taking aspirin for a headache or antibiotics prescribed by a doctor—both according to directions given on the bottle.) Then ask students to give examples of

drug abuse. Tell students not to name anyone abusing drugs. The examples should simply identify some abused drugs to show the differences between drug use and abuse. Seek examples involving both medicines and illegal drugs (like taking too many tranquilizers for the purpose of an emotional high or smoking marijuana).

escape—from life's problems, whatever they may be.

Unfortunately, when the drug is gone, the person is still left with the original problems—problems now complicated by a drug problem. The "escape" is really a trap. It prevents people from recognizing and solving their problems. People who see this clearly can better take a stand in behalf of their own well-being. The Straight Talk section at the end of this chapter, "How to Refuse Drugs without Losing Friends," offers suggestions to help teens refuse drugs while still keeping their friends.

Self-esteem is another factor. A person with high self-esteem finds it easy to refuse drugs, even when a group offers them. A person with low self-esteem needs more approval from others and may use drugs to win approval and so boost self-esteem.

Often, young people who are deceived by drug traffickers end up in detention facilities.

 KEY POINTS *People's natures affect whether they abuse drugs. Curiosity, a desire to fit in with peers, and self-esteem play major roles.*

The Nature of the Drug

In addition to the nature of the person, as just described, the nature of the drug itself partly determines whether people abuse it. Drugs that give feelings of pleasure—that is, drugs that produce **euphoria**—are most likely to be abused.

When animals are given access to a device to let them receive cocaine, they visit the device often. In fact, when they are offered either food or the drug, they choose the drug over food, until they starve. The drug itself makes them return for more, and makes them forget to eat or sleep. Cocaine can have that effect on people, too. Animals feel no peer pressure or social problems. The drug itself produces their addictive behavior.

 KEY POINTS *A drug that produces euphoria is likely to be abused.*

The Consequences from Society

A person's nature and the nature of the drug itself are not the only factors affecting the choice to abuse drugs or not. The choice is also affected by how severely the person thinks society or the family punishes people for drug abuse. A society or family that tolerates drug abuse encourages it.

MINI Glossary

drug trafficker: a person involved in the transport and sales of illegal drugs.

juvenile: a legal term meaning a person under age 18; a minor. Crimes committed by juveniles are usually punished according to the judgments of juvenile justice, and often not by adult standards.

euphoria (you-FORE-ee-uh): a sense of great well-being and pleasure brought on by some drugs; popularly called a *high*.

ASSESS

EVALUATE

To check students' refusal skills, have the students write a few short paragraphs explaining their answers to the following situation: One of your friends asks you to do cocaine. What is your reply to the persistent invitations? Repeat this exercise after students read Straight Talk on page 338. Compare their answers with what they wrote the first time.

SECTION 2 Review Answers

1. juvenile (p. 312)
2. drug trafficker (p. 312)
3. euphoria (p. 313)
4. because the feeling of pleasure blocks the feeling of need for food or sleep (p. 313)
5. People with high self-esteem find it easy to refuse drugs. A person with low self-esteem needs more approval from others and may abuse drugs to obtain others' approval. (p. 313)
6. Answers will vary.

A reproducible quiz for Section 2 is provided in the Teacher's Resource Box.

CLOSE

Have students think of songs about drug and/or alcohol abuse. Write the song titles or lyrics on the board. Is the abuse of drugs and alcohol "put down" in the songs or glorified? Is taking drugs shown to be mysterious or "cool"? Discuss.

People may think that education about the harm drugs cause is enough to prevent people from abusing drugs, but this is not true. Education alone is not effective against drug abuse. We know this because physicians, even with their superior knowledge, have narcotic addiction rates 30 times higher than the general population.

Anyone who is considering trying any illegal drug should know that harsh punishment awaits those who possess or sell such drugs, or who are even in the same room with them. The punishments range from detention in a juvenile facility to many years in jail. The dollar value of fines also varies, but can easily be an amount sufficient to buy a new car.

At the same time, entertainers, movies, songs, magazines, and books may portray drug abuse as "funny" or "cool." People may become confused and begin to think the views they see in print or other media are those of the society as a whole. This is the wrong idea. Society condemns drug abuse, but it also protects the rights of individual expression through writing and the arts. Therefore, while society severely punishes drug *abusers*, it also fiercely defends the right to make public individual points of view on drug abuse.

Don't be confused by mixed messages from different segments of society. The expression of different views is an important part of our personal freedom. However, you must be aware that society's views and the views of individuals may differ.

This chapter is about some of the most commonly abused illegal drugs. Keep in mind, though, that the most-abused drug in the United States is still the legal one, alcohol, the topic of the next chapter.

> **❝**Heaven ne'er helps the man who will not help himself.**❞**
>
> Sophocles
> Greek dramatist

KEY POINTS *A society or family that tolerates drug abuse encourages it. Harsh punishment awaits people who possess or sell illegal drugs.*

SECTION 2 Review

Answer the following questions on a sheet of paper.

Learning the Vocabulary

The vocabulary terms in this section are *drug trafficker, juvenile,* and *euphoria.*
Fill in the blank with the correct answer.

1. _____ is a legal term used to describe a person under age 18.
2. A _____ transports and sells drugs.
3. Drugs that produce _____ are most likely to be abused.

Learning the Facts

4. Drugs that produce euphoria are most likely to be abused. Why?
5. Describe what self-esteem has to do with drug use.

Making Life Choices

6. Entertainers, movies, songs, magazines, and books may portray drug abuse as funny or cool. What can you do to change this image? How can we as a society change the media's outlook on drugs?

QUICK QUIZ

Chapter 12, Section 2

The following quiz will help you assess your students' understanding of the material covered in this section of the chapter. You might use the quiz as an oral exercise, which will lead into a class discussion of the topics covered. Or, you might use it as a paper/pencil quiz to evaluate your students individually.

*If students have difficulty with the concepts covered in the Quick Quiz and the Section Review, you might suggest they review the material using the **S**urvey, **Q**uestion, **R**ead, **R**ecite, **R**eview (SQ3R) study method, which is described in detail in the introduction to this Teacher's Wraparound Edition.*

1. Scientists are studying whether a person's genetic makeup may contribute to a

SECTION 3

Addiction

Drug addiction (also called **dependence**) is unexpected. No one who starts out using a substance intends to get hooked, but it still happens. A person tries a drug for one reason, but continues taking it because addiction has set in. For example, a young teen may begin to take a drug to feel grown-up and to impress friends. Ten years later, however, the adult person is still fighting an addiction to the drug. The original reason is long gone. The addiction has taken over and may last a lifetime.

Drugs and the Brain

Drugs produce euphoria by imitating the brain's natural way of producing feelings of pleasure. The acts of eating, exercising, and relaxing produce pleasure naturally by way of **endorphins**, pleasure-producing chemicals of the brain. The lack of these chemicals produces an unpleasant feeling, known as **dysphoria**. In this way, nature encourages people to engage in health-promoting behaviors. These natural chemicals are similar to mind-altering drugs, but there is a key difference. The natural chemicals are produced in response to *healthful activities*.

The taking of mind-altering drugs produces pleasure directly in the brain, with no healthful activity associated with it. At the same time, the brain of the drug taker produces fewer and fewer of its own endorphins. Thus after each round of drug-taking, when the pleasure from the drugs wears off, the

Some people choose health-promoting activities over those that cause harm.

MINI Glossary

drug addiction (dependence): a physical or psychological need for higher and higher doses of a drug.

endorphins: chemicals in the brain that produce feelings of pleasure in response to a variety of activities.

dysphoria (dis-FORE-ee-uh): unpleasant feelings that occur when endorphins are lacking; these feelings often follow drug-induced euphoria.

SECTION 3

FOCUS

OUTCOMES

In this section students will learn about the:

1. Physical nature of withdrawal symptoms.

2. Difference between physical and psychological addiction.

FOCUS ACTIVITY

Tell students that a recent university study found that between 1991 and 1996, marijuana abuse tripled among 8th graders (from 6 to 18 percent), more than doubled among 10th graders (from 15 to 34 percent), and increased by two-thirds among 12th graders (from 22 to 36 percent). Of particular concern, nearly 1 in 20 (4.9 percent) of seniors smokes marijuana daily. Ask students whether they agree or disagree and why. Discuss their observations about the use of marijuana at school, reminding them not to identify specific people by name.

TEACH & APPLY

The background information sheet in your supplementary material entitled "Stopping Drug Addiction" will help prepare you for questions the students might ask about different strategies our society is using, could use, to help stop drug addiction.

tendency to abuse drugs. (True)

2. Personality is not a factor in drug abuse. (False)

3. Peer pressure is a major cause of drug abuse. (True)

4. A juvenile caught trafficking drugs is punished lightly by the court. (False)

5. People resort to drug abuse in order to escape from other problems. (True)

6. Drugs help people to deal with their problems. (False)

7. People with low self-esteem are especially prone to drug abuse. (True)

8. Drugs that produce euphoria are least likely to cause addiction. (False)

9. A drug itself causes addictive behavior. (True)

10. It is important to tolerate another person's drug addiction. (False)

COMPREHENSION CHECK

Have students develop their own stress-free, endorphin-releasing activities. Tell students to develop a list of ten activities that give them a natural high. Tell them that what one person enjoys, another may not like at all. Sometimes friendships between two people are based on activities that both enjoy, such as playing a particular sport. Interests like this can help students "fit in" with a group whose members enjoy doing the same kinds of things.

Have students read their lists. Write on the board the suggestions that come up most frequently. Call out each activity in turn and ask students who enjoy it to raise their hands. Tell them to look around the room to notice the other people who share the same interests. You might want to give students time to organize an outing for people who share similar interests.

DISCUSSION

Ask students if they know anyone who has gone through withdrawal. How did the person describe the withdrawal experience? Was the experience successful?

 You will find an overhead in the Transparency Acetate Binder called "The Cycle of Psychological Addiction." You may want to use this overhead for enrichment.

Many people who use drugs to chase away unpleasant feelings are unaware that eventually the unpleasant feelings may be the aftereffects of the drugs themselves.

❝*Despair is better treated with hope, not dope.*❞

Richard Asher

person is left with the unpleasant sensation, dysphoria. The person may then use more drugs to chase away the dysphoria, unaware that still more unpleasant feelings will follow, along with the desire for still more drugs—and so on.

When people take drugs to ease dysphoria, they may be headed toward drug addiction (also called dependence). Drug addiction can be either physical or psychological.

Most of the drugs that cause addictions are euphoria-producing drugs. A few drugs, though, produce addictions without euphoria. Nicotine, the active drug in tobacco, is one. Caffeine is another.

 KEY POINTS *Euphoria is produced whenever endorphins, the pleasure-producing chemicals of the brain, are released. Dysphoria is the unpleasant feeling that follows when euphoria produced by a drug wears off.*

Physical Addiction

In **physical addiction**, the body chemistry actually changes. The body must have the drug—not for pleasure, but just to be able to function normally. As the body begins to clear the drug from the system, the altered body chemistry is unable to function normally. The symptoms of **withdrawal** begin.

The symptoms of withdrawal vary from drug to drug. They may include abnormalities in vision, muscle activity, digestion, brain function, temperature regulation, or many other processes (see Figure 12–2 on pages 320–323). Withdrawal symptoms create an urgent need for more of the drug.

A physical addiction to a drug is detectable from the withdrawal symptoms it produces. Withdrawal changes brainwave patterns, affects mood, and makes the person crave the drug (just as withdrawal of food makes people crave food).

Physical addiction is also involved when the person develops a tolerance to the drug—when the person needs to take higher and higher doses. The craving created by withdrawal, and the need to take higher and higher doses, creates a spiral of physical addiction, as shown in Figure 12–1 on the next page. Recovery from addiction is described on pages 333–335.

 KEY POINTS *Physical addiction occurs when the body's chemistry adjusts its functioning to the presence of a drug. The addicted person requires higher and higher doses of the drug to ward off symptoms of withdrawal.*

Ability Levels

Basic

Ask the class if anyone has ever seen a person on TV or a character in a movie who is addicted to a drug and who is having to go

without his or her drug. Have students describe what behaviors they observed. What did the person do to get money for drugs? Read the following paragraph from the text to the students.

"In physical addiction, the body chemistry actually changes. The body must have the

Psychological Addiction

Physical addiction always has a psychological effect, too—a strong mental craving for the drug. However, **psychological addiction** can occur without physical addiction. Habits or behavior other than drug taking—such as overworking, overeating, or overexercising—can also set up a craving. People who never learned to cope with emotional pain often develop psychological addictions to drugs. This happens because these people have learned they can use drugs to relieve emotional pain for a while. However, this too can set up a cycle of worsening addiction. Psychological addictions can be, for some people, as powerful as physical addictions.

The psychological craving for a drug can last for years after the person has stopped taking the drug. Curing psychological addiction has been compared to trying to cure someone's appetite for food, except that the drug craving is stronger. Imagine to what lengths people may go to get food when they are hungry. The drug-addicted person will go much farther. Attachment to the drug becomes almost like a great love relationship with another person. Addicted people defend, cherish, and protect the drug habit as they would defend and protect a loved one.

People who experiment with drugs often want to believe that the craving won't get to them—only to others who "can't handle it." In truth, no one

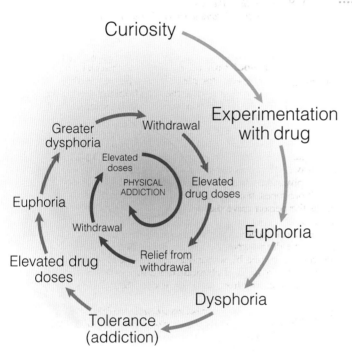

Figure 12–1 The Spiral That Leads to Physical Addiction

Glossary

physical addiction: a change in the body's chemistry so that without the presence of a substance (drug), normal functioning begins to fail, and withdrawal symptoms set in; also called *physical dependence*.

withdrawal: the physical symptoms that occur when a drug to which a person is addicted is cleared from the body tissues.

psychological addiction: a craving for something; mental dependence on a drug, habit, or behavior; also called *psychological dependence*.

drug—not for pleasure, but just to be able to function normally. As the body begins to clear the drug from the system, the altered body chemistry is unable to function normally. The symptoms of withdrawal begin.

The symptoms of withdrawal vary from drug to drug. They may include abnormalities in vision, muscle activity, digestion, brain function, temperature regulation, or many other processes. Withdrawal symptoms create an urgent need for more of the drug."

Ask if anyone thinks withdrawal symptoms would be easy to overcome. Discuss why this would or would not be true.

DISCUSSION

Tell students that the odds that a first-time user of crack cocaine will become addicted are one in three. Does this statistic frighten them? Or, does it make them think they would be part of the two-thirds that wouldn't become addicted? How could they be sure?

GUEST SPEAKER

Bring a recovering drug abuser to the class to describe the daily fight with drugs and addiction. The person should also discuss how he or she became addicted, overcame the addiction, and fought the withdrawal symptoms caused by the drug. As a class, prepare questions to ask the guest speaker.

An overhead of Figure 12–1 is provided in the Transparency Acetate Binder.

GROUP ACTIVITY

Ask students to talk their way through Figure 12–1 on physical addiction on this page, explaining in their own words what happens at each point. Have them create an imaginary character so as to explain what happens in a story-like manner. As they tell their stories, you should be able to determine whether or not they understand the terms *euphoria, dysphoria, tolerance, elevated drug doses, withdrawal,* and *addiction*. If students are having trouble, have them reread the preceding pages.

COMPREHENSION CHECK

Have students write a page explaining the difference between physical addiction and psychological addiction.

ASSESS

EVALUATE

Review Answers

1. withdrawal (p. 316)
2. psychological addiction (p. 317)
3. Endorphins (p. 315)
4. eat, exercise, and relax (p. 315)
5. condition in which the body chemistry changes and the body must have the drug to function (p. 316)
6. abnormality in vision, muscle activity, digestion, brain function, temperature regulation, etc. (p. 316)
7. overwork, overeating, overexercising (p. 317)
8. Answers will vary.

A reproducible quiz for Section 3 is provided in the Teacher's Resource Box.

CLOSE

Before moving on to the next section, check to be sure that students are able to:

1. Describe both physical and psychological addiction.
2. List ways to stimulate endorphin release in their own minds without drug use.

---

who is exposed repeatedly to an addictive drug can remain free from addiction. Remember that even laboratory animals helplessly become addicted when given such drugs. This is why sellers of drugs often give new drug takers the first few doses for free. Once the drug has a person hooked, the seller's job becomes easy.

The only sure way to escape drug addiction is never to experiment with taking drugs that produce it. Groups who invite their friends to join them in drug taking don't have the same motivation as those who sell drugs, but the effect is the same. A few doses into the habit, and the new member no longer has a choice. Groups do pressure people to join them, however, because any outsider who refuses to join in threatens the group's assumption that their behavior is OK. Get the outsider hooked, and the threat is gone.

KEY POINTS *Psychological addiction occurs when a strong mental craving for a drug sets in. The craving may last for years after the drug is gone. The only sure way to escape drug addiction is never to experiment with drugs that produce it.*

Review

Answer the following questions on a sheet of paper.

Learning the Vocabulary

The vocabulary terms in this section are *drug addiction (dependence), endorphins, dysphoria, physical addiction, withdrawal,* and *psychological addiction.*
Fill in the blank with the correct answer.

1. The physical symptoms that occur when a drug to which a person is addicted is cleared from the body tissues are called ____.
2. A craving for something; mental dependence on a drug, habit, or behavior is called ____.
3. ____ are chemicals in the brain that produce feelings of pleasure in response to a variety of activities.

Learning the Facts

4. What can people do to naturally produce endorphins?
5. Define physical addiction.
6. List the withdrawal symptoms from physical addiction.
7. List three psychological addictions mentioned in this section.

Making Life Choices

8. Your younger friend Renee has been hanging around a group of high school kids. Her attitudes about school, friends, and family have changed. She has a large amount of money in her piggy bank. You are sure that the high school kids she hangs around with use drugs. You are afraid she may be using drugs and giving them to other young teens. How will you feel if your suspicions are true? What will you do in this situation? Who can help you?

Chapter 12, Section 3

The following quiz will help you assess your students' understanding of the material covered in this section of the chapter. You might use the quiz as an oral exercise, which will lead into a class discussion of the topics covered. Or, you might use it as a paper/pencil

quiz to evaluate your students individually.

If students have difficulty with the concepts covered in the Quick Quiz and the Section Review, you might suggest they review the material using the Survey, Question, Read, Recite, Review (SQ3R) study method, which is described in detail in the introduction to this Teacher's Wraparound Edition.

1. Drug addiction is easy to predict and avoid. (False)

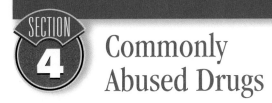

Commonly Abused Drugs

This section discusses a few commonly abused drugs and compares their actual effects with popular beliefs about them. Figure 12–2 on the following pages presents many more details about abused drugs.

Anyone considering experimenting with illegal drugs should know that no watchdog agency such as the FDA screens such drugs for safety or purity. Street drugs are unpredictable in their contents.

Each person who handles an illegal drug makes a profit. To make the most money, sellers mix drugs generously with other substances at every turn. For example, "consumer-quality" cocaine is expected to be "cut" (diluted) with some quantity of white powder other than pure cocaine, usually talcum powder or a type of powdered sugar. However, some sellers of cocaine are more greedy than others, and they add enormous quantities of powders. Then they mask the weakened effect of the cocaine with cheaper drugs, such as stimulants or anesthetics that imitate some of cocaine's effects.

As great a danger as the drugs themselves may pose to the takers, greater still may be the dangers from unknown substances they contain. Street drugs often contain nasty surprises.

You'd be surprised to hear how many people take illegal drugs without first learning about their risks. They think that illegal (street) drugs are about the same as legal ones in their purity and safety. This is completely false. With street drugs, no amount of learning can ensure that the taker knows all the risks in advance. Street drugs can contain anything, even pure poisons.

Marijuana

Marijuana is the most often abused illegal drug in the United States today. To get marijuana to market, sellers harvest and dry the plants. They then sell the flowers, as well as some of the leaves and small stems. Marijuana smokers roll the mixture into cigarettes (joints) or smoke it in pipes. They may also grind it up, mix it with food, and eat it.

The chemicals in marijuana that produce euphoria are all related to the chemical delta-9-tetrahydrocannabinol, or THC for short, which the plant produces as it grows. When inhaled by smoking, the active chemicals are rapidly and completely (90 percent) absorbed from the lungs. They then travel in the blood to the various body tissues that process them—the brain, liver, and kidneys.

THC affects sensitive brain centers. It alters hearing, touch, taste, and smell, as well as the sense of time, the sense of space, and feelings of the body. THC also produces changes in sleep patterns. Marijuana is unique among drugs because it seems to bring about great enjoyment of eating, especially of sweets ("the munchies"). It is not known how this effect occurs.

THC was once used to fight the intense nausea people suffer when they undergo treatments for cancer and AIDS. It also can reduce eye swelling from the disease glaucoma. Because marijuana is illegal, other drugs are used for these purposes.

DEA officer holding a marijuana plant.

FOCUS

OUTCOMES

In this section students will learn about:

1. The effect and dangers of commonly abused drugs.
2. The impact of drug abuse in the school and community.
3. How dangerous it is to take drugs that are bought on the street.

FOCUS ACTIVITY

Have students discuss the safety and purity of drugs of abuse compared with that of medicines. Ask them why drugs of abuse are unsafe and impure. (no FDA approval, greed motivates additions of unknown substances, no consumer protection, and so on)

TEACH & APPLY

GUEST SPEAKER

Invite a school administrator to visit your class and discuss what types of drugs are most commonly sold and abused at school. Ask the administrator to inform students about the school district's policy on controlled substances. How are students caught abusing and selling drugs and what are the consequences?

2. Dysphoria is the feeling caused by a lack of endorphins in the brain. (True)
3. Drug abuse decreases the brain's endorphin supply, causing dysphoria. (True)
4. Nicotine and caffeine are euphoria-producing drugs. (False)
5. Physical addiction occurs when the body's chemistry changes in response to a drug. (True)
6. Physical addiction occurs after the development of tolerance and is followed by withdrawal symptoms. (True)
7. Withdrawal symptoms create an urgent desire for higher and higher doses of the addictive drug. (True)
8. Psychological addiction can only occur after physical addiction to a drug. (False)
9. Psychological addiction is a mental craving for a drug. (True)
10. Psychological addiction often outlasts physical addiction by many years. (True)

DISCUSSION

Point out to students that this table covers four pages and that they should use the table for reference as they work their way through the rest of the chapter. The table does not contain as much information as is provided within the body of the text, but it does contain some supplemental information, such as street names and medical uses of drugs. Because there is so much information in the table, you may want to ask a few questions to help students familiarize themselves with the table and how to use it:

1. How many different classes of drugs are included in the table and what are the names of those classes? (seven: narcotics, depressants, stimulants, hallucinogens [psychedelics], inhalants, cannabis, other)

2. Ask if all of the drugs have a medical use. (No, most of the psychedelics do not.)

3. Tell students that not all drugs are physically addictive. Ask them to name the drugs that experts either are uncertain about or know to be nonaddictive physically. (amphetamines, LSD, amphetamine variants, psilocybin, phencyclidine hydrochloride and others in the psychedelic group, marijuana, designer drugs, clove cigarettes, ephedra herbal products)

4. Which classes of drugs potentially can cause death? (all but cannabis)

Figure 12–2 Abused Drugs and Substances[a]

	Drug Name with Selected Generic Names, Brand Names, and Street Names[b]	Medical Use	Physical/Psychological Dependence
Narcotics	**Opium** (paregoric), *Dover's Powder, Parepectolin,* "O," "black," "dream stick," **morphine** *Pectoral Syrup,* "mister blue," "morpho" **codeine** *Darvon, Empirin with Codeine, Fentanyl, Levo-Dromoran, Lomotil, Percodan, Robitussin A–C, Sublimaze, Talwin, Tussionex*	Pain reliever, antidiarrheal, cough reliever	Yes/Yes
	Heroin (diacetylmorphine), "black tar," "H," "horse," "smack"	No legal use	Yes/Yes
	Hydromorphone (hydrochloride) *Dilaudid,* (meperidine hydrochloride) *Demerol*	Pain reliever	Yes/Yes
	Methadone hydrochloride *Dolophine, Methadone, Methadose*	Pain reliever, heroin substitute	Yes/Yes
Depressants	**Barbiturates** (phenobarbitol), *Noctec* (chloral hydrate), *Nembutal* (pentolbarbital), *Seconol* (secobarbital), *Alurate, Butisol, Tuinal,* "barbies," "downers"	Anesthetic, anticonvulsant, sedative, hypnotic	Yes/Yes
	Glutethimide *Doriden, Methaqualone, Quaalude*[c], *Sopor,* "ludes,"	Sedative, hypnotic	Yes/Yes
	Benzodiazepines *Ativan, Clonopin, Dalmane, Diazepam, Equanil, Librium, Miltown, Noludar Placidyl, Serax, Tranxene, Valium, Valmid*	Anxiety, reliever, anticonvulsant, sedative, hypnotic	Yes/Yes
	Rohypnol "date rape drug," "rophy," "circles," "Mexican Valium," the "drop drug," "roofies," "rope," "R-2," "roach-2," "the forget pill"	Not sold or manufactured in the United States	Yes/Unknown
Stimulants	**Cocaine** (cocaine hydrochloride), "base," "coke," "crack," "flake," "rock," "snow"	Local anesthetic	Yes/Yes
	Amphetamines *Dexedrine* (dextroamphetamine), *Didrex* (benzphetamine), *Ionamin* (phentermine), *Preludin* (phenmetrazine hydrochloride) *Ritalin* (metylphenidate hydrochloride), *Tenuate* (diethylpropion), *Adipex, Bacarate, Cylert, Desoxyn, Plegine, Sanorex, Tepanil,* "black beauties," "speed," "uppers," "white crosses"	Control of hyperactivity in children, sleep disorders, and body weight	Possible/Yes
	Methamphetamine *Desoxyn Gradumet* (methamphetamine hydrochloride), "crank," "crystal," "ice," "meth"	Diet pill, control of hyperactivity in children	No/Yes

[a]The most commonly abused drug, alcohol, is given a chapter of its own—Chapter 13.
[b]Generic names appear in parentheses; brand names are italicized, and street names are in quotation marks.
[c]Quaalude is no longer legally sold in the United States.

COOPERATIVE LEARNING

Divide the class into ten groups. Each group will write a research report. Each report must be written, have a visual aid, and be presented orally to the class. Groups should cite their sources in their reports. Visual aids may include a video, poster, or overhead transparency. The responsibility for oral reports should be shared by all members of the group.

Suggested topics:

1. Over-the-counter medicines
2. Drugs and sports
3. Drinking and driving
4. Alcohol
5. Tobacco
6. Drug and alcohol treatment

Figure 12–2 Abused Drugs and Substances (continued)

Usual Method of Administration	Possible Effects	Effects of Overdose	Withdrawal Syndrome
Oral, smoked, injected	Euphoria, drowsiness, respiratory depression, constricted pupils, nausea	Slow and shallow breathing, clammy skin, convulsions, coma, death from sedation of vital functions	Watery eyes, runny nose, yawning, loss of appetite, irritability, tremors, panic, chills and sweating, cramps, nausea
Injected, sniffed, smoked			
Oral, injected			
Oral, injected			
Oral, injected	Slurred speech, disorientation, drunken behavior without odor of alcohol. For Rohypnol, extreme sleepiness, slurred speech, difficulty walking, confusion, increased irritability, personality changes, memory loss, dizziness, visual disturbances	Shallow respiration, cold and clammy skin, dilated pupils, weak and rapid pulse, coma, possible death. For Rohypnol, headache, extreme anxiety, loss of identity, hallucinations, convulsions, shock, death	Anxiety, insomnia, tremors, delirium, convulsions, possible death. For Rohypnol, anxiety, insomnia, tremors, racing pulse, elevated blood pressure, grand mal seizures
Oral, injected			
Oral, injected			
Oral			
Sniffed, injected, smoked	Increased alertness, excitation, aggression, euphoria, increased pulse rate and blood pressure, insomnia, loss of appetite, reduced athletic endurance, skin lesions. For methamphetamine, extreme aggression, paranoia, hallucinations	Agitation, increase in body temperature, hallucinations, convulsions, injury to the heart and its arteries, heart attack, kidney failure, death. For methamphetamine, restlessness, tremors, rapid respiration, confusion, combativeness, panic, heart problems, circulatory collapse, convulsion, coma, death	Apathy, long periods of sleep, irritability, depression, disorientation. For methamphetamine, apathy, long periods of sleep, extreme fatigue, depression, disorientation
Oral, injected			
Ingested, injected, smoked, sniffed			

7. Hallucinogens
8. Narcotics
9. Stimulants
10. Depressants

Current events would also make good report topics.

Arrange to bring your class to the school library to provide time for research. Reports should include a brief history of the subject or drug classification; a list of short- and long-term effects; a statement of how the drug affects families and communities; the economic costs to individuals, community, and law enforcement; and so on. Reports may include a stand for or against legalization of a drug, which could later be used as a debate topic for the class.

INTERDISCIPLINARY ACTIVITY: CREATIVE WRITING

Assign students to write a story about how their families would change if a family member started abusing drugs or was addicted.

TEACHER SUPPORT

Key Passage

Tell students that the percentage of THC in marijuana today is considerably higher than in the 1960s when marijuana use became popular. Today's marijuana averages 3 percent–4 percent THC with some samples exceeding 10 percent, compared with the marijuana of the 1960s, which usually contained less than 0.5 percent. Many of the studies of marijuana's effects were made using the older, weaker drug. It is unknown whether today's marijuana has the same effects as the marijuana of the 1960s.

DISCUSSION

Ask students what the word *empathy* means. What does it mean to be empathetic to someone? (trying to put oneself in someone else's shoes; seeing the world from another's point of view) Then have students tell you what qualities a good listener has. (maintains eye contact, blocks out distractions, gives feedback such as facial expressions and nods, and so on) Ask the students to listen with empathy while you read the last paragraph on page 318. Then discuss what you have read with the students. Remind them to be empathetic. Ask if

Figure 12–2 Abused Drugs and Substances (continued)

	Drug Name with Selected Generic Names, Brand Names, and Street Names	Medical Use	Physical/Psychological Dependence
Hallucinogens (psychedelics)	**Lysergic acid diethylamide**, or **LSD** "acid," "microdot," **mescaline** and **peyote** "mesc," "buttons," "cactus"	None	No/Unknown
	Amphetamine variants "2, 5-DMA," "PMA," "STP," "MDA," "MDMA," "Ecstasy," "TMA," "DOM," "DOB"	None	Unknown/Unknown
	Psilocybin and related mushroom species "mushrooms," "shrooms"	None	Unknown/Yes, Rarely
	Phencyclidine hydrochloride "PCP," "angel dust," "hog"	None in the United States	Unknown/Yes
	Others "PCE," "PCPy," "TCP," "DMT," "DET," "morning glory seeds"	None	No/Unknown
Inhalants	**Hydrocarbon vapors** from many sources, such as plastic cement, gasoline, spray can vapors "glue," "gas," "poppers," "locker room," "rush," "odor of mar," *Aspirols, Vaporal,* (amyl nitrite) (butyl nitrite) (nitrous oxide), "laughing gas"	Amyl nitrite relieves heart pain; nitrous oxide relieves anxiety	Yes/Yes
Cannabis	**Marijuana** (delta-9-tetrahydrocannabinol) "Acapulco gold," "dope," "grass," "hashish," "hash," "hashish oil," "hash oil," "pot," "reefer," "sinsemilla," "THC," "Thai sticks," "weed"	Relief of glaucoma and cancer therapy's side effects	Unknown/Yes
Other	**Clove cigarettes** rolled from high-nicotine and high-tar tobacco, clove oil, cocoa, licorice, and other ingredients *Djarum, Kreteks*	None	Unknown/Unknown
	Ephedra herbal products (ma huang) (herbal ecstasy), *Ecstacy*[a], *Ultimate Xphoria*	In Chinese medicine, relief of respiratory ailments; in Western medicine, as appetite controller and stimulant	No/Unknown

[a]Misspelling intentional in brand name

The THC from a single marijuana cigarette can linger in the body's fat for a month before being removed in the urine. Drug tests can detect trace amounts of THC for as long as six months after its use.

In addition to THC, scientists have identified at least 400 different chemicals in marijuana. Further, the chemicals vary with each genetic strain of plants, within the same strain from season to season, and even from one part to another of the same plant. These differences in chemical makeup affect the different experiences people have from marijuana.

Another factor that affects marijuana users' experiences is their expectations. How people expect to feel, along with their surroundings and their

HEALTHY PEOPLE 2000

Provide to children in all school districts and private schools primary and secondary school educational programs on alcohol and other drugs, preferably as part of quality school health education.

A quality school health education program should provide factual information about the harmful effects of drugs, support and strengthen students' resistance to using drugs, carry out collaborative drug-abuse prevention efforts with parents and other community members, and be supported by strong school policies as well as services for confidential identification, assessment, referral to treatment, and support groups (often provided through a student assistance program) for drug users.

Traditionally, alcohol and other drug education programs have focused on junior and

Figure 12–2 Abused Drugs and Substances (continued)

Usual Method of Administration	Possible Effects	Effects of Overdose	Withdrawal Syndrome
Oral, injected Oral, injected Oral Smoked, oral, injected Smoked, oral, injected, sniffed	Illusions and hallucinations, poor perception of time and distance, nausea, vomiting	Longer, more intense "trip" episodes; psychosis; organ damage; death by accident or suicide; for amphetamine variants, death from heart or kidney failure or from blood clotted in the veins	None reported
Sniffed, vapors concentrated and inhaled	Altered time sense; brief euphoria; nausea; vomiting; dizziness; headache; liver, brain, and kidney cancer	Loss of consciousness, death by suffocation or sudden sniffing death syndrome, cerebral hemorrhage	None reported
Smoked, oral	Euphoria, relaxed inhibitions, increased appetite, memory loss, disoriented behavior	Fatigue, paranoia, possible psychosis	Insomnia, hyperactivity, decreased appetite
Smoked	Vomiting, respiratory dysfunctions, and bleeding, allergic reaction	Possible death from severe lung infection	None reported
Ingested	Anxiety, nervousness, rapid heartbeat, headache, paranoia	Seizures, racing ineffective heartbeat, death from heart attack or stroke from as few as eight tablets taken over several hours' time	None reported

history of marijuana abuse, all combine to vary their reactions. Reactions range from a mild euphoria and uncontrollable laughter to **hallucinations**. Some people may feel more confident than usual. On the other hand, some may feel unfounded fears and be less confident. They may feel graceful (but act clumsy). They may feel like excellent drivers (but actually drive dangerously). They may feel brilliant or witty (but make no sense). Marijuana may dull sexual pleasure and is likely to make people feel sleepy, not sexy.

The morning after an evening of smoking marijuana is, for many, a morning of feeling tired and down. For many, this is a time to roll another

Glossary

hallucinations: false perceptions; imagined sights, sounds, smells, or other feelings, sometimes brought on by drug abuse, sometimes by mental or physical illness.

senior high school students. However, as indicated by statistics for the average age of first use of the gateway drugs, prevention must also be directed to elementary school students. It is particularly crucial to prevent or at least delay the use of alcohol and other drugs by children and teenagers because rapid growth can amplify the physiological and psychological effects.

State boards of education, governing boards of State university systems, and State legislatures can play a crucial role by mandating school drug and alcohol policies and alcohol and other drug education and prevention programs. States can also set minimum curriculum standards for drug and alcohol education and require teaching certification in the subject. States can disseminate data on effective prevention practices and assist local educational agencies and communities in surveying drug use and evaluating prevention programs.

CLASS ACTIVITY

Assign students to make posters of a particular drug. Include street names, effects, side effects, withdrawal effects, price of the drug, if known, and punishment for having or selling the drug. Students should use Figure 12–2 for information.

GUEST SPEAKER

Bring in a law officer to discuss the legal aspects of drug abuse. Ask the officer to bring a drug board that shows drugs and drug paraphernalia. Have the officer explain exactly what happens to minors and adults if they get caught selling or abusing drugs. Have the officer explain what a "minor in possession" charge is and how these situations might affect a person's future.

they understand how this might happen to someone rather suddenly and how he could come to regret the first time he ever experimented with drugs. What type of friend would get someone started on something that might eventually kill him or ruin his life? Ask students to share any bad situations experienced by (anonymous) friends or family members as a result of drug abuse. Remind students again that they are to be empathetic listeners.

DISCUSSION

DISCUSSION

Ask students if any of their thoughts on marijuana and its dangers are different after reading this section. Did they consider it a harmless drug, used just for recreational use and partying? How will this section help them say "no" to marijuana if they are ever offered it?

FAST FACTS

Hallucinogen abuse is gradually increasing among 8th, 10th, and 12th graders. Between 1991 and 1996, the increases were 2, 3, and 4 percent respectively.

Abuse of heroin gradually increased in 8th, 10th, and 12th graders between 1992 and 1996. The increase is believed to be linked to abuse by means other than injection, such as smoking, because young people falsely believe that addiction is not possible by means other than injection.

The proportion of 8th, 10th, and 12th graders abusing inhalants in 1996 was 12 percent, 10 percent, and 8 percent, respectively. This is not higher than in previous years, but still poses an enormous problem with highly dangerous drugs.

joint to get rid of the unpleasant feelings of dysphoria. This is the road to psychological addiction and habitual abuse of marijuana.

Most people who smoke marijuana have the idea that since it has been around for thousands of years, it must provide a harmless high. Unfortunately, they are wrong. Research indicates that harmful health effects are associated with marijuana. These include short-term memory loss and a shortened attention span.

Marijuana also changes the heart's action, causing rapid and sometimes irregular heartbeats. Marijuana may also impair the body's immune response. In young men, it may reduce both hormone levels and sperm count. Like other drugs, marijuana can pose the greatest hazard to those who use it most heavily and frequently.

Hashish is a concentrated marijuana resin collected from the flowering top of the plant. The resin is smoked or sometimes eaten. With hashish, the risks are higher, because the taker receives a stronger dose.

Marijuana smoking, even more than cigarette smoking, damages the lungs and so can lead to bronchitis, emphysema, or even lung cancer. Smoking three to four marijuana cigarettes damages the lungs as much as smoking more than 20 tobacco cigarettes.

Other hazards exist: marijuana may be contaminated with pesticides, poisonous molds, or herbicides. It may contain dangerous drugs. An example is the animal tranquilizer phencyclidine hydrochloride (PCP, or "angel dust") added to marijuana by sellers to trick buyers into thinking that its potency is high.

A dangerous side effect of marijuana is that it impairs driving ability. Even after a small dose, a person's reaction time and judgment are impaired. The effect lasts long after the high is gone and even into the next day.

Some people respond to long-term marijuana abuse by losing ambition and drive—the so-called **amotivational syndrome**. Others find that they've come to crave the drug and require therapy to give it up.

 KEY POINTS   *Marijuana affects hearing, touch, taste, and smell. It alters the sense of time, the sense of space, and the feelings of the body. Its use can cause abnormal heart action; reduced immunity; a lowered sperm count in men; lung damage, including cancer; and amotivational syndrome. It also impairs driving ability.*

Amphetamines

For **Y**our **I**nformation

Hyperactivity and Ritalin's effects are topics of the Straight Talk section of Chapter 5.

In this high-speed society, a drug that claims to provide some extra get-up-and-go might tempt even a cautious person. The **amphetamines** are said to be just such drugs. They are stimulants—drugs that stimulate the nervous system and so increase activity, block fatigue and hunger, and produce euphoria. Amphetamines are used to treat diseases such as constant sleeping or, in children, hyperactivity.

People may start taking amphetamines to depress the appetite or to combat fatigue so they can lose weight or stay awake at night. They may also take amphetamines to reduce the sleepiness brought on by alcohol, marijuana, or **sedatives**. Sometimes a daily cycle develops in which people take sedatives to relieve the effects of amphetamines and then take more amphetamines to pick themselves up again. The body builds up tolerance to amphetamines in just a few weeks. Soon, the taker may need several hun-

enrichment.....

Most drugs can be placed on a scale ranging from stimulation to depression. Drugs such as amphetamines stimulate the central nervous system, while drugs such as barbiturates have just the opposite effect. While some drug abusers take a variety of drugs, many tend to favor either the stimulants or the depressants.

You may want to give students some additional information about cocaine. Contrary to popular belief, cocaine is not a new drug. The U.S. experienced its first cocaine epidemic in the late 1880s. Sigmund Freud tested and praised the drug in 1884. Coca-Cola once dred times the original dose to get an effect. At this point, drug addiction is severe.

When used as medicine, amphetamines are taken by mouth. The usual route for abuse is injection into a vein. The risks from abusing any drug increase dramatically when the drug is injected. Overdoses are likely. Needles may not be sterile. The skin may not be properly cleansed. The needle puncture may carry life-threatening microbes or a fatal air bubble into the bloodstream. People who share needles share infections such as AIDS and hepatitis (a dangerous, often incurable liver infection).

A person injecting amphetamines experiences an intense, but short-lived, euphoria. The drug taker may feel unusually strong. This, combined with the drug-induced overactivity and euphoria, can lead to dangerous behavior. An addicted person may inject the drug ten times a day for days, with no sleep and very little food.

The euphoria wears off much more quickly than the drug's other effects. The abuser cannot sense tiredness until suddenly overwhelmed by it, perhaps while driving or crossing the street. Severe dysphoria and mental depression follow amphetamine abuse. Thus the person may turn again to the drug for relief. Side effects of injecting amphetamines include extreme anxiety, temporary mental illness, and malnutrition. High doses can cause convulsions, lack of oxygen, loss of consciousness, dangerously high temperature, bleeding of the brain, high blood pressure, and death.

People taking amphetamines sometimes think that the drugs make them better in some way. They think their drugged selves compare favorably with their undrugged selves. In continuing to take the drugs to maintain their illusions, they abandon real life, in which they could become genuinely more sensitive, more fun, more intelligent, more physically fit, or whatever else might improve the quality of their lives.

 Amphetamines are stimulants. They increase activity, block fatigue and hunger, and produce euphoria. Amphetamines are addictive drugs, because tolerance to them develops quickly. Withdrawal from amphetamines causes severe dysphoria and psychological depression.

Cocaine

Cocaine's effects are like those of two groups of medical drugs: the local anesthetics and the stimulants. In fact, experienced cocaine abusers cannot tell the difference between injected amphetamine and injected cocaine.

The drug cocaine is taken from the leaves of the coca bush. In coca-growing cultures, people chew the leaves to receive small doses of the stimulant in the belief that it will help them to work longer. In other cultures, pure cocaine is usually mixed with other white powders—some active, some not—before it is sold. If an unwary consumer happens upon pure cocaine and uses it in the same quantity as the diluted product, the reactions are severe or fatal.

People may use any of a number of methods to take cocaine. One route is snorting—that is, sniffing the powder into the nose. Other routes are injecting or smoking the drug. Many a person who starts by snorting a little soon increases the doses, goes on binges, and moves to the more direct routes—injection or smoking.

amotivational syndrome: loss of ambition and drive; a characteristic of long-term abusers of marijuana.

amphetamines (am-FETT-ah-meenz): powerful, addictive stimulant drugs. Because they suppress appetite, they are reserved for use in cases where overfatness threatens health. Also called *speed*.

sedatives: drugs that have a soothing or tranquilizing effect.

contained minute amounts of cocaine, enough to act as a significant stimulant, which has since been replaced by caffeine. Coca-Cola was marketed as a brain tonic that could relieve headaches, cure all nervous afflictions, and act as an antidote to toothache pain. It was offered to treat asthma and became the official remedy of the American Hay Fever Association. In 1910 President Taft presented a State Department report to Congress declaring cocaine a public enemy. In 1914 Congress passed the Harrison Act, which tightly regulated the distribution and sale of the drug.

(continued from previous page)

party. If they do decide to go to a party like this where people abuse drugs or alcohol, they should be aware that the law of "guilty by association" often applies.

It can help if students will make decisions in advance and not let peer pressure make important decisions for them. Tell students to brainstorm reasons for not abusing drugs or alcohol. Then have students brainstorm a list of reasons teenagers do abuse drugs or alcohol. ("Everyone else is doing it," or "I look like a nerd with a can of soda in my hand," or "People won't like me if I don't join.") List all ideas on the board or overhead and discuss.

FAST FACTS

Cocaine abuse in all forms is increasing very gradually among 8th, 10th, and 12th graders, but the increases are not statistically significant.

Cocaine robs babies of oxygen and nutrients while still in the womb, and causes seizures and other problems after birth.

Cocaine in its smokable forms ("base," "crack," or "rock") is an extremely addictive drug. Smokable cocaine now rivals marijuana in frequency of use in some areas of the United States. Crack opened whole new cocaine markets because of its low price. Widespread addictions and deaths from the drug followed.

The short-lived burst of euphoria from cocaine is mixed with a feeling of being out of control. It is followed by intense dysphoria. The intensity of the high and the low depends partly on the drug dose, partly on the route of administration, and partly on the abuser's expectations. Repeated abuse of the drug shuts off all drives, including the hunger and sex drives. It replaces them with a drug-seeking drive.

Cocaine stimulates the nervous system and brings on the stress response—constricted blood vessels, raised blood pressure, widened pupils of the eyes, and increased body temperature. It also drives away feelings of fatigue.

Cocaine taken into the nose destroys the nasal tissues, leaving a hole internally between the nostrils. Over half of chronic snorters report nasal problems. Many more cocaine abusers suffer chronic fatigue, inability to perform sexually, and severe headaches. Cocaine, and especially crack, causes death—usually by heart attack, stroke, or seizure. It does lasting damage to many essential body systems.

Pregnant women who abuse cocaine risk permanent birth defects and death of their infants. In hospitals throughout the country, doctors are seeing more and more cocaine- and crack-damaged babies. Many of these babies are born too small, too early. The pregnant woman who smokes crack cuts off the flow of oxygen and nutrients to her baby, stunting the baby's growth during pregnancy. Such babies may also suffer seizures and malformations of the kidneys, intestines, spinal cord, and others. Caring for these babies through childhood is expensive, with estimates approaching a million dollars per child. Some women who abused cocaine during pregnancy have been sued to pay for the damage they caused their children.

Cocaine abuse is a problem for over 1 million people in the United States. Between 60 and 80 percent of takers questioned believe themselves to be addicted, unable to turn the drug down if offered, and unable to limit their abuse of cocaine. A person who is addicted to cocaine loses the ability to work, to play, to keep a job, or to stop abusing the drug.

 KEY POINTS *Cocaine is a stimulant and an anesthetic that produces a short-term, intense high followed by extreme dysphoria. Side effects include eroding of nasal tissues, chronic fatigue, severe headaches, birth defects, and deaths of users.*

Sedatives and Barbiturates

Sedatives slow down body systems; they are depressants. Some sedatives slow the heart; some act on the brain and nervous system; some do both. They may be used to calm an upset person, to dull sensation, or to put a person to sleep. Thus they are useful tools in the hands of medical professionals. They can be dangerous, however, when taken without medical care. Some are more addictive and dangerous than others, but none are safe.

The **barbiturates** are a group of drugs that depress the central nervous system, slow the heart rate, slow the respiration rate, and lower the blood

?decision making activity?

Have student brainstorm a list of major decisions that they have to make in their lifetimes. You might receive answers such as what college to attend, who to marry, where to live, and so on. Then ask students if drug abuse might impair a person's ability to make sound and responsible decisions. Tell students that a

good decision is made when a person considers positive and negative consequences of the decision beforehand. Have them look at their lists of decisions and speculate on poor decisions that might be made by a person who is abusing drugs. Ask them if they or people they know ever make a decision without considering the consequences. Make sure they understand that they will have to live with the consequences of decisions.

pressure and body temperature. They, too, have their medical uses, but they are easily abused. Long-term abuse can cause depression, forgetfulness, reduced sex drive, and many other harmful effects, including addiction. Overdoses kill.

 KEY POINTS *Sedatives and barbiturates act as depressants, slowing the body's systems. Long-term abuse causes many dangerous effects, including addiction.*

Opiates

Opiates come from the seed pods of the opium poppy. In fact, some people who ate ordinary poppy seeds in breads and muffins and then took a drug test were shocked when their tests turned out to be positive for opiates. The poppy seeds in a single muffin are enough to cause a positive test result.

Most **narcotics**—drugs that relieve pain and cause sleepiness—are forms of opiates. Narcotics come in different strengths, from **codeine** and **opium**, which are less dangerous painkillers, to **morphine** and **heroin**, which are strong and highly addictive.

Physicians sometimes prescribe codeine for pain relief or to calm a cough. Codeine is weak, compared with other narcotics. However, codeine is still abused for the euphoria it produces, and can cause addiction. Opium is also a pain reliever, but it has side effects such as slowed breathing, slowed heart rate, loss of appetite, and loss of mental abilities.

Morphine is one of the strongest painkillers in medicine. Since it is extremely addictive, its medical use is limited to those with diseases such as cancer, who are in desperate need of pain relief. Morphine is often abused. It often causes addiction with withdrawal symptoms so painful that most addicted people need professional help to stop abusing the drug.

The narcotic abused most often in the United States is heroin, a concentrated form of morphine. It is not used as a medicine in this country because it is so addictive. In fact, heroin is illegal in the United States.

Some young people, drawn to heroin's new higher purity and lower prices, may rationalize snorting or smoking it as "safer" than injecting it. They make a serious mistake in underestimating heroin's highly addictive nature, however. Very soon, the person snorting or smoking fails to achieve the desired effect. As the craving for heroin deepens, the abuser loses any fear or loathing of needles and resorts to injecting heroin. Now the addicted person must have heroin at any cost to avoid the pain of withdrawal. Such costs are often high: loss of schooling, loss of career, loss of family, and many times, loss of life itself.

 KEY POINTS *Narcotics are drugs that are used to relieve pain, but they are also very addictive. Codeine can relieve minor pain and coughing. Morphine is used rarely in medicine. Heroin is illegal in the United States because it is so addictive.*

Hallucinogens

While many drugs can produce false sensations in the mind, **hallucinogens** produce vivid visions, sounds, smells, and other sensory

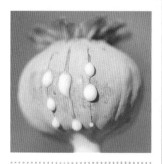

This seed pod from the opium poppy yields a powerful narcotic drug.

barbiturates: depressant drugs that slow the activity of the central nervous system.

opiates: a group of drugs derived from the opium poppy, that relieve pain and induce sleep. Also known as *narcotics*.

narcotics: habit-forming drugs that relieve pain and produce sleep when taken in moderate doses. Also called *opiates*, because most are derived from the opium poppy.

codeine: a narcotic drug that is commonly used for suppressing coughs.

opium: a narcotic drug that relieves pain and induces sleep, made from the opium poppy.

morphine: a narcotic drug that physicians prescribe as a painkiller.

heroin: a narcotic drug derived from morphine.

hallucinogens (hal-LOO-sin-oh-jens): drugs that cause visions and other sensory illusions.

 TRANSPARENCIES An overhead, "Stimulation to Depression," can be found in your Transparency Acetate Binder. It shows several drugs and their effects on a range from high stimulation to low depression.

BACKGROUND INFORMATION

In recent years many critics have charged that federal crack laws are subjecting thousands of African Americans to unfairly long prison sentences while treating whites with comparative leniency. Some studies suggest that more than 90 percent of all federal crack defendants are African American (about 5 percent are white) and many are serving mandatory prison sentences of five years or more for as little as five grams of crack. Each gram of crack is considered the equivalent of 100 grams of powder cocaine according to the federal law. To trigger the same minimum sentence for a defendant using powder cocaine, the criminal would have to be convicted of trying to sell 500 grams. (About 45 percent of powder cocaine defendants are white.) Some argue that the penalties are justified because crack is much more dangerous and addictive than powdered cocaine.

Ask students, "In what ways might a drug abuser have to live with the consequences of a decision? What decisions do drug abusers make?" Students need to realize that young people who abuse drugs alter their ability to make good decisions. Every decision students make is important and may affect their happiness.

Have students work with a decision-making model (see Chapter 2) to practice making an important decision (choosing college, buying a car, spending money, picking a place to live, and so on.

Explain how this is a responsible way to make a decision based on what is important to them. They do not have to follow a plan like this every time but this will help them make a wise decision.

Consumer SKILLS

Answers to Critical Thinking

1. Answers will vary.
2. Answers will vary.

BACKGROUND INFORMATION

Tell students about the highly addictive drug known as "ice." This is a potent, smokeable form of methamphetamine, which was recently added to the problem of stimulant abuse. Like crack, the smokeable form of cocaine, ice produces an intense high without the use of needles. Also, like crack, crystal methamphetamine leads very quickly to compulsive abuse and severe drug dependence.

BACKGROUND INFORMATION

Tell students that more people taking PCP die from injuries resulting from drug-induced behavior than from the drug itself. Auto accidents and falling from roofs and windows are some of the accidents linked to PCP. It is reported that people on PCP have drowned in shallow water because they were unable to tell which way was up. Also linked to PCP use are suicides, self-inflicted wounds, and drownings from sedation.

FAST FACTS

Nearly five percent of 10th and 12th graders abused MDMA (ecstasy) in 1996. The abuse of crystal methamphetamine (ice) by 12th graders more than doubled between 1992 and 1996.

Look-alikes

Another group of easily purchased drugs is the so-called **look-alikes**. Drug pushers, posing as companies, combine medicines, such as the potentially dangerous drug **ephedrine**, and other legal substances to produce pills and powders that look like the illegal drugs that abusers seek. For example, magazines publish ads for "legal stimulants" ("mail-order speed") that look like amphetamines, but with one important difference: the pills contain a mix of over-the-counter stimulants, decongestants, caffeine, and other drugs instead of amphetamines.

Because look-alikes are weaker than the drugs they look like, takers tend to take a lot of them and then experience sleep disturbances, abnormal heartbeat, and sudden rises in blood pressure. The most

dangerous situation is when a taker can't tell the difference between the look-alike and the real thing. When such a person gets some of the real, high-powered drugs and takes the same number of pills, a fatal overdose results.

The look-alikes are legal in many states, so there are few limits on their sale. Those who sell them make huge profits at the expense of the taker's health. So it is with all street drugs—no one is looking out for the consumer.

Critical Thinking

1. Do you think companies should be allowed to advertise "legal stimulants" in magazines? Why or why not?
2. Should look-alikes be legal? Give reasons for your answer.

experiences that are out of touch with reality. One of the best known of the hallucinogens is **LSD (lysergic acid diethylamide)**. So powerful is the pure chemical LSD that just a tiny drop of solution, ingested with sugar or other food, sends the taker on a mental "trip" of distorted visions that lasts for hours, and that cannot be stopped until the drug wears off. Some people say that trips have given them new ideas. Others, though, have experienced nightmarish "bad trips." A person having a bad trip may become irrational and do dangerous things to try to escape an imaginary pursuer. A taker of LSD may experience a temporary resurfacing of the drug's effects, called a flashback, days or even years after the original trip has subsided.

A drug that causes frightening hallucinations and violent tendencies is **PCP (phencyclidine hydrochloride)**. It was first made as a tranquilizer for animals. People who take it for its hallucinogenic effect suffer dangerous and unpredictable side effects. PCP causes some users to become so violent that they commit murder or suicide. Others suffer seizures, coma, and death.

Some hallucinogenic drugs are made in the tissues of plants. The **peyote** cactus produces the drug **mescaline**. Mescaline's effects have been compared to a mild LSD trip, but one accompanied by vomiting, sweating, and painful abdominal cramping. The taking of peyote is part of the religious ceremonies of some Native Americans of the southwestern United States. Two other hallucinogens, **psilocybin** and **psilocin**, are part of the tissues of a strain of mushrooms. Many wild mushrooms look alike, but some contain deadly poisons. Even expert mushroom hunters have been fooled by appearances.

HEALTHY PEOPLE 2000

Increase by at least 1 year the average age of first use of cigarettes, alcohol, and marijuana by adolescents aged 12 through 17. Drug use among young people appears to develop in predictable stages, consistent with the "gateway" concept. This concept suggests that experimentation with drugs usually begins with cigarettes, alcohol, or marijuana, and then

progresses to other drugs. Young people engage in relatively little experimentation with most illicit drugs before the final three years of high school. Less than 11 percent of the class of 1986 had tried any illicit drug except marijuana before they entered the 10th grade. However, 50 percent of the high school seniors who had ever used marijuana already had used it before entering high school, while an even greater percentage of pre-high school students had already used alcohol.

Drugs that produce false sensations in the mind, such as vivid and distorted visions, are called hallucinogens. LSD, PCP, mescaline, psilocybin, and psilocin are hallucinogens.

Inhalants

Three types of chemicals are sometimes inhaled to produce a high. The first type, solvents, are liquids that vaporize at room temperature. They include fumes from gasoline, glue, lighter fluid, cleaning fluid, and paint thinner. A second type, propellants, are substances added to products such as paint, deodorant, hair spray, whipped cream, and oil to make them sprayable. A third type is intended for medical use: chloroform, ether, nitrous oxide (laughing gas), and others. Amyl nitrite, a heart pain medicine, is sometimes abused this way. So is butyl nitrite, sold legally as a "room odorizer."

Products of the first two types bear labels that warn against inhaling their fumes because of the hazards they present. A person who experiments with them, even once, risks permanent brain damage or death from heart failure or suffocation. Chemicals of the third type bring on headache, dizziness, a quickened heart rate, nausea, nasal irritation, or coughing. In high doses, they may cause a heart attack or stroke.

The effects of inhalants on brain cells are unpredictable. The effects depend on the chemicals inhaled and the dose. In general, even short-term abuse disrupts vision, impairs judgment, and reduces muscle and reflex control. These effects may be permanent. Many cases of permanent brain and nerve damage have resulted from sniffing.

The cells of the brain and nerves are made largely of fat. Fats dissolve in solvents. Thus when solvent vapors reach the brain, the brain cells begin to dissolve. Brain scans of habitual sniffers of solvents often show that whole areas of the brain have been lost in this way. The kidneys, blood, liver, and bone marrow also suffer damage.

The use of inhalants can cause death. When the lungs fill with gases that contain no oxygen, or when the sniffer passes out with a plastic bag over the nose and mouth, death by suffocation results. However, most deaths from inhalant abuse are from **sudden sniffing death syndrome**, which results when a person who is sniffing experiences a sudden fright. The fright causes a surge of stress hormones that stops the heart.

 Three categories of chemicals are used as inhalants: solvents, propellants, and medicines such as chloroform and nitrous oxide. People who experiment with inhalants risk permanent disability or death.

Designer Drugs

Laboratory-made drugs that closely resemble illegal drugs in chemical structure are called **designer drugs**. Two examples are MDMA (*Ecstasy*), which mimics methamphetamines, and *fentanyl*, a synthetic narcotic commonly used in surgery, but sold on the street as synthetic heroin.

Each drug is defined as legal or illegal based on its exact chemical formula. Because designer drugs have new formulas, they are legal, at least for a while. They are similar enough to illegal drugs so that they produce similar effects in the body—at least, that is the maker's plan.

Mini Glossary

look-alikes: combinations of OTC drugs and other chemicals packaged to look like prescription medications or illegal drugs.

ephedrine: a stimulant added to look-alikes and diet pills, and found in herbs such as ma huang; has caused heart attacks, strokes, seizures, and death, especially when combined with caffeine.

LSD (lysergic acid diethylamide): a powerful hallucinogenic drug. Also called *acid*.

PCP (phencyclidine hydrochloride): an animal tranquilizer, abused by human beings as a hallucinogen.

peyote: a cactus that produces the hallucinogen mescaline.

mescaline: the hallucinogen produced by the peyote cactus.

psilocybin (sill-oh-SI-bin), **psilocin** (sill-OH-sin): two hallucinogens produced by a type of wild mushroom.

sudden sniffing death syndrome: sudden death, usually from heart failure, in a person who is startled while abusing inhalants. The fright often occurs upon discovery of the sniffer by an authority figure or when the drug produces a frightening hallucination.

designer drugs: laboratory-made drugs that closely resemble illegal drugs in chemical structure, but that are different enough to be legal until ruled illegal.

This objective is particularly important because the use of drugs at preteen ages, especially use of those gateway drugs, appears to predict both greater involvement with alcohol and with other drugs and less likelihood of recovery. The use of cigarettes, alcohol, and marijuana is correlated with other health problems including adolescent suicide, homicide, school dropout, motor vehicle crashes, delinquency, and early sexual activity. People who begin smoking in childhood are more inclined toward heavy smoking or drinking at an earlier age than those who start later. They also are more likely to abuse other drugs. Young adults are unlikely to develop alcohol and drug problems if age of first use is delayed beyond childhood and adolescence.

Marijuana use exemplifies the age-at-first-use phenomenon. Use of marijuana prior to age 15 has been associated with both heavier use after 15 and the use of other drugs.

BACKGROUND INFORMATION

One of the most disturbing characteristics of inhalants is their availability. Currently, there are in excess of 300 products offered in aerosol form. Because of the relative ease with which these products can be obtained (and abused), and to discourage abuse, many of the products have certain chemical additives, which result in unpleasant side effects in inhalants.

BACKGROUND INFORMATION

Many people experience very pronounced psychological effects from inhaling volatile substances. Among the effects experienced are tenseness, retarded motor-coordination skills, lack of behavioral control, confusion, hyperactivity, impaired judgment, and in some cases, acute psychosis and permanent brain damage.

GUEST SPEAKER

Invite an emergency room doctor or nurse to speak to your class about drug overdoses or drug-related injuries that they have seen or treated. Ask the speaker to emphasize how many patients get treated, but have no money. Those treatments are paid for by the students' parents' tax dollars.

INTERDISCIPLINARY ACTIVITY: ART

Assign students to make their own antidrug posters or notebook covers to be displayed around the classroom.

ASSESS

EVALUATE

SECTION 4 Review Answers

1. barbiturates (pp. 326–327)
2. heroin (p.327)
3. morphine
4. for a month (p. 322)
5. because the taker receives a stronger dose (p. 324)
6. extreme anxiety, temporary mental illness, and malnutrition (p. 325)
7. birth defects; death of infants; stunted growth; suffer seizures and malformations of kidneys, intestines, spinal cord, and others (p. 326)
8. LSD (pp. 327–328)
9. Answers will vary.

A reproducible quiz for Section 4 is provided in the Teacher's Resource Box.

CLOSE

Assign students to choose three types of drugs. Then have them write essays describing how the drugs would adversely affect their lives if they abused them.

A story of what actually can happen with designer drugs was told in an episode of the public television series *Nova.* A fumbling amateur chemist, using a crude basement laboratory in California, tried to produce a batch of designer heroin. His attempt at chemistry produced, instead, a substance toxic to brain cells. When the heroin addicts who purchased it injected the stuff, they were immediately and permanently paralyzed. The substance left them with Parkinson's disease—destruction of the parts of the brain that control muscle movements. When the police found and arrested the "chemist," he, too, had developed parkinsonism from his creation. He had absorbed the chemical through his skin and lungs while making it.

This story shows the problem all takers of street drugs face: lack of testing. People who take street drugs, or even simply handle them, are risking exposure to highly toxic chemicals. The Consumer Skills feature on page 328, "Look-alikes," warns of street drugs made from legal, but often dangerous substances.

 KEY POINTS *Designer drugs are laboratory-made drugs that closely resemble illegal drugs in chemical structure. Lack of testing presents an enormous risk to the taker.*

SECTION 4 Review

Answer the following questions on a sheet of paper.

Learning the Vocabulary

The vocabulary terms in this section are *hallucinations, amotivational syndrome, amphetamines, sedatives, barbiturates, opiates, narcotics, codeine, opium, morphine, heroin, hallucinogens, look-alikes, ephedrine, LSD (lysergic acid diethylamide), PCP (phencyclidine hydrochloride), peyote, mescaline, psilocybin, psilocin, sudden sniffing death syndrome,* and *designer drugs.*
Use the clues given to help you determine the term.

1. Depressant drugs that slow the activity of the central nervous system.
2. A narcotic drug derived from morphine, illegal in the United States.
3. A narcotic drug that is prescribed by physicians as a painkiller.

Learning the Facts

4. How long does THC linger in the body?
5. Why are the risks of using hashish even greater than the risks of using marijuana?
6. What are the side effects of injecting amphetamines?
7. What are the risks for the unborn baby and the newborn when the mother uses cocaine?
8. What is one of the best known hallucinogens?

Making Life Choices

9. Reread the Consumer Skills feature, "Look-alikes," on page 328. Discuss some of the problems associated with look-alike drugs. What problems do users experience? Why are look-alikes potentially dangerous?

QUICK QUIZ

Chapter 12, Section 4

The following quiz will help you assess your students' understanding of the material covered in this section of the chapter. You might use the quiz as an oral exercise, which will lead into a class discussion of the topics covered. Or, you might use it as a paper/pencil
quiz to evaluate your students individually.

If students have difficulty with the concepts covered in the Quick Quiz and the Section Review, you might suggest they review the material using the S urvey, Q uestion, R ead, R ecite, R eview (SQ3R) study method, which is described in detail in the introduction to this Teacher's Wraparound Edition.

1. The content of any street drug is absolutely unpredictable. (True)

SECTION 5

Drugs and Driving

One more hazard of all the drugs just described is their effect on driving ability. Mind-altering drugs, including alcohol, marijuana, and others, slow people's reactions and make them unable to judge how fast they are going. In simulator tests, people on drugs crash often. In the cases of alcohol and marijuana, the impairment of driving lasts for hours *after* the high from the drug has worn off—even into the next day.

You might think amphetamines would improve people's driving, because they speed up the nervous system. Accident studies show otherwise, though. Heavy amphetamine use allows fatigued people to override their feelings of exhaustion. Their driving ability, however, declines even though they think they are doing well.

Even many over-the-counter medicines can impair a person's ability to drive. In one year alone, 1995, more than 17,000 needless deaths and untold numbers of injuries could have been prevented if people taking drugs or medicines that affect driving would have stayed away from the wheel.

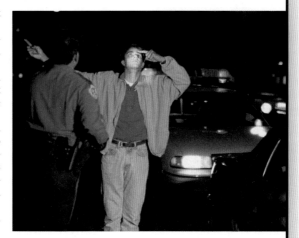

A person who is too impaired to walk should certainly not drive.

 KEY POINTS *Mind-altering drugs slow people's reactions and impair their judgment of speed. Therefore, mind-altering drugs impair driving ability.*

 Review

Answer the following questions on a sheet of paper.

Learning the Facts
1. List the effects drugs have on driving.
2. Could marijuana and alcohol have an effect on your ability to drive the next day? Explain your answer.
3. How do amphetamines impair a person's ability to drive?

Making Life Choices
4. You are visiting an aunt's house. She wants to take you out to her favorite restaurant. Before you go she has to take a diet pill. She also has been sipping on wine most of the afternoon. You have a long drive to get to this special restaurant. What are some of the problems that may occur on your way? How can you help prevent these problems? What will you do to protect yourself from danger? What can you do differently the next time you go to visit her?

2. There are no known health risks associated with taking marijuana. (False)
3. Marijuana does not impair driving ability. (False)
4. Amphetamines are highly addictive stimulants that have severe withdrawal symptoms, including dysphoria and psychological depression. (True)
5. Cocaine is a depressant. (False)
6. Sedatives and barbiturates increase the activities of the central nervous system.

(False)
7. Codeine, morphine, and heroin are narcotics. (True)
8. Hallucinogens produce false sensations in the mind. (True)
9. There are only mild health risks associated with inhalant abuse. (False)
10. Designer drugs are artificially made, and their effects are highly unpredictable. (True)

SECTION 5

FOCUS

OUTCOMES

In this section students will learn that:

1. Drugs affect judgment needed for driving.
2. Marijuana and alcohol affect driving long after the high has worn off.

FOCUS ACTIVITY

Have students brainstorm a list of OTC drugs they have at home that could affect driving. List these on the board. This will get students thinking about the drugs that could affect drivers in their own families.

TEACH & APPLY

DISCUSSION

Have students investigate how different drugs affect the nervous system and a person's judgment. Have different groups research marijuana, alcohol, OTC medications, and amphetamines.

ASSESS

EVALUATE

 Review Answers

1. slow people's reactions and makes them unable to judge how fast they are going (p. 331)

(continued on next page)

(continued from previous page)

2. Yes. In cases of marijuana and alcohol the impairment of driving lasts for hours after the high has worn off, even into the next day. (p. 331)

3. They allow fatigued people to override their feelings of exhaustion. Their driving ability has declined even though they think they are doing well. (p. 331)

4. Answers will vary; could include: discussion of aunt's driving ability, offering to drive or skip the special dinner, or calling a taxi.

CLOSE

Have students write a paragraph describing how drugs can affect driving.

Discussion

Here are some questions that should help you promote class discussion.

1. How has the drug abuse in your community affected you personally?

2. Do you think that adults are aware of the drug problems in your school?

How Has Drug Abuse Affected Your School Or Community?

We go to school with people selling drugs. The principal and teachers who know keep asking to make unexpected searches to see if you have drugs on you. When they find out that a student has drugs, they call the cops. In our community little kids can't go out and play because of all the drug traffic. There could be a cross-fire shooting or even a dealer trying to sell drugs to them.
Shay Murphy, 18,
Poughkeepsie High School, NY

Drug abuse is a serious problem in all communities, not just mine. I know of people who have used drugs, and have even sold them. Drugs have become a normal thing. It is common to hear people discussing their plans for the weekend and hear them say they are going to get high, trip, or go out drinking. Because of drug busts in our community, people have stopped, or they have become more aware. You can get drugs as easily as buying a newspaper. They are being sold on every corner.
Keith Levy, 18,
Orange Park High School, FL

Drug abuse has affected my school and community by causing an increase in crime. I think that most acts of crime are done under the influence of drugs. In school it has caused the number of dropouts to increase.
Hannah Gleason, 15,
Manzano High School, NM

Though drug abuse creates a problem everywhere drugs are accessible, I don't think it has greatly affected my community, and I have only attended my high school for one year. I live in a fairly rural community and drugs haven't played a major role in our lives here. I do, however, see that if drug abuse were to become a prevalent issue in our town it would cause a major uprising, which would offbalance our whole community. Drug abuse would burden us greatly for we're all interrelated by family, friendship, or employment and the problems of one will be taken on by our community as a whole.
Marin Hice Miller, 14,
Manzano High School, NM

Drugs consume the lives of the people who use them to the point where people neglect themselves, their responsibilities, and everything just for a fix. This has lead to chaos in my community. Children have been neglected, and people have been killed. Also, diseases spread easily. Drug abusers do not care about being sterile.
Emilee Owen, 15,
Manzano High School, NM

I have seen countless people around me wreck their lives over something they call a "drug." I think that "drug" doesn't define it accurately. "Life ruiner" would make a lot more sense. When your only purpose in life is to get something, why do you even go on? We need to reach out to these young people and show them the love and guidance my parents and God have shown me.
Josh MacDonald, 14,
Manzano High School, NM

Drug abuse has changed my community a great deal. When I was younger, it was easier growing up in my neighborhood. People were more concerned for every child. Times have changed. You have to be careful walking down the street because a crackhead might try to kill you. Little ones have to stay in the house. Everywhere you go, people are selling and using drugs. Death is everywhere, in the parks, at home, and in the schools. Drug abuse is killing innocent people. Government spends so much money on defense, but they can't invest money on America's future. Drugs in the community have brought my community down. It seems like the government doesn't care as long as drug abuse stays in the black community.
George Watson, 17,
Woodrow Wilson High School, CA

Pursuing wellness

If you or one of your students knows someone who is looking for a treatment program for a drug problem, encourage that person to discuss the following questions with a trained professional to determine the best treatment program:

1. How serious is the abuse problem? Is the person out of control and unable to stop abusing? Are large amounts of drugs being taken?

2. Is there an addiction to several drugs? If so, is detoxification necessary?

3. Has the drug abuse resulted in serious behavioral and psychiatric problems? Have medical problems resulted? Is the

Kicking the Habit

When people realize they have a drug problem, they have taken one important step: admitting it. Now comes a hard choice: suffer on and on, or quit. To quit involves suffering, too, but the suffering ends. Recovery requires much more than is presented here. The process is described in the next chapter.

Facing the Problem If you think a drug may be causing you a problem, here is a way to recognize it: give up the drug for a month. (Of course, if the drug is a medicine, the physician should decide whether it is safe to do without it.) Coffee, colas, cigarettes, herbs, OTC drugs, prescriptions, and alcohol, as well as illegal drugs, all qualify for this test. Try doing without one, and write down your responses to this chapter's Life Choice Inventory on the next page. The first step in solving a drug problem is to face the fact that you have one.

Getting Help For those who face the problem and choose to quit, the next step is to get help. Rarely do people recover from drugs on their own. Figure 12–3 lists sources of help. Help comes in many forms—hospitalization,

Many agencies stand ready to help teens with drug problems or just to answer questions. You don't have to give your name. A few examples are Covenant House, Just Say No International, National Cocaine Hotline, and National Institute of Drug Abuse. To find these agencies and others:

Look in your telephone book under Drug Abuse, Drug Addiction, Alcohol Treatment, or Rehabilitation Services.

Go to the local library, and ask the reference librarian for the addresses and telephone numbers of drug abuse agencies.

Ask someone you trust—such as your parents, a favorite teacher, or the school guidance counselor—for help in finding a drug abuse agency.

Figure 12–3 Help Resources

Enjoy Life

Pleasure is there for the taking, for those who know where to look.

▶ Run, walk, or skip across an open field or along a beach.
▶ Ask a grandparent what life is about.
▶ Play with a baby.
▶ Give a friend a gift that you made with your own hands.
▶ Work hard at something, and see it through to completion.
▶ Have a good cry about that thing you have been hiding from for too long.
▶ Learn some relaxation techniques.
▶ Eat a delicious, nourishing food.
▶ Write some poetry for yourself (it doesn't have to rhyme).
▶ Climb a mountain; or visit a river, ocean, or lake.
▶ Say "thank you" more often.
▶ Beat the feathers out of a pillow next time you are very angry.
▶ Stop biting your nails (or another bad habit).
▶ Read a good book.
▶ Give someone a long hug.
▶ Tell your parent, "I love you."
▶ Volunteer your time to help others (serve food at a soup kitchen, or collect needed items for your favorite charity).

Source: Adapted from S. J. Levy, Managing the "Drugs" in Your Life (New York: McGraw-Hill, 1983), p. 104.

person violent or suicidal?
4. Can the person still function on a daily basis? (go to work, relate to people, and so on)
5. Has the person tried and failed in other attempts at treatment?

You might want to have students talk with a local drug counselor or a group such as Narcotics Anonymous to find out if there are things in addition to this list that they look for in a person with a drug problem. If there are additional questions, have students add them to the list.

FOCUS

OUTCOMES

In this section students will learn:

1. How difficult it is to give up a drug problem.
2. That the first step to beating drug abuse is admitting to a drug problem.
3. To name agencies that help with drug problems.
4. How the revolving door of drug treatment works.

FOCUS ACTIVITY

Present this problem to the class: How do you help a drug abuser who does not want to quit or even acknowledge that there is a problem? Evaluate and discuss the students' answers. Emphasize that a person must first admit to the problem and want help.

TEACH & APPLY

DISCUSSION

We may often think the following of drug abusers, "Why don't they just make themselves give up drugs? All they need is willpower." Have students think of things in their own lives (a favorite video game, friend, dessert, television program, or comfortable bed) that would be hard to give up if someone asked them to. None of these things has the kind of physical or psychological effect on them that a drug could have. Do students now have a better appreciation of what a long road it is to recovery from drug addiction?

A reproducible copy of the Life Choice Inventory is provided in the Teacher's Resource Box.

ROLE PLAY

Ask three students to take turns pretending to be a teenager who has to admit a drug problem to his or her parents. Have them role play this situation for the rest of the class. Assign all the class to explain on paper how they would handle this situation and how their parents probably would react.

DISCUSSION

Ask students about the last time they did something wrong, even though they knew at the time that they were doing the wrong thing. Why did they do it? Explain that even though most people know that drug abuse is wrong and illegal, some people experiment, and become addicted anyway.

ASSESS

EVALUATE

Assign students to answer the following essay question: How would you help one of your friends if he or she admitted a drug problem to you and asked for your help?

334

CHAPTER 12: Drugs of Abuse

Is Any Drug or Medicine a Problem for You?

This exercise is an informal way to find out if any drug is a problem for you. Drugs can include alcohol, antacids, caffeine, OTC medicines, herbs, tobacco, or any of the drugs described in this chapter. Give up this drug for a month, and answer these questions. Your answers to the Life Choice Inventory are personal and private. Share them with others only if you are comfortable doing so.

1. Do you miss the drug?
2. Are you experiencing withdrawal effects?
3. Does life seem less full or less fun without the drug?
4. Are you suddenly aware of problems in your life that you had been ignoring?
5. Are you feeling more tense or anxious than usual?
6. Are you feeling depressed?
7. Do you feel better without the drug?
8. Do you have more problems concentrating or meeting goals and due dates than usual?
9. Do you find that you spend a lot of time thinking about the drug?
10. Did you make sure you could get some of the drug quickly, just in case you missed it too much?

SCORING

If you were unable to give up the drug for a month, you have a drug problem.

If you answered yes to many of these questions, you may have a drug problem.

If you gave up the drug for a month, you may want to kick the habit permanently now. You need not figure it out alone. You may want to get someone to help you.

Source: Adapted from S. J. Levy, *Managing the "Drugs" in Your Life* (New York: McGraw-Hill, 1983), p. 41.

A person who faces up to a drug problem has taken the important first step.

drug-quitting groups such as **Narcotics Anonymous (NA)**, psychological therapy groups, individual psychotherapy, and drug therapy.

An example of drug therapy is the use of **methadone** as treatment for heroin addiction. Methadone is an addictive drug, as heroin is. However, it is cheaper, and its effects are milder and longer lasting. Taking a "maintenance" drug such as methadone allows people addicted to heroin to recover socially. That is, they no longer must struggle to buy high-priced illegal drugs to hold off withdrawal.

Other useful drugs are the **narcotic antagonists**, which the person takes daily. The antagonists block the effects of the problem drugs. By taking the antagonists, the person commits to staying drug-free that day. This once-a-day commitment is easy to make. Then, when the urge to take the drug strikes, the person is protected from giving in to it. The same drugs are used to treat overdoses.

Problems along the Way   Few people who attempt recovery make it all the way. Most people who seek treatment get caught in something like a

special needs

Logical-mathematical

To help students gain a better understanding of the vocabulary concepts in this chapter, you may want to have them use the chapter mini glossary to create a crossword puzzle.

The following words and terms should be included: amotivational syndrome, amphetamines, barbiturates, codeine, designer drugs, drug abuse, drug addiction, drug misuse, drug trafficker, drug use, dysphoria, endorphins, ephedrine, euphoria, hallucinations, hallucinogens, heroin, juvenile, look-alikes, LSD, mescaline, methadone, morphine, narcotic antagonists, narcotics, opiates, Narcotics Anonymous, opium, PCP, peyote, physical addiction, psilocybin, psychological addiction, recreational drug use, sedatives, sudden sniffing death syndrome, withdrawal.

revolving door: getting treatment, giving up the drug, getting out of treatment, taking the drug again, going back into treatment—and so on.

When the person first becomes free of the drug, he or she faces more problems than ever, and now they must be handled without the escape of the drugs. The person who develops a support system and makes needed lifestyle changes has the best chance of staying free of drugs.

Still, some people make it. The first part is the hardest, for life seems empty without the drug. Later, looking back, the recovered person finds that the rewards of sanity and health outweigh by far whatever the drug seemed to offer. The Health Strategies section on page 333, "Enjoy Life," shows that life is full of natural highs available to everyone.

Honest talk helps people face problems.

KEY POINTS *Admitting a drug problem is the first step to overcoming it. Help comes in many forms: hospitalization, Narcotics Anonymous, psychological therapy groups, individual psychotherapy, and drug therapy. Not everyone who attempts recovery makes it all the way. Those who do, however, are always glad they did.*

 Review

Answer the following questions on a sheet of paper.

Learning the Vocabulary

The vocabulary terms in this section are *Narcotics Anonymous (NA)*, *methadone*, and *narcotic antagonists*.
Fill in the blank with the correct answer.

1. _____ oppose the actions of other drugs.
2. A 12-step program that promotes personal growth and leads to the person's helping others to recover is called _____.
3. A drug that is used to treat heroin addiction is _____.

Learning the Facts

4. What is the first step in kicking a drug habit?
5. List some of the drugs to which the Life Choice Inventory on the opposite page applies.
6. Name the different agencies that can help people with drug problems.
7. Explain what is meant by "the revolving door syndrome" in drug treatment.

Making Life Choices

8. After completing the Life Choice Inventory on the opposite page, are you satisfied with your results? Do you have a problem with any of the items mentioned in the opening paragraph? Give suggestions on how you could make more healthful choices. What benefits might you gain by making these choices?

 Glossary

Narcotics Anonymous (NA): a free, self-help program of addiction recovery. It uses a 12-step program, promotes personal growth, and leads to the person's helping others to recover.

methadone: a drug used to treat heroin addiction; it holds off withdrawal and helps people recover socially.

narcotic antagonists: drugs that oppose the actions of other drugs. The word *antagonist* means something or someone who struggles with, or opposes, another.

 Review Answers

1. Narcotic antagonists (p.334)
2. Narcotics Anonymous (p.334)
3. methadone (p.334)
4. admitting it (p. 333)
5. caffeine found in coffee and colas, cigarettes, OTC drugs, prescription (with physician's approval), alcohol, and illegal drugs (p. 334)
6. Covenant House, Just Say No International, National Cocaine Hotline, National Institute of Drug Abuse (p. 333)
7. getting treatment, giving up the drug, getting out of treatment, taking the drug again, going back into treatment, and so on, with the person failing to make lifestyle changes (pp. 334–335)
8. Answers will vary.

 A reproducible quiz for Section 6 is provided in the Teacher's Resource Box.

CLOSE

Have students take the Life Choice Inventory on page 334. Even though they might not abuse drugs, these questions might be answered for a family member or friend, or they might have relevance to other compulsive behaviors such as gambling, overeating, shopping, or overexercising.

Students should look up each glossary word in the chapter, making a note of the page(s) where each word is discussed, and then should rewrite the definition in their own words. After their definitions have been checked, have them use graph paper to create a completely connected crossword puzzle. Remind them to number the words using Across and Down clues appropriately. Have students exchange puzzles with a classmate.

To supplement this activity, you might have the students participate in a round-table discussion on drug prevention programs. An excellent premise would be having the students describe an ideal program and what treatment methods they would use. Have them discuss such issues as intervention and peer counseling. Layout and design an informational brochure describing your program to the public.

SECTION

7

FOCUS

OUTCOMES

In this section students will learn:

1. Why blame or judgment will not help give the drug abuser more will to quit.

2. To see that the drug abuser's will to quit is the only thing that will help him or her quit.

FOCUS ACTIVITY

Have the class try to convince you (a drug abuser) that you should stop abusing drugs. Be strong. Have some responses prepared in advance. Show them that the drug abuser must want to quit.

Ask students to think of habits that they have. Could someone make them quit their habits if they did not really want to quit them? Discuss.

TEACH & APPLY

ROLE PLAY

Assign students to role play. One student's job is to show that he does not approve of another student's drug abuse problem. Enforce the rules, however, that they cannot blame and they cannot judge the individual. The drug abuser is to try to justify his habit. Invite the class to interact and help both.

SECTION

7

Helping Someone Else Kick the Habit

Many agencies stand ready to help people with drug problems.

You may know someone who has a drug problem and feel the need to reach out to that person. First, you may want to take a look at Figure 12–4 on the next page, to help you determine whether the person really is a drug abuser.

Extreme caution should be used in attributing any of the signs to drug abuse. They may be caused by hundreds of other things as well. Probably the best way to find out for sure if a person is abusing drugs is to express concern and ask questions. If you care, this is a way to show it.

Another way to show you care about a person with a drug problem is to make the effort to help, even if this means being tough. You may have to risk confronting the person, standing against your peers, and maybe even losing a friend in the effort to save the person's health or life. Things you can do include:

▶ Making sure the person knows you won't approve of the drug habit.

▶ Making available all the information you can gather on the health effects of the drug.

▶ Making sure the person knows, on choosing to seek help, where to go for it.

Life without drugs has much to offer. Enjoy life!

Pursuing wellness

Denial and enabling are among the most common defense mechanisms that apply to the chemical dependency process. Denial simply involves the unwillingness to admit that a problem exists. Most everyone surrounding the chemically dependent person participates.

Common phrases may sound like some of these examples:

"He's just going through a phase."

"All teenagers do stupid things like that."

"Life has not been good to her, it's not her fault."

"Don't most kids try marijuana? I did when I was in college and I'm doing OK."

How can you tell whether someone close to you is abusing drugs? Here are some signs to look for:

- Paleness and perspiration.
- Dilated pupils.
- Runny nose and nosebleeds.
- Jitters and hyperactivity.
- Ability to go without food or sleep for long periods of time.
- Anxiety, anger, or unreasonable suspiciousness.
- Loss of memory.
- Unexplained increases in energy and talkativeness, followed by lethargy and depression.
- Sudden carelessness about personal appearance.
- Broken appointments, broken promises, lying.
- Inability to explain what happened to money.
- Tardiness, unexcused absences, declining grades.
- Trouble with the law, family or school authorities.

Figure 12–4 Signs of Drug Abuse

Drug addiction does not mean someone is a bad person. Blame is a useless concept. It can make people feel guilty, but it can't help them get better. Drug-addicted people pay heavily enough for past choices. If you want to help, you won't judge, and you won't blame.

No amount of effort on your part, however, can supply the key ingredient in someone else's choice to give up drugs: the will to quit. In fact, the toughest job for many people whose lives are affected by drug abusers is to learn to enjoy their own lives without being dragged down. Often they have to learn simply to accept the other person's choice, painful as that may be. Beyond caring, you have to let go. Live your own life as fully as possible while it is yours to live.

 KEY POINTS *You cannot make someone quit a drug habit. The person has to have the will to quit. The toughest part for those close to an addicted person is to learn to enjoy their lives without being dragged down.*

 SECTION 7 Review

Answer the following questions on a sheet of paper.

Learning the Facts
1. List the signs of drug abuse given in this section.
2. What are three things you can do to help a person with a drug problem?
3. What is the crucial ingredient needed for a person to give up drugs?

Making Life Choices
4. There are many agencies that work with drug addictions. How could you help a friend choose the right agency? What are some of the advantages and disadvantages about each of the agencies?

 Answers to FACT or FICTION Here are the answers to the questions at the start of the chapter.
1. **True.**
2. **False.** Even people who are fully aware of the hazards abuse drugs.
3. **False.** People continue abusing drugs to avoid the pain of withdrawal symptoms.
4. **False.** Psychological addictions can be as powerful as physical ones.
5. **False.** Smoking marijuana is associated with harmful health effects.
6. **True.**
7. **False.** Amphetamines impair driving ability.
8. **False.** People rarely recover from drug dependency on their own.

"The police were just waiting for him to mess up."
"The school is being unreasonable, they won't give her a chance."
"Don't most kids skip school?"
"If you knew anything about his family you'd understand."

Enabling involves a deliberate attempt to prevent the natural consequences of the chemically dependent person's behavior to occur. Making excuses, explaining and rationalizing, and covering up for the chemically dependent person is standard enabling behavior. Denial and enabling are intertwined in the process.

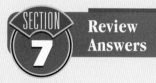 **ASSESS**

EVALUATE
Assign students to answer the following essay question: A good friend of yours is abusing drugs. How would you help? Students should include showing disapproval, making information available, and making sure the drug abuser knows where to seek help.

SECTION 7 Review Answers
1. Refer to Figure 12–4 for answers. (p. 337)
2. make sure the person knows you don't approve of the drug habit, make available all the information you can gather on the health effects of the drug, make sure the person knows where to go for help (pp. 336–337)
3. the will to quit (p. 337)
4. Answers will vary.

CLOSE
Have the class list negative consequences of drug abuse. Have several students share their lists. Ask students the following questions. Do you want to prevent these things from happening to you? Why or why not? Do you feel the need to protect your family members and friends from these things? Why or why not? What things might stand in your way as you try to protect family and friends from situations involving drug abuse?

Ask for volunteers to participate in a role playing scenario in which you ask each of the students to use some illegal drugs. When they refuse, have them give their reasons for refusing. Try to focus on valid arguments to combat peer pressure. Show students how to use refusal skills and still keep their friends by following these steps:

1. Be direct, friendly, and confident in refusing.
2. List the consequences of getting caught.
3. Offer a fun alternative that will not get you in trouble.
4. If they refuse your alternative, leave an open invitation and walk away.

Another option is to divide the class into groups to role play. Give them the following scenario and have the groups develop skits using their refusal skills. "You are walking down the street with a group of your friends. One of them pulls out and lights up a marijuana cigarette and offers it to you."

Straight Talk

How to Refuse Drugs without Losing Friends

Chapter 3 introduced a set of refusal skills as useful tools for handling all sorts of peer pressure situations. Many people find those same skills helpful in situations concerning drug abuse. To apply the skills effectively, a primary goal is to develop your confidence in yourself, and let it shine through as you deliver your message.

 I was once in a situation where I wanted to say no to my friends but I couldn't think fast enough. What is the first step in handling this situation?

You've already taken the first step—to realize that quickly making a smart decision under pressure is hard. Even harder is making a smart decision while your friends are trying to influence you.

When you speak to peers under pressure, try to sound convincing. This doesn't mean raising your voice, or becoming angry or nasty—far from it. It means calmly expressing your high regard for yourself by choosing your own behaviors, without angering or insulting others in the process.

It helps to keep the consequences of the action firmly in mind. As the chapter mentioned, the law deals out stiff punishment for smoking marijuana and taking other illegal drugs. For minors, alcohol and tobacco are against the law, too. Even more important, drugs endanger your well-being.

 How do I help make my answer convincing without raising my voice?

Be honest, and sound firm. Your mind is made up. Give short answers to direct questions (see

Figure 12–5 for examples) to avoid a lot of discussion. The more discussion that occurs, the more you open yourself to pressure from the group. Avoid wishy-washy comments like "I don't think so." Stand straight and proud, look confident and relaxed, and speak convincingly, even if you feel nervous inside. Show that you are in control. Maintain eye contact, and use a steady voice. Smile.

 But what if my friends don't listen to what I say? What else can I do?

Ignoring the offer may work. If you simply don't answer the suggestion, the person making it will probably take that as a no. Busy yourself with another activity, such as hunting for your keys, to buy yourself time. Start up a new conversation with another person.

Another tactic is to make an excuse and walk away. Here is an example:

As you are walking to your car after school, your friends say they are going to someone's house to get high, and they want you along. You quickly act as though you just remembered something and walk away to take care of it. You might call over your shoulder something like, "I see Sally ahead. I've got to ask her about a homework assignment. See you later."

If you cannot leave the situation, offer another idea of something to do. "Let's go see a movie or visit a friend." This will allow you to remain in control.

Other times, you may be able to use humor to turn the suggestion into a joke, or to act shocked in mockery. Laughter often defuses a situation, and lets you shine in the eyes of others.

338

HEALTHY PEOPLE 2000

. . . .

Reduce the proportion of young people who have used alcohol, marijuana, and cocaine in the past month, as follows:

Substance/Age	1988 Baseline	2000 Target
Alcohol/aged 12–17	25.2%	12.6%
Alcohol/aged 18–20	57.9%	29%
Marijuana/aged 12–17	6.4%	3.2%
Marijuana/aged 18–25	15.5%	7.8%
Cocaine/aged 12–17	1.1%	0.6%
Cocaine/aged 18–25	4.5%	2.3%

Note: The targets of this objective are consistent with the goals established by the Office of National Drug Control Policy, Executive Office of the President.

I'm not much of a comedian. I need suggestions to help keep me from getting nervous during such times.

You may not be able to lose all your fear, but a helpful tactic is to practice in advance what you might say in response to a conversation about drugs. Read over the suggestions of Figure 12–5. Practice them with a friend or in front of a mirror. You might even get some friends together and do some role-playing.

Also, keep in mind that friends who pressure you to do illegal or harmful things are not true friends. Choosing your friends is a way of editing your life to make it better. You may find that as you assert yourself, you may have to let go of some of those friends who no longer share your common goals. They can become acquaintances instead of friends.

 What are some other ways to stay away from drugs?

Stay busy and involved. Take up a new hobby. Play a sport or two. Volunteer your time to help those in need. When you are busy and involved in activities you love, you'll meet people who enjoy the same things you do. You'll have fun, and you'll find that drugs have no place in your life.

Be strong, and believe in yourself. Every time you say no, give yourself credit for standing up for yourself and doing what is in your best interest. It takes commitment, skill, and self-esteem to refuse to go along with the crowd. Be proud of your accomplishment.

> Here are some example situations involving peers who abuse drugs. The example responses may help you to refuse offers of drugs.
>
> *Situation:* "Come on, just try a little coke (or pot, or speed). It'll make you feel good."
>
> *Responses:* "No, I already feel just fine."
> "No, I have a test (or game or job interview) tomorrow, and I want to be at my best."
> "No, I'm driving tonight."
>
> *Situation:* "Don't be such a chicken. Try something new."
>
> *Responses:* "I'm not a chicken. I can make my own choices, and I choose not to take drugs."
> "I've already got other plans."
> "How did I pick such a weird friend?" (laugh, walk away, shake your head in mockery)
> "You usually have such good ideas. This isn't your best one. Let's think of something else to do."
>
> *Situation:* "Here, take a hit off this joint."
>
> *Responses:* "No, I'll pass. I'm going running tomorrow, and I don't want anything to slow me down."
> "No, I've had a cold, and I don't want to do anything to make it worse."
> "No, I don't like the way it tastes."
> "No, I think I'll just watch you guys get stupid."

Figure 12–5 *Practicing Your Refusal Skills*

Mind-altering and addictive substances have been shown to jeopardize physical, mental and social development during the formative years and to endanger the successful transition from school to the workplace. Moreover, use of these substances, including alcohol, is illegal for young people and thus may have long-term implications for such things as employment and schooling.

Of particular concern is drug use among school dropouts, lower income, inner-city youth whose rates of use do not appear to have declined as much as rates among general population youth. Also of particular concern is the increasing rate of use among pregnant teenagers whose pregnancies must be considered at high risk even without drug involvement.

1. a. Physical addiction produces a change in the body's chemistry so that normal functioning begins to fail without the drug, while psychological addiction is a mental dependence on a drug, habit, or behavior. **b.** Drug abuse is the deliberate taking of a drug for nonmedical reasons, while drug misuse is taking drugs for a medical purpose, but not in the correct amount, frequency, or manner. **c.** Look-alikes are a combination of OTC drugs and other chemicals packaged to look like prescription medications or illegal drugs, while designer drugs are laboratory-made drugs that closely resemble illegal drugs in chemical structure, but are still legal.
2. a. withdrawal **b.** sedatives **c.** peyote **d.** euphoria **e.** juvenile delinquent **f.** narcotics **g.** hallucinations **h.** methadone
3. Answers will vary.
4. a. Codeine **b.** dysphoria **c.** morphine **d.** amotivational syndrome

RECALL

SECTION 1

1. taking of a drug for its medically intended purpose; deliberate taking of drugs for a nonmedical purpose that could be harmful; taking of a drug for the correct medical purpose, but not in the right amount, frequency, or manner (pp. 310–311)

CHAPTER 12 Review

Summarizing the Chapter

Your ability to respond correctly to the following statements ensures your understanding of the main concepts in the chapter.

1. Explain the problems associated with physical and psychological addiction.
2. Identify the effects of marijuana and related drugs.
3. Define and discuss the abuse of stimulants, narcotics, and depressants.
4. Describe the effects of inhalants, look-alike drugs, and designer drugs.
5. List the signs of drug abuse.
6. Describe ways to enjoy a drug-free high.

Learning the Vocabulary

drug use	codeine
drug abuse	opium
drug misuse	morphine
recreational drug use	heroin
drug trafficker	hallucinogens
juvenile	look-alikes
euphoria	ephedrine
drug addiction	LSD (lysergic acid
(dependence)	diethylamide)
endorphins	PCP (phencyclidine
dysphoria	hydrochloride)
physical addiction	peyote
withdrawal	mescaline
psychological addiction	psilocybin/psilocin
hallucinations	sudden sniffing death
amotivational syndrome	syndrome
amphetamines	designer drugs
sedatives	Narcotics Anonymous
barbiturates	(NA)
opiates	methadone
narcotics	narcotic antagonists

Answer the following questions on a separate sheet of paper.

1. Explain the differences between the two terms in each of the following sets:
   a. physical addiction and psychological addiction
   b. drug abuse and drug misuse
   c. look-alike drugs and designer drugs
2. ***Matching***—*Match each of the following phrases with the appropriate vocabulary term from the list in the left column.*
   a. the physical symptoms that occur when a drug to which a person is addicted is cleared from the body tissue
   b. drugs that have a soothing or tranquilizing effect
   c. a cactus that produces the hallucinogen mescaline
   d. a sense of great well-being and pleasure brought on by some drugs
   e. a youth under age 18
   f. habit-forming drugs that relieve pain and produce sleep when taken in moderation
   g. false perceptions; imagined sights, sounds, smells, or other feelings
   h. a drug used to treat heroin addiction
3. Write a paragraph using at least ten vocabulary terms. Underline each term that you use.
4. **a.** _____ is a narcotic drug that is commonly used for suppressing coughs.
   b. An unpleasant feeling that often follows a drug-induced euphoria is called _____.
   c. The narcotic drug _____ is prescribed by doctors as a painkiller.
   d. A person who loses energy and ambition as a result of marijuana use is said to have _____.

Recalling Important Facts and Ideas

Section 1
1. Define drug use, abuse, and misuse.

Section 2
2. Name the factors that lead people to abuse drugs.
3. People who focus their attention on themselves rather than on other people or activities are likely to abuse drugs. List reasons these people abuse drugs.

340

SECTION 2

2. nature of the person, nature of the drug, and possible consequences that await the abuser from family and society (p. 312)
3. different from the rest of society, drugs fit image, drugs fill void of excitement and fun, substitute drugs for friends, parental love, an escape from life's problems (p. 312)

SECTION 3

4. Harsh punishment awaits those who possess or sell drugs, while entertainers,

movies, songs, magazines, and books may portray drug abuse as "funny" or "cool."
   Society condemns drug abuse, but also protects rights of individuals to make public individual points of view on drug abuse. (p. 314)
5. nicotine, caffeine (p. 316)
6. dysphoria (p. 315)
7. curiosity, experimentation, euphoria, dysphoria, tolerance, elevated drug doses, euphoria, greater dysphoria, withdrawal, elevated drug doses, relief from withdrawal, withdrawal, elevated doses, and

Section 3

4. How is society sending us mixed messages about drugs?

5. A few drugs produce addictions without euphoria. What are they?

6. What is the unpleasant sensation people may feel after taking drugs?

7. Describe the spiral that leads to physical addiction.

8. How does drug addiction compare to a great love relationship?

9. What is the *only* sure way to escape drug addiction?

10. Explain why a drug seller's job is so easy.

Section 4

11. THC affects sensitive brain centers. In what ways does THC affect the body?

12. Research indicates that harmful health effects are associated with the use of THC. What are they?

13. What are the medical uses for amphetamines?

14. List the effects of barbiturates on the body.

15. What can long-term abuse of barbiturates cause?

16. What is one of the strongest painkillers and why is its use so limited?

17. What is the most often abused narcotic in the United States and why is it illegal?

18. What are the three ways to take cocaine?

19. List the effects of cocaine on the nervous system.

20. Describe the various hallucinogens and the side effects each one causes.

21. What are three types of chemicals inhaled to produce a high?

22. Why are look-alike drugs so dangerous to users?

Section 5

23. How long does the driving impairment caused by alcohol or maijuana last?

Section 6

24. Explain how methadone and narcotic antagonists help in the treatment of drug addiction.

25. Of the 17 ways to "enjoy life" listed on page 333, write down the ones you've experienced.

Section 7

26. List some signs of drug abuse.

Critical Thinking

1. Suppose a friend who was anxious about getting into college confided in you that she was taking increasingly greater amounts of speed to enable her to study more hours. What advice would you offer your friend? What action would you take to help your friend?

2. The use of marijuana by young teens is on the rise. What are some of the reasons so many more young students are using marijuana? What do you think should be done to solve this problem?

Activities

1. Put together a list of community resources for people seeking help for drug problems. Provide the name, address, and phone number of each agency. Describe the services the agencies provide, the basic costs of their services, and details of services to school-age children and adolescents.

2. Make a video for your class or community about drug abuse. In your video describe the different types of drugs, ways that any drug may be misused, the physical and emotional dangers of drug abuse, and the treatments for various types of drug abuse.

3. Write a public television or radio announcement that describes the physical and emotional dangers of drug abuse. Share these announcements with your local elementary school.

Making Decisions about Health

1. One of your relatives complains of fatigue and depression. The person is also overweight and under a lot of stress at work. The person's health history indicates no regular exercise routine, and a poor diet. The doctor has run extensive tests and no physical abnormality has turned up, but in hopes of bringing the patient some relief, the doctor reaches for his/her pad to prescribe a stimulant.

  a. What might be at the root of your relative's complaints?

  b. Why might the prescription of a stimulant for your relative be an unwise decision, given the circumstances?

  c. What might you suggest to your relative so that he or she may get some relief?

  d. What can you tell your relative about the use of stimulants? What are some of the risks of stimulant use?

15. depression, forgetfulness, reduced sex drive, addiction, death in cases of overdose (p. 327)

16. morphine; it is extremely addictive (p. 327)

17. heroin; because it is so addictive (p. 327)

18. snorting, injecting, and smoking (p. 325)

19. See page 326.

20. See page 328.

21. solvents; propellants; those intended for medical use (p. 329)

22. See page 329.

SECTION 5

23. for hours after the high has worn off (p. 331)

SECTION 6

24. See page 334.

25. Answers will vary. Refer to page 333.

SECTION 7

26. See page 337.

physical addiction (p. 317)

8. Addicted people defend, cherish, and protect the drug habit as they would a loved one. (p. 317)

9. Never experiment with drugs that would produce it. (p. 318)

10. once hooked, will do almost anything to get the drug (p. 318)

SECTION 4

11. alters hearing, touch, taste, and smell; sense of time, space, and feelings of the body (p. 319)

12. short-term memory loss, shortened attention span, rapid and irregular heartbeats, reduces body's immune response, reduces hormone levels and sperm count in men, damages the lungs (p. 324)

13. constant sleeping and hyperactivity in children (p. 324)

14. depress the central nervous system, slow the heart rate, slow the respiration rate, lower the blood pressure and body temperature (pp. 326–327)

KEY POINTS

Chapter 13 is 28 pages long and divided into five sections. This chapter defines alcohol as the most widely used and abused drug in the U.S. It stresses the impact of alcohol abuse on the judgment centers of the brain and on the liver both immediately and over an extended period of time. This chapter emphasizes the effect alcohol has on everyone in society and the difficulty in overcoming alcoholism. It stresses the importance of saying no and feeling good about the decision. Some excellent tips are included to aid in entertaining without alcohol.

ACTIVITY TO INTRODUCE CHAPTER

The Life Choice Inventory (on page 348) is an excellent activity to begin this chapter. Students can answer for themselves or for a friend they are concerned about. Another effective activity for beginning the chapter is to discuss the Consumer Skills, Advertisements for Alcohol, on page 347. Discuss some of the most popular ads, shows, and entertainers that influence our thoughts on alcohol. Then use the Critical Thinking questions to provoke thoughts on our society's promotion of alcohol.

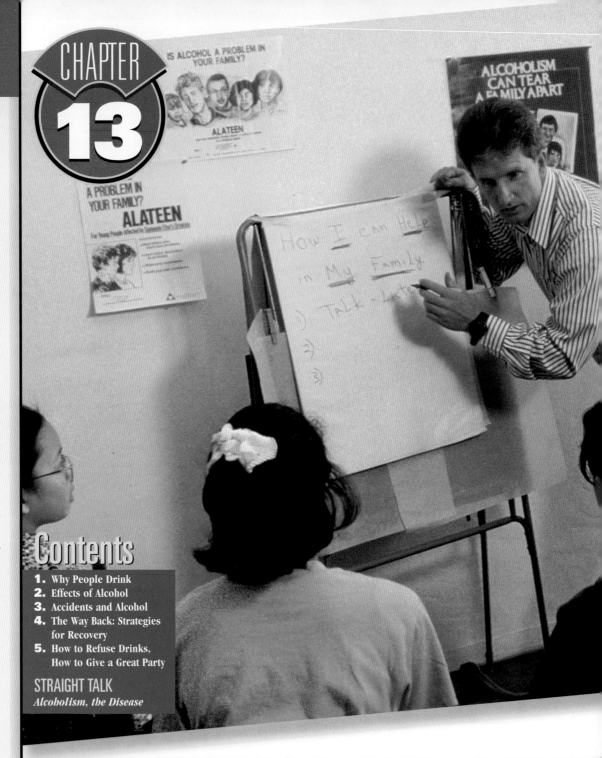

CHAPTER 13

Contents

NOT Enough Time?

Following are some suggestions to help you make sure that you cover the key topics in this chapter if you have limited time.

DAY 1 Assign students to read Sections 1 and 2 prior to class. At the beginning of class do the Fact or Fiction on page 343 to evaluate students' comprehension of the information. During class have the students do the Focus Activity on page 344 and the Learning with Visuals activity on page 353.

Alcohol: Use and Abuse

What do you think? Are the following statements true or false? If you think they are false, then say what is true.

1. Alcohol is a drug.
2. A person who drinks two drinks every day may be a moderate drinker.
3. In the body, alcohol is digested just as food is.
4. Alcohol is a depressant drug; it slows people down.
5. Impaired driving performance occurs when the blood alcohol level is 0.08 percent or higher.
6. A person who has had too much to drink should walk around so the muscles will burn off the alcohol more quickly.
7. Drinking black coffee can help a drunk person sober up.

(Answers on page 364)

Introduction

In chemistry, the term **alcohol** refers to a class of chemical compounds. One of these compounds is the active ingredient of alcoholic beverages—**ethanol**, or **ethyl alcohol**, often called just *alcohol*.

In medicine, ethanol is a drug and a toxin (it changes the way the body functions). If, however, it is diluted enough, and taken in small enough quantities, it produces effects on the body that people seek. These effects are achieved at some risk, but most people are unaware of these risks. This lack of knowledge is one reason that ethanol is the most widely used—and abused—drug in our society. Drinking alcohol is legal, however, only for those who are 21 years of age or older.

If alcohol is legal for adults, then why is it illegal for teenagers? One reason is that **alcoholism**, or alcohol addiction, sets in much more quickly in young people than in adults. Also, more teenagers die, or are permanently injured, from alcohol-related traffic accidents each year than from any other cause. Teens who drink alcohol are also more often the ones who abuse other drugs and tobacco and, in fact, who take risks of all sorts. Drinking alcohol also poses many other threats to life and health. Later sections make these threats clear.

BULLETIN BOARD IDEA

On one side of the bulletin board, pin up advertisements for alcoholic beverages—from beer to wine to hard liquor. On the other side of the bulletin board, pin up pictures that reflect the dangerous consequence of alcohol use and abuse—newspaper pictures of car accidents; illustrations of damaged livers from a medical journal; man or woman sporting a "beer belly;" person looking like they are suffering from a hangover. Title the bulletin board something like "The Myth and the Reality."

Answers to

1. **True.**
2. **True.**
3. **False.** Alcohol is not digested. It is immediately absorbed into the blood.
4. **True.**
5. **False.** Driving is impaired at blood alcohol levels lower than 0.08 percent.
6. **False.** Muscles do not use alcohol for fuel, so walking does not affect the body's rate of alcohol breakdown.
7. **False.** Coffee can wake up, but not sober up, a person who is drunk.

DAY 2 Discuss Section 3 and use the Making Life Choices in the Section 3 Review as a role-play activity. Use the Discussion activity on page 357 to get the students thinking about drinking and driving.

DAY 3 Assign students to read Sections 4 and 5 prior to class. During class have students complete the Focus Activity on page 359 and the Discussion activity on page 360. Close the lesson on alcohol by using the Group Activity on page 363 and the Discussion activity on page 366.

SECTION 1

FOCUS

OUTCOMES

In this section students will learn the:

1. Reasons people choose to drink alcohol.
2. Difference between drinking in moderation, abusive drinking, and addictive drinking.
3. Media's influence on people's drinking choices.

FOCUS ACTIVITY

Write the names of ten drugs on the board. Be sure to include alcohol and at least one pre-scription or OTC medicine. Then draw a continuum on the board. On one end write "Bad," in the middle put "Neutral," and on the other end put "Good." Ask the students to break into groups of two or three. They are to draw this same continuum on a sheet of paper and then put each drug listed on the board on the continuum where they believe it belongs. When they are done, choose a drug and ask them where they placed it. Write the drug on the continuum on the board reflecting student choices. Do this with four or five more, making sure to include alcohol and a medicinal drug. When you are done, tell students that almost all drugs belong in the middle. Ask them why. The point is that the drugs aren't the problem, people are the problem. It's the way peo-ple use the drugs that make them "bad" or "good." Penicillin, for example, can help cure dis-ease, but it can be harmful to

For Your Information

Chapter 19 includes further discussion of the effects of addictions on the family.

SECTION 1

Why People Drink

Drinkers will give lots of reasons why they drink alcohol: to celebrate, to unwind, because they like the taste of alcoholic beverages, because it's the custom. Some young people may drink because peer pressure encourages it, or because they think drinking makes them look grown-up, or because it is a way of rebelling against authority. Sometimes they drink simply because alcohol is available to them—say, at a party—and they don't yet know how to refuse drinks. (They will, after reading the last section of this chapter.) The advertisers of alcohol also promote drinking, of course. They appeal to many aspects of people's self-image. (See the Consumer Skills feature, "Advertisements for Alcohol," on page 347.)

Drinking may encourage people to relax and be social. Of course, peo-ple might benefit more from learning how to relax in the face of life's pres-sures without alcohol.

For whatever reasons people drink, they derive drug effects by doing so. Like other addictive drugs, alcohol produces euphoria, changes mood, relieves pain, and releases tension.

Drinking in Moderation   Some debate exists about whether alcohol, taken in **moderation** by healthy adults, harms health. In fact, some evidence suggests that adults taking two to six drinks a week die less often from heart attacks and other causes than people who drink more or less than this amount. Other evidence links the same amount of alcohol with an increased likelihood of cancer. While research continues, no one should drink for health's sake. Especially, young people gain no health benefits from alcohol, because heart attacks are rare for them.

Servings of alcohol equal to a standard drink. From left to right: hard liquor, wine cooler, beer, wine.

special needs

Bodily-kinesthetic

For students who have problems with alcohol themselves, or who are closely involved with friends or family with alcohol-related prob-lems, reading words on a page or discussing possible solutions may not be enough to help them realize that they can make a difference.

To give students an opportunity to practice dealing with tough situations without placing themselves or others in danger, you may want to conduct role play situations.

This chapter contains many situations that can be adapted for role play. Select from the following or devise your own scenarios based on the needs of your students. (1) Skills for Moderation list from Section 1; (2) Making Life Choices from Section Reviews in Sections 2, 3,

Most authorities recommend that people who drink, should do so in moderation. Just what does this mean? No one exact amount of alcohol per day is moderate for everyone, because people have different tolerance levels. Some people might be able to consume slightly more than one or two drinks a day. Others could definitely not handle nearly so much without danger.

What Is a Drink? Alcoholic beverages contain a lot of water and other substances, as well as alcohol. Wine and beer have relatively low percentages of alcohol. In contrast, whiskey, vodka, rum, and brandy may contain as much as 50 percent alcohol. The percentage of alcohol in alcoholic beverages is stated as **proof**. For example, 100-proof liquor is 50 percent alcohol. Proof equals twice the percentage of alcohol.

People measure alcohol in servings they call "a **drink**." However, the serving any one person considers to be a drink may not match the standard "drink" that experts use to define moderation. A standard drink delivers ½ ounce of pure ethanol:

- ▶ 1 ounce of hard liquor (whiskey, gin, brandy, rum, or vodka).
- ▶ 1 (10-ounce) wine cooler.
- ▶ 12 ounces of beer.
- ▶ 3 to 4 ounces of wine.

The photo on the preceding page shows what these servings look like.

Range of Drinking Behaviors A wide range of drinking patterns fall between not drinking at all and alcoholism. The most danger lies at the extreme of excessive alcohol intake. The more a person drinks, the closer to that dangerous extreme the person is.

Females cannot drink nearly as much alcohol as males can at a sitting without becoming drunk. The smaller female body size, smaller volume of blood, and higher percentage of body fat limit the amount of alcohol a woman's body can handle. Also, a man's stomach makes more of an alcohol-destroying compound than does a woman's stomach, so less of what he drinks actually enters into his blood. The point is, females should never try to keep up, drink for drink, with males.

People who drink must monitor and evaluate their own drinking behaviors. Figure 13–1 to the right lists terms and definitions that describe people who drink. Figure 13–2 on page 346 compares some behaviors of

A *moderate drinker* does not drink excessively. The person doesn't behave inappropriately because of alcohol. The person's health is not harmed by alcohol over the long term.

A *social drinker* drinks only on social occasions. Depending on how alcohol affects the person's life, the person may be a moderate drinker or a problem drinker.

A *binge drinker* drinks four or more drinks in a short period.

A *problem drinker*, or an *alcohol abuser*, suffers social, emotional, family, job-related, or other problems because of alcohol. This person is on the way to alcoholism.

An *alcohol addict (alcoholic)* has the full-blown disease of alcoholism. This person's problems, caused by alcohol abuse, are out of control.

Figure 13–1 Terms Used to Describe People Who Drink Alcohol

MINI Glossary

alcohol: a class of chemical compounds. The alcohol of alcoholic beverages, **ethanol** or **ethyl alcohol**, is one member of this class.

alcoholism: the disease characterized by loss of control over drinking and dependence on alcohol, both of which harm health, family relations, and social and work functioning.

moderation: an amount of alcohol that causes no harm to health: not more than one to two drinks a day for healthy adults.

drink: the amount of a beverage that delivers ½ ounce of pure ethanol—12 ounces of beer, 3 to 4 ounces of wine, 1 (10-ounce) wine cooler, or 1 ounce of 100-proof liquor.

proof: a measure of the percentage of alcohol in alcoholic beverages. *100 proof* means 50 percent alcohol, *90 proof* means 45 percent, and so forth.

someone who is allergic to it. LSD can prove harmful to many, but some psychiatrists say it has helped certain clients, including the terminally ill. Alcohol can be used socially by many without negative problems, yet it is the cause of many accidental deaths and the disease alcoholism. Even the most dangerous drugs are "neutral" if people will just say "no" to them.

TEACH & APPLY

BACKGROUND INFORMATION

Tell students that people are most likely to suffer accidents, engage in dangerous activities that they wouldn't even consider without alcohol, and be more sexually uninhibited when drinking. The minimum age for drinking is intended to keep teens from hurting themselves and others and to safeguard against the development of alcoholism.

BACKGROUND INFORMATION

Tell students that ethyl alcohol is a colorless, flammable liquid. It is obtained from fermentation and distillation of grain. Among other things, it's used as a preservative of biological specimens and in antifreeze products.

DISCUSSION

Have each student bring in an ad for an alcoholic beverage. You should have five to seven of your own. Tape the ads to the board. Ask the students to look them over and then have each student choose one to discuss. In the discussion, ask the students to answer the following:

(continued on the next page)

4, and 5; (3) Suggestions for dealing with someone who is intoxicated, from When a Friend Has Drunk Too Much, Section 3; (4) Pointers for the nondrinker from Section 5; and (5) Making Decisions about Health from the Chapter Review.

You may want to divide the class into groups and have them discuss the role play situation. They can then decide on the best way to handle a certain set of circumstances

before presenting the role play. You could also give students a specific character type to play and ask them to demonstrate how they think that type of person would act in a given situation. To conclude, ask students to think of situations they have been in and to evaluate whether or not they could have made different choices in how to handle themselves.

(continued from previous page)

1. What is the ad stating?
2. To whom is the ad appealing?
3. What does the ad NOT show?

Be sure to stress how unrealistic the ads are.

COMPREHENSION CHECK

Look for alcohol advertisements that state the proof and percentage of the alcohol. Ask students to describe the difference between the two. (Proof equals twice the percent of alcohol present. Example: 90 proof = 45 percent alcohol.) Put five items on the board and ask the students to convert them.

DISCUSSION

Develop your own drinking questionnaire (or use the "Thinking about Drinking" questionnaire in the Teacher's Resource Box) for students to answer as homework. Remind them that they should answer the questions honestly and thoroughly. Then use the questionnaire as the content for a circle discussion, allowing students to answer freely. Be sure each question is processed with a closure statement or fact before going on to the next.

COMPREHENSION CHECK

Have one student read aloud an item from one column from Figure 13–2, then have another student read the corresponding item from the other column. This should help students see the difference between moderate drinking and problem drinking.

Figure 13–2 Behaviors of Moderate Drinkers and Problem Drinkers

Behaviors typical of moderate drinkers include these:	Those who are problem drinkers have different behaviors, such as these:
• They drink slowly (no fast gulping).	• They gulp or "chug" their drinks.
• They eat before or while drinking.	• They drink on an empty stomach.
• They don't binge, and they know when to stop drinking.	• They binge on many drinks in a row and drink to get drunk.
• They respect nondrinkers.	• They pressure others to drink.
• They know and obey laws related to drinking.	• They drink when it is unsafe or unwise to do so.
• They avoid drinking alcohol when solving problems or making decisions.	• When they have problems to solve, they turn to alcohol.
• They do not focus on drinking alcohol—they focus on other activities.	• They maintain relationships based solely on alcohol.
• They do not view drunkenness as stylish, funny, or acceptable.	• They believe that drunks are funny or otherwise admirable.
• They do not become loud, violent, or otherwise changed by drinking.	• When drinking, they may become loud, angry, violent, or silent.
• They cause no problems to others by drinking.	• They physically or emotionally harm themselves, family members, or others.

Young people gain no health benefits from drinking alcohol.

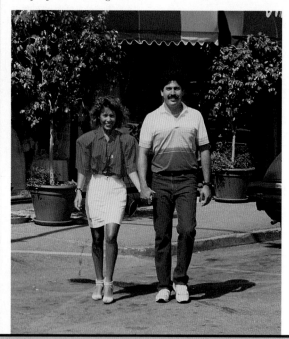

people who drink moderately with behaviors of problem drinkers.

Skills for Moderation Those people who succeed in drinking moderately drink at appropriate times and in appropriate settings only. They limit their intakes, and they enjoy being in control. Among the skills they report they've had to learn are the following:

▶ "I decide in advance how much I'm going to drink. If it's BYOB (bring your own bottle), I take only two drinks with me."
▶ "If they're serving beer by the pitcher, I still order it by the glass. That way, I don't feel I must drink more than I want to."
▶ "I allow time for my body to break down the alcohol I've drunk before I drive."
▶ "I sip my drinks; I add ice cubes or water; I drink water or soft drinks if I'm thirsty."

Pursuing wellness

The alcohol industry spends in excess of 1 billion dollars annually to convince us that if we want to be cool, close to our families, popular and celebrate life to its fullest, we must use alcohol. This effort has been so successful that many American adults believe that having fun without alcohol is not possible.

Alcohol abuse is a national health problem,

yet as a nation we continue to endorse its use, especially to young people. Many of our decision-makers are concerned about supply-side control of drugs, while confirming the demand-side and use of alcohol in our country.

The following activities will help your students focus on the effects alcohol has on our society.

1. Have students bring in current alcohol

Advertisements for Alcohol

Consumer SKILLS

Magazines, television, and other media project an image of alcohol drinkers as members of an exclusive clique. The drinkers wear expensive clothes and drive plush automobiles. They are smiling, healthy, fun, beautiful, strong, and young. The message is that everybody who's somebody drinks, and you'd better drink, too, if you want to be somebody. This is one sort of advertising appeal for alcohol.

Drinking alcohol can also be shown as a way to belong to a group. For example, drinking alcohol has become linked with certain sports, partly because famous athletes are paid large sums to appear in alcohol advertisements. Such ads glorify the athletes. Both fans and athletes are drawn to the glorious images and to the alcohol that goes with them. The tragic result: alcoholism sometimes destroys athletes early in their careers. A famous ex-baseball player who opened an alcoholism clinic says, "We just . . . winked at each other as we drank each other to death."*

Appeals to drink alcohol have found their way into almost every area of life. A sign that hangs over a bar at a golf club in New Hampshire reads: "You can't

*Ryne Duren, as quoted by L. Herberg, Alcoholism: The national pastime, *Arizona Republic*, 30 March 1980, p. f1.

trust a man who doesn't drink." Greeting cards and comedy routines make drinking and even drunkenness socially acceptable and funny.

Actually, though, alcohol use produces the opposite of all the qualities used to promote it. A person striving for rewarding social interactions needs not to lose control, but to gain it by practicing social skills. A person seeking sports success will find it not by drinking beer on the couch, but by faithfully practicing the sport.

All such appeals fail to mention any possibility of harm. All of them set you up to want to drink alcohol. Learn to watch out for advertising appeals. Remember, it's up to you to decide whether you really want what is offered.

Critical Thinking

1. *Why do you think that teenagers connect drinking with popularity?*
2. *Do you feel that athletes, as role models for many young people, should earn large sums of money promoting alcohol use?*
3. *If you were the athlete or the company wanting to pay the athlete to advertise your product, how would you feel about athletes receiving financial rewards to push alcohol?*

▶ "Now and then I skip a drink. I don't accept drinks I don't want."
▶ "I go slowly with unfamiliar drinks."
▶ "If I need sleep, I sleep—I don't drink. If I need to relax, I relax—I don't drink."
▶ "I know my capacity, and I don't exceed it."

Assessing Drinking Behaviors   How *much* people drink is not the only question to ask in determining whether people have drinking problems. Other important questions are the *reasons* for their drinking and the *conse-*

event articles or magazine advertisements, or write a description of their favorite TV beer ad. Use class time to analyze the articles or ads and identify the celebrities and/or advertising techniques used.

2. Ask the students, "What is the number one spectator sport in the U.S.? Also inquire as to whether the students think the alcohol and tobacco industries know the answer to that question. The answer is auto racing—stock, indy, funny, monster trucks,

and so on. List products endorsed by the race car teams in addition to alcohol or tobacco.

3. Have a local highway patrol or police department spokesperson or officer be a guest lecturer. Some local police departments have special programs that address alcohol and drug issues.

4. Recruit a drug and alcohol abuse counselor to be a guest lecturer about alcohol and families.

Ask students to privately complete the Life Choice Inventory. Give them three or four minutes to complete it. Ask them to read over the scoring. Remind them to be aware of the "yeah, buts" and to seriously think about their relationships with alcohol.

A reproducible copy of the Life Choice Inventory is provided in the Teacher's Resource Box.

GUEST SPEAKER

Invite a representative from the Alcoholics Anonymous organization to speak to your class on the work and mission of AA, Alanon, and related groups. Allow the speaker to present their own ideas but check with school administration before the discussion. If possible, have the speaker discuss the warning signs of alcoholism as he or she has experienced them.

Arrange the chairs in a circle and allow time for questions and answers at the end of the talk.

Does Someone You Know Have a Drinking Problem?

On a sheet of paper, answer the following questions either yes or no. Each yes answer is worth 1 point. Your answers to the Life Choice Inventory are personal and private. Share them with others only if you are comfortable doing so.

1. Does the person drink more than most people?
2. Do friends and relatives remark that the person drinks more than most people?
3. Is the person unable to stop drinking on occasion?
4. Do parents or other near relatives worry or complain about the person's drinking?
5. Has the person ever attended a meeting of Alcoholics Anonymous?
6. Has drinking ever created problems between the person and a parent, spouse, or other near relative?
7. Has the person ever gotten into trouble at work because of drinking?
8. Has the person ever neglected his or her obligations, family, or schoolwork for two or more days in a row because of drinking?
9. Has the person ever gone to anyone for help about his or her drinking?
10. Has the person ever been in a hospital because of drinking?
11. Do you hear the person ever expressing guilt about his or her drinking?
12. Has the person ever been arrested for drunken driving, driving while intoxicated, or driving under the influence of alcoholic beverages?
13. Has the person ever been arrested, even for a few hours, because of other drunken behavior?

SCORING

A score of 0 to 1 indicates no alcohol problem. A score of 2 indicates possible alcoholism. A score of 3 or more indicates alcoholism. This test is highly accurate but is for screening purposes only. Final diagnosis should be made by an alcoholism expert.

Source: Michigan Alcoholism Screening Test (MAST), developed by Dr. Melvin L. Selzer. There are longer tests, but this short one is valid. It detects from 94 to 99 percent of people with alcoholism.

quences (results) of it. This chapter's Life Choice Inventory asks questions that are used to identify alcoholism. You can apply these questions to anyone you are concerned about—even yourself. If the answer is yes to two or more of the questions listed, the person may be on the road to alcoholism.

KEY POINTS   *People may drink for many reasons. A moderate drinker differs from a problem drinker in how much the person drinks, the reasons for drinking, and the consequences of the drinking.*

Chapter 13, Section 1

The following quiz will help you assess your students' understanding of the material covered in this section of the chapter. You might use the quiz as an oral exercise, which will lead into a class discussion of the topics covered. Or, you might use it as a paper/pencil quiz to evaluate your students individually.

Like the Quick Quiz, the Section Review can also be used as an assessment tool to spark class discussion or as an individual student evaluation. It can also be used as a review in preparation for this quiz.

1. Alcoholic beverages contain water and other substances as well as alcohol. (True)
2. Proof refers to the amount of alcohol

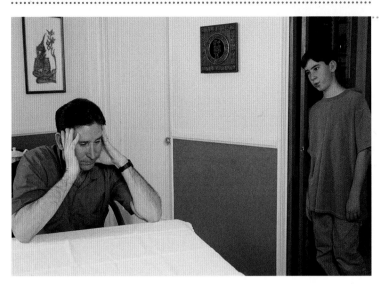

Sometimes others can see the symptoms of a drinking problem more clearly than the person suffering from them.

ASSESS

EVALUATE

SECTION 1   Review Answers

1. **a.** Proof **b.** moderation **c.** drink (pp. 344–345)
2. peer pressure encourages it, drinking makes them look grown-up, a way to rebel against authority (p. 344)
3. Answers may vary; alcohol addiction sets in much more quickly in young people than adults; more teenagers die or are permanently injured in alcohol-related accidents than from any other cause; poses other threats to life and health. (p. 343)
4. Refer to Figure 13–1 on page 345 for possible answers.
5. Answers will vary. Refer to Figure 13–2 on page 346 for possible answers.
6. Answers will vary.

A reproducible quiz for Section 1 is provided in the Teacher's Resource Box.

SECTION 1 Review

Answer the following questions on a sheet of paper.

Learning the Vocabulary

The vocabulary terms in this section are *alcohol, ethanol (ethyl alcohol), proof, alcoholism, moderation,* and *drink.*

1. Fill in the blank with the correct response:
   a. _____ is a term used to describe the percentage of alcohol in alcoholic beverages.
   b. To drink an amount of alcohol that causes no harm to health is to exercise _____ .
   c. A _____ is the amount of a beverage that delivers ½ ounce of pure ethanol.

Learning the Facts

2. List three reasons that young people give as to why they drink alcohol.
3. Give two reasons why alcohol is illegal for teenagers.
4. List and define the terms used to describe people who drink alcohol.
5. Describe the skills that moderate drinkers of alcohol use.

Making Life Choices

6. Reread the Consumer Skills feature, "Advertisements for Alcohol," on page 347. What does this tell you about our society and drinking? Describe the different ways alcohol is being advertised. What could you do to change how alcohol is being advertised?

> 66 *We drink to one another's health and spoil our own.* 99
>
> Jerome Jerome
> (1859–1927)
> English humorist

CLOSE

Before proceeding to Section 2, the students should be able to answer these questions:

1. What impact can alcohol abuse have on your life?
2. Why is abstinence from alcohol as a teenager and moderate use of alcohol as an adult important?
3. What are some signs that alcohol is becoming a problem?

contained in a beverage. (True)
3. Alcohol is not considered a mind-altering drug. (False)
4. Ethanol, the alcohol contained in alcoholic beverages, is not poisonous. (False)
5. Alcohol is the only legal, nonprescription drug that produces euphoria. (True)
6. People who drink alcohol from a young age are less prone to developing an alcohol addiction. (False)
7. Teenagers may be expelled from school, fined, and even imprisoned for drinking alcoholic beverages. (True)
8. A standard drink delivers four ounces of pure ethanol. (False)
9. On average, females can drink more than males without becoming drunk. (False)
10. Problem drinkers differ from moderate drinkers not only in the amount of alcohol they consume, but in their reasons for drinking. (True)

SECTION
2

FOCUS

OUTCOMES

In this section students will learn the:

1. Short- and long-term effects of alcohol on the body.
2. Effects of alcohol on the brain and the various thought processes.
3. Long-term effects of alcohol on unborn children. (fetal alcohol syndrome)

FOCUS ACTIVITY

Have the students write a short paragraph describing a typical "drunk" using personal experience or popular belief as depicted on TV. List some of the common descriptions of "drunks" on the board. As you discuss the chapter, continue to remind students that these characteristics result from the use of alcohol.

TEACH & APPLY

TEACHER SUPPORT

Key Passage

Tell students it is a myth that alcohol helps to warm people up when they are cold. Alcohol will open the skin's blood vessels and make the person seem warmer, but the extra blood that flows through the skin will allow extra heat from the inner body to be transferred into the air, chilling, rather than warming, the person.

SECTION
2

Effects of Alcohol

The drug alcohol has both immediate and long-term effects on the body. These effects depend on the size of the dose of alcohol. As with other drugs, all of alcohol's effects on the body occur when a person drinks it, no matter which effect the drinker is seeking.

Moderate Drinking: Immediate Effects

Alcohol is a special molecule in many ways. It is extremely small, as molecules go. It can move fast, and it can mix with both fatty and watery substances. This means that it meets with no barriers in the body. It can go anywhere. Alcohol affects every cell of the body.

Alcohol begins acting on the body the moment a person swallows it. From the stomach and intestines, it moves rapidly into the bloodstream. (Alcohol does not have to be digested.) From the blood, it enters every cell. Within minutes after the first sip of a drink, ethanol is affecting the brain, muscles, nerves, glands, and small blood vessels of the skin. It also passes through the liver.

The liver is the organ most well-equipped with the machinery to change alcohol into harmless wastes that the body can excrete. The liver goes to work on alcohol right away, but can handle only about one drink an hour. If a person drinks faster than this, the excess keeps building up, affecting all the cells more and more.

The effects the drinker can feel are from alcohol's action on the nervous system. Alcohol first depresses the action of some of the brain's fine-tuning nerves—those that usually set limits on behavior. A person slightly under the influence of alcohol will talk or laugh more loudly and gesture more widely after these controls are gone. A loud buzz of conversation starts to rise a half hour into a party where alcohol is served, because alcohol has depressed people's fine-tuning nerves.

The loosening-up effect of one drink has given people the impression that alcohol is a stimulant. It is not; it is a depressant. After drinking alcohol, a person might feel socially stimulated. However, the molecule itself never stimulates any process within the body. In fact, it acts like the anesthetics that are used to put people to sleep for surgery.

Alcohol is a poor choice among anesthetics, though. Like heroin, the amount of alcohol that causes unconsciousness is close to the amount that causes death. It does not reliably keep people under, and yet it can kill them. (It is still sometimes used in emergencies, however, when no better anesthetic is available.)

Soon after a few sips of alcohol, the drinker can feel it warming the skin. Nerves normally keep the blood vessels of the skin narrow to prevent the body's losing too much heat. Alcohol relaxes these nerves, and the blood vessels of the skin widen. The skin of a person who has been drinking may appear flushed and feel warm.

Alcohol meets with no barriers in the body; it can go anywhere.

Effects of Alcohol

Divide the class into groups of three. Have the groups read the chapter together, discuss and debate each of the sections in the chapter.
Section 1—Why do some teens choose to drink. Responses will vary but may include peer pressure, curiosity, stress or boredom. Have them also discuss reasons why some teens choose not to drink. Are those teens popular? What consequences are paid by those teens who choose not drink? Are the consequences worth it? Ask students to debate the paragraph that deals with drinking in moderation. Do they believe that it is OK to drink in moderation? Why does the book talk about adults drinking in moderation, but not teens? Finally have teens discuss the range of behavior that they have seen in people who drink. How do teens feel about these behaviors?

Another early effect of alcohol in the brain is to sedate the cerebral cortex (see Figure 13–3), where conscious thinking and learning takes place. The drinker loses certain kinds of awareness, including awareness of unpleasant recent events, worries, insecurity, discomfort, and pain. At the same time, the brain's speech and vision centers are being put to sleep.

Alcohol also disturbs sleep and reduces the ability to learn or to perform mental tasks. The brain normally helps to shut out distractions. Alcohol, however, puts this function to sleep, allowing attention to wander easily.

In addition, alcohol reduces the brain's ability to inhibit the awareness and expression of emotions. Thus the person expresses love, joy, sorrow, anger, and hatred more easily than before.

At this point, a person who decides to drink no more alcohol can easily recover from these effects. Recovery becomes complete as soon as the liver clears the last of the alcohol from the body. If the person decides to drink still more, though, alcohol's depressant effects start to add up.

 KEY POINTS *Alcohol affects every cell. In moderate amounts, it depresses the brain's fine-tuning nerves, opens the blood vessels of the skin, disturbs sleep, impairs mental abilities, dulls awareness, clouds vision and speech, and intensifies emotional expression.*

Excessive Drinking: Immediate Effects

With increasing doses of alcohol, behavior becomes unpredictable. People may act against their own desires and wishes, because their awareness of those desires and wishes is now gone. Against all reason and judgment, a person may pick a fight; or may become sexually aggressive or have unplanned, unprotected sexual intercourse; or may attempt a dangerous physical exploit—with painful or even tragic results. The reason these things can happen is clear from the map of the brain in Figure 13–3. The person's judgment might have prevented the behavior, but the judgment center has been put to sleep.

Judgment would also tell the person not to have another drink—but again, judgment is gone. This is why a person may go on to drink to the point of passing out. The person can no longer see the need to stop.

Next, speech, vision, and coordination are disabled. The drinker should not drive. However, many do so, because at this point, drinkers cannot tell that they should not drive. Everyone has seen the out-of-control driver, weaving back and forth on the highway, unable to tell how fast to go and how to steer. The driver doesn't see that the risks are life-threatening, and may be more entertained than frightened.

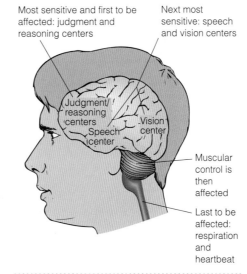

Most sensitive and first to be affected: judgment and reasoning centers

Next most sensitive: speech and vision centers

Judgment/reasoning centers
Speech center
Vision center

Muscular control is then affected

Last to be affected: respiration and heartbeat

Figure 13–3 Alcohol's Effects on the Brain. Alcohol is rightly termed an anesthetic, because it puts brain centers to sleep in the following order: first the frontal lobe (the reasoning and judgment centers), then the speech and vision centers, then the centers that govern muscular control, and finally the deep centers that control respiration and heartbeat.

Why do some people become more friendly while others become angry and violent when drinking? **Section 2**—Have students debate the immediate effects of drinking. They should discuss effects on body systems and glands for both moderate and excessive drinking. Have the groups also debate and discuss the long-term effects of both types of drinking. Conclude this section by discussing hangover cures. **Section 3**—Ask students to debate ways of preventing drinking and driving accidents. How can they stop a friend from driving when the friend has been drinking and refuses to give up his keys? How can they tell when a friend has had too much to drink? **Section 4**—Have groups discuss different treatment programs that are available for teens as well as adults with drinking problems. Have each group write out a description of a person with alcoholism. **Section 5**—Have the groups list ways to say no to alcohol and to list things to do instead of drinking.

LEARNING WITH VISUALS

TRANSPARENCIES An overhead, "Comparing Excessive vs. Moderate Drinking," in the Transparency Acetate Binder graphs the difference between a social drinker and an alcohol abuser, showing the amount of alcohol needed to achieve euphoria and how that relates to the amount of alcohol the body will tolerate. Remind students that any drinking by those under 21 is illegal, even if they are not legally drunk.

DISCUSSION

Ask students if they have ever been around someone who has had too much to drink and acted in unpredictable, irrational ways. Remind students not to name any names. How did this person's behavior make them feel? Embarrassed, uncomfortable, fearful?

LEARNING WITH VISUALS

TRANSPARENCIES In the Transparency Acetate Binder you will find an overhead of Figure 13–3 entitled "Alcohol's Effects on the Brain."

FAST FACT

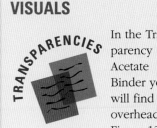

140 million Americans use alcohol, and an estimated 18 million of these people have a serious drinking problem.

GROUP ACTIVITY

Divide the class into four groups. Assign one of the following systems to each group: circulatory, respiratory, nervous, and muscular. Have each group research the assigned system and then do a class presentation on how alcohol affects that system.

BACKGROUND INFORMATION

Display a chart of the body's internal organs (see overhead "The Digestive System" in chapter 6). Explain to students how the liver is the first major organ to be affected by alcohol. Emphasize that nutrients and alcohol are absorbed into the blood from the digestive tract and travel immediately to the liver and brain and then throughout the body. Remind them of the part played by fat production in the liver. Describe "fatty liver" and "cirrhosis of the liver."

BACKGROUND INFORMATION

Your Teacher's Resource Box contains a handout "Blood Alcohol Concentration by Number of Drinks and Body Weight."

With still more drinking, the conscious brain is completely depressed, and the person passes out. Figure 13–4 on the next page shows the blood alcohol levels that correspond with progressively greater **intoxication**.

The Body's Defenses During these events, the drinker's body is processing alcohol as fast as it can. Alcohol is a toxin (a poison). The body protects itself against toxins in several ways. For one thing, the throat stings as straight alcohol goes down and triggers the choking reflex. This keeps the drinker from swallowing too much in a gulp. A second protective device is the stomach, which rejects a too-large dose. The drinker vomits and expels at least part of the dose before it can be absorbed. Third, the body breaks down any alcohol that does get into the blood as quickly as possible.

The Role of the Liver Alcohol entering the stomach and intestines is absorbed rapidly into the bloodstream unless food is present to slow down its absorption. From there, it travels directly to the liver, which filters the blood before releasing it to the rest of the body. The liver's location in the cardiovascular system permits it to remove toxic substances carried there from the intestines before they reach other body organs, such as the heart and brain. However, the liver itself faces a hazard. When a person eats or drinks too much of any toxin, the liver is the first organ to be damaged.

A hangover is a mild form of alcohol withdrawal.

KEY POINTS *Excessive drinking makes people unaware of their desires and wishes, and it steals judgment. Still more alcohol puts the conscious mind to sleep. The body protects itself from toxic doses of alcohol through the choking reflex, vomiting, and the breakdown of alcohol by the liver. The liver itself can be damaged by alcohol.*

The Hangover

The hangover—the awful feeling of headache pain, unpleasant sensations in the mouth, and nausea that a drinker suffers the morning after drinking too much—is a mild form of withdrawal. (A much worse form is a **delirium** with severe **tremors**, which warns of a danger of death and demands medical treatment.)

Hangovers are caused by several factors. One is the toxic effects of ingredients other than alcohol in alcoholic beverages—**congeners**. The congeners in gin are different from those in vodka, which in turn are different from those in bourbon or rye whiskey.

HEALTHY PEOPLE 2000

Approximately two-thirds of American adults drink alcohol at least occasionally. Of these, it is estimated that about 18 million currently experience problems as a result of alcohol use, and about 7 percent of drinkers experience moderate levels of dependence symptoms. Alcohol is a factor in approximately half of all homicides, suicides, and motor vehicle fatalities. With fetal alcohol syndrome affecting as many as 3 infants per 1,000 live births in some hospital reports, it is the leading preventable cause of birth defects. Alcohol is also responsible for numerous deaths due to liver disease. Of special concern are the problems for young people. Nine out of ten high school seniors report using alcohol at least once.

Some people are more sensitive to the congeners in some liquors than to those in others. More important than the type of congeners in bringing on hangovers, though, is the total amount of alcohol drunk.

Dehydration of the brain is a second factor causing a hangover. Alcohol causes the body to lose water. It reduces the brain cells' water content, too. When these cells rehydrate the morning after, the nerves hurt as the cells swell back to their normal size.

Figure 13–4 *Effects of Various Blood Alcohol Levels.* Note: *Data are for an average-sized person under ordinary circumstances. Effects vary greatly from person to person, from day to day, and from one circumstance to another.*

Another reason for the hangover is the effects of **formaldehyde**, a chemical familiar as the fluid biology labs use to preserve dead animals. Formaldehyde forms when the body breaks down alcohol.

Nothing helps the headache pain, the nasty taste in the mouth, and the nausea of a hangover. Popular remedies such as vitamins, tranquilizers, aspirin, drinking more alcohol, breathing pure oxygen, exercising, eating, or drinking something awful do not work. Time alone is the cure for a hangover. The problem comes simply from drinking too much.

(KEY) POINTS *A hangover is a mild form of withdrawal that causes headache, unpleasant sensations in the mouth, and nausea. The extreme form is delirium with tremors. Time is the only cure.*

Long-Term Effects of Excessive Drinking

A reason why some people can drink excessively for years and not suffer obvious damage is that they allow their systems time to recover. The damage done by each bout of drinking is repaired before the next bout. Long-term drinking in excess, without sufficient recovery periods between times, however, wrecks the health of body systems. It may damage one person's heart, another person's pancreas, and another person's brain the most. However, it always affects all organs to some extent.

Probably the most common disease to occur among abusers of alcohol is liver disease. One effect of excessive drinking is that the liver cells start to fill with fat. If time between drinking bouts is not long enough to permit this fat to be removed, then the fat-stuffed liver cells stop functioning. The liver cells die and harden, and lose their function forever.

When the liver is injured, the whole body suffers. One of the worst effects of liver damage is high blood pressure. High blood pressure makes

MINI Glossary

intoxication: literally, a state of being poisoned; often used to mean drunkenness.

delirium: a state of mental confusion, usually with hallucinations and continual movement.

tremors: continuous quivering or shaking.

congeners (CON-jen-ers): ingredients in alcoholic beverages, other than the alcohol itself, that may irritate the nervous system.

formaldehyde: a substance related to alcohol. Formaldehyde is made by the body from alcohol and contributes to hangovers.

These are the immediate health problems posed by alcohol and other drugs. Their abuse, however, is closely related to a host of other social and health problems, such as early unwanted pregnancy, delinquency, and school failure. The economic cost of problems attendant to alcohol abuse was estimated in 1990 to be $70 billion, and another $44 billion for drug problems.

Businesses, schools, parent groups, and minority organizations have developed ways to fight the pervasive dangers of alcohol and other drugs. A changing social climate has been accompanied by legislative and policy actions, particularly concerning drinking and driving.

LEARNING WITH VISUALS

You may want to use the overhead in the Teacher's Resource Box entitled "The Liver" to show how the liver works as students begin to read about the effects of alcohol on the liver. Tell students that should the liver become fatty, the second state of liver disease, fibrosis, begins and scar tissue replaces fat. The last stage of liver disease is cirrhosis, in which liver cells die and lose their function. The liver cells can no longer regenerate, and the person may die.

BACKGROUND INFORMATION

Distribute the handout entitled "The Disguises of Alcoholism," found in the Teacher's Resource Box, to the students. This handout lists several illnesses and problems that often result from alcoholism.

DISCUSSION

Emphasize that many women are pregnant for up to two months before they realize it. How does this impact the development of a healthy fetus? You may want your students to read the Straight Talk, "Drinking During Pregnancy," Chapter 20. After students have read the Straight Talk, ask them if drinking during pregnancy is the same thing as child abuse. Should a woman be punished for placing her unborn child in this danger?

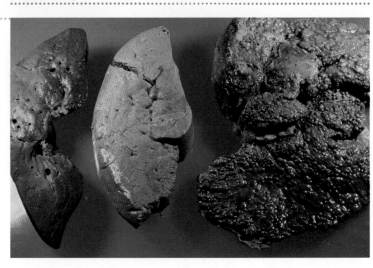

Left: normal liver. Center: liver with excess fat deposits from drinking. Right: liver beyond recovery from years of alcohol abuse.

heart attacks and strokes likely. Liver damage also weakens the body's defenses against infection.

The liver makes fat from alcohol. This fat collects in the blood vessels and heart muscle, as well as in the liver and other places. Wherever it collects, the fat interferes with function. The fat also collects in fat's regular storage sites—under the skin at the hips, belly, legs, and other fatty areas. Other times, the alcohol abuser becomes too sick to eat, and alcohol cannot nourish the body. Its toxic effects on muscle and other tissues causes them to wither. The person thus becomes bone thin as the tissues shrink away.

Nerve and brain tissues are especially sensitive to alcohol. The brain shrinks, even in people who drink only moderately. Excessive drinking over many years can cause major, permanent brain damage affecting vision, memory, learning ability, and other functions.

Alcohol abuse also increases the risk of cancer of the mouth, throat, lungs, liver, pancreas, and rectum. Abusing alcohol also directly causes the pancreas to stop producing insulin. Thus some people develop diabetes from alcohol abuse.

Other long-term effects of alcohol abuse:

► Ulcers of the stomach and intestines.
► Shrinking of all the body's muscles, including the heart muscle.
► Abnormal changes in the blood.
► Kidney, bladder, and gland damage.
► Skin rashes and sores.
► Shrinkage and damage to the testicles, causing men to become feminine and develop sexual problems.
► Failure of the ovaries and menstrual problems in women.
► Lung damage leading to flu, pneumonia, or tuberculosis.
► Psychological depression and mental illness.

Chapter 13, Section 2

The following quiz will help you assess your students' understanding of the material covered in this section of the chapter. You might use the quiz as an oral exercise, which will lead into a class discussion of the topics covered. Or, you might use it as a paper/pencil

quiz to evaluate your students individually.

Like the Quick Quiz, the Section Review can also be used as an assessment tool to spark class discussion or as an individual student evaluation. It can also be used as a review in preparation for this quiz.

1. Alcohol affects every cell of the body. (True)

2. Alcohol must be digested before it can begin to affect the body. (False)

Then there are the risks to the fetus when a pregnant woman abuses alcohol—the longest-term risks of all. The effects of **fetal alcohol syndrome (FAS)** are severe. They include mental and physical retardation and birth defects that last a lifetime. The Straight Talk section of Chapter 20 describes FAS in more detail.

In short, alcohol abuse damages health in every possible way. Even social drinking is linked with a higher-than-normal risk of death. Social drinkers who drink to excess are at risk, even though they may never appear drunk. Add, to all these risks, one other. This risk crosses over the boundaries of self-destruction to destroy the lives of other innocent people—the risk of accidents due to drinking.

 KEY POINTS *The effects of excessive drinking add up over the years to cause severe health damage. The liver, brain, and nerves suffer most. All organs suffer to some extent. The longest-term damage is suffered by the infant born to a woman who abused alcohol during pregnancy—fetal alcohol syndrome.*

SECTION 2 Review

Answer the following questions on a sheet of paper.

Learning the Vocabulary

The vocabulary terms in this section are *intoxication, delirium, tremors, congeners, formaldehyde,* and *fetal alcohol syndrome (FAS).*

1. Match each of the following phrases with the appropriate vocabulary term from the list above:
   a. a state of mental confusion
   b. made by the body from alcohol and contributes to a hangover
   c. ingredients in alcoholic beverages that may irritate the nervous system

Learning the Facts

2. Which cells are affected by alcohol?

3. List the effects of alcohol when a person is slightly under the influence.
4. Why is alcohol a poor choice for an anesthetic?
5. List the order in which brain centers are affected by alcohol.

Making Life Choices

6. How would you react to the following statements: "Steve's parents won't allow him to drink alcohol. They say it's illegal and that it can lead to other drug addictions. All of Steve's friends are drinking. He doesn't see anyone taking other drugs. Recently, he discovered his parents drinking at their parties. They are saying one thing but doing another." How can Steve make up his mind? The mixed messages he's getting are so confusing. What would you tell Steve?

MINI Glossary

fetal alcohol syndrome (FAS): a cluster of birth defects, including permanent mental and physical retardation and facial abnormalities, seen in children born to mothers who abuse alcohol during pregnancy.

3. The liver is the organ most effective in changing alcohol into harmless waste. (True)
4. Alcohol is a stimulant. (False)
5. Alcohol depresses the action of some of the brain's fine-tuning nerves and sedates the brain's cerebral cortex. (True)
6. Alcohol intensifies a person's emotional responses. (True)
7. Excessive alcohol makes people more aware of their desires and wishes. (False)

8. The body defends itself against alcohol poisoning through the choking reflex, vomiting, and the actions of the liver. (True)
9. A hangover can be cured by OTC medication. (False)
10. The long-term consequences of alcohol abuse include ulcers, shrinking of the muscles, cancer of the liver, and brain damage. (True)

ASSESS

EVALUATE

SECTION 2 Review Answers

1. a. delirium b. formaldehyde c. congeners (pp. 352–353)
2. every cell of the body (p. 350)
3. talk or laugh more loudly and gesture more widely (p. 350)
4. The amount of alcohol that causes unconsciousness is close to the amount that causes death. (p. 350)
5. reasoning and judgment centers; speech and vision centers; centers that govern muscle control; deep centers that control respiration and heartbeat (p. 351)
6. Answers will vary.

 WORKSHEETS A reproducible quiz for Section 2 is provided in the Teacher's Resource Box.

CLOSE

Before going to the next section make sure that students can explain the following:

1. Alcohol is toxic to the brain and liver and has immediate effects on all body systems, behaviors, and perceptions.
2. The liver is the organ that processes alcohol at a rate of 1 oz. per hour.
3. Hangovers are the result of toxic congeners, dehydration, and the formation of formaldehyde in the system.
4. Alcohol has many long-term effects, including Fetal Alcohol Syndrome.

SECTION 3

FOCUS

OUTCOMES

In this section students will learn the:

1. Correlation between alcohol abuse and accidents.

2. Skills in dealing with an intoxicated friend.

3. Agencies and groups available to help friends and family members.

FOCUS ACTIVITY

Bring in a number of newspapers. Have students search the newspapers for articles about accidents or arrests that are alcohol related. Discuss some of the articles.

TEACH & APPLY

BACKGROUND INFORMATION

Give students the following percentages for violent crimes in which alcohol abuse is a factor: 64 percent of murders, 41 percent of assaults, 34 percent of rapes, 29 percent of other sex crimes, 30 percent of suicides, 50 percent of fights in the home, and 60 percent of child abuse cases.

FAST FACT

Nearly 8,000 young people die each year in automobile accidents that are alcohol related. An additional 40,000 are either disfigured for life or crippled.

Accidents and Alcohol

Drinking slows reactions. It impairs coordination and dulls depth perception. Drinking before and while driving is the single greatest hazard on the road. Of all fatal automobile and motorcycle accidents on the roads today, about half involve alcohol. There is no better way to display friendship than to keep a friend who has been drinking off the road.

Drinking, Driving, Accidents, and Violence

The dangers of drinking and driving are so great that states have passed laws that forbid driving under the influence of alcohol. Under these laws, it is a crime to be **DWI** (**D**riving **W**hile **I**ntoxicated) or **DUI** (**D**riving **U**nder the **I**nfluence of alcohol or any other mind-altering substance). The "influence of alcohol" is proved if an adult driver's blood contains 0.08 percent alcohol in some states, and 0.10 in others. To reduce fatal alcohol-related crashes involving drivers under 21, many states have adopted a "zero-tolerance" limit for young drivers—actually, a 0.02 percent blood alcohol limit.

The alcohol content of the blood is reflected in the alcohol level in a person's breath. Therefore, the **breathalyzer test** is one method used to measure the blood alcohol level of a person suspected of driving under the influence of alcohol.

Lobby groups such as MADD (Mothers Against Drunk Drivers) and SADD (Students

Don't do it. Don't ever drink and drive.

HEALTHY PEOPLE 2000

Reduce deaths caused by alcohol-related motor vehicle crashes to no more than 8.5 per 100,000 people.

This objective is stated in terms of fatalities because of the availability of reliable and precise data regarding deaths caused by motor vehicle crashes. Injuries are also a serious problem. Although decreases in deaths may indicate parallel reductions in injuries, improvements in occupant protection and emergency medical services may prevent deaths while the incidence of crash-related injuries is actually increasing.

In 1987, motor vehicle crashes were the fifth leading cause of death in the U.S., and approximately half of these were alcohol-related. Alcohol-related traffic crashes are the leading cause of death and spinal cord injury for young Americans.

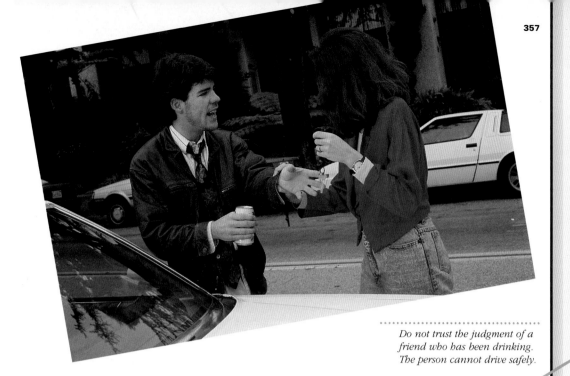

Do not trust the judgment of a
friend who has been drinking.
The person cannot drive safely.

TEACHER SUPPORT

Key Passage
To emphasize this point, tell
students that driving under
the influence of alcohol is
especially hazardous for
young drivers who are inexperienced in both driving and
drinking. Drivers younger
than 20 represent fewer than
8% of the nation's licensed
drivers, but they are involved
in more than 25% of all collisions, and drinking and driving accidents are the leading
cause of death.

Against Driving Drunk) are pressuring the government to make the laws stricter. They have lost too many cherished sons, daughters, and friends to alcohol-related accidents on the highways and are trying to prevent other needless losses.

A drinker cannot drive safely for several hours after the blood alcohol level has fallen back to zero. Even moderate drinkers are advised not to drive the *morning after* an evening of drinking. They may feel fine, but their driving ability may still be abnormal.

Not only auto accidents, but drownings, fatal falls, suicide attempts, and abuse of other drugs are all more likely when people drink alcohol. Violent crimes are more likely, too. Most are committed by people who have drunk heavily enough to produce blood alcohol levels from 0.10 to 0.30 percent. (With levels higher than that, people pass out.) Remember, these people are not necessarily violent people to begin with. Under alcohol's influence, however, they become violent. Violent behavior attributed to the effects of alcohol accounts for one third to two thirds of all murders, assaults, rapes, suicides, family violence, and child abuse.

 KEY POINTS *Alcohol makes auto accidents and other accidents much more likely. DWI and DUI laws punish people who drink or take drugs and drive. Violent behavior is strongly linked to alcohol use.*

When a Friend Has Drunk Too Much

If a friend has drunk too much, you can't speed up the recovery process by taking your friend for a walk. The muscles have to work to walk, but

MINI Glossary

DWI: driving while intoxicated with alcohol or any abusable substance—a crime by law. Intoxication is defined by blood alcohol level (a level of 0.08 percent in some states and 0.10 percent in other states).

DUI: driving under the influence (of alcohol or other mind-altering substances). See *DWI.*

breathalyzer test: a test of the alcohol level in a person's breath, which reflects the blood level of alcohol.

DISCUSSION

Write the following situations on the board:

1. The people you are baby-sitting for come home from a party smelling of alcohol and acting silly. They are supposed to give you a ride home.
2. You are watching a couple's children at your home. They come to pick up their children smelling of alcohol and acting silly and uncoordinated.
3. You are at a party that your parents told you that you could not attend. Your ride to the party is obviously drunk and you do not have enough money for a taxi ride home.
4. You and your parents have been to dinner at a friend's home. You noticed that both your mom and dad had two glasses of wine with dinner and a cocktail with dessert.

Ask students what they would do in these situations. Is dying or placing other people in danger worth sparing someone's feelings or the anger of your parents?

The alcohol-related proportion of crash deaths dropped by 10 to 15 percent between 1982 and 1986 because of the emergence of highly visible citizen activist groups, the media attention, increased enforcement of alcohol-impaired driving laws (sobriety checkpoints), and use of sanctions such as license suspensions and revocations. In 1988, the Surgeon General of the U.S. Public Health Service explicitly recognized the contribution of alcohol advertising to the problem of drinking and driving and called for increased regulation of alcohol advertising.

The levels of citizen activism, enforcement, and sanctioning activity have declined in recent years. Progress in further reducing alcohol-related crashes has slowed since 1985. These shifts in alcohol-related crash deaths show how united citizen, private business, and government concern can bring attention to a problem and develop strategies to address it.

BACKGROUND MATERIAL

The handout entitled "Attitudes About Drunk Driving" can be found in the Teacher's Resource Box.

ASSESS

EVALUATE

Review Answers

1. a. sober (p. 358) b. breathalyzer test (p. 356)

2. drinking before and while driving (p. 356)

3. breathalyzer test (p. 356)

4. don't respond to emotions stirred by alcohol; show concern; do not trust your friend's judgment about further drinking; take your friend's car keys away (p. 358)

5. Answers will vary.

CLOSE

Before proceeding to the next section, students should be able to:

1. Write the definitions of DWI and DUI.

2. Connect alcohol use and abuse with accidents and violence.

---

since they cannot use alcohol for fuel, they cannot help clear it from the blood. Time alone can do the job of making your friend **sober** again. Each person's blood is cleared of alcohol at a steady but limited rate.

It will not help to give your friend a cup of coffee. Caffeine is a stimulant, but it won't help break down alcohol. The police say, "A drunk who drinks a cup of coffee won't get sober but may become a wide-awake drunk."

Other suggestions for dealing with someone who is intoxicated:

▶ Don't respond to emotions stirred by alcohol.
▶ Do show concern.
▶ Do not trust your friend's judgment about further drinking.
▶ Take your friend's car keys away.

For someone who has had too much to drink, we repeat: time is the only real cure. One-half pint of alcohol takes 10 hours to leave the system. A person who has passed out from drinking needs 24 hours to sober up completely. Let such people sleep. (Let them lie on their sides, rather than on their backs. That way, if they vomit, they won't choke.) Don't let them drive, and never let them take a drink for the road.

A great weight of evidence shows that alcohol can harm health. The only points in its favor seem to be the social effects and a slight effect against heart attacks mentioned at the start of this chapter. There, the question of why people drink was asked. Perhaps an even more important question is, "How can people who become addicted to alcohol stop drinking?"

KEY POINTS *Time alone restores a person who is drunk to a sober state.*

SECTION 3 Review

Answer the following questions on a sheet of paper.

Learning the Vocabulary

The vocabulary terms in this section are *DWI, DUI, breathalyzer test,* and *sober.*

1. Match the following phrases with the appropriate terms:
   a. free of alcohol's effects and free of addiction
   b. a test that reflects the blood level of alcohol in a person's body

Learning the Facts

2. What is the single greatest hazard on the road?

3. What is one method for measuring a person's blood alcohol level?

4. List four suggestions for dealing with someone who is intoxicated.

Making Life Choices

5. What would happen in this situation? After a party, Tim, who has had two beers, gets into his car to drive home. He claims to feel just fine and doesn't need your advice. What would you say to him to stop him? What other action would you take?

Chapter 13, Section 3

The following quiz will help you assess your students' understanding of the material covered in this section of the chapter. You might use the quiz as an oral exercise, which will lead into a class discussion of the topics covered. Or, you might use it as a paper/pencil quiz to evaluate your students individually.

*If students have difficulty with the concepts covered in the Quick Quiz and the Section Review, you might suggest they review the material using the **S**urvey, **Q**uestion, **R**ead, **R**ecite, **R**eview (SQ3R) study method, which is described in detail in the introduction to this Teacher's Wraparound Edition.*

1. Drinking slows reaction time by impairing coordination and depth perception. (True)

SECTION 4

The Way Back: Strategies for Recovery

We know a great deal about the addictive nature of alcohol. We also know a great deal about recovery from alcohol addiction. Some of the struggles to recover from addiction apply only to alcohol. Many, though, apply to all drugs.

Costs of Alcoholism How can we add up all the misery caused by addiction to alcohol, or alcoholism? One way is to measure the impact in terms of losses to society. People who are addicted to alcohol and other drugs take many sick days from work or school. They may lose their jobs or quit school. This limits their ultimate contributions to society. Not only do they fail to contribute; they also draw heavily on society's resources. They require more hospitalization, placing a burden on insurance companies to pay for services. They cause avoidable accidents and injuries, and they commit crimes. These behaviors require the services of public support systems such as police, ambulances, courts, prisons, lawyers, and rehabilitation centers. The true dollar costs of alcoholism, if added up in this way, are colossal.

For some, the costs in dollars may be far outweighed by the other costs of alcoholism. Another way to measure the tragedy of alcoholism is to look at the effects upon one family in which a member is addicted to alcohol. The family suffers losses of income, of status in the community, of physical and mental health, and even of life itself. Both the person with alcoholism and the people close to that person suffer these losses.

However, only one individual can put an end to the misery—the addicted person. The day that person admits to having a dependency problem is the first day on a long road to recovery. With recovery, though, comes an end to the losses and miseries suffered by the family and the community.

Why Recovery Is So Difficult You may be wondering why, when faced with all these losses, the addicted person does not simply quit drinking. The reason is that a person who is addicted to alcohol is in the grip of a powerful force that nonaddicted people cannot possibly imagine.

The addicted person may want to quit drinking, may promise to do so, but may drink secretly and then feel guilty and worthless. More promises unkept and more drinking lead to physical, mental, and moral deterioration until the addiction becomes life's only reality. Finally, one day, the person may admit complete defeat in the face of physical, financial, and emotional losses. This is the point of surrender for

Clifton Perry, Detroit, MI
Grades 10-12

For Your Information

Young people who take up alcohol drinking before age 15 are four times as likely to become dependent on alcohol as those who begin drinking at age 21.

MINI Glossary

sober: free of alcohol's effects and of addiction; not drunk.

SECTION 4

FOCUS

OUTCOMES

In this section students will learn the:

1. Symptoms of alcoholism.
2. Impact of alcoholism on family, friends, and society.
3. Symptoms of enabling an alcohol addict.
4. Tools for coping with and surviving alcoholism in the family.

FOCUS ACTIVITY

Draw an outline of a person on the board. Ask students to give the symptoms of an alcohol addict. As they give the correct ones, fill in the head, arms, torso, etc., with the symptoms. Stress the difference between a functional alcohol addict and a nonfunctional alcohol addict.

TEACH & APPLY

BACKGROUND INFORMATION

Distribute the handout in the Teacher's Resource Box entitled "The Progression of Alcoholism," which shows the behavior that occurs in five stages of developing full-fledged alcoholism. Discussing the behaviors listed on the handout will help increase student interest in Section 4.

2. Alcohol is involved in nearly half of all fatal automobile accidents. (True)

3. A breathalyzer test can determine whether a person is DWI or DUI. (True)

4. A person can drive safely after drinking as soon as his/her blood alcohol level has returned to zero. (False)

5. There is no connection between violent behavior and alcohol abuse. (False)

6. Coffee can speed a person's recovery time from alcohol. (False)

7. Exercise can lower a person's blood alcohol level. (False)

8. An intoxicated person may not realize that she/he has had too much to drink. (True)

9. A person who has passed out from alcohol should be propped up on his/her side rather than allowed to sleep on his/her back. (True)

10. Only time can make a person sober. (True)

many who then seek out helping programs and begin their way back. Others may begin recovery at earlier points.

Recovery from addiction occurs in stages. First, the person has to accept that the problem exists and "own" the problem. Then the person must quit using the drug and (usually) get help. Then the person must "stay quit." This sounds simple, and it is, but it is not easy. Some people will not make it.

 KEY POINTS *People who are addicted to alcohol and other drugs not only fail to contribute to society; they also draw heavily on society's resources. People addicted to alcohol and members of their families suffer financial, physical and emotional losses. Recovery from alcohol addiction occurs in stages.*

Don't Enable

You may know someone in the recovery process. Let's assume you are another family member, or a helper such as a counselor. Let's also assume that the person with the problem is still drinking. The most important thing you can do is *not* **enable** the person to escape the problems that come along with excessive drinking.

An enabler is a rescuer—a person who tries to save the alcohol abuser from the consequences of his or her behavior. The rescuer seems good-hearted. In the case of alcoholism, however, rescuing blocks recovery. By blocking the consequences of the alcohol abuser's behavior, the enabler prevents the learning that would otherwise take place. The alcohol abuser never has to face the music as long as the enabler is around. An enabler within the same family as the alcohol abuser is sometimes called a **codependent**.

Enabling takes many different forms—coming up with money when it's owed, helping make excuses ("I'm sorry to have to tell you this, Boss, but my brother is sick today"), doing the other person's work. Enablers can be family members or helpers outside the family (religious leaders, health-care providers, counselors, lawyers, and others).

A support group for codependents, Al-Anon, is similar to Alcoholics Anonymous (for people addicted to alcohol). Al-Anon helps enablers learn how not to get in the way of lessons that lead to recovery. Alateen, a support group sponsored by Al-Anon, is for young people whose lives have been affected by alcoholism of a family member or a close friend. Figure 13–5 on page 362 lists resources for people with alcohol-related problems. The Health Strategies section on this page, "How Not to Enable," provides rules to prevent enabling.

Beyond these strategies, family members and friends should go about living and enjoying their own lives as best they can. The alcohol problem is not their problem. They cannot solve it, change it, take it away,

Health Strategies

How Not to Enable

These strategies will help you keep yourself from enabling someone else's drug-addicted behavior:

► Stay concerned. (Give the message, "I care about you. I think your behaviors are wrong, but I see you as a worthwhile person.")
► Be prompt. Speak up as soon as possible after each drinking or drug episode.
► Speak about the behavior, but do not attack the person. (Say, "You got drunk last night." Don't say, "You are a no-good, worthless drunk.")
► Be specific; name and describe behaviors. Don't judge. (Say, "You fell and broke the lamp." Don't say, "You made a fool of yourself.")
► Act as a mirror—tell what you see. ("Your eyes are red; your hands are shaking.")
► Don't try to smooth things over. (Say, "Go ahead and cry. Here's a tissue." Don't say, "There, there, it'll be all right.")
► When you are angry, cool off before you talk to the person. (Don't let the other person "make" you angry. That's letting yourself be controlled.)

BACKGROUND INFORMATION

WORKSHEETS

The Teacher's Resource Box contains an activity, "Myths about Alcoholism," that requires students to correct myths about alcoholism. Twenty myths are stated and space is provided for students to write the facts. Also included is an answer sheet with the facts to correct the myths.

DISCUSSION

Write the word *enabling* on the board. Ask students to give definitions. Then ask the following questions:

1. How do family members enable parents who are alcohol abusers? (They call work and make excuses, clean up after them, accept their apologies, and cover up for their problem.)
2. How do teens enable their friends who are problem drinkers or alcohol abusers? (They let them copy homework, lie for them, and drink with them.)
3. What is the #1 way teens enable their friends? (The Code of Silence. They keep their mouths shut even though they know there is a problem. They know facts and conceal them from adults. Teen alcoholics rely heavily on the unspoken Code of Silence.) Use this activity to lead in to a discussion of the Health Strategies, "How Not to Enable."

decision making activity?

Begin discussion by asking the students to determine who, in the following examples, has the most serious problem and why. This could lead to discussing assessment and referral for drug or alcohol abuse. It could also focus the students' attention on behavior associated with drug and alcohol abuse and the effect on family, rather than how often or how much a person drinks or uses chemicals.

1. Terri is a 40 year old divorced bookkeeper. Her two children are both out of high school and support themselves. Terri has been drinking for about two years.

Lately, Terri finds herself drinking more

or take responsibility for it. They can, though, take the responsibility for their own lives.

 Enabling feels like rescuing, but it blocks recovery. It doesn't help. Concerned people should be careful not to enable, but should make their feelings known. Family members and friends of alcohol-dependent people must live their own lives as best they can.

Recovery

Traveling the road back to normal life from alcohol addiction may take years. It's hard, and not everyone succeeds. After all, in most cases the damage done by alcohol has progressed for years. All parts of life have been changed by it. During recovery, the person must take these steps: stop drinking, become able to sleep, regain an appetite, begin to function better socially, return to work, and recover health.

A person giving up a drug goes through the same emotional stages as someone who is grieving over the loss of a loved one. An early stage is **denial**. Another is bargaining. Then come anger and guilt, and finally acceptance. The person giving up addiction needs the respect given to any grieving person.

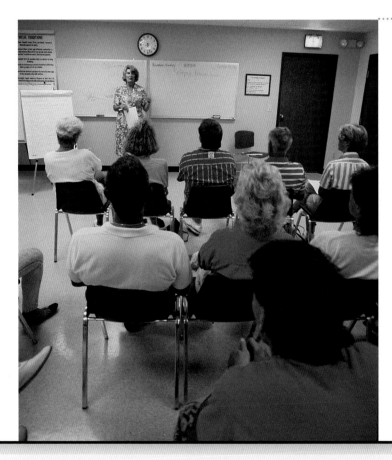

Recovery from alcohol addiction takes effort, support, and time, and not everyone makes it.

enable: make possible. In addiction, enabling means "helping" by trying to "save" the addicted person from the consequences of the behavior. This makes possible continued alcohol or other drug abuse. Also defined in Chapter 5.

codependent: an enabler who is a member of the family of, or has a close relationship with, a person addicted to a drug.

denial (dee-NIGH-al): refusal to believe the facts of a circumstance—for example, to deny that a person is a problem drinker in the face of clear evidence that it is so.

and enjoying the effect of alcohol. Alcohol helps her feel less lonely. Twice in the last two months, Terri has not been certain of how she got home after a night of drinking.

2. Gerald is a 17 year old high school student. He made A's and B's in school until the middle of his junior year. He began partying a lot, skipping school, and getting into trou-

ble often. His grades are now D's or F's.

Gerald drinks almost any alcoholic beverage. When he drinks no one is sure what Gerald is going to do. He recently lost a part-time job because of being late and calling in sick too often.

ASSESS

EVALUATE

SECTION 4 Review Answers

1. The codependent is an enabler who is a member of the family or in a close relationship with an addicted person. (p. 360)
2. Denial (p. 361)
3. losses of income, status in the community, physical and mental health, and life itself (p. 359)
4. The enabler tries to save the abuser; however, rescuing blocks recovery and the abuser never has to face the music (p. 360)
5. Al-Anon Family Group, Alcoholics Anonymous (p. 362)
6. A person giving up alcohol goes through the same emotional stages (p. 361)
7. Answers will vary.

WORKSHEETS

A reproducible quiz for Section 4 is provided in the Teacher's Resource Box.

CLOSE

Before going to the next section, students should be able to explain in their own words that:

1. We are all victims of alcoholism in some way.
2. Only the alcohol addict can take the first step to recovery, but it is up to others to show compassion without enabling.
3. The goal of a recovering alcohol addict is to enjoy life without alcohol.

362

CHAPTER 13: Alcohol: Use and Abuse

Figure 13–5 Resources for People with Alcohol-Related Problems

AL-ANON Family Group   1-757-563-1600
   Headquarters
   1600 Corporate Landing Parkway
   Virginia Beach, VA 23454-5617

Alcoholics Anonymous   1-212-870-3400
   World Service Office
   475 Riverside Drive
   New York, NY 10115

www.ALCOHOLICS-ANONYMOUS.org

❝*Water is the only drink for a wise man.*❞

Henry David Thoreau
(1817–1862)
American writer

It helps if the person is in touch with other people who have recovered. No one is as powerful in helping a person who is recovering from substance abuse as another person who has already traveled that road. The worldwide self-help recovery group Alcoholics Anonymous (AA) works this way. The AA program takes a positive approach—12 steps to recovery and spiritual growth that end in the person's helping others. In AA, thousands of people have helped one another recover from alcoholism.

In the beginning of the recovery process, the ex-user is "dry." The person doesn't drink or take drugs, but still craves the substance, and doesn't enjoy life without it. Only later does the person become "sober." The person who is sober actually prefers life without the substance.

KEY POINTS   *The road to recovery from alcohol or other drug abuse is long and hard. Not all who try to quit succeed. AA helps many people, first to overcome their grief at giving up the addiction, and then to become sober.*

SECTION 4 Review

Answer the following questions on a sheet of paper.

Learning the Vocabulary

The vocabulary terms in this section are *enable, codependent,* and *denial.*

1. What is the difference between an enabler and a codependent?
2. _____ is an early stage of recovery from addiction.

Learning the Facts

3. What losses does a family suffer when one of its members is addicted to alcohol?
4. Describe how an enabler affects a person addicted to alcohol.

5. Name two agencies that help those with alcohol-related problems.
6. What does giving up alcohol have in common with grief?

Making Life Choices

7. You have made a date with a very good-looking, popular student at your school. You have heard that this person likes to have a good time and goes to parties where other people drink alcohol and use other drugs. You are worried that you might be asked to use drugs or alcohol. How would you feel about being asked to use alcohol? What would you do? Why would you take that action?

QUICK QUIZ

Chapter 13, Section 4

The following quiz will help you assess your students' understanding of the material covered in this section of the chapter. You might use the quiz as an oral exercise, which will lead into a class discussion of the topics covered. Or, you might use it as a paper/pencil quiz to evaluate your students individually.

1. Alcohol is not an addictive substance. (False)
2. There are both economic and emotional consequences to alcohol addiction. (True)
3. Society as a whole suffers the consequences of alcohol addiction. (True)
4. Family members should do everything they can to enable an alcoholic to escape

SECTION 5

How to Refuse Drinks, How to Give a Great Party

Delicious food and good company mean great fun.

The only way to be completely protected against alcohol addiction is not to drink at all. The choice is personal. Those who choose not to drink have every right to make that choice. It is no one else's business. It is perfectly OK to say, "I don't drink because I don't want to drink."

Unfortunately, some social groups give people a hard time for refusing to drink, because drinking is a shared experience. Two useful pointers for the non-drinker are:

▶ Don't apologize.
▶ Expect others to respect your choice.

The Health Strategies section on this page, "How to Give a Great Party without Alcohol," offers suggestions.

 KEY POINTS *Each person has the right to choose not to drink. Expect others to respect your choice. Alcohol is not required to have fun.*

Health Strategies

How to Give a Great Party without Alcohol

To give a great party:

1. Make it known that this is to be a party with no alcohol.
2. Offer interesting nonalcoholic beverages, such as punch.
3. Provide plenty of food and snacks—make-it-yourself sandwiches can be fun.
4. Remember, if anyone is disappointed, that's a reflection on their drinking problem, not on your hospitality.
5. Keep the music low. Loud music makes people anxious.
6. Arrange activities, such as badminton or swimming, as the focus. Or provide a dress theme (such as entertainment or sports celebrities). Or plan games.
7. Get your guests involved—ask them to bring musical instruments or their favorite music tapes or compact discs.

SECTION 5

FOCUS

OUTCOME

In this section students will learn:

1. Skills for giving and participating in a successful nonalcoholic party.

FOCUS ACTIVITY

Have students brainstorm things that are usually done at parties they attend. List their ideas on the board and discuss.

TEACH & APPLY

GROUP ACTIVITY

Divide students into three groups, with equal numbers of males and females in each group. Ask them to draw a line down the middle of a sheet of paper. On one side, they are to list all the things that could be done to have fun at a drug-free (alcohol-free) party. On the other side they are to list the things nondrinkers need to remember or can do if criticized or pressured by drinkers. Once they have developed a list they can all agree on, give each group two pieces of poster board. Ask the groups to use markers to transfer their lists onto the poster pieces. Display the posters on the wall.

from the consequences of his drinking. (False)

5. A family member who enables an alcoholic is called a codependent. (True)

6. Al-Anon and Alateen are support groups for people who have been involved with alcoholics. (True)

7. Part of helping an alcoholic is telling that person how their drinking makes you feel. (True)

8. You should try to become heavily involved in your friends' drinking problems, and not worrying about what their drinking is doing to you. (False)

9. Denial is a very early stage of the recovery process, often followed by bargaining, anger, and guilt. (True)

10. Being "dry" is another term for being sober. (False)

ASSESS

EVALUATE

Review Answers

1. not to drink at all (p. 363)
2. don't apologize, expect others to respect your choice (p. 363)
3. Answers will vary; could include mentioning contacting Al-Anon or Alateen.

A reproducible quiz for Section 5 is provided in the Teacher's Resource Box.

CLOSE

Before going to the next chapter, students should know:

1. No amount of alcohol is legal for people younger than the legal drinking age.

2. That for adults drinking within the acceptable limits of the law or abstinence is a personal choice.

3. They should expect others to respect their choice of abstinence.

Reproducible Study Outline and Reading Close worksheets for Chapter 13 are provided in the Teacher's Resource Box.

Reproducible Chapter Tests A and B are also provided in the Teacher's Resource Box.

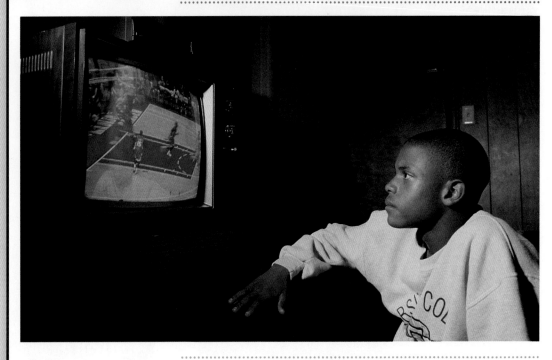

Family members and friends of alcohol abusers should enjoy their own lives as best they can.

Answers to FACT or FICTION

Here are the answers to the questions at the start of the chapter.

1. **True.**
2. **True.**
3. **False.** Alcohol is not digested. It is immediately absorbed into the blood.
4. **True.**
5. **False.** Driving is impaired at blood alcohol levels lower than 0.08 percent.
6. **False.** Muscles do not use alcohol for fuel, so walking does not affect the body's rate of alcohol breakdown.
7. **False.** Coffee can wake up, but not sober up, a person who is drunk.

Review

Answer the following questions on a sheet of paper.

Learning the Facts

1. What is the only way to be completely protected against alcohol addiction?
2. Name two useful pointers for a nondrinker.

Making Life Choices

3. Your best friend's parents are addicted to alcohol. Your friend has come to you many times about this problem. You have told her several times to go to the counselor at your school. You want to go to her parents and talk to them, but you don't really know what to say. What would you do in this situation? How can you help your friend? How would you feel if you had a similar problem? Would your responses be different?

CRITICAL THINKING

Have students role play a party at which drinks are served, after they have read Section 5. Select one person to be the "host;" then pass out slips of paper to the rest of the class, the "guests," telling them whether to accept drinks enthusiastically (most should do this) or refuse (a few should be selected to do so). The host passes a tray of glasses (pretend cocktails). Host and guests then pressure the

Straight Talk

Alcoholism, the Disease

Alcoholism is one of the nation's most serious health problems. About two thirds of all U.S. adults drink. Of these, about one in every ten is addicted to alcohol. The annual cost to the nation, including work time lost to alcohol abuse, is estimated in the tens of billions of dollars. Worse still, the rate of alcoholism is on the rise.

 I know people who drink alcohol, but I don't think I know anyone who is addicted to it.

If you know ten people who drink, chances are that at least one of them is addicted to alcohol or is on the road to addiction. Teenagers have an even higher rate of alcoholism than do adults, and they slide more quickly into addiction. One in every five teenagers who drink (aged 14 to 17) is already becoming dependent on alcohol.

 I know more than ten people who drink, but not one has the reputation of being addicted.

Many people would rather not see the problem of alcohol addiction. In fact, people can choose not to see it. They can convince themselves that it doesn't exist, or that it is a minor problem. Such blindness is even found in hospitals. Physicians may list on patients' records many alcohol-related illnesses, such as liver disease, but never suggest the possibility of alcoholism. Yet anywhere from 33 to 95 percent of all patients may be in hospitals because of alcohol-related illnesses—including diseases of every body organ, broken bones, and emotional problems. Any of these disorders may be due to other causes, but alcoholism is often a contributor.

Whenever the problem underlying any of these diagnoses is alcoholism, this has to be dealt with first. To deal with alcoholism, we have to acknowledge it and face it. Denial blocks recovery.

 Isn't alcoholism easy to recognize? Isn't it drunkenness?

No, to be drunk is not the same thing as to be a person with alcoholism. Anybody can get drunk, simply by drinking too much alcohol. However, that does not necessarily reflect alcoholism. (It may, but you would have to look at other factors to identify the disease. The key factors are listed in Figure 13–6 on the next page.)

Many misconceptions attached to the term *alcoholism* need to be corrected. For example, alcoholism is not related to the kind of beverage drunk. Even wine coolers and beer can produce it. Nor is alcoholism tied to a particular age. As mentioned, even teenagers can develop it. It is not always obvious. It is easy to hide, even in its advanced stages. People have been amazed to learn that a good friend, whom they thought they knew well, had reached a late stage of alcoholism before they found out about it. The addiction had been developing for years, but friends had no clues.

 You have told me what alcoholism is not. Now, please tell me what it is.

The American Medical Association (AMA), the American Psychiatric Association (APA), and other authorities define alcoholism as a disease of dependence on alcohol. It is chronic (long-lasting), progressive (gets worse over time), and potentially fatal. It often involves tolerance, physical addiction, and organ damage caused by alcohol.

365

refusers in various ways to go ahead and accept an alcoholic drink while refusers practice their assertiveness skills. Afterwards have the refusers describe their feelings about the experience, telling what was most difficult for them and why. Have the drinkers describe

their feelings about why it was important that the nondrinkers accept a drink and how it felt to pressure them into drinking.

BACKGROUND INFORMATION

Write down the following question on the board or overhead, then ask for volunteers to give the correct answers. "John and Sue each have had four drinks tonight. What will determine how they react to these four drinks?" Make sure students consider the following:

1. *Time:* How fast did each one drink? If John drank four drinks in one hour, and Sue drank four drinks in four hours, John will have a more severe reaction.

2. *Tolerance:* If John is used to drinking and Sue has never had a drink, then Sue will have a more severe reaction because her body has not developed tolerance to the drug.

3. *Body weight and size:* If John is 170 lbs. and Sue is 115 lbs., Sue will have the higher blood alcohol content level because she has less blood. A smaller person has less blood, and less blood causes a higher blood alcohol concentration.

4. *Gender:* Besides the fact that women often weigh less than men, their bodies do not produce a certain stomach enzyme that further breaks down alcohol that men produce.

5. *Food in the stomach:* If there is no food in the stomach, the effect will be quicker and stronger.

6. *Concentration of the drink:* Was it four shots of whiskey or four 12-oz. beers? The four shots of whiskey will give a more severe effect because there is less fluid to interfere (dilute) with absorption of the alcohol into the bloodstream.

(continued on next page)

7. *Mental disposition:* If the person is depressed to begin with, the alcohol will exaggerate the depression. If the person is anticipating getting drunk, the person will get "drunk" more quickly.

8. *Setting:* Where the person is and with whom will affect the person's reaction to alcohol. (school, home alone, at a party with friends, at a party with strangers)

DISCUSSION

Put the following on the board—one underneath the other:

1. D&D
2. D
3. D
4. DD

Start the activity by saying, "Okay, we've been talking about alcohol. Tell me what these "Ds" are about." Someone will eventually come up with Drinking and Driving for #1. Ask the students what they know about drinking and driving. Then ask them how many of them have ever ridden in a car with a driver under the influence (more than two drinks in two hours). Ask them why they did it. The reason is the second "D"— Denial. We really don't think anything will happen to us and drunk drivers definitely deny they are drunk. So, #1 D&D plus #2 D, equals #3 D—Death. People drink, they drive, they deny, and they die or cause other people's deaths. What is #4, DD? It is one prevention all drivers can agree on— Designated Drivers.

Alcoholism, the Disease (continued)

The path of worsening symptoms is well known. Alcoholism progresses from the first drink, usually in the teen years, to more involvement with alcohol. It goes on to a point where alcohol comes to dominate the person's life, damaging family ties and friendships, work life, and physical health. Alcoholism at its worst typically takes from three to ten years to develop after heavy drinking has begun. For young abusers, less time is required. Some teenagers are clearly already addicted to alcohol.

How is alcoholism identified?

Usually, the person with the problem identifies it by taking a quiz such as the one in this chapter's Life Choice Inventory. The person answers yes to three or more questions and faces the result squarely. This is

> **The presence of three or more of these conditions is required to make a diagnosis of alcoholism:**
>
> Loss of control over drinking. The person intends to have a drink or two but has 9 or 10, or the person tries to quit drinking but fails.
>
> Continued drinking despite medical, psychological, family, employment, or work problems.
>
> A great deal of time spent in obtaining and drinking alcohol, or in recovering from drinking.
>
> Increasing alcohol tolerance. The person needs higher and higher intakes of alcohol to achieve intoxication.
>
> Withdrawal symptoms. The person who stops drinking experiences anxiety, agitation, increased blood pressure, or seizures.

Figure 13–6 Key Signs of Alcoholism

important to understand, because people with alcoholism try to deny the problem exists. Someone else may see that a person has a problem with alcoholism. However, until the person has accepted that fact, nothing can be done.

What sorts of people suffer from alcoholism?

Just as people with diabetes or cancer come in all sizes, shapes, and varieties, so do people with alcoholism. The disease does not respect income, education, social class, or physical attractiveness. The person you most admire is just as likely to be addicted to alcohol as the person you most dislike. All people may be susceptible to alcoholism, but some people's genetic inheritance makes addiction especially likely if they begin drinking alcohol. This means that if one or more of your close relatives has alcoholism, you may have inherited a tendency toward developing it.

It is useful to separate the *person* from the *condition.* Think of the person as worthwhile, even though you disapprove of what the person *does.* Use words that show this attitude. Speak of "the person with alcoholism," not of "the alcoholic." After all, if treatment is successful, the person will recover (that is, the person will become a person without active alcoholism).

It is probably not correct to think alcoholism can be cured. However, the disease is treatable, and it can be arrested, as long as the person steers clear of alcohol. The person is not "an alcoholic" any more than the person with cancer is "a canceric."

How can I tell whether someone I know is becoming addicted to alcohol?

A telling event on the way to alcoholism is the occurrence of **blackouts**—episodes of **amnesia**. Some authorities say that blackouts are the single most notable sign to warn of alcoholism. This statement is open to question, but blackouts are certainly common in people with alcoholism.

366

enrichment

You may want to tell students that some researchers have observed that drinking makes people feel good as long as the blood alcohol remains at a level of about 0.05. In

this range people feel relaxed, euphoric, and sociable. At higher levels, they go from moderately intoxicated to thoroughly drunk. A 140-pound person could consume only 1¼ drinks per hour and still maintain the blood alcohol level of .05 or lower, with one drink equaling 12 ozs. of beer, 4 ozs. of wine,

A friend of my brother's drank so much that he passed out. Was that a blackout?

No. In fact, blacking out bears no resemblance to passing out. A person who has had too much to drink may pass out—that just means losing consciousness. A person having a blackout, on the other hand, may show no outward signs of it at all. The person acts normal, although drinking. The next day, however, the person is unable to remember anything that happened beyond a certain time.

An example may help make this clear. Judy eats dinner with her family and then sits down at the sewing machine with a drink by her side, to make a dress. She finishes the first drink, goes and gets a second one, and continues making the dress. Several hours later she has had five drinks, has finished the dress, has ironed it and hung it up in the closet, has put away her sewing machine, and has gone to bed. The following morning she remembers nothing beyond the time when she started to sew. To see what she has done, she has to go back and look around. She finds the completed dress in the closet and a half-empty bottle in the cabinet.

As you can see, a person's behavior can be completely normal during a blackout. Of course, some terrible thing may happen instead. Rather than simply having completed a dress, Judy might have taken the car, gone out to buy another bottle, and killed someone on the way. The following morning, as before, she would have awakened completely unaware of what had happened the evening before. A dent and some blood on the front of her car might have been her first clues to what went on.

Blackouts often mark a turning point for people on their way to alcoholism, because blackouts are scary. Realizing that their lives are out of control, people come to recognize their condition. The disease of alcoholism can progress far beyond blackouts, but people can stop drinking at any time along the way. The beginning of blackouts is one excellent place to stop.

Glossary

blackouts: episodes of amnesia regarding periods of time while drinking. The person may act normal during a blackout, but later be unable to recall anything about it. Blackouts are likely to occur in the life of a person with alcoholism.

amnesia: loss of memory.

367

2½ ozs. of brandy, or 1¼ ozs. of 80 proof liquor.

As enrichment you may want to explain to students why failure to eat prior to drinking can increase the effects of alcohol. Enzymes in the liver that metabolize alcohol are made of protein, and like all body protein, they break down when a person fails to eat. Fasting for as little as one day can reduce the rate of alcohol metabolism by half. Therefore, drinking on an empty stomach not only lets the drinker feel the effects more promptly but also raises the blood alcohol level higher for longer times and anesthetizes the brain more profoundly.

VOCABULARY

1. a. DUI **b.** sober **c.** tremors **d.** blackout **e.** codependent **f.** alcohol **g.** proof **h.** enable **i.** amnesia

2. a. formaldehyde **b.** denial

3. a. Ethanol is the alcohol in alcoholic beverages, while congeners are ingredients other than alcohol that may irritate the nervous system. **b.** Moderation is an amount of alcohol that causes no harm to health, family, and social functioning, while alcoholism is a loss of control over drinking that harms health, family relations, and social and work functioning. Moderation means a person has control over alcohol. Alcoholism means that alcohol has control over the person.

RECALL

SECTION 1

1. alcohol (ethanol) (p. 343)

2. to celebrate, to unwind, they like the taste of alcoholic beverages, it is the custom (p. 344)

3. Answers will vary. Refer to Figure 13–2 on page 346 for possible answers.

4. Answers will vary. Refer to Figure 13–2 on page 346 for possible answers.

SECTION 2

5. brain, muscles, nerves, glands, the small blood vessels of the skin, the liver (p. 350)

6. one drink an hour (p. 350)

7. Alcohol relaxes the nerves of the blood vessels of the

Summarizing the Chapter

Your ability to respond correctly to the following statements ensures your understanding of the main concepts in the chapter.

1. List three reasons why young people start to drink alcohol.

2. Explain what alcohol is and how it affects the body.

3. Identify the immediate effects of intoxication.

4. Discuss what is meant by fetal alcohol syndrome.

5. Describe the effects of drinking on driving.

6. Explain why alcoholism is a family disease.

7. Identify how an enabler's behavior affects the person with whom alcohol is a problem.

8. List what kinds of help are available to the alcohol-dependent person.

Learning the Vocabulary

alcohol	fetal alcohol syndrome
ethanol (ethyl alcohol)	(FAS)
proof	DWI
alcoholism	DUI
moderation	breathalyzer test
drink	sober
intoxication	enable
delirium	codependent
tremors	denial
congeners	blackouts
formaldehyde	amnesia

Answer the following questions on a separate sheet of paper.

1. *Matching*—Match each of the following phrases with the appropriate vocabulary term:
a. driving under the influence of alcohol
b. free of alcohol's effects and of addiction
c. continuous quivering or shaking
d. temporary amnesia linked to alcohol abuse
e. an enabler who is a member of the family of a person addicted to a drug
f. a class of chemical compounds
g. term used to describe the percentage of alcohol in alcoholic beverages
h. make possible; in addiction, to "help"
i. a loss of memory

2. a. _____ is a substance made by the body from alcohol, and it contributes to hangovers.
b. Refusal to believe the facts of a circumstance is called _____.

3. Explain the relationships between:
a. congeners and ethanol
b. moderation and alcoholism

Recalling Important Facts and Ideas

Section 1

1. What is the most widely used and abused drug in our society?

2. List four reasons that drinkers give as to why they drink alcohol.

3. List five behaviors that are typical of moderate drinkers.

4. List five behaviors that are typical of problem drinkers.

Section 2

5. Within minutes after the first sip of a drink, ethanol is affecting what body parts?

6. How much alcohol can the liver handle?

7. Explain why people think alcohol warms them up when they drink it.

8. What happens to a person who has drunk enough to affect the judgment centers of the brain?

9. Describe what happens when the conscious brain is completely depressed.

10. How does the body protect itself from toxins?

11. What are three symptoms of a hangover?

12. What are the effects of liver damage on the body?

13. Excessive drinking over many years can cause severe and permanent brain damage. What are three things most affected by this type of brain damage?

14. Identify and describe five other long-term effects of alcohol abuse.

Section 3

15. How long does it take for someone who has passed out from an alcohol overdose to sober up?

skin. These widen, making the drinker appear flushed and feel warm. (p. 350)

8. The drinker loses certain kinds of awareness. The brain's speech and vision centers are being put to sleep. People may act against their own desires and wishes, may pick a fight, may become sexually aggressive, and may attempt a dangerous physical exploit. (p. 351)

9. The person passes out. (p. 352)

10. The throat stings and triggers the choking reflex. The stomach rejects too large a dose and causes the drinker to vomit. Finally, the body breaks down any alcohol that does not get into the blood as quickly as possible. (p. 352)

11. headache pain, unpleasant sensations in the mouth, nausea (p. 352)

12. The whole body suffers. One of the worst effects is high blood pressure, which can

Section 4

16. Describe how alcoholism costs society colossal amounts of money.

17. List the seven strategies to keep from being an enabler.

18. What are the five emotional stages someone has to go through in giving up a drug?

Section 5

19. List three strategies for giving a great party without alcohol.

Straight Talk

20. List at least three misconceptions about alcoholism.

21. Alcoholism at its worst typically takes how many years to develop?

Critical Thinking

1. Movies and other entertainment media often show an intoxicated person as a funny individual having a great time. But, is this the way it really is? Do all who drink become hilariously funny, agreeable, and friendly? What can be done to change this image?

2. After reading the Straight Talk section, "Alcoholism, the Disease," why do you think so many people who are aware of the dangers of alcohol still drink? Why is it that so many people fall victim to alcoholism? How long does it take to become addicted to alcohol? Which group of people are most likely to become addicted to alcohol? What is a sure-fire sign of alcoholism? What did you learn from reading this Straight Talk section?

Activities

1. Write a report profiling a candidate for alcoholism. Include a description of the person's personality and family background.

2. Interview a local law enforcement official about the problems associated with teenage drinking. What are the problems? Has raising the legal drinking age to 21 helped alleviate the problems? What does the official think will help stop teens from drinking?

3. Attend a local Alcoholics Anonymous meeting. What happened at the meeting? What are the goals of the people who attend the meetings?

4. Write a radio announcement to convince the public not to drink and drive.

5. Identify different groups at school or in the community that encourage responsible drinking behavior. A few examples might be Students Against Driving Drunk (SADD), a safe-ride program, and Mothers Against Drunk Drivers (MADD). Call these local agencies and make a poster showing each one's name, address, phone number, and hours of operation. Display these posters around the school.

6. Plan an alcohol-free party. Give the party a clever name. Plan healthful activities and a healthful menu. Design an invitation on a sheet of poster board. Discuss the party you have planned with your class.

7. On a sheet of paper, draw a stick figure or outline figure of the human body. Reread Section 2, Effects of Alcohol. To the side of your drawing, list the effects alcohol has on the body and draw a line to the part of the body affected. For example, for the head, you might write "Loss of awareness and judgment." For the throat, you might write "Stinging, choking reflex." For the pancreas, you might write "Stops producing insulin." Be sure to include both short-term and long-term effects. You might want to make your drawing into a poster to hang in your classroom or somewhere else in your school. You might ask about giving the poster to a class of elementary students.

Making Decisions about Health

1. Randy and Colleen are both college seniors. Randy is taking Colleen to a dance in his new car. Randy's friends are drinking at a party before the dance. Randy and Colleen decide to drink with them. Randy drinks four beers in one hour and Colleen drinks one glass of champagne.

Randy and Colleen go to the dance for two hours and then go to another party, where they drink and dance for about two hours. Randy has six more beers and Colleen has two more drinks. It is getting late and Colleen is nervous because Randy has drunk too much to drive. Colleen is from out of state and doesn't have a current driver's license.

a. What advice would you give Colleen?

b. How should Colleen get home?

c. What should Randy do?

SECTION 4

16. People addicted to alcohol require more hospitalization, placing a burden on insurance companies; cause avoidable accidents and injuries; commit crimes; require the services of police, ambulances, courts, prisons, lawyers, and rehabilitation centers. (p. 359)

17. stay concerned; be prompt; speak about the behavior, but do not attack the person; be specific—name and describe behaviors—don't judge; act as a mirror—tell what you see; don't try to smooth things over; when you are angry, cool off before you talk to the person (p. 360)

18. denial, bargaining, anger, guilt, acceptance (p. 361)

SECTION 5

19. Answers will vary. Refer to the Health Strategies on page 363.

STRAIGHT TALK

20. alcoholism is not related to the kind of beverage drunk—even wine coolers and beer can produce alcoholism; alcoholism is not tied to a certain age—even teenagers can be alcoholics; and it is easy to hide. (p. 365)

21. three to ten years (p. 366)

---

lead to heart attacks and strokes. Liver damage also weakens the body's defenses against infection. (pp. 353–354)

13. vision, memory, learning ability, and other functions (p. 354)

14. Answers will vary; could include: ulcers of stomach and intestines; shrinking of all the body's muscles, including the heart muscle; abnormal changes in the blood; kidney damage; bladder damage; gland damage; skin rashes and sores; shrinkage and damage of the testicles; failure of the ovaries and menstrual problems in women; lung damage leading to flu, pneumonia, tuberculosis; and psychological depression and mental illness. (p. 354)

SECTION 3

15. 24 hours (p. 358)

KEY POINTS

Chapter 14 is 28 pages long and is divided into five sections. This chapter addresses a major health problem in our society, the use of tobacco. The chapter explains why people continue to smoke, even though they may be well informed of the dangers that accompany their bad habit. This chapter then gives specific details about how smoking affects the smoker's and non-smoker's health. The effects of smokeless tobacco are also discussed in this chapter. The last section explains why and how a person should quit smoking. The chapter focuses on tobacco as a problem of our society, and states that it should be addressed on a personal level.

ACTIVITY TO INTRODUCE THE CHAPTER

In order to get students thinking about how their life choices and behaviors affect their lives, ask them to write a paragraph describing how they plan to spend the last 20 years of their lives, or how they would like to live after they retire. After they have completed this part of the assignment, ask them to turn their papers over and write how smoking would affect their retirement plans. Remind them that smoking may cut as many as 18 years from their lives. They now have two years of retirement to write about. This will help students realize how devastating the smoking habit can be to them and their plans.

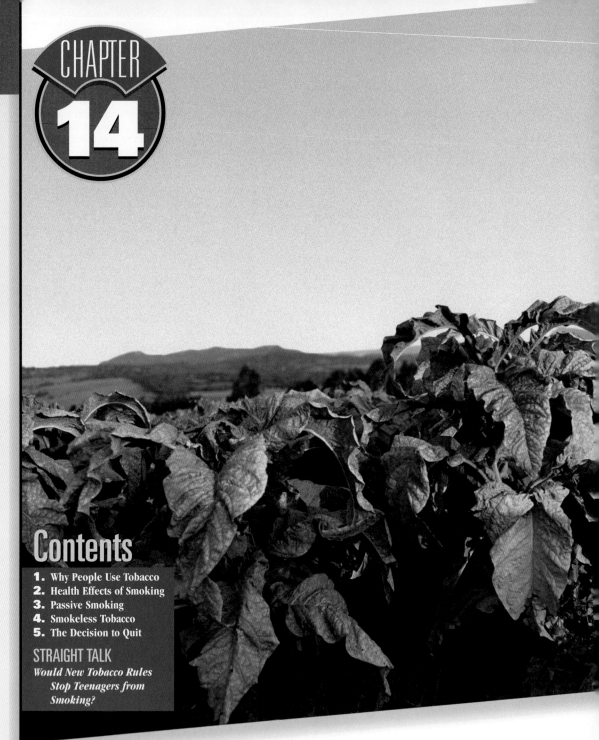

CHAPTER 14

Contents

STRAIGHT TALK
Would New Tobacco Rules Stop Teenagers from Smoking?

NOT Enough Time?

Following are some suggestions to help you make sure that you cover the key topics in this chapter if you have limited time. (Refer to the daily lesson plans in your Teacher's Resource Box for additional suggestions.)

DAY 1   Assign students to read the chapter prior to class. Ask students to answer the Section 2 Review questions on page 383 and the Section 3 Review questions on page 385. Next, assign the Section 4 Review questions

Tobacco

BULLETIN BOARD IDEAS

Recreate the table in Figure 14–3 on page 380 on the bulletin board. You might also want to show pictures of blackened lungs, people on oxygen, and other effects of tobacco on the human body. Contrast these with advertisements for cigarettes and smokeless tobacco.

What do you think? Are the following statements true or false? If you think they are false, then say what is true.

1. After someone has started smoking, enjoyment is the reason he or she continues to smoke.
2. One of nicotine's chief effects is to elicit the stress response.
3. A sign of nicotine withdrawal is an inability to concentrate.
4. Nicotine is not an addictive drug.
5. In emphysema, the lungs first become damaged not because people can't breathe in but because they can't breathe out.
6. Smoking wrinkles the skin.
7. To live with a smoker is to run the risk of contracting lung cancer.
8. One effective way to reduce the risk of getting cancer is to switch from smoking cigarettes to chewing tobacco or snuff.

(Answers on page 393)

Introduction

Without a doubt, tobacco offers something people seek. Otherwise they wouldn't use it, because, as nearly everyone knows, many health hazards accompany tobacco use. This chapter begins with the question of why people use tobacco. It then goes on to look at the health effects of smoking and smokeless tobacco. The last section tells how to quit using tobacco and how to help the quitter. It tries to present all the facts—both for and against—with honesty. The health evidence, though, is one-sided—against.

Answers to FACT or FICTION

1. **False.** The main reason for continuing to smoke is addiction to nicotine.
2. **True.**
3. **True.**
4. **False.** Nicotine is a highly addictive drug.
5. **True.**
6. **True.**
7. **True.**
8. **False.** The risks of cancer of the mouth and throat are greater for people using smokeless tobacco products than for smokers.

BACKGROUND INFORMATION

Tell students that according to the Office of Smoking and Health, Federal Centers for Disease Control, that 41.2 percent of white high school students, 32 percent of Hispanic students, and 16.8 percent of African-American students smoke or use other tobacco products.

on page 387. After students have completed the section review questions, go over their answers aloud. If reteaching activities are needed, choose some of the activities that are provided, such as the Comprehension Check on page 379, the Evaluate assessment on page 385, and the Close activity on page 387.

DAY 2 On Day 2, assign students to answer the Sections 1 and 5 Review questions on pages 376 and 393. The Quick Quiz on page 376 and the Role Play activity on page 391 will provide additional reinforcement for these sections.

SECTION 1

FOCUS

OUTCOMES

In this section students will learn that the following are causes of people using tobacco despite knowing there are problems associated with its use on a regular basis:

1. Advertising strategies aimed at a young impressionable public.
2. Physical addiction to nicotine.
3. Using tobacco to avoid nicotine withdrawal.
4. Psychological dependency on the smoking habit and the mannerisms that accompany it.

FOCUS ACTIVITY

Ask students to tell about a habit they have, such as biting their nails. Then ask the students to explain why they continue their habits, even though they may not be desirable. Explain to students that smoking is similar to these habits, only worse because of the addictive drug nicotine.

TEACH & APPLY

BACKGROUND INFORMATION

Ask students if it is possible that there are still people unaware of tobacco's drawbacks. Do students know any such people? Tell students that one poll showed that 13 to 17 percent of smokers did not know that cigarette smoking is hazardous at

SECTION 1

Why People Use Tobacco

For many years, the tobacco industry has used highly effective role models in their advertisements. Ads suggested that tobacco users were handsome, macho cowboys; cool, sexy characters; or athletic, dynamic-looking women. These images were not realistic because smoking ruins people's health, but people didn't always see through them.

Cigarette company ads deliver double messages. They are required to say that smoking harms health, but they show healthy people smoking.

Teenagers and Tobacco Advertising

The tobacco companies address young people directly, because they must attract children and young teenagers in order to replace the more than 2 million adult smokers who die each year worldwide from lung cancer and other smoking-related illnesses. The industry knows that a person who doesn't become a smoker during the teen years is most unlikely to take up the habit later on. Eighty-two percent of adults with a history of smoking took their first cigarette before age 18.

Statistics on smoking are disturbing. Each day, 5,000 children light up for the first time—some of them only seven or eight years old, in a hurry to grow up. About one in five high school seniors smokes regularly. More than 3,000 teenagers become regular smokers each day. The surgeon general warns that if the current rate of tobacco use by young people continues, 5 million of today's children will die of smoking-related illnesses in their later years.

A folder written by young people for young people describes how smokers try to explain their choice to smoke:

▶ I'm young now. I can quit later.
▶ I don't inhale. Smoking can't hurt me.
▶ Smoking makes me look grown-up.
▶ I smoke filter cigarettes. Filters protect me.
▶ My parents (friends) smoke. Why shouldn't I?
▶ If I don't spend the money on cigarettes, I'll spend it on something else.
▶ It keeps me from biting my nails, putting on weight, or being mad or bored or hurt or unhappy.

Advertising works both ways: Tobacco ads promote smoking; ads like this one promote healthy behaviors instead.

HEALTHY PEOPLE 2000

Tobacco

Tobacco use is the most important single preventable cause of death in the United States, accounting for one of every six deaths, or some 390,000 deaths annually. It is a major risk factor for diseases of the heart and blood vessels; chronic bronchitis and emphysema; cancers of the lung, larynx, pharynx, oral cavity, esophagus, pancreas, and bladder; and other problems such as respiratory infections and stomach ulcers. Cigarette smoking is responsible for an estimated 21 percent of all coronary heart disease deaths (40 percent of those under age 65), 30 percent of all cancer deaths, and 87 percent of lung cancer deaths

All of these reasons are unrealistic. However, the new smoker believes them.

 Tobacco advertising has prompted millions of teenagers and children to start smoking. Overwhelmingly, adults who smoke started before age 18. People begin using tobacco for a variety of reasons: influence of advertisements, peer pressure, or boredom.

Nicotine Addiction

A person whose mind is open to using tobacco begins by trying it once. That one time may be followed by another. In a short while, using tobacco is no longer a free-will choice, because tobacco's active ingredient, **nicotine**, is a powerfully addictive drug.

The first use of tobacco is, to most people, a sickening experience. Chewing tobacco in the mouth tastes unpleasant. The body reacts to inhaled smoke as to any smoke—by coughing to expel the irritating substance.

If this were all there were to it, no one would get hooked. Why, then, do people keep on using tobacco? Users keep coming back for more, mainly for the drug nicotine, to which they have become addicted. The addiction is so strong that when users suddenly can't get their form of tobacco, they helplessly switch to other forms—from cigarettes to a pipe, pipe to chewing, chewing to smoking.

A memo revealed during a lawsuit against a tobacco company described cigarettes this way: "The cigarette should be conceived not as a product but as a package. The product is nicotine. . . . Smoke is beyond question the [best] vehicle of nicotine and the cigarette the [best] dispenser of smoke." The memo revealed that tobacco companies were aware of their product's addictive nature.

The director of the FDA has called the tobacco use among young people "an epidemic of addiction that has enormous consequences for public health." He goes on to say that every year in the United States, "smoking kills more people than AIDS, car accidents, alcohol, homicides, illegal drugs, suicides, and fires *combined*." In addition to loss of life, medical treatments for smoking-related illnesses cost this nation $50 billion each year.

 All people who continue to use tobacco do so because they are addicted to the drug nicotine. Smoking causes enormous losses.

Nicotine's Other Effects

Nicotine has many effects on the body. It affects the body's major organ systems: the nervous and hormonal systems, the cardiovascular system, and the digestive system. It triggers the release of stress hormones, so it speeds up the heart rate and raises the blood pressure. It changes the brainwave pattern. It calms the nerves, but some people may feel stimulated. It reduces anxiety, reduces feelings of pain, helps the person concentrate, dulls the taste buds, and reduces hunger. Nicotine acts on many different brain centers, so

in the United States. The risk of dying from lung cancer is 22 times higher for men and 12 times higher for women who smoke than for lifetime nonsmokers. Passive or involuntary smoking causes lung cancer and other diseases in healthy nonsmokers and severe respiratory problems in children. Middle ear infections in children have been linked to passive smoking.

Among youth, more than half of 8th graders and nearly two-thirds of 10th graders report having tried cigarettes. More than one-fourth of 10th graders report having smoked a cigarette during the preceding month and nearly one in five reports smoking a pack or more in the previous month.

MINI Glossary

nicotine (NICK-oh-teen): an addictive drug present in tobacco.

all. A survey of more than 15,000 high school seniors revealed that nearly 50 percent did not perceive any great risk associated with smoking. Nearly half of all teenagers are unaware that nicotine is an addictive drug.

INTERDISCIPLINARY ACTIVITY: WRITING

Ask students to write about the statistic, from the following list provided by the American Cancer Society, that has the most impact on them. Make sure they explain their choices.

- Smoking is the #1 preventable cause of death in the nation.
- Every 13 seconds, someone dies from a tobacco-related illness.
- Cigarette smoking is responsible for one out of every five American deaths.
- More people die from tobacco-related illnesses than from alcohol, traffic accidents, illicit drugs, murder, and suicide.
- 85 percent of teenagers who smoke two or more cigarettes, and overcome the initial discomfort, will become addicted smokers.
- Nicotine is a deadly poison, which if taken in high doses, can kill.

DISCUSSION

Tell students to reread the sentence that says 82 percent of adult smokers began smoking before the age of 18. What does this say about the effectiveness of the cigarette ad campaigns targeted toward teenagers? Do students think any of the new advertising regulations will make a difference in the number of teens who start smoking? Will taking Joe Camel off billboards really make a difference? If so, how? If not, why not?

Teen Views

Following are some questions you may want to use to encourage discussion of the ideas expressed by the students in the Teen Views feature:

1. Ask students if they are influenced by famous athletes, musicians, and other well-known personalities. Would seeing a member of their favorite band smoking cigarettes increase the chances that they might try smoking?

2. Is curiosity more of a factor than peer pressure in causing people to try smoking?

3. Do students believe that they can become hooked by smoking just one cigarette? If not, how many does it take?

4. Do students believe that smoking increases a person's sex appeal? Why or why not?

FAST FACTS

Smoking kills more Americans *each year* than died in battle during World War II and the Vietnam War put together. *Every day* more than 1,200 Americans die from smoking-related causes, the equivalent of three or four fully loaded jumbo jets crashing with no survivors.

Teen Views: Why Do So Many Teens Think Smoking Is Cool?

Well, being a smoker I don't smoke to show off to my friends or to look older or look cool. I do it to relieve my stress because I have a lot of it. And that is the one way that helps me most. I can't count to ten and feel better or I can't get stoned or drunk and feel better when it wears off. Smoking helps me most out of the different cures for stress. I also smoke to keep my weight off. I like to eat fatty foods too much to go on a diet, so I also smoke to stay the size I am.
Jennifer Lusk, 15,
Manzano High School, NM

Many teens see in a lot of movies that the hero of the story is smoking; cigarettes to calm down when they are nervous, cigars when they reached a goal. Kids may think that if you want to be like this person, you have to smoke.

In other situations one may see older students smoke at school or in other places. They want to be like they are. But to reach that goal, do you have to smoke? The answer is no. If your friends start smoking, do you have to start it, too? No. Nobody may tell you what you have to do or not. If one has a strong self-concept, one knows by himself that it is

not necessary to copy others to improve himself. If one's self-concept is not that strong, one can prove it by saying no to it.

The movie stars may have it in their script that in this scene a little smoke is needed and they really hate smoking themselves. The last words of the man who played the happy Marlboro cowboy for years were that mankind should be informed about the danger of smoking and what may happen. He died of cancer, caused by his smoking in those cool commercials.
Joerg C. Stephan, 17,
Billings West High School, MT

I don't smoke, but some of my best friends do. They tell me that they were not pressured by their peers to start smoking. They started because they saw older teens smoking and thought, "Why not?" They thought it would make them more adult-like, and it was cool for them to do because they were not allowed. So, they tried it and got addicted. Some of them no longer think it is cool and a few of these are trying to quit.
Matthew Himrod, 17,
Wheeling Park High School, WV

For a lot of people smoking simply starts out as a small rebellion. They start smoking to prove that they, not their parents, are in control. The big problem is that

the more and more addicted the smoker becomes, the less and less control they have. Although I smoke myself, I think it's wrong and admire anyone who can successfully beat the habit.
Erika Karlsson, 17,
Orange Park High School, FL

Kids don't smoke because they think it's "cool." They do it because they tried it once and got hooked. Smoking is a waste of money, time, and energy. I choose not to smoke or do drugs because I want to live to be healthy. I have better things to do than waste all my money on something that can end up killing me.
Brenda Weiler, 15,
Fargo South High School, ND

I'm from Germany, and over there, smoking is very popular. It's not allowed, but everyone is doing it. If you talk to 100 people, 30 will say that they don't like to smoke, but they're doing it because it's "cool"! Fifty will say that they are doing it because if they don't do it, everybody will laugh at them. Ten might say they smoke because it is the only way they can relax and it tastes good. Finally, 10 might say that they feel like adults if they smoke. I can live a cool and healthy life without smoking.
Ralf Buyna, 15,
Wilson High School, CA

special needs

Linguistic

To help students understand why smoking is such a controversial issue, what the effects of smoking are on their health, and what the dangers are, to themselves and to others, you may want to stage a debate. The topic for the debate is: "Are the stricter rules recently imposed by the Food and Drug

Administration effective in stopping young people from smoking?"

To prepare for the debate, divide the class into two teams; one side will defend the "yes" position, and the other will defend the "no" position. Allow at least one week for students to research the issue. On the day of the debate, be sure to set time limits. Each side should have the same amount of time to present its position, and then each side should

Many people are quitting smoking successfully.

different people respond differently to it. As a result, the reasons why people use tobacco (other than addiction) differ.

The user of tobacco notices the pleasant effects of nicotine immediately. Even more noticeable, however, are the unpleasant effects of withdrawal as the dose wears off. Withdrawal is signaled by a slowed heart rate, lowered blood pressure, nausea, headache, irritability, restlessness, anxiety, drowsiness, inability to concentrate, and a craving for another dose.

Many users take the next dose of nicotine in order to avoid the letdown from the last one—a pattern that points to addiction. The addiction becomes so strong that they cannot quit even if they know that their health is suffering in the ways described in the next section.

Physical addiction is not the only reason people continue to use tobacco, although it is the most important reason. Psychological dependence also plays a role, because nicotine both brings pleasure and reduces pain. People enjoy the behavior itself. It provides an excuse, in a busy routine, to take a break and relax. Important, too, is that it provides an escape from small stresses. A person who is embarrassed or angry and doesn't know what to say can light up a cigarette. Many teenagers smoke to express their willingness to take risks, as the Consumer Skills feature on the next page points out. For these and many other reasons, people use tobacco, but they pay a tremendous price.

 KEY POINTS *Nicotine affects all the body's organs. It triggers release of the stress hormones; it reduces anxiety and feelings of pain; and it reduces hunger. The pleasant feelings of nicotine are followed by unpleasant ones as the drug wears off.*

best tip yet:

DON'T START!

AMERICAN CANCER SOCIETY

have an equal amount of time for rebuttal.

Possible sources of information may include: school library/media center, school nurse, teachers in the science department, public library, public health clinics, American Cancer Society, American Lung Association, the Tobacco Institute, and the Internet. Students may also wish to interview people who smoke or who have quit smoking.

Suggested points of argument:

1. Are the new laws tough enough to prevent young people from smoking?
2. Can or should the new laws be made tougher, or more restricting?
3. Should tobacco products be labeled as controlled substances?
4. Will higher tobacco product prices be a deterrent in stopping young people from ever starting to smoke?

BACKGROUND INFORMATION

Give students some more information about nicotine. When pure, it is a colorless, oily fluid with little odor but a sharp burning taste. Nicotine is one of the most toxic and addicting of all poisons. It acts as swiftly as cyanide. The fatal dose for an adult is estimated to be less than 5 milligrams per kilogram of body weight.

TEACHER SUPPORT

Key Passage

WORKSHEETS

You may want to distribute the handout from the Teacher's Resource Box entitled, "Smokers and Their Smoking Habits." This handout contains 17 questions that the students can use in interviewing smokers about their smoking habits. Be sure to discuss privacy and anonymity issues with students before assigning the survey.

Consumer SKILLS

Answers to Critical Thinking
(from page 376)

1. Their illegality, potential for addiction, and the damage they cause to health.
2. They may have "risk-taking" personalities.

ASSESS

EVALUATE

SECTION 1 **Review Answers**

1. Answers will vary.
2. more than 2 million (p. 372)
3. Answers will vary; could include: I'm young now; I don't inhale, smoking can't hurt me; I smoke filter cigarettes; my parents smoke; it keeps me from putting on weight; or being mad, bored, hurt, or unhappy, and so on (p. 372)
4. $50 billion (p. 373)
5. the nervous and hormonal systems, the cardiovascular system, and the digestive system. (p. 373)
6. Answers will vary.

A reproducible quiz for Section 1 is provided in the Teacher's Resource Box.

CLOSE

To show mastery of the information in the first section, students are to develop a plan for the following assignment. "The president just named you as the new Surgeon General. Your first assignment is to significantly lower the number of teenagers starting to smoke in America. What reasons that cause people to smoke do you attack first, and how?" After giving students time to draw up their plans, ask students to present short oral summaries of their plans to the class.

Tobacco as a Gateway Drug

Consumer SKILLS

Of all the harmful effects of tobacco, one stands out for some teenagers—tobacco is a **gateway drug**. This means that users of tobacco are much more likely than nonusers to eventually abuse other destructive substances, such as alcohol, cocaine, or heroin. In one state, Florida, children and teenagers who use tobacco products regularly are three times more likely to take cocaine, five times more likely to drink alcohol, and eight times more likely to smoke marijuana than those not using tobacco. Other states report similar findings.

Some people would like to argue that tobacco doesn't lead to anything except more tobacco use. They ridicule the gateway idea by saying that children drink sodas or even infant formula before they use tobacco, making these "gateways" as well. The truth is, for children and teenagers, tobacco, alcohol, and other drugs do not remotely resemble innocent products consumed by children. Instead, they resemble one another in terms of their illegality, their potential for addiction, and the damage they cause to health. A few people who use tobacco may never go on to other drugs, but most smokers are also drinkers, and many abuse other drugs as well.

Why do users of tobacco move on to other drugs? Some researchers believe that some teenagers may have "risk-taking" personalities. Such teens may be attracted to tobacco partly because of the danger it poses. Tobacco may be just the first in a series of risks that they will seek. Their risk-taking tendencies make them likely to commit crimes, cut classes, drive drunk, and have unprotected sexual intercourse, as well as to abuse substances.

Youngsters may get hoodwinked into thinking that smoking a few cigarettes each day won't harm them much. The trouble is, a few each day lead to a pack each day, and, for some, one illegal and risky behavior can lead to another.

Critical Thinking

1. *What characteristics do tobacco and other gateway drugs have in common?*
2. *Why might some teenagers who use tobacco move on to other drugs?*

SECTION 1 **Review**

Answer the following questions on a sheet of paper.

Learning the Vocabulary

The vocabulary terms in this section are *nicotine* and *gateway drug.*

1. Write a sentence using each of the vocabulary terms.

Learning the Facts

2. How many adults die each year from smoking-related diseases?

3. List five statements that describe how smokers try to explain their choice to smoke.
4. How much do medical treatments for smoking-related illnesses cost this nation each year?
5. Identify the major systems of the body that are affected by nicotine.

Making Life Choices

6. Make a list of the immediate effects nicotine has on the body. How might these affect health?

QUICK QUIZ

Chapter 14, Section 1

The following quiz will help you assess your students' understanding of the material covered in this section of the chapter. You might use the quiz as an oral exercise, which will lead into a class discussion of the topics covered. Or, you might use it as a paper/pencil quiz to evaluate your students individually.

Like the Quick Quiz, the Section Review can also be used as an assessment tool to spark class discussion or as an individual student evaluation. It can also be used as a review in preparation for this quiz.

1. Tobacco companies do not direct their advertisements to minors. (False)
2. The vast majority of nicotine addicts took their first cigarette before the age of 18. (True)

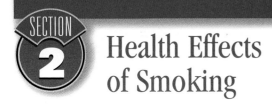

SECTION 2
Health Effects of Smoking

Anything being burned releases many chemicals not present in the original raw material. The damage people cause themselves by smoking is primarily from the *burning* ingredients of cigarettes.

What's In a Cigarette?

More than 4,000 hazardous compounds make their way into the lungs of smokers and into the air that everyone breathes. The most harmful of these are the **tars**, which are similar to the tars used on roads. These are well-known **carcinogens**, known to cause most cases of lung cancer and many cancers of other organs. Smokers who puff 20 to 60 cigarettes per day collect anywhere from ¼ to 1½ pounds of the sticky black tar in their lungs each year. Tars are also the principal cause of **emphysema**, another major disease of the lungs.

Many other ingredients in cigarettes also harm smokers. Cigarette makers select from over a thousand additives to enhance their products—flavoring agents, moistening agents, ammonia to release nicotine into the gases of smoke, agents to prevent cigarettes from going out once lighted, and others. Among the flavoring agents are cocoa, licorice, prune juice, and raisin juice. You might think these would be harmless. However, both cocoa and licorice, when burned, form carcinogens.

When people smoke, they inhale many harmful compounds. Naturally, the organ most affected by smoke is the lungs.

 KEY POINTS *More than 4,000 hazardous compounds make their way into the lungs of smokers and into the air that everyone breathes. Tars in cigarettes are the most harmful compounds.*

The Lungs

A detailed diagram of the lungs appeared in Chapter 6. Figure 14–1 on the next page serves as a reminder of the lung structures of concern here. The lungs receive blood pumped from the heart and add oxygen to it. Then the blood, with its oxygen cargo, returns to the heart to be pumped to all the body's cells. Every cell has to breathe. The lungs provide oxygen to the cells so they can stay alive.

Healthy Lungs   The lungs are huge, compared with the heart. They are rich with blood vessels, and they fill the chest. Twelve to fourteen times a minute they draw in air deeply and, like a sponge, soak up oxygen and squeeze out carbon dioxide.

Healthy **bronchi**, the major breathing tubes leading to each lung, are coated with slippery **mucus** and little waving hairs (**cilia**). The mucus catches dirt and bacteria that would otherwise lodge in the lungs. The cilia sweep the mucus in a constant stream, up to the windpipe (also lined with cilia) and then all the way up to the throat. When you clear your throat and

MINI Glossary

gateway drug: a drug whose abuse is likely to lead to abuse of other, more potent and dangerous drugs. Alcohol, marijuana, and tobacco are most often named as gateway drugs.

tars: chemicals present in (among other things) tobacco. Burning tars release many carcinogens.

carcinogens (car-SIN-oh-gens): cancer-causing agents.

emphysema (em-fih-ZEE-muh): a disease of the lungs in which many small, flexible air sacs burst and form a few large, rigid air pockets.

bronchi (BRONK-eye): the two main airways in the lungs; branches of the windpipe (trachea). The singular form is *bronchus*.

mucus (MYOO-cuss): a slippery secretion produced by cells of the body's linings that protects the surfaces of the linings.

cilia: hairlike structures extending from the surface of cells that line body passageways, including the trachea and upper lungs. The cilia wave, propelling a coating of mucus along to sweep away debris.

SECTION 2

FOCUS

OUTCOMES

In this section students will learn:

1. How smoking damages the human body.
2. How smoke affects the lungs, heart, and circulatory system.
3. Why smoking is the single greatest cause of preventable death in America today.

FOCUS ACTIVITY

Ask students to describe the physical appearance of people they know who have smoked for years. How many negative effects can they name? Also ask students if they have any relatives or friends who have died or been sick from smoking-related problems. Have them describe how the illness affected the individual, and how long the person had been smoking.

TEACH & APPLY

COMPREHENSION CHECK

Make sure that students know that the word *carcinogen* simply means something that causes cancer.

LEARNING WITH VISUALS

 Your Transparency Acetate Binder contains an overhead entitled "Normal Lung," which you may want to use during this lesson.

GUEST SPEAKER

Invite a doctor or nurse to speak to the class about the effects of smoking that he or she treats daily. Ask the speaker to focus the message on the irreversible damage and the end result caused by this bad habit. Also, ask the speaker to talk about how smoking will affect an unborn fetus.

LEARNING WITH VISUALS

To demonstrate the chemicals in cigarette paper, obtain some cigarettes. Slit the paper carefully down the length of the cigarette and pour out the tobacco. Save the tobacco for the next part of the experiment. Twist two cigarette papers together and light. Allow students to smell the smoke. Most students react as if they have smelled ammonia. This will help them realize that cigarettes contain many chemicals in addition to those used in the tobacco. Now take the discarded tobacco and sprinkle it on a petri dish for growing bacteria. Allow the tobacco to sit in the covered petri dish for a few days and then observe. The mold and bacterial growth is usually extensive and not very appealing.

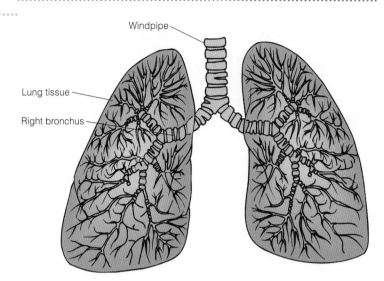

Figure 14–1 The Lungs. The windpipe branches to form the right and left bronchi. These branch again and again, finally ending in tiny passageways that conduct air into the air sacs (shown in Figure 14–2).

Windpipe

Lung tissue

Right bronchus

A lung from a person who died from smoking-related lung disease.

swallow or spit, you remove a bit of this mucus with its burden of debris from your air passages.

Smoke Damage to Lungs Smoking damages the lung tissue in many ways. The tars in cigarette smoke make the coat of mucus abnormally thick. They also slow the action of the cilia in sweeping out the mucus. Irritation builds, making the smoker feel like coughing. However, each puff on a cigarette paralyzes the cilia and numbs the throat for a while, so the smoker experiences *relief* from irritation. As a result, the need to cough feels like a need to smoke. The smoking, which harms, also soothes.

Bronchitis and Emphysema Some people who smoke ultimately get one or more chronic diseases of the lungs, such as **bronchitis** or emphysema. Bronchitis is familiar to most people as an infection of the bronchi, which become clogged with heavy mucus. The resulting irritation causes deep, harsh coughing and wheezing. Bronchitis develops in almost all cigarette smokers after about ten years.

Emphysema takes longer to develop than bronchitis, and its effects are more life-threatening. Emphysema does not strike only smokers. Some people who live in smoggy cities or who are exposed to polluted air for other reasons (for example, coal miners or workers in smoky factories) may get it, too. A few people will develop emphysema whether they smoke or not. Most, however, get emphysema from smoking.

Figure 14–2 on the next page shows normal lung tissue and lung tissue damaged by emphysema. As you can see

Ability Levels

Basic

To demonstrate the effects of smoking, obtain the following equipment:

- One-gallon jar
- Two-hole stopper
- Cigarettes (filtered and unfiltered)
- Two delivery tubes (glass)
- Cigarette holder
- Vacuum pump

(Your Teacher's Resource Box contains a diagram that explains how to set up this demonstration.)

Fill the gallon jar half full with water. Place an

Normal Lung

Tiny air sacs
Capillaries
Tiny air tubes

Passageways lined with cilia

Lung with Emphysema

Trachea

Trapped air

Tiny air sacs have merged, forming a large, rigid air pocket

① ③
②

Pressure

Large air tube (bronchus)

Normal Lung. In a normal lung, tiny sacs at the ends of the air passageways permit release of the body's carbon dioxide into the air. This is also where the blood is recharged with oxygen from the air.

Lung with Emphysema. In emphysema, air sacs have burst to form a single, rigid, balloonlike pocket (1). The tiny air tube leading to this portion of lung tissue opens to bring in air, but then closes under pressure from the surrounding tissue so that the air is trapped (2). The capillaries are breaking down (3).

Figure 14–2 Normal Lung versus Lung with Emphysema

by comparing the two, the normal tissue has many tiny, bubblelike air sacs. A tiny air tube leads to each little sac. As the lung expands, the sac expands and draws air in through the tube. As the lung deflates, the sac gets smaller and squeezes air back out.

In emphysema, the fine dividing walls between the tiny air sacs break. The sacs balloon out to become large pockets of air with hard, inflexible walls. (This is much like what happens when 50 tiny soap bubbles merge to form one big bubble.) As the lung expands, the pockets still draw air in. As the lung deflates, however, the stiffened tissue around the airways blocks air from escaping. The air trapped in the lungs bursts and tears lung tissue, making the pockets larger and worsening the condition. Lung damage occurs not because people can't breathe in but because they can't breathe out.

Emphysema makes it hard to breathe. Also, each breath delivers less oxygen to the person panting for it. The person with emphysema breathes fast—30 times a minute at rest, compared with the normal adult's 15–20 times. However, the person with emphysema never gets to take a deep breath. Emphysema is a crippling, ever-worsening condition. It ruins the quality of life, and finally it kills. Death is from slow suffocation—or from heart failure. The heart muscle itself cannot get the oxygen it needs at the same time it is asked to pump harder to provide oxygen to the other tissues.

Bronchitis, emphysema, and a few other diseases of the lungs are often termed **chronic obstructive lung disease (COLD)**, because less and less air flows in and out of the lungs. Smoking-related COLD kills an estimated 57,000 people a year in the United States. The surgeon general concludes that "the contribution of cigarette smoking to COLD deaths far outweighs all other factors."

Glossary

bronchitis (bron-KITE-us): a respiratory disorder with irritation of the bronchi; thickened mucus; and deep, harsh coughing.

chronic obstructive lung disease (COLD): a term for several diseases that interfere with breathing. Asthma, bronchitis, and emphysema are examples of COLD.

unfiltered cigarette in the holder, attached to the jar with a glass bend, and light it. Using the vacuum pump, attached to the jar with the other glass tube, draw smoke from the cigarette into the gallon jar and watch the water as the smoke enters. Continue pumping until the cigarette is completely burned. Examine the color of the water and allow students to smell it. Repeat the experiment with

a filtered cigarette and note that there is little difference in the color of the water.

(Smoking machines may be obtained from the Cancer Society or purchased from health education companies.)

INTERDISCIPLINARY ACTIVITY: MATHEMATICS

Have students who are interested in math calculate the weekly, monthly, and yearly cost of smoking for a pack-a-day smoker. Determine the amount spent over 40 years. Then make a list of the items the students could buy if they had the weekly, monthly, or yearly amount of money available. Have the students work in groups to prepare posters with pictures of all the items one could buy in a week, month, and year with the smoker's money.

COMPREHENSION CHECK

Students might need help with Figure 14–3. Using lung cancer as an example, tell them that if they smoke they are at least seven times more likely to develop lung cancer than if they did not smoke. Depending on how much they smoke, they could be as many as 15 times more likely to develop lung cancer. Make sure students read the important sentence at the bottom of the figure, which states that the smoker has risks of all of the diseases at the same time.

GUEST SPEAKER

The American Cancer Society can often provide former cancer patients to speak to classes. Some have obvious physical impairments, such as no larynx, as a result of surgery for cancer. Some may be willing to speak to classes about their experiences and their present attitudes towards smoking.

Cancer Another disease of the lungs—cancer—is much more common in smokers than in nonsmokers. The carcinogens in cigarette smoke cause cancer not only in the lungs but also in the nose, lips, mouth, tongue, throat, and esophagus. Some of the carcinogens get into the bloodstream and travel freely, so they can cause cancer in any other organ as well. Smokers have higher rates of cancer of the bladder, pancreas, and kidney than do nonsmokers (see Figure 14–3).

Figure 14–3 The Risks of Smoking

Disease	Smokers Increase Their Risks of Dying By[a]:
Lung cancer	7 to 15 times
Throat cancer	5 to 13 times
Oral cancer	3 to 15 times
Esophagus cancer	4 to 5 times
Bladder cancer	2 to 3 times
Pancreatic cancer	2 times
Kidney cancer	1½ times
Heart disease	1½ to 3 times
Emphysema and other chronic airway obstructions (including asthma)	10 to 20 times
Peptic ulcer disease	2 times

[a]The risks of a person who smokes one pack of cigarettes or less per day are at the lower end of the spectrum. Risks of those who smoke more than a pack a day are at the higher end. Most important, *the smoker has risks of all these diseases at the same time.*

> **" Cigarettes are killers that travel in packs. "**
>
> Marie S. Ott

Lung cancer now causes more deaths in women than does breast cancer. Women are said to be the victims of an "epidemic of smoking." African Americans suffer the highest rates of lung cancer of any group in the country. As a result of all this, cigarette smoking is the major single cause of cancer deaths in the United States.

Smoking combined with other risk factors for cancer creates a far greater hazard than smoking by itself. For example, the risk of developing many types of cancer increases sharply for people who smoke and drink alcohol. For another example, exposure to the insulating material asbestos, combined with smoking, adds up to a deadly hazard.

Smokers know that they are risking lung cancer, but many are sure it won't happen to them. Others believe that if they contract it, X-ray tests can catch it in time to save their lives. Unfortunately, by the time a cancerous spot in the lung is only a millimeter across—just large enough to be seen on an X-ray film—it is already too late to cure it.

 KEY POINTS *Smoking cigarettes is linked with health hazards such as bronchitis, emphysema, COLD, cancer of the lungs, and other cancers. Drinking alcohol greatly increases the smoker's cancer risk.*

HEALTHY PEOPLE 2000

Reduce cigarette smoking to a prevalence of no more than 15 percent among people aged 20 and older. (Baseline: 29 percent in 1987, 32 percent for men and 27 percent for women)

If the current trend continues, smoking prevalence among people with a high school education or less will be approximately 31 percent in the year 2000. Accelerating the rate of change for this population presents a major challenge to public health professionals, and the target of 20 percent reflects this challenge.

Smoking prevalence varies by occupational category. In 1987, 26.1 percent of white-collar males smoked cigarettes as did 26.6 percent of white-collar females. Among blue-collar workers, 36.1 percent of males and 36.6 percent of females smoked. The unusual similarity of the data between men and women within the

The Heart and Cardiovascular System

Smoking is as damaging to the heart and cardiovascular system as it is to the lungs. It causes about one-fifth of all deaths from heart disease and stroke. Smoking burdens the heart in five ways at the same time:

▶ Nicotine speeds up the heart rate. This increases the heart's workload, so the smoker's heart requires extra oxygen.

▶ Nicotine also raises the blood pressure. The heart has to push blood around the body against this pressure. This, too, increases the heart's workload and the need for oxygen.

▶ Smoking reduces the amount of oxygen the blood can carry. When the smoker inhales, the blood gets a dose of **carbon monoxide** from the smoke. The carbon monoxide takes the place of oxygen in the red blood cells. This reduces the red blood cells' ability to transport oxygen. As a result, the heart muscle receives less oxygen than it needs.

▶ Nicotine also triggers the formation of blood clots. When clots lodge in arteries that feed the heart muscle, they kill parts of that muscle—heart attacks. When they lodge in arteries that feed the brain, they kill parts of the brain—strokes.

▶ Smoking drastically reduces the blood flow in the heart's own arteries, another cause of heart attack.

To sum up, two major ingredients of cigarettes—tars and nicotine—damage the body's two major life-support systems. Tars reduce the lungs' ability to *supply* oxygen. Nicotine increases the heart's *need* for oxygen.

A health-care professional can easily tell a nonsmoker from a smoker, based on the performance of the lungs and heart.

 KEY POINTS *Smoking burdens the heart and cardiovascular system in several ways. Smoking reduces the body's supply of oxygen, but increases the heart's need for it. Smoking is strongly linked with heart disease.*

Other Effects of Smoking

Smoking damages other organs besides the lungs and the heart. In fact, it harms every organ. Smoking does the following:

▶ Shuts down circulation in the small vessels, causing cold hands and feet. In some cases, this results in a disease that requires surgical removal of limbs.

▶ Causes wrinkling of the skin, especially of the face, and graying of the hair. (Smokers in their 40s may look as if they are in their 60s.)

▶ Doubles the risk of developing colon cancer; increases the risk of cancer of the pancreas (almost always fatal) by 70 percent.

▶ Slows normal growth of lungs in smoking adolescents.

MINI Glossary

carbon monoxide: a deadly gas; a gas formed during the burning of tobacco.

blue- and white-collar working categories suggests that the work environment is an important influence on smoking status.

The prevalence of cigarette smoking has been much higher among military personnel than among the overall population. Smoking is inversely associated with military rank, and at least twice as high among enlisted personnel as among commissioned officers. According to worldwide surveys of substance abuse among military personnel conducted by the Department of Defense, smoking prevalence fell from 52 percent in 1980 to 42 percent in 1988. If the 1980 through 1988 trend continues, smoking prevalence among military personnel will be roughly 26 percent in the year 2000. The target of 20 percent is believed attainable given increased antismoking activities within the Department of Defense.

▶ Increases risks of **ulcers** (and makes dying from ulcers more likely).

▶ Increases tolerance to drugs, making larger doses needed for illness and pain relief (and can make vaccinations ineffective).

▶ Greatly increases risks of heart attack and stroke in women who take oral contraceptives (see Figure 14–4 below).

▶ In pregnant women, limits the oxygen supply to the fetus (resulting in smaller babies, premature births, miscarriages, a doubled risk of birth defects, impaired development in children up to age 11, and early death of infants).

▶ Causes women to become infertile; causes early menopause and increased bone loss.

▶ Gradually reduces oxygen supply to the brain, impairing memory.

▶ Thickens mucus, increasing the risk of chronic and painful infection of the **sinuses** (this can spread to the brain and spinal cord—a life-threatening condition).

▶ Interferes with the immune response, making colds, flu, and other infections likely.

▶ Prevents normal sleep (quitters sleep better within three nights of quitting).

▶ Exposes the chest to radiation (smoking one pack of cigarettes a day for one year is equal in radiation to having 250 chest X rays).

▶ Makes it likely that men will produce abnormal sperm (this can result in birth defects).

▶ Causes hearing and vision loss (this worsens over time).

▶ Encourages gum disease.

▶ Is associated with an increased risk of leukemia (cancer of the blood-producing organs).

Figure 14–4 Smoking and Oral Contraceptives. A woman who smokes and takes birth control pills is 10 times as likely to suffer a heart attack and 20 times as likely to have a stroke as a woman who does neither.

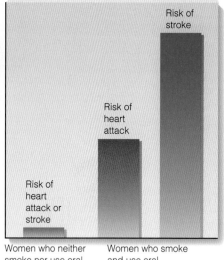

Risk of stroke

Risk of heart attack

Risk of heart attack or stroke

Women who neither smoke nor use oral contraceptives

Women who smoke and use oral contraceptives

Appearance and Odor   The effects of smoking go beyond health to personal appearance. Besides wrinkling the skin, smoking causes bad breath and yellows the teeth. The smell of stale smoke clings to the smoker's hair, clothes, home, and car. Therefore, people who find the smell unpleasant want to avoid both the person and the surroundings. Many nonsmokers refuse even to date people who smoke.

Financial Costs and Fire Danger   Then there is the cost. At upwards of $2.50 a pack, smoking can cost the heavy smoker from $1,000 to $2,000 a year. A person who collected that amount in a personal fund instead could visit Hawaii every three years.

Finally, there is the danger of fire. Fires started by dropped cigarettes cause some 2,000 deaths and 4,000 injuries a year. Altogether, smoking is the single greatest cause of preventable death in the United States today.

 KEY POINTS   *Smoking harms every organ of the body. Pregnant women's smoking harms fetuses and endangers the lives of newborns. Smoking damages appearance and attractiveness, and is expensive. It is the single greatest cause of preventable death in the United States today.*

QUICK QUIZ

Chapter 14, Section 2

The following quiz will help you assess your students' understanding of the material covered in this section of the chapter. You might use the quiz as an oral exercise, which will lead into a class discussion of the topics covered. Or, you might use it as a paper/pencil quiz to evaluate your students individually.

Like the Quick Quiz, the Section Review can also be used as an assessment tool to spark class discussion or as an individual student evaluation. It can also be used as a review in preparation for this quiz.

1. Cigarettes release carcinogens which cause many forms of cancer. (True)

2. Tar from cigarettes is the principle cause of emphysema, a critical lung disease. (True)

Are *Any* Smoking Products Safer?

Low-tar, low-nicotine cigarettes are no better than the regular kind just described. Smokers who switch to them often smoke more cigarettes, smoke to a shorter butt, puff more often, or inhale more deeply. Such smokers face the same risks as smokers of regular cigarettes.

Cigar and pipe smoking also carries high risks. Cigar and pipe smokers who do not inhale tend to have lower rates of lung and heart diseases than do cigarette smokers. However, they are likely to develop cancer of the lips and tongue. Pipe smoke is higher in tar than cigarette smoke, so those who inhale may face a higher risk of lung cancer than they would from cigarettes.

Quitting smoking is clearly the best way to avoid the ills caused by tobacco use. The sooner, the better, too. The risks of heart attacks in both men and women fall rapidly to the range of nonsmokers' risks within a few years. The risk of dying from lung cancer falls steadily in people who quit smoking. Ten years after quitting, the risk is about half of that for smokers. In short, people who quit smoking live longer than those who continue to smoke.

Still, reducing the number or the strength of the cigarettes smoked is better than doing nothing. The less a person smokes, the smaller the risks. Every cigarette counts.

KEY POINTS *Smoking tobacco in any form is unsafe for health.*

You can save enough money quitting smoking to vacation in Hawaii.

SECTION 2 Review

Answer the following questions on a sheet of paper.

Learning the Vocabulary

The vocabulary terms in this section are *tars, carcinogens, emphysema, bronchi, mucus, cilia, bronchitis, chronic obstructive lung disease (COLD), carbon monoxide, ulcers,* and *sinuses.*

1. Match the following phrases with the terms:
   a. cancer-causing agents
   b. two main airways in the lungs
   c. harmful chemicals in burning tobacco
   d. gas formed during burning of tobacco
   e. open sores in the lining of the digestive system

Learning the Facts

2. Explain what happens to the lungs of a person with emphysema.
3. List the cancers that are more likely to occur in smokers than in nonsmokers.
4. List the effects of smoking on personal appearance.
5. In what ways can smoking affect the unborn child of a pregnant woman?

Making Life Choices

6. The number of women smokers is on the rise. What is the most common type of cancer in women today?

MINI Glossary

ulcers: open sores in the lining of the digestive system.

sinuses (SIGN-us-es): spaces in the bones of the skull.

3. Carcinogens are the only harmful substance in cigarettes. (False)
4. Physical addiction to nicotine makes the need to cough feel like a need to smoke, because inhaling on a cigarette temporarily paralyzes the cilia in the lungs. (True)
5. Bronchitis and emphysema are chronic diseases of the lungs associated with smoking. (True)
6. Bronchitis, emphysema, and a few other diseases of the lungs are collectively referred to as chronic obstructive lung disease (COLD). (True)
7. Drinking alcohol greatly increases a smoker's chances of developing cancer. (True)
8. Smoking does not affect the heart and cardiovascular system. (False)
9. Smoking during pregnancy can cause massive birth defects. (True)
10. Low-nicotine cigarettes minimize the effects of smoking. (False)

SECTION 3

FOCUS

OUTCOME

In this section students will learn about:

1. The risks involved with passive smoking.

FOCUS ACTIVITY

Ask two students to role play. One is a smoker lighting up a cigarette in a car. The other is the passenger, a nonsmoker who does not want the car to smell like smoke. How does each justify his or her feelings to the other? Ask for volunteers to analyze their arguments.

TEACH & APPLY

INTERDISCIPLINARY ACTIVITY: WRITING

Form groups of three or four students to write an article entitled "Survivor's Guide to Living Around Smokers." Each group is to come up with ten tips for protecting health in an environment of smokers. Tips might relate to survival in smoke-filled washrooms, homes, job places, cars, and so on. Combine all tips and turn in the article to the school newspaper for possible publication.

FAST FACTS

A person who has not started smoking as a teenager is unlikely ever to become a smoker.

For Your Information

Passive smoking does about 40 percent as much damage to arteries as smoking does.

Figure 14–5 *Carbon Monoxide Sources Compared. Spending one hour in a smoke-filled room presents the nonsmoker with as much carbon monoxide as smoking one cigarette would. The abbreviation ppm refers to parts per million—units of carbon monoxide per million units of air.*

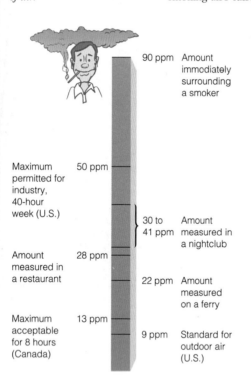

SECTION 3

Passive Smoking

The smoke that reaches smokers is a little different from the smoke that reaches those in the room with them. The **mainstream smoke** from a cigarette is the smoke that passes through the cigarette and then enters the smoker's lungs. The **sidestream smoke** is the smoke that enters the air from the burning tip of the cigarette. Together, smoke exhaled from smokers' lungs and sidestream smoke can fill a room, exposing other people to **environmental tobacco smoke (ETS)**.

ETS Health Risks   Does inhaling ETS (passive smoking), cause lung cancer? Many experts now say yes. Families and co-workers of people who smoke run an increased risk of dying from lung cancer. You may choose not to smoke. If you live or work with a smoker, however, you are a smoker, too—a passive smoker.

Passive smoking raises not only cancer risks, but also doubles the risks of heart disease. Nonsmokers who live with smokers suffer damage to their hearts. For example, passive smokers cannot exercise as well as nonsmokers, probably because smoke reduces blood flow to their hearts. Passive smoking also raises heart attack risks.

Living or working with a smoker creates other hazards, too. ETS worsens allergic symptoms, **asthma**, and sinus conditions. It irritates the eyes, especially if a person is wearing contact lenses. It causes headaches, dizziness, and nausea. In babies and children, it doubles the risk of lung infections, causes permanent lung damage, makes serious middle ear infections likely, and brings on asthma attacks. If a pregnant woman lives with a smoker during her pregnancy, her infant faces many of the same risks as the infant born to a smoking mother.

There is no question about it: other people's smoking is bad for nonsmokers. In fact, 53,000 deaths a year are linked to passive smoking. This makes passive smoking the third leading preventable cause of death in the United States, behind active smoking and alcohol drinking. As the experts say, "If you can smell it, it can harm you."

Compounds in ETS   The harm to passive smokers comes from ETS, which contains over 40 known carcinogens, as well as other compounds. One of its gases is carbon monoxide. In a closed room with smokers, a nonsmoker may suffer from the same lack of oxygen in the blood as was described for the smoker. Figure 14–5 shows that a person exposed to a smoky room may inhale more carbon monoxide than is considered safe. (A hazard of sitting in a traffic jam, as you probably know, is the high concentration of carbon monoxide in the air from the exhaust pipes of the jammed cars. As you also know, a person who breathes these fumes in a closed car dies

---

QUICK QUIZ

Chapter 14, Section 3

The following quiz will help you assess your students' understanding of the material covered in this section of the chapter. You might use the quiz as an oral exercise, which will lead into a class discussion of the topics covered. Or, you might use it as a paper/pencil

quiz to evaluate your students individually.

Like the Quick Quiz, the Section Review can also be used as an assessment tool to spark class discussion or as an individual student evaluation. It can also be used as a review in preparation for this quiz.

1. Mainstream smoke enters the smoker's lungs directly from the cigarette. (True)

2. Sidestream smoke escapes from the tip of the cigarette into the air. (True) within minutes.) Carbon monoxide has no smell, so you cannot tell if it is present. One sign of exposure, though, is yawning.

Bans on Smoking Reduce ETS Exposure Many nonsmokers rightly demand that smoking not be allowed in areas they share. Thanks to the efforts of nonsmokers' rights associations, most restaurants now have nonsmoking areas, and some ban smoking altogether. Motels provide nonsmokers' rooms, and a federal law bans smoking on most airline flights. Almost every state bans smoking in public transportation, hospitals, elevators, schools, libraries, and other public buildings.

If you object to people's smoking near you, you can practice being assertive. Without being insulting to the smoker, simply say, "Please don't smoke. It bothers me."

People who can't stand smoke find it hard to be around smokers.

 KEY POINTS *Passive smoking raises the risks of cancer, heart disease, and many other hazards. Passive smoking is the third leading preventable cause of death in the United States.*

 SECTION 3 Review

Answer the following questions on a sheet of paper.

Learning the Vocabulary

The vocabulary terms in this section are *mainstream smoke, sidestream smoke, environmental tobacco smoke (ETS),* and *asthma.*

1. Write a sentence using each term.

Learning the Facts

2. How does passive smoking affect allergy and sinus conditions?

3. What are the health problems associated with passive smoking?

4. How many deaths a year are linked to passive smoking?

Making Life Choices

5. If you could, would you change the way television portrays the images of smokers? Describe the portrait of a smoker you'd put on television. Why do you suppose television often glamorizes smokers? What does this tell you about the media and the tobacco industry?

 MINI Glossary

mainstream smoke: the smoke that flows through the cigarette and into the lungs when a smoker inhales.

sidestream smoke: the smoke that escapes into the air from the burning tip of a cigarette or cigar, or from burning pipe tobacco.

environmental tobacco smoke (ETS): the combination of exhaled mainstream smoke and sidestream smoke that enters the air and may be inhaled by other people.

asthma: difficulty breathing, with wheezing sounds from the chest caused by air rushing through narrowed air passages.

ASSESS

EVALUATE

Have each student write a well-supported essay answer to one of the following questions.

1. What health hazards are presented by passive smoking?

2. What can you do as a nonsmoker to avoid passive smoke?

 SECTION 3 Review Answers

1. Answers will vary.
2. worsens allergic and sinus conditions, irritates eyes, causes headaches, dizziness and nausea (p. 384)
3. raises the risks of cancer and heart disease. In babies it doubles the risk of lung infections, causing permanent lung damage, and brings on asthma attacks. (p. 384)
4. 53,000 (p. 384)
5. Answers will vary.

 WORKSHEETS A reproducible quiz for Section 3 is provided in the Teacher's Resource Box.

CLOSE

Assign each student to write a letter to a future spouse who smokes. Have each explain why he or she would not marry unless the potential spouse stops smoking. The letter should explain how smoking causes health risks for the couple and their future children, as well as creates other undesirable effects.

3. Environmental tobacco smoke (ETS) cannot affect your health. (False)
4. Passive smoking increases the risks of heart disease and cancer, and worsens the symptoms of allergies and asthma. (True)
5. ETS contains more than forty known carcinogens, and is the third leading preventable cause of death in the United States. (True)
6. Pregnant women who live with smokers don't risk harming their fetuses unless they smoke themselves. (False)
7. If you can smell another person's cigarette smoke, it can harm you. (True)
8. Carbon monoxide is a harmless gas associated with ETS. (False)
9. Yawning is a sign of exposure to carbon monoxide. (True)
10. You have the right to politely ask others not to smoke. (True)

SECTION 4

FOCUS

OUTCOMES

In this section students will learn about the:

1. Problems associated with smokeless tobacco and nicotine addiction.
2. Double messages of advertisements, which cause many to overlook warnings.

FOCUS ACTIVITY

Ask some volunteers to explain what effects smokeless tobacco had on them the first time they tried it. List these effects on the board. Explain that nicotine caused all these unpleasant feelings.

TEACH & APPLY

ROLE PLAY

Tell students that they have been asked to serve on a panel of experts that will devise a plan to discourage the use of smokeless tobacco in the general public, as well as among teens. What incentives and deterrents can they think of to discourage its use?

DISCUSSION

The use of smokeless tobacco is prevalent in the sport of baseball. It is not uncommon to see professional ball players with a wad of tobacco in their cheek during a game. How is this a mixed message? (Athletes, who are to be in prime physical condition, are using something that can cause great physical harm.)

386

Smokeless Tobacco

Some people use **smokeless tobacco** products—snuff or chewing tobacco. People dip snuff by holding a pinch of moist, shredded tobacco between the gum and cheek, where it gradually releases its nicotine. Chewing tobacco is chewed, and then, like snuff, is held in the cheek in a wad, or **quid**. This stimulates the release of saliva. This saliva becomes contaminated with tobacco and must be spit out, not swallowed.

Smokeless Tobacco Isn't Safer The use of smokeless tobacco by high school athletes is on the rise. Although the habit carries health risks, as many as one out of three high school athletes has tried or used smokeless tobacco. Smokeless tobacco products produce the same addiction as smoked products, because they also deliver the drug nicotine.

The tobacco industry tries to get people hooked on smokeless tobacco. A typical advertisement suggests. "Use this sparingly at first, because it will irritate the gums. After a few weeks, the irritation will lessen. Start slowly, and increase use over time, because it takes time to get used to strong products and large doses." The person who is alert to double messages will see that this one says the product is dangerous, but to go ahead and use it anyway.

Smokeless tobacco is a hazardous tradition among athletes. Better, chew gum or sunflower seeds at game time.

Health Risks of Smokeless Tobacco Smokeless tobacco use is linked to many health problems, from minor mouth sores to cancer. Snuff dipping is linked with cancerous tumors in the nasal cavity, cheek, gum, and throat. Tobacco chewing holds a *greater* risk of mouth and throat cancers than does tobacco smoking. More than half of the National League baseball players who use smokeless tobacco have developed mouth sores that lead to cancer. One of baseball's legends, Babe Ruth, was a heavy user of snuff and chewing tobacco. He died of throat cancer at the age of 53.

The dentist who examines a person's mouth for signs of oral cancer looks for **leukoplakia**. These are whitish or grayish patches that form in the mouths of tobacco chewers, and they tend to become cancerous. They develop where the quid is held.

Other drawbacks to tobacco chewing and snuff dipping include bad breath, brown teeth, and blunted senses of smell and taste. Tobacco chew-

enrichment

For enrichment you might want to share with your students the following information from the U.S. Department of Health and Human Services.

Smokeless tobacco includes primarily moist or dry snuff and chewing tobacco. Oral cancer has been shown to occur several times more frequently among smokeless tobacco users than among nonusers and may be 50 times as frequent among long-term snuff users. All smokeless tobacco products contain substantial amounts of nicotine; their use can support nicotine dependence and may lead to cigarette use.

The consumption of smokeless tobacco in the United States increased 40 percent between 1970 and 1986. Most new users of smokeless tobacco products are adolescent males. In 1988, 6.6 percent of males aged 12

Don't be fooled into thinking that smokeless tobacco means harmless tobacco. Smokeless tobacco increases your risks for many different cancers.

Cancer of the tongue occurs often in those who use smokeless tobacco.

ing also damages the gums, wears away the tooth surfaces, and eats away the jawbones. This makes it likely that users will eventually lose their teeth.

 Smokeless tobacco contains nicotine and so is addictive. Its use carries risks of mouth sores; cancerous tumors of the mouth, nasal cavity, cheek, gum, and throat; bad breath; and brown teeth.

 Review

Answer the following questions on a sheet of paper.

Learning the Vocabulary

The vocabulary terms in this section are *smokeless tobacco, quid,* and *leukoplakia.*

1. Write a sentence using each term.

Learning the Facts

2. List the health problems associated with smokeless tobacco.

3. What are the dental problems that occur with the use of smokeless tobacco?

Making Life Choices

4. The tobacco industry gets young teenagers hooked on smokeless tobacco by showing professional athletes using these products. Teenagers look up to these athletes. How can you help prevent fellow teens from using smokeless tobacco? How can health advocates' messages compete against professional athletes pushing smokeless tobacco?

 Glossary

smokeless tobacco: tobacco used for snuff or chewing rather than for smoking.

quid: a small portion of any form of smokeless tobacco.

leukoplakia (loo-koh-PLAKE-ee-uh): whitish or grayish patches that develop in the mouths of tobacco users and that may lead to cancer.

ASSESS

EVALUATE

Ask students to make posters illustrating the dangers of smokeless tobacco. Have them create large warning labels that could be placed on all packages and cans.

SECTION 4 Review Answers

1. Answers will vary.
2. minor mouth sores; cancerous tumors in nasal cavity, cheek, gum, throat; a greater risk of cancer of mouth and throat (p. 386)
3. bad breath, brown teeth, damage to gums, wearing away of tooth surfaces, eating away jawbones (pp. 386–387)
4. Answers will vary.

CLOSE

Ask students to write essays explaining how they would answer their ten-year-old brother, who asked them to buy him some snuff. What would they tell him about the effects of smokeless tobacco?

FAST FACTS

Of the 6 million people in this country who use smokeless tobacco, as many as 1 in 4 is under age 19 years.

through 17 had used some form of smokeless tobacco in the preceding month. The prevalence of smokeless tobacco use among males aged 18 through 24 was 8.9 percent in 1987.

Between 1970 and 1986, the prevalence of snuff use increased fifteenfold and chewing tobacco use increased more than fourfold among men aged 17 through 19. In contrast, the prevalence of use among men aged 50 and older declined by almost half for each type of product. Attaining the target of 4 per-

cent will be a challenge as it requires reversing an upward trend.

Smokeless tobacco use among women was less than 1 percent in 1987. Use of smokeless tobacco by minority groups varies. Black and Hispanic adolescent populations report lower usage rates than whites. In contrast, Native American schoolchildren have reported prevalences of regular smokeless tobacco use ranging from 18 to 64 percent.

FOCUS

OUTCOMES

In this section students will learn strategies for:

1. Quitting nicotine-related habits.
2. Helping someone else quit.

FOCUS ACTIVITY

Have students help you generate two lists on the board. One list is reasons to smoke. The other list is reasons to stop smoking. This will get students to realize that there are many more reasons to stop smoking than to start or continue to smoke or use smokeless tobacco.

TEACH & APPLY

Key Passage

Ask students if they have ever been around a friend, acquaintance, or relative who has tried to quit smoking. What effects did this experience have on that person? Was the person able to endure the effort, or did he or she give in and resume smoking? Has that person tried again to quit?

> **"** To cease smoking is the easiest thing I ever did. I ought to know, because I've done it a thousand times. **"**
>
> Mark Twain
> (1835–1910)
> American writer

Health Strategies

Giving Up Smoking

To give up smoking, smokers must:

1. Ask themselves whether they really want to quit.
2. Believe in their ability to succeed.
3. Review the health benefits of quitting smoking.
4. Expect to be challenged.
5. Plan their strategy.
6. Find new ways to relax.
7. Make a list of alternative activities.
8. Commit themselves.
9. Seek support.
10. Tune in to the immediate rewards.

The Decision to Quit

A smoker who couldn't quit asked a successful quitter how to do it. The quitter replied, "I just got my inner self and my outer self together. When they had agreed that we should quit, we did. It was easy."

Over 30 million people in the United States have quit using tobacco in the last 20 years or so. Many teenagers are deciding not to start. Of people who still smoke, nine out of ten would like to stop but say they "can't." Still, people do decide to quit. This section is addressed to smokers, but it applies to the users of smokeless tobacco as well.

How People Quit Smoking

A newspaper columnist invited his smoking readers to explain why they continued to smoke. He expected a flood of angry letters scolding him for his strong antismoking messages. Instead, most letters read like the one that follows:

A Fight against Addiction "Don't refer to what we do as smoking—refer to it as nicotine addiction. Nobody really likes smoking all that much. It's the nicotine that we get hooked on. I am trying to quit. It is truly the most difficult thing I've ever experienced—and I haven't had an uneventful life. If I give in to the addiction, I know I'll die with a cigarette in my hand."

In other words, people continue smoking because they are hooked. Whenever they try to quit, they face withdrawal: irritability, restlessness, anxiety, and of course, a craving for nicotine. It takes several weeks or a month of abstinence for withdrawal symptoms to fade. The Health Strategies section on this page, "Giving Up Smoking," provides some tips for the quitter.

Secrets for Success Successful quitters believe they can succeed. They know they can resist the urge to smoke. With each success, they gain more confidence and resist more easily.

Smokers must remind themselves again and again of the health benefits—both immediate and long term—of quitting. Smoking cuts life short by about 18 years. The truth is, there just are not many 85-year-old smokers. They died many years before.

Smokers trying to quit find it useful to discover what they like most about smoking. This chapter's Life Choice Inventory on page 390 enables people to find out what it is about smoking that is most important to them—stimulation, handling the cigarette, relaxation, or something else. Then, when they try to quit, they can meet those needs in other ways. The Life Choice Inventory offers suggestions for each type of smoker.

After discovering what they enjoy most about smoking, it helps for smokers to make a list of activities that will take the place of smoking. For example, smoking may be the way

Pursuing wellness

Adopt-A-Smoker. Suggest that students try to find a smoker who wants to quit, preferably a student that many of them know or a volunteer from the class. Have the entire class adopt this smoker to help him or her quit. The class members could each devise a way to help. For example:

1. Contact the smoker's brothers and sisters to help at home.
2. Make chewy snacks to substitute for cigarettes.
3. Escort the students to classes to avoid areas in the school where smoking may occur.
4. Meet the student to engage in exercise.
5. Call the student in the evening to check on progress or be available if the student needs to call someone to avoid smoking

Today, many teens oppose tobacco, and are letting the world know it.

some people relax. To replace this function, such people must find new ways to relax. A long, hot bath or some light stretching may help release tension (see Chapter 4 for more on relaxation, and Chapter 9 for stretching exercises). Other types of smokers should find other activities to replace smoking's functions.

Two Ways to Quit There are two ways to quit—tapering off or quitting all at once (cold turkey). A way to taper off is to start smoking each day an hour later than the day before. Another is to take up a fitness activity that will squeeze out the smoking. For example, many people take up jogging and notice that smoking limits their performance. This may give them the motivation to quit smoking.

While tapering off works well for some people, most are more successful quitting cold turkey. This is because the hard part is over more quickly. Two weeks after quitting, people who quit cold turkey have fewer and less intense cravings for cigarettes than those who cut back gradually.

The Pleasures of Quitting At first, quitters are keenly aware of the craving to smoke. They constantly fight the temptation to light up again. Tuning in to the pleasures of *not* smoking raises the odds in favor of success. Quitters list small and big pleasures:

▶ I can breathe deep breaths of clean air.
▶ I'm free from having to carry cigarettes and matches wherever I go.
▶ My behavior is not a threat to anyone's health. I can look my friends and family members in the eye.
▶ Food tastes delicious, and I can smell flowers.
▶ My clothes and hair smell fresh, not like smoke.
▶ I can walk easily without getting out of breath.

For Your Information

Things to do instead of smoking:
▶ Daydream
▶ Dance
▶ Draw
▶ Jog
▶ Listen
▶ Play
▶ Ride
▶ Sing
▶ Skate
▶ Smell
▶ Swim
▶ Talk

a cigarette.

6. Provide gum so the smoker is never without it.

7. Provide fruit juice instead of soft drinks and coffee.

8. Talk to the smoker's friends and get them to help by not smoking in the smoker's presence.

Be sure all are patient and not judgmental in dealing with the smoker. If the smoker

slips, forgive and go back on the program. The smoker should keep a log of progress.

Each student could then write what they did on an index card and have the smoker write whether it helped and why, on the back of the card. Cards could then be collected and used as quit tips for the next class that adopts a smoker. Be sure students continue to contact and reinforce the former smoker for the entire semester.

INTERDISCIPLINARY ACTIVITY: WRITING

Have students visit a store to investigate products that help people stop smoking. Have students write a report that includes prices, method each product uses, and how long the process takes. Ask students to look for information about success rates and money-back guarantees. Have students present a summary of all the methods found in a short oral report. This will inform students about some of the products on the market to help people fight nicotine addiction.

COMPREHENSION CHECK

Ask students to stop a habit or addiction that they have for a weekend. Some examples would be biting nails, eating candy, or chewing gum. On Monday, have students give a short oral report explaining how they did. Ask if it was as easy as they had thought it would be. Explain that a chemical addiction would be tougher to give up because of the physical and psychological addiction.

GROUP PROJECT

Assign students to work together in groups on a project to help promote the Great American Smoke-out Day. Explain that groups could make videos, posters, fliers, bookmarks, bookcovers, buttons, or stickers. Their primary goal is to come up with an original slogan or saying promoting the day set aside for people to not smoke. Have groups present their ideas to the rest of the class.

Students who are non-smokers can benefit from doing the Life Choice Inventory and answering the questions as if they did smoke. This could help them understand a friend or acquaintance who smokes. You could also have these students give the inventory to a friend or relative who does smoke. They could then read to the person the strategies suggested in the scoring section.

A reproducible copy of the Life Choice Inventory is provided in the Teacher's Resource Box.

BACKGROUND INFORMATION

Here are some helpful tips for smokers who want to quit "cold turkey."

1. Promise themselves they will not smoke at all for a week. More than a week is too much to handle.

2. Inform everyone close to them to gather support.

3. Get a friend to quit with them.

4. Ask for special consideration at first in case they are irritable.

5. Keep busy.

6. When wanting to reach for a cigarette, reach for the radio or the telephone instead—talk with someone, find substitute activities.

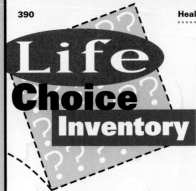

What Motivates a Smoker?

Here are some statements people make to describe what they get out of smoking cigarettes. On the scoring handout or on a piece of paper, the smoker should record the number (1, 2, 3, 4, or 5) that describes how often he or she feels this way (see below). Important: ANSWER EVERY QUESTION. (If you don't smoke, have a smoker friend take the inventory, and discuss it with you.) Your answers to the Life Choice Inventory are personal and private.

Share them with others only if you are comfortable doing so.

5 = Always   4 = Frequently   3 = Occasionally
2 = Seldom   1 = Never

Stimulation
A. I smoke cigarettes to keep myself from slowing down.
B. I smoke cigarettes to stimulate myself, to perk myself up.
C. I smoke cigarettes to give myself a lift.

Handling
D. Handling a cigarette is part of the enjoyment of smoking.
E. Part of the enjoyment of smoking a cigarette comes from the steps I take to light up.
F. When I smoke a cigarette, part of the enjoyment is watching the smoke as I exhale it.

Pleasure/Relaxation
G. Smoking cigarettes is pleasant and relaxing.
H. I find cigarettes pleasurable.
I. I want a cigarette most when I am comfortable and relaxed.

Crutch/Tension Reduction
J. I light up a cigarette when I feel angry about something.
K. When I feel upset, I light up a cigarette.

▶ I can talk on the phone without panicking if my cigarettes are out of reach.
▶ There are no dirty ashtrays around me.
▶ I don't burn holes in my clothes.
▶ I have more money to spend on other things.
▶ That attractive nonsmoker who sits next to me in class has started showing an interest in me.

No matter why people decide to quit, what makes them stick with it is that after only two or three days, they feel better physically, as well as emotionally.

The Fear of Weight Gain   Some smokers are afraid that if they quit, they will gain weight. Some people actually lose weight. However, most quitters do gain—usually about 4 to 5 pounds, but sometimes more—for two reasons. Smoking is an oral behavior, and some quitters turn to another oral

HEALTHY PEOPLE 2000

Reduce the initiation of cigarette smoking by children and youth so that no more than 15 percent have become regular cigarette smokers by age 20.

Reducing the initiation of cigarette smoking by youth is an important national priority. If 29 percent of the 70 million children now living in the United States start smoking and

continue to smoke cigarettes as adults, then at least 5 million of them will die of smoking-related diseases. Initiation is more sensitive to intervention than is quitting behavior. Preventing the initiation of smoking by youth should be a major focus of efforts to reduce the prevalence of cigarette smoking.

Experimentation with smoking is occurring at younger and younger ages and initiation now occurs almost entirely during adolescence. Two surveys of high school students

L. When I feel blue, I smoke cigarettes.

Craving/Psychological Dependence

M. When I have run out of cigarettes, I find it almost unbearable until I can get more.

N. When I'm not smoking, I am very much aware of it.

O. I crave a cigarette when I haven't smoked for a while.

Habit

P. I smoke cigarettes without being aware of it.

Q. I light up a cigarette without realizing I still have one burning in the ashtray.

R. I sometimes find a cigarette in my mouth and don't remember putting it there.

SCORING

1. On your paper, add up your scores as follows:
Stimulation score = A + B + C.
Handling score = D + E + F.
Pleasure/relaxation score = G + H + I.
Crutch/tension reduction score = J + K + L.
Craving/psychological dependence score = M + N + O.
Habit score = P + Q + R.
The highest scores indicate which aspects of smoking will be hardest for you to give up.

2. Substitute these activities for any needs previously satisfied by smoking:

▶ *Stimulation.* Brisk walking, other exercise, dancing.

▶ *Handling.* Toy with a pen or pencil. Draw. Play with a coin, a smooth stone, or plastic straws.

▶ *Pleasure/relaxation.* Substitute chewing gum, healthful snacks or beverages, or social or physical activities.

▶ *Crutch/tension reduction.* Choose physical activity, healthful snacks or beverages, chewing gum, or social activities.

▶ *Craving/psychological dependence.* Isolate yourself completely from cigarettes until the craving is gone—or use a patch or nicotine gum as described in the chapter. Giving up cigarettes may be so hard and cause so much discomfort that once you do quit, you will be strongly motivated to resist the temptation to go back to smoking. You'll know that if you do start smoking again, you will have to go through the same agony to quit again.

▶ *Habit.* Try to break your habit patterns. Become aware of each cigarette you smoke. Ask yourself, "Do I really want this cigarette?" You may be surprised at how many you do not want.

behavior to take its place—eating. People can prevent weight gain, however, by drinking fluids, snacking on crunchy vegetables, and taking up physical activity.

Even smokers who do gain a few pounds say it's worth it to give up cigarettes. Later, as ex-smokers, they take the weight off. Others have done it; you can too. Chapter 8 in this book tells how.

Help for Quitters   Some people can't make it alone, or don't choose to. Classes are offered by Smokenders, the American Cancer Society, the American Lung Association, and the American Heart Association. A class can help to identify a smoker's style and tailor a quitting plan to each person's needs.

Nicotine delivery devices, including gum, patches, inhalers, and nasal sprays are aids available to smokers as stepping stones to freedom from smoking. Both the gum and patches are readily available over the counter. The sprays and inhalers require a prescription. A dose of nicotine from the

found that for those who had ever smoked, about one-quarter had smoked their first cigarette by the 6th grade, one-half by the 8th grade, three-fourths by the 9th grade, and 94 percent by the 11th grade.

In 1988, the National Household Survey on Drug Abuse found that 23 percent of adolescents aged 12 through 17 had smoked at least one cigarette during the preceding year and 12 percent had smoked within the preceding month. In 1987, the National Adolescent Student Health Survey found that 51 percent of 8th graders (aged 13 and 14) and 63 percent of 10th graders (aged 15 and 16) reported having tried cigarettes. Sixteen percent of 8th graders and 26 percent of 10th graders reported having smoked a cigarette during the preceding month, and 8 percent of 8th graders and 18 percent of 10th graders had smoked a pack or more within the preceding month.

7. Take up some form of physical activity to get the heart and lungs in shape again. Great pleasure comes from the rapid recovery of breathing.

ROLE PLAY

Assign students to pair up and role play in front of the class. One is a smoker, the other is a friend trying to get the smoker to quit. Discuss reasons the friend should quit smoking. How do they encourage quitting? What methods do they suggest to help the smoker?

GROUP PROJECT

Have students break into groups of four or five. Each group should design a "Quitter's Box." Each box should contain the things a smoker would need to quit smoking. The students should include snacks and candies to eat instead of smoking when a craving hits, things for the smoker to "handle" to keep their hands busy when a craving hits, index cards with motivational and encouraging phrases, plenty of gum, and so on. Have the students make an inventory list of their boxes. If any of the students know someone who is trying to quit smoking and would like to cooperate in this project, the class could make a box for the person. After two weeks, the person could come and talk to the class and report if and how the "Quitter's Box" helped.

Smoking hurts sports performance.

Gum containing nicotine helps some smokers quit.

gum, patches, inhalers, or sprays equals that in two or three cigarettes. The user must stop smoking and allow the devices to deliver nicotine into their bloodstream instead of tobacco. Nicotine-free pills, also available by prescription, help curb tobacco cravings and withdrawal symptoms, without nicotine. The drug's side effects are many, though, including shakiness, skin rash, dry mouth, sleeplessness, and seizures.

All of these aids help quitters, first to lose all the habits of smoking. handling the cigarettes, puffing on them, and so forth. After that (the theory goes), it becomes much easier to taper off, since nicotine addiction is the only problem left. In the case of the pills, even the physical addiction disappears after some months of use.

KEY POINTS *The smoker must make a firm decision to quit. Many programs and strategies can help a smoker to quit. Quitting is not easy, but the rewards of a smoke-free life are worth the work.*

How to Help the Smoker Quit

What if you are a concerned bystander who wants to help a smoker quit? First, you must realize that smokers can quit only when they are ready. Your job, then, is to help them get ready. You cannot force them to quit.

The key to helping is "tough love"—a term borrowed from alcoholism treatment. The idea is this. If you really care about a person, you will not keep quiet about a dangerous habit. Assert yourself. Confront the person. At the same time, show that you care. Make it clear that you reject the behavior, not the person. Talk about the risks of the behavior. Offer research news you hear about the effects of smoking and the benefits of quitting. Focus on

QUICK QUIZ

Chapter 14, Section 5

issues that matter to the person. Tell a friend at school, for example, that smoking hurts sports performance and that it is unattractive.

Do not be surprised, though, if the smoker cannot "hear" what you are saying. The person may be committed to smoking, at least at present. The person knows about, but ignores, health warnings: "Yes, I know." If the person continues to smoke, then protect your own health. Insist, "Don't smoke around me." Someday your comments, along with others, may tip the scale in favor of health, and the person will quit.

Employers can help by banning smoking on the job. This may seem unfair to smokers. However, it is fair to nonsmokers, it protects their health, and it is legal. Studies show that smokers take more breaks and are absent from work more often than nonsmokers.

Some magazines, films, and other media can help by not advertising tobacco. This takes courage, because advertising is so profitable. Even children can help, by asking parents who smoke to stop.

The tobacco industry does what any industry must do to be successful: make profits and find new markets for its products. Unfortunately, however, to do these things, tobacco companies must start more people using tobacco. This destroys health. Thus much of the normal business activity of the tobacco industry is viewed as **unethical** by many people. The Straight Talk in this chapter focuses on the tobacco industry's efforts to promote itself, and on ways in which the Food and Drug Administration would like to limit those efforts.

 If you want to help smokers quit, remember that smokers can quit only when they are ready. Express your concern. Offer information. If they are not willing to quit, protect yourself by insisting that they do not smoke around you.

SECTION 5 Review

Answer the following questions on a sheet of paper.

Learning the Vocabulary

The vocabulary term in this section is *unethical.*

1. Write a sentence using the vocabulary word.

Learning the Facts

2. Describe the withdrawal symptoms people experience when they quit smoking.

3. List the different strategies described in this section to help a person quit smoking.
4. List seven pleasures quitters gain when they stop smoking.

Making Life Choices

5. Four nicotine delivery devices are on the market to help people quit smoking: nicotine gum, nicotine patches, nicotine inhalers, and nicotine nasal sprays. Learn from a pharmacist or physician how each of these works, and explain.

MINI Glossary

unethical: against the rules of right and wrong; not in line with accepted moral standards.

SECTION 5 Review Answers

1. Answers will vary.
2. irritability, restlessness, anxiety, craving for nicotine (p. 388)
3. Answers will vary. Refer to the section "How to Help the Smoker Quit" on these pages.
4. Refer to the bulleted points on pages 389–390 for possible answers.
5. Answers will vary.

 A reproducible quiz for Section 5 is provided in the Teacher's Resource Box.

CLOSE

In order to show that students have mastered the material in Section 5, have each of them write a letter to a friend or relative who smokes. Have them include why the person should stop smoking, and what products can help him or her stop. Students should explain that they disapprove of the habit, not the person, and that they would support any attempts to quit. This will give students a chance to use all the information learned from this section.

 Reproducible Study Outlines and Reading Cloze worksheets for Chapter 14 are provided in the Teacher's Resource Box.

Reproducible Chapter Tests A and B are also provided in the Teacher's Resource Box.

severe withdrawal symptoms. (True)
4. It takes only a few days for the syptoms of withdrawal to fade. (False)
5. There are two ways to quit smoking: by tapering off slowly or by going cold turkey. (True)
6. Taking up a fitness activity can often help people who are trying to taper off their smoking by limiting their opportunities to smoke. (True)
7. There are several delivery devices that can

ease the transition to non-smoking. (True)
8. It takes months for a person who has stopped smoking to feel the health benefits of being smoke-free. (False)
9. You help a person quit smoking by practicing "tough love," which includes confronting the person about the effects of his/her smoking. (True)
10. You can help people quit smoking by demanding that they not smoke near you. (True)

ON LINE WITH HEALTH

You may want to have your students visit the following URLs, where they will find information and additional Web site resources to enhance their study of this chapter. As with all Web sites, you should check these out first to be sure the information found there is appropriate for your students.

QuitNet
http://www.quitnet.org/

Quit4Life
http://www.quit4life. com/html/splash.html

Campaign for Tobacco-Free Kids
http://www. tobaccofreekids.org

QuitNet is sponsored by the Massachusetts Tobacco Control Program and the Boston University School of Public Health. Quit4Life is an interactive site following stories of 4 teenagers through their steps to recovery from addiction.

FAST FACTS

A new organization, the National Center for Tobacco-Free Kids, has been formed to influence society's views on smoking and to support public policies that oppose teen smoking. The phone number is 800-284-KIDS.

Straight Talk

Would New Tobacco Rules Stop Teenagers from Smoking?

Recently, the Food and Drug Administration (FDA) proposed new restrictions for the advertisement and sale of tobacco products. At first, it seemed as if the rules could mark the beginning of the end of teenage smoking in this country. Soon, questions arose about whether the rules, if enacted, would have the desired effect. As of this writing, the courts are still debating the future of the FDA's proposals. By the time you, the student, read this, much will have been settled, but the question remains of whether new rules can help teens to avoid smoking.

Why do lawmakers believe that making new laws will stop teenagers from smoking? Smoking was illegal for kids before, and you can see how well that stopped them!

It's true that laws cannot directly stop teenagers from smoking, but the FDA hopes to make it more difficult for teens to buy tobacco. For example, a proposed rule that is likely to remain on the books states that anyone younger than about 27 years must show proof of age before buying tobacco. Nationwide, many states seem eager to work with FDA inspectors to crack down on vendors who sell tobacco to young people.

Two other proposed rules might restrict how and where tobacco may be sold. The FDA would like to ban the sale of small quantity packages of cigarettes ("kiddie packs"), and place tobacco vending machines only in areas that are not accessible to underage people. These rules would greatly cut down on tobacco sales to minors, and the tobacco companies are fight-

ing them in court. Here are some other restrictions that the FDA would like to see in place to protect teenagers from being targets for tobacco advertisements:

▶ Cigarette brand names would no longer sponsor sporting or other events, nor appear on billboards in or around sports arenas and stadiums.
▶ Tobacco advertisements on billboards and in youth-oriented publications would be limited to text only (no pictures).
▶ No clothing or gear with tobacco brand decoration would be allowed.
▶ No gifts with tobacco brand logos would be allowed when proofs of purchase are redeemed.
▶ All advertisements for tobacco products would carry FDA-approved warnings.
▶ No human or cartoon images would be used in tobacco advertising or on packages.
▶ No Internet advertisements would be allowed for tobacco products.

For Your Information

Advertisements make tobacco seem sexy, cool, or fun. Proposed tobacco warnings on packages may soon tell the truth:

▶ WARNING: Cigarettes Are Addictive.
▶ WARNING: Cigarettes Cause Cancer.
▶ WARNING: Smoking Can Kill You.
▶ WARNING: Tobacco Smoke Causes Fatal Lung Disease in Non-Smokers.

COOPERATIVE LEARNING

Tobacco Debate

Recently large tobacco companies have taken a lot of criticism for their roles in the addiction of millions of people to tobacco. It is estimated that over 1,000 people die every day from diseases or disorders caused by tobacco use. Explain to students the different chemicals in tobacco and what those chemicals do.

Nicotine is the addictive drug within tobacco that stimulates the nervous system, cardiovascular system, hormonal system, and digestive system. Tar contains hundreds of cancer causing chemicals that clog the bronchial tubes and alveoli within the lungs. Carbon monoxide is the same deadly gas that comes from car exhaust.

Debate—Divide your class into groups of three or four. Have them discuss some of the new laws that relate to tobacco use by both

I guess some of those things would make it harder for teenagers to buy tobacco products. Does advertising really make that much difference, though?

It's no accident that 86 percent of teenagers who smoke choose the three most heavily advertised brands. Among adult smokers, 66 percent buy the cheapest brands, not the most expensive, heavily advertised ones. Teenagers were led by advertisers to associate particular tobacco brands with positive experiences—sports events, gear and gifts, amusing characters, or people with admirable traits. Adults, however, seek only nicotine to satisfy their addiction.

Tobacco companies paid an estimated $13 million *each day* to make advertisements work to sell their products to teenagers. They seem to have gotten their money's worth. After Camel introduced its "Joe" cartoon advertising figure, Camel sales among underage smokers jumped 400 percent.

 Wow! Advertising is more powerful than I thought. What other steps is the government trying to take to protect teenagers?

One idea is to raise the price of tobacco products by taxation. The government already receives tax money for every tobacco product sold, and a plan exists to raise this amount much higher. The hope is to make tobacco products so high in cost that they will be out of reach of most teenagers' budgets. It also might make people think twice about giving cigarettes away to underage people who ask for them. As a representative of the American Cancer Society said, "The [tobacco] industry can't repeal the laws of economics."*

 It makes me mad that teenagers have been harmed by the huge advertising campaigns by tobacco companies. What can kids do to make our voices heard?

One organization, the National Center for Tobacco-Free Kids, speaks powerfully for teenagers across the nation. The center also helps teenagers take a stand against tobacco use in their own communities. They have helped teenagers around the nation organize a "Kick Butts" day that gives teens a chance to say and demonstrate how they feel about tobacco and its advertising. Ask your teacher about how to write to them or contact them by way of the Internet.

In the end, teenagers must choose for themselves whether or not to use tobacco. As the chapter pointed out, people who do not start smoking during the teenage years will probably never start. A goal of the new rules, therefore, is to help young people get through the teenage years without ever having started smoking.

*John D. Giglio, as quoted by M. Grossman and F. J. Chaloupka in Cigarette taxes: the straw to break the camel's back, *Public Health Reports* 112 (1997): 291–297.

395

---

teens and adults. (Examples are those laws that prohibit teens from buying or possessing tobacco product until the age of 18; another topic could be whether students think there should be a ban on smoking in all businesses.)

Provide time for research and discussion before having groups choose a stand on topics that have been chosen. Then have the class debate the issues. Although it may be difficult for some groups to support sides they

do not believe in, they will be able to effectively support the issue if they attempt to look at the issue from another person's point of view. Make sure that you don't take sides in the debate, or allow false information to be supported by one side or the other. At the conclusion of the class make sure that you follow up with your own evidence and support for the topics discussed.

CNN® You can update your coverage of health and fitness topics, as well as spark lively classroom discussion and deeper understanding, by using the **CNN Health and Fitness Updates.** These video updates are produced by Turner Educational Services, using the resources of CNN, the world's first 24-hour, all-news network.

With the introduction of the **CNN Health and Fitness Updates,** West Educational Publishing is proud to be the exclusive partner of CNN for textbook/video integration in high school health. By making use of the **CNN Health and Fitness Updates** you can bring the power of CNN, the network known for providing in-depth, live coverage and analysis of breaking news events, to your health class.

For assistance in using and incorporating the **CNN Health and Fitness Updates** into your classroom presentations, see the *Classroom Guide to the CNN Health and Fitness Updates.* The **CNN Health and Fitness Updates** are available with West Educational Publishing's *Health: Making Life Choices.*

395

VOCABULARY

1. Answers will vary.

2. Mainstream smoke is the smoke that goes straight from the cigarette into the smoker's lungs; sidestream smoke is the smoke that escapes from the burning end of a cigarette, cigar, or from burning pipe tobacco that is inhaled by the smoker and others.

3. a. asthma **b.** unethical **c.** sinuses **d.** emphysema **e.** bronchitis **f.** ulcers

4. a. mucus **b.** tars **c.** leukoplakia **d.** quid

RECALL

SECTION 1

1. slowed heart rate, lowered blood pressure, nausea, headache, irritability, restlessness, anxiety, drowsiness, inability to concentrate, and a craving for another dose (p. 375)

SECTION 2

2. Anywhere from one-fourth to one and one-half pounds of sticky tar collect in the lungs each year, causing emphysema and diseases of the lung. (p. 377)

3. bronchitis, emphysema, chronic obstructive lung disease, lung cancer (pp. 378–380)

4. Lungs are filled with carcinogens, which are cancer causing. The tar makes the coat of mucus thick and slows down the action of the cilia. Each puff on a cigarette paralyzes the cilia and numbs the throat so

CHAPTER 14 Review

Summarizing the Chapter

Your ability to respond correctly to the following statements ensures your understanding of the main concepts in the chapter.

1. Describe the immediate effects of nicotine on the body.

2. Describe the effects of smoking on the respiratory system.

3. Describe the effects of smoking on the cardiovascular system.

4. List negative aspects of tobacco use other than health hazards.

5. Identify ways in which other people's tobacco smoke harms nonsmokers who are exposed to it.

6. Identify the health problems associated with the use of smokeless tobacco.

7. Describe the withdrawal symptoms that follow quitting smoking and the pleasures of doing so.

Learning the Vocabulary

nicotine	ulcers
gateway drug	sinuses
tars	mainstream smoke
carcinogens	sidestream smoke
emphysema	environmental tobacco
bronchi	smoke (ETS)
mucus	asthma
cilia	smokeless tobacco
bronchitis	quid
chronic obstructive lung	leukoplakia
disease (COLD)	unethical
carbon monoxide	

Answer the following questions on a separate sheet of paper.

1. Write a paragraph using at least ten vocabulary terms. Underline each of the terms that you use.

2. Explain the difference between mainstream smoke and sidestream smoke.

3. *Matching*—Match each of the following phrases with the appropriate vocabulary term from the list above:
a. difficulty breathing, with wheezing sounds from the chest
b. against the rules of right and wrong
c. spaces in the bones of the skull
d. disease that causes flexible air sacs to burst.
e. thickened mucus, and deep, harsh coughing
f. open sores in the lining of the digestive system.

4. a. _____ is a slippery secretion produced by cells of the body's lining.
b. Burning _____ release many carcinogens.
c. _____ are whitish or grayish patches in the mouth that may lead to cancers.
d. A small portion of smokeless tobacco is referred to as a _____.

Recalling Important Facts and Ideas

Section 1

1. List the withdrawal symptoms people experience as a dose of nicotine wears off.

Section 2

2. Explain what tar does to the respiratory tract.

3. Name four respiratory problems associated with smoking.

4. Describe why smokers are more susceptible to respiratory infections than nonsmokers.

5. List the effects nicotine has on the heart and cardiovascular system.

6. In what ways can smoking affect the unborn child of a pregnant woman?

Section 3

7. What can carbon monoxide do to a passive smoker?

8. Describe the steps that are being taken to protect nonsmokers from sidestream smoke.

Section 4

9. What are the dangers to oral health of using smokeless tobacco?

10. Describe why using smokeless tobacco is not preferable to smoking, for health's sake.

Section 5

11. How can quitting smoking improve a person's health?

the smoker experiences relief from irritation. Bronchitis usually develops in all smokers after about ten years. Emphysema takes longer to develop. (p. 378)

5. speeds up the heart rate, raises the blood pressure, reduces the amount of oxygen the blood can carry, triggers the formation of blood clots, reduces the blood flow in the heart's own arteries (p. 381)

6. smaller babies, premature births, miscarriages, a doubled risk of birth defects and impaired development in children up to age 11, early death of infants (p. 382)

SECTION 3

7. A nonsmoker may suffer from the same lack of oxygen in the blood as is typical for a smoker. (p. 384)

8. Most restaurants have nonsmoking areas, and some ban smoking altogether; motels provide nonsmokers' rooms; federal ban on smoking on most airline flights; states ban smoking in public transportation, hospitals, elevators, schools, and libraries. (p. 385)

12. Explain why smokers sometimes gain weight when they quit smoking.

13. List the different programs available for smokers who want to quit.

14. Explain how you can influence your peers not to smoke.

Critical Thinking

1. Some individuals have filed suit against the tobacco industry because family members have died due to smoking. What might be the arguments for each side of the controversy? Which side would you support and why?

2. Laws have been passed to prohibit smoking on all domestic airplanes. Where else should smoking be prohibited? What action can you take to help prohibit smoking in those places? Why will you take this action?

Activities

1. Draw a picture of the human body and label the health problems associated with smoking. What parts of the body are most affected and why?

2. Smoking causes emphysema. This activity will make you feel like a person who has emphysema. You need a straw to perform this activity. Plug your nose and put the straw in your mouth and breathe through it. Now jog in place for two minutes. Plug your nose and breathe through the straw again. Does breathing through the straw make you feel uncomfortable? In what ways are you uncomfortable? What have you learned about emphysema from this activity?

3. List ten reasons why you would not smoke.

4. Form small groups in your class and go to the elementary school and give a presentation on not smoking. How can you persuade these young kids not to smoke? What strategies might work best with these kids? Suggestions: lectures, puppet shows, plays, admired role models.

5. Find someone you know who smokes. Make charts showing what times of day the person smokes. Use the information to try to help the person quit. Convince the person to replace smoking behaviors with other positive health behaviors. Give rewards for positive progress and penalties for negative smoking behavior.

6. Write to your local chapter of the American Heart Association, Lung Association, or Cancer Society for information about ways to quit smoking. Share the information with the rest of your class.

7. Go to the library and look up ways companies market their cigarettes in our country and other countries. Compare and contrast the ways that cigarettes are marketed in several countries.

8. Make a collage of different smoking advertisements found in magazines. Change the advertisements to persuade people not to smoke. Put these collages up around the school.

9. Choose one of the following statements from the American Cancer Society and write a one-page essay on it.

► Smoking is the #1 preventable cause of death in the nation.

► Every 13 seconds, someone dies from a tobacco-related illness.

► Cigarette smoking is responsible for one out of every five American deaths.

► More people die from tobacco-related illnesses than from alcohol, traffic accidents, illicit drugs, murder, and suicide.

► 85 percent of teenagers who smoke two or more cigarettes, and overcome the initial discomfort, will become addicted smokers. .

► Nicotine is a deadly poison which, if taken in high doses, can kill.

Making Decisions about Health

1. A middle-aged friend has been a heavy smoker most of her life. The health effects are obvious to you, but not to her. She's short of breath and can walk only a few steps without wheezing. She suffers from frequent colds and her physician has warned her that she's risking severe heart trouble if she continues to smoke. Now the physician has told her family that her life is in imminent danger, "She must stop smoking or else I can't be responsible for her health care anymore." Still, she refuses to quit. "I'd rather smoke and die happy," she says "than live without my habit." What would you do and why?

13. Classes are offered by Smokenders, the American Cancer Society, the American Lung Association, and the American Heart Association. (p. 391)

14. Answers will vary; could include: by confronting the person, but showing that you care at the same time; informing them of the health risks of smoking; commenting that their smoke is harming you; by commenting that you do not think it is cool to smoke, and, in fact, it is even unattractive. (pp. 392–393)

397

SECTION 4

9. mouth sores, mouth and throat cancers, leukoplakia, bad breath, wearing away of tooth surfaces, damage to gums (pp. 386–387)

10. Answers will vary; could include: smokeless tobacco still contains nicotine, can cause cancers of the mouth and throat, causes brown teeth and bad breath like smoking, and so on. (p. 387)

SECTION 5

11. Answers will vary; could include: live longer, take deep breaths, walk easily without getting out of breath. (p. 389)

12. Smoking is an oral behavior, and some quitters turn to another oral behavior such as eating to take its place. Drinking fluids, snacking on crunchy vegetables, and taking up a physical activity can help prevent weight gain. (pp. 390–391)

	OUTCOMES	FEATURES

CHAPTER 15

Infectious Diseases

- Identify the microbes, how they develop, and common diseases they cause.
- Describe the public health system's defenses against infectious diseases.
- Describe how the body defends itself against infectious diseases.
- Describe the course of an illness.
- Outline actions a person can take to avoid infectious diseases.
- Identify types and symptoms of food poisoning and how to prevent it.
- Discuss the transmission, symptoms, detection, and treatment of mononucleosis.

Health Strategies: How to Avoid Infections (page 410)
Life Choice Inventory: How Well Do You Protect Yourself against Infectious Diseases? (page 411)
Consumer Skills: Is It a Cold or Is It Flu? (page 412)
Straight Talk: Mononucleosis—The Kissing Disease (page 415)

CHAPTER 16

Sexually Transmitted Diseases

- List barriers to reducing the number of cases of STDs in this country.
- Describe common symptoms of STDs.
- Discuss the treatment or cures for common STDs.
- Identify potential complications of STDs.
- Describe how the AIDS virus is and is not transmitted.
- Discuss ways of eliminating the risk of contracting STDs.
- List measures to reduce the chances of contracting STDs.

Health Strategies: Avoiding Contracting Sexually Transmitted Diseases (page 440)
Consumer Skills: Tricks Used to Sell STD Treatments (page 426)
Straight Talk: The Alcohol, Drug Abuse, and STD Connection (page 444)
Teen Views: Would your behavior toward a classmate change if that person contracted AIDS? If so, how would it change? (page 442)

CHAPTER 17

Lifestyle Diseases: Diabetes, Cardiovascular Disease, and Cancer

- Identify risk factors that contribute to diabetes, heart disease, stroke, and cancer.
- List the warning signs of diabetes.
- Describe the two types of diabetes and how they differ.
- Explain the long-term effects of diabetes on the body.
- Explain prevention and control of diabetes.
- Identify the parts of the cardiovascular system and their functions.
- Describe the major diseases of the cardiovascular system and some medical treatments for each.
- List the warning signs of heart attack and stroke.
- Identify the risk factors for cardiovascular disease.
- Explain how to reduce the risks of cardiovascular disease.
- Identify the four classes of cancer.
- Explain how cancer develops.
- Discuss the risk factors of cancer.
- Describe the methods of detection and treatment for cancer.
- Discuss the implications of living with cancer.
- Describe the links between nutrition and cancer prevention.

Health Strategies: Reducing the Risk of CVD (page 466)
Health Strategies: Helping a Friend with Cancer (page 480)
Life Choice Inventory: How Healthy Is Your Heart? (page 468)
Life Choice Inventory: How Well Do You Protect Yourself against Cancer? (page 478)
Consumer Skills: Deception of the Desperate (page 483)
Straight Talk: Diet for Disease Prevention (page 486)

TEACHING SUPPORT

Vocabulary: Learning Key Terms, Crossword Puzzle, Infectious Diseases Puzzle
Study Outline
Reading Cloze
Reteaching: Word Choice, Understanding Infectious Disease, Bacteria vs. Virus
Enrichment: Food Poisoning, Famous Contributors, The Course of a Disease, Public Service Message
Career Brief: Clinical Laboratory Technologists and Technicians
Life Choice Inventory: How Well Do You Protect Yourself against Infectious Diseases?

Handouts: The First Vaccine, Researching Infectious Diseases, Immunization Schedule, U.S. Public Health Service Objectives for the Nation
Teacher Information Sheet: How Fever Works
Quizzes: Sections 1–4
Tests: Chapter 15 Test A, Chapter 15 Test B
Transparencies: How Viruses Multiply and Cause Infection, How Infections Spread

Vocabulary: Learning Key Terms, Avoiding STDs Puzzle, Crossword Puzzle
Study Outline
Reading Cloze
Reteaching: Understanding AIDS and Other STDs, Word Choice, Multiple Choice, Common Sexually Transmitted Diseases
Enrichment: Getting the Word Out, Role Play
Career Briefs: Physicians
Handouts: U.S. Public Health Services Objectives for the Nation, HIV Behavior Diagrams

Quizzes: Section 1–3
Tests: Chapter 16 Test A, Chapter 16 Test B

Vocabulary: Learning Key Terms, Crossword Puzzle, Fill in the Blanks
Study Outline
Reading Cloze
Reteaching: Warning Signs of Diabetes, Heart Attack, Stroke, and Cancer; Paragraph Completion; Heart Parts and Blood Flow; Reducing Your Risk of Diabetes, Heart Attack, Stroke, and Cancer
Enrichment: Taking Control of My Heart Goals, When a Friend Has Cancer
Career Briefs: Radiologic Technicians
Life Choice Inventories: How Healthy Is Your Heart?, How Well Do You Protect Yourself against Cancer?
Handouts: Factors Beyond People's Control, U.S. Public Health Services Objectives for the Nation, Diabetes, Heart Disease, Stroke, Cancer Scenarios, Practical Tips for Teens with Diabetes

Quizzes: Sections 1–10
Tests: Chapter 17 Test A, Chapter 17 Test B
Transparencies: The Heart's Major Arteries, An Overview of the Cardiovascular System, Two Kinds of Pressure in the Capillaries, The Formation of Plaques in Atherosclerosis, A Thrombus and an Embolus, The Effect of Stroke Location, Comparing HDL and LDL, Cancer Initiators and Promoters, Cancer Cures by Surgery

MULTIMEDIA SUPPORT

- Health Video Library
- CNN Health and Fitness Update Videos
- Westest
- Student Review Software
- Diet Analysis Software
- Nutrition CD-ROM

LESSON PLANNING

You will find detailed daily lesson plans for both **traditional scheduling** and **block scheduling** in your Teacher's Resource Box.

KEY POINTS

Chapter 15 is 20 pages long and is divided into four sections. This chapter introduces students to microbes and focuses on the transmission of those microbes that cause infectious diseases. The importance of a public health system in the control of infectious diseases is stressed. Also explained fully is the defense against infectious diseases provided by the body's immune system. Students are given some health strategies they can use to minimize their risks of infection.

ACTIVITY TO INTRODUCE THE CHAPTER

Ask students how many of them have had chicken pox. Explain that chicken pox is caused by a virus and that most people get this disease only once. Ask the students why someone might never get chicken pox. Then tell students that some people do get this infectious disease twice. Why might this happen? (shingles occurring later in life) Ask students at what age they think most people become infected. Why do they suppose people tend to get the disease at that age? Also tell students that a chicken pox vaccination is available now, so chicken pox might just become a disease of the past, like mumps and measles. Ask students what the term *incubation* means and explain that for chicken pox it is 12 to 19 days. Review some symptoms. Explain that treatments might include an anti-itching lotion. Health-care providers

CHAPTER 15

Contents

NOT Enough Time?

If you have only two days to spend on this chapter, the following are some suggestions to help you make sure you cover the main objectives.

DAY 1 Assign Sections 1 and 2 to be read prior to class. Also assign the Life Choice Inventory, "How Well Do You Protect Yourself against Infectious Diseases?" on page 411 and Fact or Fiction on page 399. During class have students do the Focus Activity for Section 1 on page 400 and the first Discussion activity on

Infectious Diseases

FACT or FICTION

What do you think? Are the following statements true or false? If you think they are false, then say what is true.

1. It would be a great service to humankind if we could wipe out all microbes.
2. A healthy body is host to millions of microbes.
3. Washing with soap and water is an effective way to remove bacteria from the skin.
4. A hospital is a place where people can easily pick up infectious diseases.
5. Antibiotics are among the few medicines effective against viruses.
6. Fevers are dangerous, especially when people have infections.
7. Food poisoning can be fatal.

(Answers on page 414)

Fungal infection greatly magnified. The long strings are the fungus attacking cells.

Introduction

You are surrounded by millions of **microbes**—living things too small for the human eye to see without the help of a microscope. A microscopic zoo lives all around you—on the surfaces you touch, in the air you breathe, on the forkfuls of food that you lift to your mouth, and on the surfaces of your body.

Most microbes are harmless. Many even perform valuable services, such as decomposing wastes, making nutrients, and even making bread rise. Others, however, can cause **infectious diseases**. These microbes are known as **pathogens**. This chapter focuses on the pathogens and offers strategies you can use to protect yourself against infections.

might also suggest that the infected person's fingernails be cut. Discuss why this might be necessary.

Vocabulary worksheets are provided in the Teacher's Resource Box.

BULLETIN BOARD IDEAS

Recreate the Health Strategies, "How to Avoid Infections" (p. 410), on the bulletin board. If you are artistic, draw a person suited up in a protective suit, with a gas mask, (like something from the film *Outbreak*) or look for an advertisement with something like this. Position the strategies around the figure.

Answers to FACT or FICTION

1. **False.** Many microbes are harmless and provide services needed for life.
2. **True.**
3. **True.**
4. **True.**
5. **False.** Antibiotics are useful against bacteria but useless against viruses.
6. **False.** Fevers are part of the body's defense against infection, and low fevers are not dangerous.
7. **True.**

page 401. Also have students do the Focus Activity for Section 2 on page 404.

DAY 2 Assign students to read Sections 3 and 4; the Consumer Skills, "Is It a Cold or Is It Flu?" on page 412; and the Straight Talk, "Mononucleosis—The Kissing Disease" on

page 415. During class have students do the Role Play activity on page 407, the last Comprehension Check on page 407, and the first Discussion activity on page 411.

FOCUS

OUTCOMES

In this section students will learn the:

1. General classes of microbes that cause infectious diseases.

2. Modes of transmission of microbes.

FOCUS ACTIVITY

Place several microscopes around the classroom with samples of water taken from local creeks or ponds. A concave slide can be used. Next to the microscope, place a glass container with a larger sample of the same water. Attach an index card that reads, "What do you see?" Explain to the students that the water under the microscope is the same as that in the glass container. Discuss the differences in what they see.

TEACH & APPLY

BACKGROUND INFORMATION

You might want to tell students that the normally harmless bacteria that live on the skin, in the digestive tract, and elsewhere in the human body are called endogenous bacteria. Some normally harmless, endogenous bacteria can become pathogenic, given the opportunity. These bacteria are often called opportunists because they take advantage of the opportunities that come their way.

Meet the Microbes

The **bacteria** and the **viruses** are two types of microbes. Some bacteria can be beneficial. For example, those normally found in the human digestive tract protect *against* some diseases and help digest food. If a person's immune system becomes weakened, though, even these normally helpful bacteria may cause illness. As for viruses, they specialize in causing illness. They have no known beneficial functions.

Bacteria and viruses cause many different diseases. The next two sections discuss a few of the more common disease-causing bacteria and viruses.

In addition to bacteria and viruses, **fungi**, **protozoa**, **worms**, and other **parasites** also cause illness. These are all general classes, within which exist both innocent and harmful varieties.

Bacteria

Many bacteria grow and multiply best in environments like the human body: warm, dark, moist, and nutrient-rich. Bacteria thrive inside deep puncture wounds, where medicines applied to the surface cannot reach. Normally, ordinary soap makes bacteria slippery so that they are easy to wash away with water. A puncture wound, however, requires medical attention.

Tetanus A type of bacterium especially likely to invade a puncture is the one that causes **tetanus**. This disease is serious and often fatal, even when the person receives medical help. Tetanus bacteria produce a poison that causes uncontrollable muscle contractions. When the muscles that work the lungs and heart become involved, tetanus kills the person. Tetanus shots provide immunity against the tetanus poison.

Tuberculosis Worldwide, one bacterium has recently gone on a rampage. **Tuberculosis (TB)** infects a new person every second of every day, and kills millions each year. The World Health Organization has declared a global state of emergency for TB, a disease that 20 years ago was thought to be under control. In developing countries, TB causes more than a fourth of all adult deaths. In the United States, in spite of modern public sanitation and advanced medical treatments, TB is spreading and is killing more and more people each year.

Of particular worry are new **drug-resistant** strains of TB that fail to respond to even the most powerful antibiotics. Some place blame for creating such fierce strains of TB on ill people who fail to complete their prescribed antibiotic therapy. The course of therapy for TB can last up to a year, but some people take the drug just until the worst symptoms are gone. At this point, the drug has killed off only the most sensitive of the bacteria. The ones remaining are a sort of "superstrain" that are less affected by the antibiotic. Once the drug is gone, these resistant bacteria multiply rapidly, causing a renewed infection that must be treated with a different antibiotic. If the patient repeats the mistake of cutting the antibiotic therapy short, the result is a strain of TB against which *two* antibiotics are useless. As the resistant TB

enrichment

You might want to share the following information with your students.

Because antibiotics are overused in the

United States, antibiotic-resistant bacteria are becoming a great threat to health. For example, suppose a person is taking an antibiotic for a particular condition. This person has a large population of normally harmless bacteria in the digestive tract. While the antibiotic is gles can pass the virus to others, who will get chicken pox if they have not previously had it.

Another illness possibly caused by a virus, **chronic fatigue syndrome**, makes its presence known only through a severe, never-ending tiredness that disrupts normal life completely. People who feel worn out shouldn't jump to the conclusion that they suffer from this illness, though. Some more common causes of fatigue are too much stress, caffeine addiction, mental depression, too little sleep or physical activity, and boredom. These and other causes of fatigue are more easily treated than the syndrome.

 Viruses are not cells. Viruses cause diseases by invading cells and forcing them to reproduce viruses. Some remain in the body for life.

Other Pathogens

In addition to bacteria and viruses, pathogens include the fungi—both **yeasts** and **molds**. Fungi cause an amazing variety of illnesses, from **athlete's foot** to dangerous and incurable lung infections.

Next in the pathogen lineup come protozoa, single-celled creatures that cause diarrhea and other ills. As for worms and other parasites, the most dangerous of these are fairly rare in the United States. Some worms and parasites, such as **pinworms** and **head lice**, are common and easily cured.

 Fungi (yeasts and molds), protozoa, worms, and other parasites cause a variety of diseases.

Answer the following questions on a sheet of paper.

Learning the Vocabulary

The vocabulary terms in this section are *microbes, infectious diseases, pathogens, bacteria, viruses, fungi, protozoa, worms, parasites, tetanus, tuberculosis (TB), drug-resistant, Lyme disease, cold, flu, shingles, chicken pox, chronic fatigue syndrome, yeasts, molds, athlete's foot, pinworms,* and *head lice.*

1. Write a paragraph using at least ten vocabulary terms. Underline the terms you use.

Learning the Facts

2. What is the difference between viruses and bacteria?

3. List five types of microbes.

4. Which type of bacterium commonly invades puncture wounds?

5. What are the symptoms of Lyme disease?

6. List three common causes of fatigue.

Making Life Choices

7. Young children get a greater number of infections than adults. List as many reasons as you can think of why children are more susceptible to pathogens. As a teenager, have you found that you are more or less susceptible to pathogens than when you were a young child? Why do you suppose that this is so?

Glossary

- **cold:** an upper respiratory tract infection.

- **flu:** short for **influenza** (in-flew-EN-za), a highly contagious respiratory infection caused by any of a variety of viruses.

- **shingles:** a painful skin condition caused by the reemergence of the chicken pox virus in later life.

- **chicken pox:** a usually mild, easily transmitted viral disease causing fever, weakness, and itchy blisters.

- **chronic fatigue syndrome:** unexplained repeated bouts of extreme fatigue that bed rest does not cure and that last at least six months; caused by a virus.

- **yeasts:** one-celled fungi, some of which cause diseases.

- **molds:** many-celled fungi, some of which cause diseases.

- **athlete's foot:** a fungal infection of the feet, usually transmitted through contact with floors.

- **pinworms:** small, visible, white parasitic worms that commonly infect the intestines of young children.

- **head lice:** tiny, but visible, white parasitic insects that burrow into the skin or hairy body areas.

3. Many kinds of bacteria are harmless or even beneficial. (True)
4. Certain kinds of viruses have beneficial functions. (False)
5. Bacteria cause tetanus, Lyme disease, and tuberculosis (TB). (True)
6. Fungi, protozoa, worms, and other kinds of parasites can also cause illness. (True)
7. Thanks to modern medicine, tuberculosis is no longer a life-threatening disease. (False)

8. Many diseases, such as tuberculosis, malaria, pneumonia, and many sexually transmitted diseases, are becoming increasingly drug resistant. (True)
9. Viruses cause disease by taking over normal cells. (True)
10. Fungi and molds are viruses. (False)

SECTION 2

FOCUS

OUTCOME

In this section students will learn:

1. The defenses against infectious diseases offered by the public health system.

FOCUS ACTIVITY

Ask the students to list ways the school district attempts to provide protection against infectious diseases. Encourage students to include help provided by custodial crews, cafeteria staff, bus drivers, teachers, school nurses, and administrators. If available, distribute the school district's immunization requirements. Discuss students' lists in class. Also mention their responsibility to stay home when they are truly sick with an infectious disease.

TEACH & APPLY

Key Passage

Your Transparency Acetate Binder contains an overhead, "How Infections Spread," which illustrates the process described in this paragraph.

SECTION 2
Public Defenses against Infectious Diseases

With so many pathogens bombarding everyone every day, why aren't people ill from infection most of the time? Actually, they would be, except that people have defenses. Public programs to control infections provide one line of defense. People's own barriers and immune systems provide another.

How Diseases Spread   To understand how diseases are prevented, it helps to know how they spread. One way to view the spread of disease is as a cycle. An infected person (the host) contaminates the air, food, or objects near another, who breathes the air or eats the food or handles the objects and transfers the pathogen to his or her body. Chances are that, once inside, the pathogen will grow and multiply in the body of the new host, causing disease.

An example might help to illustrate the cycle. Not long ago, students at a certain high school were coming down with the dangerous liver disease **hepatitis** in record numbers. Health officials hurried to test the school's water, its cafeteria food, and adult employees to find a person who carried the hepatitis virus. They had no luck. Finally, someone noticed that all the sick students had something else in common—they all liked to stop at the same neighborhood bakery for glazed doughnuts and other baked goods. Have you guessed how the students contracted hepatitis? A baker at the shop was suffering from an active case of hepatitis, but thought it was only flu. Through unsanitary food-handling practices used at the bakery, he had contaminated the glaze that coated most of the sweet items in the shop. Because glaze is not cooked and is kept for use from day to day, the virus lurking there survived to infect many. Once the host had been identified, the cycle of infection was broken, and the threat of new cases vanished.

Public Programs against Pathogens   Public sanitation measures provide some protection against infections. Government agencies chlorinate public water supplies and treat sewage to kill pathogens that could otherwise contaminate drinking water. Where sanitation is poor, sick people pass on diseases such as **cholera** through untreated water. People who travel to countries with poor public health systems must take precautions against infections that may be common to a particular area. Travelers should avoid raw fruits, vegetables, meats, and seafood. In addition, they should boil local water for at least five minutes before using it.

In public pools and other shared facilities, **disinfectants** are applied to surfaces to kill microbes before they can spread. Even simple bathing and washing each day with soap and water washes many bacteria away and protects against some infections. In case of a cut or other wound, **antiseptics** prevent bacterial growth on the skin.

Immunization   Public health programs often control viral diseases by destroying animal and insect carriers of viruses, and by immunizing household pets. For example, **rabies** is spread to people through bites or scratches from infected animals. To protect against rabies, health departments require that pets be immunized and that infected animals be destroyed.

Some illnesses in people can also be prevented by immunizing people. This involves injecting a **vaccine**—a drug made from the pathogen or from a

MINI Glossary

hepatitis: a liver disease caused by any of several types of viruses transmitted by infected needles (drug use, tattoos, blood transfusions), by eating raw seafood from contaminated water, and by any contact (including sexual contact) with body secretions from infected people.

cholera (KAH-ler-uh): a dangerous bacterial infection causing violent muscle cramps, severe vomiting and diarrhea, severe water loss, and death.

disinfectants: chemicals that kill microbes on surfaces. Bleach is a disinfectant.

antiseptics: agents that prevent the growth of microorganisms on body surfaces and on wounds.

rabies: a viral disease of the central nervous system that causes paralysis and death.

vaccine: a drug made from altered microbes or their poisons injected or given by mouth to produce immunity.

QUICK QUIZ

Chapter 15, Section 2

The following quiz will help you assess your students' understanding of the material covered in this section of the chapter. You might use the quiz as an oral exercise, which will lead into a class discussion of the topics covered. Or, you might use it as a paper/pencil

quiz to evaluate your students individually.

Like the Quick Quiz, the Section Review can also be used as an assessment tool to spark class discussion or as an individual student evaluation. It can also be used as a review in preparation for this quiz.

1. The immune system provides an important barrier against infection and disease. (True)

2. A person who has been infected with a

poison it produces, which trains the body's immune system to recognize the active disease agent when it invades. Just as an airplane pilot in training practices on a flight simulator before trying out a real plane, the body practices on the vaccine as a sort of pathogen simulator. If the real invader arrives, the practiced reaction is so fast that the disease never has a chance to develop.

Status of Infectious Diseases   The status of infectious diseases is constantly changing. At present, the U.S. Public Health Service is working hardest to control the following infectious diseases: tuberculosis; hepatitis; **pneumonia**; **polio (poliomyelitis)**; **measles**; **rubella**; **mumps**; AIDS; and **hospital infections**, which may include any of these or others. Many people are admitted to hospitals because of infectious diseases. The diseases spread easily to others, causing much preventable illness and expense.

While public health systems can control diseases, they can seldom completely eliminate a disease. One disease, **smallpox**, may be an exception. For all others, though, control is the best outcome to hope for. Even **bubonic plague**, spread by rats in ancient days, has not been wiped out completely.

The "controlled" diseases are simply that—they are under control. Their causes are alive and with us today, waiting in the wings for public health systems to break down, or for drugs to lose their effectiveness. Just as TB has made a dramatic comeback, these other diseases could easily become uncontrollable today if conditions became right once again.

 KEY POINTS   *Public health measures such as chlorination of water, treatment of sewage, and immunization of people and animals are all used to control infectious diseases.*

SECTION 2 Review

Answer the following questions on a sheet of paper.

Learning the Vocabulary

The vocabulary terms in this section are *hepatitis, cholera, disinfectants, antiseptics, rabies, vaccine, pneumonia, polio (poliomyelitis), measles, rubella, mumps, hospital infections, smallpox,* and *bubonic plague.*

1. The intestinal disease _____ can be contracted from infected water or foods.

2. To prevent the spread of infectious agents, you can spread _____ on surfaces and use _____ on your skin.

3. Immunization can prevent some illnesses in people and involves injecting a _____.

4. The disease _____, which is spread by rats, has not been wiped out completely.

Learning the Facts

5. Why are public water supplies chlorinated?

6. How do public health programs control viral diseases?

7. List five infectious diseases that the U.S. Public Health Service is working hard to control.

Making Life Choices

8. In recent years, some groups have challenged the right of government to make laws requiring immunizations of children for entry into school. If you were given the task of justifying the need for these laws, what would you say? Why do you think so many parents fail to have their children immunized? What could be done to encourage people to be vaccinated?

MINI Glossary

pneumonia: a disease caused by a virus or bacterium that infects the lungs, with high fever, severe cough, and pain in the chest; especially dangerous to the very old or young.

polio (poliomyelitis): a viral infection that produces mild respiratory or digestive symptoms in most cases but that may produce permanent paralysis or death; preventable by immunization.

measles: a highly contagious viral disease characterized by rash, high fever, sensitivity to light, and cough and cold symptoms; preventable by immunization.

rubella: a viral disease that resembles measles but that lasts only a few days and does not cause serious complications, except in pregnancy; preventable by immunization.

mumps: a highly contagious viral disease that causes swelling of the salivary glands and, occasionally, of the testicles; preventable by immunization.

hospital infections: infectious illnesses acquired during hospitalization.

smallpox: a severe viral infection with skin eruptions; once often fatal, it is now believed to be wiped out world wide, thanks to immunizations.

bubonic plague: a bacterial infection causing swollen lymph glands and pneumonia, frequently fatal.

virus or bacteria is called a host. (True)

3. The cycle of an epidemic can often be stopped by identifying the host of a virus. (True)

4. Public sanitation measures provide no protection against infectious diseases. (False)

5. Chlorinated water is an example of a public sanitation measure. (True)

6. Cholera is a disease spread through raw meat. (False)

7. Travelers in foreign countries should take precautions against common local infections, for example, by boiling drinking water and receiving immunizations. (True)

8. Disinfectants and antiseptics prevent bacterial growth. (True)

9. Soap and water have no effect in preventing bacterial infection. (False)

10. Immunizations are given through the injection of a vaccine. (True)

FOCUS

OUTCOME

In this section students will learn about the:

1. Defenses against infectious diseases offered by the human body.

FOCUS ACTIVITY

Ask the students to create a list of ten tips for building resistance to disease and tell why these tips could work.

TEACH & APPLY

TEACHER SUPPORT

Key Passage

Tell students that during the maturing process of each T cell, the T cells are programmed to recognize one specific enemy: the antigen. Of course, there are millions of potential antigens, so millions of T cells are programmed. After programming, these cells have the ability to tell the difference between sick body cells and well ones, between cells already infected with bacteria and those not yet infected, and between cells that are acting cancerous and their innocent neighbors. When T cells destroy enemies, they save portions of the undigested antigens and attach them to the outsides of their own coatings to show other cells of the immune system what the enemy looks like.

1. Body is challenged by foreign invaders (antigens).

2. Immune system cells record shape of invaders.

Antibodies

3. Cells use this memory record to make antibodies.

4. Later, antibodies destroy foreign invaders.

5. Memory remains to make antibodies faster the next time this foreign invader attacks.

Figure 15–1   Antigens and Antibodies

The Body's Defenses and Infectious Diseases

The body has many barriers against infectious diseases. When a disease does get past the first barriers, the body can often still fight it off.

Barriers to Diseases

One way the body controls pathogens is to bar their entry into the tissues by way of barriers such as skin and membranes.

Skin   The skin is beautifully designed to protect the body. The skin produces salty, acidic sweat secretions (most microbes don't like salt or acid). It also has one-way pores that let things out but won't let microbes in.

Scientists have also found a natural antibiotic protein made by the skin with a unique killing action. Instead of killing chemically, it works mechanically by punching lethal holes in bacterial cells, causing them to leak like a sieve. The scientists hope to use the newly discovered strategy to treat infections from bacteria that have developed drug resistance.

The Body's Membranes   The membranes that line the body chambers are also barriers to pathogens. The membranes have even more defenses than the skin. These include a layer of mucus that traps microbes, cilia (beating, hairlike structures) that sweep them out, and cells and chemicals of the immune system that destroy them. These internal membranes fend off great numbers of pathogens every day. Together with the skin, they are the body's first line of defense against diseases.

Components of the Immune System   If a pathogen passes through the body's outer membranes, the immune system takes over fully. Usually, the immune system can destroy invaders in time to prevent diseases. If you are healthy now, thank your immune system for serving as your personal bodyguard. It fights off invaders every day.

It is hard to say just where in the body the immune system is located, because parts of the system are everywhere (see Chapter 6). An important part of the system is the bone marrow, which grows white blood cells called **lymphocytes**. Another part of the system is the **thymus gland**, which incubates some of the lymphocytes and changes them into **T cells** (*T* for *thymus*). The T cells then have the ability to recognize enemies. Other lymphocytes become **B cells**. B cells make **antibodies**, large molecules that serve as ammunition to kill invaders. The invaders are known as **antigens** (see Figure 15–1).

How the Immune System Fights Back   The lymphocytes travel in body fluids. During an infection, they are drawn to the lymph nodes, and make them swell. You can feel the small, lima bean– shaped lymph nodes in your throat swell up when you are getting a cold.

COOPERATIVE LEARNING

Jigsaw Study

Divide the class into groups of four. Assign each member of the group a letter. (A, B, C or D). After each member of all the groups has been assigned letters, instruct the class to separate into jigsaw groups. All the A's form one group, the B's form one group, the C's form one group, and D's form one group. Assign each group one of the four sections of Chapter 15. A's—Section 1, Meet the Microbe; B's—Section 2, Public Defenses against Infectious Diseases; C's—Section 3, The Body's Defenses and Infectious Diseases; D's—Section 4, Taking Action. Have the jigsaw groups read their sections together, complete the questions at the end of the section, and come up with a brief plan of how to explain it to their original groups. Students who struggle in the understanding of the

When a cold strikes, lymph nodes in the throat swell up.

For **Y**our **I**nformation

B (in B cells) is for *bursa*, an organ in the chicken in which B cells were first observed.

Another type of swelling is produced by the action of **histamine**, a chemical produced by some lymphocytes. Histamine inflames the site of attack and attracts defenders to it. During a cold, your nasal passages swell and become inflamed from histamine's action. In allergy, histamine's effects are unwanted, because they bring no benefits—only discomfort. The drugs called antihistamines work by reversing histamine's effects. They relieve the symptoms of unwanted swelling and inflammation from allergy.

The strike force of T and B cells works as a unit. If one of the T cells spots an enemy it recognizes, it sends out an alert (a chemical message). B cells respond to the alert by making antibodies that destroy the invader.

When T cells have identified an enemy and B cells have fired antibodies at it and killed it, still other lymphocytes (we'll call them scavenger cells) capture and devour the dead invader. In the background are still other cells (memory cells) that "remember" the invader so that the system can quickly destroy it, should it show up again.

As you might suspect, all of this death and destruction could be hazardous if it got out of hand. Therefore, the body has developed a shutoff system to control it. The immune response is shut down and other cells become active as the battle comes to an end.

Immunity   When the action is over, only some antibodies and memory cells remain, but they carry the history of what has happened. Memory cells live on for many years. They are responsible for the immunity that follows many infections or immunizations.

You may wonder why people can't develop immunity to colds, flu, or cold sores. Why do people get these illnesses over and over again? Why don't the memory cells do their job? Actually, it is likely that the symptoms of sickness we call "a cold" represent many *different* colds, each caused by a different pathogen. Also, some flu viruses can hide from the immune cells just well enough to keep the cells from recognizing them when they reinfect the person. The reason why a person who gets cold sores (fever blisters) will have

MINI Glossary

lymphocytes (LIM-fo-sites): white blood cells, active in immunity.

thymus gland: an organ of the immune system.

T cells: lymphocytes that can recognize invaders that cause illness.

B cells: lymphocytes that make antibodies.

antibodies: large protein molecules produced to fight infective or foreign tissue.

antigens: foreign substances in the body, such as viruses or bacteria, that stimulate the immune system to produce antibodies.

histamine (HIST-uh-meen): a chemical of the immune response that produces inflammation (swelling and irritation) of tissue.

COMPREHENSION CHECK

On posterboard, have students illustrate the way the body fights invasion by pathogens.

ROLE PLAY

Select students to role play the immune system and how it reacts when a pathogen gets into the body. Select students to play the role of T cells, B cells, antibodies, lymphocytes, and a pathogen. When the pathogen comes into the class, show the actions the immune system would take.

COMPREHENSION CHECK

Have students write a description of the course of an illness through the eyes of a specific pathogen (see pages 408–409). Be sure to identify which diseases they are.

GROUP ACTIVITY

Working in pairs, the students should select an infectious disease and trace the course of that disease through the five periods (see Figure 15–2 on page 408). Research time will be needed to obtain the proper incubation period, the correct symptoms, any medical treatment, and total recovery time. The final product can be an oral presentation, a poster, or a written report.

COMPREHENSION CHECK

Ask the students to explain why it might be a bad idea to try to reduce a slight fever during an infection. Discuss how a fever fights disease (see page 409).

material will benefit from the other students who have a good idea of how to explain the information to others. Another requirement for the jigsaw groups is to come up with a chart or poster that will help them teach their section to their original groups. A good example of a chart or poster may be diagraming a germ entering the body and the parts of the immune system that attack the germ. Germs and attackers should be labeled and described on the poster (see Figure 15–1). Another good

chart may be one that lists many different germs and a list of the diseases caused by the different germs with a treatment following each disease.

After the jigsaw groups have completed their sections, have them return to their original groups and share their ideas and findings with the other members of their groups. By doing this, all members of the group will be given information about the chapter in a relatively short period of time.

COMPREHENSION CHECK

Have students write a fictional case study of a person with an infectious disease. They should include information about each stage of the illness.

BACKGROUND INFORMATION

Tell students that if a person was vaccinated earlier against a disease, the immune system will launch a full attack and stop the progression of the disease during incubation. In the clinical period, the symptoms have progressed to the point that a health-care provider can connect the symptoms with a particular disease (earlier, the symptoms were general, and as stated in the prodrome period explanation, they are the same for many diseases). To simplify the information in this chart, give students the following brief descriptions:

1. Incubation—microbes multiply in the body
2. Prodrome—onset of general symptoms
3. Clinical period—symptoms are specific to the disease
4. Decline—symptoms are subsiding
5. Convalescence—body repairs damage

BACKGROUND INFORMATION

The Teacher's Resource Box contains background information, "How Fever Works."

Figure 15–2   The Course of a Disease

Period	Events
1. Incubation	The period after invasion of pathogens, when they multiply in the body. The person may be unaware of the infection at this stage and may infect others without knowing it. The immune system may begin to detect the invaders. The immune system often wipes out the pathogens in this stage and stops the disease. If the immune system fails in this task, the disease progresses to the next phase.
2. Prodrome	The onset of symptoms, such as fever, sneezing, and coughing. These are the same for many diseases. In this stage, the disease is easily transmitted. The immune system is stepping up its fight.
3. Clinical	The period of symptoms known to be caused by the disease. The immune system is in full battle. (Medical treatments could possibly shorten this and succeeding stages.)
4. Decline	The period when the immune system has almost won the fight against the infection, and symptoms are going away. Memory cells form.
5. Convalescence (con-va-LESS-ence) or death	The period when the body either repairs damage and returns to normal, or dies from the effects of the illness. Upon recovery, the pathogen may or may not remain in the body. If it does, the person may remain a carrier of the disease, able to infect others even if no symptoms are evident.

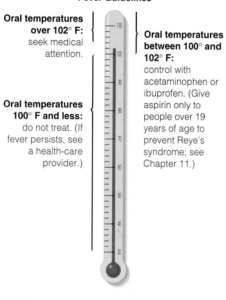

Fever Guidelines

Oral temperatures over 102° F: seek medical attention.

Oral temperatures 100° F and less: do not treat. (If fever persists, see a health-care provider.)

Oral temperatures between 100° and 102° F: control with acetaminophen or ibuprofen. (Give aspirin only to people over 19 years of age to prevent Reye's syndrome; see Chapter 11.)

Figure 15–3   Fever Guidelines

repeated outbreaks is that the virus takes up residence in the nerves of the face and hides there. When the virus becomes active again, the immune system doesn't fully recognize the old enemy fast enough to prevent an outbreak.

 KEY POINTS   *The body defends itself against infections. Skin and membranes offer a barrier to microbes. The immune system fights infections that make it past this barrier.*

Recognizing the Course of an Illness

Occasionally, pathogens break through the body's defenses and produce illness. Not all diseases develop the same way, but many do. A person who recognizes the early phases of an infection can take action right away. The five phases are described in Figure 15–2 above.

The **prodrome** symptoms listed in Figure 15–2 are ones you might have with any of a number of infections, many of them minor. One warning: if any of the prodrome symptoms listed in Figure 10–10 in Chapter 10 are present, do not delay seeking help. These symptoms can mean the disease is serious.

Antibiotics   A person who has developed a bacterial infection can often assist the immune system's defenses by taking antibiotics—drugs that prevent bacterial growth. With bacterial numbers in check, the immune system can overpower and eliminate the pathogenic bac-

QUICK QUIZ

Chapter 15, Section 3

The following quiz will help you assess your students' understanding of the material covered in this section of the chapter. You might use the quiz as an oral exercise, which will lead into a class discussion of the topics covered. Or, you might use it as a paper/pencil

quiz to evaluate your students individually.

Like the Quick Quiz, the Section Review can also be used as an assessment tool to spark class discussion or as an individual student evaluation. It can also be used as a review in preparation for this quiz.

1. The skin takes an active part in fighting off infection and diseases by releasing salty, acidic secretions. (True)
2. There is a natural antibiotic protein made

teria. Each type of antibiotic is useful only against certain kinds of bacteria, however. Therefore, it takes a trained health-care provider to select the right one and to get the dosage right.

Antibiotics are useless against viruses, because antibiotics work by preventing cell growth, and viruses are not cells. The immune system has to work by itself to wipe out the virus. All that can be done for most viral infections is to relieve symptoms until the disease runs its course.

Fever If you develop a fever, think twice before you reach for fever-relief medicine. Fever has long been feared because it often develops with dangerous diseases. However, fever itself may actually assist the immune system in its fight against infection. For example, cold viruses thrive and multiply at temperatures between 86 and 95 degrees Fahrenheit, but die off at higher temperatures. Fever also helps to activate the immune system. Figure 15–3 on the opposite page provides fever guidelines.

 Many illnesses follow a predictable course. Antibiotics act against bacterial diseases, but are useless against viruses. A mild fever can help the immune system fight an infection.

> 66 *Sickness is felt, but health not at all.* 99
>
> Proverb

SECTION 3 Review

Answer the following questions on a sheet of paper.

Learning the Vocabulary

The vocabulary terms in this section are *lymphocytes, thymus gland, T cells, B cells, antibodies, antigens, histamine,* and *prodrome.*
Fill in the blank with the correct answer.

1. When a disease attacks the body, cells known as _____ recognize the invaders, and cells known as _____ produce antibodies to fight the disease.
2. Antihistamines work by reversing _____'s effects: they relieve irritation of mucous membranes.
3. The stage of a disease when the symptoms are appearing is the _____.

Learning the Facts

4. Why are your skin and internal membranes important in defending you against infections?
5. How does the body's immune system know when a disease agent has attacked the body?
6. Why does your throat sometimes swell up when you are getting a cold?
7. How does inflammation help you to fight off a cold?
8. Identify the steps in the course of a disease. Why is it useful to know them?

Making Life Choices

9. The body's immune system is speedy and accurate in its responses to infection. In view of how "smart" the body is, what do you think of someone who hurries to take medicine every time a minor health problem sets in? When is it wise to take medicine, and when is it not wise? How can you be sure to do the right thing in each case?

MINI Glossary

prodrome: the onset of general symptoms common to many diseases, such as fever, sneezing, and coughing.

SECTION 4

FOCUS

OUTCOMES

In this section students will learn:

1. Ways people can protect themselves from infectious disease.
2. How food poisoning can be prevented.

FOCUS ACTIVITY

From a local pediatrician or from a public health office, obtain an immunization chart. Distribute copies of the chart to each student and discuss when shots should be given, how long they are good for, and if booster shots are necessary. As an assignment, have students take the chart home to record the dates of all the vaccines they have received since birth. If parent(s) cannot locate a record of immunization, the student may want to get the information from the school's office. What did students discover? Were any booster shots due? (Be sensitive to any students who may not want to share personal, private information.) Ask the students if they can think of any additional vaccines that might be needed if they were to travel to an undeveloped country.

TEACH & APPLY

DISCUSSION

Ask students if they agree with the following statements: "If food tastes and smells fine, it is OK to eat," and "It's OK to drink water from a stream if it's clear." Discuss their opinions.

SECTION 4

Taking Action

One of the most important steps a person can take to avoid infectious diseases is to keep immunizations up to date. (Chapter 10 provides a schedule of recommended immunizations.) What more can people do to prevent infections? Keep your resistance up by taking care of your immune system. It works best when given a balanced diet. Related to diet is alcohol intake. Alcohol and many other drugs are directly toxic to the immune system, weakening resistance.

Regular physical activity supports the immune system. If you don't exercise, start.

Stress also makes illness likely. You may have noticed that when you are worried or nervous about something, your throat tends to get sore. This is a warning that before long, unless you manage the stress better, the pathogens you encounter can make you ill.

The principles of self-protection against colds and other infections are summarized in the Health Strategies section on this page, "How to Avoid Infections." To see how well you protect yourself, refer to the Life Choice Inventory.

Airborne Infections

You can often avoid viral and other infections by remembering that for pathogens to cause disease, they must be transferred from a person or an object to you. Millions of pathogens are sprayed into the air by uncovered sneezes and coughs.

Imagine that the viruses or bacteria are a quart of red paint that has been sprayed all over your classroom, and is still wet. What would happen if you touched the surfaces and then touched your mouth, eyes, or nose? You would have red paint on your face. This is how bacteria and viruses are transferred to you from your surroundings.

In public places, stay a good distance away from anyone who is carelessly sneezing or coughing into the air, and touch no "red" surfaces. Wash yourself, including your hair and even your clothes, if you think you've been sprayed. Comfort sick people with soothing words from across the room instead of with hugs or kisses.

This advice holds for cold and flu viruses and for many other microbes as well. This chapter's Consumer Skills feature on page 412 explains how to tell whether your sniffle is a cold or the flu, and what to do about either one.

KEY POINTS *To minimize their risks of infection, people can keep immunizations up-to-date, keep their immune systems strong, and maintain distance when others are ill.*

Health Strategies

How to Avoid Infections

1. Take measures against bacterial growth, both on your body and in your surroundings. Maintain a cool, well-lit, dry, clean environment.
2. To remove bacteria from skin, use soap and water. To kill bacteria, use antiseptics on skin and disinfectants on surfaces and objects.
3. Obtain medical treatment for deep wounds.
4. Stay current with immunizations to develop necessary immunity before infection sets in.
5. Avoid unnecessary contact with people who are ill.
6. Do not share objects with people who are ill.
7. Wash your hands often throughout the day, especially before eating.
8. Keep away from people who are coughing or sneezing into the air.
9. Select a diet that supports immune system health, such as was described in Chapter 7.
10. Do not drink alcoholic beverages.
11. Exercise regularly.
12. Do not use tobacco.
13. Control stress.
14. Get adequate rest.

---

special needs

Interpersonal, Spatial, Musical, and Linguistic

It is commonly believed that the best way to learn something well is to teach it to someone else. In order to help your students internalize the concepts regarding infectious diseases, you may want to have them complete one or all of the following activities. These can be specifically based on the list of fourteen ways to avoid infections from the Health Strategies on this page, or you can choose other information on which to base activities. These activities are designed to help students share what they have learned with other students at your school and in the community. You will need to get the permission of the principal in order to complete these activities.

Assign artistically talented students the task of creating a comic-strip style set of posters or

How Well Do You Protect Yourself against Infectious Diseases?

On your own paper, answer the following questions with either yes or no. A no answer to any of these questions indicates a way to improve defenses

against infection. Your answers to the Life Choice Inventory are personal and private. Share them with others only if you are comfortable doing so.

1. Do you keep your environment cool, clean, dry, and well lit?
2. Do you wash your hands several times during the day and before mealtimes?
3. Are your immunizations up to date?
4. Do you heed the advice of public health departments during times when people should receive special immunizations?
5. Do you avoid sharing food, beverages, utensils, towels, and other objects with people who have symptoms of contagious infections, such as colds, cold sores (fever blisters), flu, or others?
6. Do you, whenever possible, place yourself at a distance from people who are coughing or sneezing into the air?
7. Is your diet balanced and adequate—the kind of diet your immune system needs?
8. Do you abstain from drinking alcohol?
9. Are you including exercise in your daily routine?
10. Do you make time for rest and fun?
11. Is stress under control in your life?
12. Do you abstain from using tobacco?
13. If you do get sick, do you follow the full course of treatment to prevent a relapse?

A reproducible copy of the Life Choice Inventory is provided in the Teacher's Resource Box.

DISCUSSION

Have students rate themselves on each of the 14 strategies for avoiding infections on page 410. For each one, they should rate their behavior as Excellent, Fair, or Poor. What is the one strategy that they could implement that would most improve their resistance to disease? As another way for students to assess their behavior, have them do the Life Choice Inventory.

DISCUSSION

In each of the following situations, ask the students to identify how the individual could reduce the risks of getting an infection and why the suggested behavior would reduce risk:

1. Rhonda has to work tonight and does not know how she is going to write the paper that is due tomorrow. She is very worried and may have to pull an all-nighter.
2. Ellen is sick a lot. When she goes to the doctor, he notices that she chews her fingernails.
3. John is always tired. He comes home every day, watches TV, and eats his favorite snack food—potato chips.

Food Poisoning

If you had awakened this morning with abdominal cramps, a headache, vomiting, diarrhea, and a fever, would you have suspected yesterday's meatball sandwich as the cause? Maybe you should have. At least one-third of people living in the United States are treated for food poisoning each year. It may be that almost everyone experiences a touch of some type of food poisoning in a year's time. However, most people mistakenly pass the incidents off as "stomach flu." The truth is that while some viruses do cause intestinal distress, food poisoning is a much more likely cause.

Pathogens growing in foods can make people sick in two ways: by infecting them or by poisoning them.

Pathogen Infection   In the first case, a pathogen such as the ***Salmonella*** bacterium can infect the digestive tract, causing the symptoms just mentioned. In people weakened by illness or in the very old or very young, *Salmonella* infections can be fatal.

Glossary

Salmonella: a common food-borne pathogen causing digestive system infections in many people each year.

bulletin board. They should find a way to visually/graphically represent each of the fourteen listed strategies. Remind them that they must find a way to get and keep people's attention if they want to get their message across.

Ask one group of students to write short radio-style public service announcements that can be broadcast over the school's public address system. One or more of the fourteen strategies should be included in each

announcement. Again, remind students that they must get and keep the attention of their intended audience if they want their message to get through.

A third group of students could be assigned to make the recordings. Encourage them to be creative, using music, sound effects, and their voices in order to effectively communicate.

Consumer SKILLS

Answers to Critical Thinking

1. They throw money away if they spend it on antibiotics that do them no good. Another drawback to using antibiotics to fight what is probably a virus is that the body can develop antibiotic-resistant cells that can cause the person harm later.

2. Answers will vary. Students will hopefully see a middle ground with regard to this question. Many people do overreact to symptoms, thus increasing their medical bills needlessly when the body could take care of the disease.

BACKGROUND INFORMATION

Tell students that studies show that the chances are one in three that a chicken sold in the supermarket is infected with salmonella. Tell students this is why it is important that all poultry be cooked thoroughly and kept from contact with any other foods.

BACKGROUND INFORMATION

A handout in the Teacher's Resource Box gives the U.S. Public Health Service objectives from the U.S. Department of Health and Human Services for immunization and infectious diseases.

Is It a Cold or Is It Flu?

Consumer SKILLS

Almost everyone suffers from an **upper respiratory infection** at least once each year. A person whose eyes begin to water, nose starts to run, or throat gets scratchy thinks of little else but obtaining relief from these symptoms. When this happens to you, the most important step is to decide what you have, so that you can use effective treatments. After all, what feels like the start of a cold may turn out to be something worse—even **infectious mononucleosis** or pneumonia.

Influenza, or flu, is almost always caused by a virus. Thus antibiotics bring no relief. Flu usually spreads as an **epidemic** in the spring or fall of the year. It sweeps through a population, and nearly everyone in the area suffers at least a mild attack. Flu symptoms develop one or more days after exposure to the virus. The early symptoms are identical to some of those of a cold: possible fever and chills, runny nose, sneezing, and nasal congestion. Unlike colds, though, flu brings a sudden muscle weakness and aches and pains in the arms, legs, and back. A dry, hacking cough, which produces no mucus but which may cause chest pain, is another telling sign of flu. Some people report suffering psychological depression from the flu, lasting up to a week beyond full recovery from the other symptoms.

Flu strains bear the names of the locations where they are thought to have originated—Hong Kong flu, Russian flu, Asian flu, and so on. Flu shots taken in the fall can provide immunity to some of them. However, flu shots go out-of-date each year as new strains of virus develop.

Colds can be viral or bacterial. Symptoms that characterize a cold are a sore throat; watery eyes; hoarseness; and a thick, greenish yellow nasal discharge. Some people believe that exposure to drafts or having wet feet is a sure way to bring on a cold. In reality, exposure to viruses, not wet feet or drafts, will bring on a cold.

Sometimes, though, a cold or flu turns out to be dangerous. You should definitely see a health-care provider immediately if any of the following symptoms occur:

▶ A cold or flu that is accompanied by headache or facial pain (indicating sinus infection).
▶ A deep, "honking" cough; wheezing; or shortness of breath (indicating bronchitis or pneumonia).
▶ High fever (above 102 degrees Fahrenheit).
▶ Pain in the ears.

Colds and flu are usually harmless and cannot be medicated away, even with antibiotics. Some, though, are not so ordinary. The right treatment can be life-saving.

Critical Thinking

1. *Why do you think it is important to know that flu and most colds are caused by viruses?*
2. *Some people see a physician for every sniffle, "just in case." Do you agree or disagree with this course of action? Why?*

Poisoning　Pathogens also cause illnesses by giving off poisons into food as the numbers of pathogens grow. For example, a person unfortunate enough to eat canned food contaminated with the poison **botulin toxin** faces severe, often fatal nervous system damage unless medical treatment is prompt. Symptoms of **botulism** come on fast, many times while the person is still at the table. If you or someone you're with experiences double vision,

Pursuing wellness

The following are some questions you may want to use to encourage discussion.

1. How many students get flu shots? Do they seem to help?
2. Do some students seem to catch more colds than others? Why?
3. Reasons given as to why people might catch colds more frequently are not wearing warm clothes, not keeping dry, being

muscle weakness, or difficulty swallowing or breathing after eating canned food, get medical help right away.

Preventing Food-Borne Illness
Some people have come to accept a yearly bout or two of intestinal illness. In truth, though, most of these illnesses can be prevented. To protect yourself, insist that the food you eat be prepared according to three simple rules: keep hot food hot, keep cold food cold, and keep the kitchen clean.

Rule #1. Keep hot food hot, because microbes die at temperatures above about 140 degrees Fahrenheit— piping, steaming hot. (Figure 15–4 in the margin lists other important temperatures.) Refuse hot dishes such as meatballs, cream soups, casseroles, and other foods that have been allowed to stand at room temperature or that feel just warm. Spoiled food often tastes fine, because the pathogens or toxins may have no taste or smell. However, they will still make you sick. Certainly, if the food smells or tastes bad, throw it out.

Rule #2. Keep cold food cold, because microbes divide and produce poisons very slowly at temperatures below 40 degrees Fahrenheit. Refuse cold dishes that have been allowed to stand at room temperature for two hours or more. Macaroni salad; cold meats; egg, ham, or chicken salads; and many others should be served refrigerator-cold.

Rule #3. Eat only foods that have been prepared and served on clean surfaces by clean hands. Avoid foods served with utensils that previously held raw meats or that are dirty from other uses.

Figure 15–4 Important Temperatures for Food Safety

°F

212° Boiling	210	
Cooking	200 190 180	Kills most bacteria
165°	170	
Warming	160 150	Prevents most bacterial growth
140°	140	
125°	130 120	Allows some bacterial growth
Danger	110 100 90	Rapid bacterial growth Toxins produced
	70	
60°	60	
Thawing	50	Allows some bacterial growth
40° Refrigerating	40	Slows bacterial growth
32°	30	
	20	Stops bacterial growth, but does not kill bacteria
Freezing	10	
0°	0	

SAFE TEMPERATURES / **DANGER**

Glossary

upper respiratory infection: an infection of the membranes of the nasal cavities, sinuses, throat, and trachea, but not involving the lungs.

infectious mononucleosis (MON-oh-new-klee-OH-sis): a viral infection involving mononucleocytes, a type of white blood cell. The symptoms vary from mild, coldlike symptoms to high fevers, swollen glands, and spleen and liver involvement. Also called *mono*.

epidemic (EP-ih-DEM-ick): an infection that spreads rapidly through a population, affecting many people at the same time.

botulin toxin: a potent poison produced by bacteria in sealed cans, plastic packs, or jars of food.

botulism: the often fatal condition of poisoning with the botulin toxin.

DISCUSSION

Explain to students that the best way to fight pathogens is by practicing sanitation. Ask them to make a list of some basic aids to sanitation. (Possible answers: refrigeration, heat, disinfectant, antiseptics, ultraviolet rays)

COMPREHENSION CHECK

On the board write the following:

Leading Causes of Death in the U.S. in 1900	*Leading Causes of Death in the U.S. Today*
1. Pneumonia and Flu	**1.** Heart Disease
2. Tuberculosis	**2.** Cancer
3. Inflammation of the Digestive Tract	**3.** Stroke

Compare the three leading causes of death in the United States today and those in the early 1900s. Discuss what advances have occurred to cause such a change in the first list. What impact has lifestyle had on today's list? (You may want to refer students back to the beginning of Chapter 1 where this topic is covered in more detail.)

around people who are infected, not getting enough sleep, being overly stressed, not eating right, and not washing at appropriate times. Do students think any of these reasons are more of a factor than the others? If so, which ones?

4. How do students treat their colds or flu? Do they go to the doctor, use over-the-counter medicines, use home remedies, or wait it out?

5. What recommendations would students give for avoiding colds or flu?

ASSESS

EVALUATE

Divide the students into groups of three or four and have them develop a list of ways to avoid food poisoning. Have each group read its list to the class.

SECTION 4 Review Answers

1. upper respiratory infection
2. epidemic
3. infectious mononucleosis
4. Salmonella is an actual bacteria that causes digestive system infections, while botulin toxin is the poison produced by bacteria in sealed cans, plastic packs, or jars of food. (pp. 411–412)
5. Answers will vary. Refer to the Health Strategies, "How to Avoid Infection," on page 410 for possible answers.
6. sore throat, watery eyes, hoarseness, thick, greenish-yellow nasal discharge (p. 412)
7. Answers will vary; could include: a cold or flu accompanied by headache or facial pain; deep "honking" cough, wheezing or shortness of breath; high fever above 104 degrees Fahrenheit; and pain in the ears. (p. 412)
8. Answers will vary.

CLOSE

Students should be able to answer the following questions:

1. What are some ways to prevent infections?
2. What are the symptoms of food poisoning?
3. What are some ways to protect yourself from food poisoning?

Something as simple as washing your hands can make a difference between getting sick and staying well.

Answers to FACT or FICTION Here are the answers to the questions at the start of the chapter.
1. **False.** Many microbes are harmless and provide services needed for life.
2. **True.**
3. **True.**
4. **True.**
5. **False.** Antibiotics are useful against bacteria but useless against viruses.
6. **False.** Fevers are part of the body's defense against infection, and low fevers are not dangerous.
7. **True.**

One last rule: toss out any cans of food that bulge out on top or that appear to be leaking. Even a taste of such food can cause deadly botulism. The risk of this illness far outweighs whatever pleasure you might find in the food.

If you follow these rules, you may have to skip a meal once in a while, but you can make up for it later. At least, aside from feeling hungry, you will be fine.

KEY POINTS *Food poisoning is a likely cause of intestinal distress. Pathogens growing in foods can make people sick by infecting them or by poisoning them. To protect yourself from food poisoning, keep hot food hot, keep cold food cold, and keep the kitchen clean.*

SECTION 4 Review

Answer the following questions on a sheet of paper.

Learning the Vocabulary

The vocabulary terms in this section are Salmonella, *upper respiratory infection, infectious mononucleosis, epidemic, botulin toxin,* and *botulism.*

1. At least once a year almost everyone suffers from an _____, which affects the nasal cavity, sinuses, throat, and trachea.
2. An _____ is an infection that spreads rapidly through a population, affecting many people at the same time.
3. _____ is a viral infection involving mononucleocytes.
4. What is a difference between *Salmonella* and botulin toxin?

Learning the Facts

5. List four steps a person can take to avoid infectious diseases.
6. What are some common cold symptoms?
7. List three symptoms that would require a visit to a health-care provider.

Making Life Choices

8. Take the Life Choice Inventory on page 411 to determine how well you protect yourself against infectious diseases. Identify those habits you need to change. What other health practices can you add to the list that would prevent the spread of infection?

Chapter 15, Section 4

The following quiz will help you assess your students' understanding of the material covered in this section of the chapter. You might use the quiz as an oral exercise, which will lead into a class discussion of the topics covered. Or, you might use it as a paper/pencil quiz to evaluate your students individually.

*If students have difficulty with the concepts covered in the Quick Quiz and the Section Review, you might suggest they review the material using the **S**urvey, **Q**uestion, **R**ead, **R**ecite, **R**eview (SQ3R) study method, which is described in detail in the introduction to this Teacher's Wraparound Edition.*

1. Immunization is a vital step in preventing many diseases and infection. (True)

Straight Talk

Mononucleosis— The Kissing Disease

ON LINE WITH HEALTH

You may want to have your students visit the following URLs, where they will find information and additional Web site resources to enhance their study of this chapter. As with all Web sites, you should check these out first to be sure the information found there is appropriate for your students.

National Immunization Program
http://www.cdc.gov/nip/

Infections and Immunizations
http://www.drreddy. com/shots/

Both sites are chock-full of information about diseases, shots, and so on. The first is sponsored by the National Center for Disease Control and the second by a practicing pediatrician. (Though both are good sites, the second is a lot more fun!)

Beginning at about age 15, teenagers are likely to come down with infectious mononucleosis, or "mono." Recovery from this viral attack is usually complete, and complications are rare. However, the illness can make some people feel sicker than ever before.

Why do they call mono the kissing disease?

The name "kissing disease" is related to a theory about activities of the age group most likely to get the disease—15- to 30-year-olds. People in this age range are most active in courting, and therefore in kissing, the theory goes, and mono is thought to be spread through oral contact.

Interestingly, mono sometimes sweeps through a school population as an epidemic, indicating one of two things: that mono spreads by modes other than kissing or that students in some school populations are extraordinarily fond of all of their classmates. Nevertheless, people who are married for many years hardly ever get mono, because they are only kissing each other. This makes them less likely to pick up infections.

What are the symptoms?

Mono is difficult to diagnose from symptoms alone, because it can imitate so many other conditions. One person may be infected and develop only a mild sniffle. Another may experience weakness, a severe sore throat, fever, swollen glands, an enlarged spleen,

and an infected liver with symptoms like those of the dangerous liver infection hepatitis. Mono may come on slowly or quickly. Once the first attack subsides, it can come on again with even more ferocity. Most bouts last from three to six weeks, although some cases can last even longer.

How can physicians tell whether someone has mono?

A blood test that takes just minutes can accurately diagnose mono. The test studies the white blood cells known as mononucleocytes, from which the disease gets its name. This test is the only way to distinguish mono from many other infections ranging from colds to hepatitis.

How dangerous is mono?

Luckily, few people suffer serious side effects from a bout of mono. The spleen may become sensitive and, very rarely, may rupture, requiring surgery. This is why people diagnosed with mono are advised to take it easy. Rest is the best treatment for mono. Athletes with mono are told to warm the bench instead of playing hard at a sport that may injure the spleen.

After a person recovers from mono, can it come back?

The immune system develops immunity to mono after one bout. That one course of the illness can last as long as a few months. After full recovery, mono will not strike the same person again.

415

2. A balanced diet strengthens the immune system. (True)
3. Alcohol has no effect on the immune system. (False)
4. Physical activity boosts the immune system. (True)
5. Stress stimulates the immune system and helps to prevent infection. (False)
6. You can minimize the risk of airborne infection by distancing yourself from a coughing or sneezing person. (True)
7. Frequently washing your hands is another way to minimize the risk of infection. (True)
8. Food poisoning is an unlikely cause of intestinal distress. (False)
9. Pathogens hiding in food can cause illness by infecting the digestive tract or by poisoning the food itself. (True)
10. Spoiled food is always revealed by an odd taste and smell. (False)

VOCABULARY

1. a. athlete's foot **b.** hepatitis **c.** fungi **d.** T cells **e.** head lice **f.** worms **g.** flu **h.** B cells **i.** pathogens **j.** rabies **k.** tuberculosis **l.** infectious diseases

2. a. Yeasts are one-celled fungi, while molds are many-celled fungi. **b.** Rubella only resembles measles, lasting a few days and causing no serious complications for the sufferer, except in pregnancy. Measles causes rash, high fever, sensitivity to light, cough, and cold symptoms for the sufferer.

3. a. lymphocytes **b.** Lyme disease **c.** tetanus **d.** pneumonia

RECALL

SECTION 1

1. warm, dark, moist, and nutrient rich (p. 400)

2. Answers will vary; could include: wearing high socks, wearing long pants, using tick repellent (especially on the ankles, legs, and groin area). (p. 401)

3. Answers will vary; could include: colds, flu, chicken pox, shingles, and chronic fatigue syndrome. (pp. 402–403)

SECTION 2

4. An infected person contaminates the air, food, or objects near another who breathes the air or eats the food or handles the objects and transfers the infection to his or her body. (p. 404)

CHAPTER 15 Review

prodrome
Salmonella
botulin toxin
botulism

upper repiratory infection
infectious mononucleosis
epidemic

Summarizing the Chapter

Your ability to respond correctly to the following statements ensures your understanding of the main concepts in the chapter.

1. Identify the microbes, how they develop, and common diseases they cause.
2. Describe the public health system's defenses against infectious diseases.
3. Describe how the body defends itself against infectious diseases.
4. Describe the course of an illness.
5. Outline actions a person can take to avoid infectious diseases.
6. Identify types and symptoms of food poisoning and how to prevent it.
7. Discuss the transmission, symptoms, detection, and treatment of mononucleosis.

Learning the Vocabulary

microbes	head lice
infectious diseases	hepatitis
pathogens	cholera
bacteria	disinfectants
viruses	antiseptics
fungi	rabies
protozoa	vaccine
worms	pneumonia
parasites	polio (poliomyelitis)
tetanus	measles
tuberculosis (TB)	rubella
drug resistant	mumps
Lyme disease	hospital infections
cold	smallpox
flu (influenza)	bubonic plague
shingles	lymphocytes
chicken pox	thymus gland
chronic fatigue syndrome	T cells
yeasts	B cells
molds	antibodies
athlete's foot	antigens
pinworms	histamine

Answer the following questions on a separate sheet of paper.

1. Matching—*Match each of the following phrases with the appropriate vocabulary term from the list above:*
  a. a fungal infection of the feet
  b. a disease of the liver caused by several types of viruses transmitted by infected needles and other means
  c. living things that absorb and use nutrients of organisms they invade
  d. lymphocytes that can recognize invaders that cause illness
  e. tiny but visible parasitic insects that burrow into the skin or hairy body areas
  f. visible parasites that burrow into the blood supplies of victims
  g. a viral respiratory infection that can become epidemic
  h. lymphocytes that make antibodies
  i. microbes that cause diseases
  j. spread by bites or scratches of infected animals
  k. a bacterial disease of the lungs
  l. diseases caused and transmitted from person to person by microorganisms or their toxins

2. a. What is the difference between yeasts and molds?
  b. What is the difference between measles and rubella?

3. a. _____ are white blood cells active in immunity. They include both T cells and B cells.
  b. The bacterial infection that is spread by deer ticks is called _____.
  c. A disease caused by a toxin produced by bacteria deep within a wound is called _____.
  d. _____ is a condition caused by an infection of the lungs with high fever, severe cough, and pain in the chest.

Recalling Important Facts and Ideas

Section 1
1. In what type of environment do bacteria grow and multiply best?

416

2. Name some precautions you can take against tick bites.
3. Name three diseases caused by viruses.

Section 2

4. Describe how infections spread.

Section 3

5. How does the body defend itself against pathogens?
6. How do T and B cells work together to destroy disease-causing invaders?
7. What is the role of the memory cells?
8. During which phase of infection is the immune system in full battle?
9. Why aren't antibiotics effective against viruses?
10. How does a fever assist the immune system?

Section 4

11. Name one thing that weakens the body's resistance and one thing that strengthens resistance.
12. How can you avoid contracting airborne infections?
13. What are some symptoms of *Salmonella* infection?
14. Name three rules that should be followed when preparing food.

Critical Thinking

1. In 1979 the U.S. Surgeon General stated that "the health of the people has never been better." Taking into account recent changes in the infectious disease pattern, what kind of statement do you think the Surgeon General might have made in 1989? What statement do you think will be made in 2000? Justify your answers.

Activities

1. Find a newspaper or magazine article less than one year old that discusses some aspect of infectious diseases. Write a one-page summary and reaction to the article. Include a copy of the article with the date and source.
2. Interview a local public health official to obtain the following information: how the local public health unit keeps track of local incidences of infectious diseases, what the most common infections are in the area, and what reports must be made to higher levels of government. Identify the name of the person interviewed and the agency the person works for.

3. Choose a developing country and find out which infectious diseases are common in that country. Discuss what is being done to control the diseases.
4. On the left half of a poster board, make a collage of advertisements for cold remedies. On the right half, collage your own non-drug alternatives for treating a cold.
5. Identify some of the community programs in your area that are aimed at preventing disease. List the name, address, and phone number of each program and the services they provide to help reduce the spread of infectious disease.
6. Choose a foreign country you would like to visit and find out what health precautions are necessary to travel to that country. What vaccines are necessary and why?
7. Choose one of the infectious diseases mentioned in the chapter such as cholera, hepatitis, mumps, measles, and so on. Do additional research on the disease you choose. After your research, write a one-page essay on the methods you would use to control or wipe out the disease.
8. Find out more about parasitic worms: flatworms, tapeworms, roundworms, pinworms, and hookworms. How do they invade the human body? How can they be destroyed? What problems and symptoms do they cause? Write down your findings and share the results with the rest of the class.

Making Decisions about Health

1. Your friend is really looking forward to going to a big dance at school tonight. Unfortunately he has had a headache all day, his throat is feeling a little bit sore, and he has the chills. Would you advise him to take an aspirin substitute and go to the dance or stay home and rest? Explain your reasoning.
2. Your friend has been working part-time after school in a day care center. Since she has been working there, she has had the flu several times and has had many colds. It seems that every time one of the children gets sick, your friend gets sick, too. What could you tell your friend about how pathogens are spread? How could she help protect herself from the infectious diseases?

417

SECTION 3

5. bars entry by way of skin and membranes and the immune system (p. 406)
6. If the T cells spot an enemy, they tell the B cells so that the B cells can produce antibodies to destroy it. (p. 406)
7. To "remember" the invader so that the system can quickly destroy it, should it show up again. They are responsible for the immunity that follows many infections or immunizations. (p. 407)
8. clinical (p. 408)
9. Antibiotics work by preventing cell growth, and viruses are not cells. (p. 409)
10. Cold viruses die off at temperatures above 95 degrees Fahrenheit and fever helps to activate the immune system. (p. 409)

SECTION 4

11. Answers will vary; could include: weakness—alcohol, many other drugs, and stress; strengthens—exercise and balanced diet. (p. 410)
12. Wash yourself, including your hair, and even your clothes, if you think you've been sprayed with a cough or sneeze. Do not comfort ill people with hugs and kisses. (p. 410)
13. Answers will vary; could include: abdominal cramps, headache, vomiting, diarrhea, and fever. (p. 411)
14. keep hot food hot; keep cold food cold; eat only foods that have been prepared and served on clean surfaces by clean hands. (p. 413)

KEY POINTS

Chapter 16 is 30 pages long and divided into three sections. This chapter introduces students to some of the most common STDs, including AIDS. It provides information on the transmission, causes, symptoms, complications, treatments, and preventative actions for each disease. The chapter also stresses the importance of individual choices regarding abstinence, sexual behavior, and drug usage in order to avoid STDs. The necessity for good communication between partners about sexual values, possible infection, and limits for sexual contact is discussed.

ACTIVITY TO INTRODUCE THE CHAPTER

Since the topic of this chapter is sometimes difficult for students to discuss in a mature fashion, begin with a pretest to help students separate fact from fiction on STDs. This is a safe way for students to uncover their own false beliefs without revealing them to classmates. Use the Fact or Fiction feature as the pretest. The Fact or Fiction feature might also be used by students at the end of this chapter to check their understanding and prepare them for the final test. An extension of this activity might be to have students give the Fact or Fiction statements to others, such as family members and students in other classes to determine the most common myths believed by these groups of people.

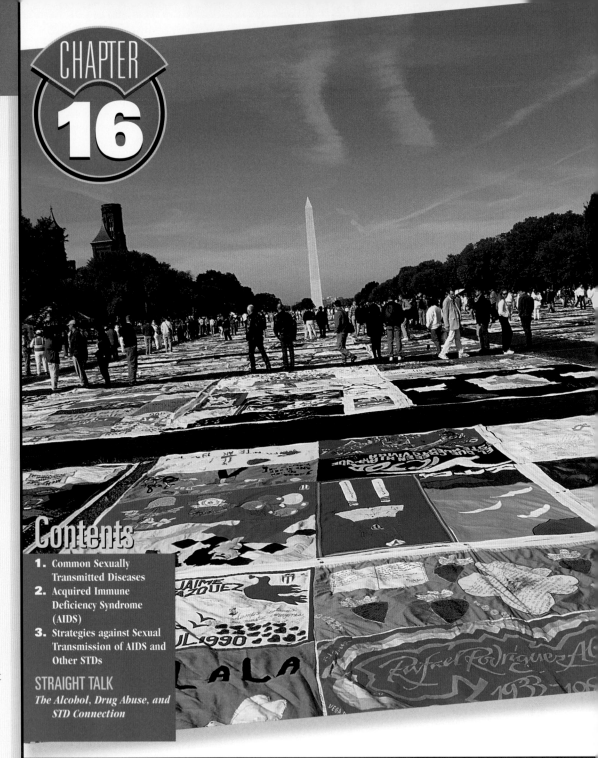

CHAPTER 16

Contents

NOT Enough Time?

Following are some suggestions to help you make sure that you cover the key topics in this chapter if you have limited time. (Refer to the daily lesson plans in your Teacher's Resource Box for additional suggestions.)

DAY 1 Assign Section 1 to be read at home before class. On Day 1, begin with the Focus Activity on page 420. Have students take the Fact or Fiction pretest on page 419. Then do the Group Project on page 422.

DAY 2 Presentations planned the previous day during the Group Project should be given, limiting each group to three minutes. Do the Comprehension Check on page 421. Assign Sections 2 and 3 to be read prior to Day 3.

DAY 3 Begin class with a discussion of

Sexually Transmitted Diseases

What do you think? Are the following statements true or false? If you think they are false, then say what is true.

1. A sexually active woman who takes birth control pills to prevent pregnancy is also protected against most forms of sexually transmitted diseases.
2. People who know what symptoms to look for can tell if they have contracted sexually transmitted diseases.
3. If someone develops an STD, the most considerate thing that person can do for his or her partner is to keep quiet about it and cease to have sexual relations with the person anymore.
4. A reliable strategy for preventing STDs is to ask potential partners about their past sexual experiences.
5. The use of condoms always protects the user from contracting STDs.

(Answers on page 443)

Introduction

The pathogens that cause **sexually transmitted diseases (STDs)** can all be transferred from person to person by way of sexual contact. That is, a person who has sexual relations with someone else who is infected can come down with one or more of these diseases. Once in the body, STDs cause symptoms ranging from rashes and bumps to blindness and death.

Some STDs are caused by bacteria. These are curable with antibiotic drugs that help the body kill off bacterial infections. Others are caused by viruses that the body cannot fight off completely, and so remain incurable, because antibiotics are useless against viruses.

The most threatening of the viral STDs is **acquired immune deficiency syndrome (AIDS)**. As the last section of this chapter shows, however, one defense, abstinence from sexual intercourse, is 100 percent effective against AIDS and all other STDs.

This discussion refers to many parts of the body. For pictures and explanations of these body parts, you may want to review Chapter 6. Looking ahead to Chapter 20 will provide you with additional information on the reproductive organs. You may also wish to review the information in Chapter 15 on infectious diseases.

BULLETIN BOARD IDEAS

Recreate Figure 16–1, found on page 420. Condense the information so that you can make it large enough to easily be read.

Answers to

1. **False.** Birth control pills do not protect a woman against any form of sexually transmitted disease.
2. **False.** Sexually transmitted diseases often progress with no outward symptoms. An example is chlamydia.
3. **False.** If you develop an STD, the considerate thing to do is to inform your partner. This protects you from reinfection, protects the health of your partner, and protects others.
4. **False.** Asking potential partners about past sexual partners or past sexual experiences does not ensure that you will learn the truth about whether they are free of STDs.
5. **False.** Condoms may provide an effective barrier to body fluids, but they sometimes fail to protect against STDs.

FAST FACTS

The phone number for the National STD Hotline is: 1-800-227-8922.

AIDS with a few student responses to the Focus Activity on page 433. After ten minutes of discussion, use the Straight Talk on page 444 to explain how AIDS attacks the body. Have the cards prepared for the Discussion activity on page 436 and hand out to the class. Complete this activity and tell students there will be a brief quiz at the beginning of class on Day 4 to see if they understand AIDS (Quick Quiz, pages 438–439). You may assign the Close activity on page 439 to reteach the material.

DAY 4 Begin with the Quick Quiz on pages 438–439. Then do the Focus Activity on page 440. Complete the Decision Making Activity on pages 428–429. Select either the Role Play activity on page 440 or the Discussion activity on page 437, depending on the needs of your students. The Evaluation assessment or the Close activity on page 443 may be assigned as homework.

FOCUS

OUTCOMES

In this section students will learn:

1. The symptoms, treatments, complications, and prevention measures for several different STDs.

2. The effects of STDs on fertility, pregnancy, and the unborn child.

3. About other infections of the genital and urinary tract that are not sexually transmitted.

FOCUS ACTIVITY

Present students with a fictitious story about two adolescents who have been dating each other for four months. The girl, Tina, has never had sexual intercourse with anyone before, but she does not know the sexual history of her boyfriend, James. As they have grown closer emotionally, they have also grown closer physically, and Tina thinks they will soon be making a decision about intercourse. Tell the students to imagine that Tina has come to them for advice. She wants to hear the pros and cons of becoming sexually active, and she is especially concerned about STDs. They are to list three items of advice they would give Tina.

Students should write their advice on blank paper with no names and you should collect them personally. Write a few of the students' answers on the board. Emphasize those that deal with obtaining a sexual history, or the idea that from the standpoint of STDs, having sex with James is like having it with everyone with whom he has

The great threat from STDs remains hidden because of embarrassment, fear, ignorance, and undertreatment due to poverty.

Figure 16–1 The Hidden Epidemic: Curable STDs

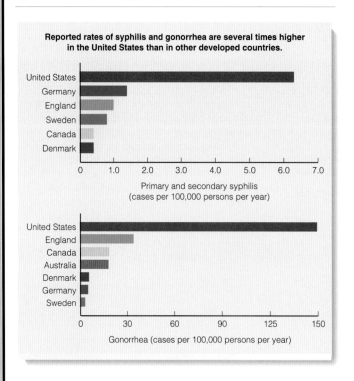

Reported rates of syphilis and gonorrhea are several times higher in the United States than in other developed countries.

Primary and secondary syphilis
(cases per 100,000 persons per year)

Gonorrhea (cases per 100,000 persons per year)

Common Sexually Transmitted Diseases

Many people suffer the effects of STDs, but few ever talk about them, because they fear embarrassment or social rejection. Meanwhile, the numbers of cases of curable STDs in this country far exceed those of other developed countries (see Figure 16-1). Teenagers, especially, seem to act as though they are not at risk. They are, though, and the numbers prove it. Teenagers account for more than a fourth of all STD cases reported in the United States each year.

STDs are so common among some groups of people that they rival the common cold in frequency. So many varieties of STDs exist in the world that space limits this section to mentioning only the most common ones. Figure 16–2 on pages 422 and 423 briefly describes the common STDs. The next few sections are arranged to present the most widespread STDs first, and to provide some details about their symptoms, harmful effects, and available treatments.

Clearly, poverty acts as a barrier to stopping the spread of STD in this country. People who lack education, health insurance, routine health care, or transportation to clinics also lack materials and knowledge that would allow them to prevent or obtain cures for STDs. Abuse of alcohol and other drugs worsens the STD problem, too, as the Straight Talk section of this chapter makes clear.

Media such as television, magazines, and movies bear some of the blame, too. They pour out a constant stream of sexual suggestions without an inkling of the associated risks or responsibilities. Medical experts have asked the media to put forth a new healthy norm of sexual behavior in the United States.

Some people hold false ideas about how to prevent STDs. They believe that simple measures such as washing the reproductive organs after intercourse or taking birth control pills can prevent STDs. These ideas are false. You will see by the end of this chapter that STD prevention requires knowledge, thought, and effort—not guesswork—to be effective.

HEALTHY PEOPLE 2000

Increase to at least 95 percent the proportion of schools that have age-appropriate HIV education curricula for students in 4th through 12th grade, preferably as part of quality school health education.

AIDS information and education programs have increased public knowledge and influenced attitudes about HIV and AIDS. However, some misinformation still persists at all levels of society. The first step toward reducing high-risk behaviors is for people to be able to use information about how HIV is transmitted to assess their own risk of becoming infected. Only when people know that they are at risk will they change their behavior.

Although intensive education has reduced high-risk sexual and drug abuse behaviors

Effective STD prevention includes regular health care.

Chlamydia

An STD that threatens the health of millions of people in the United States, but often causes no symptoms to warn them, is **chlamydia**. Men with this bacterial infection may feel a little burning when urinating or notice some mucus-like white discharge from the penis. Some may feel pain in the testicles. A few others may develop greatly enlarged lymph glands in the groin or may become infertile from a long-standing infection. Many men, however, have no symptoms at all.

Women with this infection may have some discharge from the vagina. Many, though, have no symptoms. A few have burning pain when urinating, pain in the lower abdomen, fever, bleeding or pain with sexual intercourse, or irregular menstrual periods.

With or without symptoms, chlamydia can progress to injure the reproductive organs. This is one reason why regular physical examinations that include STD tests are recommended for sexually active people. Many STDs can be silently progressing without symptoms to alert the person of their presence.

In advanced cases, chlamydia spreads to the deeper pelvic structures of women—a dangerous condition known as **pelvic inflammatory disease (PID)**. Girls age 19 and younger may run a 10 times greater risk of PID than women a few years older. The immature reproductive tissues of teenagers are believed to be more susceptible to infection leading to PID. More than any other condition, PID has the ability to cause sterility in women. Men, too, may become sterile when chlamydia spreads to the testicles.

Because most people have no symptoms, they seek no treatment and allow the disease to do its damage unopposed. Without routine testing, sexually active men and women may unknowingly suffer damage from chlamydia. Equally unknowingly, they may spread it to others.

When chlamydia damages a woman's reproductive tract, she becomes likely to experience an extremely dangerous and potentially fatal condition—**ectopic pregnancy**. In this condition, scar tissue blocks one or both fallopian tubes, the passages through which fertilized eggs must travel to enter the uterus. The embryo cannot implant and grow normally in the uterus. Instead, it may grow in one of the tubes, and eventually ruptures the tube. Ectopic pregnancy is shown in Figure 16–3 on page 424.

MINI Glossary

sexually transmitted diseases (STDs): diseases that are transmitted by way of direct sexual contact. An older name was *venereal diseases*.

acquired immune deficiency syndrome (AIDS): a fatal, transmissible viral disease of the immune system that creates a severe immune deficiency, and that leaves people defenseless against infections and cancer.

chlamydia (cla-MID-ee-uh): an infection of the reproductive tract, with or without symptoms; a frequent cause of ectopic pregnancy or failure to become pregnant.

pelvic inflammatory disease (PID): an infection of the fallopian tubes and pelvic cavity in women, causing ectopic pregnancy and pregnancy failures.

ectopic pregnancy: a pregnancy that develops in one of the fallopian tubes or elsewhere outside the uterus; a dangerous condition.

among some people, there is an urgent need to continue this trend and to ensure that low-risk behaviors are sustained. The public is generally aware of the linkage between intravenous drug abuse and HIV infection and of the risk for the spread of HIV infection from intravenous drug abusers to their sexual partners and children. Less well known is the risk of HIV infection among crack cocaine abusers, caused in part by the practice of exchanging sex for crack cocaine or by the

rape of drugged victims.

It is important to maintain and expand awareness for several reasons. First, educating children in school is a means of reaching the family members and sexual partners of intravenous drug abusers and crack cocaine abusers who are often difficult to contact through more focused outreach. Second, sexually active people should consider the possible drug-using practices of their current and potential sexual partners.

had contact. Explain that anybody can contract an STD, and some could have an STD and be unaware of it. Teachers should suggest that Tina ought to seek advice from her parents, a pastor, or a health-care provider.

WORKSHEETS Vocabulary worksheets are provided in the Teacher's Resource Box.

TEACH & APPLY

COMPREHENSION CHECK

Before assigning the reading in this section, put the following words on the board: *pathogen, symptom, antibiotics, discharge, infertile, bacteria, virus, lymph glands, sterility, cervix, genitals, abstinence, condom, vaginal, fetus.*

Ask students to copy each word, and rank it according to the following scale:

0—I don't know what it means.

1—I've heard the term, but I'm not sure I can explain it.

2—I am fairly certain I understand this term well enough to explain it to someone else. Explain any terms that were not ranked a "2." Students should write the definitions and use this vocabulary list to help them read the section.

BACKGROUND INFORMATION

Emphasize the point that regular check-ups are important because symptoms of an STD are not always visible. They will read repeatedly of STDs that do not announce themselves. The complications caused by these illnesses can only be avoided if health-care providers know they're there.

BACKGROUND INFORMATION

This chart contains a great deal of information about the common STDs. Its primary value will be as a reference for students as they work through the chapter. Students should be aware that the different categories of information have been condensed and that they can learn much more about the different factors for each disease in the text explanations and descriptions.

BACKGROUND INFORMATION

One of the things you'll want to do with this chart is focus students' attention on the preventive measures given for the different STDs. A conscious attempt was made by the authors to emphasize the abstinence message. While different specific measures are given for the different diseases, abstinence is mentioned first for each one.

GROUP PROJECT

Divide the class into eight groups. Each group will be assigned one STD to research. Each group will be given class time to prepare a 3–5 minute talk on its assigned disease. Students should be encouraged to create visual aids such as transparencies (drawn by students and made by you), posters, models, or chalk drawings. Each group must include information on cause, symptoms, treatment, complications, and prevention. Each group must also make a set of flash cards that teach about this disease. Cards should contain a question on one side and the answer on the other, such as: "What are three symptoms of chlamydia?" Answer, "burning during urination, a discharge, and abdominal pain."

Figure 16–2 Common Sexually Transmitted Diseases

	AIDS	Chlamydia	Genital Herpes	Gonorrhea
Symptoms	Swollen lymph glands, diarrhea, pneumonia, weight loss, other infections, night sweats.	In men, usually mild burning on urination. In women, vaginal discharge, abdominal pain, or no symptoms.	Painful, blisterlike sores on or near penis, anus, vagina, cervix, or less commonly, the mouth.	Possibly no symptoms; vaginal/penile discharge. In males, painful urination, tender lymph nodes, testicular/abdominal pain, fever. In females, heavy or painful menstruation or painful urination, bleeding after intercourse. Also called "clap", "drip", or "dose."
Treatment or cure	Treatment aimed at curing secondary infections, relieving symptoms, and prolonging life. No cure for AIDS exists.	Antibiotics for both partners simultaneously.	No cure; prescription medication may lesson severity and frequency of outbreaks.	Antibiotics for both partners simultaneously.
Potential complications	Immune system failure, severe illness leading to death, eight to ten years to see signs of infection, infection of infants leading to death.	In women, pelvic inflammatory disease (PID) with abnormal pain, fever, excessive menstrual bleeding, ectopic pregnancies, infertility. In men, dangerously enlarged lymph glands of the groin or infection of testicles leading to sterilization. Infection during birth can cause blindness or illness in newborn.	Recurrence, herpes eye infection, infection of newborn during birth.	Sterility, skin problems, PID, arthritis, infection of heart lining, infection of eyes of newborns leading to blindness.
Prevention measures	Abstinence from sexual intercourse and from use of intravenous drugs; mutual sexual monogamy with uninfected partner; some protection provided by condoms.	Abstinence from sexual intercourse; mutual monogamy with an uninfected partner; some protection provided by condoms.	Abstinence from sexual intercourse; mutual monogamy with uninfected partner; some protection provided by condoms only if sores are absent from groin and thighs.	Abstinence from sexual intercourse; mutual monogamy with uninfected partner; some protection provided by condoms.

Ability Levels

Basic, On Level, Advanced

You might want to have students work individually, in pairs, or in groups, for this activity. Each group will need a maximum of 45 index cards. Students will make sets of study cards to learn about the sexually transmitted

diseases listed in the chart on this page.

- All students should list the names of the sexually transmitted diseases on nine index cards, one name per card.
- Basic level students should write the symptoms and prevention measures of the sexually transmitted diseases on 18 additional index cards, one symptom and one preven-

Figure 16–2 Common Sexually Transmitted Diseases, continued

Hepatitis B	Human Papilloma Virus Infections	Pubic Lice	Syphilis	Trichomoniasis
Possibly no symptoms; may have a low-grade fever, nausea, vomiting, fatigue, muscle and joint pain, cough, sore throat, dark urine, jaundice, tender liver.	Often no symptoms. With some varieties dry, wartlike growths on or near penis, anus, cervix, or vagina. Other varieties cause no outward symptoms, but in a woman create cancerous or precancerous cervical cells that register positive on Pap tests.	Itching; lice in pubic hair; eggs, possibly visible, clinging to hair strands. Also called "crabs."	Primary (3 weeks after exposure): chancre on penis, vagina, rectum, anus, cervix. Secondary (6 weeks after primary): rash on feet and hands; flulike symptoms, including appetite loss, fever, sore throat, nausea, headache. Tertiary (10 to 20 years later): severe nerve damage.	Possibly no symptoms in men. In women, frothy, thin, greenish discharge; genital itching and pain. Also called "trick."
No cure; treatment aimed at relieving symptoms.	No cure; controlled by removal of growths or abnormal cervical cells.	Prescription or over-the-counter shampoo, lotion, or cream used by both partners simultaneously.	Antibiotics for both partners simultaneously.	Antibiotics for both partners simultaneously.
Chronic liver disease, liver damage (cirrhosis), potential for development of liver cancer.	Recurrence; cervical cancer; penile cancer; possible obstruction of cervix, vagina, anus.	Skin irritation.	Brain damage; heart disease; spinal cord damage; blindness; infection of fetus, causing death or severe retardation.	Bladder and urethra infections; increased risks of PID in women, and of premature birth in pregnant women.
An effective vaccine is available and recommended during adolescence. Avoidance of intimate contact with infected persons (spread through infected blood, body fluids, saliva, and breast milk); abstinence from sexual intercourse and from use of intravenous drugs; mutual monogamy with uninfected partner; some protection provided by condoms. Avoidance of tattooing and body piercing unless performed under sanitary conditions and with sterile equipment.	Abstinence from sexual intercourse; mutual monogamy with uninfected partner; little protection provided by condoms.	Abstinence from sexual intercourse; mutual monogamy with uninfected partner; not sharing towels or bedclothes with others; good personal hygiene; no protection provided by condoms.	Abstinence from sexual intercourse; mutual monogamy with uninfected partner; some protection provided by condoms.	Abstinence from sexual intercourse; mutual monogamy with uninfected partner; some protection provided by condoms.

tion measure per card.
- On-level students should make cards with symptoms and prevention measures, and they should add treatment or cure on another nine cards.
- Advanced students should do symptoms, prevention measures, treatment or cure, and potential complications, for a total of 45 cards.

Students can work individually, in pairs, or in groups to match the symptoms, treatment or cure, potential complications, and prevention measures to the correct sexually transmitted diseases.

These cards may be used by the class to help in studying for the test on this section or the entire chapter. You should retain them once completed by each group.

CLASS ACTIVITY

Have a student research and report on the development and use of the Pap test for cervical cancer. Some hospital labs may be able to supply slides of normal and abnormal Pap tests, so students can see the difference between normal cervical cells and malignant cells.

COMPREHENSION CHECK

Write two words on the board: *canker* and *chancre*. Ask students to explain the difference between these words. Canker sores, which appear in the mouth for unknown reasons, have no relation to syphilis. Canker sores are painful while chancres from syphilis are not.

COMPREHENSION CHECK

Once students have studied the chart, you might have them list the STDs that are curable on one side of a paper and those that are not on the other. Discuss the following questions: What do the curable diseases have in common? What do the incurable ones have in common? (The curable diseases are caused by bacteria or parasites and respond to antibiotics, but the incurable ones are caused by viruses—AIDS, herpes, genital warts—for which there are no cures.)

Drops placed in a baby's eyes at birth can help protect the eyes against STD infection.

Even in a normal pregnancy, chlamydia causes trouble. During birth, the bacteria can infect the lungs or eyes of the newborn baby, causing pneumonia or blindness. Health-care providers can prevent these tragedies by treating infected pregnant women with antibiotics before delivery.

Although chlamydia is treatable with antibiotics, only a health-care provider should make the choice of which drug to use. Self-prescribed treatments are dangerous and ineffective (see the Consumer Skills feature, "Tricks Used to Sell STD Treatments," on page 426).

KEY POINTS *The common STD chlamydia can damage the reproductive organs, often without any symptoms to warn the person. Untreated chlamydia infections can lead to ectopic pregnancies or infections of newborns during birth. Antibiotics effectively treat chlamydia infections.*

Gonorrhea

As with chlamydia, some people infected with **gonorrhea** do not feel any symptoms. Also as with chlamydia, the damage from the bacteria that cause gonorrhea can advance silently, bringing permanent damage to many organs of the body. This makes periodic testing for gonorrhea especially important for sexually active people.

Men are most likely to have warning symptoms with gonorrhea infections—a thick, pale yellow discharge from the penis and a burning feeling when urinating. Women who have symptoms may notice a yellow-green vaginal discharge and pain when urinating. However, most women have no symptoms at all.

Figure 16–3 *An Ectopic Pregnancy*

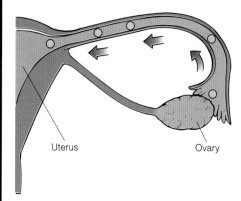

Normal pregnancy

Uterus   Ovary

Normally, a fertilized egg travels freely through the fallopian tube and lodges and develops in the uterus.

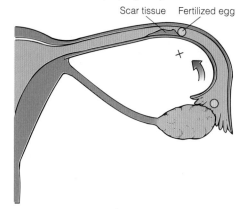

Ectopic pregnancy

Scar tissue   Fertilized egg

In PID, scar tissue partly blocks the tube leading to the uterus. Although tiny sperm can swim up the tube, the large fertilized egg is trapped and lodges to begin developing in the tube.

CRITICAL THINKING

Use the following questions to prompt discussion among your students about sexually transmitted diseases.

1. Do students believe that education is the key to stopping the transmission of sexually transmitted diseases? If so, how can education help? If not, why do they think it won't help?

2. What role should parents play in providing their children with information about sexually transmitted diseases? Should they be doing more to inform their children?

3. Some people feel that the responsibility of sexually transmitted diseases, including AIDS, rests on those involved in sexual

If left untreated, the gonorrhea bacteria can spread all over the body. They can attack the joints, leading to arthritis; attack the skin, leading to sores and other problems; attack the heart, weakening it; and attack the reproductive system, leading to sterility in both men and women. Gonorrhea can cause PID in women and can infect infants' eyes at birth, a common cause of blindness. To protect babies born in the United States against blindness from gonorrhea, public health laws require that a gonorrhea-killing antibiotic be applied to every infant's eyes within minutes after birth.

In people who seek treatment for gonorrhea infection, antibiotics effectively cure most cases. However, more and more cases of the disease each year are reported to be resistant to antibiotics. For these cases, combinations of drugs or special antibiotics may be able to wipe out the infection before it can seriously damage the person.

While the infection is curable, no treatment known can restore health to an organ damaged by gonorrhea. The longer a person has the infection, the higher the risks to health.

 Gonorrhea is a bacterial STD that attacks many organs of the body when left untreated. Antibiotic drugs are usually effective in treating it, but more and more resistant cases are reported each year.

Genital Herpes

Another common STD, **genital herpes**, is caused by a virus, not by bacteria. Thus it cannot be cured once it sets in. The disease is different from those discussed so far in another way, too—it is not known to cause internal organ damage. Testing for herpes is expensive and is not usually recommended as part of a routine STD screening.

The virus causes clumps of painful blisters to appear on the skin (see the photo in the margin). The blisters last for as short a time as a few days or for as long as several months. The blisters can occur in several areas of the body:

▶ On the penis.
▶ In and around the vaginal area.
▶ In the mouth or on the lips.
▶ On the thighs or abdomen.
▶ Around or in the anus.

The sores cause pain, burning, or itching. They closely resemble those of a related condition—cold sores or fever blisters on the mouth. The mouth infection is most often caused by the herpes simplex I virus, while the genital infection is usually caused by the herpes simplex II virus. The two viruses can take each other's places, though, causing the same sorts of sores in either location.

A person need not have obvious sores to transmit the virus. A woman may have internal blisters and not be aware of them. She then can unknowingly transmit the virus to others. It also may be possible for men without active sores to transmit the virus by way of semen. Typically, though, the virus is passed to others by active blisters. After blisters have completely healed, the risk of passing the virus to someone else drops dramatically, but not completely to zero.

Herpes blisters.

Mini Glossary

gonorrhea (gon-oh-REE-uh): a bacterial STD that often advances without symptoms to spread though the body, causing problems in many organs.

genital herpes (HER-peez): a common, incurable STD caused by a virus that produces blisters. The symptoms clear up on their own, but the virus remains to cause future outbreaks.

intercourse and not on society or the community. Do students agree or disagree with this statement? Have them explain their reasons.

4. Should society promote abstinence instead of the use of condoms in an effort to keep sexually transmitted diseases under control? Why or why not?

5. Many people are afraid or uncomfortable talking about sexually transmitted diseases. What can be done to help rid society of this fear?

6. Ask students where most of their information on STDs has originated. From where do they think most of their information should come?

Consumer SKILLS

Answers to Critical Thinking

1. There are many possible reasons—one being that the drugs may not actually be antibiotics. Another is that if they are antibiotics, there is no way of knowing whether or not the antibiotic is the one most likely to help the patient.

2. Answers may vary. Students might say that the one from the physician is what it's supposed to be, whereas the pusher's drug may be "doctored up" with unwanted chemicals.

3. Answers will vary. People become desperate and try almost anything when faced with difficult situations. A quack would reinforce the patient's hope for a miracle cure to make a profit.

GROUP ACTIVITY

Discuss the possible outcomes of having an untreated STD. Each row of students should work together to prepare a brief list of negative outcomes for someone who has an untreated case of:

1. Gonorrhea/Chlamydia
2. Syphilis
3. Trichomoniasis
4. Pubic lice

Be certain students consider the effects on future fertility, as well as the likelihood of continuing the chain of infection by passing the diseases on to future sexual partners.

426

CHAPTER 16: Sexually Transmitted Diseases

Tricks Used to Sell STD Treatments

Consumer SKILLS

STDs can be embarrassing. Some people who suspect they may have an STD may feel so embarrassed that they seek treatment on their own, outside the medical community. Drug pushers make large profits selling antibiotics. However, the chances of being cured from taking street drugs are very small. More likely, the attempt will delay needed medical attention, allowing the disease time to progress and to damage the body. Meanwhile, the misuse of antibiotics give *other* bacteria present in the body a chance to develop antibiotic resistance.

Especially for STDs such as genital herpes, genital warts, and AIDS—for which no real medical cures exist—tricksters with fake "cures" are everywhere. The desire for privacy is understandable. Reaching for any hope of cure is also natural.

Still, only health-care professionals have access to reliable treatments. People should not let shame or fear keep them from seeking the best possible medical help. Health-care providers do not waste time pointing fingers at people who are sick. They are more likely to congratulate them for seeking help.

Critical Thinking

1. Why are pills sold on the street as antibiotics not likely to cure even a bacterial STD?
2. How does a drug from a physician compare with one obtained from a pusher?
3. Why would a person with an STD for which there is no cure be especially vulnerable to the lies of quacks?

Herpes blisters.

With the first outbreak, a person may feel ill with fever, headache, muscle aches, painful urination, and swollen glands. Thereafter, the virus hides in nerve fibers, where it is safe from attack by the body's immune system. Later, the virus can become active again, and again cause sores. Some people experience only one episode in a lifetime. Others suffer outbreaks many times a year for 10 to 15 years or even longer.

Among the more rare, serious effects of herpes are dangerous eye infections that can result from touching the eyes after touching the blisters. The open blisters can also serve as entrances into the body for other microbial infections, including the viruses that cause AIDS or hepatitis.

The newborn baby of a woman suffering her first outbreak of herpes is at extreme risk if blisters are present during the baby's birth. Herpes infections in newborns can cause blindness, severe mental retardation, and even death. Newborns of women with outbreaks of older herpes infections often resist infection during birth, because they received the mother's antibodies to the virus while still in the womb. Still, women with severe blisters at the time of labor may be advised to give birth by surgical means rather than take a chance of infecting the newborn.

enrichment

Assign students research reports on sexual attitudes in other cultures. You might have students choose their own culture or assign cultures to be sure of a good variety. In the reports, students should provide answers to the following questions:

1. Are the behavior standards the same for males and females?
2. How are people who "break the rules" treated or punished in the culture?
3. Do some cultures have a "double standard"?

While not curable, herpes is treatable with an oral antiviral drug that reduces the frequency, duration, and severity of outbreaks. A prescription cream applied to the blisters may shorten an outbreak. However, questions about the cream's effectiveness have not been fully answered.

 KEY POINTS   *Genital herpes is an incurable viral STD that can cause repeated outbreaks of painful blisters. Herpes can infect newborns, causing severe mental retardation, blindness, and death.*

Human Papilloma Virus (HPV) Infection

Another common STD infection is **human papilloma virus (HPV)**. Over 50 forms of this virus are known to infect the genitals. The symptoms vary with the forms of the virus. Some cause no detectable symptoms. Others cause **genital warts**, contagious warty growths on the genital and surrounding skin. The worst of all cause dangerous cell changes that can lead to cancer of the cervix. Some varieties may cause both warts and cancer. HPV causes many more cancer deaths in women each year than any other STD, and twice as many as AIDS (Figure 16–4 on page 428). As is true for herpes, infections with HPV viruses are not curable by drugs.

Once in the body, the infection may remain for life. Treatment consists of removal of the growths or abnormal cervical tissue by surgery or by freezing; or for external growths, by applying a prescription medication (*not* the liquid available for regular warts). Even after treatment, the virus remains in the body, and the warts tend to grow back. Only special laboratory procedures can detect the existence of the virus.

The story of the discovery of the link between HPV and cervical cancer shows that scientists are often called upon to think like detectives. A few years ago, researchers knew only that some form of viral STD was linked to cervical cancer in women. They at first thought the herpes virus was the culprit. Then a story became known of a man who had the unfortunate experience of marrying five times, only to have each wife die of the same disease—cervical cancer. After studying the history of this man and his wives, researchers concluded that he carried HPV, and that each wife had become infected with it. Acting on this information, many more researchers completed experiments that later proved HPV did actually cause cervical cancer.

Infection with HPV is now named as the leading cause of death from cervical cancer worldwide. The virus may be responsible for an epidemic of cervical cancer in the United States. The virus is also linked with anal cancer and may be linked with cancer of the penis in men, but this is rare.

Many sexually active people have the virus, but most never know it. Only 10 percent of people who carry it ever develop the warts that reveal the virus's presence in the body. A woman may discover her infection when a routine **Pap test** detects abnormal cervical cells.

HPV may reside on the skin of the genitals, invisible and symptomless, or it may be present in semen of infected men. People who have had sexual intercourse with more than one partner are at greatest risk for carrying the virus. Even young women who have had no more than one sex partner, however, may have become infected with this common virus. Thus these women should have Pap tests taken on schedule, without fail, to detect abnormal cervical cells. Without detection and treatment, the abnormal cells may turn cancerous and endanger the lives of these women.

Genital warts.

MINI Glossary

human papilloma virus (HPV): any of over 50 related viruses whose effects include genital warts and cervical cancer. Members of this virus family also cause skin warts, commonly found on the hands.

genital warts: contagious wartlike growths on infected areas, caused by HPV viruses. Sometimes called *condyloma* (con-di-LOW-ma). The viruses that cause genital warts can also cause cervical cancer in women.

Pap test: a test for cancer of the cervix (the lower part of the uterus). A few cells are removed painlessly and examined in a laboratory.

4. Are the most restrictive cultures the ones with the lowest incidences of AIDS and other sexually transmitted diseases? Why or why not?

want to share information of a sexual nature, and be prepared to share the information for them.

You might want to have students share their information with the rest of the class. Be sensitive to those students who might not

BACKGROUND INFORMATION

Many historians and anthropologists believe that Columbus and his men introduced syphilis to Europe upon their return from America, where they had been infected. In the year 1500, an epidemic of syphilis erupted in Europe. European physicians said it was a disease that they had never seen before. However, other experts say that syphilis had been in Europe since ancient times, but it had been confused with leprosy. Researchers have examined skeletons, both in Europe and North and South America, looking for signs of syphilis. While interpretations vary, the consensus seems to be that no definite effects of syphilis can be found among the remains of early Europeans.

DISCUSSION

Ask students to explain why syphilis might be called "The Great Imitator." (because the symptoms of syphilis in its three stages mimic many other disorders) Have students brainstorm some other diseases a syphilis victim might believe he or she has contracted. The symptoms come and go, leading victims to believe the disease has gone away. Sometimes the victim may not make a connection between the symptoms and a sexual contact that took place months previously.

Syphilis chancre.

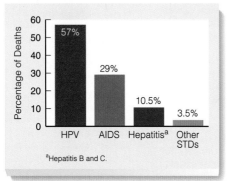

Figure 16–4 *Percentages of Deaths from STD-Related Cancers in U.S. Women. Among STD-related cancer deaths in women, cervical cancer is most common by far.*

Source: Data from Committee on Prevention and Control of Sexually Transmitted Diseases, Institute of Medicine, *The Hidden Epidemic: Confronting Sexually Transmitted Diseases*, eds. T. R. Eng and W. T. Butler (Washington, D.C.: National Academy Press, 1997), p. 50.

 KEY POINTS *Human papilloma virus can cause genital warts and is a major cause of cervical cancer worldwide. The virus is most often present without growths and is thought to infect many sexually active people.*

Syphilis

In the years before the discovery of antibiotics, many people suffered for years from the brain damage and other symptoms of advanced **syphilis** before they died of its effects. Some of the people suspected of having had or having died of syphilis include Al Capone, Julius Caesar, Cleopatra, Napoléon Bonaparte, Catherine the Great, Peter the Great, Henry VIII, Mary Tudor, John Keats, Franz Schubert, Oscar Wilde, Ludwig van Beethoven, and Adolf Hitler. For complete cure of a syphilis infection today, a person who is diagnosed with this bacterial infection may need only a physician's prescription and a trip to the corner drugstore. The number of new cases has dropped slightly, but syphilis remains a major public health problem.

Syphilis announces its presence within a few weeks after infection with a hard, painless sore called a **chancre** that disappears in a few weeks on its own. This sore can help people recognize and treat syphilis before spreading it to others. Some women, however, may not notice the chancre, especially if it occurs deep within their internal tissues. The margin photo shows what a chancre looks like. Notice how different in appearance it is from the sores of genital herpes (shown earlier) and the growths of genital warts, shown on page 427.

If a person infected with syphilis allows the chancre stage to pass by without treatment, the sore will heal, but the infection moves on to the next stage. The next stage of syphilis brings swollen glands, a skin rash, hair loss, or flulike symptoms. These symptoms may seem ordinary to the sufferer and may not cause sufficient alarm for the person to seek help. If the person fails to seek medical help at this stage, these symptoms, too, clear up by themselves in a few weeks. Untreated, the disease progresses to its **latent** stage, a period of symptomless advancement of the disease.

The latent stage of syphilis is long—as long as 10 to 20 years. During this stage the infected person feels well but can transmit the disease to others. With few outward clinical signs, the infection begins to silently attack the internal organs.

In the final stage of syphilis, the infection destroys whole organs. The results are permanent: blindness, deafness, brain damage, skin damage, and heart disease. Without treatment, death is likely. Even in the final stage, a syphilis infection can still be cured and its progression stopped. By that time, however, permanent organ damage has already been done. To escape the worst of syphilis, then, early diagnosis and treatment are critical.

Possibly the saddest effects of syphilis are those on the **fetus** of a pregnant woman with the infection. Syphilis easily enters the bloodstream of the fetus. Unless the woman is treated early in her pregnancy, her fetus is sure to be infected. Syphilis may kill the fetus or cause severe brain damage. Many severely retarded inmates of mental hospi-

decision making activity ?

In the Focus Activity on page 420, a story was presented about Tina, who wanted to know about the sexual history of her boyfriend prior to agreeing to have sex with him. To expand the story, tell students that Tina has questioned her boyfriend and it is possible that he could have a sexually transmitted disease. Have students help Tina decide what to do. Their decisions should include answers to the following questions.

1. How can Tina convince her boyfriend

tals, who are 20, 40, 60, and even 80 years old today, are there because they were infected with syphilis before they were born.

 Syphilis is a dangerous bacterial STD. Although the infection is easily cured by antibiotics, its early symptoms may go unrecognized. This permits the disease to progress silently to cause irreversible organ damage and death. Syphilis attacks the fetus of an infected woman, causing severe mental retardation and other effects.

Hepatitis B

A less common but highly dangerous STD is **hepatitis B**. Teenagers often fall victim to this virus. Once in the body, hepatitis B attacks the liver, causing severe illness. It can lead to incurable liver cancer and death later on.

The word *hepatitis* means "inflammation of the liver." Four different viruses cause it. The relatively mild one, hepatitis A mentioned in the last chapter, often spreads by way of consuming the virus in contaminated food or water.

Hepatitis B, however, enters the body by way of contact with infected body fluids. This can happen in any of the following ways:

▶ By having sexual activity with an infected person.
▶ By sharing a needle with an infected intravenous drug abuser.
▶ By receiving a tattoo or having ears or other body parts pierced with unsterilized equipment.
▶ Less likely, by receiving infected blood from a blood transfusion.

These routes are known, but in more than a third of cases, the cause of the infection remains mysterious.

Once hepatitis B sets in, there is no curing it. The virus may also remain in the body to cause trouble, and possibly to infect others, throughout life.

The key to avoiding the illness, therefore, is prevention. The best weapon by far is the effective vaccine now recommended for all teenagers. Another weapon is the commonsense avoidance of those situations known to transmit the virus.

 Hepatitis B is caused by infection with a virus that attacks the liver. This STD is spread by contact with infected body fluids and is preventable by immunization.

Trichomoniasis

The STD **trichomoniasis** is caused by a parasite. Most often, trichomoniasis is acquired by sexual activity. On rare occasions, it has been acquired by trading wet clothes or towels with an infected person. In women, this infection causes an unpleasant-smelling, foamy, yellow-green or gray discharge; abdominal pain; pain when urinating; or itching in the genital area. Most men have no symptoms. A few have a watery discharge or burning when urinating. Men often unknowingly transmit the disease to their partners. Antibiotics are an effective treatment.

 Trichomoniasis is caused by a parasite and is treated effectively with antibiotics.

For **Y**our **I**nformation

The open chancre of syphilis also makes a convenient entry port to the bloodstream for HIV, the virus that causes AIDS. See page 433.

MINI **Glossary**

syphilis: a bacterial STD that, if untreated, advances from a sore (chancre) to flulike symptoms, then through a long symptomless period, and later to a final stage of irreversible brain and nerve damage, ending in death.

chancre (SHANG-ker): a hard, painless sore; chancres develop early in syphilis infections.

latent: temporarily unseen or inactive.

fetus: a developing human being before birth (see Chapter 20).

hepatitis B: a viral STD that causes loss of liver function and severe liver disease. Hepatitis B is preventable, but not curable.

trichomoniasis (trick-oh-mo-NEYE-uh-sis): an STD caused by a parasite that can cause bladder and urethral infections.

to be tested for a sexually transmitted disease?

2. What should she do if he refuses to be tested and treated?

3. What decisions does she need to make about herself and this relationship?

4. In what ways might this situation be different if it was the boyfriend questioning

Tina's sexual past?

You might add other questions for students to answer based upon your familiarity with your students and their knowledge of sexually transmitted diseases.

> **These symptoms mean that medical help is needed right away:**
>
> - Unusual discharge from vagina, penis, or rectum.
> - Pain or burning while urinating.
> - Pain in the abdomen (women), testicles (men), or buttocks and legs.
> - Blisters, open sores, warts, rashes, or swelling in the genital area or sex organs.
> - Flulike symptoms: fever, headache, diarrhea, aching muscles, swollen glands.

Figure 16–5 Common Symptoms of STDs

Multiple STDs

A person who has one STD may very well have others. This is of special concern, because one STD may mask another, more dangerous one. Syphilis, for example, is a serious second infection. Its early symptom, the chancre, easily hides in, say, a cluster of herpes blisters. If the herpes alone is diagnosed, the syphilis will go untreated and will silently spread through the body. A person who contracts any STD should see a health-care provider and request a test for syphilis—and, possibly, for several other STDs. All of the STDs listed in Figure 16–2 presented earlier in the chapter are likely second infections, even **pubic lice**. The symptoms listed in Figure 16–5 to the left mean that medical help is needed right away.

 KEY POINTS *STDs often occur together. Anyone who contracts one STD should be tested for others.*

Getting Help and Protecting Others

Anyone who suspects the presence of an STD should get help. Among possible sources of help are parents, school health services, public health departments, community STD clinics, or the offices of private physicians. Most organizations keep information about individuals, such as names, confidential. (They may report the incidence of the diseases for tracking purposes.) Treatments may be free of charge in some clinics.

Anyone diagnosed with an STD must notify any sexual partners. Otherwise, the partners may end up passing the disease back and forth several times. They may suffer needless harm, and they may pass the disease to someone else.

The best way to notify a partner about an STD is simply to do it as directly as possible—in person or on the phone, when only that person is

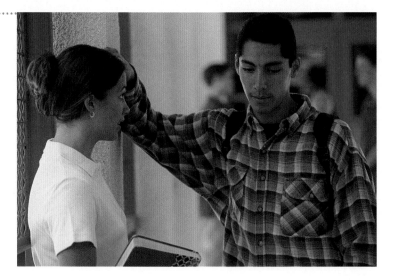

In mature relationships, partners can talk freely about STD prevention—a reason to postpone sexual intercourse until a relationship matures.

HEALTHY PEOPLE 2000

Almost 12 million cases of sexually transmitted diseases occur annually, 86 percent of them in people aged 15 through 29 years. By age 21, approximately one out of every five young people has required treatment for a sexually

transmitted disease. Because only some teenagers are sexually active, this amounts to an effective rate of at least 25 percent among those who are.

Women and children suffer an inordinate amount of the sexually transmitted disease burden. Apart from acquired immunodeficiency syndrome (AIDS) and subsequent

The yeast of candidiasis, magnified over 6,000 times.

listening. A letter is a bad idea because letters have a way of getting opened by other people or lost in the mail.

 KEY POINTS   *A person with a diagnosis of an STD should be treated immediately and inform others who may have the infection.*

Other Infections

The STDs just described are usually transmitted by sexual contact. Other infections of the genital and urinary organs that are *not* transmitted by sexual contact are also common. Like STDs, they should be treated right away to maintain the health of the reproductive or urinary tract organs.

Yeast Infections (Candidiasis)   Most girls and women suffer from vaginal yeast infections at some time in life. A **yeast infection**, or **candidiasis**, is caused by a yeast that normally lives in the vagina. (The same yeast also causes diaper rash in babies.) This yeast usually causes no problem but may multiply out of control to cause intense itching, burning, irritation, and swelling of the outer genitals and a whitish, lumpy vaginal discharge. A woman who is pregnant, takes birth control pills, has diabetes, takes antibiotics, or uses douches is especially likely to develop candidiasis.

Be aware that other, more serious infections share some symptoms with yeast infections. Contact your physician if you have any of the signs listed in the margin of page 430.

Over-the-counter antifungal vaginal inserts and creams relieve symptoms and help cure yeast infections. For prevention, wearing loose-fitting cotton—not nylon—underwear or panty hose with cotton panels is best. Should yeast infections occur frequently or not respond to treatment, a woman should see a physician.

Urinary Tract Infections   Another common complaint occurs when bacteria invade the urinary tract, causing **urinary tract infections (UTIs)**.

MINI Glossary

pubic lice: an STD caused by tiny parasites that breed in pubic hair and cause intense itching.

yeast infection, or **candidiasis** (can-did-EYE-a-sis): an infection caused by a yeast that multiplies out of control in the vagina; not an STD.

urinary tract infections (UTIs): bacterial infections of the urethra that can travel to the bladder and kidneys; not a sexually transmitted disease.

death, the most serious complications are pelvic inflammatory disease (PID), sterility, ectopic pregnancy, blindness, cancer associated with human papilloma virus, fetal and infant death, birth defects, and mental retardation. The medically underserved (e.g., the poor, racial and ethnic minorities) also shoulder a disproportionate share of the sexually transmitted disease problem, experiencing higher rates of disease and disability than the population as a whole. The total societal cost of sexually transmitted diseases exceeds $3.5 billion annually, with the cost of PID and PID-associated ectopic pregnancy and infertility alone exceeding $2.6 billion.

SECTION 1 Review Answers

1. **a.** genital herpes **b.** latent **c.** sexually transmitted diseases (STDs)

2. curable: chlamydia, gonorrhea, pubic lice, syphilis, trichomoniasis; incurable: AIDS, genital herpes, human papilloma virus infections, hepatitis B (pp. 422–423)

3. During birth, the bacteria can infect the lungs or eyes of the newborn, causing pneumonia or blindness. (p. 424)

4. Gonorrhea bacteria attack the joints, causing arthritis; attack the skin, leading to sores; attack the heart, weakening it; attack the reproductive system, leading to sterility; cause PID in women; cause blindness in babies born to women with gonorrhea. (p. 425)

5. on the penis, in and around the vaginal area, in the mouth or on the lips, on the thighs or abdomen, around or in the anus (p. 425)

6. notify any sexual partner (p. 430)

7. Answers will vary.

CLOSE

Have students explore why women tend to have fewer symptoms of many STDs, including gonorrhea, than men. Discuss anatomical differences that make it much easier for a man to see his genitals, as well as any sores or discharge, than it is for a woman, whose organs are on the inside of her body. For this reason, what should a male do once he discovers he has an STD? (He should tell his partner to be treated.) What might be the result if he remains silent?

The urethra (the tube through which urine leaves the body) leads to the bladder and makes a convenient route for invading bacteria.

Most UTIs cause frequent, urgent, and painful urination. Some people notice a dull, aching pain above the pubic bone or blood in the urine.

UTIs are easily treated with antibiotics. If left untreated, however, infection of the bladder may progress to a possibly fatal infection of the kidneys. People who get UTIs often may be able to reduce the frequency by drinking extra fluids; urinating frequently; and for women, wiping from front to back after urination or bowel movements.

Jock Itch Ringworm of the inner thigh and groin, nicknamed **jock itch**, causes intense itching. It is caused by a fungal infection. This condition is common among athletes who sweat heavily and whose clothes stay wet for long periods. Over-the-counter medications usually clear it up. Other preventive measures include staying dry, not sharing towels with others, and not allowing clothing to touch the floor.

For Your Information

Warning signs of something more serious than yeast infection:

▶ Abdominal pain, fever, or a foul-smelling discharge.
▶ No improvement within three days of treatment.
▶ Symptoms recur within two months.

KEY POINTS *Yeast infections and urinary tract infections are infections of the genitals and urinary organs that are not sexually transmitted. These can sometimes be prevented by routine self-care. They are easily treated.*

SECTION 1 Review

Answer the following questions on a sheet of paper.

Learning the Vocabulary

The vocabulary terms in this section are *sexually transmitted diseases (STDs), acquired immune deficiency syndrome (AIDS), chlamydia, pelvic inflammatory disease (PID), ectopic pregnancy, gonorrhea, genital herpes, human papilloma virus (HPV), genital warts, Pap test, syphilis, chancre, latent, fetus, hepatitis B, trichomoniasis, pubic lice, yeast infection (candidiasis), urinary tract infections (UTIs),* and *jock itch.*

1. Match each of the following phrases with the appropriate term:
   a. a common, incurable STD caused by a virus that produces blisters
   b. temporarily inactive
   c. diseases that can be transmitted by direct sexual contact

Learning the Facts

2. Which STDs are curable? Incurable?
3. Describe the health problems of a newborn baby whose mother has chlamydia.
4. Describe the physical problems that occur in people who are not treated for gonorrhea.
5. List and identify the areas of the body on which genital herpes blisters occur.
6. What should people do if they are diagnosed with STDs?

Making Life Choices

7. Reread the "Common Sexually Transmitted Diseases" chart in Figure 16–2 on pages 422–423. How serious do you consider the risks associated with STDs as compared with the risks from smoking, drug or alcohol abuse, or other risky behaviors?

QUICK QUIZ

Chapter 16, Section 1

The following quiz will help you assess your students' understanding of the material covered in this section of the chapter. You might use the quiz as an oral exercise, which will lead into a class discussion of the topics covered. Or, you might use it as a paper/pencil quiz to evaluate your students individually.

1. Sexually transmitted diseases (STDs) are caused by pathogens transferred during sexual contact. (True)
2. The STDs caused by bacteria can be cured by antibiotics, but those caused by viruses, such as acquired immune deficiency syndrome (AIDS), are incurable. (True)
3. There is no one-hundred percent effective way to prevent the spread of sexually transmitted diseases. (False)

SECTION 2

Acquired Immune Deficiency Syndrome (AIDS)

A disease of enormous concern worldwide is acquired immune deficiency syndrome (AIDS). First observed in the late 1970s, AIDS has spread rapidly to more than 100 countries and every inhabited continent of the globe. Health-care authorities are working hard to stop AIDS from becoming an even bigger problem. Figures 16–6 and 16–7 show the advancement of AIDS among U.S. teenagers and adults and those around the world. The number of those infected but not yet ill is thought to be ten times greater than the number of people diagnosed with AIDS.

Teenagers are currently the most rapidly growing group for both infection with **HIV** (the virus that causes AIDS) and AIDS. In the United States, in every hour of every day and night, one to two teens are infected with HIV.

Within the last few years, the number of teens who test positive for the AIDS virus has doubled and even, in some areas, tripled. People who think that they are too young to get AIDS, not the right type to get it, or are somehow excused from getting it are its most likely next victims.

HIV Infection and AIDS

Infection with HIV and the disease AIDS are not the same thing. A person with an HIV infection may live normally for years with the virus present in the cells of the body. A diagnosis of AIDS comes with the destruction of the immune system and development of the disease typical of AIDS: a form of pneumonia, fungal infections, and cancers rarely seen in people with a healthy immune system.

How HIV Destroys Immunity   HIV is unique among infections—the virus attacks the very cells and tissues that provide the body with immunity and disables its defenses. When a person first becomes infected with HIV, the virus incubates in the body for several weeks but causes no symptoms. Then, a period of illness may set in with fever, headache, night sweats, rash, sore throat, swollen lymph nodes, and a general ill feeling that resembles the flu. If the person is tested for HIV during this time, the test is likely to turn out negative, because the antibodies detected by the test take several months to form.

HIV invades the immune system's white blood cells, the T cells. Because it hides inside the cells, it remains safely out of reach of immune defenses.

Once inside the T cells, the virus tricks the cells into acting like tiny virus factories. Each cell begins churning out millions of copies of the AIDS virus. The new viruses then break free from the "parent" cell to find other T cells to infect.

After months or years of silently infecting T cells and reproducing, the HIV infection begins to destroy immunity. More accurately, the immune system destroys itself in its attempt to rid the body of HIV. The self-destruction occurs when cells of the immune system find the infected T cells and kill

For Your Information

Chapter 15 described the incubation, prodrome, and other typical stages of an illness. See page 408.

MINI Glossary

jock itch: a fungal infection of the groin and inner thigh; not a sexually transmitted disease.

HIV: an abbreviation for *human immunodeficiency virus*, the virus that causes AIDS.

---

4. Poverty prevents the widespread cure of sexually transmitted diseases. (True)
5. Chlamydia is a STD which frequently causes no symptoms, but if untreated can result in pelvic inflammatory disease or an ectopic pregnancy. (True)
6. Gonorrhea is a viral STD that cannot be treated. (False)
7. Genital herpes is incurable, but can be treated with an oral antiviral drug which reduces its severity and duration. (True)

8. A Pap test can detect the abnormal cervical cells which signal HPV, the leading cause of death from cervical cancer. (True)
9. Syphilis is easily cured by antibiotics, but can cause organ damage and death if allowed to progress untreated. (True)
10. Yeast infections and urinary tract infections are commonly sexually transmitted diseases. (False)

SECTION 2

FOCUS

OUTCOMES

In this section students will learn:

1. The way HIV invades and attacks the body.
2. Methods of transmission of the virus that causes AIDS.

FOCUS ACTIVITY

Students are asked to imagine that a new student is joining their class. This student has been diagnosed as HIV positive. (Others in the class may be HIV positive, but not know it.) Discuss the following questions.

1. Should the family of this student inform the school about his or her HIV status?
2. Should the school inform the parents of other students of this student's HIV status, and should the student's identity be revealed?
3. What rights of privacy does the student have in regard to others knowing his or her medical condition?
4. How would you react to the inclusion of this student in your class? How would you treat him or her?

It would be best not to draw any conclusions on these questions until after the class has completed Section 2. Then the students may want to rethink their answers.

FAST FACTS

The phone number for the National AIDS Hotline is: 1-800-342-AIDS.

TEACH & APPLY

COMPREHENSION CHECK

Explaining to students how HIV behaves in the body can be difficult. Your supplementary material contains an activity that includes four diagrams that will help students see how HIV affects the immune system and the results that occur. The diagrams graphically compare germs to a fire, white cells (T cells) to a fire alarm, antibodies to water, and so on.

COMPREHENSION CHECK

You may want to break down the AIDS acronym. *Acquired* means something that is obtained; *immune* and *deficiency* are words that students have learned earlier; *syndrome* means a group of signs or symptoms that, collectively, indicate a disease or disorder or other abnormal condition.

BACKGROUND INFORMATION

You may want to refer students back to the discussion and illustration of the immune system in Chapter 6.

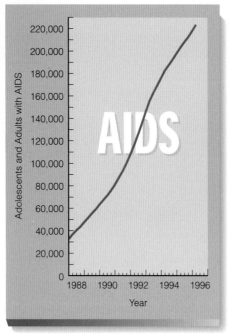

Figure 16–6 **U.S. Teenagers and Adults Living with AIDS**

Source: U.S. Department of Health and Human Services and Centers for Disease Control and Prevention, *HIV/AIDS Surveillance Report.*

A photomicrograph of the AIDS virus

them off as they would any other infected cells. As the T cells are relentlessly attacked and destroyed, the T cell fighting force loses it effectiveness as part of the immune system.

In a healthy immune system, the T cells spring into action when infections set in. They direct B cells to produce disease-fighting antibodies (see Chapter 15). With the onset of AIDS, T cells dwindle to about a fifth of their original number. They cannot effectively signal the B cells, which then sit idle while infections of all kinds thrive unchecked.

The Disease of AIDS As AIDS sets in, the first symptoms are usually troublesome, but vague. Fatigue, appetite loss, weight loss, and nagging cough are typical. As the disease progresses, AIDS patients almost always have persistent yeast infections of the mouth, throat, or vagina. A diagnosis of AIDS is often first made when a health-care provider detects the presence of one of the diseases typical of AIDS. Blood tests revealing low levels of T cells and the presence of HIV genetic material complete the diagnosis.

The disease that first brings most people with AIDS to a physician is an otherwise rare form of pneumonia, called **PCP**. Other defining diseases include a fungal infection of the linings of the brain and spinal cord, a skin cancer called **Kaposi's sarcoma**, tuberculosis and other lung diseases, and persistent diarrhea.

HIV also makes its way to the brain and nervous system, causing the severe mental disorder **AIDS dementia complex**. The symptoms include agitation, anxiety, confusion, depression, hallucinations, increased sex drive, loss of will, memory loss, mood swings, and social withdrawal. Some victims become suicidal or homicidal (they want to kill themselves or others). HIV's attack on the nerves can cause numbness in the hands and feet. It also reduces control over the muscles, causing leg weakness, poor coordination, and unsteady walking.

HIV damages the body's tissues, but people with AIDS do not die of HIV itself. They die of the other diseases against which they become defenseless.

 KEY POINTS *HIV invades the T cells of the immune system, forcing them to make new viruses and weakening the immune system. AIDS begins when immunity fails and other diseases set in. HIV attacks the nervous system, causing mental disorders. Victims die of the infections that overpower their bodies.*

Treatment and Life with AIDS

With new treatments of drugs, radiation, and surgery, some people with AIDS are living longer than others before them. An important discovery was that antivirus drugs such as AZT (zidovudine) reduce the level of HIV in the

enrichment

To provide students with some background information about AIDS, you might share with them the following information.

Scientists and researchers don't know for sure where the AIDS virus came from, but

they have some good ideas. They believe that AIDS originated on the African continent, specifically in the Congo region. The first known human case was that of a Bantu tribesman living in the Congo region. A sample of his blood, which was taken in 1959, was analyzed and found to contain traces of HIV. The man had gone to a clinic for treat-

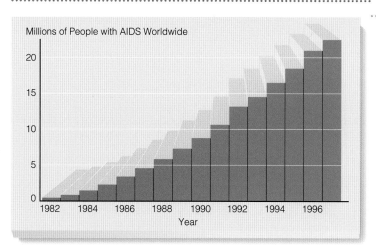

Millions of People with AIDS Worldwide

Figure 16–7 Advancement of the AIDS Epidemic Worldwide

blood. The lower the level of HIV in the tissues and blood, the slower the progression of AIDS. Unfortunately, AZT's effects last only about a year, because the virus becomes resistant to the drug.

Combination Treatments   Today, the best medical treatment for HIV infection is a combination of drugs, including those of the AZT drug family, a group known as **protease inhibitors**, and others. The therapy is known as highly active antiretroviral therapy, or HAART (HIV is a member of a group called the *retroviruses*). The therapy consists of giving three drugs that stop HIV reproduction at various stages. HAART gets results: it reduces HIV levels, increases T cells, and prolongs life in 65 to 85 percent of patients using it perfectly.

A key to success with these drugs, however, is the ability of the AIDS patient to stick with a complicated schedule of taking 20 to 50 pills a day, at four-, six-, and eight-hour intervals, around the clock, seven days a week without holidays. Researchers are optimistic that if HAART is used aggressively enough, and started early enough in the course of the infection, that the disease may be controlled completely. The earlier the therapy begins, the better the chance of preventing irreversible damage to the immune and nervous systems.

AIDS patients may take up to 50 pills a day, each timed precisely, to combat the disease.

Glossary

PCP: the pneumonia characteristic of AIDS; *Pneumocystis carinii* pneumonia.

Kaposi's (cap-OH-zeez) sarcoma: a normally rare skin cancer causing a purplish discoloration of the skin, seen commonly among people with AIDS.

AIDS dementia complex: the mental disorder resulting from an attack by HIV on the brain and nerves.

protease inhibitors: drugs that stop the action of an enzyme which ordinarily helps HIV to reproduce. The drugs help slow HIV reproduction, but takers run an increased risk of developing diabetes.

The Threat of Resistance   Of great concern to health-care providers is the astonishing ability of HIV to become resistant to medications, a lesson

ment of symptoms that were similar to those of sickle cell anemia, which is a fairly common disease of the blood suffered by Africans. However, researchers now believe he actually had AIDS and not sickle cell anemia.

Researchers can only speculate how HIV, which was originally found in monkeys in Africa, was transmitted to humans. One theory

is that the uncooked flesh of an infected monkey was eaten by a human who then became infected. During the 1980s and early 1990s, AIDS became an epidemic in Africa. Researchers think that the rapid spread of the disease might have been caused by the use of unsterilized needles for vaccinations.

DISCUSSION

On index cards, print in large letters ways that AIDS could be spread from one person to another (one idea on each card). Also, print ways AIDS is not spread. (Figure 16–8 on page 438 would be a good beginning, but you may also want to include other behaviors students incorrectly believe to be means of transmission, such as eating in a restaurant that has an employee who is HIV positive, or dry kissing.) Prepare enough cards so that every student has one. Draw a long line on the chalkboard. At one end write "High Risk" and at the other end "No Risk." Have each individual student read what is on his or her card, then come up and place it in the chalk tray at the point he or she believes it falls on the continuum between a high-risk behavior and a no-risk behavior, in regard to transmission of HIV. Make no comments on the placement of the cards until all are placed. Then students may discuss which cards they feel should be moved to more accurately reflect the risk of each activity. You may interject information when students do not seem to have a clear idea of the risk. Once the cards are properly placed, it will be clear that AIDS is spread in only four fluids: blood, semen, vaginal fluids, and breast fluids. In addition, a mother can infect her unborn baby during pregnancy. Any behavior that allows transmission of these fluids should be considered "high risk." By avoiding the behaviors at the "high-risk" end of the chalkboard, students can avoid AIDS.

Because this activity provides students with a graphic view of the transmission of AIDS, it is particularly effective with students with learning disabilities.

For **Y**our **I**nformation

Chapter 15 explained how microbes develop drug resistance. See pages 400–401.

The AIDS quilt is a tribute to loved ones lost to AIDS.

learned from AZT. Should a patient taking the HAART medications be prone to forgetting a pill here and there, chances are great that the therapy will soon lose its effectiveness because the virus will become resistant to the drugs. In general, about half of all medical patients fail to take the medications as they are prescribed. The complicated nature of the HAART regime makes such failures almost a certainty.

Other Concerns The drugs used to treat HIV infection and AIDS are expensive, costing tens of thousands of dollars each year. Without adequate insurance, few people can afford to buy them. Indeed, this situation applies to the great majority of infected people worldwide. Sadly, most of the world's people with AIDS receive no treatment at all.

Without effective treatments, some people who are infected with HIV sicken and die within six months of infection. Others may live without symptoms for years. Once AIDS symptoms set in, however, most die within two to five years. Researchers are hoping for an effective, inexpensive vaccine to prevent HIV infections and end the epidemic, but such a vaccine is slow in coming.

Living with AIDS A person diagnosed with an HIV infection must accept many heavy losses. First the person must accept the diagnosis. Then the person must decide how and whom to tell. Soon follow the losses of finances, sexual activity, health, and some social support. Day-to-day living changes dramatically. The person may face endless medical examinations, begin complicated drug therapies, and adopt strict eating habits to prevent food poisoning and other infections. Alcohol enhances the reproduction of HIV, and so alcoholic beverages are strictly forbidden.

The disclosure of HIV infection may result in discrimination concerning housing, employment, child custody, insurance benefits, or potential employment. People who later develop AIDS can expect to lose physical strength, mental sharpness, control of life activities, self-esteem, and in the end, life itself.

Many people react to these losses with courage. One young woman who believes she must have contracted HIV as a teenager has committed the rest of her life to traveling and speaking to teen groups about AIDS. Basketball star Magic Johnson has become a powerful voice for groups trying to stop the spread of HIV. Many others work in quieter ways. They join local education efforts. They support those who have been newly diagnosed. They work in AIDS food banks, or they answer calls for a helping hotline. They may be facing losses, but even so, their self-esteem stays high as they find new, meaningful roles.

 POINTS *Many new drug treatments can extend life and health for many AIDS patients. However, the drugs are expensive and therefore unavailable to many people worldwide who need them. With the progression from HIV infection to AIDS, many losses occur, including losses of health, finances, and social support.*

COOPERATIVE LEARNING

Pass It Around

This activity will help students understand how quickly HIV can spread, and also that there is no real way of identifying a person with HIV.

Without any preparation, ask students to stand and face the center of the room. Walk to the center of the class, and shake hands with the three students closest to you. Ask those three to shake hands with three others, and pass on the instruction to shake hands with still another three. Give the students about a

Transmission of the AIDS Virus

People who feel and look healthy can be infected with HIV and can transmit it to others. They can pass on the virus before they develop any signs of illness, during the incubation stage. Often, people who become ill with AIDS in their 20s were infected with the virus when they were teenagers.

Sexual Transmission   Most people with HIV acquired their infections by way of sexual intercourse. These people can then pass the virus on to others by way of blood, semen from the penis, fluids of the vagina, or other body fluids. Steady sex partners of people with AIDS take the greatest risks of contracting HIV. However, it takes just one contact with an infected person to acquire the virus. This means a single sexual encounter can infect a formerly healthy person with HIV.

The presence of STDs can also increase the risk of contracting HIV. The open sores of herpes or syphilis give the HIV virus easy access to the bloodstream. STDs like gonorrhea draw immune cells, such as T cells, to the areas of infection.

Needles   The sharing of needles among people who practice **intravenous (IV) drug abuse** is the second most common path by which HIV travels from person to person. Programs that allow the exchange of used needles for sterile ones have reduced the spread of blood-borne illnesses in other countries. Such programs are not favored in the United States, however, because of fears of encouraging drug abuse. So little blood is needed to pass on the virus that even being scratched by an infected needle can transmit AIDS. Unsterilized needles used for any purpose are dangerous, including the needles of acupuncture, tattooing, ear or body piercing, and electrolysis (the removal of hair by electricity using a needle).

The announcement by basketball star Ervin "Magic" Johnson that he was HIV-positive helped to focus national attention on the AIDS crisis.

HIV-infected mothers who receive drug therapy stand a fifty-fifty chance of protecting their newborns from the virus.

Mini Glossary

intravenous (IV) drug abuse: the practice of using needles to inject drugs of abuse into the veins. (The word *intravenous* means "into a vein.")

minute to complete some handshaking. Interrupt the activity, and ask all students who did not shake hands with anyone to remain standing, while the handshakers sit down. Point out that the people who are standing are the only ones who did not have contact with your initial handshake. Often, AIDS and other STDs can travel as rapidly as the handshake did. Also, people with STDs often appear healthy, so there is no real way of identifying them in advance.

BACKGROUND INFORMATION

Experts estimate that one-third of the nation's AIDS cases originate from IV drug use. Specifically, 71 percent of all females with AIDS are linked directly or indirectly to IV drug use. In a two-year study done in New Haven, Connecticut, it was demonstrated that a needle exchange program can dramatically slow the rate of infection without encouraging new IV drug use. In the New Haven study, more than 90 percent of the needles confiscated and exchanged for clean needles were contaminated with the AIDS virus.

Awareness, accurate information, and medical tests are three important defenses against AIDS.

Figure 16–8 Ways HIV Is Transmitted and Ways It Is Not Transmitted

Pregnancy, Childbirth, Breastfeeding HIV can be transmitted to infants in three ways. Women who have AIDS or carry the virus can infect their offspring during pregnancy, during birth, or by way of breastfeeding. Effective antivirial drugs given to the pregnant woman with HIV or AIDS can sometimes protect her infant from being infected. As a rare exception to the rule that breastfeeding is best for babies, new mothers who are HIV-positive are urged not to breastfeed their infants.

Blood Traces Only traces of whole cells are needed to convey the virus from person to person. Semen commonly carries HIV, but so can blood—the amount you see sometimes when brushing your teeth, for example. Passing this tiny amount of blood to a partner through intense, open-mouthed kissing could possibly pass on the virus. Ordinary kissing poses little danger, especially in people with healthy mouths.

Ways HIV Is NOT Transmitted HIV appears not to be transmitted by casual contacts such as sharing meals, shaking hands, coughing, or sneezing. It also seems not to be transmitted by mosquitoes or other insects, by saunas, by pools, or by food handled by HIV carriers. HIV is also not transmitted to people who donate blood using sterilized needles; to those being vaccinated using sterilized needles; or by contact with unbroken, healthy skin. HIV does not appear to be transmitted by touching shared objects, such as toilet seats. Intimate sexual activity or contact with blood—not casual contact—transmits HIV. Figure 16–8 reviews the ways HIV is transmitted and ways that it is not transmitted.

Blood Transfusions and Tissue Transplants Another way people have acquired HIV infections is by way of blood products used in medical treatments or transplanted tissues or organs. Those who received blood or tissues in the years before 1985 risked being infected with the virus, because medical products were not screened as they are today. Thanks to the advances in screening of potential donors, testing of the donated products, and more accurate tracking of information, today's blood, tissue, and organ supplies are almost always safe to use.

Routine Medical Care A few years ago, a story of a young woman who was infected with HIV by her dentist was cause for great concern. It

HIV is known to be transmitted by:	HIV has not been transmitted by:
• Any form of sexual intercourse with an infected partner. • Sharing infected needles. • Ear or body piercing with an infected needle. • Acupuncture using an infected needle. • Tattooing using an infected needle. • Removal of hair by electrolysis using an infected needle. • Infected blood transfusions. • Infected organ transplants. • Pregnancy, childbirth, or breastfeeding by an infected mother (virus transmitted to infant).	• Casual contact. • Mosquitoes or other biting insects. • Eating food prepared by HIV-infected people. • Blood donation. • Vaccinations using sterilized needles. • Contact with unbroken, healthy skin. • Contact with tears, saliva, or sweat from an HIV-infected person. • Touching shared objects, including towels. • Wearing clothes of an HIV-infected person. • Using a toilet used previously by an HIV-infected person. • Hugging or lightly kissing an HIV-infected person. • Swimming with an HIV-infected person.

QUICK QUIZ

Chapter 16, Section 2

The following quiz will help you assess your students' understanding of the material covered in this section of the chapter. You might use the quiz as an oral exercise, which will lead into a class discussion of the topics covered. Or, you might use it as a paper/pencil quiz to evaluate your students individually.

*If students have difficulty with the concepts covered in the Quick Quiz and the Section Review, you might suggest they review the material using the **S**urvey, **Q**uestion, **R**ead, **R**ecite, **R**eview (SQ3R) study method, which is described in detail in the introduction to this Teacher's Wraparound Edition.*

1. Infection with HIV and the disease AIDS are the same thing. (False)

2. AIDS is diagnosed after the deterioration

appeared that she had contracted the virus during a routine dental procedure. As the case unfolded, however, evidence seemed to indicate that her infection may not have been accidental. No one may ever know the truth, but this case helped to bring national attention to the importance of sanitation measures for all health-care providers.

The best protection against acquiring any infection from the office of a health-care provider is to notice whether the provider uses precautions such as those listed in the margin. If you find a health-care provider who doesn't, leave right away, and report the problem to your parents or the school nurse.

The Risk to Health-Care Professionals Young people considering careers in the medical fields often ask about the risk of contracting AIDS in the performance of medical jobs. Very rarely do health-care workers contract AIDS by being accidentally stuck with an infected needle. Because the risk is well known, they take every precaution to protect themselves and their patients. Only when health workers become tired, careless, or hurried do accidents happen.

Millions of people have highly rewarding careers in the health-care field and remain free of contagious diseases. The chances of dying from almost any other cause are enormous compared with the chance of dying from AIDS acquired by offering routine health care. This is true even for health-care providers who specialize in caring for people with AIDS. After all, no one knows better how to stop the spread of disease than a health-care professional.

 KEY POINTS *AIDS is a fatal disease caused by infection with a virus, HIV. HIV is readily transmitted by way of sexual contact or exchange of blood. HIV does not appear to be transmitted through casual contact and is rarely transmitted to health-care professionals in the workplace.*

SECTION 2 Review

Answer the following questions on a sheet of paper.

Learning the Vocabulary

The vocabulary terms in this section are *HIV, PCP, Kaposi's sarcoma, AIDS dementia complex, protease inhibitors,* and *intravenous (IV) drug abuse.*

1. Match each phrase with the appropriate vocabulary term from the list above:
   a. the virus that causes AIDS
   b. a normally rare skin cancer causing a purplish discoloration of the skin
   c. a normally rare type of pneumonia

Learning the Facts

2. What is the difference between HIV and AIDS?
3. What does the AIDS virus do, after it gets into the body?
4. What are the first physical symptoms of AIDS?
5. What is the treatment for AIDS?

Making Life Choices

6. Look at Figure 16–8. Which items did you already know? Have you heard of other ways AIDS is transmitted or not transmitted? How can we correct misconceptions?

of the immune system has begun. (True)
3. HIV invades the immune system's white blood cells and tricks them into reproducing millions of the virus. (True)
4. The body's immune system begins to destroy massive numbers of its T cells with the onset of AIDS. (True)
5. HIV is a direct cause of death. (False)
6. HIV attacks the nervous system, causing AIDS dementia complex. (True)
7. Highly active antiretroviral therapy (HAART) is a relatively effective combination treatment for HIV infection. (True)
8. The HAART regime is generally successful because it is simple and easy to follow. (False)
9. Sexual intercourse is the most common means of transmission of the AIDS virus. (True)
10. AIDS can be transmitted through casual contact. (False)

 ASSESS

EVALUATE

SECTION 2 Review Answers

1. a. HIV **b.** Kaposi's sarcoma **c.** PCP
2. HIV is the virus that causes AIDS, while AIDS is the actual disease that causes the immune system to be defenseless against infections and cancers. (p. 433)
3. attacks the immune system, disabling its defenses (p. 433)
4. Fatigue, appetite loss, weight loss, and a nagging cough are typical. (p. 434)
5. drugs, radiation, and surgery (p. 434)
6. Answers will vary.

 A reproducible quiz for Section 2 is provided in the Teacher's Resource Box.

CLOSE

Instruct students to write three true statements describing the progress of AIDS in the body, and three true statements describing how AIDS is spread. Statements could be written on cards and then exchanged at random. If students receive statements that do not seem correct, they should raise their hands and read them out loud. The class will then decide if the statements are true or false. Collect the cards to evaluate student understanding at the end of this section.

SECTION 3

FOCUS

OUTCOMES

In this section students will learn:

1. Behaviors that will eliminate the risk of acquiring an STD.
2. Behaviors that will reduce, but not definitely eliminate, the risk of acquiring an STD.

FOCUS ACTIVITY

Write the following statement on the board: "AIDS is a disease you don't have to get." Ask students to comment on this statement. Do they agree that AIDS is an avoidable disease? If so, how does one avoid it? Students may be able to determine that the major ways to avoid AIDS are abstinence, mutual monogamy with an uninfected person, and avoidance of IV drugs.

TEACH & APPLY

ROLE PLAY

Since refusal skills are a big part of practicing abstinence, have two students role play a situation in which a boy is trying to convince a girl to have sex with him, and the girl believes in abstinence. In this role play situation, have a male student take the part of the girl and have a female student take the part of the boy. It will be interesting for the class to witness the various "lines" males use to convince girls, and the various statements the girl can use to refuse his sexual advances without putting him down.

For Your Information

Remember to never let anyone stick you with a needle, to pierce your ears or skin, to give you a tattoo, or to remove hair unless you are certain that the needle has been steam-heat-sterilized for 15 minutes, or is a disposable needle that has never been used.

Health Strategies

Avoiding Contracting Sexually Transmitted Diseases

*People can **completely** protect themselves from sexual transmission of STDs by:*

1. Practicing sexual abstinence.
2. Having a responsible, mature, mutually monogamous sexual relationship with an uninfected partner. (Teens are rarely mature enough to be sure that their relationships fall into this category. See the text discussion.)

*People can **reduce** their STD risks by:*

1. Avoiding contact with the partner's body fluids.
2. Using latex condoms with **spermicide** throughout every sexual act to keep body fluids from being exchanged.
3. Refusing alcohol or other drugs.
4. Avoiding high-risk behaviors, and avoiding relations with others who engage in high-risk behaviors.

SECTION 3

Strategies against Sexual Transmission of AIDS and Other STDs

The rest of this chapter gives details about how people must adjust their sex lives to protect themselves from contracting AIDS and other STDs. It describes those practices that *eliminate* the risk of acquiring a disease through sexual behaviors. These behaviors promise that people who follow them consistently will not contract an STD through sexual contact. Total commitment to **abstinence** or to a mutually **monogamous** relationship (such as marriage) with an uninfected partner are the only strategies that eliminate the risk of STDs entirely.

The chapter goes on to describe **safer-sex strategies**—behaviors that will reduce STD risk but that cannot promise complete protection. The Health Strategies feature on this page, "Avoiding Contracting Sexually Transmitted Diseases," summarizes these guidelines.

Eliminating the Risk of STDs

Only two strategies, if practiced consistently, reduce the risk of sexually acquired infections to zero. Keep in mind, though, that AIDS and other infections of the blood can be passed by nonsexual means. The strategies you are about to study prevent *sexual* transmission only.

The most effective way to protect against STDs is not to have sexual relations with other people (abstinence). Abstinence from sexual activities is the most effective strategy for preventing STDs.

Limiting sexual relations to one uninfected partner only, who is also monogamous, also provides protection from STDs. Safety here depends on knowing the partner's infection status and on knowing that the partner is monogamous. The problem is, though, that people can have many STDs, including HIV, without knowing it. People who look and feel healthy can be infected. You cannot tell by looking. Before using the strategy of mutual monogamy, partners must determine two things:

▶ The prospective partner's infection status.
▶ The prospective partner's sexual faithfulness.

Until the partner's infection status is known, it is not safe to have sex.

It's OK to ask about a potential partner's sexual history. Unfortunately, though, people do not like to reveal their sexual pasts, and so they may be tempted to lie. A physician reported that he had asked an AIDS-infected client whether

HEALTHY PEOPLE 2000

Increase to at least 50 percent the proportion of sexually active, unmarried people who used a condom at last sexual intercourse.

Abstinence from sexual intercourse, monogamous sexual relations with an uninfected partner, and avoidance of intravenous drug use are the most effective means of pre-

venting HIV infection. Proper use of condoms, reducing the number of sexual partners, and abstinence from drug abuse decrease, but do not eliminate risk of HIV infection.

Although there is no absolute guarantee that using a condom will prevent people from getting sexually transmitted diseases, including HIV, risk can be greatly reduced if condoms are used properly. Failure of condoms to prevent the transmission of disease is more often caused by improper use than by product fail-

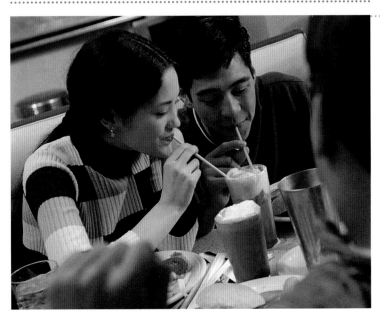

Many teens today are committing to abstinence from sexual intercourse.

For Your Information

Some people who are diagnosed with an STD say that they had "intended" to be abstinent, or "hoped" that their partner was monogamous or healthy. True STD protection is based on complete commitment and total certainty; intentions and hopes can be easily shattered and expose people to risks.

he had told his sex partner of the AIDS infection. The client responded, "No, Doctor, it would have broken the mood."

Asking about STDs may not be enough. Medical testing, especially for AIDS, is not unreasonable. Both partners must be willing to be tested. Blood tests detect either the antibodies to HIV or the HIV genetic material itself. For privacy, a home test can also reliably detect HIV genetic material. The user scrapes cells from the lining of the mouth and submits them for examination by a laboratory. The results are obtained by way of a recorded phone message, identifiable only by a code from the test package. A parent or pharmacist can help explain the test kit instructions.

A caution about AIDS testing—the blood or cells of people who are newly infected may register as negative for the virus, especially during the early months. That is, if a person was infected just last week, last month, or several months ago, then there is some chance that the person might test negative for the virus today. This is just one more reason why abstinence from sexual intercourse is a good idea.

 KEY POINTS *Abstinence or mutual monogamy with an uninfected partner are the only safe sexual practices.*

Reducing the Risk of STDs

Some strategies can greatly reduce—but not eliminate—risks of acquiring an STD. With these strategies, the goal is to avoid any exchange of body fluids. Condoms made of latex material (not natural skin) and treated with a **spermicide**, if properly used, are effective in reducing the risks of STDs. A

abstinence: refraining completely from sexual relations with other people. Also called *celibacy* (SELL-ih-ba-see).

monogamous: having sexual relations with one partner only, excluding all others. These relationships are usually long-term relationships.

safer-sex strategies: behavior guidelines that reduce STD risk, but that do not reduce the risk to zero.

spermicide: the compound nonoxynol-9, intended for birth control, that also kills or weakens some STD organisms.

DISCUSSION

Tell students of a movement among teenagers today to commit to abstinence. Interested teenagers may attend an official ceremony at their churches or temples where they commit to themselves, their families, and their spiritual leaders that they will remain virgins until marriage. What do students think of this? Would promising to someone else to abstain from sex before marriage make it easier to say "no" when facing pressures to have sex? What are the advantages of this commitment? The disadvantages?

COMPREHENSION CHECK

Mutually monogamous is a term that will sound difficult to students and is one with which they probably are unfamiliar. Monogamous is defined in the Mini Glossary. Ask them to define *mutually.* (having to do with both parties; same for both people involved) They should see that it is not enough for one person to be monogamous to avoid contracting an STD; both must be.

BACKGROUND INFORMATION

Tell students that according to a University of Southern California study, the more sexual partners an HIV-infected man has had, the less likely he is to try to notify them of the risk. What does this say about the level of responsibility and morals of the person involved?

ure in the United States, where condoms must adhere to quality control standards set by the Food and Drug Administration.

To be most effective in reducing the spread of HIV, condoms and instructions for their proper use should be made more widely available through health care providers who offer services to sexually active men and women, particularly in sexually transmitted disease clinics, family planning clinics, and drug abuse treatment centers. Counselors at

these facilities should become more confident in counseling patients on infection prevention and should emphasize age-appropriate assertiveness skills. Instructions in correct condom use can be obtained from *Condoms and Sexually Transmitted Diseases . . . Especially AIDS* or the National AIDS Hotline, 1-800-342-AIDS.

Follow-Up Questions:

Here are some questions to help promote class discussion of the Teen Views comments.

a. Matthew Himrod talks about trusting the person with AIDS. What about the infected person? What part would trust play in his or her relationships?

b. Would how a person contracted AIDS make a difference to you as it would to Aasima Afsar and Marin Miller? Why or why not?

c. Natalie Leary would make friends with someone with AIDS to show that she cares. Would you go out of your way to make friends with someone with AIDS?

d. Danielia Williams very honestly says she would probably act differently toward someone with AIDS. She says she would probably "freak out if the person cut himself or herself." Do you think you would act similarly?

e. Emilee Owen would be more careful around a person with AIDS. Do you think this would be necessary?

Would Your Behavior Toward a Classmate Change If That Person Contracted AIDS?

My behavior toward a classmate would not change if that person contracted AIDS, because that classmate would still be the same person. He or she would most likely still be able to do everything that all of my other classmates do and have just as much fun doing so. Because of this, I would, in effect, forget that the person has AIDS. I also would trust that the person would not do anything to infect me or any of my other classmates.

Matthew Himrod, 17,
Wheeling Park High School, WV

If a classmate of mine contracted AIDS, I would not act or behave any differently around them. I'm sure, subconsciously, I would be more careful around them, but I would still treat them as my equal. If I was trusted enough to know about their disease, then I would be mature enough to accept it at face value and move on. I'm sure they wouldn't want any pity or special treatment, anyway. I think it would be bad enough to have AIDS as it is.

Emilee Owen, 15,
Manzano High School, NM

I don't consider myself a biased person, but I do believe that I would probably act differently toward a person who had AIDS. I wouldn't be completely different. For instance, I wouldn't ignore the person by not speaking to him or her or by trying to keep my distance. Instead, I would feel sorry for the person. I would try to be closer to the person. But I must admit that if the person would cut himself or herself, I would probably freak out.

Danielia Williams, 17,
Wheeling Park High School, WV

My behavior toward a student with AIDS wouldn't change, because of the fact that they are people too. You can't get AIDS by touching someone, kissing someone, or even sitting beside them. AIDS is a disease caused by sexual contact or blood transfusion. A person with AIDS would stay my friend, if they already were. Even if they were not my friend, I'd try to make friends with them, to show them I care. AIDS is not a disease that you would want a loved one to have, but regardless of who has it, a caring attitude is important.

Natalie Leary, 15,
Northeastern High School, NC

If a classmate contracted AIDS, my behavior towards them would depend on how they had contracted the virus. Had it been a fairly innocent act such as sex or even accidentally coming in contact with another person's body fluids (blood), I could never think less of them than I had before. However, if the virus was contracted due to their use of drugs or not taking safety measures during sex, I would be forced to question their judgment and reevaluate my opinion of them.

Marin Miller, 14,
Manzano High School, NM

My behavior towards a classmate would be the same if that person contracted AIDS because it's what's inside that counts. But if the person contracted it by having unprotected sex and slept around, I would probably think less of that person.

Aasima Afsar, 15,
Manzano High School, NM

Our society should put more money into the schools to help teach younger kids about the disease and the responsibility they have to stop the spread of HIV [the AIDS virus]. We need to get rid of the ignorance and the fear. AIDS is forever.

Shaterra Marshall, 17,
Wilson High School, CA

Parents and guardians need to talk to their kids about the dangers of unprotected sex and of contaminated drug needles.

Jennie Miller, 15,
Duluth East High School, MN

Chapter 16, Section 3

The following quiz will help you assess your students' understanding of the material covered in this section of the chapter. You might use the quiz as an oral exercise, which will lead into a class discussion of the topics covered. Or, you might use it as a paper/pencil quiz to evaluate your students individually.

Like the Quick Quiz, the Section Review can also be used as an assessment tool to spark class discussion or as an individual student evaluation. It can also be used as a review in preparation for this quiz.

1. Abstinence or a mutually monogamous relationship with an uninfected partner are the only ways to absolutely eliminate the risk of infection from an STD. (True)

2. Safe-sex strategies only minimize the risk of contracting a sexually transmitted condom may provide an effective barrier to body fluids, and the spermicide may kill some bacterial cells and weaken some viruses. Before choosing condoms for protection, though, people should be aware that some types are more reliable than others and that all types require special care after purchase.

How effective are condoms in preventing STDs such as AIDS? Researchers are uncertain, since few reliable studies have been done. In these limited studies, however, the failure rates in preventing HIV transmission have ranged from 0 to 17 percent, depending on how consistently and effectively the condoms have been used. Of course, even a 1 percent failure rate can be fatal in the case of AIDS.

Common sense and good judgment are powerful weapons against STDs. Chapter 13 made clear that alcohol robs a person of judgment. Other mind-altering drugs do, too. The Straight Talk section that follows makes the point that the person wishing to avoid STDs needs to remain in control of clearheaded thinking.

Lastly, be aware of groups at high risk for STDs. Avoid becoming sexually involved with:

▶ Intravenous drug abusers.
▶ Anyone who has had previous sexual partners and who has not, since then, been tested for STDs.

 KEY POINTS *A preventative measure that will reduce—but not eliminate—the risks of STDs is the use of latex condoms with spermicide (from 0 to 17 percent failure rate, depending on how they are used). Alcohol and other mind-altering drugs rob people of the judgment needed to avoid STDs.*

SECTION 3 Review

Answer the following questions on a sheet of paper.

Learning the Vocabulary

The vocabulary terms in this section are *abstinence, monogamous, safer-sex strategies,* and *spermicide.*

1. Match each of the following phrases with the appropriate vocabulary term:
  a. having sexual relations with one partner only, excluding all others
  b. refraining completely from sexual relations with other people
  c. a compound that kills sperm and may weaken some STD organisms

Learning the Facts

2. What are the two ways to eliminate the risk of STDs?
3. Describe what two things must be determined before mutual monogamy is effective.
4. What type of condom is most effective against STDs?

Making Life Choices

5. Reread the Health Strategies feature, "Avoiding Contracting Sexually Transmitted Diseases," on page 440. How can you be completely protected from STDs? Explain how avoiding alcohol and other drugs may reduce the risks of STDs.

 Answers to FACT or FICTION Here are the answers to the questions at the start of the chapter.

1. **False.** Birth control pills do not protect a woman against any form of sexually transmitted disease.
2. **False.** Sexually transmitted diseases often progress with no outward symptoms. An example is chlamydia.
3. **False.** If you develop an STD, the considerate thing to do is to inform your partner. This protects you from reinfection, protects the health of your partner, and protects others.
4. **False.** Asking potential partners about past sexual experiences does not ensure that you will learn the truth about whether they are free of STDs.
5. **False.** Condoms may provide an effective barrier to body fluids, but they sometimes fail to protect against STDs.

disease. (True)
3. Abstinence absolutely eliminates the possibility of contracting AIDS. (False)
4. It is possible for you or your partner to have a sexually transmitted disease without knowing it. (True)
5. You should assume that your partner will tell you anything you should know about his/her sexual history. (False)
6. Anonymous AIDS testing is available. (True)
7. AIDS testing is 100 percent reliable. (False)
8. The goal of safe sex is to avoid any exchange of body fluids. (True)
9. All condoms are equally reliable and require no particular care or handling after purchase. (False)
10. The use of spermicide can increase the effectiveness of a condom in preventing the transmission of STDs. (True)

ASSESS

EVALUATE

Have students divide a piece of paper into two columns. At the top of the first column, have them write "Eliminating the Risk of STDs." At the top of the second column write "Reducing the Risk of STDs." Have students list information they can recall from this section that belongs in each column.

SECTION 3 Review Answers

1. a. monogamous **b.** abstinence **c.** spermicide
2. abstinence; mutually monogamous sexual relationship with an uninfected partner (p. 440)
3. the prospective partner's infection status, and the prospective partner's faithfulness (p. 440)
4. latex (p. 441)
5. Answers will vary. Avoiding alcohol and drugs helps you to make wise decisions and avoid having sex against your better judgment.

CLOSE

Have each student write a paragraph detailing his or her official plan to avoid AIDS and STDs. Tell them that during sexual activity in the heat of the moment is NOT the time to have to think of a clear plan of action for avoiding STDs. The time is NOW!

ON LINE WITH HEALTH

You may want to have your students visit the following URLs, where they will find information and additional Web site resources to enhance their study of this chapter. As with all Web sites, you should check these out first to be sure the information found there is appropriate for your students.

An Introduction to STDs
http://www.niaid. nih.gov/factsheets/ stdinfo.htm

AIDS and HIV
http://www.healthfinder. gov/tours/aids.htm

HIV InSite
http://hivinsite.ucsf.edu/

CDC National AIDS Clearinghouse
aidsinfo@cdcnac. aspensys.com

Tips for Teens about AIDS
http://www.health.org/ pubs/tips/teenaids.htm

These sites are well organized and easy to understand. They each offer comprehensive information on key HIV, AIDS, or STDs topic areas.

The Alcohol, Drug Abuse, and STD Connection

When Dr. Wah, a respected gynecologist, makes an STD diagnosis in her office she asks the patient, "Had you been drinking alcohol or taking illegal drugs at the time you were exposed to this disease?" More often than not, the answer is yes. Experts would urge teenagers to take this finding seriously. Strong links exist between teenagers who experiment with drugs or alcohol and those who acquire an STD.

I know that people who inject drugs can get AIDS and hepatitis from sharing needles. I wouldn't ever inject drugs, so none of this applies to me, right?

You are right in saying that sharing needles is extremely risky for the diseases you mention, and you are wise to exclude yourself from the group that does so. The links between substances and STDs, though, go far beyond the danger of injecting drugs. Research finds that those teenagers who drink alcohol or who smoke crack cocaine are also very likely to contract STDs such as gonorrhea, HPV, herpes, and syphilis, as well as HIV. In other words, people involved with any mind-altering substances are at risk.

That sounds strange. How can drinking or smoking something cause STDs?

Of course, these activities don't cause STDs directly. Sexual activity is responsible for passing on the STD-causing microbes. However, people who engage in drug or alcohol abuse often engage in the risky sexual behaviors that make STDs likely.

The reasons why substance abuse and STDs occur together is a topic of debate among health researchers. One school of thought holds that teenagers who grow up with certain factors in their lives may be more likely to engage in both substance abuse and in risky sexual behaviors. These factors may include:

► An unsupportive, unstable, or abusive home life.
► One or more parents who abuse substances.
► Peer groups who abuse alcohol and other drugs, commit crimes, or are truant from school.
► Poverty and the social disadvantages it brings.
► Inborn personality traits that may make the person prone to taking risks.

A teenager with one or more of these factors may begin sexual activities early in life, before having a chance to learn of the health threats from STDs. By adulthood, such a teenager may have had more sexual partners than most people do in a lifetime, while being less likely than most to take precautions against STDs. The Health Strategies section on page 440 listed those precautions.

I've seen people make all sorts of dumb decisions when they've been drinking or taking drugs. Does drinking alcohol or abusing drugs make people more careless about STDs?

The observations of physicians like Dr. Wah and of other experts suggest that this is true. The mental effects of drugs and alcohol seem to encourage

444

special needs

Interpersonal, Linguistic

There is general agreement that the topic of STDs can be embarrassing, so embarrassing that it is usually avoided as a topic of conversation. As a result, too many young people are completely unaware of the dangers they may be facing. The Teen Views feature on

page 442 gives students the opportunity to read the opinions of other teens regarding the question, "Would your behavior toward a classmate change if that person contracted AIDS? If so, how would it change?"

Give your students the opportunity to share their opinions on this question. You may divide the class into small groups to give more students the chance to brainstorm. Ask students to share ideas on what they think teenagers to throw caution to the wind. Many a teenager who began an evening by experimenting with alcohol or marijuana ended up regretting the result: unplanned and unprotected sexual intercourse that resulted in an STD.

Mind-altering drugs and alcohol reduce a person's ability to make sound judgments. Even a small amount of alcohol, say the amount in one drink, reduces inhibitions and relaxes a person's resolve. A teenager who has resolved to abstain from sexual activity, but who takes a drink of alcohol or a puff of marijuana, may suddenly lack the judgment necessary to keep that commitment. Risky situations suddenly seem less risky. With more alcohol or drugs, self-

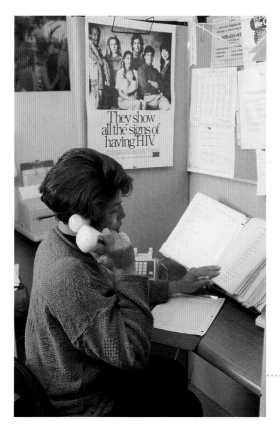

In small and big ways, people work toward eliminating the suffering of AIDS.

control erodes further, until cautious people are likely to take unbelievable risks.

An even worse problem is one of addiction. An addiction can strip people of all previous resources. It robs them of money, employment, and other supports. They may be driven to do anything, including having sexual intercourse with strangers, to obtain money to buy the drugs that can hold off the pain of withdrawal. So powerful is the force of addiction that its victims are likely to ignore even the deadly threat of AIDS, if it means that they can get the drug they crave.

 That's interesting. Luckily, those things could never happen to me or my friends. We're too smart to become addicted or infected by STDs.

Most teenagers feel just as you do. They think that STDs only infect other people—perhaps only older people, or those who are different from themselves, or those less able to handle life. Yet, the facts speak otherwise. AIDS today is a leading cause of death among teenagers, and ten times more teenagers than those who receive a diagnosis are believed to be HIV-positive.

Teenagers also make up an enormous proportion of those who are infected with many of the other STDs each year. Tragic stories abound of young adults who lost their health or their ability to bear healthy children as a result of an STD acquired during their teen years. An easy mistake is to think that because you never hear about STDs among your peers, the diseases are absent. The first page of this chapter made clear that a conspiracy of silence hides the giant problem of STDs. Nobody is talking about them, so the problem grows. However, with or without your awareness of them, STDs are a threat. The best way to avoid that threat is to abstain from sexual intercourse. Avoiding drugs and alcohol is important for all the reasons given in Chapters 12 and 13. Another reason is to help prevent STDs.

445

CNN® You can update your coverage of health and fitness topics, as well as spark lively classroom discussion and deeper understanding, by using the **CNN Health and Fitness Updates.** These video updates are produced by Turner Educational Services, using the resources of CNN, the world's first 24-hour, all-news network.

With the introduction of the **CNN Health and Fitness Updates,** West Educational Publishing is proud to be the exclusive partner of CNN for textbook/video integration in high school health. By making use of the **CNN Health and Fitness Updates** you can bring the power of CNN, the network known for providing in-depth, live coverage and analysis of breaking news events, to your health class.

For assistance in using and incorporating the **CNN Health and Fitness Updates** into your classroom presentations, see the *Classroom Guide to the CNN Health and Fitness Updates.*

The **CNN Health and Fitness Updates** are available with West Educational Publishing's *Health: Making Life Choices.*

could or should be done to inform more teens about the risks of STDs and AIDS. The result could possibly even save lives of young people in your own community.

After brainstorming, you may ask students to write a letter to the editor of your school and/or local newspaper. Included in the letter should be the reason for writing along with ideas students have generated to help stop the spread of AIDS and other STDs. You could

sponsor a contest to determine which letter will actually be sent to the paper(s). You might also phone the paper to make them aware of the letter and to find out about a possible publication date. If the letter is printed, make sure your students see a copy of the paper to help them learn that they really can make a difference.

ANSWERS TO CHAPTER 16 REVIEW

VOCABULARY

1. Answers will vary.
2. **a.** fetus **b.** pelvic inflammatory disease **c.** intravenous drug users **d.** gonorrhea **e.** chlamydia **f.** syphilis
3. **a.** Pap test **b.** ectopic pregnancy **c.** pubic lice **d.** Safer-sex strategies

RECALL

SECTION 1

1. chlamydia (p. 421)
2. A gonorrhea-killing antibiotic is applied to every infant's eyes within minutes of birth. (p. 425)
3. A woman may have internal blisters and not be aware of them. (p. 425)
4. feeling ill with fever, headache, muscle aches, painful urination, swollen glands (p. 426)
5. cancer of the cervix (p. 427)
6. removal of the growths or abnormal cervical tissue by surgery; by freezing; by applying prescription medication to external growths (p. 427)
7. detection of abnormal cervical cells, which may cause cancer of the cervix (p. 427)
8. The chancre stage begins with the presence of a hard, painless sore that disappears on its own in a few weeks. The next stage, brings swollen glands, skin rash, hair loss, and flu-like symptoms that clear up by themselves in a few weeks. The latent stage is the

CHAPTER 16 Review

Summarizing the Chapter

Your ability to respond correctly to the following statements ensures your understanding of the main concepts in the chapter.

1. List barriers to reducing the number of cases of STDs in this country.
2. Describe common symptoms of STDs.
3. Discuss the treatments or cures for common STDs.
4. Identify potential complications of STDs.
5. Describe how the AIDS virus is and is not transmitted.
6. Discuss ways of eliminating the risk of contracting STDs.
7. List measures to reduce the chances of contracting STDs.

Learning the Vocabulary

sexually transmitted diseases (STDs)
acquired immune deficiency syndrome (AIDS)
chlamydia
pelvic inflammatory disease (PID)
ectopic pregnancy
gonorrhea
genital herpes
human papilloma virus (HPV)
genital warts
Pap test
syphilis
chancre
latent
fetus

hepatitis B
trichomoniasis
pubic lice
yeast infection
candidiasis
urinary tract infections (UTIs)
jock itch
HIV
PCP
Kaposi's sarcoma
AIDS dementia complex
protease inhibitors
intravenous (IV) drug abuse
abstinence
monogamous
safer-sex strategies
spermicide

Answer the following questions on a separate sheet of paper.

1. Write a paragraph using at least ten vocabulary terms or phrases. Underline each term or phrase that you use.
2. *Matching*—Match each of the following phrases with the appropriate vocabulary term from the list above:
   a. a developing human being before birth
   b. an infection of the fallopian tubes and pelvic cavity in women
   c. the practice of using needles to inject drugs of abuse into the veins
   d. a bacterial STD that often advances without symptoms to spread through the body
   e. an infection of the reproductive tract; a frequent cause of ectopic pregnancy
   f. a bacterial STD that, if untreated, advances from a sore to flulike symptoms and, years later, to severe nerve damage
3. **a.** A _____ is a test for cancer of the cervix.
   b. An _____ is a pregnancy that has begun to develop in one of the fallopian tubes or elsewhere outside the uterus.
   c. An STD caused by tiny parasites that breed in pubic hair and cause intense itching is called _____.
   d. _____ are behavior guidelines to reduce STD risk.

Recalling Important Facts and Ideas

Section 1

1. Which STD threatens the health of millions of people in the United States?
2. Explain what the United States does to protect newborn babies' eyes against gonorrhea.
3. Why is it easier for women than for men to transmit the herpes virus?
4. List and identify symptoms of the first outbreak of genital herpes.
5. What can the worst forms of human papilloma virus cause in women?
6. Describe the treatment for human papilloma virus.
7. What is the purpose of a Pap test?
8. List and identify the stages of syphilis and the symptoms of each stage.

advancement of the disease. In the final stage, organs are infected, causing blindness, deafness, brain damage, skin damage, and heart disease leading to death. (p. 428)
9. possible death or very severe mental retardation (p. 428)
10. unpleasant-smelling yellow-green or gray discharge; abdominal pain; pain when urinating; itching in the genital area (p. 429)

11. women who are pregnant, using birth control pills, have diabetes, take antibiotics, or use douches (p. 431)

SECTION 2

12. Fatigue, appetite loss, weight loss, and nagging cough are typical. (p. 434)
13. agitation, anxiety, confusion, depression, hallucinations, increased sex drive, loss of

9. What could happen to the fetus of a woman with syphilis?
10. List the signs of a trichomoniasis infection in women.
11. Which women are especially likely to develop candidiasis?

Section 2
12. Describe the first symptoms of AIDS.
13. What are the mental symptoms of AIDS?
14. Describe the ways in which the AIDS virus is transmitted in adults.
15. Name the three additional ways that the AIDS virus is transmitted to infants.
16. List and identify ways in which HIV is not transmitted.

Section 3
17. What is the most effective way to protect against STDs?

Critical Thinking

1. Do you think a school should let the public know if someone with AIDS is going to the school? What would you do if you found out someone with AIDS was in your class? Explain how you would react to being assigned to work with a lab partner with AIDS.

Activities

1. Make a collage of all the famous people you know that have died from AIDS. Display these around the school.
2. Cut out at least five articles from magazines and newspapers about AIDS research. Write a one-page report on your findings.
3. Have a class debate about Magic Johnson. Do you think an athlete infected with HIV should play basketball in the NBA? Who is at risk if he plays? Would you play against him?
4. Take a class survey about AIDS patients in hospitals. Do you and your classmates think AIDS patients should all be in an isolated area? If you were a nurse or a doctor, would you treat AIDS patients? Why, or why not?
5. Work with a group of three to five students to prepare a research project on one of the STDs listed in Figure 16–2. In addition to the research, your group will be responsible for preparing a 3–5 minute talk to give to the class. Visual aids should be prepared for use during

the talk. You might develop transparencies, posters, models, or drawings to use. The information you present to the class should include the following: cause, symptoms, treatment, complications, and prevention of the STD.
6. Choose one of the STDs described in Figure 16–2 and prepare a set of flash cards that will teach someone about this disease. Each card will have a question on one side and the answer on the other side. For example, the question could be, "What are three symptoms of chlamydia?" Answer, "Three symptoms are burning during urination, a discharge, and abdominal pain." When flash cards are finished, use them to work with a partner or group to study STDs.
7. Create a poster or write a newspaper article that influences others to avoid the high-risk behaviors of intravenous drug use and sexual activity. If you create a poster, ask permission to display your poster somewhere around your school. If you write an article, ask to have it published in the school newspaper.
8. Write a dialog between two people; one thinks he has an STD; the other is trying to convince the first to go for testing. In the dialog, the infected person should give all the reasons for not being tested. The other person should give all the reasons for being tested. If time permits, role play the dialog with a partner.
9. Many historians believe that Christopher Columbus and his men introduced syphilis to Europe at the return of their voyage to the New World. Research syphilis or another STD to find where it is believed to have originated. How did it spread? Is it currently spreading out of control in any areas of the world? If so, why? What measures are being taken to stop the spread? Share the information you find with the rest of your class.

Making Decisions about Health

1. Your friend volunteers at a hospital after school. He has become concerned because he has been asked to help out with some AIDS patients. He is afraid that he'll somehow "catch" AIDS from being around the patients. What advice would you give your friend?

447

saliva, or sweat from an infected person, touching shared objects, wearing an infected person's clothes, using a toilet previously used by an infected person, hugging or lightly kissing an infected person, swimming with an infected person. (p. 438)

SECTION 3

17. abstinence from sexual activities (p. 440)

will, memory loss, mood swings, and social withdrawal (p. 434)
14. sexual intercourse, by the transmission of blood, semen, fluids of the vagina or other body fluids; possibly through open-mouthed passionate kissing; sharing of needles among intravenous drug users; unsterilized needles used for acupuncture, tattooing, ear piercing, and electrolysis;

blood transfusions and tissue transplants (pp. 437–438)
15. during pregnancy, during birth, by way of breastfeeding (p. 438)
16. casual contact, mosquitoes and other biting insects, eating food handled by infected persons, blood donation, vaccinations with sterilized needles, contact with unbroken, healthy skin, contact with tears,

KEY POINTS

Chapter 17 is 44 pages long and divided into ten sections. Briefly, this chapter introduces students to the concept of relating lifestyle habits to the development or prevention of disease, focusing on diabetes, cardiovascular disease, and cancer. It stresses the importance of knowing the risk factors of lifestyle diseases, as well as the alternatives for reducing such risks. The chapter also gives a brief overview of how cancer develops, controllable risk factors, screening and early detection, and cancer treatments. It includes some "hands-on" information, including suggestions on what you can do when someone close to you has cancer.

ACTIVITY TO INTRODUCE THE CHAPTER

Have students review the definition of "lifestyle diseases" in Chapter 1 and list all of their behaviors and those of their parents that they feel might contribute to the possibility of developing a lifestyle disease someday. (Answers will vary.) Now have the students imagine giving up these habits or behaviors. How would their lives change? How would their lives change physically? Financially? Mentally? Discuss their answers. Some might include: "I'd save a lot of money if I didn't smoke." "I wouldn't have as many wrinkles, freckles, or sunburns if I used sunscreen."

BULLETIN BOARD IDEAS

The American Heart Association is a rich resource for posters and other educational information

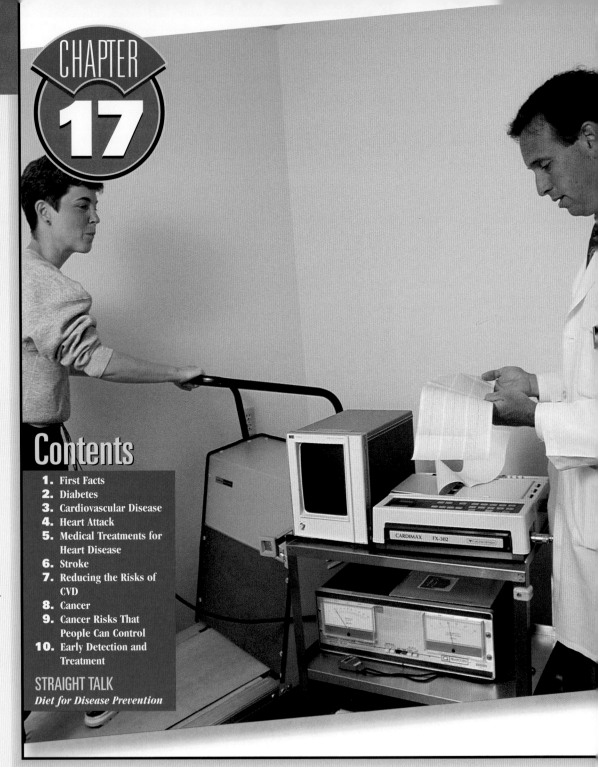

CHAPTER 17

Contents

STRAIGHT TALK
Diet for Disease Prevention

NOT Enough Time?

Following are some suggestions to help you make sure you cover the key topics in Chapter 17 if your teaching time is limited.

DAY 1   Have students read Sections 1 and 2 prior to class. Use the Activity to Introduce the Chapter on page 448. Discuss Sections with students. Do the Learning with Visuals

activity on page 453.

DAY 2   Have students read Sections 3 and 4 prior to class. During class do the Class Activity on page 457 and the Class Activity on page 460. For Section 4, do the Discussion activity on page 462. For both sections, use the Section Reviews to evaluate students' understanding of the material.

DAY 3   Have students read Sections 5 and

Lifestyle Diseases: Diabetes, Cardiovascular Disease, and Cancer

What do you think? Are the following statements true or false? If you think they are false, then say what is true.

1. A family history of diabetes, cardiovascular disease, or cancer can act as a warning sign for the younger generation.
2. Type 1 diabetes affects children and teenagers.
3. Obesity has no effect on Type 2 diabetes and its prevention.
4. A diet very low in bread, sugar, potatoes, and other carbohydrates while high in fat and protein is best for diabetes management.
5. The heart muscle receives all the nutrients and oxygen it needs from the blood in its chambers.
6. The sound of the heartbeat can tell much about the health of the heart.
7. For a person who has had a heart attack, it is too late for lifestyle changes to be of any help.
8. You can tell whether your blood pressure is high by the way you feel.
9. You can prevent most cancers by choosing healthful ways to live.
10. People with darkly pigmented skin are naturally protected against skin cancer and so do not need sunscreen products.
11. People who would like to tan without risking skin cancer can do so in tanning booths or with lamps.
12. The detection of many common cancers requires routine tests and self-examinations.

(Answers on pages 484)

Introduction

The infectious diseases of the last two chapters are major health problems of humankind. The diseases that we more often face, however, are of a different kind. They are lifestyle diseases, brought on partly by the choices we make each day. This chapter takes a look at three of these diseases: diabetes, both Type 1 and Type 2; cardiovascular disease, including heart attack, heart disease, and stroke; and cancer.

on the heart and heart disease. It can be reached by calling 1-800-AHA–USA1. This will route you to the closest AHA office. Contact the AHA for current posters to use for bulletin board displays for this unit.

Answers to FACT or FICTION

1. **True.**
2. **True.**
3. **False.** Of the two types of diabetes, Type 2 is most preventable by controlling body fatness.
4. **False.** A diet of fresh, low-fat, high-fiber, high-nutrient food is best for controlling diabetes.
5. **False.** The blood that passes through the heart's chambers brings no nourishment or oxygen to the heart's tissues. The heart muscle depends on its own network of arteries and capillaries, just as other muscles do.
6. **True.**
7. **False.** Lifestyle factors can be helpful not only in prevention but also in reversal of heart disease.
8. **False.** High blood pressure does not feel abnormal.
9. **True.**
10. **False.** While people with fair complexions who burn easily are at greater risk, everyone needs to use sunscreen to prevent skin cancer from sun exposure.
11. **False.** Tanning booths and lamps are no safer than sunbathing, as far as cancer risks are concerned.
12. **True.**

6 prior to class. During class do the Focus Activity on page 463 and the Close activity on page 465. If time allows, do the Ability Levels activity at the bottom of pages 464 and 465.

DAY 4 Have students read Sections 7 and 8 prior to class. During class do the second Class Activity on page 467 and the Life Choice Inventory on page 468. Discuss answers with students and do the Life Choice Inventory activity on page 468. Do the Class Activity on

page 474. Check students' understanding of Section 8 by giving the Quick Quiz on page 474.

DAY 5 Have students read Sections 9 and 10 prior to class. Do the Life Choice Inventory on page 478. Discuss students' answers. Use the Quick Quiz on page 478 to check students' understanding of the material in Section 9. Do the Class Activity on page 481 in Section 10.

SECTION 1

FOCUS

OUTCOMES

In this section students will learn:

1. The difference between infectious diseases and lifestyle diseases.
2. Common risk factors relating to lifestyle diseases.

FOCUS ACTIVITY

Ask students to name as many diseases as they can while you write them on the board. After you have a workable number listed, focus on causes. Divide the diseases into groups: infectious (caused by bacteria, viruses, or other microbes) and noninfectious. Discuss the diseases under each heading. How many noninfectious diseases are related to poor diet, lack of exercise, smoking, alcohol, and the like?

TEACH & APPLY

COMPREHENSION CHECK

Ask students to define *risk* and discuss their answers. Reach a class consensus on an appropriate definition. Have each student write an example of a risky activity to support the definition. Now ask students to offer definitions for *risk factor*. Discuss risk factor. Then, for the risky activity students wrote about, have them list as many things as they can that are risk factors related to that activity. Finally, ask students to identify those risk factors on their lists that can be eliminated, modified, or reduced.

450

CHAPTER 17: Lifestyle Diseases: Diabetes, Cardiovascular Disease, and Cancer

F or Y our I nformation

The term *lifestyle disease* was defined in Chapter 1. Lifestyle diseases are often included in the group called *degenerative diseases*.

F or Y our I nformation

The top ten diseases of today were listed in Figure 1–1 of Chapter 1.

SECTION 1

First Facts

Teenagers often believe (wrongly) that they have little to fear from lifestyle diseases. They think that older people—people their grandparents' or parents' ages, not teenagers—have lifestyle diseases. To a point, these beliefs are valid, because lifestyle diseases most often set in after years of behaviors that injure health. A danger lies in this reasoning, however, because the behaviors that bring about disease in later life start when people are young—very young.

For example, in this country, almost everyone has some degree of heart and artery disease. Even children only four or five years old have early traces, which steadily worsen through the years. Autopsies on teenagers as young as 15 have shown that their arteries were already clogged with fat.

Disabling disease is not inevitable, though. In fact, over the last two decades, the number of deaths from the nation's number-one killer of adults, heart disease, has shrunk by a third. About half of the decline resulted from improved treatments. Credit for the other half goes to people's efforts to avoid heart disease and heart attacks in the first place.

The choices young people make have everything to do with their health in later life. You can take action now to promote the health of your body before diseases take their toll on your health and quality of life.

Risk Factors for Lifestyle Diseases   Infectious diseases can each be blamed on a distinct bacteria, virus, or other microbe. This is not true with lifestyle diseases. These diseases tend to have clusters of suspected causes known as **risk factors**. Risk factors often include poor diet, physical inactivity, smoking, alcohol, unrewarding social interaction, other diseases, or inherited genetic traits (family history). In many cases, the presence of one risk factor increases the likelihood of others.

Young people who adopt healthy habits are less likely than others to develop lifestyle diseases later on.

special needs

Logical-mathematical

Since lifestyle diseases—diabetes, cardiovascular disease, and cancer—tend to occur more often in later life, many teenagers think of them as diseases that only affect old people. To emphasize the fact that many young people may have misconceptions about lifestyle

diseases and their causes, cures, and effects, you may want to have students conduct a survey and then chart the results.

The survey should include information from each section of the chapter, and have ten to twenty questions. (An alternative would be to have students use the Fact or Fiction questions at the beginning of the chapter as the basis for the survey.) Assign each student a set number of surveys to have completed. An-

Among risk factors, poor diet, physical inactivity, smoking, alcohol intake, and social interaction are largely under people's control. They are changeable. If a change can't hurt, and might help, why not make it.

Family History The choice to change is doubtless more important for some people than for others. People who are genetically prone to developing certain diseases would benefit most. A way to begin to decide which lifestyle changes might benefit you is to take a look at your family's medical history to see which diseases are common in your family. If any condition listed in the margin shows up in several close relatives, that condition may be of special concern to you.

Your family's medical history can give you clues to lifestyle changes that might benefit you most.

For **Y**our **I**nformation

A family history with any of the following lifestyle diseases may be a warning sign for the younger generation:

► Cancer.
► Diabetes.
► Heart attacks.
► Heart disease.
► Hypertension.
► Liver disease.*
► Obesity.†
► Osteoporosis.‡
► Strokes.

*Liver disease relates to alcoholism (see Chapter 13).
†Obesity was discussed in Chapter 8.
‡Osteoporosis is a topic of Chapter 23.

 KEY POINTS *People who adopt healthy habits when they are young lower their risks of lifestyle diseases when they are old. Risk factors for lifestyle diseases include poor diet, physical inactivity, smoking, alcohol, unrewarding social interactions, and family history.*

SECTION 1 Review

Answer the following questions on a sheet of paper.

Learning the Vocabulary

The vocabulary term in this section is *risk factors.*

1. Write a sentence using the vocabulary word.

Learning the Facts

2. When do lifestyle diseases most often set in?

3. When do the behaviors that bring about lifestyle diseases begin?

4. List seven risk factors for lifestyle diseases.

5. Which of the risk factors are under people's control?

Making Life Choices

6. If you were to discover lifestyle diseases in your family history, what steps would you take to help ensure future good health for yourself?

MINI Glossary

risk factors: factors linked with a disease by association but not yet proved to be causes.

other option would be to have students in all health or physical education courses complete the survey.

When the surveys have been completed, you may want to divide the class into groups to tabulate the results. Data can then be charted or graphed in several ways: 1) total number of correct and incorrect answers for each question; 2) total number of correct and incorrect answers by gender; 3) total number

of correct and incorrect answers by age; and so on. Students can present their findings on a bar graph, a double bar graph, line graph, and so on. You may decide to use other categories or methods.

As an enrichment to this project, you could have students develop other health-related opinion polls.

FOCUS

OUTCOMES

In this section students will learn:

1. To distinguish between Type 1 and Type 2 diabetes.
2. To identify dangers involved with diabetes.
3. Three key methods of controlling diabetes.

FOCUS ACTIVITY

Write the word *diabetes* on the board. Then give students three minutes to write down everything they can think of about diabetes. Discuss their answers. (This will give you some idea of how much knowledge students have. Do they simply relate diabetes with people having to give themselves shots, or do they have some basic understanding of the cause and progression of the disease?)

TEACH & APPLY

COMPREHENSION CHECK

Ask students some of these questions to refresh their memories about glucose and hormones: What is glucose, and why is it important to the body? (It is a sugar, and one of the body's main fuels—particularly for the brain and nervous system.) What foods contain glucose? (carbohydrates—fruits and vegetables are good sources of glucose) What are hormones? (chemical messengers sent through the bloodstream to particular target organs) If necessary, refer to Chapter 6, Section 10 and Chapter 7, Section 3.

SECTION 2 — Diabetes

Figure 17–1 Warning Signs of Diabetes

- Excessive urination and thirst.
- Glucose in the urine.
- Weight loss with nausea, easy tiring, weakness, or irritability.
- Cravings for food, especially for sweets.
- Frequent infections of the skin, gums, vagina, or urinary tract.
- Vision disturbances; blurred vision.
- Pain in the legs, feet, or fingers.
- Slow healing of cuts and bruises.
- Itching.
- Drowsiness.
- Abnormally high glucose tolerance test results.

For Your Information

Chapter 7 described glucose as the body's carbohydrate fuel (see page 171).

For Your Information

The pancreas performs two main functions:

▶ To produce digestive juices, which aid digestion.
▶ To produce the hormone insulin, which controls blood glucose.

Chapter 6 listed the pancreas with both the digestive and hormonal systems.

Diabetes, or officially **diabetes mellitus**, is among the top ten killers of U.S. adults and is the leading cause of blindness in the United States. Diabetes also contributes greatly to heart disease. Both major types of diabetes, Type 1 and Type 2, are caused by problems in the body's use of its blood sugar, glucose. Of the two types, Type 1 is less common and more often affects children and teenagers. Type 2 accounts for 80 percent of cases, and most often affects people of middle age or older. Both types produce the same warning signs that can signal their presence (see Figure 17–1).

Normally, blood glucose is under tight hormonal control. In diabetes, the concentration of blood glucose soars far beyond the normal level. When this happens, a classic symptom of diabetes shows up—glucose can be detected in the urine. The kidneys, which normally *prevent* glucose losses, allow some of the excess glucose to spill into the urine. This is why a urine test can point to diabetes: diabetic urine contains glucose, but normal urine does not. A special blood-testing method confirms the diagnosis.

The Pancreas and Its Insulin

The hormone **insulin**, made by the pancreas, lies at the heart of the problems of both types of diabetes. Insulin conducts glucose from the blood into the body's cells, which need glucose for energy. Without enough insulin, the glucose level in the blood builds up, even while the body's cells are starving for glucose. It helps to think of insulin as a key that fits a lock in a cellular doorway. To enter the cell, glucose from the blood must pass through that doorway, which remains locked until opened by insulin. No other key can unlock the door; insulin alone can do the job.

Type 1 Diabetes In Type 1 diabetes, the person's own immune system attacks the pancreas and destroys the cells that make insulin. The reason why this happens is not clear. It could be that toxins, allergies, or a virus trigger the attack. A person's genetic inheritance also may make it likely that the immune system will misbehave in this way.

enrichment

You might want to share the following information with students.

Travel usually can be a very rewarding experience if a little advanced planning is

done. People with diabetes and who are dependent on insulin, however, have to plan and prepare more carefully than most of us for any type of lengthy trip. For example, travel may bring changes in their usual sleeping, eating, exercising, and fluid intake routines, which could disturb their diabetes

Diabetes Type 1	Diabetes Type 2
Usually sets in during childhood or adolescence	Usually sets in during adulthood
Pancreas makes too little or no insulin	Pancreas makes enough or too much insulin
Body cells respond to insulin action	Body cells resist insulin action
Insulin shots required	Insulin shots generally not required, but other drugs may be of help
Low to average body fatness	High body fatness

Figure 17–2 Diabetes Types 1 and 2 Compared

Whatever the cause, the pancreas soon no longer produces enough insulin. Without insulin, each meal brings a large, long-lasting surge of glucose to the bloodstream.

Type 2 Diabetes   The blood of a person with Type 2 diabetes also builds up glucose to an abnormally high level, but for a different reason. Instead of a lack of insulin (the pancreas usually produces plenty), the fault lies with the body's cells, which fail to respond to insulin. The cellular locks have been changed, so to speak, so that insulin cannot open them. A gain of body fat may have this effect; excess fat makes cells less responsive to insulin's effects. Indeed, obesity, or even just modest weight gain, often occurs just before Type 2 diabetes set in. Obesity is a major risk factor for diabetes. The two types of diabetes are compared in Figure 17–2.

 In both Type 1 and Type 2 diabetes, the body's cells fail to handle glucose in normal ways. The pancreas of a person with Type 1 diabetes does not produce enough insulin. The body cells of a person with Type 2 diabetes do not respond to insulin.

The Dangers of Diabetes

Some of the dangers of diabetes are immediately apparent, as when blood glucose goes out of control. Other dangers occur over time, as damage from diabetes accumulates in the body.

Diabetic Coma   An immediate threat to those who fail to control their diabetes is **diabetic coma**. When body tissues are starving for glucose (even though glucose in the *blood* remains high), the tissues are forced to use more fats than normal for energy. Under these conditions, fat molecules are broken down only part way, and fragments of fat, known as **ketones**, build up to toxic levels in the blood. This causes tiredness, dry or flushed skin, abdominal pain, nausea or vomiting, difficulty breathing, confusion, and ultimately, loss of consciousness and death.

diabetes (DYE-uh-BEE-teez) **mellitus** (MEL-ih-tuss): a condition of abnormal use of glucose, usually caused by too little insulin or lack of response to insulin.

insulin: a hormone produced by the pancreas and released in response to high blood glucose following a meal. Insulin promotes the use and storage of glucose by the body's tissues.

diabetic coma: a loss of consciousness due to uncontrolled diabetes and the resulting buildup of toxic ketones in the blood.

ketones: fragments formed by the tissues during incomplete use of fat for energy, and released into the blood.

treatment plans. They must take extra precautions against such things as motion sickness, which can disrupt fluid balance and normal eating schedules and lack of exercise, which can inhibit proper circulation. The different foods of other countries also are a cause for concern. They must be analyzed to ensure that the proper amounts of protein and carbohydrate are being ingested. Even foot care can be a problem. Because people with diabetes often have difficulty with their feet and travel often involves a lot of walking, extra care must be taken to ensure that no problems develop with the feet.

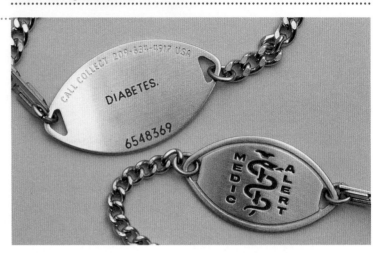

Medical identification bracelets and necklaces can mean the difference between life and death.

For Your Information

Across the nation, the emergency number is 911.

For Your Information

Carry these items with you if you have diabetes:

▶ Identification, such as a medical wallet card, bracelet, or necklace.

▶ Phone or emergency money.

▶ Blood glucose testing strips.

▶ Glucose tablets or other high-sugar food if you use insulin injections or diabetes pills.

▶ A watch with an alarm to remind you when a snack or dose of insulin is due.

Insulin Shock   The opposite case is **insulin shock**. When meals are skipped, when too much insulin is given, or when exercise has used up too much glucose, blood glucose levels can fall dangerously low. Symptoms including shakiness, dizziness, hunger, sweating, headache, pale skin, rapid heart rate, jerky movements, confusion, and a tingling sensation in the mouth signal the start of insulin shock. The person needs glucose quickly to avert disaster. Glucose tablets, candy, or fruit juice are good sources.

Medical Emergencies   Loss of consciousness in a person with diabetes is a red-hot medical emergency. If a well-meaning helper were to misdiagnose the cause of the situation and give wrong treatment, it could be a fatal mistake. The treatment for diabetic coma worsens insulin shock, and treatment for insulin shock deepens diabetic coma. No one but a medical professional or other trained person should inject insulin or put anything into the mouth of an unconscious person with diabetes. Anyone else should call for help instead.

Long-Term Effects   Diabetes's long-term effects, while less immediate, can be severe. The damage from diabetes slowly steals the health of the body's organs, often even while drugs control blood glucose. The root cause of all the problems of diabetes (listed in Figure 17–3) is probably the same. Diabetes causes blockage or destruction of small blood vessels that feed body organs such as the eyes, heart, and kidneys. It also blocks the blood flow to the legs and feet. Without blood flow through the tissues, they die from lack of oxygen and nourishment. This is why diabetes is named as a risk factor for many other diseases.

Some teenage girls with diabetes face delayed growth and maturation. This is especially true in young athletes who do not regulate their blood glucose accurately enough. Once they regain control over blood glucose, growth proceeds normally.

Pursuing wellness

Have students consider the following situation.

You're walking home with a friend who suddenly becomes dizzy and passes out. You call an ambulance and then try to contact the friend's family but are unable to reach them. At the hospital, the doctor discovers that your friend has an infection and is about to administer penicillin. Suddenly the doctor stops. Why? She has seen the Medic Alert necklace around your friend's neck. It tells the doctor that your friend is allergic to penicillin and should not be given the drug.

Too little insulin or lack of response to insulin leaves blood glucose levels high and cells starved for glucose energy. Poor control of diabetes causes damage to blood vessels in many parts of the body. Diabetes in some teenage girls may delay growth and maturation.

Prevention and Control of Diabetes

Of the two types of diabetes, Type 2 is most preventable. It tends to run in families, especially ones where obesity is prevalent. With family history to warn family members of the danger, they can take weight control seriously to reduce their chances of developing the disease. While most cases of Type 2 diabetes occur in overweight middle-aged adults, even children and teenagers who are overweight can develop it. Figure 17–4 on the next page shows that diabetes and obesity worsen each other. Older people must also watch their alcohol intakes. Heavy use of alcohol makes development of Type 2 diabetes likely.

Once diabetes is diagnosed, its control is essential to health. Like a juggler who keeps three circus balls constantly in motion, the person with diabetes must constantly balance three lifestyle factors—medication, diet, and physical activity. The person with diabetes who fails in these three controls opens the door to all of the medical consequences mentioned earlier.

Medication   Because the pancreas of a person with Type 1 diabetes does not make enough insulin, the person must receive insulin from shots or from an implanted pump at certain times each day. Pills taken by mouth cannot deliver the needed insulin. Insulin is a protein and would be digested before it could be absorbed into the bloodstream. Researchers hope to soon be able to transplant healthy tissue into the pancreas of people with Type 1 diabetes to get it working again.

Treatment of Type 2 diabetes may involve drugs that stimulate the pancreas to release extra insulin. The extra insulin sometimes helps the tissues to respond and to remove glucose from the blood more quickly. Other drugs work in other ways to stimulate body tissues to use up more glucose from the bloodstream.

Diet   As for diet, a balanced diet of fresh, high-fiber vegetables, whole grains, low-fat meats and milk products, and other high-nutrient food is best for controlling diabetes. Sweets such as sugar, honey, syrups, soft drinks, and sugar-sweetened foods should be strictly controlled. The amount of sugar allowed varies with an individual's blood glucose response to it.

The same diet is also low in calories, and so helps in controlling weight. It is high in complex carbohydrates, and so supports physical activity best.

Diabetes, especially when poorly controlled, can cause these serious problems:

- Impaired circulation.
- Disease of the feet and legs that often leads to amputation.
- Kidney disease that often requires hospital care or kidney transplant.
- Impaired vision or blindness due to cataracts and damaged retinas.
- Nerve damage.
- Skin damage.
- Strokes and heart attacks.

*Figure 17–3 **The Destructive Results of Diabetes***

Mini Glossary

insulin shock: the result of too much insulin, which causes a dangerous drop in blood glucose. Also called *hypoglycemia*.

COMPREHENSION CHECK

Have students refer to the text for the probable root cause for the destructive results of diabetes. (blockage or destruction of small blood vessels that feed body organs such as the eyes, heart, and kidneys) Ask students to relate this probable root cause to the various destructive results listed in Figure 17–3. (For instance, blockage or destruction of these small blood vessels would reduce the circulation within the body.)

DISCUSSION

Have students study Figure 17–4 on page 456. Discuss how the problem of obesity and Type 2 diabetes can be self-feeding. Where does a person need to break the cycle? Why does it help to know that increased appetite is a factor in this cycle? Why does this make weight loss more difficult?

Medic Alert bracelets and necklaces carry engraved warnings against using certain drugs or about particular conditions the wearer has. When a person cannot communicate in an emergency, the Medic Alert emblem conveys important information. If you or a friend or family member has a medical condition such as diabetes or an allergy to certain medications, you should consider getting a Medic Alert bracelet or necklace. It could save your life. For more information, contact the Medic Alert Foundation. Phone: 1-800-825-3785. Web site: http://www.medicalert.org/

ASSESS

EVALUATE

SECTION 2 Review Answers

1. diabetic coma
2. insulin shock
3. ketones
4. diabetes
5. insulin
6. diabetes (p. 452)
7. problems in the body's use of its blood sugar, glucose (p. 452)
8. Answers may vary; refer to Figure 17–1 for answers (p. 452).
9. blockage or destruction of small blood vessels that feed body organs such as the eyes, heart, and kidneys; it blocks the flow of blood to the legs and feet (p. 454)
10. Answers will vary.

A reproducible quiz for Section 2 is provided in the Teacher's Resource Box.

CLOSE

Give students the following list of terms and ask them to use these terms properly in a paragraph describing diabetes and its treatment. (pancreas, insulin, glucose, Type 1, Type 2, diet, medication, exercise)

Figure 17–4 The Obesity-Diabetes Cycle

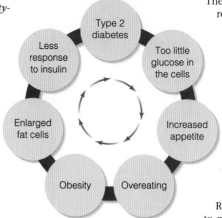

Type 2 diabetes → Too little glucose in the cells → Increased appetite → Overeating → Obesity → Enlarged fat cells → Less response to insulin → Type 2 diabetes

The Straight Talk section on page 486 reveals the nature of the diet thought best for protecting against diabetes and other lifestyle diseases.

Teenagers with diabetes often face special problems. Friends get together for a pizza, ice cream, or other treats. It can be hard for a teenager with diabetes to look on and say, "No, thank you." It helps to know that with planning, almost any food is acceptable. Even a small piece of birthday cake at a party might be allowable. The trick is to eat it as part of a meal, and to keep track of it as a source of glucose. Registered dietitians have all sorts of tips to make life more pleasurable for teenagers with diabetes.

Physical Activity Physical activity is important, too. It not only helps to control body weight, but also helps use up blood glucose. Some people with diabetes find that they need less insulin or other drugs when physical activity becomes part of their daily routine.

KEY POINTS *Maintaining appropriate body weight is an important strategy for preventing diabetes. Medication, diet, and physical activity are the three tools for controlling diabetes and its consequences.*

SECTION 2 Review

Answer the following questions on a sheet of paper.

Learning the Vocabulary

The vocabulary terms for this section are *diabetes, insulin, diabetic coma, ketones,* and *insulin shock.*
Match the following phrases with the appropriate term from the list above:

1. a loss of consciousness due to uncontrolled diabetes
2. the result of too much insulin
3. fragments formed by the tissues during incomplete use of fat for energy, and released into the blood
4. a condition of abnormal use of glucose
5. a hormone produced by the pancreas and released in response to high glucose following a meal

Learning the Facts

6. What is the leading cause of blindness in the United States?
7. What is the cause of both types of diabetes?
8. List five warning signs of diabetes.
9. What are the long-term effects of diabetes?

Making Life Choices

10. What advice would you give someone who has diabetes?

QUICK QUIZ

Chapter 17, Section 2

The following quiz will help you assess your students' understanding of the material covered in this section of the chapter. You might use the quiz as an oral exercise, which will lead into a class discussion of the topics covered. Or, you might use it as a paper/pencil quiz to evaluate your students individually.

Like the Quick Quiz, the Section Review can also be used as an assessment tool to spark class discussion or as an individual student evaluation. It can also be used as a review in preparation for this quiz.

1. Diabetes is the leading cause of blindness in the United States. (True)
2. Diabetes is unrelated to the incidence of heart disease. (False)

SECTION 3

Cardiovascular Disease

MINI Glossary

The number-one killer of adults is **cardiovascular disease (CVD)**. Many people become sick and die of CVD long before they reach retirement age. One in every four people living in the United States is ill with some form of this disease. Most others are in some stage of developing it. Fortunately, however, everyone can take steps to reduce the risks of developing CVD.

Disease of the heart and blood vessels—cardiovascular disease (CVD)—develops slowly over a lifetime. Of the three kinds of blood vessels—the **arteries**, **capillaries**, and **veins**—the disease is most noticeable in the arteries. Therefore, properly speaking, we should be referring to *heart and artery disease*.

The Cardiovascular System

The body system that provides all the tissues and cells with all that they need to live is the **cardiovascular system**—the heart and blood vessels (see Chapter 6). Also called the *circulatory system,* it pumps the equivalent of 4,000 gallons of **blood** around the body each day, driving this blood with over 85,000 heartbeats.

The Heart's Chambers The heart, at the center of the cardiovascular system, is almost all muscle. Four hollow **chambers** inside collect blood and then pump it out again into tough, elastic arteries. The heart can be compared to an import-export business. Just as an importer receives and distributes goods, the heart receives and distributes blood. Two of the heart's four chambers function as receiving areas and two, as shipping areas. The receiving chambers, the **atria**, pool the blood as it arrives from the body. The shipping chambers, the **ventricles**, contract powerfully to send the blood on its way again.

Coronary Arteries The heart does not benefit from the blood within its chambers. That blood is simply passing by, and does not nourish or cleanse the heart's tissues. The heart relies on its own network of vessels—the **coronary arteries** and capillaries—for nourishment and cleansing blood flow. The coronary arteries branch into capillaries that weave all over the heart's outer surface and feed it with nutrients and oxygen (see Figure 17–5 on the next page). This fact becomes important to understanding how the heart is affected by disease of the arteries.

The Heart's Valves You have probably listened to your own or someone else's heartbeat and noticed its two-step rhythm, sometimes called *lub-dub.* The first beat ("lub") is the sound made when the atria contract to send the blood they have pooled to the ventricles below them. The second beat ("dub") is the sound made when the powerful ventricles contract to send the blood on its way to the lungs and to the body. (The atria relax and pool more blood during the "dub.")

You may be wondering why the contraction of the heart muscle should make any sound at all. In reality, it does not. The sound comes from the

cardiovascular disease (CVD): a general term for all diseases of the heart and blood vessels.

arteries: blood vessels that carry blood from the heart to the tissues.

capillaries: the smallest blood vessels, which connect the smallest arteries with the smallest veins. Nourishment and fluid normally trapped in thick-walled arteries and veins can easily pass through the delicate walls of the capillaries.

veins: blood vessels that carry waste-containing blood from the tissues back to the heart.

cardiovascular system: the system of structures that circulate blood and lymph throughout the body. Also called the *circulatory system.*

blood: the thick, red fluid that flows through the body's blood vessels and transports gases, nutrients, wastes, and other important substances around the body. Blood also plays roles in body temperature regulation.

chambers: rooms; in the heart, large, hollow areas that receive incoming blood from the lungs and tissues and ship it out again.

atria (singular, **atrium**): the two upper chambers of the heart—the receiving areas that pool incoming blood.

ventricles: the two lower chambers of the heart—the shipping areas that send blood on its way to the lungs or the tissues.

coronary arteries: the two arteries that supply blood to the heart muscle.

---

3. A person with diabetes has a blood glucose level high above normal. (True)

4. In Type 1 diabetes, the pancreas produces too much insulin. (False)

5. In Type 2 diabetes, the body's cells fail to respond to insulin. (True)

6. Obesity may cause the onset of Type 2 diabetes. (True)

7. Diabetic coma occurs when keetones build up to toxic levels in the blood. (True)

8. Insulin shock is caused by an excess of glucose in the blood. (False)

9. Because diabetes causes blockage or destruction of the small blood vessels it has been named as a risk factor for many other diseases. (True)

10. Medication, diet, and exercise must be carefully controlled in order to maintain health after the onset of diabetes. (True)

SECTION 3

FOCUS

OUTCOMES

In this section students will learn:

1. That the cardiovascular system provides each body cell with all it needs to live.

2. That the heart, blood vessels, blood, and lymph play important roles in keeping cells alive and well.

3. The frequency of CVD in the U.S. today.

4. The relationship between atherosclerosis and CVD.

FOCUS ACTIVITY

List the following causes of death on the board: heart disease, cancer, accidents, suicide, and AIDS. Ask students to consider the list and pick the one they think the most people die of every year in the U.S. Count the number of students choosing each and record it on the board next to their choices. Stress that heart disease is the number-one killer. Are they surprised?

TEACH & APPLY

CLASS ACTIVITY

Ask your students to stand next to their seats. Count off the students, one through four. Ask all of the fours to sit down. Tell them that one in every four people living in the U.S. is ill from some form of CVD. Ask students how this information makes them feel. Would they like to be able to do something to avoid becoming a statistic?

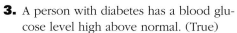

CHAPTER 17: Lifestyle Diseases: Diabetes, Cardiovascular Disease, and Cancer

CLASS ACTIVITY

Bring a stethoscope to class and allow students to listen to their own heartbeats and to a partner's heartbeat to identify the "lub-dub," two-step rhythm. Ask which chambers create the lub sound and which create the dub sound. Discuss the real source of the sound. (the closing of the valves) Ask how you murmur when you talk. (mouth slightly open) Discuss how this is related to a heart murmur.

The transparency, "The Heart's Major Arteries," (Figure 17–5) is provided in the Teacher's Resource Box.

CLASS ACTIVITY

Atherosclerosis can be a difficult word to pronounce for many students. Have them practice aloud with each other.

BACKGROUND INFORMATION

As enrichment, you may want to remind students that the heart is a muscle. Explain that as it tries to respond to the extra strain of high blood pressure, it becomes larger and stronger, especially in its left ventricle. More and more research indicates that an enlarged left ventricle reflects advancing heart and artery disease. This heart abnormality can be detected by a test that compares the mass of the left ventricle to the other portions of the heart. This comparison produces a score known as the *left ventricle mass index.*

Figure 17–5 The Heart's Major Arteries. The coronary arteries feed the heart muscle itself. The heart derives no nourishment from the blood inside its chambers.

Right Coronary Artery

Left Coronary Artery

slapping shut of the heart's **valves**—flaps of tissue located at the entrances and exits of the chambers. The heart's valves are illustrated in Figure 6–7 on page 145, in Chapter 6. (You may wish to turn back there to review the cardiovascular system as you read this chapter.) Normally, the valves allow blood to flow in only one direction on its way through the heart. If the valves are damaged or unusually shaped, however, some blood will flow backward. This changes the heartbeat sound (a **heart murmur**). Heart murmurs usually do not indicate trouble. Sometimes, though, they can mean that the heart requires medical attention.

A heart examination includes a physician's listening to the heartbeat and, possibly, an **electrocardiogram**. An electrocardiogram is a record of the electrical activity of the heart.

The Workings of Capillaries   As blood moves through the tiniest vessels, the capillaries, much of its fluid **(lymph)** is strained out into the tissues. The fluids flow around the cells of the tissues, providing them with nutrients and oxygen and collecting their wastes. Then, the used fluids seep back into the bloodstream to be carried away for cleaning and renewal. In this way, the tissues are nourished and cleansed.

Heart Disease   Disease in any part of the cardiovascular system affects many of the body's tissues, of course, because the blood nourishes all the tissues. Any disease that affects the heart muscle or other working parts of the heart is called **heart disease**. The term *cardiovascular disease* refers to diseases of all parts of the cardiovascular system, including both the heart and blood vessels. The onset of these diseases can be postponed or prevented by changes in people's lifestyles. Therefore, these diseases can often be controlled by individuals.

 The cardiovascular system consists of the heart and the blood vessels. Also called the circulatory system, it serves as the tissues' supply line for both nutrients and oxygen, as well as their waste disposal system. The working parts of the heart include its four chambers and the valves that connect them. The coronary arteries nourish and cleanse the tissues of the heart.

The Dangers of Atherosclerosis

The disease **atherosclerosis**, or hardening of the arteries, is the most common form of CVD. It begins with an accumulation of mounds of soft fat along the inner walls of all the arteries of the body. Such mounds gradually enlarge and harden with mineral deposits to form **plaques**. Plaques make the passageway through the arteries narrower than normal (see Figure 17–6 on page 460).

Ability Levels

On Level, Advanced

Ask a student to begin this activity by drawing a diagram of the heart on the board. Ask other students, one at a time, to add, correct, or delete from the picture, and label all of the structures as the diagram progresses. At minimum, labeling should include: left atrium, right atrium, left ventricle, right ventricle, aorta, inferior and superior vena cava, septum, pulmonary artery, pulmonary vein, and valve locations. Arrows should be used to indicate

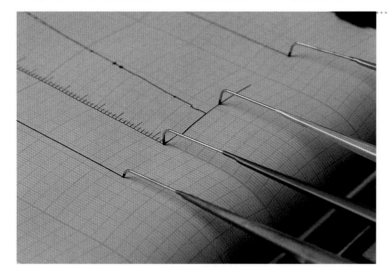

An electrocardiogram records the heart's electrical activity.

MINI Glossary

valves: flaps of tissue that open and close to allow the flow of blood in one direction only. The heart's valves are located at the entrances and exits of its chambers.

heart murmur: a heart sound that reflects damaged or abnormal heart valves.

electrocardiogram: a record of the electrical activity of the heart that, if abnormal, may indicate heart disease.

lymph: the clear fluid that bathes each cell and transfers needed substances and wastes back and forth between the blood and the cells. Lymph also plays a role in immunity.

heart disease: any disease of the heart muscle or other working parts of the heart.

atherosclerosis (ATH-uh-roh-scler-OH-sis): the most common form of CVD; a disease characterized by plaques along the inner walls of the arteries.

plaques (PLACKS): mounds of fat, mixed with minerals, that build up along artery walls in atherosclerosis.

aneurysm (AN-your-ism): the ballooning out of an artery wall at a point where it has grown weak.

aorta (ay-OR-tah): the largest artery in the body; it conducts freshly oxygenated blood from the heart to the tissues.

platelets: tiny, disk-shaped bodies in the blood, important in blood clot formation.

As mentioned, the heart muscle depends on blood flow through its own arteries for nourishment and oxygen. In atherosclerosis, the arteries that supply the heart begin to narrow and harden, depriving the heart of its health and strength. Arteries that feed other organs and tissues narrow and harden, too, cutting off their supplies of nutrients and oxygen.

High Blood Pressure   Atherosclerosis not only weakens the heart, but also leads to high blood pressure. Normally the arteries expand with each heartbeat to allow blood to pass, and they then contract again. Arteries hardened by plaques cannot expand, so the pulses of blood must squeeze through them. This causes pressure to build up, because the blood backs up at the narrowed areas while the heart strains to push it through.

This high blood pressure in the arteries, or hypertension, is a major contributor to CVD. Hypertension damages the artery walls and can even cause them to go into spasms, further blocking blood flow. Also, as pressure builds up in an artery, the arterial wall may become weakened and balloon out, forming an **aneurysm**. An aneurysm can burst. When this happens in a small artery, it leads to death of the tissue surrounding it. In a major artery such as the **aorta**, a ruptured aneurysm leads quickly to massive bleeding (hemorrhage) and death. Figure 17–7 on page 461 illustrates an aneurysm and a hemorrhage.

Blood Clots   Abnormal blood clotting is another threat caused by atherosclerosis. Under normal conditions, clots form and dissolve in the blood all the time. Small, cell-like bodies in the blood, known as **platelets**, cause clots to form whenever they detect injuries. This normal function protects the body against blood losses by plugging minor wounds. Clots also form accidentally inside the blood vessels when the platelets encounter rough spots such as plaques. Normally, these clots soon dissolve again. In atherosclerosis, however, platelets encounter many plaques and begin the clotting process more often than normal.

the path of the flow of blood into, through, and out of the heart, to the lungs, back to the heart, and out to the body. Two chalk colors could be used for arrows, heart chambers, and blood vessels to differentiate oxygenated and deoxygenated blood flow. Check each correct item as the diagram progresses. Refer

students to Figure 17–5 and Figure 6–7 on page 144 in Chapter 6 to make final additions or deletions. If students are not knowledgeable enough to keep this activity moving along, you may wish to have them use Figures 17–5 and 6–7 as a guide at the beginning of the activity.

The transparency, "The Formation of Plaques in Atherosclerosis," (Figure 17–6) is provided in the Transparency Acetate Binder.

COMPREHENSION CHECK

Review with students the process of hardening of the arteries to be sure they understand how hardening of the arteries can harm the individual in many ways other than weakening the heart. (Hardening of the coronary arteries weakens the heart; hardening of the other arteries damages the organs and tissues throughout the rest of the body.)

CLASS ACTIVITY

Obtain several long, skinny balloons that are small and that will blow up in one area on initial inflation. (This usually works best with very cheap or poor-quality balloons.) Use one to simulate an aneurysm. Have students look at Figure 17–7. Give them five minutes to review the chapter information on aneurysms and be able to: 1. Explain how or why an aneurysm develops. 2. Give a cause for an aneurysm developing. 3. Tell what can result from an aneurysm. Ask for volunteer answers and award extra credit.

Figure 17–6 *The Formation of Plaques in Atherosclerosis*

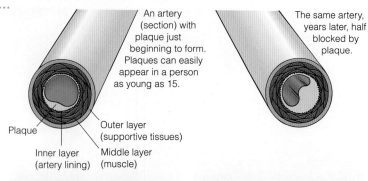

An artery (section) with plaque just beginning to form. Plaques can easily appear in a person as young as 15.

The same artery, years later, half blocked by plaque.

Plaque
Inner layer (artery lining)
Outer layer (supportive tissues)
Middle layer (muscle)

A healthy artery provides an open passageway for the flow of blood.

Plaques along an artery narrow its diameter and interfere with blood flow. Clots can form, making the problem worse.

Artery Blockages   Atherosclerosis can cause blockage of an artery in any of three ways:

1. The plaques themselves can enlarge enough to block the flow of blood.
2. A blood clot may form, stick to a plaque, and gradually grow until it cuts off the blood supply like a plug (a **thrombus**). In the arteries of the heart, such a blockage is called a **coronary thrombosis** (a type of **heart attack**). In a vessel that feeds the brain, the blockage is called a **cerebral thrombosis** (a type of **stroke**).
3. A clot may also break loose, become a *traveling* clot (an **embolus**), and circulate until it reaches an artery too small to allow its passage. The sudden blockage of the vessel is an **embolism**.

When an artery is blocked, the tissue normally supplied by the blocked vessel may suddenly die. Tissue death can occur gradually, too, resulting in organ damage.

QUICK QUIZ

Chapter 17, Section 3

The following quiz will help you assess your students' understanding of the material covered in this section of the chapter. You might use the quiz as an oral exercise, which will lead into a class discussion of the topics covered. Or, you might use it as a paper/pencil

quiz to evaluate your students individually.

Like the Quick Quiz, the Section Review can also be used as an assessment tool to spark class discussion or as an individual student evaluation. It can also be used as a review in preparation for this quiz.

1. Cardiovascular disease (CVD) is the number-one cause of death in adults. (True)
2. CVD refers to disease of the heart and

The development of atherosclerosis reaches a **critical phase** when more than half of the inner surfaces of the arteries are covered with plaques. Once in the critical phase, a person faces a high risk of heart attacks or strokes.

An aneurysm   A hemorrhage

Figure 17–7 An Aneurysm and a Hemorrhage

KEY POINTS *Atherosclerosis is the formation of plaques in the arteries. It worsens hypertension and makes blood clots likely. Atherosclerosis can cause blockage of arteries that feed critical organs, such as the heart or brain.*

SECTION 3 Review

Answer the following questions on a sheet of paper.

Learning the Vocabulary

The vocabulary terms for this section are *cardiovascular disease, arteries, capillaries, veins, cardiovascular system, blood, chambers, atria, ventricles, coronary arteries, valves, heart murmur, electrocardiogram, lymph, heart disease, atherosclerosis, plaques, aneurysm, aorta, platelets, thrombus, coronary thrombosis, heart attack, cerebral thrombosis, stroke, embolus, embolism,* and *critical phase.*

Match the following phrases with the appropriate term from the list above:

1. system of structures that circulates blood and lymph throughout the body
2. flaps that allow the body's fluids to flow in one direction only
3. small, cell-like bodies in the blood that are important in clot formation
4. a stationary clot that blocks a vessel that feeds the brain

Learning the Facts

5. What is the difference between an embolus and a thrombus?
6. The equivalent of how many gallons of blood are pumped around the body each day?
7. How does the heart obtain the nutrients and oxygen it needs?
8. What makes the heartbeat sound?
9. What has happened to the arteries of someone diagnosed with atherosclerosis?

Making Life Choices

10. Why do people think that cardiovascular disease won't happen to them? How does this thinking cause people to make poor health choices and to continue unhealthy behaviors?

MINI Glossary

thrombus: a stationary clot. When it has grown enough to close off a blood vessel, this dangerous event is a *thrombosis.*

coronary thrombosis: the closing off of a vessel that feeds the heart muscle by a stationary clot, or *thrombus.*

heart attack: the event in which vessels that feed the heart muscle become blocked, causing tissue death.

cerebral thrombosis: the closing off of a vessel that feeds the brain by a stationary clot, or *thrombus.*

stroke: the shutting off of the blood flow to the brain by plaques, a clot, or hemorrhage.

embolus (EM-bow-luss): a clot that breaks loose and travels through the bloodstream. When it causes sudden closure of a blood vessel, this dangerous event is an *embolism.*

embolism: the sudden closure of a blood vessel by a traveling blood clot, or *embolus.*

critical phase: in atherosclerosis, the stage when plaques cover more than half of the inner surfaces of the arteries.

ASSESS

EVALUATE

blood vessels, but is most noticeable in the capillaries. (False)
3. The cardiovascular system is also called the circulatory system. (True)
4. The heart's ventricles pool the blood as it arrives from the body. (False)
5. The heart consists almost entirely of muscle. (True)
6. The coronary arteries provide nourishment to the heart. (True)
7. A heart murmur is caused by blood flowing backward through the heart's valves. (True)
8. The capillaries deliver lymph to the tissues. (True)
9. One of the symptoms of atherosclerosis is low blood pressure. (False)
10. Thrombus, embolism, and coronary or cerebral thrombosis are all potential results of atherosclerosis. (True)

SECTION 4

FOCUS

OUTCOME

In this section students will learn:

1. Causes and symptoms of heart attack.

FOCUS ACTIVITY

Ask students if they know anyone who has had a stroke or heart attack. Discuss their experiences.

TEACH & APPLY

DISCUSSION

Discuss with students the warning signs for stroke or heart attack. Ask students if they would know what to do. (see Figure 17–8)

ASSESS

EVALUATE

Review Answers

1. Answers will vary.
2. Heart muscle tissue dies for lack of oxygen.
3. Refer to Figure 17–8.
4. Answers will vary.

CLOSE

Ask students to outline what happens in a heart attack. Discuss the paragraphs.

Figure 17–8 Warning Signs of Heart Attack and Stroke

The warning signs of heart attack:

Even though not every heart attack is announced by clear-cut symptoms, you should get help immediately if you or someone you are with:

1. Feels uncomfortable pressure, fullness, squeezing, or pain in the center of the chest lasting for more than two minutes.
2. Experiences pain that spreads to the shoulders, neck, or arms.
3. Becomes dizzy, faints, sweats for no apparent reason, or has nausea or shortness of breath—especially when other symptoms are present.

The warning signs of stroke:

Report to a physician immediately any of the following:

1. Sudden, temporary weakness or numbness in any part of one side of the body.
2. Temporary loss of speech or of understanding of speech.
3. Dizziness, unsteadiness, or unexplained falls.
4. Temporary dimness or loss of vision, particularly in one eye.

Heart Attack

Heart attacks are the most common of the life-threatening events brought on by atherosclerosis. A heart attack occurs when blood flow to the heart becomes so restricted that some of the heart's muscle tissue dies for lack of oxygen. When heart muscle tissue dies, it is replaced by scar tissue that cannot do the heart's pumping work. The remaining muscle tissue must work harder to make up for the loss.

Another problem of reduced oxygen to the heart is pain. A sudden exertion or emotional upset can bring on a pain in the chest, called **angina**. Angina is not always a symptom of a heart attack, but it can be. A person experiencing angina may deny that a heart attack is occurring and blame the symptoms on "indigestion." Many heart attack victims might have been saved had they only taken their pain seriously. If you or someone nearby suffers any of the heart attack symptoms listed in Figure 17–8, get medical help fast. Chapter 23 offers first-aid procedures for heart attack victims.

Often, a person has no pain before a first heart attack occurs and so may not be warned of the coming attack. Even medical tests designed to predict future heart attacks often fail to do so. Many heart attack deaths are sudden and unexpected.

KEY POINTS *A heart attack occurs when blood flow to the heart becomes so restricted that part of the heart muscle dies for lack of oxygen. Symptoms often include pain. They demand prompt attention.*

Review

Answer the following questions on a sheet of paper.

Learning the Vocabulary

The vocabulary term for this section is *angina.*

1. Write a sentence using the vocabulary term.

Learning the Facts

2. What occurs when someone has a heart attack?
3. List the three warning signs of a heart attack.

Making Life Choices

4. What would you do if someone in your family appeared to be having a heart attack but denied it and insisted on continuing with whatever he or she was doing?

enrichment

Students may find it helpful to know that the term *angina* comes from the Latin word *angere,* which means *choke,* and is characterized by a suffocating sensation.

Technically, *angina* is any disease which causes spasmodic squeezing pain. *Angina pectoris* is angina of the chest. It is caused by constriction of the blood supply traveling to the heart muscle through the coronary arteries.

SECTION 5
Medical Treatments for Heart Disease

Heart attacks do not always end in death or disability. Many times a person who suffers a minor heart attack can recover fully. The heart in heart attack may go into **fibrillation**. The heart muscle contracts in quivering, rapid spasms that lack power to pump blood through the body. The person quickly loses consciousness, lacks a pulse, and may die unless a normal heartbeat is restored quickly. Electric shocks delivered to the chest by a defibrillator can reorganize the heart's normal electric signals and restore a normal heartbeat. One drug given within a few hours after the onset of a heart attack triggers the clot-dissolving action of the blood and thus stops a heart attack in its tracks, preventing much tissue damage.

Other drugs may be used to strengthen and stabilize the heartbeat. A **pacemaker** is an implanted device that provides electrical stimulation for a failing heartbeat.

A common surgery for a failing heart is **coronary artery bypass surgery**. This involves replacing the blocked coronary arteries with sections of the person's own veins or with synthetic tubing. In another form of

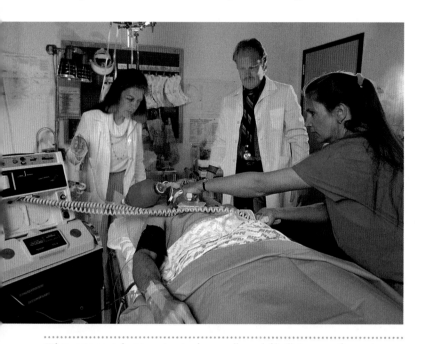

When a person's heart contracts abnormally, a defibrillator can often restore a normal beat.

MINI Glossary

angina (an-JYE-nuh or ANN-juh-nuh): pain in the heart region caused by lack of oxygen.

fibrillation (FIH-brill-AY-shun): extremely rapid contractions of the heart that lack the power needed to pump blood around the body.

pacemaker: a device that delivers electrical impulses to the heart to regulate the heartbeat.

coronary artery bypass surgery: surgery to provide an alternate route for blood to reach heart tissue, bypassing a blocked coronary artery.

Since it is a symptom, not a cause, the critical factor is to determine the cause. It could be a spasm of the artery, it could be atherosclerosis, or it could be something else entirely.

Students who have heard of the use of nitroglycerin in treating heart disease will be interested to know that nitroglycerin is used specifically in the treatment of angina. Nitroglycerin dilates the coronary arteries.

SECTION 5

FOCUS

OUTCOME

In this section students will learn:

1. Several treatments available in medicine today for dealing with heart disease.

FOCUS ACTIVITY

Have students watched any television shows relating to emergency medicine? Have they seen on these any treatment of heart problems? Do the words fibrillation or defibrillator mean anything to them? Can anyone describe defibrillation? What other treatments have they seen on these shows?

TEACH & APPLY

DISCUSSION

Ask students what they remember about the function of the heart from Chapter 6, Section 6. Have them look back to see how the right atrium functions as the heart's pacemaker. (acts almost as a spark plug by sending an electrical impulse through the heart that causes both atria to contract) Discuss what would happen if this natural pacemaker began to function erratically.

CLASS ACTIVITY

Collect newspaper and magazine articles about heart transplants and artificial hearts. Ask students to read and share something special about their articles. Time needed will vary according to the length of the articles. If possible, collect articles that are similar in length.

surgery, instruments inserted into the arteries flatten, scrape, or vaporize the plaques and so widen the passageways.

Sometimes the heart is so badly damaged that it cannot recover its ability to pump enough blood to meet the needs of blood. In such cases, the person's life can often be saved by a **heart transplant**. Transplants are not a sure cure, and are a last resort for several reasons. A person who needs a new heart may have to wait years for one to become available. Even then, rejection of the new heart by the body's immune system is a constant threat. Under development is an **artificial heart** that would have the advantage that the human immune system would not recognize it as foreign and so would not reject it.

Even the most progressive medical techniques are only temporary repairs, though. Nothing has been found that will cure atherosclerosis. Blockages recur, and people may require repeated treatments. Because medicine isn't perfect, people with heart trouble may be lured into the hands of quacks and receive treatments that are frauds.

Lifestyle factors such as proper diet and physical activity have proved helpful in preventing or postponing CVD, and in hastening recovery from heart attacks. Medical advances are exciting, but in the end, everyday health habits may well turn out to be most reliable for preventing—and even sometimes reversing—heart disease.

Even if damaged, the heart keeps pumping.

 KEY POINTS *Heart attacks do not always end in death or disability. Treatments of heart attacks and heart disease range from clot-dissolving drugs to heart transplants.*

SECTION 5 Review

Answer the following questions on a sheet of paper.

Learning the Vocabulary

The vocabulary terms for this section are *fibrillation, pacemaker, coronary artery, bypass surgery, heart transplant,* and *artificial heart.*

Match the following phrases with the appropriate term from the list above:

1. surgical replacement of a diseased heart with a healthy one
2. a device that delivers electrical impulses to the heart to regulate the heartbeat
3. surgery to provide an alternate route for blood to reach heart tissue
4. extremely rapid contractions of the heart
5. a pump designed to fit into the human chest cavity and perform the heart's function

Learning the Facts

6. Explain what a defibrillator does.
7. When might a heart transplant be performed?
8. List the cures for atherosclerosis.

Making Life Choices

9. What would you tell someone who doesn't pay attention to lifestyle factors that affect his health and thinks that whenever something goes wrong with his heart medicine can take care of it?

Ability Levels

Basic, On Level

Create a blood vessel with a loosely rolled piece of posterboard. Line the inside with a cloth that has a nap or rough surface. Obtain as many ping-pong balls a possible. Attach a small square of Velcro to each ball. Allow the students to demonstrte blood clots (a thrombus and an embolus) by rolling balls inside the tube. Ask students to identify which con-

SECTION 6
Stroke

Strokes occur in the same way as heart attacks do—by the blocking of arteries—but the arteries are located in the brain. Strokes can also arise from the bursting of aneurysms (hemorrhages) in the small vessels of the brain.

Strokes are not as common as heart attacks. However, they still claim many of the lives lost to atherosclerosis each year. Sometimes a person will suffer a small stroke—a warning that a blockage is forming. A minor stroke may have no lasting effect except to startle a person into taking action to reverse damaging habits.

When a major stroke occurs, a part of the brain is starved for blood and dies. This dead tissue interferes with the person's mental and physical functioning. The location of the damage determines the nature of the impairment, as shown in Figure 17–9.

Victims of severe strokes are robbed of their former abilities. They must start from scratch to relearn even simple personal hygiene measures or how to walk. Most stroke victims can recover some functioning. However, recovery is always an exhausting test of will for the victim, medical professionals, and family.

Like heart attacks, strokes require immediate medical attention. Prompt treatment can often stop a stroke in progress. Act quickly, should any of the warning signs of stroke occur (see Figure 17–8 on page 462).

KEY POINTS *Strokes are blockages or hemorrhages in the vessels that feed the brain. Strokes often result from atherosclerosis and can impair a person's functioning.*

Figure 17–9 **The Effect of Stroke Location.** *Damage on one side of the brain affects the opposite side of the body.*

Brain damage affects opposite side of body

Right brain damage — Left brain damage

Paralyzed right side — Paralyzed left side

Speech, language problems — Sensory problems

Behavioral style—slow, cautious — Behavioral style—quick, impulsive

SECTION 6 Review

Answer the following questions on a sheet of paper.

Learning the Facts
1. How and where do strokes occur?
2. What happens when a major stroke occurs?
3. What are the effects of damage to the right side of the brain?
4. List the warning signs of a stroke.

Making Life Choices
5. If you know someone who has been diagnosed with atherosclerosis and is at risk for stroke, what lifestyle factors would you suggest the person change to reduce the risk of stroke?

MINI Glossary

heart transplant: the surgical replacement of a diseased heart with a healthy one.

artificial heart: a pump designed to fit into the human chest cavity and perform the heart's function of pumping blood around the body.

SECTION 6

FOCUS

OUTCOME

In this section students will learn:

1. The cause and effect of strokes.

FOCUS ACTIVITY

Have students speculate on the results if the blood supply to a portion of brain tissue were shut off.

TEACH & APPLY

COMPREHENSION CHECK

Stroke was defined earlier in the chapter on page 461. Ask students to define it here.

ASSESS

EVALUATE

SECTION 6 Review Answers

1. They occur by the blocking of arteries in the brain.
2. a part of the brain is starved for blood and dies
3. paralyzed left side, sensory problems, behavioral style—quick, impulsive
4. Refer to Figure 17–8.
5. Answers will vary.

CLOSE

Make sure students see that damage to one side of the brain affects the opposite side of the body.

figurations of the ping-pong balls represent a thrombus, a thrombosis, an embolus, and an embolism. (Refer students to pages 460–461.) This may be done in groups of two to four students, one group at a time, or simultaneously if you have been able to construct more than one blood vessel model. (Extra credit could be given to students who volunteer to construct blood vessel models.) This activity could be used as a demonstration by the teacher or one or two students.

SECTION 7

FOCUS

OUTCOMES

In this section students will learn that:

1. CVD develops slowly over a lifetime.

2. CVD is directly linked to lifestyle habits and often to other CVDs.

3. Improving personal choices can enhance the quality of their lives and their longevity.

FOCUS ACTIVITY

Ask students to define *lifestyle*. Discuss their definitions. Ask them if they think some diseases may be primarily lifestyle diseases (lifestyle diseases or degenerative diseases are defined on page 450). Have them give examples of what these diseases might be and discuss students' opinions and reasons.

TEACH & APPLY

COMPREHENSION CHECK

To make sure students did not miss any of the several ways in which smoking damages the heart, ask them to name as many of these ways as they can.

SECTION 7

Reducing the Risks of CVD

When people find out they have CVD, they may be as surprised as if they had just come down with the measles. Yet many of their own personal choices—repeated day after day, year after year—may have made the disease almost a certainty.

The many risk factors linked to CVD are listed in Figure 17–10 on the next page. Some of the risk factors are powerful predictors of CVD. The Life Choice Inventory on page 468 shows one way of calculating your risk score. This system isn't perfect. A few people with many risk factors live long lives without disease. A few people with only a few or none die young of CVD. On the average, though, the more risk factors in a person's life, the greater that person's risk of disease.

Many diseases—not just heart and artery disease—share the same risk factors. This means that if you scored high on risk factors for heart and artery disease, you also may have an increased risk of developing hypertension, obesity, diabetes, and certain cancers. The Health Strategies section on this page, "Reducing the Risk of CVD," briefly describes actions you can take to counter each of the risk factors for CVD.

Of all the risk factors, heredity and gender are unchangeable, but can alert you to the need for extra diligence in controlling *other* risk factors. The four factors that respond best to lifestyle changes and that have emerged as major predictors of risk of CVD are smoking, hypertension, high blood cholesterol, and diabetes. Diabetes was discussed earlier as a disease of major consequences to health. The next sections discuss the other three factors: smoking, hypertension, and high blood cholesterol.

KEY POINTS *Major risk factors for heart disease are heredity, gender, smoking, hypertension, high blood cholesterol, and diabetes. Lack of physical activity, obesity, and stress also play roles. People can reduce their risks by controlling their risk factors.*

Smoking

When tobacco smoke enters the lungs, it delivers to the blood a load of nicotine, a stimulant that triggers the stress response. This raises the blood pressure, increases the heart rate, and greatly increases the heart's need for oxygen. At the same time, carbon monoxide from the smoke is mistaken for oxygen and picked up by the blood. Carbon monoxide provides no oxygen to tissues. It simply rides in the blood, starving the tissues of oxygen. Not only that, but nicotine directly damages blood platelets, making clot formation likely.

Health Strategies

Reducing the Risk of CVD

To reduce the risk of CVD:

1. Learn about your heredity, and use the information. Control the lifestyle factors that may affect you.

2. Don't smoke. If you do smoke, stop.

3. Keep your blood pressure below 125/80 if you are a teenage girl; 130/80 if you are a teenage boy.

4. Keep your blood cholesterol within the normal range (below 170 milligrams per deciliter for teenagers).

5. If you have diabetes, keep your blood sugar under control.

6. Exercise vigorously for at least 20 minutes three or more times weekly.

7. Maintain appropriate body weight.

8. Control stress. Learn to relax.

Source: Adapted from R. E. Olson, How to reduce your risk of coronary heart disease (CHD), *Priorities,* Spring 1990, p. 21.

Hypertension: The Silent Killer

You may want to share the following information with your students.

In many cases the cause of hypertension is unknown. Excessive elevated blood pressure can damage arteries, which can contribute to heart attack, stroke, congestive heart failure, vision problems, and kidney diseases. While there may be some symptoms of hypertension in some people, in many cases there are no obvious physical indications of the problem. In fact, for some, the first symptom of hypertension may be death, and that is *not* a good first symptom. Because of this fact, it is very important to have regular checks for hypertension.

No combination of factors could better set the stage for heart attacks. The action needed to reduce the risk of CVD from smoking is obvious. Don't smoke. If you do, plan to stop. Even people who have smoked for years can reduce their risks by quitting.

 KEY POINTS *Smoking damages the heart. To reduce risks of CVD, don't smoke.*

Hypertension

A certain blood pressure is vital to the trading of materials between tissues and the bloodstream. The pressure of the blood against the capillary walls is what pushes fluids out into the tissues.

The term *hypertension* refers to excess pressure of the blood in the arteries. Hypertension has a link to heredity; it runs in families. People who are middle-aged or elderly, black, obese, heavy drinkers, users of oral contraceptives, or suffering from kidney disease or diabetes often develop hypertension.

The most effective single step you can take to protect yourself from CVD is to know whether your blood pressure is high or not. A person who feels healthy may be shocked to hear that he or she has dangerously high blood pressure. High blood pressure does not feel abnormal. Teenagers should heed the advice to have their blood pressure checked, because heart disease starts early. A health-care professional can give you an accurate blood pressure reading.

When blood pressure is measured, two numbers are important: the pressure during contraction of the ventricles of the heart and the pressure during relaxation of the ventricles. The first number is the **systolic pressure** (during the "dub" of the heartbeat). The second number is the **diastolic pressure** (during the "lub"). Figure 17–11 shows what a blood pressure reading means.

When the blood pressure is taken, two measures are recorded: the systolic pressure first, and the diastolic pressure second (example: 120/80). High blood pressure is defined differently for different purposes. For teenage boys, a systolic reading over 130 or a diastolic reading over 80 generally indicates a too-high blood pressure. For teenage girls, a systolic reading over 125 or a diastolic reading over 80 generally indicates a too-high blood pressure.[a]

120 ← This is the systolic pressure
80 ← This is the diastolic pressure, the most sensitive indicator of hypertension

[a]Heavier or taller adolescents have higher blood pressures than smaller individuals of the same age. Therefore, a health-care provider should assess the meaning of a teen's blood pressure reading.

Figure 17–11 How to Interpret Your Blood Pressure

Figure 17–10 *Risk Factors for Heart and Artery Disease*

- Heredity (history of CVD prior to age 55 in family members).
- Gender (being male).
- Smoking.
- Hypertension.
- High blood cholesterol, high LDL, and/or low HDL (see page 470).
- Glucose intolerance (diabetes).
- Lack of exercise.
- Obesity (30 percent or more overweight).
- Stress.

MINI Glossary

systolic (sis-TOL-ic) **pressure:** the blood pressure during that part of the heartbeat when the heart's ventricles are contracted and the blood is being pushed out into the arteries.

diastolic (DYE-as-tol-ic) **pressure:** the blood pressure during that part of the heartbeat when the heart's ventricles are relaxing.

Hypertension can be identified by measuring the body's blood pressure using a device called a sphygmomanometer. This procedure is quick, painless, cheap, easy, and quite accurate. You can have your blood pressure taken in a matter of a few minutes at the doctor's office, the school nurse's office, a health fair, or anywhere you have a sphygmomanometer and someone who knows how to properly operate it. If a problem is found with elevated blood pressure, it should be brought to the attention of your family doctor. Your doctor may recommend controlling the problem by diet, exercise, or medication.

Assign the Life Choice Inventory, "How Healthy is Your Heart?" Each student should read the inventory and score themselves to determine their risk of heart attack. Point out that at their ages they should have a score from zero to nine—very remote.

Ask students to identify the risk factors that contributed to a less than perfect score for them. On paper, the students should put their names, the risk factors they identified, and state one lifestyle choice they would be willing to change or improve to better their scores. Give the students a 5 × 7-inch card on which they can print their names and the statement: "I am willing to _____ to improve the quality and longevity of my life as well as reduce my risk for developing heart disease."

For extra credit, have students take their books home and ask their parents to score themselves on the Life Choice Inventory to determine their current risks of heart attack. Tell students to ask parents to make a pledge as students did.

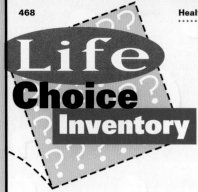

How Healthy Is Your Heart?

Every disease has risk factors. Those for heart disease are among the best known. The better you know the nature of the risks you face, the better you can decide what preventive measures may be appropriate for you. To determine your risk of heart disease, pick the item in each category that most nearly describes you. Record your answers on a piece of paper, and then score yourself as directed. Your answers to the Life Choice Inventory are personal and private. Share them with others only if you are comfortable doing so.

1. *Gender.* If you are: Female, 0 points; Male, 4 points.
2. *Family heart disease history.* (Consider just heart attacks and strokes as heart disease here.) If you have:
   No relatives with heart disease, 1 point.
   One relative with heart disease over 60 years old, 2 points.
   Two relatives with heart disease over 60 years old, 3 points.
   One relative with heart disease under 60 years old, 4 points.
   Two relatives with heart disease under 60 years old, 6 points.
3. *Smoking.* If you smoke:
   Not at all, 0 points. A cigar or pipe, 1 point.
   10 cigarettes or fewer per day, 3 points.
   11 to 30 cigarettes per day, 4 points.
   30 or more cigarettes per day, 6 points.
4. *Blood pressure.* If you are a teenager and your diastolic blood pressure (the lower of the two numbers on a blood pressure reading) is:
   Less than 80, 0 points.
   80 to 84, 1 point.
   85 to 89, 2 points.
   90 to 94, 4 points.
   95 or more, 5 points.
   (If you don't know your blood pressure, give yourself 5 points.)
5. *Blood cholesterol.* (If you don't know your cholesterol level, guess at the amount of fat in your diet.) If you have:

Hypertension can usually be controlled by medication or by means of lifestyle strategies. Limiting salty, fatty foods while choosing more nutrient-rich, high-fiber, low-fat foods; losing weight; exercising aerobically; and reducing stress may help lower blood pressure. In severe hypertension, or when other factors increase CVD risks, drugs that lower blood pressure can be a life-saving treatment.

In some cases, control of hypertension is a matter of reducing body fatness. In addition to diet, regular aerobic activity seems to help keep blood pressure in the normal range. In many people, physical activity can be as effective as drugs in lowering blood pressure.

 Hypertension is high blood pressure. Hypertension worsens atherosclerosis. To fight hypertension, first know your blood pressure. If it is high, take steps to control it.

CRITICAL THINKING

After students have learned the meaning of blood pressure (including the proper technique for measuring), resting heart rate, and exercise heart rate, divide the class into small "statistic gathering" groups. Assign a group to each of the following age groups: 20–30 years old, 31–40 years old, 41–50 years old, and 51 years old and older.

Have the groups collect the following information from people in their assigned age group: resting heart rate, exercise heart rate, and blood pressure.

Make sure the people being studied in

Cholesterol below 170 or almost no fat in diet, 0 points.

Cholesterol 170 to 185 or a low-fat diet, 1 point.

Cholesterol 186 to 199 or a moderately low-fat diet, 2 points.

Cholesterol 200 to 239 or a typical American diet, 4 points.

Cholesterol 240 to 300 or a high-fat diet, 5 points.

Cholesterol over 300, 6 points.

6. *Diabetes.* If you have:
No relatives with diabetes, 0 points.
One relative with diabetes, 2 points.
Two relatives with diabetes, 3 points.
Diabetes in yourself beginning before age 20, 6 points.

7. *Exercise.* If you engage in:
Strenuous exercise both at work and at leisure, 0 points.
Moderate exercise both at work and at leisure, 1 point.
Sedentary work and intense leisure-time activity, 2 points.
Sedentary work and moderate leisure-time activity, 3 points.
Sedentary work and light leisure-time activity, 4 points.
Little or no activity, 6 points.

8. *Body weight.* (Use the weight you selected for yourself in the Life Choice Inventory of Chapter 8.) If you are:

5 or more pounds below appropriate weight, 0 points.

Up to 5 pounds above appropriate weight, 1 point.

6 to 19 pounds above appropriate weight, 2 points.

20 to 39 pounds above appropriate weight, 3 points.

40 to 60 pounds above appropriate weight, 4 points.

More than 60 pounds above appropriate weight, 6 points.

9. *Stress.* If you are:
Almost always relaxed, 0 points.
Sometimes tense or depressed, 1 point.
Frequently tense or depressed, 2 points.
Almost always tense, 4 points.
Constantly anxious/depressed, 5 points.

SCORING

Add the points for the nine answers. Your current risk of heart attack is:

0 to 9: Very remote.
10 to 19: Below average.
20 to 29: Average; consider lowering your score.
30 to 39: High; reduce your score.
40 to 50: Danger—reduce your score!

Elevated Blood Cholesterol

Like hypertension, high blood cholesterol is a symptomless risk factor for cardiovascular disease. High blood cholesterol is much talked about but little understood. Cholesterol is a type of fat (see Chapter 7). It is found in foods and is also made and destroyed in the body.

Blood cholesterol may be high in some people who are born with the tendency to make it too fast or destroy it too slowly. Many teenagers in this country have high blood cholesterol for lifestyle reasons: they eat too much fat, exercise too little, are obese, or all of these. A blood test can tell you your blood cholesterol level. Figure 17–12 on the next page shows how to interpret it. Cholesterol levels are important for everyone, from the youngest toddler to older adults.

each age group include a variety of exercisers and nonexercisers such as: weight lifters, runners, walkers, aerobic dancers, couch potatoes, and people who use wheelchairs.

Have the groups present the information they collect in graph and written form. Students will summarize and draw conclusions from the information relating to the fac-

tors listed above.

To personalize this activity, have students collect the same information on themselves three different times during the course of the semester. Students should then evaluate and draw conclusions about themselves and classmates as they relate to exercise.

CLASS ACTIVITY

Ask the students to number 1 to 10 on a piece of paper and respond true or false after each statement. This activity is not to be graded, since many of these facts were not covered in the chapter. Use the questions for discussion.

1. The heart pumps 5.3 quarts of blood per minute. (T)

2. At first, an experience of fear lowers the heart rate. (T)

3. The cardiovascular system pumps the equivalent of 4,000 gallons of blood around the body each day. (T)

4. The heart beats continuously from the fifth month before birth until death. (T)

5. The heart rate is at its highest in the early afternoon and at its lowest in the morning. (T)

6. The human heart weighs about ½₀₀ of the total body weight. (T)

7. The human heart beats about four billion times during an average lifetime. (T)

8. Each heartbeat lasts about ⁸⁄₁₀ of a second. (T)

9. The heart beats over 85,000 times a day. (T)

10. In one minute the heart pumps from 8 to 10 pints of blood. (T)

Figure 17–12 Cholesterol Values for Teenagers

	Total Cholesterol (mg/dL[a])	LDL Cholesterol (mg/dL)
Acceptable	<170	<110
Borderline	170–199	110–129
High	≥200	≥130

[a]Blood cholesterol is measured in milligrams per deciliter of blood.

The heart prefers fiber to saturated fat.

Cholesterol, being a fat, does not mix well in the blood, which is watery. However, proteins mix so well with watery substances that they can carry fats along with them in the blood. To ship cholesterol and other fats from place to place in the body by way of the bloodstream, the liver first wraps the cholesterol and fat with protein in packages called **lipoproteins**.

Two kinds of lipoproteins carry cholesterol (as well as other fats) around the body. These are **low-density lipoproteins (LDLs)** and **high-density lipoproteins (HDLs)**. The LDLs carry cholesterol from the liver (where it is made) to the tissues, which use it to make hormones, to build cell membranes, and to make vitamin D. These are all beneficial uses of cholesterol. However, harm from cholesterol may also occur. When the tissues have all the cholesterol they need, LDLs tend to deposit excess cholesterol along the artery linings, forming plaques. HDLs, on the other hand, work to gather up excess cholesterol from the artery linings and carry it back to the liver to be disposed of.

Whatever a person does that raises the LDL concentration in the blood also raises that person's risks of developing CVD. In contrast, raised HDL levels are associated with a lowered risk of CVD. The thing to remember about the blood level of HDL is "the higher, the better."

Several factors affect the blood cholesterol level. Some of the factors you can control, and some you can't. First, being female helps. Women have higher HDL levels than men. Second, nonsmokers have higher HDL levels than smokers. Maintaining appropriate body weight is helpful. Diet and physical activity also affect blood cholesterol. Regular aerobic activity seems to lower LDL and raise HDL in the blood. The role of diet is complex, but the complexities are worth learning and applying. The next section shows you why.

KEY POINTS *Elevated blood cholesterol predicts CVD. Two types of blood cholesterol are important in CVD: LDL and HDL. LDLs are harmful, because they carry cholesterol to the tissues and can deposit cholesterol in artery walls, worsening atherosclerosis. HDLs are beneficial, because they carry cholesterol away from the arteries for disposal. Physical activity raises HDL and lowers LDL levels.*

Diet and Cholesterol

People are often confused about the role of diet in connection with high blood cholesterol. They think that cholesterol in foods raises blood cholesterol. It does, but regular dietary fat—especially saturated fat—raises it much more. The key to lowering blood cholesterol seems to be to eat as little total fat as possible while still eating a balanced diet. The fat you do eat should be mostly the unsaturated type. Also, one or two fish meals a week provide fish oils that alter the blood's chemistry so as to favor a healthy heart.

Choosing low-fat food is becoming easier for teens who eat in a school cafeteria. Government regulations require that all schools that receive gov-

HEALTHY PEOPLE 2000

Reduce coronary heart disease deaths to no more than 100 per 100,000 people.

The death rate for coronary heart disease has declined by 40 percent over the past 15 years. Despite this progress, coronary heart disease continues to be the leading cause of death in the United States. It affects about 7 million Americans, causes over 500,000 deaths annually, and costs the Nation approximately $43 billion per year in direct and indirect costs.

Further reductions in coronary heart disease mortality may be achieved through advances in treatment. Early intervention (prompted by early recognition of an impending heart attack) has the potential to reduce or postpone some of the mortality due to this condition. But the greatest potential for reducing coronary heart ernment money must serve low-fat meals that meet teenagers' nutrient needs.

Dietary fiber also offers protection against heart disease. High-fiber foods move quickly through the digestive tract, and carry cholesterol with them. Diets high in fiber are typically low in fat and cholesterol anyway—another fiber advantage. Some people's elevated blood cholesterol does not respond to changes in lifestyle. Such people may need cholesterol-lowering drugs.

 KEY POINTS   *Dietary fat raises blood cholesterol much more than dietary cholesterol does. High-fiber foods can offer protection against heart disease.*

Dietary fiber helps protect against heart disease.

Emotions and the Heart

When people get angry, anxious, or depressed, these emotions may affect much more than just the other people nearby. They may also turn inward to damage the heart. Everyone has seen someone overreact to everyday stressors such as traffic jams or tests. These people, called "hot responders," are very likely to have a heart attack, to undergo heart surgery, or to die from heart disease. Men who describe themselves as grumpy and prone to angry outbursts are two to three times as likely as calmer men to have heart

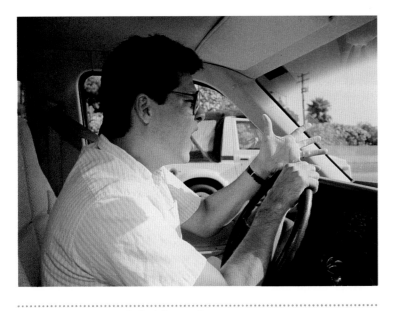

Losing your temper can be bad for your heart.

MINI Glossary

lipoproteins (LIP-oh-PRO-teens): protein and fat clusters that transport fats in the blood.

low-density lipoproteins (LDLs): lipoproteins that carry fat and cholesterol from the liver, where they are made, to the tissues where they are used. LDLs also deposit cholesterol in arteries, forming plaques.

high-density lipoproteins (HDLs): lipoproteins that carry fat and cholesterol away from the tissues (and from plaques) back to the liver for breakdown and removal from the body.

disease morbidity, disability, and mortality appears to rest with prevention.

Many factors influence not only whether a person will develop coronary heart disease, but also how rapidly atherosclerosis progresses. Genetic predisposition, gender, and advancing age are recognized factors over which individuals have little control. Key modifiable factors include cigarette smoking, high blood cholesterol, high blood pressure,

excessive body weight, and long-term physical inactivity. Control of each of these factors is important in the prevention of coronary heart disease. People with diabetes, who are especially prone to vascular disease, may benefit by controlling these other risk factors. Risk factor reduction in those who already suffer from coronary heart disease and are at increased risk of having another coronary event is also of great importance.

Ask students to identify which statements are examples of the heart's incredible ability to perform its functions. (1, 3, 7, 8, 9, and 10.) Ask students to figure the approximate weight of their own hearts based on their own weights and statement 6.

CLASS ACTIVITY

Ask students to list and examine ten food labels brought from home or available in your classroom. (Fill a box with food labels that you've brought from your home.) The students should read the ingredients and information available and decide whether the foods belong in the saturated or unsaturated fat categories. Have students mark them as mostly saturated, mostly unsaturated, all saturated, or all unsaturated. Point out key words to look for such as hydrogenated, cocoa butter, coconut, or palm oil. (Refer to For Your Information on page 180 for saturated and unsaturated fat sources.)

ASSESS

EVALUATE

SECTION 7 Review Answers

1. high-density lipoproteins (HDL)
2. systolic
3. lipoproteins
4. diastolic
5. low-density lipoproteins (LDL)
6. See Figure 17–10.
7. smoking, hypertension, high blood cholesterol, and diabetes (p. 466)
8. Nicotine raises blood pressure, heart rate, and the heart's need for oxygen. It also damages blood platelets, making clot formation likely. Carbon monoxide from the smoke starves tissues of oxygen. (p. 466)
9. limiting salty, fatty foods while choosing more nutrient-rich, high-fiber, low-fat foods; losing weight; exercising aerobically; and reducing stress (p. 468)
10. Answers will vary.

CLOSE

Before going on to the next section, students should be able to:

1. List six risk factors of CVD.
2. Mark each of the risk factors as controllable or noncontrollable.
3. List five ways to reduce the risk of CVD and give an example of how to accomplish each of these.
4. List ten healthy food choices to reduce the risk of CVD.

CHAPTER 17: Lifestyle Diseases: Diabetes, Cardiovascular Disease, and Cancer

---

disease. Those who suffer from depression and feelings of hopelessness also develop heart disease more often than people with an upbeat outlook.

The idea that anger might increase heart disease makes sense. When tempers flare or anxiety arises, a surge of stress hormones causes diseased coronary arteries to constrict. This raises the blood pressure and greatly reduces blood flow to the heart. Also, intense stress can interrupt the activity of the nerves that control the heartbeat, causing the heart to beat rapidly and ineffectively—a main cause of death during heart attack.

It used to be thought that highly motivated achievers, or people with so-called Type A personalities, ran a greater risk for heart disease. However, years of research has revealed no connection between heart attacks on the one hand and attaining high achievements and being busy on the other.

If you see yourself as a "hot responder," if you tend to fly off the handle and lose your temper, you would be well-advised to learn how to take life in stride. An optimistic view of the world not only can improve your mental health, but may protect your physical health, as well. Counseling or therapy can help to change destructive attitudes. Plain old love and affection, given and received, can also positively affect the heart and arteries. Even just owning a pet may bolster heart health. No doubt the mystery of CVD—like all the great human mysteries—involves the mind and spirit, as well as the body.

KEY POINTS *Tendencies toward anger, hostility, anxiety, and depression are linked with increased rates of heart attack. Those with negative responses to the world are advised to relax and adopt a more positive life view.*

SECTION 7 Review

Answer the following questions on a sheet of paper.

Learning the Vocabulary

The vocabulary terms for this section are *systolic pressure, diastolic pressure, lipoproteins, low-density lipoproteins (LDLs),* and *high-density lipoproteins (HDLs).*
Match the following phrases with the appropriate term from the list above:

1. carries cholesterol away from the tissues
2. blood pressure when the blood is being pushed out into the arteries
3. protein and fat clusters
4. blood pressure when the heart's ventricles are relaxing
5. carries fat and cholesterol from the liver

Learning the Facts

6. List the risk factors for cardiovascular disease.
7. What four factors have emerged as major predictors of risk of cardiovascular disease?
8. What happens in the body after tobacco smoke enters the lungs?
9. What lifestyle strategies help control hypertension?

Making Life Choices

10. What recommendations would you make to someone with high blood cholesterol?

QUICK QUIZ

Chapter 17, Section 7

The following quiz will help you assess your students' understanding of the material covered in this section of the chapter. You might use the quiz as an oral exercise, which will lead into a class discussion of the topics covered. Or, you might use it as a paper/pencil quiz to evaluate your students individually.

1. The onset of cardiovascular disease can often be predicted by an examination of your risk factors. (True)
2. Many diseases share the same risk factors. (True)
3. Heredity, smoking, hypertension, and high blood cholesterol are the major predictors of risk of CVD that respond best to lifestyle changes. (False)

SECTION 8

Cancer

Years ago, the future for someone diagnosed as having **cancer** was bleak. Today, millions of people are fighting battles against cancer and winning. Still, preventing cancer is far easier than curing it. Most cancers result from conditions in people's lives, many of which they can control themselves. For example, the number-one cancer in both men and women is now lung cancer, which is closely linked to smoking. The great majority of lung cancer cases occur in people who smoke.

Over a hundred diseases are called cancer. Each has its own name and symptoms, depending on its type and location in the body. Some cancers are named for the body tissues in which they arise, with the suffix -oma (meaning **tumor** or other **malignancy**) added on. For example, cancer of the pigmented cells of the skin, the melanocytes, is called **melanoma**. A tumor of the bone marrow is a **myeloma**—*myelos* means "marrow." Other cancers are named in other ways.

Generally, all cancers can be assigned to one of four classes, depending on tissue type:

▶ Cancers of the immune system organs are **lymphomas**.
▶ Cancers of blood-forming organs are **leukemias**.
▶ Cancers of the glands and body linings—such as the skin, the lining of the digestive tract or lungs, or other linings—are **carcinomas**.
▶ Cancers of connective tissue, including bones, ligaments, and muscles, are **sarcomas**.

How Cancer Develops

Cancer begins with a change in a normal cell. After the change, the cell begins reproducing itself out of control. The steps in the development of many cancers are thought to be:

1. Exposure to a carcinogen (an **initiator**).
2. Entry of the initiator into a cell.
3. Change of the cell's genetic material. The change may be a **mutation**.
4. Possible speeding up of cancer formation by a **promoter**.
5. Out-of-control multiplication of the cells.
6. Tumor or other malignancy formation.

Initiators and promoters work together, an effect shown in Figure 17–13 on the next page. Alcohol and tobacco work this way in the development of cancers of the mouth, throat, and esophagus. Normally, these cancers are rare. In a person who smokes two packs of cigarettes a day, the risk of developing them is one and a half times greater than for the nonsmoker. Should that smoker also drink two alcoholic drinks each day, the risk would become

Mini Glossary

cancer: a disease in which abnormal cells multiply out of control, spread into surrounding tissues and other body parts, and disrupt normal functioning of one or more organs.

tumor: an abnormal mass of tissue that can live and reproduce itself, but performs no service to the body.

malignancy: a dangerous cancerous growth that sheds cells into body fluids and spreads to new locations to start new cancer colonies. (The word *malignant* means "growing worse.")

melanoma: an especially dangerous cancer of the pigmented cells of the skin, related to sun exposure in people with light-colored skin.

myeloma: a cancer originating in the cells of the bone marrow.

lymphomas (limf-OH-mahs): cancers that arise in organs of the immune system.

leukemias (loo-KEE-me-ahs): cancers that arise in the blood cell–making tissues.

carcinomas (car-sin-OH-mahs): cancers that arise in the skin, body chamber linings, or glands.

sarcomas (sar-KOH-mahs): cancers that arise in the connective tissue cells, including bones, ligaments, and muscles.

initiator: a carcinogen, an agent required to start the formation of cancer.

mutation (myoo-TAY-shun): a change in a cell's genetic material. Once the genetic material has changed, the change is inherited by the offspring of that cell.

promoter: a substance that assists in the development of malignant tumors, but does not initiate them on its own.

SECTION 8

FOCUS

OUTCOMES

In this section students will learn:

1. To define cancer and differentiate between benign and malignant tumors.
2. The stages in the development of cancer and the meaning of the word *metastasized*.

FOCUS ACTIVITY

Put the following quote by Cervantes on the board and leave it up while you study the chapter: "The beginning of health is to know the disease." Have a class discussion using these questions: What do you know about cancer? What is your reaction when you hear the word cancer? List on the board the six stages of cancer development. Emphasis should be on "knowing cancer" and that each student has lifestyle choices to make that may determine whether or not he or she contracts cancer.

4. Inhaling cigarette smoke triggers the stress response, raises the blood pressure, increases the heart rate, and increases the heart's need for oxygen. (True)
5. Smoking does not directly damage the heart. (False)
6. Hypertension can be detected by measuring systolic and diastolic pressure. (True)

7. High blood cholesterol and hypertension are both symptomless risk factors for cardiovascular disease. (True)
8. High-density lipoproteins (HDL) are a beneficial form of cholesterol. (True)
9. Regular dietary fat is not an important cause of cholesterol. (False)
10. Short-tempered people are more prone to develop cardiovascular disease. (True)

Figure 17–13 *Cancer Initiators and Promoters.* *Initiators and promoters work together to produce many more tumors than initiators alone would produce.*

Initiator only

A few tumors develop.

Promoter only

No tumors develop.

Initiator plus promoter

Many tumors develop.

TEACH & APPLY

TRANSPARENCIES

Transparency 17–8, "Cancer Initiators and Promoters," (Figure 17–13) is available in the Transparency Acetate Binder.

TEACHER SUPPORT

Key Passage

It might be helpful to write *benign* and *malignant* on the board together and point out to the students that they are opposite in meaning. Tumors can be either malignant or benign. If they are benign they are not cancerous.

CLASS ACTIVITY

Have the students make a list of all substances or materials that they know to be carcinogenic, or cancer causing. Their list can be general or broken down into particular substances. Have students put a "C" beside the carcinogens that can be controlled by an individual's lifestyle choices and an "NC" by carcinogens over which individuals have little or no control. Have a class discussion on the lists themselves, specific breakdowns, and lifestyle choices affecting the intake of or exposure to carcinogens.

Two factors that work together as carcinogens: tobacco and alcohol.

15 times greater. Alcohol alone may also increase the risk of these particular cancers, and it promotes them, once they have started. Tobacco smoke probably acts in both ways too: it initiates and promotes the cancers.

All of the changes that lead to cancer happen inside an individual's cells, so cancer itself is not contagious—that is, it cannot be passed from person to person. Once started inside the body, cancer can grow and damage any tissue, from the solid bone to the fluid blood.

Normally, cells divide only when new cells are needed. A cancerous cell, though, does not respond to the command to stop dividing. It divides continuously. The result may be a lump of tissue (a tumor).

KEY POINTS *Cancers are classified according to the types of tissue they affect. Cancer develops in stages.*

Harmless and Cancerous Tumors

Sometimes a tumor may be harmless, or **benign**. It does not spread. Rather, it is a well-defined, solid mass contained in an external membrane. A benign tumor poses no threat and can simply be removed.

Cancerous tumors, on the other hand, are malignant. They present a threat to health. As a cancerous tumor gains in size, it competes with normal tissues around it for nutrients, oxygen, and space. With time, the cancer interrupts the normal functions of the tissues or organs into which it grows. In cancer of the large intestine, for example, the tumor may block the passage of the intestinal contents. In cancer of the brain, the growing tumor threatens thought processes and control of the body.

The Spread of Cancer In addition to invading surrounding tissues, cancer cells break loose from the original site and ride the rivers of body fluids to colonize new areas. When a cancer is just beginning, it sheds only a few cells. As it enlarges, however, more and more of these wild cells escape and start new growths in other body parts. At this point, the cancer is said to have **metastasized**. Cancer causes death when it interrupts the functioning of vital organs, such as the blood-building organs, lungs, or brain.

QUICK QUIZ

Chapter 17, Section 8

The following quiz will help you assess your students' understanding of the material covered in this section of the chapter. You might use the quiz as an oral exercise, which will lead into a class discussion of the topics covered. Or, you might use it as a paper/pencil quiz to evaluate your students individually.

*If students have difficulty with the concepts covered in the Quick Quiz and the Section Review, you might suggest they review the material using the **S**urvey, **Q**uestion, **R**ead, **R**ecite, **R**eview (SQ3R) study method, which is described in detail in the introduction to this Teacher's Wraparound Edition.*

1. There are more than one hundred distinct diseases that are called cancer. (True)

The Role of the Immune System   The immune system is on the watch for escaped cancer cells. The system works to stop these dangerous travelers before they lodge in body tissue, but it can catch only a certain number of cancer cells at any one time. When the immune defenses fail, cancer treatment is needed. The success of treatment often depends on whether or not it gets under way before the cancer has metastasized.

After the initiating event, some cancers take as long as 20 years to develop. By the time a health-care provider detects a cancer, the initiator and promoters that caused it are long gone. This is why it is hard to know what the original causes of cancer are.

 Cancer is dangerous in that it can interrupt the functioning of vital organs.

For Your Information

In the past 20 years, for men and women younger than age 55:

▶ All cancer deaths have decreased by one-fourth.

▶ Breast cancer deaths have decreased by about one-fourth.

▶ Lung cancer deaths have decreased slightly.

▶ Colon cancer deaths have decreased by 15%.

Review

Answer the following questions on a sheet of paper.

Learning the Vocabulary

The vocabulary terms in this section are *cancer, tumor, malignancy, melanoma, myeloma, lymphomas, leukemias, carcinomas, sarcomas, initiator, mutation, promoter, benign,* and *metastasized.*

1. What is the difference between melanoma and myeloma?
2. What is the difference between carcinomas and sarcomas?
3. A _____ assists in the development of a malignant tumor.
4. An abnormal mass of tissue that can live and reproduce but performs no service to the body is called a _____.

Learning the Facts

5. What are the four classes of cancer?
6. How does a cancer cell differ from a normal cell?
7. What type of tumor does not spread and is usually removed with no threat?
8. When does cancer cause death?
9. How does the immune system help fight cancer?
10. Why is it difficult to determine what the original causes of cancer are?

Making Life Choices

11. The American Cancer Society believes that ignorance and fear often prevent people from seeking medical attention for cancer early enough. To help solve this problem, the American Cancer Society asks famous people to appear in public service announcements. Do you think this is an effective technique? Why or why not? What measures would you suggest to inform as many people as possible of the necessity of prompt medical attention? What method do you believe would be most likely to sway you, and why?

MINI Glossary

benign (be-NINE): noncancerous; not harmful; a description of a tumor that is not able to spread from one area to another.

metastasized (meh-TASS-tuh-sized): when speaking of cancer cells, a term that means the cancer cells have migrated from one part of the body to another, and started new growths just like the original tumor.

2. Most cancers are the result of genetics and other unchangeable risk factors. (False)
3. The suffix -oma indicates a cancer resulting from a tumor or some other malignancy. (True)
4. A cancer of the immune system is called a lymphoma. (True)
5. Cancers of the lungs are called carcinomas. (False)
6. Cancers that develop in the blood-forming organs are leukemias. (True)
7. Sarcomas are cancers of the connective tissues. (True)
8. A carcinogen is a virus that initiates a cancer. (False)
9. Tumors that are not malignant are called benign. (True)
10. A cancer that has metastasized poses no risk to the body. (False)

FOCUS

OUTCOMES

In this section students will learn the:

1. Environmental risk factors for cancer that people can control.

2. Ways to evaluate and to reduce their risks of getting cancer.

FOCUS ACTIVITY

Have students take the Life Choice Inventory "How Well Do You Protect Yourself against Cancer?" on page 478. Then have them look at all the "no" answers and discuss what can be done to change those "no" answers to "yes" or "sometimes." Students should pick out two "no" answers and write a way in which they could change their lifestyles in order to reduce their chances of contracting cancer.

TEACH & APPLY

A handout entitled "Factors beyond People's Control" is provided in the Teacher's Resource Box. This material provides information on the causes of cancer that are beyond people's control.

SECTION 9

Cancer Risks That People Can Control

Risks of cancer fall into three categories. Some risks, you can control totally—the ones that have to do with your own behavior. Some risks, you can control partially—for example, the risks posed by environmental pollutants. You can learn about these and minimize your exposure to them.

Some risks, you cannot control at all. For example, if a major disaster should occur in your area and expose everyone to a carcinogen (a cancer-causing agent), that would be a risk you couldn't control. You also cannot control your gender, your genetic inheritance, and your age, and these affect your risks of cancer. This section focuses on the risks you can control—your smoking behavior, your exposures to radiation, and your choices of diet, alcohol, and physical activity. The Life Choice Inventory on page 478 can help you evaluate your cancer risks regarding the known controllable factors.

Tobacco

Almost everyone knows of the link between smoking and cancer, and with good reason. The evidence for the link is firm. Eighty percent of hospitalized lung cancer victims are smokers. In any community of the world, an increase in smoking is followed by a jump in numbers of lung cancer cases. When researchers spread chemicals from tobacco smoke on a patch of living skin, cancer develops at the site.

About a third of all cancer deaths are linked to tobacco use. Not only lung cancer, but also cancers throughout the body, follow smoking. Cancer of the larynx (voice box), mouth, esophagus, urinary bladder, kidney, pancreas, and many other organs have all been linked to tobacco use.

 KEY POINTS *Tobacco use is a preventable cause of cancers of the larynx, mouth, esophagus, bladder, kidney, and pancreas, as well as of the lungs.*

Radiation

Radiation from many sources bombards people every day. Whether or not they are affected by it depends on the type of radiation and their length of exposure.

The Sun's Rays   Overexposure to the sun's ultraviolet (UV) rays, for example, causes most cases of skin cancer. Today, more and more of these rays are hitting the earth's surface as pollution from human activity destroys

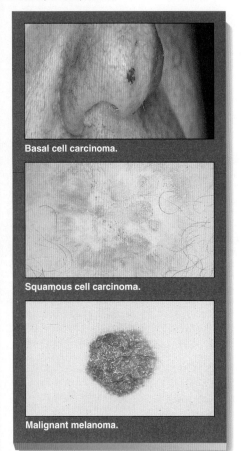

Figure 17–14 Forms of Skin Cancer. Report skin spots that resemble any of these three to a physician immediately.

Source: Courtesy of The Skin Cancer Foundation, New York, New York.

Basal cell carcinoma.

Squamous cell carcinoma.

Malignant melanoma.

≡ **Ability Levels**

On Level

To help students review, play the memory game. The first person reads the first step in how cancer develops and says it aloud: "Exposure to a carcinogen." The second person says the second one: "Entry of the initiator into a cell," then says the first step and the second step. The third person reads the third step: "Change of the cell's genetic material.

the atmospheric shield (the ozone layer) that used to filter them out. Chapter 24 tells more about this effect.

Skin cancers come in several varieties. A major distinction is between the fast-spreading, lethal skin cancer known as melanoma and other, less-threatening surface cancers of the skin. Only one blistering sunburn, if received during the teen years, may be enough to double a person's risk of melanoma. In contrast, working or playing in the sun daily makes people likely to develop the more easily treated forms of skin cancer. This means that people who let themselves in for occasional large doses of sun are taking the greatest risks of contracting the most serious type of skin cancer. Such people include indoor workers on summer vacation in the South and pale-skinned, weekend sunbathers. Figure 17–14 on page 476 shows the different forms of skin cancer.

While no one is immune to the sun's damaging effects, skin color can help predict who is most at risk for cancer. The pigment **melanin** in dark-skinned people protects against UV damage. The protection is limited, however. People with dark skin can still get cancer. The amounts of melanin in all but the lightest-colored skin increase with sun exposure. The resulting tan is the body's defense against the dangerous rays—but not against the cancers they cause. Another reason to cover up: nothing ages and wrinkles the skin so fast as overexposure to the sun.

Should a would-be tanner tan indoors, then? No. All sunlamps and tanning booths bombard the skin with UV radiation. Cancer risks from sunlamps and booths are just as high as those from sunbathing.

Choosing Sun-Protection Products   People can take precautions to avoid dangerous overexposure to the sun. One way is to stay indoors between 10 A.M. and 4 P.M., when the sun's rays are strongest. For those who must be in the sun, sun-protection products block ultraviolet radiation and prevent burning, and so are a wise investment. The higher a product's sun protection factor (SPF), the more protection it provides (but brand names don't matter at all). Learn the differences among sun products available on the market. The Miniglossary can help you to choose among **suntan lotion**, **sunscreen**, and **sun block**.

Use sunscreen and stay in the shade to protect against dangerous sunburn.

mation when they hear it a minimum of seven times. Also point out that this activity shows that everyone can learn if they know how to study.

For **Y**our **I**nformation

Sun facts:

▶ The strongest sun rays shine from 10 A.M. until 4 P.M.

▶ Fair-skinned people with blond, red, or light brown hair and blue, green, or gray eyes are most at risk for skin cancer.

▶ Freckles mean burns are likely.

▶ By age 18 most people have accumulated most of their lifetime sun exposure. No more exposure is necessary for cancer to develop.

▶ Medications that increase skin sensitivity to the sun include: acne medications, antidepressants, antihistamines, antibiotics, diuretics, and some pain relievers. Ask a physician or pharmacist whether medication you take has this effect.

MINI Glossary

melanin (MELL-eh-nin): the protective skin pigment responsible for the tan, brown, or black color of human skin; produced in abundance upon exposure to ultraviolet radiation.

suntan lotion: lotion that may or may not have any sunscreen protection.

sunscreen: a partial block against the cancer-causing rays of the sun (gamma radiation).

sun block: a total block against the cancer-causing rays of the sun. A sun block has an SPF (sun protection factor) of 50 or greater. Zinc oxide is an example of a sun block.

BACKGROUND INFORMATION

In discussing cancer and tobacco, you may want to refer students back to Chapter 14, which has additional information on cancers whose risks are increased by smoking. You may also want to remind students that people who use smokeless tobacco are still at risk for cancer.

TEACHER SUPPORT

Key Passage

You may want to tell students that sunlamps create risks in addition to skin cancer. If they are not properly filtered, they can also damage blood vessels, cause cataracts, and cause a deadly form of eye cancer.

CLASS ACTIVITY

On a piece of 8½ × 11-inch paper have each student write the answer to this question: What are some precautions that can be taken to avoid dangerous overexposure to the sun? Have a class discussion. Make a master list of students' answers on the chalkboard or on an overhead transparency. Answers should include:

1. Use of a waterproof sunscreen; the higher the SPF (sun protection factor), the better.

2. Protect the lips with a sunscreen lip balm.

3. Enjoy the sun for short periods on many occasions rather than staying out in the sun all day.

4. Take along a big hat.

5. Wear sunglasses that are marked as blocking out UV rays.

DISCUSSION

Discuss as a class the four dietary factors that are strongly linked to high cancer risks: high meat intake, high fat intake, low vegetable intake, low grain intake. In the discussion, stress ways that students can cut down on meat without giving it up and how to cut down on fat intake. Discuss fiber and how to increase vegetable intake in their diets as painlessly as possible.

BACKGROUND INFORMATION

As enrichment, you may want to tell students that the mixture of vitamins in fruits and vegetables may also block the progress of certain cancers. For example, the vitamin C in oranges may stop the formation of certain carcinogens and the vitamin A in vegetables and fruits such as sweet potatoes and peaches is important in preventing cancer in the body's external and internal linings. The fibers of plant foods, such as whole grains, fruits, and vegetables may play roles as well.

Life Choice Inventory

How Well Do You Protect Yourself against Cancer?

You cannot eliminate all cancer risks from your life. You can, however, take steps to reduce them. On a separate piece of paper, answer the following questions with either yes or no. Questions answered no indicate ways you can improve. Your answers to the Life Choice Inventory are personal and private. Share them with others only if you are comfortable doing so.

1. Are you a nonsmoker? Do you avoid using tobacco in any form? Do you request that those around you not smoke?
2. Are you careful not to sunburn? Do you avoid tanning salons? Do you wear sunglasses that block out ultraviolet rays when outdoors? Do you obtain regular eye exams?
3. Do you question the necessity of X-ray examinations?
4. Have you had your home tested for radon and taken any necessary steps to prevent exposure?
5. Do you read and follow instructions on the labels of chemicals that you use in the home, in the garden, or on the job?
6. Do you choose a variety of foods from a balanced diet that supply adequate fiber, vitamin A, and vitamin C, without too much fat? Do you eat vegetables from the cabbage family often?
7. Do you keep your weight within the normal range for your height?
8. Do you limit your intakes of cured and smoked meats?
9. Do you abstain from drinking alcohol?
10. Do you exercise regularly?
11. Do you perform breast or testicular self-examination regularly?
12. Do you, or will you, seek employment with low occupational hazards?

All people—even people with dark skin—should use waterproof sunscreens of at least SPF 15 during sunny or warm weather. To be protected, a person wearing a bathing suit needs to use a full ounce of product spread on the skin with each application. Enjoy the sun for short times rather than on all-day trips. Take along a big hat. Finally, be aware that ultraviolet rays penetrate clouds, so burns are likely even on cool, cloudy days.

X-ray Radiation People are exposed to more radiation than just from sunlight. A great deal of background radiation bombards us from the cosmos, from the soil, and from the air and water. Human-made radiation comes from medical and dental X rays and from above-ground nuclear weapons testing anywhere on earth. X-ray examinations are often required for proper medical care. However, wise clients inform their health-care providers that they wish to avoid X rays when possible.

Radon Gas You can also be exposed to radiation from a gas, **radon**, that forms naturally in the ground and escapes through cracks and vents. This can present a risk of cancer to people whose homes are built over ground where radon is escaping. People in radon-rich areas should have their homes tested. If radon is present, they should arrange for ventilation so that harmful levels of the gas will not accumulate.

QUICK QUIZ

Chapter 17, Section 9

The following quiz will help you assess your students' understanding of the material covered in this section of the chapter. You might use the quiz as an oral exercise, which will lead into a class discussion of the topics covered. Or, you might use it as a paper/pencil

quiz to evaluate your students individually.

1. Risks of cancer are categorized according to whether or not they are controllable. (True)
2. Tobacco has not been conclusively linked to the development of lung cancer. (False)
3. Tobacco use can cause cancers of the larynx, mouth, esophagus, urinary bladder, kidney and pancreas. (True)

Sun overexposure ages the skin and promotes skin cancer. Sunscreen filters the harmful rays and lowers cancer risks. Radiation from too many X rays or from radon can increase cancer risks.

Diet, Alcohol, and Physical Activity

Four dietary factors link strongly with high cancer risks: high meat intakes, high fat intakes, low fruit and vegetable intakes, and low grain intakes. Details about the foods that make up such a diet are in this chapter's Straight Talk section, along with answers to questions people ask about additives and supplements.

Alcohol, when consumed in large amounts, leads to poor nutrition, which in turn lowers the body's defenses against cancer. Alcoholic beverages also contain toxins that may initiate cancer of the liver, esophagus, mouth, throat, rectum, lungs, and breast. The evidence against alcohol is incomplete. It is safe to say, however, that people who take in alcohol on a daily basis probably increase their risks of some kinds of cancer.

Physically active people, in contrast, enjoy a reduced risk of cancer, especially colon cancer. People who fail to work out regularly suffer more cancers of this type. This effect may be related to constipation—a problem common in sedentary people but rare in physically active people. The stools contain carcinogenic material. The longer they stay in the colon, the more the chance of their changing the cells of the colon's lining. Physical activity strengthens the muscles used to move the bowels and massages the intestines to help move their contents along. With regular bowel movements, the contents of the stools spend little time in contact with the colon lining.

 A diet low in fat and meat and high in grains, fruits, and vegetables may minimize the risks of certain cancers.

SECTION 9 Review

Answer the following questions on a sheet of paper.

Learning the Vocabulary

The vocabulary terms in this section are *melanin, suntan lotion, sunscreen, sun block,* and *radon.*

1. Write a sentence using each vocabulary term.

Learning the Facts

2. What percentage of lung cancer victims are smokers?

3. What causes skin cancer?

4. Name the four dietary factors that link strongly with high cancer risks.

Making Life Choices

5. Determine how well you protect yourself against cancer by taking the Life Choice Inventory on the opposite page. Do you feel you are doing enough to protect yourself against cancer? Why or why not? List the steps you need to take to reduce your risk of cancer.

MINI Glossary

radon (RAY-don): a gas that arises from the earth where radioactive materials are present.

4. Over-exposure to the sun's ultraviolet (UV) rays is the major cause of skin cancer. (True)

5. One bad sunburn is not enough to increase the risk of developing melanoma. (False)

6. People who are in the sun every day are less likely to develop melanoma than those who get bad sunburns from time to time. (False)

7. Melanin is a pigment which protects the skin from UV damage. (True)

8. Sunlamps and tanning booths minimize the risk of UV damage. (False)

9. Radon is a natural gas which can cause cancer. (True)

10. A diet high in meat will minimize the risk of cancer. (False)

ASSESS

EVALUATE

SECTION 9 Review Answers

1. Answers will vary.
2. 80 percent (p. 476)
3. overexposure to the sun's ultraviolet (UV) rays (p. 476)
4. high meat and fat intakes, low fruit, vegetable, and grain intakes (p. 479)
5. Answers will vary.

 A reproducible quiz for Section 9 is provided in the Teacher's Resource Box.

CLOSE

Before going on to the next section, students should be able to answer these questions:

1. How can you cut down on the amount of exposure to radiation (UV rays) from the sun?
2. What are some risk factors for melanoma?
3. How do diet and exercise play a role in cancer prevention?

Discuss the answers to these questions in class.

FOCUS

OUTCOMES

In this section students will learn the:

1. Eight warning signs that could aid in the early detection of cancer.

2. Kinds of self-exams that can lead to early detection of cancer.

3. Types of laboratory tests that can be used to detect and diagnose certain kinds of cancer.

4. Types of cancer treatments.

FOCUS ACTIVITY

Ask students if they have ever known anyone who has had cancer. Did this person do self-exams? If not, did ignorance and fear play a part in the failure to do self-exams or to undergo certain laboratory tests? Stress that early detection can mean a much higher percentage of cancer cures. Explain that students can accept the responsibility for learning and practicing self-exams and being aware of the eight warning signs as they apply to changes in their bodies. Discuss how self-esteem, fear, ignorance, and responsibility help determine our ability to take charge of making wise choices, such as doing self-exams and thereby detecting cancer early and enhancing chances of survival.

Health Strategies

Helping a Friend with Cancer

To help a loved one with cancer:

1. Be there. Don't avoid your friend, who needs your presence now more than ever before.

2. Touch the person. A hug or other physical gesture oftentimes can say more than words.

3. Let the person talk. Don't avoid the word *cancer*. Ask if your friend wants to talk about the illness. If so, expect negative emotions, and accept them.

4. Make specific offers of help. Ask if you can mow the grass, help with schoolwork, go shopping, fix a snack, baby-sit, or do any other task that needs to be done—and then do it.

5. Help the friend's family. They are suffering, too. Tell family members you can stay with your friend for a few hours while they run errands or care for personal needs that may have been neglected.

6. Recognize limitations. Involve your friend in as many of your normal activities as possible, but remember that people with cancer tire easily. Don't be offended if your friend cancels an outing or cuts a visit short because of pain or fatigue.

7. Be positive. No matter what the future holds, everyone with cancer needs laughter, hope, and talk of plans for tomorrow.

Source: Adapted with permission from the *University of Texas Lifetime Health Letter*, Houston, January 1990, p. 2.

SECTION 10
Early Detection and Treatment

The treatment of cancer involves sophisticated equipment, powerful drugs, and specialized medical staff. The detection of common cancers, however, requires mostly routine tests and self-examinations. The sooner a cancer is detected, the better the chances for a complete cure.

Cancer Detection

Figure 17–15 on the next page lists cancers, such as **Hodgkin's disease** and others, that most often cause deaths among young people. It also describes the symptoms associated with each. Any of the symptoms listed should be checked by a health-care provider immediately.

Cancer "Caution" Signs Often, cancer gives some warning to the person who is developing it. Cancer can develop without symptoms, but it is wise to heed all the messages your body sends you, particularly the following warnings:

- **C**hange in bowel or bladder habits, such as diarrhea or constipation.
- **A** sore that does not heal.
- **U**nusual bleeding or discharge.
- **T**hickening or lump that suddenly appears anywhere in the body.
- **I**ndigestion or difficulty swallowing.
- **O**bvious change in a wart or mole.
- **N**agging cough or hoarseness.
- **S**udden weight loss.

To remember this list, recall that the first letters in the warning signs spell the word *CAUTIONS*. Having one of these symptoms does not necessarily mean that you have cancer. A cold or eating too much might bring about some of them, for example. Just remember that when symptoms last for more than a week, or when they occur more than once, they require the attention of a health-care provider.

Medical Exams A professional can detect a lump in places not easily examined through home self-exams (described next). Laboratory tests are important, too. The most accurate test for early breast cancer is the **mammogram** (an X-ray examination). Because mammograms involve radiation, which itself can cause cancer, they are used sparingly.

Genetic testing can play a role in identifying inherited traits that make some people likely to develop certain cancers. The hope is that with early warning, such people can take action to prevent cancers from getting started.

HEALTHY PEOPLE 2000

Reverse the rise in cancer deaths to achieve a rate of no more than 130 per 100,000 people.

Cancer is the second leading cause of death in the United States. Cancer strikes more frequently with advancing age, but many cancer deaths are premature. In 1987, 18 million years of potential life before age 65

were lost from cancer compared to 15 million years for heart disease.

Although there are many different types of cancer, a few major types account for more than half of all cancer-related illness and death. For men, the leading causes are lung cancer (35 percent), colorectal cancer (11 percent), and prostate cancer (11 percent). For women, they are lung cancer (21 percent), breast cancer (18 percent), and colorectal cancer (13 percent).

Figure 17–15 *Cancers Most Often Causing Deaths in People Ages 15 to 34*

Disease	Early Symptoms	Survival with early Diagnosis and Prompt Treatment[a]
Brain and nervous system cancer	Personality changes; bizarre behavior; headaches; dizziness; balance and walking disturbances; vision changes; nausea, vomiting, or seizures	Poor to good
Breast cancer	Unusual lump; thickening in, change in contour in, dimple in, or discharge from, the nipple	Good (about 50 percent)
Hodgkin's disease	Swelling of lymph nodes in neck, armpits, or groin; susceptibility to infection	Good (54 percent)
Leukemia	Acts like infection, with fever, lethargy, and other flulike symptoms; may also include bone pain, tendency to bruise or bleed easily, and enlargement of lymph nodes	Poor to good (up to 50 percent), depending on the type of leukemia
Skin cancer	Unusual discoloration, swellings, sores, or lumps; change in color or appearance of a wart or mole; tenderness, itching, or bleeding from a lump or mole	Excellent (up to 90 percent)
Testicular cancer	Small, hard, painless lump; sudden accumulation of fluid in the scrotum; pain or discomfort in the region between the scrotum and anus	Good to excellent (66 to 86 percent)

[a]The survival rates are estimates based on five years of disease-free survival. For all cancers, survival rates drop dramatically after metastasis.

Tests that 18-year-olds should have include, for young women, a Pap test, a pelvic examination, and a breast examination (by a physician). Young men 18 years old should have a testicle and prostate examination (by a physician). Both genders need examinations of the thyroid, lymph nodes, mouth and throat, and skin. For every advantage in early detection of cancer, these tests (and others) should continue on schedule throughout life.

A medical professional who sees a person only once a year or so may not notice small changes that would be obvious to a person familiar with his or her own body. Many thousands of cases of cancer have been cured, thanks to early detection through self-exams.

Breast Self-Exam   Once a month a young woman should check her breasts for cancer. If you start testing now, while you are young, it will be a habit that will serve you well throughout life. The breast test is easy, especially when done in the shower while the skin is slippery (see Figure 17–16).

Lumps in the breast are most often not cancerous. However, they should be checked by a health-care provider nonetheless. You'll soon easily tell the "normal lumpiness" that occurs before the menstrual period from an unusual lump. Many times, a cancerous lump feels like a little pea buried in the breast. Report anything unusual to a health-care provider right away.

Testicular Self-Exam   If you are a young man, you can help protect yourself from cancer of the testicles through self-examination (Figure 17–17). Although it occurs less frequently than breast cancer, cancer of the testicles can be deadly, because it advances rapidly. It most commonly strikes young

Glossary

Hodgkin's disease: a lymphoma that attacks people in early life and is treatable with radiation therapy.

mammogram: X-ray examination of the breast, a screening test for cancer.

Lifestyle, environment, and genetic factors, individually or in combination, can increase an individual's risk of developing cancer. The contribution of lifestyle and environmental factors to cancer mortality has been estimated as follows: diet (approximately 35 percent of cancer deaths), tobacco (30 percent), reproductive/sexual behavior (7 percent), occupation (4 percent), alcohol (3 percent), geophysical factors (3 percent), pollution (2 percent), industrial products (1 percent), and medicines and medical procedures (1 percent). Reductions in tobacco use and dietary modifications to reduce excessive fat consumption and increase consumption of fruits, vegetables, grain products, and therefore dietary fiber, hold the greatest promise as strategies to reduce cancer incidence and ultimately cancer mortality.

TEACH & APPLY

COMPREHENSION CHECK

After students have looked at Figure 17–15, have them close their books and see how much of the information from the figure they can generate. Begin by having them list the six types of cancers most often causing death in people aged 15 to 34. Then see how many symptoms they can remember for each disease. Finally, write the text statistics for survival on the board and see if they can match those to the proper types of cancer.

CLASS ACTIVITY

Write the word C-A-U-T-I-O-N-S vertically on the board or on a transparency. After each letter write the warning sign starting with that letter. (See the text material under Cancer "Caution" Signs on page 480.)

Leave space between each letter of the word so that you can cover the warning signs with a piece of paper and slide the paper down as you talk about each one for review. Give a brief overview of the warning signs. Then go over them one by one. Call on a student to give you the first warning sign, then move the paper down so the first warning sign can be seen and ask for the second one. Have the student continue until an incorrect answer is given. When one is missed, call on someone else to start with number one again and to go through all eight warning signs.

BACKGROUND INFORMATION

Both women and men should be aware of the possibility of skin cancer and should visually inspect their skin in a mirror every month, looking for changed moles or spots. Also emphasize the value of a self-exam because the person doing it becomes familiar with his or her own body. That person is more likely to notice an abnormality. It's also true that no one will care more about detecting a problem than the person doing the self-exam.

A handout on medical tests available for the early detection of symptomless cancer is provided in the Teacher's Resource Box.

GROUP ACTIVITY

Have students imagine the following: You have just been told that you have had a change in a mole and that it has become cancerous. The doctor gives you some advice but you would like more information and perhaps a second opinion.

Divide the class into groups of five to eight. Give each group a phone book. Have them look up the numbers they could call to get more information about their conditions. They may also use their textbooks. Give them approximately ten minutes. Ask each group for the names and numbers they found. On an overhead transparency, write the names and numbers they give you.

Figure 17–16 Breast Self-Examination

1. Stand before a mirror. Inspect both breasts for anything unusual, such as any discharge from the nipples or puckering, dimpling, or scaling of the skin.

2. Watch closely in the mirror. Clasp hands behind your head, and press hands forward. The purpose of these steps is to find any changes in the shape or contour of your breasts. As you do them, you should be able to feel your chest muscles tighten.

3. Next, press hands firmly on hips and bow slightly toward the mirror as you pull your shoulders and elbows forward.

Parts 4 and 5 of the exam are easy to do in the bath or shower, where fingers glide over soapy skin.

4. Raise your left arm. Use three or four fingers of your right hand to explore your left breast firmly, carefully, and thoroughly. Beginning at the outer edge, press the flat part of your fingers in small circles, moving the circles slowly around the breast. Gradually work toward the nipple. Be sure to cover the entire breast. Pay special attention to the area between the breast and the armpit, including the armpit itself. Feel for any unusual lump or mass under the skin.

5. Gently squeeze the nipple and look for a discharge. Repeat the exam on your right breast.

6. Repeat Steps 4 and 5 lying down. Lie flat on your back with your left arm over your head and a pillow or folded towel under your left shoulder. This position flattens the breast and makes it easier to examine. Use the same circular motion described earlier. Repeat on your right breast.

Figure 17–17 Testicular Self-Examination

Roll each testicle between the thumb and fingers. The testicles should feel smooth, except for the normal raised organ located on the back of each. Report any hard lump, enlargement, or contour changes to your health-care provider.

Lump is likely to be here.

men between the ages of 15 and 22. Report any large lump, enlargement, or change in shape to a health-care provider.

Skin Self-Exam One more test to perform at bath time is a visual check of your entire skin. Skin cancer is a real threat. The more familiar you become with any moles or freckles you may have, the better you will be able to detect changes in them that could mean the start of cancer.

Stand in front of a large mirror, and take a look at your skin. Use a hand mirror to help with the back view. If a mole has changed its shape or color or has begun bleeding, have it checked right away. And remember to protect your skin from the sun.

Detection tests are important, but even more important is to discover how to prevent cancer's occurrence. No disease has ever been cured out of existence. As is now the case with smallpox and polio,

CRITICAL THINKING

Put these two life situations on the board or a prepared transparency. Have the students write answers to the questions at the end of

each life situation. After they have finished, have a class discussion.

Life Situation #1—You are a 14-year-old male high school student. While taking a shower you feel a lump on your neck. It feels hard but it is not painful. You do not want to

Deception of the Desperate

Consumer SKILLS

Not all cancer treatments called "cures" are effective. Frauds in health are always cruel. Those aimed at cancer victims are especially so, because they prey on people who are already suffering. Laetrile is a cancer-cure hoax. Another such hoax is immuno-augmentative therapy, or IAT. This one involves traveling to foreign countries for dangerous blood transfusions that not only fail to fight cancer, but also spread AIDS and hepatitis to the already sick victims. Countless other vitamin, mineral, and drug "therapies" offered to cancer victims are scams.

Sometimes people report that a phony cancer cure worked. Famous quack-buster Victor Herbert has listed five possible reasons for this:

▶ The person never had cancer.
▶ The cancer was cured by conventional therapy, but the quack took the credit.
▶ The cancer is still silently progressing, but the person *thinks* that it has been cured.

▶ The person has died of cancer, but is reported as cured.
▶ The person's cancer went away by itself, and the quack took the credit.

The sellers of bogus treatments capitalize on people's fear of cancer and scare them into believing that medical doctors frown on their methods for dishonest reasons. "The doctors don't care if you die," they say. "They just want your money first." Loving life, wanting to trust someone, and wanting to hope that a cure is possible, victims of cancer easily fall prey to this sort of deception. So do relatives and friends who are willing to try anything to help their loved ones get well.

Critical Thinking

1. *Why do people's fears of cancer make them easy targets for quacks?*
2. *Why do you think someone with cancer might take chances by trying unproven therapies?*
3. *What motivates quacks to sell fake cancer cures?*

Consumer SKILLS

Answers to Critical Thinking

1. Their fear overwhelms their ability to reason; they become so afraid of dying that they will try anything.
2. They think they have nothing to lose. They may also be persuaded that health-care providers are not really concerned about them and that the people who claim to have cures are really the ones who want to help them.
3. Answers will vary.

TRANSPARENCIES

The transparency, "Cancer Cures by Surgery," is available in the Transparency Acetate Binder. This transparency illustrates the progression of cancer and the likelihood of an effective cure by surgery at the different stages of the cancer's progression. This transparency should help students see the importance of early detection.

---

widespread success can be claimed only when the disease is prevented from occurring. Still, the technology for curing cancer remains important to individuals who have developed the disease.

KEY POINTS *Professional examinations can detect early cancers. Self-examinations of the breasts, testicles, and skin can also detect cancer in early stages.*

Cancer Treatment

As soon as cancer is diagnosed, a person should seek treatment—not just any treatment, but the treatment most likely to be successful. This means finding medical experts, not quacks. Because cancer is scary, people may become irrational and seek help that promises miracles and delivers nothing but heartache. This chapter's Consumer Skills feature describes how cancer frauds are peddled.

For Your Information

The National Cancer Institute's information service number is **1-800-4CANCER** and its internet address is **http://www.nci.nih.gov** The American Cancer Society's number is **1-800-ACS-2345** and its internet address is **htttp://www.cancer.org**

---

worry your parents so you are hesitant to tell them. However, you are concerned about the lump. How would you deal with this problem?

Life Situation #2—You are a 14-year-old female high school student. Your mother tells

you that your grandmother died of breast cancer and that she is going yearly for a mammogram. What can you deduce from this new information? What are your concerns? What action would you take in view of the information you have just been given?

DISCUSSION

Have students list side effects that people develop as a result of cancer treatments. Have a class discussion on the side effects. Stress that today health-care professionals make every effort to keep the patient as comfortable as possible during treatment. There are drugs that prevent or reduce the nausea. Also, pain and diarrhea are treated. The only side effects that some cancer patients have to adjust to are loss of hair and fatigue.

ASSESS

EVALUATE

Review Answers

1. mammogram
2. chemotherapy
3. polyps
4. self-exams and lab exams (p. 480)
5. by removal of the malignant tissue and by destruction of cancer cells (p. 484)
6. Some cancer cells may lie outside the beam area and remain unaffected, while some healthy tissue that lies within the beam area is destroyed. (p. 484)
7. surgery, radiation therapy, and chemotherapy (p. 484)
8. They must retain wellness in those areas that remain open, cope with fears, and move emotionally through stages of grief before taking part in their own treatments. (p. 485)
9. Answers may vary. (see Health Strategies on p. 480)
10. Answers will vary.

Answers to FACT or FICTION   Here are the answers to the questions at the start of the chapter.

1. **True.**
2. **True.**
3. **False.** Of the two types of diabetes, Type 2 is most preventable by controlling body fatness.
4. **False.** A diet of fresh, low-fat, high-fiber, high-nutrient food is best for controlling diabetes.
5. **False.** The blood that passes through the heart's chambers brings no nourishment or oxygen to the heart's tissues. The heart muscle depends on its own network of arteries and capillaries, just as other muscles do.
6. **True.**
7. **False.** Lifestyle factors can be helpful not only in prevention but also in reversal of heart disease.
8. **False.** High blood pressure does not feel abnormal.
9. **True.**
10. **False.** While people with fair complexions who burn easily are at greater risk, everyone needs to use sunscreen to prevent skin cancer from sun exposure.
11. **False.** Tanning booths and lamps are no safer than sunbathing, as far as cancer risks are concerned.
12. **True.**

Being diagnosed as having cancer can be a frightening experience, but people should try to put their fears aside. Fear can interfere with the body's healing response, and hope can help with cure. Hope is possible, because tremendous numbers of treatments end in success, thanks to advances in cancer treatment research. For more information about cancer, people can call a cancer hotline number such as those given in the margin on the previous page.

Cancer treatments destroy cancers in two ways: by removal of the malignant tissue from the body and by destruction of cancer cells within the body. If the cancer has metastasized, surgical removal or destruction of a tumor may not eliminate all the cancer cells. Cancer *cure* comes when every cancer cell is either removed from the body or wiped out by treatments.

Surgical Treatment   Many cancers are treatable through surgery alone. Removal of a tumor can stop the cancer growth at a site, especially if the cancer is still small. The cure rate drops off, however, as the tumor invades surrounding tissues and metastasizes to other body parts. For example, the large intestine may contain precancerous growths called **polyps**. Removal of polyps protects against cancer. If the polyp begins to invade just a few millimeters into the tissue, however, its surgical removal no longer guarantees complete freedom from cancer at that site.

A small tumor on the skin or other external membrane can sometimes be destroyed by freezing with liquid nitrogen. Such a procedure is often performed in the physician's office and causes little inconvenience or pain.

Radiation Treatment   A treatment for cancer, sometimes used together with surgery, is **radiation therapy**. Medical professionals use several methods to kill tumors with radiation. A beam may be focused on the area known to be cancerous. Radioactive materials may be implanted in the tumor or, in some cases, injected into the bloodstream (when it is known that they will be absorbed only by the tumor). Under bombardment from the radioactivity, the fast-growing cells of the cancer become disrupted and die off.

Unfortunately, when a beam of radiation is used, some cancer cells may lie outside the beam area and remain unaffected. Also, some healthy tissue that lies within the beam area is destroyed. The problem cannot be solved by exposing the whole body to radiation, because the body cannot tolerate so much radiation.

Chemotherapy   In addition to surgery and radiation, a third approach is chemical treatments of cancer, called **chemotherapy**. These offer a major advantage when a tumor has metastasized. Once in the body, the drugs seek out and destroy the escaped cancer cells, as well as tumors in all locations. More than 40 drugs are now used against cancer in different ways—to cure, to inhibit cancer growth, to relieve pain, and to allow the person to lead a more normal life. Often, radiation and chemotherapy are used together.

Treatment Side Effects   Both radiation and anticancer drugs that kill cancer tissue also kill normal tissues, although more slowly. Rapidly dividing cells in the body are affected the most. The cells of the digestive tract, for example, normally divide rapidly, so treatments produce diarrhea, nausea, and vomiting. Other side effects are skin damage, hair loss, and fatigue. New blood cells also arise from a rapidly dividing tissue, so people being treated for cancer may develop blood problems.

Described here are only a few treatments for cancer. Many more have proved effective. More still are under development. A person who gets cancer has reason to be hopeful about possibilities for a cure.

QUICK QUIZ

Chapter 17, Section 10

The following quiz will help you assess your students' understanding of the material covered in this section of the chapter. You might use the quiz as an oral exercise, which will lead into a class discussion of the topics covered. Or, you might use it as a paper/pencil quiz to evaluate your students individually.

Like the Quick Quiz, the Section Review can also be used as an assessment tool to spark class discussion or as an individual student evaluation. It can also be used as a review in preparation for this quiz.

1. A sore that does not heal, an unusual lump, bleeding or discharge, or an obvious change in a wart or mole can all be symptoms of cancer. (True)
2. A mammogram is an important tool for

Cancer treatments aim to remove cancerous tissue and to destroy cancer cells. Common treatments include surgery, radiation therapy, and chemotherapy.

Living with Cancer

In the battle against a seemingly inhuman tissue, physicians tend to focus on machines, drugs, and techniques. The tissue, though, is within a living, feeling human being. Treatments often invade the person's life in intimate ways. People diagnosed with cancer must struggle to retain wellness in those areas that remain open, and meanwhile deal with the disease. They have fears to cope with. They may need to move emotionally through the stages of grief before they can take part in their own treatments and recoveries.

Some people find ways to face the crisis with courage. They are spurred into action, not despair. They cultivate a sense of humor in the midst of fear. Such people maintain strong family bonds and bonds of friendship throughout the illness. They also have an invaluable asset to recovery—the will to live. The Health Strategies section on page 480, "Helping a Friend with Cancer," offers ways you can help a friend or loved one with cancer.

 Dealing with a diagnosis of cancer takes courage. The will to live is an important asset to recovery.

SECTION 10 Review

Answer the following questions on a sheet of paper.

Learning the Vocabulary

The vocabulary terms in this section are *Hodgkin's disease, mammogram, polyps, radiation therapy,* and *chemotherapy.*
Fill in the blank with the correct answer.

1. A _____ is an X-ray examination of the breast.
2. _____ is the administration of drugs that seek out and destroy escaped cancer cells as well as tumors in all locations.
3. Tumors that grow on a stem, bleed easily, and tend to become malignant are called _____.

Learning the Facts

4. Name two ways to help detect cancer early on.
5. What are the two ways cancer treatments destroy cancer?
6. What is the disadvantage of using radiation therapy?
7. Name three common treatments for cancer.
8. What are some of the struggles faced by those with cancer?
9. List three strategies for helping a friend with cancer.

Making Life Choices

10. Look over the Health Strategies feature, "Helping a Friend with Cancer," on page 480. Imagine that you are fighting your own battle with cancer. What strategies would you add to the list for people who are close to you to follow? Now imagine someone close to you has cancer. Which suggestions on the list would you find easy to follow?

MINI Glossary

polyps: tumors that grow on a stem, resembling mushrooms. Polyps bleed easily, and some have the tendency to become malignant.

radiation therapy: the application of cell-destroying radiation to kill cancerous tissues.

chemotherapy: the administration of drugs that harm the cancer cells, but that do not harm the client, or at least do not harm the client as much as the disease does.

WORKSHEETS A reproducible quiz for Section 10 is provided in the Teacher's Resource Box.

CLOSE

Students should be able to answer these questions:

1. What are the eight warning signs of cancer?
2. What are some "protective factors" and "preventable risk factors" against cancer?
3. What body organs can be self-examined for early detection of cancer?
4. Name the basic types of cancer treatments.
5. List some of the major side effects of chemotherapy or radiation.
6. List the two ways cancer treatments destroy cancer cells.

Discuss the answers to these questions in class.

---

detecting lung cancer. (False)
3. Frequent mammograms can increase the risk of cancer. (True)
4. Teenagers should perform regular self-examinations for cancer and be tested by a physician. (True)
5. Young women should perform breast self-exams once a year. (False)
6. Young men should immediately report any large lump, change in shape, or enlargement of the testicles to a health-

care provider. (True)
7. A cancer is cured when every cancerous cell in the body has been removed or destroyed. (True)
8. Surgical treatment is especially effective on cancers that have metastasized. (False)
9. Radiation treatment and chemotherapy both produce painful side effects. (True)
10. Maintaining the will to live is a vital aspect of recovering from cancer. (True)

Straight
Talk

Diet for Disease Prevention

Background Information

Researchers have not established strong links between foods and cancer in the way that they have with tobacco. To make this point, tell students that Japanese people living in Japan develop more stomach and less colon cancer than people in the United States. However, when Japanese people come to the U.S., their children develop both stomach and colon cancer at a rate like that of U.S. citizens. Japan and the U.S. are both industrial countries. Something in the environment must be causing the changed cancer patterns. The change in diets is an obvious culprit.

Let students know that it may be certain forms of fat that are related to increased cancer rates. Some findings point to linoleic acid, the essential omega-6 fatty acid of vegetable oils. Polyunsaturated fats are more often associated with tumor growth than are saturated fats. In laboratory experiments with animals, fat does not initiate the cancers, but after exposure from a known carcinogen, a high-fat diet does make more cancers develop.

A surgeon general said that for Americans who do not smoke or drink excessively, "your choice of diet can influence your long-term health prospects more than any other action you might take." The diet choices associated with good health are well known. A warning: Popular books and magazines make many claims regarding diet and diseases. They know people will buy publications that promise control over lifestyle diseases, and not all of their claims are well founded.

 How can diet prevent all of the lifestyle diseases? That seems impossible.

You are right to say that no diet, by itself, will positively prevent diseases. Some cases of lifestyle diseases will occur no matter what a person eats. However, for most people, food choices greatly alter their risks for developing Type 2 diabetes, heart disease, or certain kinds of cancer. Also, the diet that prevents any one lifestyle disease closely resembles a diet to prevent the others. The same diet, well chosen, also boosts the immune system.

 What sort of foods do I have to eat to stay healthy? I don't want to eat a lot of strange foods.

No single food is essential to include in the diet. None has magic powers to prevent disease. You need only apply some general principles when choosing among familiar foods, and to stay physically active. These principles are displayed on the umbrella of Figure 17–18. They are from recommendations put forth by two leaders in disease prevention—the

American Heart Association and the American Cancer Society.

 Fat seems to be a big issue. What do they mean when they say to limit fats?

Every legitimate nutrition authority urges Americans to cut down on fat intakes. With few exceptions, anywhere in the world where people eat diets high in the saturated fats of animal products and processed foods, rates of heart disease and cancer are high. Conversely, groups of people who eat diets low in fat, and especially low in animal fats, have low rates of diseases. Part of the reason why many vegetarians have low rates of diseases may be that they consume little or no animal fat and few highly processed foods. They choose mostly fruits, vegetables, and whole grains.

 Do you mean that to be healthy I have to give up meat? I don't care to be a vegetarian.

You need not give up meat completely, but most Americans eat dramatically more meat than guidelines suggest. Reducing meat portions has the effect of reducing saturated fat intake and increasing fiber—two healthy outcomes.

Choosing a healthy diet isn't as simple as omitting one food group from the diet. For instance, even a vegetarian can eat a diet exceptionally high in fat, if it is based on cheese, whole milk, cream, and other fatty dairy products.

 OK. I can live without one of my daily burgers. How else can I make my diet moderate in fats?

486

CRITICAL THINKING

Cholesterol is a key factor in the development of heart disease, even in young adults. Since the American diet is dangerously high in fat, which turns to cholesterol in the body, it is important for students to internalize information relating to cholesterol, diet, heart disease, and exercise.

Have students keep a three-day diary of everything they eat and drink. Encourage them to also involve a parent in this activity. Arrange, where possible, to have students' cholesterol levels measured. Watch for health fairs or other opportunities to obtain the tests free or at reduced cost, or sponsor a health fair at your school and ask a local hospital to give the tests.

Divide the class into these groups:

To reach a moderate intake, most people must strictly limit just a few foods—the pure fats, such as sour cream, butter, oil, and margarine. Also limit or find substitutes for high-fat foods such as mayonnaise, cheese, and cream cheese. Save for special occasions, and choose small portions of, such high-fat foods as convenience foods with sauces, fried foods, burgers, steaks, chops, meat with visible fat, sausages and cold cuts, whole milk, and pastries.

 What about salad dressing and other fats?

When you use salad dressing, pick one based on olive oil or canola oil, since these don't affect the heart. Use them in moderation, though, because they are as high in calories, and as fattening to the body, as any other fats.

Sometimes fat hides in foods, mixed into the other ingredients. Examples are breads, such as croissants, biscuits, dinner rolls, and some cereals. To find the fat in such foods, take up the art of label reading. You'll be amazed at the amount of fat lurking in your foods. For health, each 100 calories of food should provide no more than about 3 grams of fat.

 So far, this advice seems like a lot of don'ts. Are there any foods left to eat?

Yes, indeed. So many, in fact, that if you busy yourself getting all of the recommended items, you'll have little time or hunger left for the other foods. Getting enough fish is important. Two or three meals of fish (broiled or baked—not fried) a week provide the heart benefits of fish oil and fish. Don't take fish oil capsules, though, because they often contain toxins.

Possibly the most urgent advice is to choose *at least 5* servings of a wide variety of fruits and vegetables each day. These foods are champions of health,

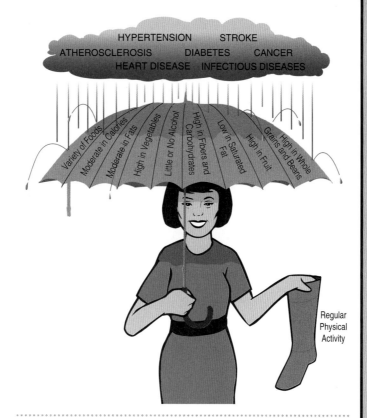

not just for their abundant vitamins, minerals, and beneficial fiber, but for their **phytochemicals** that defend against heart disease and cancer.

 How do the phytochemicals work?

Some work the way antioxidant vitamins do, to defend against harmful chemical reactions in the body. (This was described in Chapter 7.) Others seem to prepare the body to fight off cancerous cells when they arise. Still others interfere with hormones that stimulate cancer growth.

Figure 17–18 The Protective Diet. The same diet that helps protect the body against many lifestyle diseases also helps to keep the immune system strong.

487

---

1. Those already on exercise programs.
2. Those who are basically sedentary.
3. Those who would be willing to adhere to a diet of fresh fruits and vegetables, while omitting foods high in fat.
4. Those students who will begin an exercise program for the first time.

Every Friday, evaluate and share progress. At the end of the semester, have cholesterol levels checked again. Analyze results and draw conclusions.

Note for the instructor: It is difficult for teenagers to involve parents. However, encourage them to do so in activities such as this. Besides good public relations for your profession, it can personally benefit many adults who need help with their current state of wellness.

For enrichment, you may want to tell students that vegetarians have lower mortality rates from cancer than the rest of the population, even when cancers related to smoking and alcohol are removed from the comparisons. These findings match up with general findings that high vegetable and grain intakes correlate with low cancer rates.

CLASS ACTIVITY

Have students write a summary after listening to a news report, or bring in newspaper or magazine articles on lifestyle diseases, treatments, and prevention of these diseases. Make a bulletin board around a reproduction of Figure 17–18 and include pictures of healthy lifestyle activities for disease prevention (people exercising, plates of healthy foods, pictures of health fairs with monitoring equipment, relaxation scenes, clean environments, and so on). Arrange photos in the shape of an umbrella in the center, with articles surrounding it. Make "lightening bolts" of colored paper that name the lifestyle diseases. Aim the bolts at the umbrella.

Straight Talk

Diet for Disease Prevention (continued)

Do researchers know which vegetables are best for health?

Figure 17–19 can help you get to know some of the players in the phytochemical game. Among them are fruits and vegetables rich in vitamin C and vegetables of the cabbage family, the **cruciferous vegetables**—cabbage, broccoli, and brussels sprouts. Others, the ones rich in carotene, may help protect against both heart disease and cancer. The bright orange, yellow, or deep-green-colored ones, along with all dark leafy greens, are the ones to choose most often. Garlic; onions; soybeans; other beans; hot peppers; celery; herbs such as parsley, basil, and oregano; and other foods are under study as possible disease fighters.

Can't I just take supplements to get what I need from fruits and vegetables? It's hard for me to find fresh foods sometimes.

Research on supplements has been disappointing. Vegetables and fruits contain many phytochemicals and types of fiber that supplements cannot match. One exception is vitamin E for middle-aged people. A daily low-dose supplement may help to

delay a heart attack in that group. Concerns about side effects prevent authorities from recommending vitamin E supplements to the public, however.

While you should make every effort to eat fresh fruits and vegetables often, don't overlook dried, frozen, and canned fruits and vegetables. They provide many of the same benefits, and they are always available.

Also, fiber-rich whole-grain cereals, bread, or pasta; brown rice; and beans of any kind have plenty of evidence in their favor as protectors against both heart disease and cancers. Oatmeal has become famous for its heart-protecting fiber. Fibers of other whole grains, beans, fruits, and vegetables are just as effective, but less well advertised.

Do food additives cause cancer?

Food additives have little to do with cancer. Many compounds are added to foods to preserve them, or to enhance their color, flavor, or texture. They are present in such small amounts, and evidence about their safety is so abundant, that they are deemed appropriate for use in foods. Even saccharine was almost banned when evidence showed that extremely high doses caused tumors in rats. Saccharine is probably safe for people, though, in amounts used in foods. Still, it must bear a warning label, so that people may avoid it if they wish.

What about cancer from nitrites (cured meats) and charbroiled meats, and irradiated foods, and the fat-replacer olestra, and salt, and coffee, and tea, and pesticides, and herbicides, and engineered tomatoes, and . . .

So many interesting details about nutrition and disease deserve attention that we could write a book about them. Watch the news, and follow the stories on these topics. None of the concerns you mention are

488

COOPERATIVE LEARNING

This activity is a great review. It resembles the TV game show, Jeopardy. You can have two

rounds followed by a final challenge round. Produce an overhead for the first round that resembles this chart.

For round two, double the point value and change the categories. The next group of

First Facts	Diabetes	Cardiovascular	Heart Attack	Heart Disease Treatments
10	10	10	10	10
20	20	20	20	20
30	30	30	30	30
40	40	40	40	40
50	50	50	50	50

Foods to Fight Diseases

Foods High in Carotenes
Apricot, Asparagus, Broccoli, Cantaloupe, Carrots, Green onion, Greens (all varieties), Lettuce (dark green), Mango, Oriental cabbage, Papaya, Parsley, Spinach, Squash (hard, winter), Sweet potato

Cruciferous Vegetables
Bok choy, Broccoli and broccoli sprouts, Brussels sprouts, Cabbage (all varieties), Cauliflower, Greens (collards, mustards, turnips), Kale, Kohlrabi, Rutabaga, Turnip root

Foods that Contain Other Phytochemicals
Barley, Basil, Berries, Brown rice, Celery, Chives, Citrus fruit, Cucumber, Fennel, Flax seed, Garlic, Ginger, Guava, Lettuce (dark green), Mango, Oats, Onion, Oregano, Papaya, Parsnip, Potato, Soybeans and soy products, Spinach, Squash (summer), Tarragon, Tea (green and black), Thyme, Tomato, Turmeric, Whole wheat

Figure 17–19 Foods to Fight Diseases. Choose at least 5 servings of fruits and vegetables each day, from as wide a variety as possible.

thought to increase people's cancer risks significantly. Each must be treated with respect, however.

To remove or reduce pesticides that might be left on fruits and vegetables, wash them well before eating them. As for salt, coffee, cured or charbroiled meats, or fat replacers, these seem not to be significant cancer risks in the United States, although you may want to use them sparingly. Foods that are treated by **irradiation** or that are the products of **genetic engineering** seem to carry no significant disease risks. Drinking tea may even protect against some cancers.

Of the many foods available for purchase in this country, the simplest, freshest foods are still the best. Vary your choices. Don't let your diet become monotonous. Whenever you switch from food to food, you are diluting whatever is in one food with what is in the others.

489

MINI Glossary

phytochemicals: chemicals in plant-based foods that are not nutrients but that have effects on the body.

cruciferous vegetables: vegetables of the cabbage family.

irradiation: ionizing radiation applied to food to kill microorganisms and other pests. Ionizing radiation disrupts the internal molecular workings of cells, killing them.

genetic engineering: a science of manipulating the genes of living things to instill some desirable trait not present in the original organism. An example is a tomato given a gene to delay its rotting.

ON LINE WITH HEALTH

You may want to have your students visit the following URLs, where they will find information and additional Web site resources to enhance their study of this chapter. As with all Web sites, you should check these out first to be sure the information found there is appropriate for your students.

The National Heart, Lung, and Blood Institute
http://www.nhlbi.nih. gov/nhlbi/nhlbi.htm

Wellness, Inc.
http://www. wellness-inc.com/

Information, including research and educational activities, as well as links to other sites, is fairly extensive. The Wellness site, dedicated to early detection and disease prevention, is commercially sponsored, but the information and links it offers make it a very useful site.

categories should be Stroke, Reducing the Risks of CVD, Cancer, Cancer Risks that People Can Control, and Early Detection and Treatment. For the final challenge pick a topic that you have discussed in class. The questions can be from the section reviews in the chapter, or your own test questions. You may use the exact question or change the wording or, as in the TV show, give the answer and have students answer with a question.

To play the game, divide your class into three or four equal teams. One team picks a category and point value and that team has one minute to answer the question. If they answer correctly they will receive the points from the category. If they do not answer correctly, any of the other teams can answer. The person who raises their hand first, gets the first chance to answer. During the final challenge, each team wagers points and each team writes its answer on paper. Offer extra credit points to the team that wins the game.

ANSWERS TO CHAPTER 17 REVIEW

VOCABULARY

1. **a.** artificial heart **b.** electrocardiogram **c.** pacemaker **d.** capillaries **e.** embolism **f.** blood **g.** risk factors **h.** heart attack **i.** angina **j.** heart murmur **k.** chambers **l.** cardiovascular disease **m.** metastasized **n.** sarcomas **o.** leukemias **p.** mutation **q.** malignancy **r.** melanin **s.** benign **t.** myeloma **u.** cancer **v.** cruciferous vegetables **w.** carcinomas

2. **a.** Low-density lipoproteins carry fat and cholesterol from the liver to the tissues, while high-density lipoproteins carry fat and cholesterol away from the tissues back to the liver. **b.** Atherosclerosis is caused by the accumulation of plaques on the inner walls of the arteries. **c.** Atria receive the incoming blood into the heart, while the ventricles send blood out of the heart. **d.** A heart attack is when the vessels that feed the heart muscle become blocked, while a stroke is when the vessels leading to the brain become blocked. **e.** lymphomas

RECALL

SECTION 1

1. poor diet, physical inactivity, smoking, alcohol intake, and social interaction (p. 451)

SECTION 2

2. In a person with Type 1 diabetes, the pancreas does

CHAPTER 17 Review

Summarizing the Chapter

Your ability to respond correctly to the following statements ensures your understanding of the main concepts in the chapter.

1. Identify risk factors that contribute to diabetes, heart disease, stroke, and cancer.
2. List the warning signs, long-term effects, prevention, and control of diabetes.
3. List the warning signs of heart attack and stroke.
4. Explain how to reduce the risks of cardiovascular disease.
5. Describe the methods of detection and treatment for cancer.
6. Describe the links between nutrition and cancer prevention.

Learning the Vocabulary

risk factors	atherosclerosis
diabetes mellitus	plaques
insulin	aneurysm
diabetic coma	aorta
ketones	platelets
insulin shock	thrombus
cardiovascular disease (CVD)	coronary thrombosis
	heart attack
arteries	cerebral thrombosis
capillaries	stroke
veins	embolus
cardiovascular system	embolism
blood	critical phase
chambers	angina
atria	fibrillation
ventricles	pacemaker
coronary arteries	coronary artery bypass surgery
valves	
heart murmur	heart transplant
electrocardiogram	artificial heart
lymph	systolic pressure
heart disease	diastolic pressure

lipoproteins	benign
low-density lipoproteins (LDLs)	metastasized
	melanin
high-density lipoproteins (HDLs)	suntan lotion
	sunscreen
cancer	sun block
tumor	radon
malignancy	Hodgkin's disease
melanoma	mammogram
myeloma	polyps
lymphomas	radiation therapy
leukemias	chemotherapy
carcinomas	phytochemicals
sarcomas	cruciferous vegetables
initiator	irradiation
mutation	genetic engineering
promoter	

Answer the following questions on a separate sheet of paper.

1. **Matching**—*Match each of the following phrases with the appropriate vocabulary term from the list above:*
   a. a pump designed to fit into the human chest cavity and perform the heart's function
   b. a record of the electrical activity of the heart
   c. a device that delivers electrical impulses to the heart to regulate the heartbeat
   d. tiny blood vessels that form a net and weave in and around in tissues
   e. the sudden closure of a blood vessel by a traveling blood clot
   f. a thick red fluid that flows through the body's blood vessels
   g. factors that are linked with a disease by association but are not yet proved to be causes
   h. the event in which vessels that feed the heart muscle become blocked
   i. pain in the heart region caused by a lack of oxygen
   j. a heart sound that reflects damaged or abnormal heart valves
   k. large hollow areas in the heart
   l. a general term for all diseases of the heart and blood vessels
   m. cancer cells that have migrated from one part of the body to another
   n. cancers that arise in connective tissue cells

490

not produce enough insulin. In a person with Type 2 diabetes, the body cells do not respond to insulin. (pp. 452–453)
3. medication, diet, and exercise (p. 455)

SECTION 3

4. atherosclerosis (p. 458)
5. the ballooning out of an artery wall at a point where it has been weakened by deterioration (p. 459)
6. Answers will vary; could include: the plaques can enlarge enough to block the flow of blood; a blood clot may form, stick to a plaque, and grow until it cuts off the blood supply like a plug; and a clot may break loose and circulate until it reaches an artery too small to allow its passage. (p. 460)

SECTION 4

7. Answers will vary; could include: sudden temporary weakness or numbness in any part of one side of the body; temporary loss of speech or of understanding of

o. cancers that arise in the blood cell-making tissues

p. a change in a cell's genetic material

q. a dangerous cancerous growth that sheds cells into body fluids and spreads to new locations to start new cancer colonies

r. a brown pigment in human skin

s. noncancerous

t. a cancer originating in the cells of the bone marrow

u. a disease in which abnormal cells multiply out of control, and spread into surrounding tissues and other body parts

v. broccoli, brussels sprouts, cauliflower, and cabbages

w. cancers that arise in the skin, body chamber linings, or glands

2. a. What is the difference between low-density lipoproteins and high-density lipoproteins?

b. What is the relationship between atherosclerosis and plaques?

c. What is the difference between atria and ventricles?

d. What is the difference between a heart attack and a stroke?

e. What are cancers that arise in the immune system called?

Recalling Important Facts and Ideas

Section 1

1. What risk factors for lifestyle diseases are within a person's control?

Section 2

2. Explain the difference between Type 1 diabetes and Type 2 diabetes.

Section 3

3. What are the three tools for controlling diabetes and its consequences?

4. What is the most common form of CVD?

5. What is an aneurysm?

6. List two ways atherosclerosis can cause blockage of an artery.

Section 4

7. Name three warning signs of a stroke.

Section 5

8. List four medical treatments for heart disease.

Section 6

9. What are the effects of damage to the left side of the brain?

Section 7

10. Name four health strategies for reducing the risk of CVD.

11. How does dietary fiber offer protection against heart disease?

Section 8

12. What is the number one type of cancer in both men and women?

13. How do alcohol and tobacco work together to promote cancer?

Section 9

14. Name two cancer-causing factors people can control.

15. What types of cancers are most common in smokers?

Section 10

16. What does CAUTIONS stand for with regard to the warning signs of cancer?

17. When is a person considered to be cured of cancer?

Critical Thinking

1. Many public places now ban smoking in common areas. Do you think the health benefits justify this restriction? Why or why not? Do you feel that these laws infringe on the rights of the individual? Why or why not? What other restrictions would you place on smoking?

Activities

1. Develop two case histories. In one, describe someone at risk for CVD; in the other, describe someone with hardly any risk for heart disease.

2. Keep a diary of all the lifestyle risk factors for heart disease and cancer to which you are exposed for a full week. Develop a list of ways to avoid these risk factors.

3. Design an educational pamphlet aimed at high school students to inform them about cancer.

Making Decisions about Health

1. Lately, your grandfather has been experiencing sharp chest pains and has felt as though he couldn't breathe when playing actively with his grandchildren. What might your grandfather be experiencing, and what should he do about it?

491

teenager; keep your blood cholesterol within the normal range; if you have diabetes, keep your blood sugar under control; exercise vigorously for at least 20 minutes three or more times weekly; maintain appropriate body weight; control stress; and learn to relax. (p. 466)

11. High-fiber foods move quickly through the digestive tract, and carry cholesterol with them. (p. 471)

SECTION 8

12. lung cancer (p. 473)

13. Tobacco is the initiator of mouth, throat, and esophagus cancers, while alcohol is the promoter of these cancers once they have started. Smoking makes these cancers one-and-a-half times more likely, but coupled with alcohol they become 15 times more likely. (pp. 473–474)

SECTION 9

14. Answers will vary; could include: smoking behavior, exposure to sun's ultraviolet rays, and choosing proper diet and physical activity. (p. 476)

15. lung, larynx, mouth, esophagus, urinary bladder, kidney, pancreas (p. 476)

SECTION 10

16. Refer to text on page 480.

17. A person is cured of cancer when every cancer cell is either removed from the body or wiped out by treatments. (p. 484)

speech; dizziness, unsteadiness, or unexplained falls; and temporary dimness or loss of vision, particularly in one eye. (p. 462)

SECTION 5

8. Answers will vary; could include: drugs, pacemaker, coronary artery bypass surgery, heart transplant, artificial heart. (pp. 463–464)

SECTION 6

9. paralyzed right side; speech, language problems; behavioral style—slow, cautious (p. 465)

SECTION 7

10. Answers will vary; could include: learn about your heredity, and use the information and control the lifestyle factors that may affect you; don't smoke; keep your blood pressure below 130/80 if you are a

	OUTCOMES	FEATURES

CHAPTER 18
Pairing, Commitment, and Marriage

- Describe the differences between love and infatuation.
- List the advantages of sexual abstinence.
- Discuss responsible ways to cope with sexual pressures.
- Identify and describe ways of developing a healthy intimate relationship.

Health Strategies: Meeting New People (page 500)
Life Choice Inventory: Will the Marriage Work? (page 508)
Consumer Skills: Love and Sex in Advertisements (page 503)
Straight Talk: Rape Prevention (page 509)

CHAPTER 19
Family Life

- Explain how family influences a person's self-image and outlook on the world.
- List the stages of a family.
- Describe some ineffective and effective responses to family conflict.
- List characteristics of functional and dysfunctional families.

Health Strategies: The Essence of Conflict Resolution (page 527)
Health Strategies: Ground Rules for Arguing (page 528)
Consumer Skills: The Marketing of the Family (page 523)
Straight Talk: Parents as People (page 540)

CHAPTER 20
From Conception through Parenting

- List the consequences and risks of teen pregnancy for the mother, father, and child.
- Describe the signs of pregnancy and the tests used to confirm it.
- Describe the development of the fertilized egg.
- Describe the birth process.
- Discuss the responsibilities of being a parent.

Health Strategies: How to Keep a Pregnancy Safe (page 564)
Life Choice Inventory: Are You Ready to Have a Child? (page 549)
Straight Talk: Drinking during Pregnancy (page 572)

CHAPTER 21
Understanding Sexuality

- Identify the stages of the sexual response.
- List and describe examples of sexual myths.
- Describe various sexual orientations.

Consumer Skills: Pills and Potions (page 585)
Straight Talk: What About Me? Am I Missing Out? (page 589)

CHAPTER 22
Preventing Pregnancy and Sexually Transmitted Diseases

- Discuss the risks of using contraceptives.
- List all of the contraceptive methods, and state the effectiveness rate of each.
- Identify which methods of contraception also help prevent sexually transmitted diseases.
- Explain how to use each method of contraception.
- Identify the methods not recommended for contraception.

Health Strategies: Avoiding Pregnancy (page 600)
Straight Talk: Why People Don't Use Contraception (page 619)

CHAPTER 23
Mature Life, Aging, and Death

- List characteristics of people who age successfully.
- Discuss some healthful behaviors to follow in planning for good health in old age.
- Describe the physical and mental changes that occur during aging.
- Describe the stages a person goes through in accepting death.

Consumer Skills: Longevity Frauds (page 629)
Straight Talk: Helping Others Deal with Death and Grief (page 640)
Teen Views: What Makes Your Favorite Senior Citizen Your Favorite? (page 634)

TEACHING SUPPORT

Vocabulary: Learning Key Terms, Crossword Puzzle
Study Outline; Reading Cloze
Reteaching: Conflict Resolution
Enrichment: Stop, The Advice Column, Choices in Marriage, Controversial/Difficult Relationships
Life Choice Inventory: Will the Marriage Work?

Handouts: What is Your Capacity for Intimacy?, Myths and Truths about Healthy Relationships, Attitudes I Consider Important in a Prospective Partner, Writing a Marriage Contract
Teaching Information Sheet: Relationship Compatibility: The Myers-Briggs Type Indicator
Tests: Chapter 18 Test A, Chapter 18 Test B

Vocabulary: Learning Key Terms, Crossword Puzzle, Fill in the Blank
Study Outline; Reading Cloze
Reteaching

Enrichment
Quizzes: Sections 1–4
Tests: Chapter 19 Test A, Chapter 19 Test B

Vocabulary: Learning Key Terms, Crossword Puzzle, Fill in the Blank
Study Outline; Reading Cloze
Reteaching: Conception and Pregnancy, Reproduction and Conception, Risk Factor Match
Enrichment: Teenage Pregnancy
Life Choice Inventory: Are You Ready to Have a Child?

Handouts: Reproductive System Labeling
Teacher Information Sheet: Effects of Malnutrition During Critical Periods of Development
Tests: Chapter 20 Test A, Chapter 20 Test B
Transparencies: Sperm Production; The Menstrual Cycle; Fertilization; Cell Division

---

Vocabulary: Learning Key Terms, Code Fill-in
Study Outline; Reading Cloze
Reteaching: Condom Catch-Up, Myth Busters
Enrichment: Attitudes about Sexuality
Quizzes: Sections 1–4
Tests: Chapter 21 Test A, Chapter 21 Test B

Vocabulary: Learning Key Terms, Crossword Puzzle, Fill in the Blanks
Study Outline
Reading Cloze
Reteaching: Matching, Degrees of Effectiveness

Enrichment: Birth Control, The Pill Story, Adrianne's Situation, Pregnancy Scenarios, Sample Welfare Expenses, Abstinence vs. Sexual Intercourse
Quizzes: Sections 1–5
Tests: Chapter 22 Test A, Chapter 22 Test B

Vocabulary: Learning Key Terms, Crossword Puzzle
Study Outline; Reading Cloze
Reteaching: Helping Grandma
Enrichment: The Dilemma of Death, What's Your Opinion
Career Brief: Homemaker-Home Health Aides

Teacher Information Sheet: Anti-Aging Strategies; Nutrition, Aging, and Disease; Malnutrition Among the Elderly; Food and Assistance Programs for Older People
Quizzes: Section 1–3
Tests: Chapter 23 Test A, Chapter 23 Test B
Transparency: The Effects of Bone Loss

MULTIMEDIA SUPPORT

- Health Video Library
- CNN Health and Fitness Update Videos
- Westest
- Student Review Software
- Diet Analysis Software
- Nutrition CD-ROM

LESSON PLANNING

You will find detailed daily lesson plans for both **traditional scheduling** and **block scheduling** in your Teacher's Resource Box.

KEY POINTS

Chapter 18 is 22 pages long and is divided into three sections. The chapter deals primarily with the issue of relationships. Section 1 allows the students to explore the differences between mature love and infatuation. Section 2 helps the students identify what to look for in a potential partner for a relationship. Students will discuss issues in dating, abstinence, and sexual pressures. The important elements for a successful partnership, as well as the stages in the development of a healthy relationship, are highlighted. Section 3 gives the students guidelines for dealing with conflict in a constructive manner. In the "Straight Talk," some frank facts are given concerning rape.

ACTIVITY TO INTRODUCE THE CHAPTER

It is important to establish an environment that allows the students to ask questions and state their opinions. This activity will set the tone for open, frank discussions of the sensitive issues covered in this chapter. Use the "Fact or Fiction" questions. You may want to add the following questions:

1. Distrust is never a part of mature love relationships.
2. Beginning a relationship with someone who is on the rebound is asking for trouble.
3. If two seniors have been in a close relationship for a year, continuing abstinence will ruin the relationship.

CHAPTER 18

Contents

1. **Infatuation or Mature Love?**
2. **How to Develop a Healthy Relationship**
3. **Working through Conflict**

STRAIGHT TALK
Rape Prevention

NOT Enough Time?

Following are some suggestions to help you make sure that you cover the key topics in this chapter if you have limited time. (Refer to the daily lesson plans in your Teacher's Resource Box for additional suggestions.)

DAY 1 Assign Sections 1 and 2 prior to beginning the chapter. On Day 1 do the Enrichment activity at the bottom of pages 494–495 to initiate a discussion on relationships. Follow this up with the Enrichment activity on the bottom of pages 502–503. Have a prepared handout with all the information from this activity ready to give the students at the end of class. They are to review it for the next day.

Pairing, Commitment, and Marriage

FACT or FICTION

What do you think? Are the following statements true or false? If you think they are false, then say what is true.

1. You can tell when love is real because it hits you in an instant, whether or not you want to be in love.
2. To be intimate means about the same thing as to have sexual relations.
3. The best way to learn how to date may not be by dating but by attending social functions.
4. Teen pregnancy is a national tragedy.
5. Sexual activity begins early in healthy, intimate relationships.
6. To cope with a breakup, experts recommend finding another relationship as soon as possible.
7. Couples in healthy, intimate relationships spend all their free time together.
8. To make a marriage work, couples need only to love each other.

(Answers on page 506)

Introduction

All people need close relationships with others. It is important to share even simple daily life events with someone else. It is important to talk about problems, to voice our opinions, and to hear others' opinions. People who live without such relationships more often suffer poor mental and physical health than do people who maintain these relationships.

Loving, close relationships with family and friends are extremely important. It is not necessary, however, to have an exclusive, couples-type **love** relationship with a special person. Such relationships can be fulfilling, but much of a young person's self-growth and healthy development can be better achieved without such a relationship. Love relationships can keep people from focusing their energy inward. This inner focus is needed so that a person can accept, improve, love, and nurture the self. Some relationships that are not loving, or that are abusive, can even destroy emotional health and interfere with personal growth.

People spend much time and effort looking for love relationships. This chapter looks at these relationships from dating through commitment. It explores both the rewards and the problems of the relationships of couples.

4. If a girl is dressed seductively, she's just "asking" to be raped.

Ask students to answer the questions honestly, then discuss in class. As you discuss each question, ask how many said *True* and how many said *False*. Then ask students to volunteer their reasons for their answers. Do not say that any of the answers are right or wrong—leave each question open-ended. When you are finished, tell the students that these topics will be covered in this chapter and that they should check their answers again at the end of the chapter to see if their opinions have changed.

Answers to FACT or FICTION

1. **False.** You can tell when love is real because it develops slowly through the conscious choices of both partners.
2. **False.** People may be intimate psychologically as well as sexually.
3. **True.**
4. **True.**
5. **False.** Healthy, intimate relationships require time to grow before initiating sexual activity.
6. **False.** To cope with a breakup, it is best to give yourself six months to a year to heal and build up support.
7. **False.** Couples in healthy intimate relationships maintain separate interests, as well as shared ones.
8. **False.** To make a marriage work, couples need love and mutual agreements on some of life's basic issues.

DAY 2 On Day 2 begin with the Ability Levels activity at the bottom of pages 508–509. Then begin a discussion on the major points of Section 2. The discussion should cover the important factors necessary for a successful relationship. Assign Section 3 to be read for the following day.

DAY 3 On Day 3 invite a guest speaker (see the Guest Speaker activity on page 509) to come to class. Be sure the person is prepared to give facts and guidelines for rape prevention. Or, have a marriage counselor come in to discuss major issues causing divorce and how to increase the chances for a successful marriage.

FOCUS

OUTCOMES

In this section students will learn the:

1. Difference between infatuation and mature love.

2. Role of psychological intimacy in a relationship.

Vocabulary worksheets are provided in the Teacher's Resource Box.

FOCUS ACTIVITY

Ask students if they agree with the statement that people who do not have close relationships will suffer poor mental and physical health more often than people who have such relationships. Without naming names, can they think of examples that support their opinions one way or another?

TEACH & APPLY

DISCUSSION

Ask students to quietly review the list of qualities for mature love in the book. As they look at each quality, they are to ask themselves if that quality has been part of their relationships. Tell them to ask themselves why not. Stress that each person deserves the best in a relationship. What will they settle for in a relationship?

Infatuation or Mature Love?

The first step in learning how to have a strong, close love relationship is learning what one is. "Am I really in love, or is this just **infatuation**?" If you have ever asked yourself this question, you're not alone. Take a look at Figure 18–1 to find some clues.

It is natural to feel infatuation at times, especially in the teen years, when the feelings of attraction are brand new. Infatuation can be part of learning about love. Some relationships that begin as infatuation later develop into love. However, relationships built solely on infatuation usually

Figure 18–1 Is It Love or Just Infatuation?

Infatuation	Mature Love
Usually occurs at beginning of relationship	Develops gradually through learning about person
Sexual attraction is central	Sexual attraction is present, but warm affection and friendship are central
Characterized by urgency, intensity, sexual desire, and anxiety	Characterized by calmness, peacefulness, empathy, support, and tolerance of partner
Driven by excitement of being involved with a person whose character is not fully known	Driven by deep attachment; based on extensive knowledge of both positive and negative qualities
Extreme absorption in another	Wanting to be together without obsession
Insecurity, distrust, lack of confidence, feeling of being threatened	Security, trust, confidence, unthreatened feeling
Nagging doubts and unanswered questions; partner remains unexamined so as not to spoil the dream	Thorough knowledge of partner; mature acceptance of imperfections
Based on fantasy	Based on reality
Consuming, often exhausting	Energizing in a healthy way
Low self-esteem (looking to partner for validation and affirmation of self-worth)	High self-esteem (each person has sense of self-worth with or without partner)
Each needs the other to feel complete	Relationship enhances the self, but person can feel complete without relationship
Discomfort with individual differences	Individuality accepted
Each often tears down or criticizes the other	Each brings out best in partner; relationship is nurturing
Partners need to rush things, like sex or marriage; sense of urgency so as not to lose partner	Partners are patient and feel no need to rush the events of relationship; sense of security; no fear of losing partner
One is threatened by other's individual growth	Each encourages other's growth
Relationship not enduring, because it lacks firm foundation	Relationship is enduring, sustaining—based on strong foundation of friendship

enrichment...

This activity promotes listening skills and encourages students to voice their opinions. Before class list five to seven statements on the board.

1. "Love at first sight" can really happen.

2. Physical intimacy makes a relationship last.

3. Teenagers don't really know how to be in a mature, loving relationship.

4. The most important qualities necessary in a healthy relationship are _____.

5. A person in a relationship with a chemically dependent person should _____.

6. In order to love someone else, you must love yourself first.

7. There are more advantages than disadvantages to sexual abstinence in a relationship.

8. There is no such thing as healthy conflict in a relationship.

Mature love takes time to develop, and is based on friendship and sharing.

After students have studied Figure 18–1, have them close their books. Ask a student to state one of the characteristics, either from mature love or infatuation, without designating it as one or the other. Then ask volunteers to tell whether that characteristic is one of mature love or infatuation and give the corresponding characteristic for the other category. For example, a student says "based on reality." The volunteer would say that this is a characteristic of mature love and that the corresponding characteristic of infatuation is "based on fantasy." Continue the exercise until all of the characteristics have been identified.

Your supplemental material contains the student activity entitled "What is Your Capacity for Intimacy?" This activity sheet will help students evaluate whether or not they are able and willing to be psychologically intimate. You may want to distribute this activity after students have completed Section 1.

do not work out well. They usually end when the fantasies on which they are built fade away.

Unlike infatuation, **mature love** is a strong affection for, and an enduring, deep attachment to, a person whose character the partner knows well. The person accepts and tolerates the partner's negative qualities. Mature love involves a *decision* to be devoted to a person. It also requires psychological **intimacy**. This is *not* the same thing as physical, sexual intimacy, as you will see.

Psychological intimacy is probably the most important part of a love relationship. This kind of intimacy builds slowly as two people become familiar with, and close to, each other. Two intimate people reveal, a little at a time, the parts of themselves that they keep hidden from others. They share both the parts they are proud of, and those they are ashamed of. Both people are open and trusting with each other.

Before people can become intimate, both must feel that, even with their faults honestly displayed, they are worthy of love. That is, they must have high self-esteem and feel good about themselves.

The idea that some things must develop slowly seems foreign to people in our fast-paced society. Most times, therefore, they rush relationships. They may make the mistake of trying to substitute physical, sexual intimacy, which can be available right away, for psychological intimacy, which takes time to grow. This doesn't work. Hot chocolate can be "instant," and food can be fast food, but intimacy takes time to develop. Time, along with open sharing, permits a relationship to develop in its natural stages, as described in the next section.

MINI Glossary

love: affection, attachment, devotion.

infatuation: the state of being completely carried away by unreasoning passion or attraction; addictive love.

mature love: a strong affection for, and an enduring, deep attachment to, a person whose character the partner knows well.

intimacy: being very close and familiar, as in relationships involving private and personal sharing.

9. Marriage means ———.

Show students a small sponge ball, then tell them this activity is based on listening to each other's opinions. Explain that only the person holding the ball can speak. When that person is done, the ball will be passed to someone whose hand is raised. The first student will choose a topic and agree or disagree with it. The class will stay on that topic until all who want to speak about it have had a chance.

Someone may then change the topic. Remind students that everyone is entitled to his or her opinion. When someone disagrees, he/she *may not* attack the person, just voice an opinion about the topic.

You might want to repeat the activity after finishing the chapter to see if students' opinions and knowledge have changed.

ASSESS

EVALUATE

Pop Quiz

Ask the students to write definitions of the following words: *intimacy, mature love, infatuation.*

SECTION 1 Review Answers

1. **a.** mature love
   b. love
   c. intimacy
   d. infatuation
2. They usually end when the fantasies on which they are built fade away. (p. 495)
3. Answers will vary; could include: it builds trust as two people share both the bad and the good things of themselves that they do not share with others; it causes people to be able to be open and trusting with each other; and so on. (p. 495)
4. Physical, or sexual, intimacy can be available right away, while psychological intimacy takes time to grow. (p. 495)
5. Answers will vary.

WORKSHEETS A reproducible quiz for Section 1 is provided in the Teacher's Resource Box.

CLOSE

Ask each student to write an essay describing his/her perfect relationship. They must include the qualities *they* deem to be high priorities and also what they expect each person to bring into this ideal relationship.

When considering whether a person might be compatible with you, observe how the person interacts with others.

LYNDON WAS INFATUATED WITH THE FAMOUS FEMALE HOCKEY PLAYER, PATTY "THE HACKER" BOODROU...

Infatuation is an excited state and thrives on illusion.

Love is an honest state and thrives on clear vision.

KEY POINTS *Infatuation is an all-consuming desire for a partner. It is based on fantasy and is often mistaken for love. Mature love is a strong attachment to someone a person knows very well. It is based on psychological intimacy.*

SECTION 1 Review

Answer the following questions on a sheet of paper.

Learning the Vocabulary

The vocabulary terms in this section are *love, infatuation, mature love,* and *intimacy.*

1. Match each of the following phrases with the appropriate term:
   a. a strong affection for, and an enduring, deep attachment to, a person
   b. affection, attachment, devotion
   c. being very close and familiar in a relationship
   d. the state of being carried away by unreasoning passion or attraction; addictive love

Learning the Facts

2. What is the problem with relationships built solely on infatuation?
3. Explain why intimacy is so important in a love relationship.
4. Describe the difference between physical intimacy and psychological intimacy.

Making Life Choices

5. After studying Figure 18–1, "Is It Love or Just Infatuation?", think of someone you know well. Do you think most of the person's relationships are mature love or infatuation? Why do you think the person's relationships are this way? Do you think the person should change his or her relationships? If so, how?

•multicultural issues•

Although many countries are becoming more Westernized in their dating and marriage practices, traditions remain in many cultures.

In contemporary Japan for example, where half of the marriages are self-arranged, many couples still prefer a marriage in which they are matched. The go-betweens, usually a husband and wife referred to as a *nakado,* act together as mediators to introduce a couple, assist in negotiating arrangements between the two families, run the wedding and reception, and counsel the married couple if problems arise in their relationship.

Even couples who marry for love in Japan have an honorary go-between. The go-between arranges a meeting, known as a *miai,* between a man and a woman who have similar social status, education, and hobbies. The go-between usually initiates the

SECTION 2

How to Develop a Healthy Relationship

No two relationships are exactly alike or develop in just the same way. However, healthy relationships have some things in common. First, each partner in a healthy relationship must have a positive self-image. Once you feel strong and sure of yourself, you are better able to know what to look for in a partner.

Second, you should be aware, always, that love develops in stages, such as those listed in Figure 18–2 on the next page. Love cannot be rushed. Once you find an appropriate partner, do not give in to the temptation to try to "hurry things along" by skipping the early phases of development. These early times provide the foundation of a strong relationship later on. Be patient.

 KEY POINTS *Healthy intimate relationships grow in stages that shouldn't be rushed.*

What to Look for in a Partner

In thinking about a person who interests you, make sure that the person has time and energy available for love. Such people:

▶ Are not involved in other love relationships.
▶ Are well over heartaches; have not just recently broken up with someone else.
▶ Are open to being in a relationship with you.
▶ Are free of chemical or psychological addictions. (People with addictions to alcohol or other drugs, people who gamble, or people with eating disorders cannot function well in love relationships.)
▶ Have time to devote to a relationship.
▶ Have high self-esteem.
▶ Are close to you geographically—they live in your city or state.

In addition, the person must be compatible with you in terms of social values and beliefs. To evaluate these factors, see if you can honestly answer yes to the following questions:

▶ *Does the person have several close friends?* A person who has learned to keep and enjoy close friendships can put this talent to work in a love relationship.
▶ *If the relationship folded, would you still want that person as a friend?* Without friendship, the relationship may crumble during times of conflict.
▶ *Are you happy with the way the person treats other people?* Watch how the person deals with school employees, waitresses, maids, sales clerks, parking-lot attendants, telephone operators, and close friends. If you wouldn't want to be on the receiving end of that behavior, don't get involved. You may be an exception during courtship, but you won't be later on.

SECTION 2

FOCUS

OUTCOMES

In this section students will learn:

1. The stages of a love relationship.
2. Ways to identify people who might be "available for love."
3. Advantages and disadvantages of dating and going steady.
4. Advantages of sexual abstinence.
5. Consequences of early sexual involvement.
6. Facts involved in external and internal sexual pressure.
7. Skills involved in developing a healthy committed relationship.
8. Qualities necessary for a successful marriage.

FOCUS ACTIVITY

Key Passage
Before students read this section on dating, ask them to list factors that should be considered in evaluating compatibility. How do their lists compare with the factors listed here? Which of these factors would they add to their own lists? Why?

relationship by sending a letter from the man to the woman. The two families often hire detectives to check backgrounds and interview people who know the man and the woman.

Customs in India are similar to those in Japan, but also include the stipulation that the woman's educational level be no higher than the man's. Matchmakers sometimes consult horoscopes when arranging marriages in India. The groom's representative often exchanges gifts with the bride's family, thus

adding to the obligation of the relationship.

Have students discuss arranged marriages. To promote discussion, ask students the following questions.

1. How would matchmaking practices work in our country? How would they affect the lives of teenagers?
2. Do you think matchmaking would result in more stable families? Why or why not?

497

TEACH & APPLY

CLASS ACTIVITY

Refer students to Figure 18–2. Have them analyze a relationship—one in which they have been involved personally; a relationship between friends, acquaintances, or relatives; or a relationship in a movie they've seen or a book they've read. They should then list the five stages shown in the illustration. Under each stage they should briefly describe, in no more than three paragraphs, events that took place in their chosen relationship that represent characteristics of that particular stage. Students can use fictional names. Ask for volunteers to read different sections of their descriptions. Conclude by asking students if they believe most relationships do develop according to these stages. Could any of the stages be omitted?

BACKGROUND INFORMATION

In your supplementary material you will find a detailed explanation of the Meyers-Briggs Type Indicator and how the four basic temperaments used in this assessment relate to compatibility and relationships. You may find this information interesting and useful prior to discussing compatibility with students.

Figure 18–2 The Stages of a Love Relationship

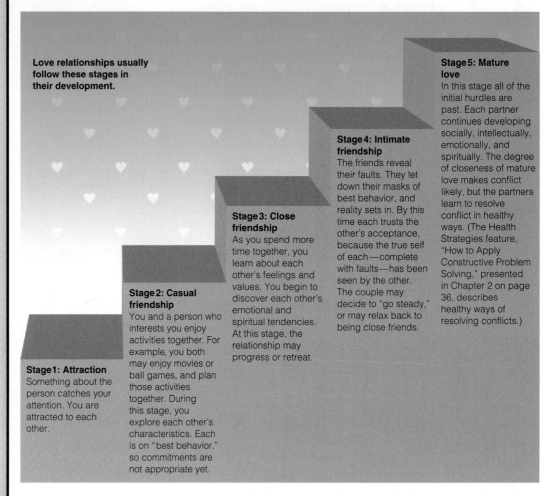

Love relationships usually follow these stages in their development.

Stage 1: Attraction
Something about the person catches your attention. You are attracted to each other.

Stage 2: Casual friendship
You and a person who interests you enjoy activities together. For example, you both may enjoy movies or ball games, and plan those activities together. During this stage, you explore each other's characteristics. Each is on "best behavior," so commitments are not appropriate yet.

Stage 3: Close friendship
As you spend more time together, you learn about each other's feelings and values. You begin to discover each other's emotional and spiritual tendencies. At this stage, the relationship may progress or retreat.

Stage 4: Intimate friendship
The friends reveal their faults. They let down their masks of best behavior, and reality sets in. By this time each trusts the other's acceptance, because the true self of each—complete with faults—has been seen by the other. The couple may decide to "go steady," or may relax back to being close friends.

Stage 5: Mature love
In this stage all of the initial hurdles are past. Each partner continues developing socially, intellectually, emotionally, and spiritually. The degree of closeness of mature love makes conflict likely, but the partners learn to resolve conflict in healthy ways. (The Health Strategies feature, "How to Apply Constructive Problem Solving," presented in Chapter 2 on page 36, describes healthy ways of resolving conflicts.)

You can be friends with people who lack these qualities, but beware of deeper relationships until these problems are resolved.

Also, be sure that *you* are available for a relationship. For example, suppose you baby-sit, study, work at an after-school job, hold offices in clubs, and volunteer in the community. You may be too busy at the moment to give a relationship the time and energy it needs to grow.

 KEY POINTS *Some people are available for relationships, but others are not. Choose carefully.*

CRITICAL THINKING

Choosing to date is not a process done in isolation. Family systems theory suggests that any action by one system affects, and is affected by, all other systems. The decision of a teen couple to date affects both of their families and the community as a whole. Conversely, the family and community have some effect on the couple's dating processes.

Ask students to discuss the following questions.

1. When should parents begin discussing values related to the dating process?

Dating

Single people of all ages like to **date**—that is, to enjoy leisure activities with other people to get to know them better. In the later half of the teen years, dating takes on more importance, while peer groups lose some of their appeal. Teens can be said to move from cliques to couples, as peer groups loosen their grip and couples begin to pair off.

While dating may be fun, it is not entirely free of stress. A couple's first date, for example, may lead to thoughts of self-doubt and worry that the person may not like you. Those are normal thoughts and feelings. Don't let them discourage you from dating. The person who practices assertive behavior and maintains high self-esteem stands to gain much from dating others. Most dates are fun—or at least not disastrous. Also, those who date learn how to communicate with many different types of people—a useful skill throughout life.

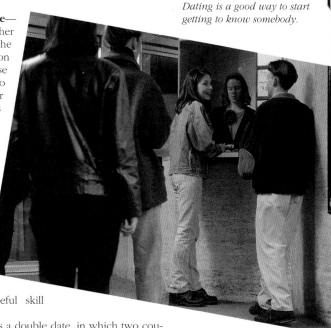

Dating is a good way to start getting to know somebody.

An especially useful form of dating is a double date, in which two couples go out together. This creates a casual and safe environment in which to check out people whom you do not know well. A sad fact is that many rapes each year occur in dating situations (see this chapter's Straight Talk section). Double dating provides safety and reduces stress. With four people talking and having fun, it's not hard to feel at ease.

People of both sexes may feel uncertain about the "proper" way to date. Who should ask the other out? Who should phone? Who should pay? In years past, the rules of dating were rigid. Today, though, these rules are more relaxed. The best approach may be one that fits in with the values both people developed at home.

It is natural to feel nervous when going out with someone for the first time. However, try to remember that even if this date doesn't go well, there will be many others in the future. The best way to ensure that a date will go well is to be open to the possibility that you will be forming a friendship, not a lifelong relationship. Possibly the best way of learning how to date is not through dating at all, but through attending social gatherings in group settings. Check the Health Strategies section on the next page, "Meeting New People," for some ideas on expanding your possibilities.

Some who have dated for a while decide to go steady or become a couple with a favorite date. Going steady has some advantages. It provides relief from the stress of dating new people and freedom from the worry of not having a date for important occasions. However, it brings many disadvantages as well. While young people who go steady may feel secure, they may also feel tied down. They lose the opportunity to date a variety of others. They also may focus on the growth of the steady relationship instead of

MINI Glossary

date: to engage in social events designed to allow people to get to know each other. A double date (two couples) is a safe arrangement for early dates with people you do not know well.

- **a.** the day of the first date
- **b.** at age 13
- **c.** from the time the child is able to understand the concept of dating
2. What personal values are important to consider in relationship to dating? (suggestions to consider: honesty, trust, love, commitment)

3. What role does the community have in dating?
4. Does the community have a responsibility to provide dating activity options? If so, what types of options should be available?

DISCUSSION

Ask students for suggestions to add to the list of ways to meet new people (in addition to those in the Health Strategies). After you have a complete list, ask them to rate the strategies from most likely to be effective to least likely. Which strategies do most students think will be most effective?

DISCUSSION

Ask if engaging in abstinence would promote a healthy intimate relationship rather than detract from it. Would this always be the case or would it vary from one relationship to another? Would any students argue against the proposition that postponing sexual intercourse will in all cases promote a longer lasting, healthier, more intimate relationship?

FAST FACTS

While the likelihood of having intercourse increases steadily with age, one in five teens do not have intercourse during their teenage years.

56 percent of young women and 73 percent of young men today have had intercourse by age 18, compared with 35 percent of young women and 55 percent of young men in the early 1970s.

on their own growth. If preserving the pair becomes more important than the emotional health of the individuals, this can lead to diminished self-esteem.

Another disadvantage of going steady is sexual pressure. This topic will be discussed at length later in this chapter. Sexual pressure may be especially strong when two people who are attractive to each other spend all their spare time together.

Another pressure may come into play: false feelings of obligation to another person. Many times teens will fear that if they refuse **sexual intercourse**, their partners will go with someone else. In fact, it may be that the partner would agree to abstinence from sexual intercourse, and take pride in that choice. If not, this probably indicates a serious flaw in the relationship—the values of the partners appear to conflict.

 KEY POINTS *Possibly the best way of learning how to date is not through dating at all, but through attending social gatherings in a group setting. Going steady has some advantages and some disadvantages.*

Health Strategies

Meeting New People

These suggestions are just a few out of dozens you can use to meet new people. Once you start thinking along these lines, you'll come up with many more ideas of your own.

1. Join a youth group (try religious and service clubs or a school activity).
2. Take up a hobby, such as dancing or collecting baseball cards. Attend meetings with others who share the same interest.
3. Create a group around a common theme—for example, a foreign language group or a comedy video group.
4. Learn to play a sport after school. Play on, or watch, local teams. Be a fan.
5. Volunteer time in an organization you believe in, such as the American Cancer Society or Habitat for Humanity.
6. Learn to play a musical instrument, and join a school or community band or orchestra.
7. Get physically fit, and attend to nutrition and sleep needs. High-level wellness gives you the energy you need for leisure activities.
8. Be friendly; reach out to others. Be yourself; don't try to impress anyone.

Advantages of Sexual Abstinence

Some high school students say that it seems as if everyone around them has become sexually active. The reality is that only some teens become sexually active before leaving high school. Those who do become involved sexually often find that it can interrupt the normal growth of a relationship. Immature partners may focus on sexual activity but neglect their intellectual, emotional, social, and spiritual growth.

Sexual activity can cloud a person's judgment. A relationship that is unhealthy or abrasive, but meets sexual needs, can be more difficult to end than a friendship gone bad. Becoming sexually involved is a way of declaring to the world your choice of a mate. Should a relationship end, the world then knows that the choice was not a sound one.

Early sexual involvement can also cause distrust of a partner's inner qualities. If a partner becomes sexually involved easily, doubts arise about the person's values and ability to be faithful. A person who easily becomes sexually involved may be judged to lack self-control, a necessary quality, if a person is to move his or her life in the desired direction.

Teenage sexual activity is a concern not just for teens, but for everyone in our society. Sexual intercourse poses risks. Teens who are sexually active often suffer sexually transmitted diseases and have become a fast-growing risk group for infection with the AIDS virus.

A famous research group, the Alan Guttmacher Institute, reports, "Each year one-quarter of the sexually active women between 15 and 19 seek treatment for a sexually transmitted disease." This figure includes only those who seek treatment. Many more suffer infections and fail to be treated. The only sure way to prevent sexually transmitted diseases is to abstain from sexual activity.

CRITICAL THINKING

A great way to discuss relationships is to let students discuss, argue, and come to agreement on a variety of issues that they are facing or may face in their lives. During this activity, ask students to bring up issues that are controversial and that they believe to be misunderstood or ignored by members of the opposite sex.

Have all the students put their desks in one large circle, ask them to sit boy/girl around the circle. Set some rules for them to follow, in case the discussion gets a little heated. Tell students they can bring up any issues that they feel are needed, but they must not direct any comments to any one person in the room. They cannot blame any one person or ridicule anyone.

Teen pregnancy is another national tragedy. The effects on the lives of both the girl and the boy can be enormous. Here are some of the frequent and serious problems resulting from teen pregnancies:

▶ Interruption of education.
▶ Early marriages with a high likelihood of divorce.
▶ Continuing legal responsibility to support a child.
▶ High risks of poverty.
▶ Low infant survival rates.
▶ Lifetime tendencies toward having more than the average number of children.

A psychologically intimate relationship is most fulfilling.

The costs to society in terms of lost education, lost earning power, and increased need for support of the individuals are staggering. Again, abstinence from sexual intercourse is the only guarantee against teen pregnancy.

Few teenagers are mature enough to develop lasting and committed sexual relationships. For teens, as for many others, sexual abstinence can reduce worry and can create a feeling of freedom. Abstinence allows teens to grow and develop without interruption by diseases or pregnancy. Abstinence also allows time for the growth of a healthy intimate relationship. Thus, for reasons of both emotional and physical health, abstinence is becoming more popular than ever before in this century.

 Abstinence is necessary for a new relationship to grow in a healthy way. Early sexual involvement can prevent personal growth of the partners and carries serious risks to health and life goals.

How to Cope with Sexual Pressures

You often hear people talk about the "pressures" to have sexual intercourse. They focus on peer pressure; pressures from images of sexiness in the movies, in popular music, and on TV; or the pressure from a partner who wants to have intercourse. Another source of pressure comes in the form of product advertisements (see the Consumer Skills feature in this chapter). All of these **external pressures** can be difficult to deal with.

Even more difficult to deal with are pressures that come from inside. Human beings have a natural, biological drive to reproduce. This normal drive builds up **internal pressures** that can be hard to deal with. During the teen years these pressures can be especially intense and can be equally strong in people of both sexes.

People with healthy self-esteem don't allow others to bully or convince them to do things they do not wish to do. All of the ideas on resisting peer pressure first presented in the Straight Talk section of Chapter 3 apply here.

The real problem of abstaining from sexual intercourse is not the battle with the wills of other people. Instead, it is the battle between a person's conscious will and the person's own biological drives. This is the meaning of

MINI Glossary

sexual intercourse: the reproductive act between the sexes. The term *intercourse* means communication of any kind—talking, for example. Sexual intercourse between human beings is termed *coitus* (CO-ih-tus). Between animals it is termed *copulation* (cop-you-LAY-shun).

external pressures: regarding sexual feelings, messages from society, peers, and others that pressure people to have sexual intercourse.

internal pressures: regarding sexual feelings, a person's internal biological urges toward having sexual intercourse.

Discussions will vary, but all should relate to topics in the chapter. Start the discussion by asking students some questions like these. What makes a good date? What makes a bad date? Should couples make any rules about dating? What makes students nervous about dating? What do they think about blind dates? How can people ease into the dating experience? When is a couple ready to have sex? What is meant by emotional maturity? How

can a person tell when they are emotionally mature? How do they know when they are in love and how do they know it will last? When is a couple ready for marriage? What are some reasons people give for marriage? Should two people ever get married if they don't love each other? Allow adequate time at the end of the discussion to summarize information and emphasize the positive statements.

(continued from previous page)

research. Each person in each group must have something to say. While the groups are working, prepare the two role-players, explaining that their characters are considering whether or not to have sex.

Day 2: Ask Groups 1 and 2 to face each other and Groups 3 and 4 to face other. The groups need to leave enough space for the couple to walk through. (Prepare ahead a stop sign such as the one shown in Figure 18–3.) Instruct the couple to *slowly* walk through the "walls of indecision" while each student speaks her or his case. The couple is to listen carefully. When the couple reaches the end, hold up the sign, STOP! Ask the class to listen to the couple answer these questions: What was the most convincing argument they heard from the voices? What sticks in their minds? What decision is each character leaning toward? Then ask the whole class, "Whose decision and pressure is it really in the end?" (each individual's) Each person has the physical ability to say NO or YES. NO ONE, NOTHING makes them say it. Hold up the stop sign again. Review what each letter on the sign stands for, stressing that each person must be absolutely sure before making such an important decision. This STOP method can effectively help people deal with the internal and external pressures in decision making.

the phrase *will power*—the power of exerting your own will over any other force, even that of your own basic drives.

The internal drive to have sexual relations is a fact of life for almost all sexually mature people. Teens may find the drive especially hard to handle, because it is new to them. They may even confuse feelings of the sex drive and those of love. People often want to express sexual feelings, especially when they fall in love.

The challenge to couples who are not yet mature and committed is to find ways of expressing love and sexual feelings so that both people benefit. Any activity that makes the other person feel loved, and that takes some extra thought or effort on the part of the giver, is satisfying for both. Think of how you felt the last time a friend gave you a hug, gave you a small gift, did you a favor, or confided in you. The good feelings those gestures brought were a genuine form of love. You can express your love in all sorts of caring ways without having sexual intercourse.

To express sexual feelings in appropriate ways, it is necessary to decide *in advance* what course of action is right for you. People who approach a situation without a clearly determined plan may find themselves tempted to "throw caution to the wind," just for the thrill of a moment. People who tend to seek out excitement—**thrill seekers**—must fight especially hard against these temptations.

Figure 18–3 *The STOP Method for Maintaining Sexual Abstinence*

S—Stop. Stop the activity that threatens to get out of control. This first step may be difficult but is critical for remaining in control.

T—Think. Analyze what is happening. Does your present behavior agree with your values? Would your parents approve? Develop in advance a list of questions meaningful to you.

O—Other activities. If your behavior feels out of control—if it conflicts with your values—direct the energy of the moment into other activities (going out for ice cream or to a movie, for example).

P—Plan. Make the next time easier by planning how to remain in charge. Decide not to plan dates that involve too much time alone (for example, plan to double date or date in public places). Commit to using this method every time you begin to feel out of control.

enrichment

Write these four categories across the top of the board (or on newsprint): *Infatuation, In Like, Dependency, In Love.* Divide the class into four groups, each with an equal number of boys and girls. Ask the groups to brainstorm the qualities describing each category of relationships. Once the groups are finished, go over each category by asking a spokes-person from each group to take a turn giving *one* quality. As one group speaks, check the other three groups to see if they agree. Be sure you have your own prepared list of qualities of which you want the students to be aware. Derive your "Infatuation" and "In Love" lists from pages 494–496. Some characteristics for "In Like" are: buddies, no strings attached, convenient, better than nothing, a relationship where the romance has ended but the partner is fun to be around.

Love and Sex in Advertisements

Consumer SKILLS

Most people want to be part of special love relationships. Advertisers use this desire for love to help sell their products. They try to make consumers think that certain products can make people more attractive, sexier, more self-confident, and therefore more likely to be loved. Many such ads are aimed directly at teenagers. A certain brand of toothpaste claims, "Want love? Get our brand!" A chewing gum commercial shows two sets of physically beautiful twins getting to know one another over sticks of gum. A breath mint is sold as "social insurance." The ads say that you never know when you'll meet someone special, so why take a chance on having less-than-sweet breath?

Some advertisers even go beyond using the need for love. They capitalize on people's sexual feelings by using subconscious sexual suggestions to make using their products seem sexy. For example, a close look at an image of a bottle in an ad for a certain brand of liquor reveals a shadowy figure of a nude woman within the bottle. The image is just clear enough for the subconscious mind to detect it, but not so clear as to be obvious.

Buying a product may be easier than working to improve self-esteem. However, the only way to become truly more attractive involves work—the work of developing self-esteem to a highly polished level. The sparkle of high self-esteem outshines physical attributes every time.

Critical Thinking

Name some characteristics of people who are influenced by advertisements that promise increased attractiveness. Why do you think people with these characteristics are most likely to be influenced?

Consumer SKILLS

Answers to Critical Thinking

Answers will vary, but should reflect the idea that people who are influenced by these advertisements often have low self-esteem and low self-confidence. These consumers are more likely to be influenced because the advertisers promise to make them sexier, more attractive, and more likely to be beloved.

DISCUSSION

Ask students if they believe the STOP strategy could help people abstain from sexual intercourse. Ask them to develop one or two questions each that they would use in the *Think* state. Write all the questions on the board. If students are not sure what type of questions apply here, tell them the questions should be ones that would help them remember what's important to them—questions that would help them see that what they're about to do may be something that they would regret later. Ask students to develop a list of activities that they could have ready to take the place of sexual activity.

To cope with strong sexual desires, it helps to channel the sexual energy into other activities. Instead of using will power to oppose the sexual drive, use it to shift gears to another activity. Dancing, sports, walking, or other activities requiring movement can release sexual energy. Some people feel that writing, speaking, singing, painting, or other expressive activities can also serve this purpose.

When a situation threatens to get out of control, some find it helpful to say mentally to themselves the word *STOP*—*S*top, *T*hink, *O*ther activities, *P*lan to abide by your vow of abstinence (see Figure 18–3 on the opposite page). That way, they never have to look back and say, "I don't know why. It just happened." Sexual intimacy is too important to just let happen. Remember STOP, to give yourself time to think.

 KEY POINTS *Pressure to have sexual intercourse arises both internally and externally. Internal pressures are hard to deal with. Doing so requires a preplanned strategy and will power.*

MINI Glossary

thrill seekers: people who are especially likely to take chances in exchange for momentary excitement.

Some characteristics for "Dependency" are: "I need him/her for my own identity security;" "No one else would ever want me so I'd better stick with him/her even though he/she does hit me;" "He/she *makes* me happy, he/she *makes* my life worth living." In a dependent relationship, jealousy is generally very high because both parties are very insecure. Thus, there are many rules in this relationship as to who can talk to whom and where each is allowed to go. Aggressive people tend to enter dependent relationships with passive people. Fighting and making up dominates the relationship, with little conversation or fun with other couples.

If students see themselves in anything other than a love relationship, emphasize the positive actions students could take to change their relationships or start new ones. (Refer to Figure 18–2 on page 498 and Health Strategies on page 504.)

ROLE PLAY

Have students role play breaking up. Stress to each person the importance of taking ownership of the breakup. Stress that threats ("I'll kill myself if you leave me") should not be given in to; that anger and accusations only push the person farther away; that promising to change for the person strips an individual of his/her pride, identity, and self-esteem. By accepting the breakup and admitting it was coming, a person can move on with life.

BACKGROUND INFORMATION

Tell students that unresolved grief from a past relationship will interfere with the ability to form a new relationship. Getting involved "on the rebound" will likely result in the breakup of the new relationship, thus creating two relationships to grieve about. Self-esteem is usually low following a breakup, even for an emotionally healthy person. When self-esteem is low, people often are attracted to, and attract, new partners with low self-esteem.

FAST FACTS

Anyone suffering from a breakup could benefit from reading *How to Survive the Loss of a Love* by M. Colgrove, et. al. (Prelude Press, 1991).

Breaking Up and How to Cope

More often than not, the relationships formed in early life break up. This is true for many reasons. Immature people may hide their true selves at first, only to discover that they cannot keep up a false act for long. Both partners end up resenting each other for being less than perfect in real life. It also happens that partners who are sincere but young may change and outgrow certain relationships. Most times, breakups are best for both partners, although it may not feel that way at the moment.

While no one really dies of a broken heart, the pain, depression, and stress that can follow breaking up may make people physically ill. Stress weakens the immune system and so can make illness likely. The breakup of a special love relationship can be difficult to cope with. You feel lonely, rejected, and depressed. What do you do?

One thing you can do is to prepare to experience grief—whether for the loss of the loved one, or for loss of the fantasy of love. The Straight Talk section at the end of Chapter 21 presents the stages of grief to expect. Give yourself the time you need to grieve fully. It is natural and normal to feel intense loneliness and pain. However, those feelings fade with time. A Health Strategies section in Chapter 5 (page 112), "Coping with Mild Depression," offers tips that can help with the feelings of loss from a breakup.

A mistake a person may make during this painful time is to quickly seek a new partner. The temptation to do so may be strong, but resist it. You may not have vision clear enough to judge a new partner. Give yourself six months to a year to heal.

People in grief often need affection. Activities and friends can fill the void. When you feel like your old self again, you may be ready for a new relationship.

Health Strategies

Developing a Healthy Intimate Relationship

To establish a healthy intimate relationship:

1. Learn the difference between a healthy intimate relationship and infatuation.
2. Build your self-esteem.
3. Make sure your partner has time and energy for love. Make sure you do, too.
4. Give yourself time to get to know new people socially, intellectually, emotionally, and spiritually.
5. Spend some of your free time alone with your partner and some with other friends. Maintain your identity.
6. Let sexual involvement wait for commitment in the relationship. Marriage is the highest form of commitment.
7. Know the meaning of commitment.
8. Explore your expectations of marriage.
9. Learn to work through conflict in healthy ways.

 KEY POINTS *When coping with a breakup, expect to feel grief. Avoid seeking a new partner too soon.*

Commitment

Anyone choosing to have a long-term monogamous relationship must do something extraordinary—make a commitment to another person. A commitment is a promise to make a long-term choice, in the face of many possible options, with the knowledge that all will not always go well. Some think that commitment is the highest form of maturity in relationships.

Choosing a life partner is a tricky business. Many people choose wrongly. Developing a long-term, intimate bond that truly satisfies both partners involves much more than simply loving each other, the wish to do so, or stating that such a bond exists.

What *does* hold a partnership together? Psychologist Carl Rogers put it this way: "We each commit ourselves to working together on the changing process of our present relationship, because that relationship is currently enriching our love and our life and we wish it to grow." Every word in

special needs

Intra-personal and Linguistic

Ask students to apply what they have learned by analyzing some of their own feelings about pairing, commitment, and marriage. The section on marriage on page 506 poses the questions, "Did you ever wonder what happened to Cinderella and the Prince after they mar-

ried? Did they really live happily ever after?"

Most students should be very familiar with this fairy tale. If they are not, you might want to bring in several copies. You may even choose to read aloud from the children's story, discussing the way the relationship between Cinderella and the Prince develops. When you are sure that all your students have a good understanding of the fairy tale, ask them to imagine themselves as the main charthis statement is significant. Figure 18–4 below shows what the words mean.

To this list of elements of partnership we would add *independence*. The person who finds ways to meet many of his or her own needs *outside* the paired relationship will be most successful at pairing. Recall the needs described in Maslow's scheme (Chapter 3). You cannot ask your partner to provide total security—whether emotional, financial, or physical. You must stand on your own feet and provide your own security. You, yourself, are the only person you will never lose. Understanding and practicing self-sufficiency is a major factor in maintaining healthy, lasting relationships.

In a real marriage, people work things out.

 KEY POINTS   *Love requires each partner to commit and work together, to accept change in the current relationship, and to be enriched by it.*

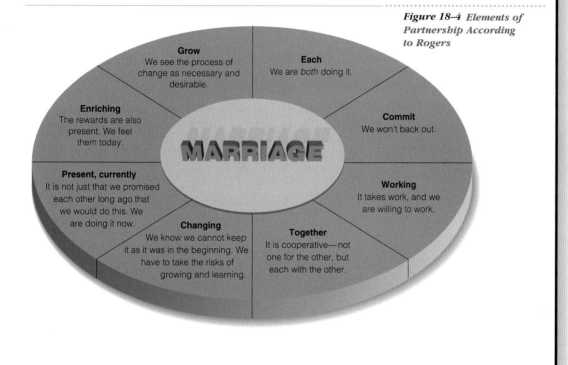

Grow
We see the process of change as necessary and desirable.

Each
We are *both* doing it.

Enriching
The rewards are also present. We feel them today.

Commit
We won't back out.

MARRIAGE

Present, currently
It is not just that we promised each other long ago that we would do this. We are doing it now.

Working
It takes work, and we are willing to work.

Changing
We know we cannot keep it as it was in the beginning. We have to take the risks of growing and learning.

Together
It is cooperative—not one for the other, but each with the other.

Figure 18–4 Elements of Partnership According to Rogers

acters: boys become The Prince, girls are Cinderella. Now, ask them to do a bit of character analysis. How would they feel if they met someone in such a way? Can they imagine what life might be like after the carriage carries off the happy couple? Ask your students to write the sequel by putting themselves into the story. After five, ten, or twenty years how are Cinderella and the Prince doing?

An alternative assignment could include asking students to rewrite or update fairy tales, possibly by writing new endings. They might also be required to use the vocabulary words and terms for this chapter: love, infatuation, mature love, intimacy, date, sexual intercourse, external pressures, internal pressures, thrill seekers, marriage, stranger rape, date rape.

DISCUSSION

Students may have a difficult time seeing how important a positive view of themselves is in developing a healthy relationship with someone else. Ask them if they can think of reasons why the more self-esteem and self-sufficiency a person exhibits, the stronger that person's relationships will be with others. (Some reasons are that the person will be more able to compromise; the person will be more open and direct and not have to pretend or cover up feelings and ideas; and the person will tend to have fewer feelings of insecurity, doubt, and jealousy about the partner—all of which can lead to problems in a relationship.)

 WORKSHEETS   At this point you may want to distribute the activity in your supplementary material that asks students to describe the characteristics they consider important, in a dating situation and then in a marriage partner.

 WORKSHEETS   Your supplementary material contains an activity that calls for students to write a marriage contract. If you choose to use this activity, it is suggested that you use it as a follow-up to the Life Choice Inventory on page 508.

ASSESS

EVALUATE

Have students review the STOP method for maintaining sexual abstinence.

Section 2 Review Answers

1. sexual intercourse
2. marriage
3. abstinence
4. external pressures
5. Each partner has a positive self-image and is aware that love develops in stages. (p. 497)
6. Answers will vary. See Figure 18–2 for possible answers. (pp. 498–500)
7. External pressures: peer pressures; pressures from images of sexiness in the movies, in popular music, and on TV; pressures from a partner who wants to have intercourse; pressure from product advertisements. Internal pressures: the natural biological drive to reproduce (pp. 501–502)
8. the idea that marriage will magically make people happy (p. 506)
9. Answers will vary.

CLOSE

Make sure that students understand the differences between serious dating and marriage. Many students will see them as the same relationship without cohabitation. Discuss.

A reproducible quiz for Section 2 is provided in the Teacher's Resource Box.

506

CHAPTER 18: Pairing, Commitment, and Marriage

Marriage

Did you ever wonder what happened to Cinderella and the Prince after they married? Did they really live happily ever after? The idea that **marriage** will magically make people happy is probably the most destructive idea that partners can have. Marriage is never the *end* of the story, as in fairy tales. It is the beginning.

The highest form of commitment between two people in our society is marriage, a relationship based on these ideas:

▶ The relationship is permanent, or at least permanence is something the partners will work for.
▶ The partners will be most important to each other. No other relationship with another person will take a higher place.

Before they marry, people would do well to look honestly at what they expect. One way to do this is to answer together the questions in this chapter's Life Choice Inventory (see page 508). Clearly, it is essential to find out what a potential partner means when the word *marriage* comes up.

The Health Strategies section on page 504, "Developing a Healthy Intimate Relationship," sums up this chapter's points about developing healthy relationships. The next section gives tips on weathering disagreements within the relationship.

KEY POINTS *Marriage is the highest form of commitment in our society.*

Answer the following questions on a sheet of paper.

Learning the Vocabulary

The vocabulary terms for this section are *date, sexual intercourse, external pressures, internal pressures, thrill seekers,* and *marriage.*
Fill in the blank with the correct answer.

1. _____ between human beings is termed *coitus.*
2. _____ is the institution that joins a man and woman by agreement for the purpose of creating and maintaining a family.
3. _____ are people who take chances in exchange for momentary excitement.
4. _____ are messages from society, peers, and others that pressure people to have sexual intercourse.

Learning the Facts

5. What two things do healthy relationships have in common?
6. List one advantage and one disadvantage of going steady.
7. Describe the pressures teenagers face to have sexual intercourse.
8. What is the most destructive idea people have about marriage?

Making Life Choices

9. Your friend, Sally, is thinking about dropping out of high school to get married. What advice would you give Sally? Why would you give her that advice? Would your advice be different if Sally were a guy named Jim?

Answers to FACT or FICTION

Here are the answers to the questions at the start of the chapter.
1. False. You can tell when love is real because it develops slowly through the conscious choices of both partners.
2. False. People may be intimate psychologically as well as sexually.
3. True.
4. True.
5. False. Healthy, intimate relationships require time to grow before initiating sexual activity.
6. False. To cope with a breakup, it is best to give yourself six months to a year to heal and build up support.
7. False. Couples in healthy, intimate relationships maintain separate interests, as well as shared ones.
8. False. To make a marriage work, couples need love and mutual agreements on some of life's basic issues.

Chapter 18, Section 2

The following quiz will help you assess your students' understanding of the material covered in this section of the chapter. You might use the quiz as an oral exercise, which will lead into a class discussion of the topics covered. Or, you might use it as a paper/pencil quiz to evaluate your students individually.

Like the Quick Quiz, the Section Review can also be used as an assessment tool to spark class discussion or as an individual student evaluation. It can also be used as a review in preparation for this quiz.

1. It is important to allow a love relationship to develop slowly through the necessary stages. (True)
2. You should consider the emotional state, time commitments, social values, and

SECTION 3
Working through Conflict

Partners may think that anger and conflict have no place in a "happy," committed relationship and so may try to hide their negative feelings. In reality, every human relationship has conflicts. How partners handle those conflicts can determine whether the relationship grows or dies.

Destructive things happen when people fail to address their feelings of anger. These people may find other, unhealthy outlets for their anger, such as drinking alcohol, abusing drugs, overeating, or gambling. They may tell friends about their anger instead of telling the one who needs to know—the partner. They may become depressed or develop other psychological problems.

Some people believe (falsely) that hitting or other physical aggression can help to "clear the air." Actually, partners withdraw in response to such events. Assertion, not aggression, is the path to clear air (see Chapter 2). Equally useless tactics are leaving when a conflict starts, refusing to talk, not taking the other person seriously ("He's just had a hard day"), or not giving the other person time to respond. Saving up hurts is useless. They come spilling out in a confusing mess at some later date.

People can handle differences constructively. The Health Strategies section of Chapter 2 (page 36), "How to Apply Constructive Problem Solving," described the process.

Every relationship has conflicts.

 KEY POINTS *Work through conflict by clearly defining and addressing each problem while honoring the other person.*

SECTION 3 Review

Answer the following questions on a sheet of paper.

Learning the Facts
1. What happens when people fail to address their feelings of anger?

2. Explain why physical aggression doesn't clear the air.

Making Life Choices
3. Give an example of a conflict you might experience in a relationship or a friendship. How would you handle the situation?

MINI Glossary

marriage: the institution that joins a man and a woman by agreement for the purpose of creating and maintaining a family.

geographical location of a person before becoming involved with him/her. (True)
3. The way a person treats casual acquaintances does not indicate whether or not she/he will be a good partner. (False)
4. Many rapes occur in dating situations. (True)
5. People who are going steady can often focus on the development of the relationship at the expense of their own personal growth. (True)

6. A feeling of sexual obligation can indicate a serious flaw in a relationship. (True)
7. Sexual intercourse is a quick way to strengthen a relationship. (False)
8. External sexual pressures include the natural, biological drive to reproduce. (False)
9. It is normal to feel intense loneliness and depression immediately after a breakup. (True)
10. Independence is a necessary part of any healthy relationship. (True)

SECTION 3
FOCUS

OUTCOME
In this section students will learn:
1. The difference between constructive and destructive conflicts.

FOCUS ACTIVITY
Ask students if they usually work through conflicts or keep their feelings inside.

TEACH & APPLY

ROLE PLAY
Have two students role play a couple working through a conflict both positively and negatively. Discuss.

ASSESS

EVALUATE

SECTION 3 Review Answers

1. Answers will vary; could include: find unhealthy outlets for anger, such as drinking alcohol or abusing drugs
2. Partners withdraw in response to such events.
3. Answers will vary.

CLOSE
Have students discuss positive ways to work through conflicts.

A reproducible copy of the Life Choice Inventory is provided in the Teacher's Resource Box.

Group Activity

It might be a good idea to have the students fill out the Life Choice Inventory either at home or some place where they can be assured of their privacy (library, study hall, and so on). The information presented should give students a better understanding what possible conflicts can arise in a committed relationship. Are they surprised with some of the topics that are presented here? Are there any others that they would include?

While there is no scoring system for this Life Choice Inventory, students should take it seriously to get a better understanding of what is important to them. It will help them to create better relationships.

CLASS ACTIVITY

Have students collect rape awareness brochures, newspaper articles, rape statistics, phone numbers of help lines and rape counselors, and so on for a Rape Prevention bulletin board. Include information from Figures 18–5 and 18–6 and the Healthy People 2000 box, all on pages 510–511. Have the students post their bulletin board in the classroom or in a visible location around the school (like outside the Guidance Office).

Will the Marriage Work?

Will the marriage work? Differences of opinion will pepper an otherwise bland relationship with challenges—but these differences can also destroy the relationship. It helps to know ahead of time where the major differences will be. The more of these questions the two people agree on, the more likely the marriage will work. Your answers to the Life Choice Inventory are personal and private. Share them with others only if you are comfortable doing so.

Money
1. Should both partners work? Should one stop working after children come?
2. Should we keep all our money in a shared bank account? If so, who should pay the bills?
3. What should the limits be on the use of credit cards?
4. Who decides on big purchases?
5. Should we follow a written budget?
6. If one of us wants to do something more rewarding personally than financially, will that be all right?
7. If one of our careers requires a move, will the other consider moving?
8. How much of our income should we save, invest, and spend on insurance?
9. Who will own the home, car, and other property? One of us? Both of us?

Children
1. Do we want to have children? How many? When?
2. Should children's needs be put before one of our needs?
3. How much money shall we save for, or spend on, the children's needs?
4. Who should discipline the children, when, and how?

In-Laws
1. How close is each of us to our families? Will it be important to see them frequently?
2. Is each of us willing to be advised by the other's parents?
3. Can we or should we accept financial help from our families? How much, for what, and from which family?

Religious Traditions
1. Are our religious beliefs similar? If not, can we each accept the other's beliefs?
2. Does either of us feel strongly that the other must attend religious services?
3. Should children be raised with particular religious beliefs?
4. Should religious practices be part of every day's routine? How will religious holidays be spent?
5. How much money, energy, or time should we spend on religious and charitable organizations?

Miscellaneous
1. Is profanity acceptable? Under what conditions?
2. Is alcohol drinking acceptable? If so, how much drinking? Will drinking in front of children be OK?
3. Is smoking acceptable? When and where?
4. Should both of us go to bed at the same time? Who should get up first?
5. Who should do the shopping? Who should choose major purchases, such as houses and automobiles?
6. Should each of us be willing to tell the other everything we think, feel, and do?

Ability Levels

On Level

This activity will help reinforce the ideas presented in the Life Choice Inventory.

On a bulletin board, draw a large circle with room for eight puzzle pieces that you have cut from paper). Above the circle write, "Who's Available for Love?"

On each puzzle piece write one of the seven qualities listed on page 497 under the heading, "What to Look for in a Partner." Put each quality into question form and add the following as number eight: "Is the person compatible with you in social values and beliefs?"

Begin the lesson by reminding students to keep an open mind about their past, present, and future relationships. Ask for eight

Rape Prevention

Rape is a serious crime that occurs all too frequently. One of every four women will suffer a rape in her lifetime. Most people know about **stranger rape**—a woman who is in a public place or in her own home is sexually assaulted by an unknown attacker. No less dangerous, and much more common, is rape by an attacker who is known to the victim. She may even be dating him. This kind of rape is **date rape** (also called *acquaintance rape*).

 Isn't stranger rape completely different from date rape?

No, both are crimes of violence. The only difference between rape by an unknown attacker and date rape is that in the latter type, the attacker and victim know each other. In both instances, the attacker forces sex on the victim. Any forced sexual activity is a crime. Figure 18-5 on page 510 offers tips to prevent rape by strangers.

 I know that women and girls are raped, but can boys be raped?

Ten percent of all rape victims are male. Any form of forced invasion of any body part by another person in any way is rape.

 How serious is rape?

Legally, rape is considered very serious, deserving jail penalties and fines. Rape is also serious physically. The rapist may be armed and may kill or injure the victim. The rapist may carry sexually transmitted diseases—even AIDS—and inflict them on the victim. The attack itself may be painful and physically damaging, and the victim may require medical treatment. A female victim also faces the threat of pregnancy as a result of the attack.

Beyond the physical threats, rape is a serious threat to the victim's mental health. Rage, shock, terror, and emotional pain that can last for years are all common in victims of rape. A writer for *Time* once put it this way: "When the body is violated, the spirit is maimed. How long will it take, once the wounds have healed, before it is possible to share a walk on a beach, a drive home from work, or an evening's conversation without always listening for a quiet alarm to start ringing deep in the back of the memory of a terrible crime?"

 Are date rapes really rape?

Yes, but they are hard to prove in court. Consider how a date rape report reads, after the fact. Two people got together socially for an evening, and they went to a private place. Then they had sexual intercourse. One of them says that the intercourse was forced. The other claims it wasn't. The problem is that no one else was there. Only the two people involved know what really happened. Cases end up being one person's word against another's.

 I heard someone say that a woman who gets mad at a man might just say he raped her to get even. Does that happen?

It may, but these false stories usually come to light during a trial. In fact,

MINI Glossary

stranger rape: sexual assault by a stranger. Also called *street rape*.

date rape: sexual assault by a known person in a dating situation. Also called *acquaintance rape*.

509

volunteers who are comfortable talking about what to look for in a partner. Shuffle the puzzle pieces and hand one to each volunteer. Ask each of the eight students to take turns tacking their piece on the board while explaining that quality to the class. Once all eight pieces are up, ask the class for examples of relationships they know of in which one of these qualities was missing and the relationship failed. (example: going out with someone who recently broke up with someone)

Reminder: No names should be given when discussing personal experiences.

In closing, write the three italicized questions from page 497 around the outside of the circle, stressing the importance of each. Remind students that all these questions apply as they determine their readiness for relationships.

Students may have heard the term *statutory rape*. Tell them that *statutory* refers to statutes, or laws, which say that it is illegal to have sexual relations with a girl under the age of 16 or 18, depending on the state. Statutory rape laws are based on the idea that young girls are not mature enough to make a decision about whether they should have sex and that a male that has sex with a girl this age is taking advantage of the girl's immaturity. This type of rape differs from other rapes in that there is no violence—the girl consents to the sexual activity.

ON LINE WITH HEALTH

You may want to have your students visit the following URL, where they will find information and additional Web site resources to enhance their study of this chapter. As with all Web sites, you should check this one out first to be sure the information found there is appropriate for your students.

Relationship Survival Guide
http://relationshipweb.com/odat/

The Relationship Survival Guide site offers daily, indexed and searchable, readings as well as online discussions.

Figure 18–5 Stranger Rape Prevention Tips

To avoid becoming a victim of rape:	If efforts fail, and you are followed:
• Do not go anywhere alone after dark, call a friend or service that offers safety escorts.	• Ring the nearest doorbell.
• Always run with a partner, and even then, never run in the dark.	• Move out of shadowy areas into the open.
• Always ask who is at your door before opening it. Do not open your door to strangers.	**If you are approached:**
• Leave word with family or friends of where you plan to go and when you will return.	• Stall for time. Someone may come along.
• Stay alert to suspicious-looking people.	• Scream "fire" (not "police," since others are then likely to avoid becoming involved).
• Keep your arms free for defense. Use backpacks, shoulder bags, and the like.	• Pull a fire alarm, if possible.
• Stay on busy, well-lit streets.	• Break a window. Someone is likely to respond to the noise.
• Have your keys in your hand before you get to your front door or car door.	• Use your key or a stickpin to aim forcefully for the attacker's eyes, temples, Adam's apple, or ears. Stab hard, without warning.
• Lock the car door as soon as you are inside.	• Try to disgust your attacker by urinating or by gagging yourself to induce vomiting.
• Keep your car full of gas and well-maintained.	• Tell the attacker you have a sexually transmitted disease.
• Carry a hatpin or stickpin in your hand. You will not have time to fumble for it.	
• Carry a whistle.	

the whole purpose of a trial is to establish the truth about what happened. False reporting of rape is a crime in itself and is treated harshly by the justice system.

How big a problem is date rape?

Date rape is the most common form of rape in our society. Compared with the incidence of rape in many other countries, the United States has a high rape frequency. Evidently, something about the way we live makes date rape likely.

The social costs of rape are enormous. Not only do victims suffer all the outcomes already mentioned, but courts, jails, and law enforcement systems are straining with the burden of rape prevention and its punishments.

Why is date rape so common here?

One theory blames the media. Movies, television, music videos, and romance novels written in this country often suggest that women want to be raped. The media plant the idea that when a woman says no, she will change her mind and say yes if a man overpowers her. This idea is completely false. No normal person wants to be raped, and *no* means *no*.

Another problem is that, in our society, girls learn early to be indirect about sex, to dress and look

sexy, but not to have sexual intercourse. As women, they may say no verbally, but their clothes or body language may seem to say yes. This is no excuse for rape, but it can confuse some men. They think that a woman who looks sexy wants to have sexual relations, regardless of what she says. Most boys are taught to be aggressive—to go for what they want without restraint. As men, they may use physical power to force sexual intercourse.

If a girl is dressed in a tight miniskirt, a cutoff top, lots of makeup, and high-heeled shoes, isn't she asking for it?

No one ever asks for rape. A girl dressed as you describe may be "asking for" attention or admiration, or she may be totally unaware of the effect of her appearance on others. The law protects a woman's right to choose clothing for herself, so long as she is decently covered. No amount of makeup nor shortness of skirt is an invitation to rape.

What if a guy gets so "turned on" that he can't stop himself?

Rape is an act of violence, not of passion. In fact, the only role of sex in rape is as a weapon. Rapists are usually unstable, aggressive men who hold strong feelings of anger—not desire—toward women. Rape expresses their anger.

510

HEALTHY PEOPLE 2000

Reduce rape and attempted rape of women aged 12 and older to no more than 108 per 100,000 women. (Baseline: 120 per 100,000 in 1986)

Young, unmarried, and low-income women are the most frequent victims of rape and rape attempts. Women between the ages of 12 and 34 are particularly vulnerable, with victimiza-

tion rates more than twice as high as women in other age categories. Most rapists are unarmed and operate alone. Reported offenders are usually strangers to the victim, but this may reflect the reluctance of victims of acquaintance and date rape to report their experiences. Most sexual assaults occur at night and are attempts rather than completed rapes.

A number of widely accepted false beliefs exist about sexual assault (e.g., rape is always

Figure 18–6 Date Rape Prevention Tips

Be aware that people you know can hurt you. To prevent date rape:

1. Get to know any potential date well as a friend before going anywhere alone with him.

2. Never accept a ride home from a social function with someone you've just met.

3. If you are interested in dating a person, go out with him in a group, and be on the lookout for warning signs. These are warning signs that suggest a risk of rape—the person:

   - Abuses you verbally (insults you, ignores you, or blows up at you).
   - Tries to boss you around by telling you who your friends should be or how to dress.
   - Talks as if he hates or dislikes women.
   - Gets jealous for no reason.
   - Tries to get you to drink alcohol, take drugs, or go someplace alone with him.
   - Acts physically cruel to you, other people, or animals.
   - Gets too close; invades your personal space.
   - Acts aggressively toward you when you don't want him to (sits too close, touches you, blocks your way with his body).
   - Has a fascination with weapons.

4. Do not let anyone you don't trust get you alone in a room or building.

5. If you open a soft drink in a public place, keep your eye on it until you finish it, or throw it away. "Guard it or discard it."

6. If you fear someone, tell an adult in a position of authority about your fears. If that person refuses to help you, find another. Don't take no for an answer.

I remember reading about a connection between drugs and alcohol, and rape. How are these connected?

The abuse of drugs or alcohol seriously impairs people's judgment. This results in two effects that make rape more likely. First, alcohol and many drugs reduce inhibitions—even inhibitions against rape in someone considering the idea. Second, drugs and alcohol make people groggy. If a high enough dose is consumed, an extremely dangerous situation occurs when the person passes out. Someone who didn't plan a rape might commit one if a potential victim falls unconscious from drugs or alcohol.

Another danger lies simply in being in the company of strangers. Rapists are known to slip a "date rape" depressant drug, such as Rohypnol (see Figure 12-2 in Chapter 12), into the drinks of young women. When the woman loses consciousness from the drug overdose, the rapist fakes assisting, and instead drives away with her to rape her. In a tragic report, a potential rapist slipped a date rape drug into the cola of a 16-year-old girl who was attending a "teen night" at a local music hall. She died from the drug dose in her cola before the rapist had a chance to act.

Hundreds of thousands of date rapes occur each year. To protect yourself, don't agree to go out alone with people you don't know well. Accept drinks only from people you know you can trust. Once a soft drink is opened in a public place, don't let it out of your sight.

Are most rapists caught?

Sadly, it is likely that fewer than 10 percent of rapes are ever even reported. Some rape victims do not report the crimes because they fear the police will treat them badly. Others do not report attacks because they feel embarrassed, as though they somehow brought the attack on. Even if a case goes to court, the victim undergoes still more trauma by attacks on her character from the opposing attorneys.

If more rapes were reported, more rapists would be convicted. It takes courage, but reporting rapes is important. Even if the victim does not want to press charges against the rapist, the rape should be reported. That way, the statements will be on record in case the victim decides to prosecute later.

How can a woman protect herself from becoming a victim of rape?

First of all, just keep it in mind as a possibility. Figure 18–6, "Date Rape Prevention Tips," sums up other precautions you should take. Figure 18-5, "Stranger Rape Prevention Tips," gives precautions against stranger rape. Finally, reread the section of this chapter called "What to Look for in a Partner." By observing closely, you can pick up clues to potential problems, and avoid them.

Rape is a serious crime that causes emotional trauma. The best protection is prevention. Should rape occur, report it, and seek medical treatment immediately.

511

a violent crime and one cannot be raped by someone familiar). One such false belief—that forced kissing, fondling, or sexual intercourse is acceptable behavior in the context of dating relationships—is an important factor underlying sexual assault in our society. A survey of students in the sixth to ninth grades in Rhode Island found that 65 percent of boys and 57 percent of girls believed it was acceptable for a man to force a woman to have sex if they have been dating for more than 6 months.

Similarly, 51 percent of boys and 41 percent of girls believed it was acceptable for a man to force a woman to have sex if he had spent a lot of money on her.

Sexual assault awareness programs for adolescents should be initiated to change or modify beliefs that condone sexual assault. The effectiveness of these programs in modifying such beliefs and in subsequently reducing sexually assaultive behavior in dating relationships should also be evaluated.

®You can update your coverage of health and fitness topics, as well as spark lively classroom discussion and deeper understanding, by using the **CNN Health and Fitness Updates.** These video updates are produced by Turner Educational Services, using the resources of CNN, the world's first 24-hour, all-news network.

With the introduction of the **CNN Health and Fitness Updates,** West Educational Publishing is proud to be the exclusive partner of CNN for textbook/video integration in high school fitness. By making use of the **CNN Health and Fitness Updates** you can bring the power of CNN, the network known for providing in-depth, live coverage and analysis of breaking news events, to your health class.

For assistance in using and incorporating the **CNN Health and Fitness Updates** into your classroom presentations, see the *Classroom Guide to the CNN Health and Fitness Updates.* The **CNN Health and Fitness Updates** are available with West Educational Publishing's *Health: Making Life Choices.*

VOCABULARY

1. a. internal pressures **b.** sexual intercourse **c.** external pressures **d.** thrill seekers **e.** marriage **f.** abstinence **g.** intimacy
2. a. Mature love **b.** date

RECALL

SECTION 1

1. Poor mental and physical health (p. 493)
2. Refer to Figure 18–1 on page 494 for possible answers.
3. Refer to Figure 18–1 on page 494 for possible answers.

SECTION 2

4. The stages are attraction, casual friendship, intimate friendship, and mature love. Refer to Figure 18–2 for complete definitions of each stage. (p. 498)
5. Look for people who are not involved in other love relationships, are well over heartaches, have not just recently broken up with someone else; are open to being in a relationship with you; are free of chemical or psychological addictions (people with addictions cannot function well in love relationships); have time to devote to a relationship; have high-self-esteem; and are close to you geographically. (p. 497)
6. Social values and beliefs (p. 497)

CHAPTER 18 Review

Summarizing the Chapter

Your ability to respond correctly to the following statements ensures your understanding of the main concepts in the chapter.

1. Describe the differences between love and infatuation, and thus be able to clarify your values and beliefs concerning sexuality.
2. Describe the stages of a love relationship.
3. List the advantages of sexual abstinence.
4. Discuss responsible ways to cope with sexual pressures.
5. Identify and describe ways of developing a healthy intimate relationship.

Learning the Vocabulary

love	external pressures
infatuation	internal pressures
mature love	thrill seekers
intimacy	marriage
date	stranger rape
sexual intercourse	date rape

Answer the following questions on a separate sheet of paper.

1. Matching—*Match each of the following phrases with the appropriate vocabulary term from the list above:*
a. a person's internal biological drive that urges the person toward having sexual intercourse
b. the reproductive act between the sexes
c. messages from society, peers, and others that pressure people to have sexual intercourse
d. people who are likely to take chances in exchange for momentary excitement
e. institution that joins a man and a woman by agreement

f. relationships involving private and personal sharing
2. a. _____ is a strong affection for and an enduring deep attachment to a person whose character is well known.
b. A social event designed to allow people to get to know one another is called a _____.

Recalling Important Facts and Ideas

Section 1

1. People who live without relationships are likely to suffer what?
2. List five signs of infatuation.
3. List five signs of mature love.

Section 2

4. List and define the stages of a love relationship.
5. Identify and describe characteristics to look for in a potential partner.
6. In what areas should partners be compatible with each other?
7. Describe the sort of person who can gain the most from dating.
8. How is double dating especially useful when you just begin to date someone new?
9. List four ways to meet new people.
10. What problems are associated with sexual activity in a high school relationship?
11. What risks are associated with teenage sexual activity?
12. It is said that abstinence gives freedom to the people in a relationship. What sorts of freedom does abstinence give?
13. Identify the pressures associated with sexual intercourse.
14. Give examples of activities that can make people feel loved without having sexual intercourse.
15. List activities that can release sexual energy.
16. In what ways do people become physically ill following breakups?
17. About how long does it take to heal after a relationship has failed?
18. What is the highest form of maturity in a relationship?
19. Describe how to establish a healthy intimate relationship.

Section 3

20. List both useless and effective ways to handle conflicts.

512

7. The person who practices assertive behavior and maintains high self-esteem (p. 499)
8. By creating a casual and safe environment in which to check people whom you do not know well. (p. 499)
9. Answers will vary; could include: Join a youth group; learn to play a sport after school; play on, or watch, local teams; get physically fit and attend to nutrition and sleep needs; be friendly, reach out to others; be yourself, don't try to impress anyone. (p. 500)

21. List the warning signs that suggest a risk of acquaintance rape.

Critical Thinking

1. The Life Choice Inventory in this chapter deals with whether a marriage will work. Do you think couples who are going to marry should take this inventory? If so, why? If not, why not? How do you think this inventory would help the success rate of marriages? Do you think a couple about to be married should agree on a certain number of the questions before getting married? If so, how many? Why? If not, why not?

2. Acquaintance or date rape is a growing problem in society today. Reread the Straight Talk section on pages 509 to 511. Why are men getting mixed signals from women? How are the media at fault? What are we being taught about sexual behaviors and how does that lead to date rape? Discuss how education can help stop this serious violent crime.

Activities

1. Complete the following sentence on a piece of paper: Love is . . . . Write all of the class members' answers on the board and compare the many ways love is defined. Discuss your response with the rest of your class.

2. Cut out the personal advertisements in the paper. Discuss why you think this is a good way to meet people or why you think it is a bad way to meet people. List the pros and cons to share with your class.

3. Design your own dating service for high school. How would you pair up students? What would you call your service? What days and times would you work?

4. Write an editorial for your school newspaper on date rape. Be sure to include how to prevent date rape in your paper.

5. Interview two happily married couples: one couple that has been married at least 30 years and another couple that has been married under five years. Ask them what the keys are to their happy marriages. Are their lists similar?

What conclusions can you draw about happy marriages?

6. Describe the characteristics you consider important, first in a dating situation, then in a marriage partner. Use attributes like looks, personality traits, educational background, age, religious beliefs, ethnic group or race, values (political, ethical), and interests. Are your lists for dates different from your lists for marriage? If so, how and why are they different?

7. Go to your local law enforcement agency and write down the number of rape cases that were reported in your community for the year. Are the numbers surprising to you? Report this to the rest of your class.

8. Write a one-page essay on the perfect relationship. In your essay include qualities and values on which you place high priority and which you would expect the other person to value highly as well. Describe what you would bring to the relationship and what you would expect the other person to bring to the relationship. At the end of the your essay, tell whether you think the relationship you described is realistic. Explain why you think the way you do.

9. Work together in a group to complete this activity. Reread the Health Strategies feature in this chapter entitled, "Meeting New Friends." As a group, brainstorm additional ideas for meeting new people. Generate as many ideas as you can. When your list is complete, print the ideas on a piece of poster board and display them in the classroom.

Making Decisions about Health

1. Jerome hasn't had a date in a long time. He thinks to himself that he must be the loneliest person on earth tonight. He feels jealous when he hears about his friends' relationships. They aren't all perfect, but at least they provide some companionship. There must be something wrong with Jerome; he's just not the likable type. He's facing another night of watching television alone in his room. How might Jerome build up his self-esteem at a time like this? What changes in his attitude might he make and how? What constructive actions could he take to ease his loneliness?

513

13. peer pressure; pressure from images of sexiness in the movies, in popular music, and on TV; or the pressure from a partner who wants to have intercourse; the biological drive to reproduce (p. 501)

14. Answers may vary; could include a hug, giving a small gift, doing a favor, confiding in others. (p. 502)

15. Dancing, sports, walking or other activities requiring movement, writing, speaking, singing, painting, or other expressive activities. (p. 503)

16. The pain, depression, and stress that can follow breaking up may make people physically ill. Stress weakens the immune system, making illness more likely. (p. 504)

17. Six months to a year. (p. 504)

18. Commitment (p. 504)

19. Refer to the Health Strategies on page 504 for possible answers.

SECTION 3

20. Answers will vary; could include useless: telling friends, physical aggression, leaving when conflict starts, refusing to talk, not taking person seriously, not giving other person time to respond, saving up hurts; useful: assertion; see Health Strategies, page 36 (p.507)

STRAIGHT TALK

21. Answers will vary; refer to Figure 18–6 on page 511. (pp.509–511)

10. Answers will vary, could include: it can interrupt the normal growth of a relationship; neglect intellectual, emotional, social, and spiritual growth; can cloud a person's judgment; and can cause distrust. (p. 500)

11. Sexually transmitted diseases, including AIDS; teen pregnancies. (p. 500)

12. It gives the freedom to grow and develop without interruption by diseases or pregnancy. Abstinence also allows time for a healthy intimate relationship to develop. (p. 501)

KEY POINTS

Chapter 19 is 30 pages long and divided into four sections. Briefly, this chapter introduces students to the importance of families, how families provide for the basic needs of an individual, including the need for belonging, and also how families help shape the personality of the individual. The chapter discusses quality family time and how to effectively resolve conflict within families. The chapter also looks into how society affects families, and problems in families such as divorce, abuse, and dysfunctional families.

ACTIVITY TO INTRODUCE THE CHAPTER

Ask each student to write the following on a sheet of paper:

1. his or her definition of family;
2. his or her picture of an ideal family—either a description or perhaps the name of a fictional family;
3. what he or she would like the family to be like when he or she is a parent.

Have students share their definitions of family. How close are their definitions to one another? What crucial information do most definitions share? Discuss the students' responses to the other questions.

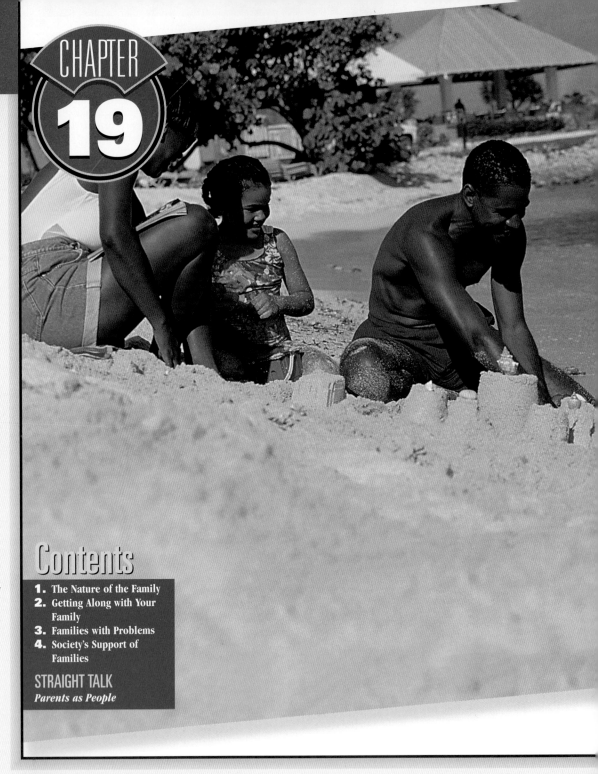

CHAPTER 19

Contents

STRAIGHT TALK
Parents as People

NOT Enough Time?

Following are some suggestions to help you make sure that you cover the key topics in this chapter if you have limited time. (Refer to the daily lesson plans in your Teacher's Resource Box for additional suggestions.)

DAY 1 Assign Sections 1 and 2 to be read prior to class. Open class with a discussion of family and the needs that families meet for their members. Have students complete the Activity to Introduce the Chapter on page 514. Review Figure 19–2 on page 520 with students to help them see how families change. Do the

Family Life

FACT or FICTION

What do you think? Are the following statements true or false? If you think they are false, then say what is true.

1. Most people consider the family to be more important than anything else.
2. Children who grow up in unsupportive homes rarely overcome their poor starts in life.
3. A person's values are most powerfully influenced by the values of his or her family.
4. The order of a child's birth in a family—being the youngest, a middle child, or the oldest—may influence the child's personality.
5. It's natural for parents to distrust their teenage children.
6. Watching television together is a great way to develop relationships among family members.
7. A closed door means "Knock before entering."
8. A reason why some brothers and sisters argue so much is that they feel secure in their relationships with each other.
9. In today's world, divorce is easily obtained and causes few problems.
10. People who abuse their own children are most likely to have been abused themselves during childhood.

(Answers on page 538)

Introduction

Recently, some researchers asked people in the United States to name the most important part of society. Overwhelmingly, their answer was that **family** is more important than schools, the military, religion, or anything else. So powerful a force is worth thinking about.

What is your family like? Have you any **siblings**, or are you an only child? Do both your parents live with you? Stepparents? Grandparents? Who else is there? What activities do family members share? Does your family value hard work? All of these things and more define the nature of your own unique family.

This chapter begins by describing types of families and the ways in which they meet their members' needs as they change with time. Next, it takes up issues of respect, trust, and communication, which serve as the foundation stones of a healthy family life. The love and support that define many families are not universal, however. Some families are living through problems such as divorce, addiction, codependency, or abuse, and they are in need of help. The last section makes clear that families need society's support through changing times.

Class Activity on page 524 and the Key Passage on page 525. Finish up with Figure 19–4 on page 529 and review with students the importance of effective communication within families. Role play the responses if time permits. Assign Section 3 and the Straight Talk to be read for homework.

DAY 2 Begin class with the Focus Activity for Section 3 on page 531. Define *dysfunctional family* and discuss Figure 19–7 on page 534, covering the Discussion Activity. Also go over Figure 19–8 on page 535 to help students compare the characteristics of functional and dysfunctional families. Finish up with a brief discussion of how families are changing today.

FOCUS

OUTCOMES

In this section students will learn:

1. That families help mold the personalities of their members.

2. The basic human needs that families provide their members.

3. How a family identity is developed and maintained.

4. The various stages that families move through.

FOCUS ACTIVITY

Give students one minute in which to write down all the benefits they can think of that families provide. When the minute is up, have students volunteer the benefits they thought of as you list them on the board to create a class list. Discuss.

TEACH & APPLY

TEACHER SUPPORT

Key Passage

Ask each student to think of three ways in which his or her family has shaped him or her. Have them put a plus sign beside each influence for which they are grateful, and a minus beside each one which they consider a handicap. Have each student then write a brief essay on how his or her family has shaped him or her.

The Nature of the Family

When people say the word *family*, what exactly do they mean? After all, families come in all shapes and sizes. Figure 19–1 describes only some of the many possibilities. Wherever on earth people live together, they form some type of family. No matter what they look like, families form the building blocks from which each society is made. Without their families, societies could not exist.

The Power of the Family

Just as families help to mold human societies, they help to mold the personalities of their members, too. For better or for worse, the influence of a child's family reaches far into the future, affecting the rest of that person's life story. Parents, siblings, aunts, uncles, and even baby-sitters are a child's first teachers. They teach the child about being human, about their values, and about whether or not others are to be loved and trusted among other things. Years later, in adulthood, early family experiences still affect most people's outlooks on themselves and on the world.

Even adults who break off communication with their families are still influenced by them. A person who remembers childhood as a painful time may experience lifelong difficulties, but may never fully understand why. An adult who grew up with an addicted or abusive parent, for example, may

For **Y**our **I**nformation

Values were discussed in Chapter 2.

Figure 19–1 A Glossary of Families

> **blended family:** a family created by remarriage after the death or divorce of a spouse; blended families include a biological or adoptive parent and a stepparent, along with the children of one or both of them.
>
> **extended family:** a family of parents, children, and other relatives, such as grandparents or aunts and uncles. The relatives may live in one household, or they may live close by and share responsibilities, such as childraising.
>
> **foster family:** a family formed when a government agency places a child in the temporary care of an adult or couple. The child's own parents may have died or for some reason cannot care for the child.
>
> **married couple:** a family consisting of two married adults.
>
> **nontraditional family:** a group of unrelated people who live together and offer support to one another.
>
> **nuclear family:** a mother and father and their natural or adopted children.
>
> **single-parent family:** one parent and his or her natural or adopted children.

• multicultural issues •

To involve your class with the community, try one of the following extra activities.

You should have a wealth of speaker options in your community. Ask members of a three-, four-, or five-generation family to talk with your class about the differences and similarities in family life between generations.

Are there recent immigrant families in your community who can speak about cultural differences? Or, try to identify possible speakers from families who immigrated 100 or more choose a series of unsupportive or abusive mates, repeating a familiar but destructive pattern learned during childhood. With the help of therapy or counselors, such a person may come to recognize these choices as part of a destructive pattern. With help, these patterns can be changed.

Of course, not every child from an unsupportive family suffers throughout life. Stories abound of the human power to overcome even painful childhood neglect, to grow strong and stable, to excel, and to emerge as adults on whom others depend. In contrast, some people who lacked nothing during youth grow up to be weak and selfish adults, blown this way and that by every ill wind. Those who triumph over poor starts do so by choosing to do so. They move on and live up to their potential.

The difficulties faced by children from unsupportive homes are enormous. To improve, such children must struggle with the ordinary problems faced by everyone, while they also combat negative feelings of low self-esteem resulting from negative family experiences. They must create for themselves the positive attitudes and values that their families, for whatever reason, did not provide for them. An important difference between those who overcome an unsupportive childhood and those who do not is an unshakable belief in their own ability to succeed. This belief lies at the heart of personal change, and seems to be basic to most forms of success in life.

 Families have far-reaching effects upon their members. Many who start out with unsupportive families may feel negative effects and experience problems later on. Many, through hard work and faith in themselves, also overcome poor starts to excel as adults.

The Benefits of Family

Why do we need our families? What benefits do they bring us? Our families meet needs that are so basic to our existence that unless those needs go unmet, they are easily overlooked and taken for granted. An example of such a basic need is family loyalty. For those who have the faith and trust of their families, it is one of life's greatest treasures. The issues of trust and honesty are taken up in a later section.

Families also meet the human need for belonging. They teach values to the younger generation. In addition, most families meet their members' needs for:

▶ Affection.
▶ Food.
▶ Clothing.
▶ Safety.
▶ Security.
▶ Sexual activity between married adults.
▶ Shelter.

We need our families, and our families need us.

Meeting the Need for Belonging   People everywhere share a common need for belonging. One of the nicest things about being part of a family is the feeling of having a place, permanently, in a group. Each family develops a **family identity**, a unique sense of being "us," distinct and dif-

family: a group of people who are related by adoption, blood, or marriage, and are committed to each other; especially a father, mother, and their children. All blood relatives and ancestors of a family.

siblings: two or more people with one or more parents in common; brothers or sisters.

family identity: a unique sense of belonging together as a unit, distinct and different from other people or groups.

years ago. Many keep alive the family and cultural traditions from the "old country."

Do you have ethnic community centers in or near your school? Students could visit one of these centers to better understand ethnic diversity. Or, you could ask the director of the center to speak in your classroom.

Watch local or regional newspapers for events that will help students understand different families. These might include Chinese New Year celebrations, Octoberfest in German communities, and Native American celebrations.

INTERDISCIPLINARY ACTIVITY: HISTORY

Have students, working individually or in groups, research families in different historical times and cultures. (societies to study might include Sparta, Rome, French nobility of the Middle Ages, sixteenth century Scotland, and so on) They should consider formation of the family (how many generations were included), values instilled, functions of the various family members, and so on. Have the students or groups of students share their knowledge, and discuss as a class what they have learned about families in these various time periods. In what society would students have preferred to live? Why? In which would they least have liked to live? Why?

GROUP PROJECT

Divide the class into small groups and assign each group a region, nation, or culture to research. Ask each group to compile information on the structure and importance of family in that culture, and changes that may be affecting the family structure. Have the groups report their findings to the class. What can students learn about features of families that are common across cultures? How do families differ across cultures?

CLASS ACTIVITY

Ask each student to write out what they believe to be the three most important values their parents are teaching them. Then encourage students to share this list with a parent. Are these the values the parent wants most to impart? What would the parents consider the three most important values they want to teach their children?

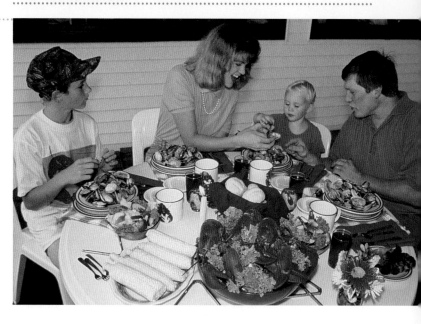

A family's identity springs from daily rituals, such as taking meals together.

ferent from anyone else. Almost without awareness, family members participate in the family's ways of doing things.

A family identity is maintained by:

▶ Keeping rituals, such as wishing each other a good night before sleeping, joining together at mealtimes, or hugging when members greet each other.
▶ Celebrating special occasions together in the family's chosen ways.
▶ Living with give and take, and realizing that a family member's attitudes and behaviors affect the nature of the whole family, just as the family affects the individual member.
▶ Spending time together, and sharing activities and experiences.

For **Y**our **I**nformation
Gangs and other groups were discussed in Chapter 3.

Belonging is so basic a need that people often join other groups to help meet it. Circles of friends, social or hobby groups, or even gangs exist because people feel the need to belong. Families meet this need in ways that other groups cannot match, through rituals, celebrations, traditions, love, and day-to-day give and take that combine to make each member feel an essential part of the whole structure.

Teaching Values Sometimes, parents formally teach values to their children. They sit them down and spell out the rules. More often, however, older people teach values to young people by the examples they set. Parents who attend religious services with their children convey the value of organized religion. Parents who work to protect the environment offer lessons in living responsibly, and so forth.

A serious mistake that some adults make is to underestimate the importance of their examples to young people. Seeing is believing, however. No matter how many times an adult tells a child that he values honesty, if the

•multicultural issues•

Today many people are trying to learn more about their family roots and looking for strength in their cultural diversity. By interviewing older members of the family, sifting through old photographs, and spending hours reading records in courthouses and libraries, they develop a clear sense of pride in who

they are and who their families are.

Students will be interested in family names when they discover the meanings that lie behind them. They can easily see that those names that have "son" or "sen" at the end carry the meaning "son of" (Anderson, Petersen, and Williamson). Endings that mean *son of* in other languages include *ez* (Spanish), *tse* (Chinese), *wicz* (Polish), and *ov* (Russian and other Slavic languages). Some adult is caught cheating on his taxes, the young person gets the message that cheating is OK (unless you get caught). Whether or not the child becomes a cheat depends on many factors, of course, including her own tendencies and the values of other important adults.

Children learn values from many sources other than their families. Schools, peers, magazines, and television may each convey a set of values, and each set of values may conflict with one of the others. Children who face this confusing situation may be left to wonder which set of values is best for them. The most powerful voice in this regard is still the family's, and it usually falls to the parents and other adult family members to clear up the confusion.

The Extras   In addition to meeting the basic needs discussed in this section, many families go much farther. They emphasize spiritual and intellectual schooling. They give instruction in social skills. They may also make sure that everyone has some fun along the way. A healthy family also acts as a refuge from the outside world, a protected place to rest and relax, where members can just be themselves.

 Families provide for many physical and emotional needs of their members. In addition to providing for food, shelter, and other physical necessities, families act as advocates, meet the human need for belonging, and pass on traditions and values. Some families also provide advanced schooling, social instruction, and fun. Families also provide their members with a refuge from the outside world.

The Life Stages of a Family

Few families stay the same from year to year. Instead, they change and evolve with passing time.

Forming a Family   Most new families form in the same way: a couple meets and falls in love. Their story often continues with marriage and unfolds as new characters arrive, grow up, and finally leave home. No one can predict what twists and turns the plot in the family story will take. One thing is sure: families are always interesting. Individual stories help to define each family as unique. Figure 19–2 on page 520 traces a family's progress through some typical stages.

Does your own family fit neatly into one of the stages in Figure 19–2? It would be unusual if it did. Because you are a teenager, your family qualifies for Stage 4. However, you may have brothers or sisters who qualify your family for Stage 2, 3, or 5.

Family Goals   Figure 19–2 also lists goals that accompany each chapter of the family story. Through the years, a family must constantly seek new ways of meeting the changing needs of its members. Parents of a toddler must provide constant supervision to ensure the child's safety. As the child grows, however, they must loosen their control or risk stifling the child's developing independence. The child, in turn, helps to meet the parents' needs for affection and loyalty. Each choice made by a family member contributes to or detracts from how well the family meets the needs of its members.

Family members must also attend to their own needs. For example, adults may save for their retirement (financial goals), teenagers may volunteer

examples would be Rodriquez = son of Rodrigo (Roger), and Ivanov = son of Ivan (John).

Many last names are associated with a person's line of work, such as Carpenter, Farmer, Baker, Miller, and Smith (blacksmith). Characteristics of a person often lead to the use of other names, such as Young, Black, Long, White, and Little. The "Mc" and "Mac" names originated in Ireland and Scotland.

You might tell students that different cultures have different rules for last names or family names. In English-speaking countries, most children take the last name of the father. Some countries use both the mother's and father's names (this custom is growing in the U.S.). A Spanish surname, for example, would consist of the father's family name followed by the mother's family name (Teresa Perez Gutierrez).

GROUP ACTIVITY

Divide the class into seven groups. Assign each group one of the seven stages of a family listed in Figure 19–2. Ask each group to look at the goal for the stage assigned to it and list ways in which parents can work toward meeting that goal. Can group members provide "success stories" that they know of for families that have met that goal well? You might want to select a three-generation television family from a popular television show, and ask the groups to evaluate that family in the appropriate stages. Discuss the findings of the various groups as a class.

DISCUSSION

Have students study Figure 19–2, which parallels Figure 3–1 on page 54, The Eight Stages of Life According to Erikson. In what stage do their families currently fall? What do they remember of past stages? Have students try to remember methods their parents used to meet the goals of the various stages. How similar or different are the methods used by the various parents? Which of these methods do students believe are cultural in nature? Which do they feel are individual to their families? Which would they like to remember for their own parenting experience?

COMPREHENSION CHECK

Review Figure 19–3 with students. Have each student list the three or four statements which they consider truest in their experience. Why did they select the ones they did? Allow students who wish to do so to share and discuss their statements.

Figure 19–2 The Stages and Goals of a Family

	Stage	Main Goal
1	Couple without children; creating a family.	Develop trust in each other.
2	Family bearing children and rearing newborns, toddlers, and preschoolers.	Develop independence and self-direction in children.
3	Family with schoolchildren.	Develop in children a sense of industry, to allow them to work with steady effort.
4	Family with adolescent children.	Guide adolescent role development, assist identity development in teenagers.
5	Family with young adults at home or leaving home.	Maintain relationships with children who leave; renew the couple's relationship.
6	Couple without children, moving toward retirement; grandparenting.	Share talents and resources with others; take pride in accomplishments.
7	Aging couple; widows and widowers; grandparenting.	Maintain satisfaction with life; enjoy fulfillment and serenity.

Source: Adapted from E. Janosik and E. Green, *Family Life: Process and Practice* (Boston: Jones and Bartlett Publishers, 1992), p. 29.

for good causes (spiritual and service goals), grandparents may make time to exercise each day (physical fitness goals), and so forth. Families may have many goals, but meeting the basic ones listed in Figure 19–2 goes a long way toward supporting the emotional well-being of the family members.

The Importance of Birth Order An interesting idea is that each member's experience in a family is somewhat different from anybody else's, and that those experiences affect personality development. You may have heard bits of wisdom about how people who are born first, middle, or last in a family share traits with others with the same **birth order**. It may be that parents treat the oldest, youngest, or in-between children differently, and that this influences their personalities.

Are oldest children most often the leaders because they receive more parental attention without competition? Are youngest children free and creative because their parents dote on "the baby"? Are middle children followers because they are largely ignored? Indeed, birth order may exert these effects to some degree. However, genetic makeup, gender, early experiences, and guidance from others also influence a child's personality development. Figure 19–3 demonstrates that no birth order in a family is preferable to any other, and that a child's responses do not follow any simple formula.

For **Y**our **I**nformation

Chapter 3 is devoted to the topic of personality development.

KEY POINTS *Families change and move through predictable stages. Each stage presents goals for the family to support each member's emotional growth and health. Personality development depends on many things, including a person's birth order.*

Chapter 19, Section 1

The following quiz will help you assess your students' understanding of the material covered in this section of the chapter. You might use the quiz as an oral exercise, which will lead into a class discussion of the topics covered. Or, you might use it as a paper/pencil

quiz to evaluate your students individually.

Like the Quick Quiz, the Section Review can also be used as an assessment tool to spark class discussion or as an individual student evaluation. It can also be used as a review in preparation for this quiz.

1. Families are the foundation of society. (True)

2. The family's effects on a person last until early adulthood. (False)

Figure 19–3 Which Birth Order is Best?

These are true statements:	And so are these:
1. A child may delight in the birth of a younger sibling.	1. A child may resent a younger sibling's arrival.
2. Parents often lavish attention on their first-born child.	2. Parents often lavish attention on "the baby."
3. Parents are more attentive to the rearing of the first-born child.	3. Parents are more relaxed and easygoing with second and later children.
4. The youngest feels most favored because he is the center of attention.	4. The youngest feels least favored because the older siblings are more competent while she is still learning, and they receive new things while she gets hand-me-downs.
5. A younger sibling looks up to the older ones and imitates them.	5. A younger sibling strives for individual identity, and chooses behaviors different from siblings'.
6. Older siblings nurture the younger ones, almost as an extra set of parents.	6. Older siblings, striving for maturity, avoid younger ones, whose childishness embarrasses them.

SECTION 1 Review

Answer the questions on a sheet of paper.

Learning the Vocabulary

The vocabulary terms in this section are *family, siblings, family identity,* and *birth order.*

1. Brothers and sisters are _____.
2. A _____ is maintained by families spending time together and celebrating special occasions in the family's chosen way.
3. The order in which children enter the family is the _____.

Learning the Facts

4. List three influences a family has on individuals.
5. What are two main functions of families?
6. Through what sources do values enter the lives of children?
7. List seven stages of family life.

Making Life Choices

8. People sometimes join church groups, social or hobby groups, or even gangs to meet needs that are not being met by their families. What needs might be met by these groups? How would the groups meet the needs? Are there other ways these needs might be met? If so, what are they?

MINI Glossary

birth order: the placement of a child among his or her siblings, such as oldest, middle, or youngest child.

ASSESS

SECTION 1 Review Answers

1. siblings
2. family
3. birth order
4. how the child feels about being human, whether or not the child develops a positive self-concept, and whether or not the child loves and trusts others. (p. 516)
5. Answers may vary; may include: families are advocates, meet the human need for belonging, provide the young with a set of values to help guide them. (p. 517)
6. schools, peers, magazines, television, and family (p. 519)
7. couple without children, creating a family; family bearing children and rearing newborns, toddlers, and preschoolers; family with schoolchildren; family with adolescent and teenage children; family with young adults at home or leaving home; couple without children, moving toward retirement, grandparenting; aging couple, widows and widowers, grandparenting (p. 520)
8. Answers will vary.

CLOSE

With their books closed, ask each student to write out as many ways as they can remember in which the family molds members and meets their needs. Have them number these ways in order of importance, from most important to least important. Have students compare their lists.

521

3. A person's relationship with his or her parents may determine the kind of relationship that person has with his or her spouse. (True)
4. Families provide their members with basic human needs such as clothing, food, and shelter. (True)
5. The family does not contribute substantially to an individual's sense of belonging. (False)
6. Rituals and other habitual behaviors help to form a family's group identity. (True)
7. The family provides the child's only opportunity for learning values. (False)
8. The family can serve as an essential support network for its members. (True)
9. The structure of a family is rigid and stays the same through time. (False)
10. Birth order may be a factor that influences an individual's personality development. (True)

SECTION 2

FOCUS

OUTCOMES

In this section students will learn:

1. The meaning of quality family time.
2. Ways to share quality time with family.
3. Effective and ineffective responses to family conflict.

FOCUS ACTIVITY

Write the following statement on the board. "In a healthy family, there is no disagreement, since all the members share common dreams and goals." Ask each student to write a brief reaction to this statement, then encourage students to discuss the statement.

TEACH & APPLY

DISCUSSION

Ask students to brainstorm qualities they believe help make a family strong. How important do they believe each quality is, relative to the other qualities? Have them rank the qualities they have suggested in order from most important to least important. Have students write down the completed list, or have one student record it for the class, and refer to it at the end of the section.

522

SECTION 2

Getting Along with Your Family

Being part of a family isn't always easy. Conflicts are almost certain to arise among people who live close to one another. Questions like these commonly arise: Which needs should be given highest priority? What task is most important? Is everyone being honest? Do we trust one another?

Interactions among family members can be more important than you might think. A squabble with a family member can serve as a sort of dress rehearsal for more threatening conflicts with people in the larger world. In a family, you learn to give and take, to communicate your own needs while respecting those of others. These are skills that, once developed, prove invaluable through life—at work, at school, with friends, and eventually, with a future mate and family. Interactions affect the present, too. Each kind word or supportive action by one member uplifts the whole family group. Each negative word or action brings it down a notch.

For Your Information

Four secrets to being honest:

1. Never promise more than you can deliver.
2. Allow for emergencies.
3. Let others know what's going on.
4. Plan ahead.

Issues of Trust and Honesty

A teenager was overheard saying, "How can I get my parents to trust me? They're always checking up on me!" This question may seem to be unanswerable. After all, how do you get parents to do anything? In truth, most parents *want* to trust their teenagers. Parents want to think of their children as honest and trustworthy.

Those interested in gaining trust must learn this principle: trust grows in direct proportion to a person's honesty. This principle also operates in reverse: people who are not entirely honest quickly lose the trust of others.

It's difficult to know how to react to someone who hasn't always been honest in the past. When a teenager has a history of dishonesty, a parent has no choice but to doubt the teen. How could a parent know whether or not the teenager is telling the truth on any one occasion? Dishonesty—that is, intentionally hiding or changing the truth—plants doubt that grows and damages the parent-child relationship.

Here is an example. Say that your neighbor has agreed to play softball with your team to fill in for an absent player. Game time rolls around, but your substitute doesn't show up. Your teammates are furious, and you must forfeit the game. On your way home, you see your neighbor riding around drinking soda, dressed in tennis clothes, and laughing with other friends. Later, when you ask why the neighbor missed the game, the person replies, "Oh, I got sick." Would you feel angry? Betrayed? Would you ever fully trust this person again?

Luckily, family members are most likely to forgive one another for such a slip in honesty, especially when the person apologizes and shows regret. With time, and with demonstrations of honesty, trust may eventually be restored. This healing of trust requires plain talk on the part of everyone. Especially, full admission to the dishonesty is needed to clear the air. Trust and honesty are the twin foundation stones of good communication. A later section provides some tips on how to communicate honestly and effectively.

special needs

Interpersonal

Family members who must provide care on a regular basis for those with special needs (such as a handicapped child or a person with Alzheimer's disease) face ongoing stresses. Discuss these special challenges to healthful ways of coping with stress. (See Chapter 4.) The following points can be used to get you started:

1. Don't become upset over situations you can't control. If a child is born with a physical or mental handicap, family members often blame themselves. Families with special-needs members need to understand that they can control the present, but not the past. Brainstorm ways family members can turn frustration over the extra time required for special care into positive feelings between family members.
2. Manage the events in your life. Time and

The Marketing of the Family

Consumer SKILLS

"Family Restaurant," says a sign hanging above a steakhouse. "Shoes for your family!" reads a newspaper advertisement. "A toothpaste for the whole family!" barks a television announcer. Today, market-wise advertisers use the word *family* to sell everything from automobiles to underwear. They know that just adding the word *family* to advertising slogans attracts consumer attention.

Of course, most people know that toothpaste suitable for family members is not different from toothpaste for single people. So, how does mentioning the family increase sales of toothpaste and other products? One answer might be found in people's desire to take care of their families. A parent who is busy at work and spends little time at home might feel better knowing that the "best family toothpaste" is riding in the grocery cart. The toothpaste, the parent hopes, will meet at least one of the family's needs. Clean teeth are important, of course, but products are a poor substitute for a parent's time and attention.

Most people associate the word *family* with childhood memories or ideals (mental images of "perfection"). When they read the word on a label, they may unconsciously link the product with love, the freedom of childhood, parental care, and support. For example, a bread wrapper may announce that the loaf within is "family-recipe bread." It may not matter that this particular loaf was one of ten thousand a day

ejected from a bread-making machine, delivered by conveyor belt, bagged by a wrapping machine, and trucked to a supermarket. The word *family* on the label is enough to make people think about the idea of "home" and buy the bread.

The word *family* may also convey an image of concerned, protective, supportive parents. The executives of a company may or may not have the best interest of the consumer at heart, but their use of the word *family* on their product implies that they do. (*To imply* means to get the message across without actually saying it.) People assume that the product can be trusted and is safe enough to use with children. However, the appearance of the word *family* on a label is no guarantee of a safe or trustworthy product.

In truth, most people respond to family-based advertising because most have positive mental images about what it means to be part of a family. Unfortunately, the needs of real families are not easily met by buying products, even "family" products. What family members most often need are the things that money cannot buy, but that must be freely given.

Critical Thinking

1. *What do you think of when you hear or see the word family?*
2. *Would seeing the word family on a package affect whether or not you would buy the product? Why or why not?*

A secret to always being honest and reliable is to try never to promise more than you can reasonably deliver. If someone asks something unreasonable, don't agree to do it. Instead, explain why it isn't possible. Three other secrets to being reliable: make allowances for emergencies, let others know what's going on, and plan ahead.

 KEY POINTS *Being completely honest is the way to gain people's trust. If trust has been breached, then an apology and commitment to future honesty can help to overcome distrust. Effective communication is essential to trust.*

energy are at a premium in special-needs families. Often these families must open up their boundaries and bring in outside resources as a way to manage. Brainstorm ideas families could use to establish good relationships with new people coming into the home. List tasks that family members can perform to help manage the work load.

3. View problems constructively. The Chinese symbol for a change is a combi-

nation of crisis and opportunity. Family members with special needs can teach us much about seeing the world differently. Brainstorm a list of positive statements to be used when problems seem to be overwhelming.

4. View problems realistically. The families of special-needs individuals need a clear and realistic understanding of the disability and a plan of action for helping this person live the fullest life possible.

Consumer SKILLS

Answers to Critical Thinking

1. Answers will vary; could include some of the following: childhood memories or ideals; mental images of perfection; love; freedom of childhood; parental care and support.
2. Answers will vary.

COMPREHENSION CHECK

Ask students to define *trust* and *honesty*. Then have them explain the link between the two. Why are they related?

DISCUSSION

Ask the students if they have heard the phrase, "Honesty is the best policy." What do they think that means? Do they agree or disagree with the statement? Are they always honest with their parents? In what situations are they not honest with them? Do they think that everything would turn out okay if they were honest with their parents from the beginning?

DISCUSSION

Have students ever lost their parents' trust? Have they ever lost trust in their parents? Discuss situations where these problems could occur. What can be done to reestablish the trust once it has been lost?

DISCUSSION

Do students know of any families that have consciously decided to live on less income in order to have more time together? If they don't know of any, propose a hypothetical family in which one parent stays home and is there for the children all the time. This means that money for extras is short—the children don't have many new, fashionable clothes or toys, older teens may be required to earn scholarships for college, and family members may need to learn how to repair cars and mend clothing.

Ask students to discuss pros and cons of such a family's lifestyle. What benefits would the family members enjoy? What pressure would the parents face from other parents? What pressure would the children face in the grade school years? During their teens? How might ownership of a television make such a situation more difficult? Less difficult? What factors do students feel are most important in making such a family situation successful?

CLASS ACTIVITY

Poll your class. How many students have at least one sit-down family meal per week? How many have at least one family meal per day? Have the students find the class average. What factors do they think keep families from having meals together? How could these factors be rearranged to promote more family time? Which family members would need to make sacrifices for this to happen? What would they need to give up? What might they gain?

Spending Time Together

Satisfying family relationships do not "just happen." They take time, commitment, and energy to develop and maintain. Some people try to take shortcuts, hoping to meet family members' needs without much effort. However, these shortcuts never work for long. Especially, buying things for family members cannot take the place of time and energy. The Consumer Skills feature on the previous page, "The Marketing of the Family," points out that marketers often try to sell the idea that products can meet the needs of the family. Instead of products, family members need each other. People who make it a point to share time with parents, brothers, sisters, and others in their families find that the results are well worth their efforts.

Relationships depend upon time spent together. To know someone well you must share ideas together, enjoy activities together, seek each other's counsel when life gets tough, and share the joys life has to offer. For many people, pressures at work, obligations at school, and social activities eat up the lion's share of their time. Without careful planning, family members may have to make do with the leftovers.

A huge problem faces many families today. The desire for more and more of the goods that money can buy makes many parents commit more and more hours to their paying jobs. These overworked parents may be richer in dollars, but they feel cheated of leisure time with their families. They have become "time poor," and they see no way to restore the balance between work and home.

Indeed, the demands of most households today require two full-time wage earners just to pay for necessities. When these exhausted workers finally arrive home, they can barely put dinner on the table, oversee homework, and attend to other family needs before falling

A discussion of the ideas seen in TV shows can turn television viewing time into quality family time.

It's sometimes surprising to discover how many activites family members can enjoy together.

Pursuing wellness

It could be argued that wellness is a strictly personal matter. It is, however, important for students to consider that everything in their lives has an effect on their families and communities; and, conversely, their families and communities affect them. Theories about family systems are helpful in understanding these relationships.

Discuss traits shared by people with a high degree of wellness, such as expressing emotions appropriately, feeling that life is meaningful, living by their values, managing their stress, taking care of their bodies, having satisfying relationships with family and friends, avoiding tobacco, alcohol and drugs, practicing safety in daily living, and being able to have fun. Ask what influence *family* can have on wellness. To prompt discussion, have students consider:

asleep. What these families gain in terms of money often costs dearly in terms of their relationships.

Some families are overheard saying, "Oh, we all watch *hours* of TV together each night. Surely our family spends enough time together!" In reality, time spent sitting in the same room watching TV does not enhance family relationships, unless the shows spark conversation lasting longer than a 60-second commercial break. When their focus is riveted to the television, each person might as well be alone in the room. They hardly notice who else is there.

What is lacking in most families today is **quality time**. This is time spent together, paying attention to one another for long enough to permit an exchange of ideas. Quality time is the kind of time that bonds family members together and enhances their relationships.

Waiting to find the time to spend together never works. Quality time isn't found; it's planned. A way to do this is to get everyone together and plan a whole-family event, such as a weekday supper or a Saturday morning ride in the country. The plan can include a special meal that everyone helps to prepare. It can include learning a new game, or making presents for others. It may require turning off Sunday afternoon football and heading for a nearby park.

Sharing hobbies with family members is another way to plan quality time. Sisters may find that they both love to garden. A dad and son might develop their cooking skills. A grandmother may teach a child to work with needles and thread. Brisk walking, golfing, paddling a canoe—these all provide the kind of peaceful time together that allows the participants to share their thoughts. The activities are limited only by imagination. They all provide a bounty in terms of improved family relationships. The margin lists just a few of the activities that family members can share.

 Many families are time poor, and spend little quality time together. Time shared among family members benefits their relationships and must be planned ahead of time.

Spending Time Apart

As important as time spent with family members is time spent alone. Teenagers, especially, need some time alone to think, to recharge their batteries, to reflect on who they are, and to imagine who they might become. Filling the pages of a diary, repeating details of an event to someone on the phone, or just plain daydreaming can be useful. These activities help the thinker to reflect on family and other interactions and to make sense of the events of the day. Some teens may play computer games or shoot hoops alone. In any case, alone time can be a sort of quality time in which you get to know yourself. Learn to respect others' need for solitude, too.

A caution is in order, however: solitude can easily be overdone. Teenagers who spend excessive amounts of time alone are often found to be suffering from depression. A healthy balance among four areas seems ideal for robust emotional health: time spent with family, time spent with peers, time spent at school and work, and time spent in solitude. Strive for balance.

 Everyone needs time alone to reflect on life and make sense of it. Solitude can be overdone, however, and excessive solitude is linked with psychological depression.

For Your Information

Here are a few activities that family members enjoy. Make your own list. Invite family members to join you in them.

► Bowling.
► Building houses with Habitat for Humanity.*
► Carving pumpkins.
► Collecting coins, shells, rocks, bottles, stamps, or anything of interest.
► Decorating for holidays.
► Cooking.
► Feeding the homeless.
► Going to the beach.
► Going to a health fair.
► Having a picnic.
► Hiking in the woods.
► Working out for exercise.
► Holding a garage sale.
► Ice skating or roller blading.
► Making candles.
► Planning a party.
► Planning grocery shopping trips.
► Riding bikes.
► Painting a room.
► Visiting relatives.
► Working with wood.
► Working in the yard.

*The organization Habitat for Humanity builds houses with volunteer labor and sells them at a low cost to lower-income families who participate in the building program.

MINI Glossary

quality time: time spent with another, of sufficient duration to allow a meaningful exchange of ideas.

DISCUSSION

Write the words *quality* and *quantity* on the board. Have students define the two, then have a student read the dictionary definition. Discuss which of the two is most important. Do students believe the two are completely independent, or is a combination of the two important? You might enjoy an abstract discussion of the two in relation to homework or study time. (Does five minutes of really high-quality study time qualify as adequate? After all, it was really quality. The question would be, was the task accomplished? Quality needs some quantity in order to perform the required function.)

TEACHER SUPPORT

Key Passage
The text states that "time spent sitting in the same room watching TV does not enhance family relationships . . ." Have students discuss why this is the case. Then have the class develop a list of guidelines for making TV watching quality family time. Which shows do they think would tend to provide quality time? Which would not? Why? What needs to happen in addition to watching the shows together?

COMPREHENSION CHECK

Ask students why it is important to spend time alone. (to recharge, reflect, and imagine) Ask students to estimate how much time they spend alone in a week. How do they spend that time? Do they enjoy it? Is it something they choose, or is it just because their friends are busy? Remind them that watching television does not count as spending time alone.

1. The methods family members use to deal with stress.
2. The use of tobacco, alcohol, and drugs in their families.
3. Methods used by their families to "have fun."
4. The use of, or failure to use, devices such as seat belts as an indication of practicing safe living.

The *community* also influences personal well-ness. Have students think of specific examples of the following:

1. Hotline availability for drugs or teen pregnancy.
2. Community commitment to chemical-free teen activities.
3. Strong codes of conduct for athletes.
4. Recreation programs for teens.
5. Active community involvement in DARE or similar programs.

DISCUSSION

Take a poll in the classroom as to how many brothers and sisters each student has. Keep a tally of the number of siblings for each student. Then ask the students these questions: What are some advantages/disadvantages of being an only child? What are some advantages/disadvantages to having brothers and sisters? Which would you prefer?

ROLE PLAY

Ask the students to respond to this question: What are some reasons for rivalry among siblings? Make a list on the board of the reasons they present. Have the students pair off and then role play siblings for each of the topics. After every pair has performed once or every reason from the board has been covered, discuss as a group how these confrontations are resolved. Can they be resolved positively for both sides?

Getting Along with Siblings

Have you noticed that some people argue more with their brothers and sisters than with their friends or even strangers? Psychologists who study **sibling rivalry** say that friction is normal between sisters and brothers.

Sibling Rivalry It may sound strange, but a reason why some brothers and sisters argue so much is that they feel *secure* in their relationships with each other. Siblings often say cruel things to each other and act in ways they wouldn't dream of acting among their friends. The difference is that they feel safe and do not fear losing their siblings' affection. With friends, they must work harder to maintain their affection.

Of course, family members cannot get away with saying or doing anything at all just because they are among family members. Far from it. A family's communication style is the heartbeat of the emotional peace of its members. It drives how and whether family members cooperate with each other. When minor struggles turn into battles, life can become miserable for everyone.

Siblings often quarrel because they feel they must compete for the attention of their parents. Even fair and loving parents find it almost impossible to dole out affection and attention in exactly equal portions. Brothers and sisters should expect that their parents will show different levels of affection to each of their children at times. To expect otherwise is to set oneself up for disappointment.

Some of the worst arguments occur among siblings who feel cheated of their parents' affection. If you find yourself measuring and comparing the

Siblings can learn much from each other—especially about communicating with others.

MINI Glossary

sibling rivalry: competition among sisters and brothers, often for the attention or affection of parents.

enrichment

The following activities might help your students better understand their feelings about their own families.

1. Ask each student to list his or her place in birth order. Do they like that place, or do they wish they were in some other place? Why? Have them write a brief essay, or deliver a short speech to the class beginning, "If I could choose, I would like to be (the oldest child, the youngest child, a middle child, an only child) because . . .

love each of you receives from a parent, stop. Instead, think about, and concentrate on, the loving actions and words shown to you. These are yours to keep, and are not made less by love shown to others.

Acceptance of New Arrivals   The relationship between siblings begins with the entrance of a new child into the family. Acceptance of a new brother or sister is one of the most demanding tasks a child faces. Most children have mixed emotions about the newcomer. They may feel excited and proud to become an older brother or sister, but also worry that they might be displaced from the favored position in the family.

Young children, especially, may even fear that they'll be given away, or traded in like an old car, for a new baby. Small children can be comforted by parents and older siblings who establish rituals, such as bathing, storytelling, playing favorite games, and so forth, that can be continued after the arrival of a new baby. Such attention raises the child's self-esteem and can help with acceptance of new family members. Many good books exist to help families prepare for the arrival of a new baby.

Struggles among Teenagers   Older children, and especially teenagers, have needs that may conflict with those of other family members. Often, issues of control over personal space, privileges, and privacy cause clashes. Most people develop a sense of ownership over a certain territory, including physical space they consider as theirs. Their sense of ownership also includes their privacy and privileges. A good rule to remember for keeping peace is that a closed door means *keep out.*

As mentioned, a territory is not always physical space. It may also include rights or possessions, or access to a favorite amusement. The telephone wars of two brothers, Josh and Daniel, provide an example. These teens must share a telephone with the rest of the family, and each is allowed one hour of phone time per night. Each night, Josh uses up his hour right away, while Daniel does his homework.

Here's where the trouble starts: Josh's friends call him later on, during Daniel's phone hour. Josh doesn't say a quick hello and goodbye, either. Instead, he grabs the portable phone, runs to his room, locks the door, and chats for 10 to 15 minutes, effectively stealing some of Daniel's rightful phone hour. This makes Daniel furious. He pounds on the door and yells. When his brother finally comes out, he physically attacks him. Finally, their parents notice the ruckus, break up the fight, and send both boys to their rooms for the night.

Josh and Daniel want to settle their conflict. They really do not want to fight. A starting point on the path to peace might be to decide to follow the conflict resolution guidelines offered in Chapter 2 of this book. The basic ideas are repeated in the Health Strategies section, "The Essence of Conflict Resolution." The boys need to accurately describe the conflict from both points of view. Also, they should sit down and brainstorm as many solutions as possible.

For **Y**our **I**nformation

To keep the peace, remember, a closed door means "Keep Out."

The Essence of Conflict Resolution

1. Identify the problem:
   ▶ Is it a conflict?
   ▶ Is it a different viewpoint?
   ▶ Is it a past grievance (complaint)?
2. If it is a conflict, then both people must:
   ▶ Desire resolution.
   ▶ Join in teamwork.
   ▶ Strive for a solution in which both parties win.
   ▶ Honor the relationships.
   ▶ Be flexible in *how* to meet needs.
   ▶ Be *firm* in meeting their own needs.
   ▶ Apologize when appropriate.
   ▶ Face the problem courageously; not back down.
3. Brainstorm and keep an open mind. (See Chapter 2 for details about brainstorming).
4. Decide on a solution.
5. Carry out the solution.
6. Evaluate the results, and revise the solution as needed.

2. Ask students which sibling they feel receives the most parental attention in their families. Why do they believe that child receives more attention? Ask the students to poll their siblings on the question. Do their siblings see things the same way? Why or why not? Do the siblings the students think get more attention actually believe that they are getting more attention? Why would this be? Discuss in class the factors which can cloud perception of relationships within a family.

BACKGROUND INFORMATION

You may want to give the students some additional information about sibling rivalry, a topic in which most of the students will probably be interested:

- Rivalry and conflict between siblings, while normal and common, is not inevitable, as people may fear.
- The parents' behavior after the birth of the second child affects the presence or absence of rivalry and conflict. If the parents include the older child in the care of the baby, the two children tend to be more friendly.
- The gender of the siblings appears to have a bearing on whether or not there will be conflict. The opposite-gender siblings usually engage in more rivalry and conflict than do same-gender siblings.
- The older sibling's angry behavior is often directed at the parent, rather than the sibling, while the parent is tending to the needs of the younger sibling.

GROUP ACTIVITY

Divide the class into groups of four or five and provide a family conflict for each group to resolve. The conflicts might have to do with performance of chores, curfew, dating, allowance, family time versus time with friends, and so on. Have each group use the information presented in the Health Strategies box to provide a resolution to the conflict. Then ask each group to present its conflict and resolution to the class. Discuss the conflicts and their resolutions.

DISCUSSION

Ask students to list on a sheet of paper three areas of conflict within their families. Collect the papers without names. Then read the responses while a student recorder writes them on the chalkboard. Where there are duplicated statements, note each occurrence of that area of conflict. When you have read all the papers, have the class rank the top three areas of conflict within families, based on the number of times students listed them. Discuss the reasons for conflict in these areas.

CLASS DISCUSSION

Ask students to relate personal experiences in which they either were or were not assertive. What were their feelings after both kinds of behavior?

ROLE PLAY

Give students some situations in which they can role play assertiveness. (Refer students to the Health Strategies on this page and Figure 19–4.) Some possible situations are: someone cuts in front of the lunch line, someone walks into the room and changes the TV channel while you're already watching something, a friend who has stayed overnight pulled out almost all of your CDs from their cases and is about to leave without having put any of them back. Monitor the role plays, pointing out the advantages of assertive behavior versus aggressive or passive behavior.

For Your Information

Emotions may come and go, but you alone are in control of, and are responsible for, your actions.

Health Strategies

Ground Rules for Arguing

Siblings normally argue. When the bickering becomes constant, however, it makes life difficult for everyone. Take these actions to reduce the wear and tear of sibling rivalry.

1. Don't blame. Don't accuse. Use *I* statements: "I'm angry because you're using up the telephone time that belongs to me and I've asked you three times to stop it."
2. Think in terms of a solution, not in terms of a war to be won. Ask, "Which hours of the day can you plan to stay off the phone?" "Will you please use E-mail to shorten your phone time or go visit your friends some of the time?"
3. Don't drag up old complaints during an argument. Don't complain about dirty clothes in the bathroom while trying to solve the present complaint about the telephone.
4. Take extra care not to call names or attack the person. Say, "I'm furious that you continue to steal my telephone hour." Don't say, "You're an inconsiderate jerk."
5. Try to anticipate and avoid situations that trigger arguments. If your sibling receives calls between seven and eight o'clock, then use that time to do some outdoor chores or to work out.

Solving the Conflict   The boys need only to come up with one solution to which they both agree. For example, since Josh's friends like to call late, the boys might agree to trade phone hours, with Daniel's hour coming first. The brothers might decide to take on extra household chores to earn money to pay for an extra phone line. Any of a number of different solutions might work, so long as both boys agree to abide by it.

One important point to keep in mind is the difference between feelings and actions. Daniel may *feel* angry enough to punch his brother, and his feeling is acceptable. However, he crosses the line when he acts out those feelings in an unacceptable way—punching. Daniel needs to remember that while emotions come and go, he alone is responsible for his actions. The second Health Strategies feature, "Ground Rules for Arguing," provides some guidance for keeping a lid on arguments. The next section shows how an assertive communication style can help you to sway people to your way of thinking.

 KEY POINTS   *Sibling rivalry is expected and normal among children who compete for parental affection. Young children may feel threatened by the birth of a new baby in the family. Older children may argue to compete for territory and privileges. Conflict resolution techniques can help siblings resolve problems without attacking the other person.*

Communicating Effectively

The secret to communicating effectively, and swaying people to your way of thinking, is to use an assertive communication style. Teens and their parents often disagree about house rules, chores, and curfews. It's normal for them to haggle over details of their agreements to make these arrangements fit changing circumstances. The more skilled family members become at communicating their wishes, the more likely that differences can be settled to meet everyone's needs.

Here's a surprising fact about using assertiveness to get what you want: the more you try to meet the needs of the other person, the more that person is likely to try to meet your needs. This chapter's Straight Talk section explains how this works with parents, but the technique can be used with just about everyone.

Remembering to use assertiveness is especially important just when it's hardest to use. When daily life becomes hectic, when financial pressures close in, or when members must deal with their own issues, small differences can explode into big problems. The following situations help to clarify how different communication styles can alter a family's interaction, even when life's stressful events seem to make problems worse.

Situation 1. Devon's father works hard at his construction company all day. He also struggles to keep their home clean and tidy. Devon has a

enrichment

Select two typical television families, one from the 50s or 60s, one current. You could use comedies or dramas. If possible, bring in videos of one or two episodes of the shows.

Whatever you select, ask students, individually or in groups, to list the types of problems faced by each of the two families. What constituted a family crisis in the ideal TV family of the 50s and 60s? What constitutes a family crisis for today's TV families? What sorts of problems confronted the TV children of 40 years

Responses	Situation 1
Passive response	Devon's Dad: Says nothing; cleans up the mess, making noise in hopes of being heard, but steams inwardly.
Aggressive response	Devon's Dad (yelling): "What a slob you are, Devon! You always mess up this house! Why can't you be more like your brother?"
Assertive response	Devon's Dad: "You left a newspaper on the couch and dishes in the sink. Please toss out the papers and wash your dishes." Devon's father watches to make sure that Devon does the chores.

Responses	Situation 2
Passive response	Angela: Vows to keep her secrets from her mother, but still wishes she could tell her some things. This makes Angela feel sad and lonely.
Aggressive response	Angela (yelling): "You traitor!! You were so mean to tell everyone about my problem! I'll never trust you again!"
Assertive response	Angela (calmly, but firmly): "Mom, Mrs. X talked to me about the private conversation I had with you the other day. Please don't repeat our secrets."

Responses	Situation 3
Passive response	Spencer: Ignores the comments; tries to spend as little time as possible in the house with Yvette; misses out on family fun.
Aggressive response	Spencer (screaming): "Yvette, I'm gonna pound you!! You little so-and-so!!" He listens in on Yvette's telephone conversations to "give her a taste of her own medicine."
Assertive response	Spencer: (forcing himself to stay calm): "Mom and Dad, please tell Yvette to stop listening in on my phone conversations. I've asked her to stop, but she won't." Then, if it continues, he sticks up for himself by telling his parents again whenever it occurs, until they effectively stop the eavesdropping.

Figure 19–4 Assertive versus Nonassertive Responses

history of sloppiness, and today his father comes home to find an all-too-familiar messy trail of newspapers and dirty dishes.

Situation 2. Angela has shared private information with her mother in a conversation that she believed was confidential. Angela is horrified when her mother's friend approaches her with the funny story about Angela's personal concern and offers unwanted tips on how to handle it.

For Your Information

Assertiveness was first explained in Chapter 2.

ago? What problems confront today's TV children? How do siblings relate to one another in the two time periods? How do parents relate to one another? To their children? What conclusions can students draw about changes taking place in families over the past 40 years? Remember that while the TV families do not

necessarily present an accurate picture of family life in either time period, they do give insight into the difference in material considered "family" entertainment. Also, changes in family structure and roles on television will reflect actual historical changes.

ROLE PLAY

Have students read the situations that go with Figure 19–4 and study that figure. Then have student volunteers role play the assertive responses for each situation, including a probable response from the other person or persons involved. Discuss the responses with the class. How well do they think these responses would work? Would they suggest any alternate assertive responses?

COMPREHENSION CHECK

Review the sections on assertiveness in Chapter 2. This would be a good time to discuss with the students if they have used what they learned in Chapter 2 in their everyday lives.

ASSESS

EVALUATE

Have students explain the following:

1. The meaning of quality family time.
2. Ways to share quality time with family.
3. Effective and ineffective responses to family conflict.

SECTION 2 Review Answers

1. sibling rivalry
2. quality time
3. Answers will vary.
4. conflicts with people in the larger world (p. 522)
5. never promise more than you can reasonably deliver (p. 523)
6. bonds family members together and enhances their relationships (p. 525)
7. They need time to think, to recharge their batteries, to reflect on who they are, and to imagine who they might become. (p. 525)
8. They feel cheated of their parents' affection. (p. 526)
9. Identify the problem: Is it a conflict? Is it a difference of opinion? Is it a past grievance? (p. 527)
10. Answers will vary.

A reproducible quiz for Section 2 is provided in the Teacher's Resource Box.

CLOSE

Refer to the list of qualities of a strong family developed by the class early in the section (see Discussion on page 522). Have the class review the list. What changes would they make to the list now, in terms of qualities listed and/or order of importance?

Situation 3. Spencer's younger sister, Yvette, eavesdrops on a private phone conversation. She then taunts Spencer with sarcastic jokes about what she heard.

In each of these situations, the responder can choose to be passive, aggressive, or assertive with family members. Figure 19–4 on the previous page presents some possible responses. As you can see from these examples, it is unlikely that a passive reaction will get any sort of response at all. Chances are that the other person won't even know that a problem exists. Aggressive responses are also unlikely to obtain a desired outcome, but are highly likely to provoke a conflict. In each case, the effective response is the assertive one.

The beauty of assertiveness is that it expresses your needs (helps you get what you want) in a way that doesn't threaten others. People who have trouble being assertive often share a problem: they let their resentments build up for so long that when they do speak, they express not a simple wish of the moment, but an age-old gripe. Some do it slow-burn style (passively), and others by way of a loud explosion (aggressively). Both are painful to express and painful to witness. Both are taken as threats by the receivers. Better to take a deep breath, think about what you are going to say, and present your case clearly and calmly before resentment has a chance to build.

KEY POINTS *Assertive communication helps family members to negotiate with one another. The more skilled they become at communicating effectively, the greater the chances of everyone's needs being met.*

SECTION 2 Review

Answer the questions on a sheet of paper.

Learning the Vocabulary
The vocabulary terms in this section are *quality time* and *sibling rivalry.*

1. Competition among sisters and brothers, often for the attention of their parents, is called _____.
2. _____ is time spent with another. The time is long enough to allow a meaningful exchange of ideas.
3. Use each vocabulary term in a sentence.

Learning the Facts
4. For what do family squabbles act as a dress rehearsal?

5. What is a secret to always being honest and reliable?
6. What two things does quality time do for a family?
7. Why do teenagers need time alone?
8. What is the cause of some of the worst arguments that occur among siblings?
9. What is the first step in conflict resolution?

Making Life Choices
10. Reread the Health Strategies section, "Ground Rules for Arguing." Think about the arguments you might have had in the past. How does your behavior during arguments compare to the ground rules given here? What improvements can you make in the way you argue?

---

quiz to evaluate your students individually.

Chapter 19, Section 2

The following quiz will help you assess your students' understanding of the material covered in this section of the chapter. You might use the quiz as an oral exercise, which will lead into a class discussion of the topics covered. Or, you might use it as a paper/pencil

1. Trustworthiness depends on honesty and the ability to communicate effectively. (True)
2. The best way to make up for any breach of trust is to admit the mistake and apologize. (True)
3. Satisfying family relationships happen naturally and do not require time or effort to maintain. (False)

Families with Problems

Sometimes, families have problems beyond those solvable by the members themselves. Family members often begin to find help when they begin to talk things over with school counselors, mental health counselors, religious leaders, and others, to get a clear picture of the situation. It also may help to find out how others have handled similar situations.

Living through Divorce

If current trends continue, about half of the marriages that form today will eventually end in divorce. Among children who live with parents, almost a third live in one-parent families, most times because their parents have divorced. Figure 19–5 describes some conditions that tend to make divorce likely. Of course, the presence of these factors in a marriage does not make divorce unavoidable. Many a couple celebrating their 50th wedding anniversary look back and laugh at the trials and tribulations of their early years of marriage. However, the factors listed here often strain a relationship and can worsen other problems.

Making Adjustments In cases where conflict between parents causes extreme anxiety and pain to family members, divorce may prevent some further injury. Regardless of the circumstances, however, divorce requires every-

> **"** *Happy families are all alike; every unhappy family is unhappy in its own way.* **"**
>
> Leo Nikolaevich Tolstoy (1828–1910) Russian philosopher, novelist, and mystic, in *Anna Karenina*

Figure 19–5 Factors That Often Surround Divorce

These factors are often seen in couples who divorce. The more factors that apply, the greater the risk of divorce.

Lower social class. When money is short, people often feel frustrated, which, in turn, makes small conflicts seem worse.

Less commitment to religion. Religious teachings often hold marriage as sacred, and condemn divorce.

Great differences in values and backgrounds. People who have grown up in different social settings possess different values and may think and act in unharmonious ways.

Young age at marriage. Young people may not have matured sufficiently to weather the storms expected in a marriage.

Come from divorced families. People whose parents divorced may be afraid to trust a relationship, and may be quick to discard it. Divorce may also seem familiar and "acceptable" to them.

Short time being married. As time passes, people learn how to better overcome small obstacles and compromise with each other.

Early childbearing. Partners need time to become partners before they become parents.

Source: Adapted from L. Beeghley, *What Does Your Wife Do? Gender and the Transformation of Family Life* (Boulder, Colo.: Westview Press, 1996).

---

4. It is very easy in today's society to make time for the family. (False)
5. The need for both parents to work full time has made many families time poor. (True)
6. Watching television is a good way to spend quality time with your family. (False)
7. A person's free time should be balanced between time spent alone and time spent socializing. (True)
8. Sibling rivalry can actually be a sign of the siblings' sense of security. (True)
9. Siblings often compete for territory and privileges as well as for their parents' affection. (True)
10. Assertive communication does not involve attempting to meet the other person's needs. (False)

TEACH & APPLY

BACKGROUND INFORMATION

For enrichment, tell students that the qualities listed below are often observed in healthy families and can serve as goals for their own families.

1. *Commitment*—Family members demonstrate commitment to promoting each other's happiness and welfare.

2. *Appreciation*—Family members often appreciate one another and contribute to each other's self-esteem.

3. *Good communication patterns*—Strong families tend to talk to each other, and their members are often good listeners.

4. *Desire to spend time together*—Even with individual time commitments, members desire each other's company.

5. *A strong value system*—Family members often agree on basic issues.

6. *Ability to deal with crisis and stress in a positive manner*—Strong families are resilient and capable of bouncing back from adversity.

Have students relate this list to what they have learned in the previous two sections.

GROUP ACTIVITY

Divide students into groups. Have them develop a package of materials that would help a new student in their school. Have them imagine that the new student may be going through a difficult family situation, such as a divorce. Have each group report to the class the materials and strategies they have developed as resources for the new student.

one to adjust to it. Those involved must rearrange everything from home addresses and school locations to emotional ties and future plans. Most children eventually adapt to the changes and live normally. Some, however, do not adjust quickly and are thrown into long-term problems such as depression.

Imagining the workings of a mobile (see Figure 19–6) helps to clarify the idea that even though it is the parents who divorce, everyone else can also feel out of place for a while. When an object hanging in a mobile changes its position, all of the other objects are left swaying this way and that until each object in the constellation finds a new balance.

Happily, while objects of a mobile must hang helplessly wherever gravity pulls them, people can choose their new positions and attitudes for themselves. When they choose positively, they change themselves and the whole system for the better.

Dealing with Hurt Feelings Both parents and children can feel hurt, shocked, lonely, or angry over a divorce, even if the previously intact family unit was destructive. It can help children to remember that people may divorce their spouses, but never their children. Both parents are still parents to their children regardless of what else happens or whom else they marry.

In advance of a divorce, parents should tell their children where they will live and with whom. Children need to get prepared for changes that affect them: new schools, new ways of getting around, new friends, and any other issues of concern. Most of all, children need to know that they will be safe and loved and that they are not at fault in the breakup.

Providing these assurances during a time of personal crisis is a tall order for the adults involved. The rewards in terms of well-adjusted children, however, are worth all efforts.

Sometimes parents do not or cannot give such assurances. Some parents use children's affections to injure each other, or they battle openly for the child as a prize to be won. The children in such situations will end up feeling insecure, anxious, angry, or guilty. In these negative conditions, children are likely to experience discipline problems, to earn low grades in school and on aptitude tests, and to possibly tend toward emotional problems.

Figure 19–6 The Family Mobile. *The positions of objects in a mobile change when its balance is disturbed. In the same way, relationships among family members change when something alters their familiar ways of interacting. Soon, a healthy family adjusts and establishes a new balance.*

Focusing ON Self-Esteem

Divorce strongly affects almost all children it touches. These effects may last into adulthood and significantly reduce self-esteem.

It should be stressed that divorce is never the children's fault. Children cannot do anything to prevent a divorce. Even though children are not responsible for divorce, they should have rights regarding the divorce.

Ask your students to consider what rights should be given to children before, during, and following legal divorce. The following list will get them started.

Allowing Time to Heal Given time, most children come to accept the split. It helps to know that children of all ages **grieve** over a parent who has left the family, just as they would if the person had died. It is normal to grieve for the family that is gone, too.

It takes time to build new families, especially with **stepparents** that may marry into the family. Stepparents may seem like intruders at first, each bringing his or her own set of thoughts and family rules. Most times, though, new balances of power can be worked out as long as everyone is permitted a say. Teenagers with good assertiveness skills can make sure that their views are heard. No family, even one that stays together, is perfect. All families require effort and cooperation to succeed.

Divorce requires adjustments on everyone's part.

 Marriages sometimes end in divorce causing families to change. Although divorce may require a difficult adjustment, most family members soon resume normal life.

Dysfunctional Families

For some teens, family conflicts are not the ordinary, day-to-day irritations that arise from living closely. For them, every day is filled with battles. Angry voices and slamming doors may be the only sounds they hear, and violence is a common occurrence. Invasions of privacy—stealing, sexual advances, prowling through possessions—are daily problems. Each day, they wake up feeling angry, frightened, confused, or trapped by the never-ending stress of conflict. They know things aren't right, but they don't know how to change them.

A family that does not cope effectively with its problems, a **dysfunctional family**, weakens its children by failing to support them. This type of family has abnormal ways of dealing with problems and erodes the self-esteem and emotional health of its members. Teenagers who see their own families described here should be reminded that they are not alone. They should also know that solutions exist, and that relationships can change into happier, more supportive ones.

Dysfunctional Family Traits All families face problems sometimes. Families are neither perfectly healthy nor totally unhealthy. Healthy families may behave in unhealthy ways during hard times. However, healthy families do not remain upset. They return to a normal healthy state. Dysfunctional families tend to grow worse. The unhealthy ways of coping grow more frequent and more severe. Dysfunctional families often have members who:

▶ Have alcoholism or other drug addictions, or long-term mental or physical illnesses.
▶ Fail to abide by society's laws and values.
▶ Lack parenting skills or social skills.
▶ Fail to engage in productive work.

MINI Glossary

grieve: to feel keen emotional pain and suffering over a loss.

stepparents: people who marry into a family after a biological parent departs through death or divorce.

dysfunctional family: a family with abnormal or impaired ways of coping that injure the self-esteem and emotional health of family members.

1. Children should have the right to answers to their questions about divorce.
2. Children should be spared from hearing negative comments from one parent about the other.
3. Children should have the right to see their non-custodial parent and grandparents.
4. Children should have the right to be children and not be expected to take on adult roles following divorce.
5. Children should have the right. . .

GROUP ACTIVITY

Divide the class into groups of four or five. Give each group a large sheet of paper. Have students divide the paper into three columns and label them "Problem," "Creates," and "Results." In the first column, students should list a problem, such as alcoholism, which is common in many families. In the "Creates" column, students should list possible actions, such as violence, that the problem could cause. In the third column, students should list physical, mental, and social results such as hitting, low self-esteem, and introversion. If more than one group listed the same problem, have those groups compare answers. Then have group members present their charts to the class.

GROUP ACTIVITY

Divide the class into groups of four or five. Give each group a large sheet of paper. Have students divide the paper into three columns and label them "Problem," "Creates," and "Results." In the first column, students should list a problem, such as alcoholism, which is common in many families. In the "Creates" column, students should list possible actions, such as violence, that the problem could cause. In the third column, students should list physical, mental, and social results such as hitting, low self-esteem, and introversion. If more than one group listed the same problem, have those groups compare answers. Then have group members present their charts to the class.

COMPREHENSION CHECK

Ask students to list developmental tasks that might not be accomplished by a child in a dysfunctional family. Students should be able to recall some of the tasks discussed in Chapter 3. Refer them back to the discussions of Erikson and Maslow in Chapter 3 (see pages 52–56).

CLASS ACTIVITY

To have students compare the traits of functional and dysfunctional families, reproduce the traits in Figure 19–8 on a sheet of paper, cut them out, scramble them, and have students arrange them in the proper pairs.

▶ Engage in **active abuse**: physical or sexual **child abuse**, **spouse abuse**, or **elder abuse**.

▶ Engage in **passive abuse**—withholding affection or physical necessities from children, spouse, or elders.

With these unhealthy coping methods, families cannot meet their children's emotional needs. This has lasting effects that may stretch into future generations (see Figure 19–7). Addictions and their effects are the focus of several other chapters of this book.

Parenting in a dysfunctional family may be unpredictable—sometimes loving, warm, caring, interested, and involved, and at other times unloving, cold, unavailable, and distant. The more severe the family problem, the greater the potential for emotional damage to the children.

How can you tell if a family is dysfunctional? Such a family usually has rigid rules such as those listed below:

▶ Don't feel—do not admit to unpleasant feelings such as sadness and anger.

▶ Don't talk—do not discuss problems or unpleasant feelings.

▶ Don't trust—because you cannot trust those who care for you.

A dysfunctional family may also keep family secrets, such as alcoholism or physical abuse; may have no sense of humor or use humor cruelly; may value ideals more than individuals; and may lack togetherness or unity. In

Figure 19–7 How a Dysfunctional Family Can Affect Future Generations

Parent has dependency problems, and so

who grows up with unmet needs because the child's

Child

fails to meet needs of child.

Child with unmet needs

fails to accomplish developmental tasks and grows up to be an

Emotionally undeveloped adult.

The emotionally undeveloped adult marries and becomes codependent (see next section, p. 536), or seeks relief in the form of alcohol or other drugs. Has a:

COOPERATIVE LEARNING

The structure of families comes in many different forms in today's society. Over the past few decades the family structure within our communities has changed in many ways. Some changes have been for the better and some have been for the worse. Explain to students what some of the changes have been (fewer children, mothers working, professional opportunities for females, more single parent families, and so on).

The following activity will help students understand the changes in family structure that have taken place and give them an opportunity to discuss whether those changes are good or bad.

Divide the class into groups of three. In each group, one member has a text book open, one member has notebook paper and a pen or pencil, and one person takes the task

Functional Family	Dysfunctional Family
Establishes rules for the sake of smooth functioning; rules are appropriate, consistent, and flexible.	Establishes rules for the sake of control; rules are rigid and irrational.
Encourages its members to develop well-rounded personalities.	Assigns rigid roles to each member, such as the hero, the scapegoat, the mascot, and the lost child.
Accepts its problems and strives to solve them.	Has deep, dark secrets that no one may admit to or work on.
Welcomes outsiders into the system.	Resists allowing outsiders to enter the system.
Values and exercises its members' sense of humor. Keeps humor positive.	Expects members to be serious, or uses humor to belittle them.
Honors personal privacy, so members can develop a sense of self.	Permits no personal privacy, so that members have difficulty defining themselves as individuals.
Fosters a "sense of family" so that members may leave and re-enter the system at will.	Enforces loyalty to the family; members may not leave the system.
Allows and resolves conflict between members.	Denies and ignores conflict between members.
Welcomes beneficial changes.	Fights against changes.
Enjoys loyalty and a sense of wholeness.	Has no real unity, is fragmented.

Figure 19–8 Characteristics of a Functional versus a Dysfunctional Family

contrast, the functional family shares and accepts feelings, and it strives for a sense of caring, support, and trust. Functional and dysfunctional families are compared further in Figure 19–8.

Exaggerated Roles of Children   Children in a dysfunctional family often develop somewhat exaggerated traits in the attempt to supply for themselves forms of support that normal parents would supply. One child may become a sort of hero, shouldering much more responsibility than is appropriate for a child. Another may take on the role of scapegoat, accepting the blame for everything that goes wrong. A third role is that of mascot, the one everybody thinks is cute and funny. A fourth role is that of lost child, the one who always needs everyone's help.

In families where people have to play roles, no one can change, grow, or adapt. No one can just be ordinary. People who adopt these roles as children often find it helpful during adulthood to discover the causes, work out their problems, and shed the roles. Dysfunctional families have recently received a great deal of public attention. Celebrities have spoken out about how the experiences of their young years affected them in their adult years. Such public statements may have a healing effect on those who finally face and admit their problems. Other victims may need more help in the form of therapy to recover completely.

Glossary

active abuse: abuse involving one person's aggression against another, such as hitting or sexually abusing the victim.

child abuse: verbal, psychological, physical, or sexual assault on a child.

spouse abuse: verbal, psychological, physical, or sexual assault on a spouse.

elder abuse: verbal, psychological, physical, or sexual assault on an elderly person.

passive abuse: abuse involving not taking needed actions, such as neglecting to provide food or shelter to a dependent victim.

of being the questioner. To make sure that all members of the groups participate equally, have them switch roles in the group after they finish each section in the chapter.

To help groups study the chapter, have the person with the book read aloud the information in the book from one of the sections. The person with the paper and pen or pencil is to write down all notes as well any questions he or the questioner may have. The questioner is to come up with as many questions as she

can think of for the group to discuss. The questioner may also facilitate questions that help the group understand all the information in the chapter. After the group has finished one section, have members switch roles and read and discuss the next section of the chapter. After all the sections have been covered, have the groups summarize all the information that was discussed and share their findings with the class.

COMPREHENSION CHECK

Write the characteristics from Figure 19–8 on index cards. Have students take turns drawing a card. After reading the characteristic aloud, have them do one of the following: state whether the characteristic is from a functional or dysfunctional family, name a well-known character from movies, TV, or literature who has that characteristic, name the opposite characteristic, or give an opinion as to why that characteristic is positive or negative.

GROUP ACTIVITY

Divide the class into groups of six. Ask half of the groups to write letters from a teen who lives with a parent who is a drug addict, feels sad, and wants to run away. Have the other half of the class write letters from a teen who is the family scapegoat and can't stand it anymore. Finally, have the groups switch letters and write advice-oriented answers to each letter. Share the letters and advice with the entire class.

DISCUSSION

Have the students brainstorm as many characters and characteristics as possible for the following terms: hero, scapegoat, mascot, lost child. An example for scapegoat might be: characteristics—takes blame, always apologizes, gives up easily, has the last choice; characters—Charlie Brown, Bud Bundy, Gilligan, Steve Urkel.

CLASS ACTIVITY

Using Figure 19–8, have students write a common home situation for each characteristic. Discuss the situations given by students.

BACKGROUND INFORMATION

One cause of problems associated with codependency is the intense shame that arises when family members are unable to control the dependent person's problems. The family hides the problem, trying to keep it a secret. The adult child of one alcoholic reported, "In our family, there were two very clear rules: there is nothing wrong here, and don't tell anyone." The exaggerated shame can be as damaging to children as the disease itself is to the addicted person. A predisposition to shame may occur in the first 18 months of life. A mother may say to her child, "If you are a good girl, Daddy won't be angry." The unspoken message is that the father's drinking results from the girl's behavior. If the drinking continues, the child feels increasingly ashamed.

COMPREHENSION CHECK

Codependency was discussed in Chapter 5 on page 123. In that chapter, a codependent person was defined as "being so focused on the needs of others that one's own needs are neglected." Dependency on drugs and alcohol was discussed in Chapters 12 starting on page 309 and 13 starting on page 343. Many of these types of dependency could be causing the problems shown in Figure 19–7. Students should realize that dependency means excessive, absolute, uncontrollable reliance on something or someone outside one's self.

 Dysfunctional families fail to provide a solid foundation for normal childhood development. These families may engage in abuses of many kinds, deny feelings, hide secrets, and fail to trust anyone.

Codependency

Suppose that you lived with (or were raised by) someone who suffered from an addiction or other dependency problem. Could you remain emotionally healthy? Few ever manage to do so. More commonly, the people close to someone with a dependency develop codependency. Codependency diminishes both the addicted person and the codependent person, so that neither is appreciated, loved, or supported on their own merits.

People with codependency want to help, but they become so focused on the addicted loved one that they forget to tend to their own needs. If asked "How do you feel?", people with codependency will often respond by saying how other people feel or by saying what they think the asker wants to hear. It is as though people with codependency aim bright spotlights outward onto other people and things. This leaves them hiding alone with their unmet needs in the darkness.

A codependent parent is no more able to nurture children than is an addicted parent. Such a parent suffers deeply, and focuses all attention on the seeming cause of all their misery—the addicted partner. Codependent people say things like "If only he would change, I could be happy. If things weren't so bad, I would do better. If only I had X, I could do Y." Meanwhile, everything and everyone else suffer from abuse or lack of attention.

Emotionally healthy people, in contrast, know that happiness lies within each individual, that no time is ever perfect, and that each day must be lived fully. It's been said, "Today is not life's dress rehearsal, but the performance of life itself." To break the chains of codependency, just one person must change for the better—and one can only change oneself.

For Your Information

Codependency is the characteristic of being focused on the needs of others to the point of neglecting one's own needs.

 Codependent people focus all their energy on helping addicted loved ones. They neglect everyone and everything else, including themselves. To recover, such people must begin to focus on themselves.

Family Violence and Abuse

More than a million children are abused each year by their parents, guardians, or other adult caregivers. More than a thousand children die each year at the hands of their abusers. Aside from physical beatings, many more children suffer repeated sexual assaults and the constant emotional abuse of unreasonable expectations, humiliation, and unmet needs.

People who abuse children are emotionally disturbed. They have low self-esteem and little power among adults. Such people may try to bolster themselves by bullying those who are weaker. It's not just children who suffer at their hands. Each year over a million wives seek medical attention for injuries from attacks by their husbands. An estimated half a million to one million elderly people are physically abused each year as well.

Family violence most often occurs when other problems worsen an existing emotional problem. Very young parents, single parents, those who are unemployed, those who fail to manage stress, and those who have few

QUICK QUIZ

Chapter 19, Section 3

The following quiz will help you assess your students' understanding of the material covered in this section of the chapter. You might use the quiz as an oral exercise, which will lead into a class discussion of the topics covered. Or, you might use it as a paper/pencil quiz to evaluate your students individually.

1. Divorce and single-parent families are rare in our society. (False)
2. Divorce often has a long-lasting and profound impact on a child's emotional development. (True)
3. Most children eventually recover from divorce and resume normal lives. (True)
4. A family that is going through a difficult, short-term period of adjustment is called

social contacts are especially likely to abuse their children. Alcohol and other drugs are strongly linked with child abuse. If the tendency to abuse exists, intoxication triggers it.

Most important, the cycle of abuse is likely to repeat. People who abuse their own children are most likely to have been abused themselves during their childhoods. Abuse runs in families and is passed on from each older generation to the next until someone breaks the chain by seeking and receiving help. A child who is rescued from an abusive situation and who is supported in working through the resulting emotional injuries can recover completely, and can achieve high-level emotional health.

By nature, human beings are capable of dramatic life changes that amaze everyone who witnesses them. Stories abound of folks who, once committed to a course of action, have found the will and perseverance to change completely and permanently. In this way, the cycle of abuse can be broken for good.

Government agencies exist to protect children from abuse, but they cannot do the job alone. People who know of child abuse should report it. You can do this without giving your name.

> 66 *Nobody who has not been in the interior of a family can say what the difficulties of any individual of that family may be.* 99
>
> Jane Austen
> (1775–1817)
> British novelist

 KEY POINTS *Child abuse and abuse of women and the elderly are all too common in the United States. Outside stressors may worsen existing emotional problems, making abuse likely. Alcohol and other drugs also trigger abuse. The cycle of abuse can be broken, but this takes commitment and effort.*

Using Figure 19–8 on page 535, have students apply these characteristics to some television families. For example, they could use the Cosby family as the functional family and the Bundy family as the dysfunctional family. While it is important that students learn to apply this information to their own lives, the teacher must be careful not to imply any criticism of the students' own families.

SECTION 3 Review

Answer the questions on a sheet of paper.

Learning the Vocabulary

The vocabulary terms in this section are *grieve, stepparents, dysfunctional family, active abuse, child abuse, spouse abuse, elder abuse,* and *passive abuse.*

1. Abuse involving one person's aggression against another is called _____.

2. _____ are people who marry into a family after a biological parent departs.

3. A _____ has abnormal and ineffective ways of coping that may cause injury to family members.

4. Verbal, psychological, physical, or sexual assault on an elderly person is called _____.

Learning the Facts

5. When might divorce prevent some injury to a family?

6. How does a dysfunctional family weaken its children?

7. List four roles that children in a dysfunctional family are likely to take on.

Making Life Choices

8. Your friend has shared with you that when her father is drunk, he hits her and her brother. She is afraid to say anything to anyone for fear her father will hit her more. What advice would you give your friend?

SECTION 3 Review Answers

1. active abuse
2. Stepparents
3. dysfunctional family
4. elder abuse
5. in cases where conflict between parents causes extreme anxiety and pain to family members (p. 531)
6. by failing to support them (p. 533)
7. hero, scapegoat, mascot, and lost child (p. 535)
8. Answers will vary.

 WORKSHEETS

A reproducible quiz for Section 3 is provided in the Teacher's Resource Box.

Have students list the characteristics of a dysfunctional family. Have the students put a star next to the characteristics they personally feel would be the most difficult to cope with and explain why.

dysfunctional. (False)

5. Dysfunctional families often fail to follow society's laws and values. (True)

6. Dysfunctional families often include parents with alcohol or drug addiction. (True)

7. Active abuse includes withholding affection or physical necessities from children. (False)

8. A codependent person often uses an addicted loved one as a shield for his or her problems. (True)

9. Abusive tendencies run in families and are passed on through generations. (True)

10. Child abuse, spouse abuse, and abuse of the elderly are major problems in our society. (True)

SECTION 4

FOCUS

OUTCOME

In this section students will learn:

1. How society can help meet the changing needs of today's families.

FOCUS ACTIVITY

Bring to class a picture of a family group from at least 50 years ago. Tell students the general date it represents and ask them to discuss what family life was probably like for such a family.

TEACH & APPLY

CLASS ACTIVITY

Have students compare the family lives in sitcoms today to those of sitcoms 30–50 years ago. Are the problems the same? Do they deal with the problems in the same manner?

ASSESS

EVALUATE

With books closed, have students write out as many of the problems facing families today as they can recall.

Answers to FACT or FICTION Here are the answers to the questions at the start of the chapter.

1. True.
2. False. Children who grow up in unsupportive homes may face challenges, but many overcome them to become successful adults.
3. True.
4. True.
5. False. Parents want to think of their children as honest and trustworthy, but may learn to distrust them in response to dishonesty.
6. False. Watching television, even in the same room with other people, is a solitary activity that does not enhance family relationships.
7. False. A closed door means "Keep Out."
8. True.
9. False. While divorce is easily obtained, most family members suffer from its effects, and must work to overcome the problems caused by divorce.
10. True.

SECTION 4

Society's Support of Families

Some people today worry that the family in the United States is breaking down. They fear that without its strong network of families to support it, society itself will crumble. Other people have an optimistic faith about families. They believe that the family, although undergoing changes, will endure. For the family to thrive, however, our nation must commit wholeheartedly to meeting the needs of the family as times and needs change.

The Changing Family Without a doubt, society has changed dramatically in the last 40 years. As mentioned, in most families today, both parents must work to earn enough money to make ends meet. Many teenagers today work, too, and contribute financially to the family. Forty years ago, this wasn't the case. Then, one wage earner was often sufficient. As women have entered the workplace, other institutions are taking over more and more of the tasks once performed exclusively by the family.

In the past, the nation depended upon women to perform much of the work involved in keeping a home and rearing children. Today, the nation's former caregivers are in the workplace during the day, and many struggle to perform the traditional roles as well. Men and women have been slow to recognize the need to shift the workload at home to a more equal distribution.

How can our society best meet the changing needs of its own basic units, its families? Some people fear that soon society will bear the whole burden for raising its children. They see a world where television is trusted to amuse the children; churches and schools to instill them with values and manners; government agencies to provide life's necessities; nannies, **day care**, malls, sports teams, and video arcades to keep them out of trouble; the police to discipline them; and no one at all to teach them about the value of family. Fortunately, evidence shows these fears to be exaggerated. Most parents care deeply about their children and try their best to be involved in their lives and provide for their needs.

Today's Problems Families across society face many common problems. Solutions to some of these are essential if families are to thrive. As just one example, quality day care for very young and very old family members is in very short supply. When it is available, the cost often exceeds the family budget. This shortage poses real problems for working families that include both toddlers and aged parents in need of care. A related child-care problem is what to do about after-school care for school-aged children while parents are at work.

One solution might be for society to support the development of facilities to care for dependent members of the family. Another might be to combine the day care needs of all ages, and allow the able elderly to become involved in caring for the young. Another solution might be for employers to develop flexible work schedules that allow families to care for their members in their own homes.

Society has made some progress in its support of today's families. In 1993, the Family and Medical Leave Act required owners of large businesses

---

enrichment

A significant portion of the public policy debate surrounding the abuse of children is the question of "place of family." Is the family a *private* or *public* institution? Are families able to live private lives, unaffected by public opinion; or, does the public sector have the right to impose certain standards on family life? Ask your students to debate the issue of community involvement in child abuse and neglect. If your school has a debate team, you may wish to ask them to participate in the discussion of this issue.

Here are two possible topics for students to debate:

1. *Family as a public institution:* The

Where would society be without its families?

to allow employees to take time off when they become parents or must care for sick family members. Employers are also beginning to institute their own family-supporting regulations as they realize that employees who are able to provide for their family's needs are more productive on the job.

Conclusion   Families are seldom perfect. Despite their many problems, however, the relationships formed among family members last a lifetime. It is worth every effort to ensure that your own family enjoys a happy, supportive, and functional atmosphere. The support you offer to your family today comes back to you many times over throughout your future.

KEY POINTS   *The United States must commit to meeting the changing needs of its basic unit, the family. Quality day care programs for young and old, as well as other family-supporting programs are needed.*

Answer the questions on a sheet of paper.

Learning the Vocabulary
The vocabulary term in this section is *day care.*

1. Write a sentence using the vocabulary term.

Learning the Facts
2. What must our nation do in order for the family to thrive?

3. List two common problems faced by families across society.
4. List three possible solutions for the problems listed in question 2.

Making Life Choices
5. You and your spouse have been married for a few years and you now have a new baby. You are used to having two incomes to meet all of your financial demands. What will you do? Will one of you stay home with the baby? Or, will you find child care for the baby? Give reasons for your answer.

MINI
Glossary

day care: supervision, usually at a facility, for preschool children or elderly people who must be supervised during daytime working hours.

For **Y**our **I**nformation

In 1998, the cost of sending a child to licensed day care for a year exceeded the cost of a year's tuition at many state universities.

SECTION 4   **Review Answers**

1. Answers will vary.
2. commit wholeheartedly to meeting the needs of the family as times and needs change. (p. 538)
3. Quality day care for very young and very old family members is in very short supply; and what to do about after-school care for school-aged children. (p. 532)
4. One solution might be for society to support the development of facilities to care for dependent members of the family. Another might be to combine the day care needs of all ages, and allow the able elderly to become involved in caring for the young. Another solution might be for employers to develop flexible work schedules that allow families to care for their members in their own homes. (pp. 538–539)
5. Answers will vary.

CLOSE

Refer the class to the list of problems facing today's families that they developed for the "Evaluate" activity on page 538. Divide the class into groups, one group for each of the problems the class cited as most immediate. Have each group determine reasons why this is a problem and develop possible solutions. Evaluate the solutions as a class.

community has a responsibility and right to step inside the family to insure the safety and well-being of children.
2. *Family as a private institution:* The family has a responsibility and right to treat children as they see fit.

As a conclusion to the debate you may invite a representative of the local Human Services/Child Protection agency to discuss

government regulations regarding procedures for identifying and reporting child abuse in your community and state. If it is possible to identify someone from a community organization that advocates family sovereignty and limited or no government intervention, invite that person to offer the opposing viewpoint.

539

Straight Talk

Straight Talk

Parents as People

Some teenagers, in their scramble to establish an identity, seem to forget that their parents are people, with needs, wants, and problems of their own. This is a mistake for at least two reasons. First, teenagers who attempt to understand their parents' points of view are in a much better position when it comes to bargaining for privileges, for money, and so forth. Second, teenagers who strive to meet the needs of their parents maintain their parents' goodwill, gain their trust, and increase the harmony of the whole family.

That sounds interesting. But how can I meet my parents' needs? I'm just a kid!

If you think about it, you'll see that meeting your parents' needs isn't too complicated. Parents have simple needs. While simple, though, these needs may not be easy to meet, especially at first. For example, the chapter already made the point that honesty is a major need of parents. A simple (but maybe not easy) way to start meeting parents' needs is to be totally honest with them, so that they can trust you.

Along with honesty, parents need reliability on your part. That is, they need to be able to depend on you to do what you say you'll do. Add to honesty and reliability a healthy dose of courtesy, and you have a fairly good start on a universal list of the needs of parents.

Ok. Now how do I go about using that information?

For starters, try treating your parents as though they were the people you most admire at your school. You wouldn't barge into a conversation and interrupt the people at school, so don't do that to your parents. You'd probably do some extra-nice things for those people at school, so try doing them for your parents.

Also, tell your parents that you love them. This becomes easier after the first time, and it generates warm feelings in almost everyone, including yourself. What many teenagers have learned is that keeping parents happy is the quickest road to gaining more of what they want at home, and especially to creating a loving home life.

I don't know about that honesty part. I don't think my parents will ever trust me.

You may think that you have lost your parents' trust forever, but remember from the chapter, your parents *want* to trust you. If you don't believe it, try this: be totally honest, and tell your parents that you are being honest, for two weeks. Then, when the two weeks is up, observe the changes in your parents' attitudes as they begin to trust you.

How do I know that all of this will work for me? How do I know that my parents will even notice?

They'll notice, because parents are people, and people usually respond positively to someone's honesty. An example may help make this clear. Suppose you need some money for a school function, say, $18.50. Your parents have only a $20 bill, and offer it to you to cover the costs of the event. Now you are faced with a decision: Should you return the $1.50 that is left?

Absolutely, and here's why. It shows your parents that you are fully responsible in handling their hard-earned money. This makes them feel great, and it

540

HEALTHY PEOPLE 2000

Increase to at least 75 percent the proportion of people aged 10 and older who have discussed issues related to nutrition, physical activity, sexual behavior, tobacco, alcohol, other drugs, or safety with family members on at least one occasion during the preceding month.

The World Health Organization characterizes the family as the "primary social agent in the promotion of health and well-being." The family, no matter how loosely defined—even as household—is a place where lifestyle patterns are initiated, maintained, and altered over time. It is where risk factors tend to cluster, and in most cases, members share a genetic history. It is the most basic consumer unit for foods, products, and services that influence health status. It is a major source of earns you credit for honesty and maturity. Since they know you will spend it wisely, they will be likely to feel generous in giving you money in the future.

I guess I've never thought of things from my parents' point of view. So what you are saying is that the more I try to meet my parents' needs, the more they will want to meet mine?

Exactly. Parents of teenagers face a tough task. They must strike a balance between setting limits on your behavior and allowing you to control your own affairs as you demonstrate readiness to accept responsibility. Parents generally notice your readiness in these areas:

- ▶ You follow the house rules.
- ▶ You perform required tasks reliably and consistently.
- ▶ You act responsibly at school and elsewhere.

If you want more control over relationships, more privacy, more telephone time, or other items or privileges you must bargain for, then your wisest action is to squelch the urge to stomp, whine, or beg. Instead, take a good, hard, honest look at how you'd grade yourself in the key areas just mentioned. If you can see ways of improving, go ahead and do them.

Give me some examples.

Do you crank your stereo up after hours, or do you respect the requests of others for quiet? Do you let your parents know where you are, or must they play a game of "Where's Waldo?" whenever they need you? Is the lawn mowed and the laundry washed, or are your chores piled up? Are your studies under control, or is your teacher working up a lower category than "failing" for your grade?

I see what you mean. Maybe if I figure out how to meet my parents' needs, they'll listen to me more.

That's right, they very well may. The better you can identify and meet your own parents' needs, the easier your task in convincing them of your point of view. Try this: study the three areas of readiness listed above, and go ahead and demonstrate how ready you are to be trusted. Then stand back and

watch as your parents react positively, just as other people would.

You may not be able to influence your parents' every decision, but it's almost a certainty that you will notice a difference in the way you are treated. A final bit of advice: be patient. Remember from the chapter that trust builds over time. So does belief in your maturity. With enough repetition, your parents will be convinced that you are ready to handle whatever life hands you.

Your parents will notice good deeds, because parents are people, too.

541

ON LINE WITH HEALTH

You may want to have your students visit the following URLs, where they will find information and additional Web site resources to enhance their study of this chapter. As with all Web sites, you should check these out first to be sure the information found there is appropriate for your students.

Family Resource Online
http://www. familyresource.com/

family.com
http://family. disney.com/

Family Resource Online is a nonprofit organization. Its site lets families plug in to current information, look out to online resources and speak up about their concerns and interests. Family.com is a comprehensive site sponsored by Disney and devoted to family issues.

Ask them to write that down. Now ask them to plan how to achieve this goal. What will they do differently in the next two weeks? Have students keep these papers in a safe place and refer to them each day to help them practice the change they have decided to make.

stress and social support.

In 1985, a Gallup survey demonstrated the influence of the family upon health-related behavior patterns. Gallup interviewed 1011 adults, asking them how they changed their behavior and who helped them change. They found that a spouse or significant other was more likely to influence a person's health habits than anyone else, including the family doctor. Husbands were twice as likely, for instance, to quit smoking (22 percent versus

11 percent) and more likely to lose weight (42 percent versus 31 percent) than single men.

Research on the family's impact on health provides empiric evidence that family patterns influence such conditions as coronary heart disease, hypertension, diabetes, substance abuse and mental disorders, anorexia nervosa, childhood illnesses, asthma, schizophrenia, and depression.

VOCABULARY

1. a. siblings
  b. birth order
  c. family
  d. grieve
  e. day care
  f. active abuse
  g. stepparents
  h. passive abuse
2. a. dysfunctional family
  b. spouse abuse
  c. child abuse
  d. elder abuse
3. Answers will vary.

RECALL

SECTION 1

1. parents, siblings, aunts, uncles, baby-sitters. (p. 516)
2. They teach the child about being human, about their values, and about whether or not others are to be loved and trusted. (p. 516)
3. It is maintained by keeping rituals, celebrating special occasions together, living with give and take, realizing that family member's attitudes and behaviors affect the nature of the whole family, and spending time together. (p. 518)
4. families, schools, peers, magazines, and television (p. 519)
5. Stage 1—develop trust in each other; Stage 2— develop independence and self-direction in children; Stage 3—develop in children a sense of industry, to

CHAPTER 19 Review

Summarizing the Chapter

Your ability to respond correctly to the following statements ensures your understanding of the main concepts in the chapter.

1. Explain how family influences a person's self-image and outlook on the world.
2. Discuss some of the needs that family fulfills for a person.
3. Describe how a family identity is developed and maintained.
4. List the stages of a family and the main goal of each stage.
5. Define quality time and discuss ways to share quality time with family.
6. Describe some ineffective and effective responses to family conflict.
7. List characteristics of functional and dysfunctional families.
8. Describe some ways society can help meet the changing needs of today's families.

Learning the Vocabulary

family	dysfunctional family
siblings	active abuse
family identity	child abuse
birth order	spouse abuse
quality time	elder abuse
sibling rivalry	passive abuse
grieve	day care
stepparents	

Answer the following questions on a separate sheet of paper.

1. Matching—*Match each of the following phrases with the appropriate vocabulary term from the list above:*
  a. two or more people with one or more parents in common
  b. the placement (oldest, middle, or youngest) of a child among his or her siblings
  c. a group of people who are related by adoption, blood, or marriage, and are committed to each other
  d. to feel emotional pain and suffering over a loss
  e. supervision, usually at a facility, for preschool children or elderly people during daytime working hours
  f. abuse involving one person's aggression against another
  g. people who marry into a family after a biological parent departs through death or divorce
  h. abuse involving not taking needed actions
2. a. A family that deals with things in abnormal ways which can injure self-esteem, is a ____.
  b. ____ is verbal, psychological, physical, or sexual assault on a marriage partner.
  c. ____ is verbal, psychological, physical, or sexual assault on a child.
  d. ____ is verbal, psychological, physical, or sexual assault on an elderly person.
3. Use at least ten vocabulary terms in a paragraph.

Recalling Important Facts and Ideas

Section 1
1. Who are a child's first teachers?
2. What do a child's first teachers teach the child?
3. How is a family identity maintained?
4. From what sources do children learn values?

Section 2
5. List the goals of each family stage.
6. What principle must those interested in gaining trust learn?
7. List four secrets to always being honest and reliable.
8. Explain the meaning of the phrase "time poor."
9. What three things are needed to develop satisfying family relationships?
10. What is the secret to communicating effectively, and swaying people to your way of thinking?

Section 3
11. List the seven factors that often surround divorce.
12. List three rigid rules that a dysfunctional family is likely to have.
13. What is codependency?

542

allow them to work with steady effort; Stage 4—guide adolescent role development, assist identity development in teenagers; Stage 5—maintain relationships with children who leave, renewing the couple's relationship; Stage 6—share talents and resources with others, take pride in accomplishments; Stage 7—maintain satisfaction with life, enjoy fulfillment and serenity. (p. 520)

SECTION 2

6. Trust grows in direct proportion to a per-

Section 4

14. Some people fear that soon society will bear the whole burden for raising its children. What do these people see?

Critical Thinking

1. In what ways are families different from other groups?

2. How would you describe an ideal family?

3. How would you help a friend whose parents are getting a divorce? Make a list of things you would say or actions you would take.

4. In what ways is your family helping to prepare you for life on your own?

5. List each member of your family. Beside each name, list at least one way you could help that person.

6. How do you think parents should handle conflicts with their teenagers?

Activities

1. Look through your local telephone book for services and agencies that focus on families. Make a list of your findings. Your list might include such things as day care centers or counseling centers.

2. Work individually and then as a class to compile a list of family traditions. Are there any traditions on your final list that are shared by all members of your class? If so, what are they? Why do you think some traditions are shared by so many?

3. Create a television or radio advertisement about an organization that offers services to families with problems.

4. Survey a number of people to get their opinions of what an ideal family would be like. Analyze the results to find what answers people have in common. Share your results with the rest of the class.

5. Watch a television program about a family. Do you consider the family portrayed to be healthy or dysfunctional? Give reasons for your answers.

6. Ask an elderly person to describe the changes he or she has seen in families over the years. Make a list of the changes and try to determine whether the changes are positive, negative, or neutral.

7. Make a collection of cartoons about families. Mount the cartoons on a poster board and write a statement about the need for humor in families.

8. Work with a group of three or four other students to design a bulletin board. The board should be in two parts. One part should show a functional family. The other part should show a dysfunctional family. Use drawings, lettered signs, photos from magazines, newspapers, and so on to complete your bulletin board. Be ready to explain your display to the rest of the class.

9. Work with a partner to brainstorm and describe the qualities that you see in your relationships with friends at school, coworkers, teammates, teachers, and so on. Are the qualities you describe also qualities that you would expect to see in relationships within a family? Why or why not?

10. Make a list of the advantages and disadvantages of the following family situations:

▶ Small families
▶ Large families
▶ Being an only child
▶ Being a twin

Get together with a partner and combine your lists. Make posters of the advantages and disadvantages to hang on your classroom wall.

Making Decisions about Health

1. When Rico started to date, his parents' rule was that he be home by 11 p.m. For six months he was always on time. Then, one Saturday night, he didn't get home until midnight. His parents were furious. For the next several months, they reminded him of the incident. It was as if his six months of getting home on time hadn't happened. All they could remember was the one time he was late. The situation has caused a lot of resentment and bad feelings between Rico and his parents. What could Rico have done differently? How could his parents have handled the situation differently? What could be done now to correct the situation and restore good feelings between Rico and his parents?

SECTION 3

11. lower social class, less commitment to religion, great differences in values and backgrounds, young age at marriage, come from divorced families, short time being married, and early childbearing (p. 533)

12. Don't feel—do not admit to unpleasant feelings such as sadness and anger; don't talk—do not discuss problems or unpleasant feelings; don't trust—because you cannot trust those who care for you. (p. 533)

13. It is the characteristic of being focused on the needs of others to the point of neglecting the person's own needs. (p. 536)

SECTION 4

14. They see a world where television is trusted to amuse the children; churches and schools instill them with values and manners; government agencies to provide life's necessities; nannies, day care, malls, sports teams, and video arcades to keep them out of trouble; the police to discipline them; and no one at all to teach them about the value of family. (p. 538)

son's honesty. The opposite is also true; people who are not entirely honest quickly lose the trust of others. (p. 522)

7. try never to promise more than you can reasonably deliver, make allowances for emergencies, let others know what's going on, and plan ahead (p. 523)

8. Time poor means parents may be richer in dollars but they feel cheated of leisure time with their families because they are overworked. (p. 524)

9. time, commitment, and energy (p. 524)

10. using an assertive communication style (p. 528)

KEY POINTS

Chapter 20 is 32 pages long and divided into eight sections. In this chapter students will learn about the reproductive system and its functions, stages of pregnancy, fetal development, the birth process, birth defects, and other associated problems. Students will also study the positive and negative aspects of parenting and will learn to identify abuse.

ACTIVITY TO INTRODUCE THE CHAPTER

These activities will give the students an idea of how much there is to learn about being a parent.

1. Have each student write a short essay entitled, "As a Parent I Will Be . . ." Make sure the students do not write their names at the top, to ensure confidentiality.
2. Shuffle, redistribute the papers, and have them read aloud. You may want to have the students vote on the best future parent.
3. At the end of the chapter, have the students write the same essay again.
4. As these essays are read to the class, ask the students to note the differences between the first set and the second set.

BULLETIN BOARD IDEAS

1. Have students bring in one of their baby pictures. Display them on the bulletin board, numbered individually. Have a contest to see who can identify the greatest number of their classmates.

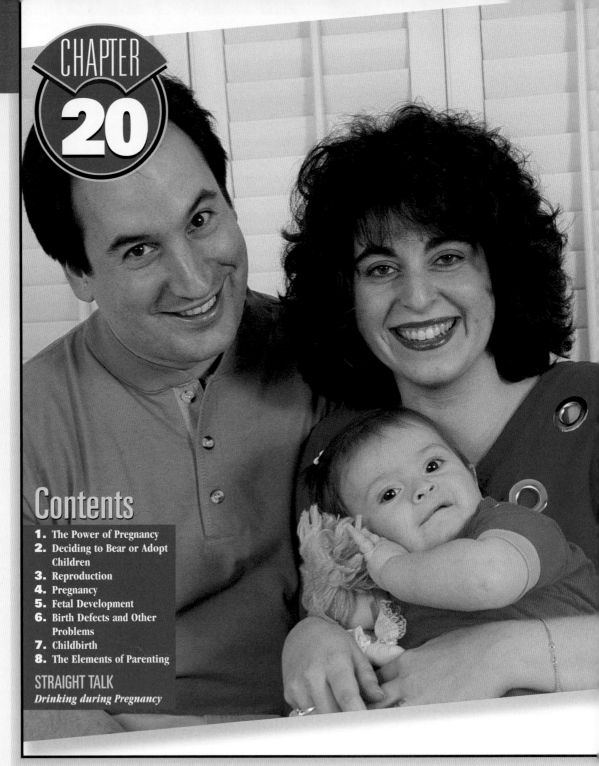

CHAPTER 20

Contents

STRAIGHT TALK
Drinking during Pregnancy

NOT Enough Time?

Following are some suggestions to help you make sure that you cover the key topics in this chapter if you have limited time. (Refer to the daily lesson plans in your Teacher's Resource Box for additional suggestions.)

DAY 1 Assign Sections 1, 2, and 3, and the Fact or Fiction (page 545) and Life Choice Inventory (page 549) features to read prior to class. During class, have students do the Activity to Introduce the Chapter on page 544, the Discussion activity on page 549, and the Focus Activity on page 551. Assign Sections 4, 5, and 6 to be read prior to Day 2.

From Conception through Parenting

What do you think? Are the following statements true or false? If you think they are false, then say what is true.

1. The lifestyle choices a couple makes in the weeks *before* pregnancy can affect their future child's development.
2. A missed menstrual period is a sure sign of pregnancy.
3. A woman can have a miscarriage (spontaneous abortion) without being aware of it.
4. Pregnant women should not be physically active.
5. A woman who is pregnant should "eat for two."
6. Possibly the single most important task in parenting is to help the child develop positive self-esteem.

(Answers on page 571)

Introduction

When people become parents, they change their lives forever. The younger the people, the more impact children will have on their future. In this chapter you will learn about the reproductive process and some basic elements of parenting.

Each student should number a paper according to the number of photographs and then write the name of the classmate next to the appropriate picture number.

2. Start a bulletin board project of the entire chapter, showing the progression from the thought of being a parent to the actual birth. Add new pictures as each section of the chapter is completed to show the growth and development of the child and the family.

Vocabulary worksheets are provided in the Teacher's Resource Box.

Answers to FACT or FICTION

1. **True.**
2. **False.** Nonpregnant women may miss periods because of other factors, and a pregnant woman may have a menstrual period.
3. **True.**
4. **False.** Physical activity during pregnancy may reduce discomfort and help to ensure a quick recovery from childbirth.
5. **False.** A pregnant woman should not "eat for two," or she will gain unneeded fat.
6. **True.**

DAY 2 On Day 2 have the students complete the Focus Activity on page 554, the Discussion activity on page 588, and the Close activity on page 565. Assign Sections 7 and 8 to be read prior to Day 3.

DAY 3 On Day 3 have students complete the Learning with Visuals activity on page 566 and the Group Activity on page 569.

SECTION 1

FOCUS

OUTCOMES

In this section the student will learn:

1. To identify some of the negative consequences of pregnancy.

2. That abstinence from sexual activity can bring certain freedoms.

FOCUS ACTIVITY

Have the students list activities in which they participate. List them all on one half of the board and then ask the students to list all of the things that parents do for their children. List these on the other half of the board. Compare the two lists in terms of time commitments.

TEACH & APPLY

DISCUSSION

Ask students if they have younger siblings. What changes occurred in their lives and the lives of their parents after the birth of their younger sisters and brothers?

COMPREHENSION CHECK

Make sure students understand the key point mentioned in the introduction—the younger they are when they have children, the more the children will change their lives. Can students think of any reasons why this would be so? Ask them to express the meaning of these two sentences in their own

The Power of Pregnancy

The power of pregnancy to affect people's lives is dramatic. Unwed teenage mothers and fathers are deeply affected, and many are taken unawares by the full force of pregnancy on their lives (see Figure 20–1). For the girl, an unplanned pregnancy may alter most of the rest of her life story. She may become isolated from her peers during her pregnancy. If she returns to school afterwards, her schoolmates will have moved on without her. Former boyfriends may now avoid her.

As for the father of a child, he bears legal responsibility for the child's financial support for the next 18 years. Unless the couple gives the baby up for adoption, both his and her freedom to go on to further education and hoped-for careers can be forever lost. Unwed teenage parents are likely to end up with more children than their peers will ever have. Busy from that time on with providing for their children, both parents are forced to neglect their own personal growth. Statistically, children born to teenage parents or to unmarried mothers are far more likely to lead troubled lives themselves later on.

Eleven percent of all teenage girls, or just under 1 million girls, and their partners face unwanted pregnancies each year. In the past, girls were often left to face the burden alone. Today, however, more and more fathers are being held legally responsible. Most states punish nonsupportive parents harshly.

Figure 20–1 Teen Beliefs and Realities about Pregnancy

Belief	Reality
94% believe they would stay in school.	70% eventually complete high school.
51% believe they would marry the mother/father.	81% of teenage births are to unmarried teens.
26% believe they would need welfare.	56% need public assistance to cover the cost of delivery and about a quarter of teen mothers receive public assistance by their early 20s.
32% believe they would consider abortion.	50% of pregnancies to unmarried teens end in abortion.

Source: This report was reprinted with permission of the Henry J. Kaiser Family Foundation of Menlo Park, California. The Kaiser Family Foundation is an independent health-care philanthropy and is not associated with Kaiser Permanente or Kaiser Industries.

Physical risks almost always accompany adolescent pregnancies. The health of both the mother and infant may suffer. These risks are explained in later sections.

The power of pregnancy affects people in less obvious and less dramatic ways, too. Just the fear of pregnancy can damage relationships. Many couples worry and disagree about readiness to bear a child, and they sometimes must make hard choices. When unwanted pregnancies occur, unstable relations are likely to crumble.

For all of the reasons just named, many teenagers find that the

COOPERATIVE LEARNING

Many teens do not understand the impact having a child can have on a young couple. Besides monetary costs (hospital bills, health care, feeding, diapers, day care, clothing, and so on), there are personal costs for the couple (loss of freedom and personal sacrifices).

Having a child during the teen years puts a lot of strain on the social development and personal growth of each young parent.

Divide your class into male/female pairs. Have each pair research the cost of having a baby, beginning with the hospital bill. You may want students to include the costs of complications such as premature delivery, C-sections, and so on. Pairs should figure

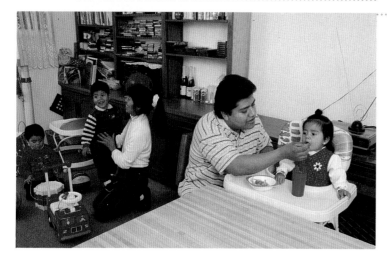

Parenting changes a person's life forever.

choice to abstain from sexual activity brings freedoms—from stress, from worry, and from unnecessary complications. The rest of this chapter assumes that pregnancy is an event welcomed with joy by mature, ready, and loving parents.

 KEY POINTS *Teenagers are often unaware of the many negative consequences of pregnancy. For teenagers, pregnancy often means losses of freedom, education, and financial potential, along with physical risks to both mother and child.*

❝ The value of marriage is not that adults produce children but that children produce adults. ❞

Peter de Vries
(1910–1993)
Journalist

 Review

Answer the following questions on a sheet of paper.

Learning the Facts

1. How many teenage girls and their partners face unwanted pregnancies each year?
2. How many years is a father legally responsible for the financial support of his child?
3. What are the freedoms that come from abstaining from sexual activity?

4. Why are teenage parents forced to neglect their own personal growth?

Making Life Choices

5. Jane is 17 years old, unmarried, and pregnant. Write her a letter explaining what she will likely experience in the months and years to come with regards to treatment by people, goals that will probably not be reached, and so on. Be realistic, but not harsh.

expenses for the obstetrician and pediatrician, baby check-ups, and health insurance.

Next, ask students to determine the income the couple might be able to expect. Have them budget money for rent, utilities, car payment and insurance, and items needed for the baby (crib, car seat, high chair, formula, baby food, clothing, medicine, and so on). Remind students to include child care expenses. (They

cannot say the grandparents will take care of the baby. It is the couple's responsibility.) How much money will be left after all the expenses have been paid?

Mention to students that should a couple decide not to marry, it is still the legal responsibility of both parents to provide the child's financial support.

SECTION 2

FOCUS

OUTCOME

In this section the student will learn:

1. How adoption compares to bearing children.

FOCUS ACTIVITY

Ask if anyone in the class is adopted or knows someone who is adopted. Ask if they would share their personal feelings about being adopted. If no one can personally share, either invite a school administrator or teacher who is adopted to speak or have the class imagine what it might be like to have been adopted. Make a list on the board as students share their ideas.

TEACH & APPLY

BACKGROUND INFORMATION

Some Hawaiians still practice the ancient custom of *hanai,* in which couples with several infants give infants to couples unable to have children. Hanai takes place openly among family and friends, unlike more modern adoption procedures.

SECTION 2

Deciding to Bear or Adopt Children

The decision whether or not to have a child is affected by personal beliefs, needs, and wishes. For example, people may base their decisions on childhood memories or romantic fantasies of what families are like. People need to love and to be loved. They may wish to participate in the human chain of life. Outside pressures—such as a spouse's needs, or parents' or friends' expectations—can also affect these decisions. Finally, people may simply wish to experience being parents. Most decisions, however, should be based on this single question: How would it affect my life if I had a child to raise? After all, children are "forever"—even more so than marriage partners.

Children Are Forever To get an idea how "forever" children are, you can try the following exercise. Pretend an egg is a baby, and that you are its parent. Don't put it down. Carry it from place to place, even while shopping or showering. Bathe it every day. Keep an eye on it at all times. Sleep with it close by. Set your alarm for 2 A.M., and check the egg. Never let it out of

For parents who are ready to accept the responsibility, babies are a joy.

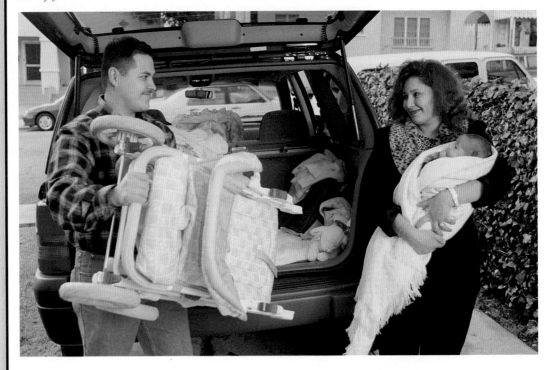

•multicultural issues•

One of today's most heated debates, and one that you may want to present to your students, concerns transracial and cross-cultural adoptions (the placing of a child of one race or culture in a family of another race or culture). Those opposed to these adoptions say that the child's basic identity is diluted by the process. Will these children develop the racial and cultural identities they need? Will they have suitable racial and cultural role models? Will they be sufficiently educated about their cultural and racial history? Will they have the skills to cope with racism?

The adoption community appears to be in agreement that the preferred match unites children with an adoptive family of the same racial and cultural background. The realities to

Are You Ready to Have a Child?

The answers to these questions will help you grasp the impact on life of bearing a child. Your answers to the Life Choice Inventory are personal and private. Share them with others only if you are comfortable doing so.

1. How will having a child affect your schooling or career? It is hard to work full-time and be a full-time parent, too.

2. Someone has to be aware of the child's whereabouts and needs, 24 hours a day, for 18 or so years. During the hours that you can't do it, who will?

3. If your partner is unable to carry the responsibility of parenthood, how will you carry it by yourself?

4. How will having a child affect your relationships with others? Will your partner be willing to share your attention, energy, and love with a baby?

5. Where will you be able to get help (for example, baby-sitters or relatives) when you need to get away? You cannot raise a child without help.

6. Will you be willing to give up much of your free time to devote yourself to the needs of a child? Will your partner? Children limit your freedom to play.

7. Are you willing and able to pay for proper prenatal (before-birth) and newborn care? Pregnant women, new babies, and new mothers have needs that are costly. Can you meet these needs?

8. Are you willing and able to invest your money for years in the well-being of your child? The cost of raising a child to adulthood varies. On the average, however, the cost in the late 1990s was about $150,000.

9. How well would you be able to adjust to raising a less-than-perfect child? Parents always run a small risk of having a child with disabilities.

10. Are you willing to make a new baby the center of attention? The new family member will grab the spotlight, and you may feel neglected.

11. Have you vented anger and frustration on pets or children in the past? If so, wait to have children until you receive help in learning to redirect hostility—important in stopping the pattern of child abuse.

A reproducible copy of the Life Choice Inventory is provided in the Teacher's Resource Box.

your sight unless you can get another person to agree to tend to it as you are doing. Try this for one week, and you will get some sense of what it would be like to care for a child. Multiply the week by 52 for a year, and then by 18 for the duration of active parenthood.

If you find this exercise difficult, remember that rearing a child is more difficult still. An egg requires neither food nor discipline. It does not cry, soil diapers, or get sick. This chapter's Life Choice Inventory offers further insight into how you may be affected by your choice to become a parent.

Adoption and Foster Parenthood   Some mature people are ready to parent. For them, one possible route to parenthood is to adopt. People may

consider, however, are that there are fewer white babies to adopt than babies of other races. At the same time, there are more white families than families of other races who either wish to adopt or are allowed to adopt. Marketing campaigns have encouraged more minority adults and kin to adopt. Some income, housing, and age requirements that served as barriers to adoption in the past have been reduced. Americans have adopted

babies from foreign countries for decades, but government officials have recently made the process more difficult. Countries now are choosing to promote lower birth rates and more in-culture adoptions to prevent cultural genocide.

One point is agreed upon by all—the best interest of the child is met by having a loving family of any race or culture to provide nurturing.

DISCUSSION

Divide the class into small discussion groups. Ask the groups to analyze the issue of adopting versus bearing children. Have students select a leader, recorder, and spokesperson in each group. The leader is responsible for guiding the discussion, following the directions, and staying on task. The recorder is responsible for the group's written work. The spokesperson will share the group's consensus with the entire class. Instruct the recorder to label a piece of paper "Adoption versus Bearing Children." Under each heading create two columns: label these "Advantages" and "Disadvantages." On the reverse side of the paper, have them record final decisions and rationales. Tell the groups to list as many items as they can under the advantages and disadvantages. Then discuss which option they feel is the best choice and why.

BACKGROUND INFORMATION

Tell students that *to foster* means to give parental care to; to nurture. Adoption is permanent, whereas foster care is temporary.

ASSESS

SECTION 2 **Review Answers**

1. spouse's needs, parent's or friends' expectations (p. 548)
2. to offer a home to a homeless child or because they have been unable to bear a child themselves (p. 550)
3. those with medical problems and children of certain other countries (p. 550)
4. Answers will vary.

WORKSHEETS

A reproducible quiz for Section 2 is provided in the Teacher's Resource Box.

CLOSE

Instruct the students to list all the advantages and disadvantages they have learned for each of the following: adoption, teen parenting, being a parent, and choosing not to have children. Have them compare their lists and discuss any different items.

Opening one's home to a foster child can be especially challenging and rewarding.

choose adoption because they want to offer a home to a homeless child or because they have been unable to bear a child themselves.

Adoption is not quick. It requires persistence, patience, and the willingness to work with an agency. Such agencies may seem to "sit in judgment," but they take seriously their job of matching parents and children. They do ask questions about people's private lives, but only so that they can be sure the match is a good one.

Babies with medical problems are usually the easiest to adopt, as are children of certain other countries. Foster parenthood offers an opportunity to care for older children with special needs. Foster children need homes but may not be able to stay permanently. Opening a home—and life—to them is especially challenging and rewarding.

 KEY POINTS *The decision to become parents is often affected by romantic ideas and pressures from others. Those considering parenting must realistically assess how a child would change their lives. Adoption is one route to parenting.*

SECTION 2 Review

Answer the following questions on a sheet of paper.

Learning the Facts

1. What outside pressures do people encounter while deciding whether or not to have a child?
2. Why might people choose adoption?
3. Which children are the easiest to adopt?

Making Life Choices

4. Reread the Life Choice Inventory on page 549, and answer the questions. Do you feel you are ready for parenthood? Why or why not? Do you want to have children? If so, when? What do you want to accomplish before you begin a family? How was this inventory helpful?

HEALTHY PEOPLE 2000

Increase to at least 90 percent the proportion of pregnancy counselors who offer positive, accurate information about adoption to their unmarried patients with unintended pregnancies.

Adoption provides families for children born to couples who are unprepared to raise a child and seek a loving, stable home for their child and is an important method of family planning for infertile couples. Although many prospective parents are waiting to adopt children, there are relatively few infants available for adoption due to the small number (about 25,000) of infants placed for adoption each year. Of the approximately one million adolescent pregnancies annually, fewer than four percent of the children born are placed for adoption. Forty-three percent of adolescent pregnancies end in abortion.

SECTION 3

Reproduction

The beginning of a whole new human being takes place in a single moment. That event is **conception**. Because many complex events lead up to conception, let's review the male and female reproductive systems before proceeding with an explanation of how conception occurs.

Reviewing Reproduction

You have probably already studied the male and female reproductive systems in this course and in earlier health and biology courses. To review some of the changes that take place in your body as the reproductive system develops, you may want to reread the "Physical Maturation" section in Chapter 3. You may also want to reexamine the sections on the reproductive systems in Chapter 6. Following your review, read the next section in this chapter, which describes an extremely important chain of events—the **menstrual cycle**—that directly affects conception.

 KEY POINTS *Earlier chapters in this text will help you review the reproductive process before you undertake a more careful study of pregnancy and parenting.*

The Menstrual Cycle

Among the many ways in which men and women differ is the way they each produce reproductive cells—the **sperm** and the **ova**. In the male body, a constant flow of the hormone testosterone stimulates sperm cells to mature in a steady flow. Sperm mature daily. In the female system, though, only one (or sometimes two or three) ova ripen and are released each month. This cyclic ripening depends on hormonal changes that occur in a monthly rhythm—the menstrual cycle.

Once each month, or every 28 days on the average, the uterus prepares itself to host a pregnancy. The cycle begins with the building up of the uterine lining with soft tissue and a rich blood supply. Sometime after this, often about midcycle, the ripened ovum bursts from the ovary. This is **ovulation**.

The ovum is gently swept into the tubes leading to the uterus. What happens next depends on whether or not sperm cells are present in the reproductive tract—whether or not a man and woman have had sexual intercourse. If the egg encounters sperm cells, it may become fertilized. If fertilized, it may embed itself in the prepared uterine lining, beginning a pregnancy.

The other possibility is that the egg is not fertilized or that the fertilized egg does not embed in the uterine lining. In this case, it passes out of the body unnoticed. With no pregnancy, the uterine lining weakens in the two weeks following ovulation, and is eventually shed. This shedding of the uterine lining is menstruation. Following menstruation, the whole cycle begins anew in preparation for a future pregnancy. The cycle is summarized in Figure 20–2 on the next page.

MINI Glossary

conception: the union of an ovum and a sperm that starts a new individual.

menstrual cycle: the cyclic ripening of an ovum and the preparation of the uterus for pregnancy. Also called the *ovulatory cycle*.

sperm: the male cells of reproduction.

ova (singular, **ovum**): the female cells of reproduction. Ova are also called *eggs*.

ovulation: the ripening and release of an ovum.

While a number of factors influence whether or not a woman faced with an unintended pregnancy places the child for adoption, it is clear that despite positive attitudes toward adoption, pregnancy counselors are often poorly informed about adoption. Many pregnancy counselors do not routinely discuss the adoption option with their clients who are faced with unintended pregnancies. This failure to discuss adoption may stem from the counselor's assumption that clients will react unfavorably to the idea of adoption.

Adoption is a practice with a very long tradition in western society. It should be recognized among providers of prenatal care and pregnancy counselors that adoption can work to the benefit of biological parents, the adoptive parents, and most importantly, the child.

SECTION 3

FOCUS

OUTCOMES

In this section the student will learn:

1. The steps of the menstrual cycle and how it relates to the reproductive process.

2. How conception and fertilization take place.

FOCUS ACTIVITY

Give the students drawings of the male and female reproductive systems, provided in the Teacher's Resource Box. Have students label each part in the systems with the correct term. Have students record the function of each part on the back of the paper, identifying each as they go.

TEACH & APPLY

TEACHER SUPPORT

Key Passage

You may want to tell students the name for the first menstruation—*menarche*. It means the beginning of menstruation. The average age of menarche is 12 or 13, although it could be as early as 9 or as late as 17. Another word they may encounter that means the same as menstruation is *menses*. Both terms come from the Latin word *menses,* meaning month.

LEARNING WITH VISUALS

The transparencies "The Menstrual Cycle," "Sperm Production," and "Fertilization" are provided in the Transparency Acetate Binder.

BACKGROUND INFORMATION

Although the 28-day cycle is regarded as the norm, only about 40 percent of menstruating women actually have a 28-day cycle, and even among these women the length of the cycle may vary. Pubescent girls often experience cycles lasting several months in their first year and a half after the beginning of menstruation.

COMPREHENSION CHECK

To check comprehension, ask students how long the egg can live. (12–24 hours) How long can sperm live? (up to three days) Can intercourse a few days before ovulation produce pregnancy? (yes) Can intercourse two days after ovulation produce pregnancy? (No, the egg would no longer be alive.)

FAST FACTS

A study showed that one-third of the girls and women polled in the survey did not know what was happening to them when they got their first menstrual periods.

Figure 20–2 The Menstrual Cycle. *The cycle begins with bleeding. The lining of the uterus then begins to thicken to become ready to support pregnancy. If no pregnancy occurs, the lining weakens and is shed in menstrual bleeding to start the cycle over.*

Ovulation typically occurs at midcycle, but timing varies

Lining of uterus

1 5 7 11 14 17 21 28 days Day 5 of next cycle

Menstrual flow   Pregnancy may occur   Uterine lining thickens   Menstrual flow

In menstruation, a few tablespoons of blood and fragments of the uterine lining flow from the vagina. Menstruation lasts four to five days on average. These few days of menstrual flow are only the outward sign of the amazing events that have taken place in the body in the earlier four weeks.

Menstruation normally varies from time to time. It may be a little late or early, with lighter or heavier flows. It may last for more or fewer days than expected. Also normal during menstruation are contractions of the muscular uterus—menstrual cramps.

If cramping is uncomfortable, treatment with the over-the-counter drug ibuprofen is usually effective in relieving it. Should cramping become severe or menstrual irregularities become extreme, a health-care provider should check for problems.

 KEY POINTS *The menstrual cycle involves a cyclic shifting of hormones that promote a monthly ripening of an ovum and the preparation of the lining of the uterus for pregnancy. If pregnancy does not occur, the lining is shed in menstruation.*

Conception

What follows is a description of conception. Imagine a family—wife, husband, and baby-to-be. Inside the woman's body, an ovum, tinier than the period at the end of this sentence, has grown ready for **fertilization**. The man has produced millions of even tinier, microscopic sperm cells, as he has done every day since puberty.

Now the man and woman have had sexual intercourse. Sperm swim up the vagina, propelled by their long, whipping tails. The ovum powerfully attracts them to its surface. One sperm finally enters the ovum, triggering an instant change in the ovum's surface so that no more sperm can penetrate (see Figure 20–3). The genetic material of the two cells unite within the fertilized ovum. The ovum implants itself in the uterine wall (**implantation**) and begins to develop. About 60 percent of all fertilized ova either fail to implant or dislodge later, to be lost from the body.

For conception to occur, sexual intercourse must take place within a certain time limit. An ovum lives for just 12 to 24 hours, and living sperm must arrive during this brief life span if they are to fertilize the ovum. Sperm can live for up to three days within the female reproductive tract, so if they

Chapter 20, Section 3

The following quiz will help you assess your students' understanding of the material covered in this section of the chapter. You might use the quiz as an oral exercise, which will lead into a class discussion of the topics covered. Or, you might use it as a paper/pencil

quiz to evaluate your students individually.

*If students have difficulty with the concepts covered in the Quick Quiz and the Section Review, you might suggest they review the material using the **S**urvey, **Q**uestion, **R**ead, **R**ecite, **R**eview (SQ3R) study method, which is described in detail in the introduction to this Teacher's Wraparound Edition.*

1. The creation of a new human being occurs at conception. (True)

Figure 20–3 Fertilization. Sperm from the penis (1) begin the journey toward a ripened ovum, released earlier from the ovary (2). The sperm work together to weaken the ovum's outer layer, but only one sperm can enter (3). (Both sperm and ovum have been greatly enlarged for this illustration.)

get there first, they can wait. Intercourse within a few days before ovulation can easily lead to conception.

A couple who wants to conceive can use the **fertility awareness method**. This method is related to the rhythm method used to prevent pregnancy. It is used to help a woman determine the time of ovulation. The couple can then time sexual intercourse so as to make sure sperm are available at the right time to fertilize the ovum. Drug stores sell at-home urine-testing kits that show a woman when she is ovulating.

 KEY POINTS *In conception, an ovum and a sperm unite to form a fertilized ovum. The fertilized ovum may then implant itself in the wall of the uterus and start a pregnancy. Couples can increase their chances for pregnancy by using the fertility awareness method.*

SECTION 3 Review

Answer the following questions on a sheet of paper.

Learning the Vocabulary

The vocabulary terms for this section are *conception, menstrual cycle, sperm, ova, ovulation, fertilization, implantation,* and *fertility awareness method.*

1. Match each of the following phrases with the appropriate term from the list above:
   a. male cells of reproduction
   b. ripening and release of an ovum
   c. joining of an ovum and a sperm

Learning the Facts

2. Describe how men and women produce reproductive cells.
3. What happens to the egg after one sperm penetrates it?
4. How long do sperm live in the female reproductive tract?

Making Life Choices

5. The menstrual cycle is an important part of reproduction. Why do you think it is important for a girl to understand menstruation? Why is it important for guys to understand the process of menstruation?

MINI Glossary

fertilization: the joining of an ovum and a sperm.

implantation: the lodging of a fertilized ovum in the wall of the uterus.

fertility awareness method: a method of charting ovulation. It involves tracking menstrual periods, body temperature, and types of cervical mucus.

2. The ova is the male reproductive cell. (False)
3. Male reproductive cells, stimulated by testosterone, are produced and mature in a constant daily flow. (True)
4. The female reproductive cell matures once a month according to the menstrual cycle. (True)
5. The monthly building up of the uterus with soft tissue and blood is called ovulation. (False)
6. An unfertilized egg will embed itself in the uterine lining. (False)
7. Cramping and slight irregularities in the menstrual cycle are normal. (True)
8. Menstruation occurs whether or not the ovum has been fertilized. (False)
9. Sexual intercourse up to three days before ovulation can lead to pregnancy. (True)
10. The fertility awareness method is commonly used to avoid conception. (False)

SECTION 4

FOCUS

OUTCOMES

In this section the student will learn the value of:

1. Preparing for pregnancy.
2. Pregnancy tests.

FOCUS ACTIVITY

Before the students read this section, have them brainstorm a list of do's and don'ts for males and females prior to childbearing. Their lists should include any lifestyle behaviors that could possibly benefit or harm their future children.

TEACH & APPLY

GROUP ACTIVITY

Have the students form small groups and prepare posters for a "Prepare Now for Future Children" campaign. The posters should specify do's and don'ts for lifestyle habits.

LEARNING WITH VISUALS

Bring various pregnancy tests into class for the students to see. Discuss the differences among them—accuracy rates, ease of use, availability, and so on.

DISCUSSION

Ask students if they knew that the health of both parents affects the baby. Did they know that the use of drugs by the parents prior to conception could harm the infant?

SECTION 4

Pregnancy

Preparation for a healthy pregnancy begins far in advance. When someone decides, "Yes, I'm ready to have a baby now," that person is in an excellent position to make choices that will give the baby-to-be every possible advantage.

Concerns before Pregnancy

During the three months prior to conception, the ovum of the mother and the sperm of the father go through a maturing process that includes cell division. Anything that prevents or disrupts cell division can damage those new cells at a tender stage. A newly recognized fact is that the man's health habits before conception, as well as the woman's, are important. For at least three months before pregnancy, *both* parents should be free from drugs of all kinds—over-the-counter medications; prescription medications (with the physician's OK); and mind-altering drugs, including alcohol.

Both prospective parents should be well nourished. Nutrition affects the ova and sperm, and good nutrition supports the hormone balance needed for conception. Before pregnancy, a diet that follows the advice of Chapter 7 would well cover the nutrient needs of the future parents.

When a woman whose nutrition has been poor becomes pregnant, she may not have stored the nutrients she needs to produce a healthy baby. For example, the vitamin folate must be in good supply in a woman's diet *before*

Both parents can prepare in advance for a healthy pregnancy.

Pursuing Wellness

Most communities have a number of resources from which you can obtain interesting and informative guest speakers on topics related to teen pregnancy. Suggestions for speakers include:

1. *Social worker:* Ask a local human services professional who deals with adoption or child protection to discuss the effects of teen pregnancy on the child.

2. *Medical professional:* It should be beneficial to have students understand the effects of pregnancy and birth on young girls. Nutrition and prenatal care could also be included in this discussion.

3. *Teen pregnancy hotline director:* Does

she becomes pregnant. Otherwise, her baby has a greater chance of being born with a birth defect affecting the spinal cord or the brain.

Women may be poorly nourished for many reasons. A woman who chooses a poor diet in order to lose weight or who snacks on candies, high-fat snacks, and soda pop may not have full nutrient stores. She may not know how to choose a good diet, or she may not have enough money to buy nourishing food. (Help for these problems is available to those who seek it.) If pregnancy is in a woman's future, she should develop healthy eating habits now. She should also be physically active. Then, once pregnancy is confirmed, she can continue eating and exercising as she did before, and her baby-to-be is likely to be healthy.

 Health habits of both parents prior to pregnancy affect the probable health of the baby-to-be.

Pregnancy Tests

Long before any tests are taken, a woman may suspect that she is pregnant. A typical sign is a missed menstrual period. However, periods are missed for many reasons, and one or two periods can also occur during early pregnancy. For these reasons, missed periods are not an accurate indicator of pregnancy. More reliable are subtle color changes in the woman's cervix and outer genital area, which darken with a bluish cast. Another sign is that the breasts may become tender and full, and the nipples may darken.

A chemical test can confirm that a woman is pregnant. All such tests rely on detecting one of the many hormones present during pregnancy. Home pregnancy test kits are available and are widely used. However, the instructions for using them may not be clear, or the results may be hard to figure out. The tests performed by a medical lab are more accurate.

 Indicators of pregnancy include missed menstrual periods and changes in the woman's body. Chemical tests detect one of the hormones of pregnancy.

SECTION 4 Review

Answer the following questions on a sheet of paper.

Learning the Facts

1. What health habits should both parents be maintaining if they think they may be within three months of starting a pregnancy?

2. Describe the most likely reasons why women might be poorly nourished in our society.

3. List the visible signs of pregnancy in a woman's body.

Making Life Choices

4. Pregnancy tests are expensive. Many women use over-the-counter pregnancy test kits. What are some of the problems in using these kits? Do you think they are effective in diagnosing a pregnancy?

your community have a pregnancy hot-line? Workers at the hotline may be able to offer good information to your students.

4. *Teen parents:* The best information about teen pregnancy and parenthood can come from teens who have experienced it. You will want to have both mothers and fathers participate in the discussion. You

may want to include recent parents, as well as those who have matured and can look back on the experience.

Ask students to develop a series of questions to ask the speakers prior to any of these presentations.

ASSESS

EVALUATE

Assign grades to the "Prepare Now for Future Children" posters (Group Activity, page 554). Criteria for grading:

1. extensiveness of information
2. correctness of content
3. creativity
4. use of color and materials
5. attractiveness

SECTION 4 Review Answers

1. be free from drugs of all kinds and be well nourished (p. 554)
2. by choosing a poor diet in order to lose weight or by snacking on candies, high fat snacks, and soda pop (p. 555)
3. missed menstrual period, bluish cast in the woman's cervix and outer genital area, full and tender breasts, darkening of nipples (p. 555)
4. Answers will vary.

CLOSE

Have each student briefly summarize, in an impromptu speech, the characteristics of a healthy prechildbearing lifestyle, and the best pregnancy tests available (in their opinion). Give them a two-minute time limit. Tell them to make about three main points on each topic.

 A reproducible quiz for Section 4 is provided in the Teacher's Resource Box.

SECTION 5

FOCUS

OUTCOMES

In this chapter the student will learn:

1. The stages of pregnancy from conception to birth.
2. Proper nutritional guidelines for pregnant women.
3. Factors that identify high- and low-risk pregnancies.

FOCUS ACTIVITY

To help students better understand pregnancy (even the boys), let each spend some time wearing an empathy belly.

The Empathy Belly is a 33-pound garment that enables the wearer to experience more than 20 pregnancy symptoms. It comes with an instructional video on its use. It is distributed by Birthway, Inc., 14804 N.E. 75th St., Redmond, WA 98052, 1-800-882-3559.

TEACH & APPLY

GROUP ACTIVITY

Divide the class into groups of two or three. Assign each group to research one of the nine months of pregnancy. Then have each group design a segment of a large bulletin board to show fetal development during their assigned month of pregnancy. Encourage students to use charts, pictures, or drawings to illustrate that stage of pregnancy. When groups have completed their sections, the bulletin board will be a large visual of the stages of pregnancy.

Fetal Development

A day after fertilization, the fertilized egg—even while it is still traveling toward the uterus through the fallopian tube—begins to divide. If the first two new cells become detached at this stage, two babies—identical twins—will begin to develop. (In contrast, if two eggs have been released and fertilized at the same time, the two babies will be fraternal twins, not identical twins.)

In each stage of **gestation** thereafter, the developing future infant is given a name—first **zygote**, next **embryo**, and finally **fetus**. Figure 20–4 displays each stage.

The Zygote

The fertilized egg, upon its first division, becomes a zygote. After the zygote becomes implanted in the uterine wall, cell division goes on and on. Each new set of cells divides again to create a ball of many smaller cells. These cells sort themselves into three layers that eventually form the various body systems.

From the zygote's outermost layer of cells, the nervous system and skin begin to develop. From the middle layer, the muscles and internal organ systems form. From the innermost layer, the glands and linings of the digestive, respiratory, and urinary tract systems form.

KEY POINTS *In the first stage of development, the zygote becomes a three-layered ball of cells. Each layer forms different organ systems of the body.*

The Placenta and Other Structures

After implantation, a whole new organ—the **placenta**—grows within the uterus, shown in Figure 20–5. Two other new structures form. One is the **amniotic sac**, a sort of fluid-filled balloon that houses the developing fetus. The other is the **umbilical cord**, a ropelike structure stretching from the fetus's "belly button" to the placenta. The umbilical cord contains blood vessels that conduct the fetus's blood to and from the placenta. The placenta is a sort of pillow of tissue in which fetal and maternal blood flow side by side. The two bloods never mix. The mother's blood delivers nutrients and oxygen to the fetus's blood across the walls of the vessels. Fetal waste products are carried away by the mother's blood, to be excreted by the mother.

From fertilization through week 2: zygote.

From week 3 through week 8: embryo.

From week 9 through the end of pregnancy (usually the 40th week): fetus. From 8 weeks to birth, the fetus grows 20 times longer and 50 times heavier.

A newborn infant.

Figure 20–4 *Stages of Gestation*

Pursuing wellness

Assign each student a lifestyle habit or other activity that can be harmful during pregnancy. Instruct students to research the effects that habit can have on children. Specify that they should name disorders and complications that could come from the lifestyle habits of one or both parents. They may wish to include information they can secure from interviewing a doctor, nurse, medical resource, or a parent who has had experiences with certain complications due to his or her own personal habits prior to childbearing. Have the student write a report using his/her own research and present

Figure 20–5 *The Placenta*

The trans-parency "The Placenta" is provided in the Transparency Acetate Binder.

The placenta is a highly active organ. It gathers up hormones, nutrients of all descriptions, large proteins such as antibodies, and other needed items and pumps them into the fetal bloodstream. The placenta also releases hormones that maintain pregnancy into the maternal blood.

The placenta must develop normally if the future infant is to grow properly. Should the placenta break down, the fetus would be left with no source of nutrients or oxygen. One reason why nutrition before pregnancy is so important is that the placenta is built largely from nutrient stores already in the mother's body at the start of pregnancy.

 KEY POINTS   *The placenta provides nutrients, other materials, oxygen, and waste disposal for the developing fetus. The placenta maintains pregnancy by producing hormones. Proper placental development is essential to a successful pregnancy.*

The Embryo

An embryo goes through many astonishing changes. The number of cells in the embryo doubles approximately every 24 hours. In comparison, this rate slows to only one doubling during the final ten weeks of pregnancy. The embryo's size changes very little. However, the events taking place are of enormous importance.

At eight weeks, the embryo is only a little more than an inch long. However, it already has a complete (although immature) central nervous system and digestive system, a beating heart, well-defined fingers and toes, and

MINI Glossary

gestation (jes-TAY-shun): the period from conception to birth. For human beings, normal gestation lasts from 38 to 42 weeks.

zygote: the product of the union of ovum and sperm, so termed for two weeks after conception. (After that, it is called an *embryo.*)

embryo (EM-bree-oh): the developing infant during the third through eighth week after conception.

fetus (FEET-us): the developing infant from the ninth week after conception until birth.

placenta (plah-SEN-tah): an organ that develops during pregnancy; it permits exchange of materials between maternal and fetal blood.

amniotic (am-nee-OTT-ic) **sac:** the "bag of waters" in the uterus, in which the fetus floats.

umbilical (um-BIL-ih-cul) **cord:** the ropelike structure through which the fetus's veins and arteries extend to and from the placenta.

BACKGROUND INFORMATION

For enrichment you may want to tell students that one of the functions of the placenta is the preparation of the mother's breasts for lactation (the making of milk). The placenta also shields the fetus from its mother's immune system, which would otherwise perceive the fetus's blood as foreign and would attack it. The placenta serves as a biochemical barrier; it allows dissolved substances to pass to the fetus, but blocks blood corpuscles and large molecules. If you want to give the students more specific information about the hormones involved, tell them that the placenta also serves as an endocrine gland, producing large amounts of progesterone and estrogen, the hormones that maintain pregnancy.

FAST FACTS

The single cell from which we all begin divides to become the 75 trillion cells that constitute an adult human being.

the report to the class.

You might share the following information with students as an example.

According to research at the Boston University School of Medicine, women should not use hot tubs or saunas during the first three months of their pregnancies. Intense heat increases the odds of a baby developing

spinal cord defects such as spina bifida. Using a hot tube or sauna just twice during the first trimester of pregnancy triples the risk.

Use the handout, "Effects of Potentially Harmful Substances on the Fetus," from the Teacher's Resource box with this activity.

GROUP ACTIVITY

Make bingo cards for the class by using all the terms in this section with one term on each square. Make the cards different by mixing up the placement of the terms, like on real bingo cards. (If all cards are the same every student can bingo at the same time.) The teacher will need a set of cards with the description of every term that appears on the student cards. Distribute the cards, one to each student. Students will need markers, like beans or paper. The teacher will draw one description card at a time, and read it aloud. The students must think of which term is being described and look for that term on their cards. If they have the correct term, they use a marker to cover that square. Once a student has markers in a row, column, or diagonally, he or she shouts "bingo!" Have the student read aloud the terms marked on his or her card. A prize or grade points can be given as rewards for winners.

DISCUSSION

Prepare a list of terms dealing with pregnancy. Make a copy of the list for each student, each copy with a different term highlighted. Tell students to study the highlighted term and prepare to teach the class about its meaning. As the student teaches, the rest of the class should take notes.

the beginnings of facial features. Anything that disrupts the embryo's rapid development alters the structure of the body permanently.

 KEY POINTS *The embryo develops rapidly, forming the early stages of all the major organ systems of the body.*

The Fetus

The fetus is the developing infant from the ninth week after conception until birth. The tasks of the fetus are to gain in size and weight. Each organ grows to maturity with its own timing. Each organ has certain **critical periods** during its growth—critical in the sense that the events taking place during those times can occur only then and not later.

Outside events can affect an organ's critical period. If, during the critical period, an organ's cell division is limited by some factor, that organ will be damaged. Forever after, the damaged organ will not function as well as it might have otherwise. Later recovery is impossible. Thus, exposure to a harmful chemical, a nutrient deficiency, or other injury during one stage of development might affect the heart. During another stage, it might affect the developing limbs.

The brain and central nervous system are first to reach maturity in the developing fetus. During its critical period, the fetal brain increases by 100,000 cells *a minute.* Problems during the brain's critical period can limit brain development permanently. Mental functioning throughout life can be subnormal. Pregnancy, then, is clearly a time for a woman to take special care of her health.

 KEY POINTS *The organ systems that started developing earlier grow and develop to make the fetus ready for birth. Each organ has a critical period of rapid growth during which it is especially likely to be injured by negative external factors.*

Spontaneous Abortion

Not all fertilized eggs develop to become infants. About 10 percent fail to implant in the uterus and are shed without anyone's ever knowing they were there. Of those that implant, about half are shed in **spontaneous abortion**, or **miscarriage**. Spontaneous abortion is a natural and expected part of fertility. Many times it prevents imperfect embryos from becoming full-term infants.

Most spontaneous abortions take place early, with no more sign than a heavy menstrual flow. The woman's hormones change, and she may feel depressed but not even know why.

A spontaneous abortion late (after three months) in pregnancy resembles a birth and presents greater hazards. An infection may start in the uterus and spread throughout the body unless caught and treated early. A woman who experiences a late spontaneous abortion may feel grief as intense as if a child had died after full-term birth.

 KEY POINTS *Spontaneous abortion (or miscarriage) is the loss of a zygote, embryo, or fetus from the uterus. It is a natural event in normal fertile women.*

enrichment

You might want to share the following information with students.

The normal gestation period for human beings is 40 weeks. It is difficult, however, to obtain accurate and objective data on the exact length of gestation; therefore, the birth weight of 5.5 pounds or less has been accepted in the medical community as the clinical criterion of prematurity, regardless of the period of gestation. Other measures suggested for prematurity are the crown-to-heel

The Woman's Experience

While the great changes of pregnancy take place in her body, a pregnant woman's life seems to go on much as before, at least outwardly. However, she experiences it differently. Here's an imaginary story to help you understand what the mother-to-be is feeling.

In one family, the mother-to-be, Gina, doesn't want to go out after work anymore. Her pregnancy barely shows, yet she always feels tired. Pablo, the young father-to-be, wonders if she is overreacting. (Pablo is used as an example here of Gina's chief support person. People other than the father may fill this role.)

Pablo doesn't realize that the changes he can see are trivial compared with the dramatic events taking place inside Gina's body. She is producing more blood. Her uterus and its supporting muscles are increasing in size and strength. Her joints are becoming more flexible in preparation for childbirth. Her breasts are growing and changing in preparation for **lactation**. The hormones creating all these changes may also affect Gina's brain and change her mood. She may be having problems with constipation, shortness of breath, frequent urination, backaches, or **morning sickness**.

The nausea of "morning" sickness actually comes at any time of the day or night. It may be a healthy sign, because it results from the many hormones needed to support pregnancy. Sometimes, nibbling on crackers before getting out of bed or snacking on small meals throughout the day helps to relieve it.

Gina needs to be fit now, just as she did before. Physical activity may reduce some of her discomforts and help to ensure a quick recovery from childbirth later on. Most types of physical activity are approved, as long as the abdomen is protected against injury. Gina should progress slowly in an exercise routine if she is just starting one. If she was physically active before pregnancy, she can continue as before, so long as she is comfortable in doing so.

As pregnancy stretches the skin over a woman's abdomen, buttocks, and breasts, the skin's lower layers may begin to painlessly separate, forming scars. The tendency to develop these "stretch marks" runs in families. Perhaps the most a woman can do to control them is to keep her weight gain within the recommended limits. An acne cream has some promise for improving the appearance of stretch marks, but only if applied early, when they are forming.

During pregnancy, as at other times, a woman needs to deal skillfully with stress. Studies suggest that stress can cause changes in the nerve cells of embryos. Pregnant women should practice the relaxation techniques described earlier, in Chapter 4.

Some final advice to Pablo: treat Gina with respect for the changes she must handle. Give her extra love and understanding. Gina, keep Pablo informed as to how you feel. Encourage him to share his feelings, too. Communication between the partners during this time will lay a strong foundation for the shared parenthood ahead.

Relaxing for two.

 KEY POINTS *External changes during pregnancy are minor, compared with the internal changes. Many discomforts can be relieved through physical activity. Pregnant women should relax.*

MINI Glossary

critical periods: periods during development when a body organ is especially sensitive to harmful factors. A critical period is usually a period of rapid cell division.

spontaneous abortion, or **miscarriage:** the expelling of a zygote, embryo, or fetus from the uterus, not induced by medical means.

lactation: the production of milk by the mammary glands of the breasts for the purpose of feeding babies.

morning sickness: the nausea (upset stomach) a pregnant woman may suffer at any time of the day; thought to be related to the hormones that maintain pregnancy.

length (47 centimeters or less), crown-to-rump length (32 centimeters or less), and the ratio of the thorax circumference to the head circumference (less than 93 percent).

While the majority of premature infants develop normally, others develop problems that extend beyond the first few weeks of their lives. Learning difficulties, lower intelligence, physical awkwardness, and vision and hearing impairment are some common problems among premature infants.

GROUP ACTIVITY

Nutrition during Pregnancy

An earlier part of this chapter pointed out that malnutrition *before* pregnancy can affect the health of a future fetus. Malnutrition *during* pregnancy not only can reduce the infant's number of brain cells but also can impair every other body organ and system.

Nutrient needs during pregnancy are greater than at any other time of life. When the baby is born, its body will contain bones, muscles, blood, and other tissues made from nutrients the mother eats. For a pregnant teenage girl, nutrient needs are extraordinary. This is because the food she eats must supply the nutrients not only to support her growing baby but also her own growth. A diet that includes a variety of foods is the best source of all the needed nutrients.

All pregnant women need professional advice on supplements. Experts recommend iron supplements for all pregnant women. Some may need other nutrients. Only a trained health-care provider can recommend a set of supplements that will be right for any one woman. Self-chosen supplements may not meet the pregnant woman's needs or may even be toxic (poisonous).

A woman's nutrient needs increase tremendously in pregnancy, but her energy (calorie) needs increase just a little. A pregnant woman should not "eat for two." If she does, she will gain unneeded fat and give birth to a fat baby. She needs foods with high nutrient levels but low calorie levels. That means she needs a diet about the same as the one recommended in Chapter 7, but with one more serving of milk and vegetables daily, and one more daily serving of meat or meat alternates.

Most women should gain about 25 to 35 pounds—mostly of lean tissue—during pregnancy. This weight gain supports normal growth of the placenta, the uterus, the breasts, and a 7½-pound baby, as well as an increased blood and fluid volume. Figure 20–6 shows an example of how a weight gain of 31 pounds is distributed. Pregnant teens should strive for gains at the upper end of the range, because some of the weight gained is that of their own maturing bodies. Obese women should gain less—about 15 pounds. Their weight gain should not be of fat, but of lean tissue built from nutrient-dense foods.

Most women should gain between 25 and 35 pounds during pregnancy.

Development	Weight Gain (pounds)
Infant at birth	7½
Placenta	1
Mother's added blood	4
Mother's added fluid	4
Growth of uterus	2½
Growth of breasts	3
Fluid to surround infant	2
Mother's fat stores	7
Total	31

Figure 20–6 Example Weight Gain during Pregnancy

 KEY POINTS *Nutrition in pregnancy is critical to health. The pregnant teenager needs nutrients to support both her growth and the pregnancy. Pregnant women need advice from their health-care providers on supplements. A weight gain of 25 pounds or more is advised.*

special needs

Intra-personal

Factor	Effect on Risk[a]
Maternal weight	Too low weight and too high weight increase risk.
Maternal malnutrition	Nutrient deficiencies and overdoses increase risk. Food fads increase risks of malnutrition.
Socioeconomic status	Poverty, lack of family support, and lack of education increase risk.
Lifestyle habits	Smoking, as well as drug and alcohol use and abuse, increases risk.
Age	The youngest and oldest mothers have the greatest risk.
Pregnancies	
Number	The more previous pregnancies, the greater the risk.
Timing	The shorter the time between pregnancies, the greater the risk.
Outcomes	Previous problems predict risk.
Multiple births	Twins or triplets increase risk.
Maternal blood pressure	High blood pressure increases risk.
Sexually transmitted diseases	Many such infections, including AIDS, can attack the fetus and greatly increase risk.
Chronic diseases	Diabetes, heart and kidney disease, certain genetic disorders, and others increase risk.

[a]Among the risks associated with these factors are low birthweight, mental retardation, and a collapsed umbilical cord.

Figure 20–7 Factors Affecting Pregnancy Outcome

High-Risk Pregnancies

Most babies are born healthy, but some are not. Some pregnancies are riskier to the life and health of the mother and fetus than are others. Figure 20–7 lists factors that identify a **high-risk pregnancy**. Many of the factors that threaten pregnancy are easy to control once they are discovered. This is why early **prenatal care** is so important.

Prenatal care supplied by health-care providers is important to the health of pregnant women. Prenatal care affords the opportunity to test for risk factors throughout pregnancy. Many clues to abnormalities are present in samples of maternal blood or urine.

A pregnant teen is considered at special risk. As already mentioned, the demands of pregnancy compete with those of her own growth. Furthermore, pregnant teens have more complications during pregnancy than do older women. A pregnant teen is likely to become anemic (because of low iron stores combined with rapid growth and lack of medical care). She is also likely to experience prolonged labor (because of her physical immaturity).

Glossary

high-risk pregnancy: a pregnancy more likely than others to have problems, such as premature delivery (prior to the 38th week of gestation) or a low birthweight. Many factors contribute to pregnancy risks.

prenatal care: medical and health care provided during pregnancy.

3. *Grief and loss:* Parents may feel they have lost the "perfect" child or "perfect" family life they have always dreamed of.
4. *Fear:* Parents fear the unknown—not knowing what will happen to their child.
5. *Guilt:* Many parents blame themselves for the child's condition. This blame is often justified.
6. *Confusion:* Caring for a special-needs child can be much different from regular child care. Many parents experience over-

load and stress.
7. *Weariness:* New demands and the unknown can cause extreme fatigue.

Many parents are able to deal with these more negative feelings through a process of adjusting expectations and adapting to the situation. Ask students to go through their lists, evaluate them, and see if they came up with ideas that would help to adjust and adapt in positive ways.

Review Answers

1. zygote
2. amniotic sac
3. lactation
4. premature
5. nutrients and oxygen (p. 557)
6. only a little more than an inch long, but already has a complete central nervous system, a beating heart, a complete digestive system, well-defined fingers and toes, and beginnings of facial features (pp. 557–558)
7. See third paragraph on page 559.
8. The demands of pregnancy compete with those of her own growth. A pregnant teen is likely to become anemic and to experience prolonged labor. A pregnant teen is more likely to bear a low birth weight infant, (more likely to experience health problems or die during early infancy than an infant of normal birthweight). (pp. 561–562)
9. Answers will vary.

CLOSE

Have the students complete a creative writing assignment, imagining they are a sperm or an egg. Have them describe the trip from the ovary or testicles, how they met their mates, and what happened after their union. Tell them to use specific descriptions that demonstrate their knowledge of the conception process and stages of pregnancy.

Perhaps the greatest risk, though, is death of the teenage mother's infant. Teenage mothers are more likely than any other age group to bear **low-birthweight** infants.

Many women with high-risk pregnancies give birth to low-birthweight babies (those who weigh less than 5½ pounds at birth). An infant's birthweight is a predictor of the baby's future health. Low-birthweight infants often face illness and early death. Many die before their first birthday. They may be too weak to suck to obtain milk or to cry to win attention. Therefore, their conditions often worsen.

Low birthweight can arise from two causes. One is early birth. When the infant is born early, it is called a **premature infant** (born before the 38th week). Such babies are the right size for the number of days they have spent in the uterus, and their development is normal. They may be small, but they catch up if given proper care. The other cause of low birthweight is growth failure in the uterus. Babies who are small for this reason are called **small for date**. These infants do not catch up as well.

 KEY POINTS *Any of a number of factors can increase the risk level of a pregnancy. One common outcome of a high-risk pregnancy is a low-birthweight baby, who is less likely to survive than is a baby of normal weight.*

SECTION 5 Review

Answer the following questions on a sheet of paper.

Learning the Vocabulary

The vocabulary terms for this section are *gestation, zygote, embryo, fetus, placenta, amniotic sac, umbilical cord, critical periods, spontaneous abortion (miscarriage), lactation, morning sickness, high-risk pregnancy, prenatal care, low-birthweight, premature,* and *small for date.*
Fill in each blank with the correct answer.

1. The product of the union of the ovum and sperm for two weeks after conception is called the _____.
2. The _____ is the "bag of waters" in the uterus, in which the fetus floats.
3. The production of milk by the mammary glands of the breasts for the purpose of feeding babies is called _____.
4. A _____ baby is a baby born before the end of the normal nine months.

Learning the Facts

5. What does the mother's blood deliver to the fetus?
6. Describe an embryo at eight weeks.
7. Describe what is taking place inside Gina's body when she is pregnant.
8. Why is a pregnant teen at special risk?

Making Life Choices

9. Why is early prenatal care so important to pregnant teens?

quiz to evaluate your students individually.

1. In the first stage of gestation the fertilized egg becomes a zygote. (True)
2. The placenta, uterus, and umbilical cord are three new structures that develop within the womb during the early stages of pregnancy. (False)
3. The placenta produces hormones and provides nutrients which support the developing fetus. (True)

Chapter 20, Section 5

The following quiz will help you assess your students' understanding of the material covered in this section of the chapter. You might use the quiz as an oral exercise, which will lead into a class discussion of the topics covered. Or, you might use it as a paper/pencil

SECTION 6
Birth Defects and Other Problems

Although most infants are born normal, some have **congenital** abnormalities—*congenital* meaning "from birth." Some of these conditions are diseases. Others involve abnormally formed body parts, and these are known as **birth defects**. Congenital abnormalities can arise from many causes. Two of them, genetic inheritance and exposure to harmful chemicals or radiation before or during the development of the fetus, are discussed here. Others include accidents during childbirth, severe nutrient imbalances, and exposure to excessive heat, to name a few.

Inherited Problems

Certain abnormalities run in families. A **genetic counselor** can advise a family on the odds of bearing a child with a congenital abnormality and help them choose whether to bear or adopt children.

Down Syndrome A risk associated with pregnancies of older-age parents is bearing a child with **Down syndrome**. Down syndrome is an inherited condition that causes the child to be born with many physical abnormalities and mental retardation. The condition starts at fertilization, when an error in the transfer of genetic material occurs. The error is then repeated and passed on to every cell of the child's body.

PKU Many other inherited conditions affect offspring. For example, **PKU (phenylketonuria)** is the inherited inability of the cells to handle one of the amino acids (parts of protein). Brain damage causing severe mental retardation can result if PKU goes untreated. At birth, every baby born in the United States is tested for PKU by the medical attendant so that PKU babies may be given a special diet right away to prevent brain damage.

Many inherited problems can be prevented or controlled with special diets or drugs. Thanks to appropriate prenatal care and tests such as **amniocentesis**, the overwhelming majority of babies are born healthy.

 KEY POINTS *Congenital abnormalities are inborn conditions that last throughout life. Down syndrome and PKU are examples of abnormalities caused by genetic inheritance.*

Harmful Chemicals and Other Factors

Chemicals, radiation, and many other factors cause birth defects. Such factors may damage developing organs directly. They also may act by limiting the supply of oxygen or nutrients to the fetus. Many attack the genetic material of the dividing cells. When the genetic material in a cell of a developing embryo or fetus is damaged, the damage multiplies with every division. The final, completed organ of which those cells are a part remains abnormal throughout life.

Alcohol and Other Drugs Many drugs, including alcohol (see this chapter's Straight Talk section), are known to damage developing fetuses.

MINI Glossary

low birthweight: a birthweight of less than 5½ pounds (2,500 grams), used as a predictor of poor health in the newborn infant.

premature infant: an infant born before the 38th week of gestation.

small for date: a term used to describe an infant underdeveloped for its age, often because of malnutrition of the mother.

congenital (con-JEN-ih-tal): present from birth.

birth defects: physical abnormalities present from birth.

genetic counselor: an advisor who predicts and advises on the likelihood that congenital defects will occur in a family.

Down syndrome: an inherited condition of physical deformities and mental retardation.

PKU (phenylketonuria): a congenital disease causing severe brain damage with mental retardation if left untreated; now detected and treated at birth.

amniocentesis (am-nee-oh-cen-TEE-sis): a test of fetal cells drawn by needle through the woman's abdomen.

SECTION 6

FOCUS

OUTCOMES

In this section the student will learn about:

1. Common congenital abnormalities and birth defects.
2. Tests to detect possible problems or abnormalities with the fetus.
3. The adverse effects of drug use before pregnancy on a child's development.

FOCUS ACTIVITY

Ask the class to list any birth defects and abnormalities that they can think of. Write these on the board. The students should make their own lists at the same time at their desks. Ask them to share where they heard about these, and what they know about them.

TEACH & APPLY

CLASS ACTIVITY

Assign each student one of the defects or problems that the class brainstormed in the Focus Activity. Have students read and study the topic, and be prepared to report to the class all they can find out about that defect. Allow the students to make oral presentations several days later.

FAST FACTS

If a woman contracts rubella (German measles) during the first three months of pregnancy, her child has a 50 percent chance of suffering brain, eye, ear, or heart abnormalities.

4. The fetus is the term which describes the developing infant from the ninth week after conception until birth. (True)
5. Organs that do not develop properly during their critical period may reach maturity at a later stage. (False)
6. Spontaneous abortion is another term for miscarriage and is a natural part of fertility. (True)
7. Very few of the changes that occur during the early months of pregnancy are visible externally. (True)
8. Prenatal care is ineffective in offsetting the dangers of a high-risk pregnancy. (False)
9. A teenage mother must meet the nutritional needs of both her infant and her own developing body. (True)
10. Teenage mothers are especially at risk to bear low-birthweight and premature infants. (True)

FIELD TRIP

Arrange a tour of the local hospital's labor and delivery area. Arrange to have the tour conducted by a health-care professional who can point out specific care areas for babies born with defects or abnormalities. Allow the students to ask questions and receive answers from the tour guide. Have the students take notes during this tour and write a summary of the main points they learned concerning birth disorders and problems.

BACKGROUND INFORMATION

As enrichment tell students about the *Rh factor*. Blood tests performed early in pregnancy establish whether or not a woman's blood contains the Rh factor. If a woman with Rh-negative blood conceives a child with Rh-positive blood (inherited from the father), her body may detect the Rh factor's presence in the fetus and develop antibodies against it.

Your supplementary material contains a handout listing some of the more common tests that health care providers use during pregnancy to detect potential problems. For enrichment you may want to distribute the handout in your supplementary material entitled "Effects of Potentially Harmful Substances on the Fetus."

FAST FACTS

Only 15 percent of birth defects have a known genetic cause.

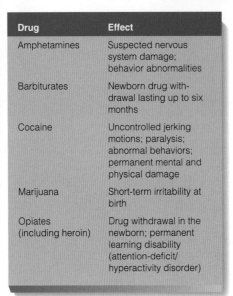

Drug	Effect
Amphetamines	Suspected nervous system damage; behavior abnormalities
Barbiturates	Newborn drug withdrawal lasting up to six months
Cocaine	Uncontrolled jerking motions; paralysis; abnormal behaviors; permanent mental and physical damage
Marijuana	Short-term irritability at birth
Opiates (including heroin)	Drug withdrawal in the newborn; permanent learning disability (attention-deficit/hyperactivity disorder)

Figure 20–8 Some Negative Effects of Drugs of Abuse on Pregnancy

How to Keep a Pregnancy Safe

1. Avoid drugs, smoking, and alcohol.
2. Exercise moderation in other things, such as physical activity and caffeine use.
3. Avoid environmental toxins.
4. Skip unnecessary X rays.
5. Obtain proper nourishment.

Most drugs of abuse also harm developing fetuses. Their effects are still under study. Some of the known ones are listed in Figure 20–8.

Nutrition and Spina Bifida Even large doses of some nutrients can be harmful in pregnancy—especially large doses of vitamins A, B_6, C, and D; the mineral iodine; and other minerals. A diet lacking fruits and vegetables can also be harmful. This diet is also likely to lack an important vitamin, folate. Such a diet, eaten *before* pregnancy occurs, jeopardizes the nerve development of a fetus conceived later. Normal development of the brain, nerves, and spine depends on folate to prevent **spina bifida** (shown in Figure 20–9) and other **neural tube defects**. These common defects range from a child born with a mild defect of the spine that causes little trouble to one who lacks a brain and dies shortly after birth.

About half of all neural tube defects are believed to be preventable by an adequate intake of folate before and during pregnancy. For this reason, all cereals, breads, rice, pasta, and other foods already enriched with other nutrients must now also contain extra folate. That way, the future infants of women who eat few vegetables and fruits are protected.

Smoking and SIDS Pregnant women should not smoke. Smoking limits the delivery of oxygen and nutrients to the growing fetus. The more a mother smokes, the smaller her baby will be. The pregnant woman who smokes risks retarded development of her infant and complications at birth. The effects can last throughout childhood.

In addition, **sudden infant death syndrome (SIDS)**—the sudden, unexplained death of an infant—may be linked to a woman's cigarette smoking during pregnancy. SIDS may even be linked to smoking by others in the household—the environmental tobacco smoke discussed in Chapter 14. Finally, the surgeon general has warned that maternal cigarette smoking causes death in otherwise healthy fetuses and newborns.

Caffeine Should pregnant women give up coffee, tea, and colas because of the caffeine they contain? Too much caffeine may lower infant birthweight. However, the caffeine in a cola or two is well within safe limits. When people give too much attention to relatively safe practices, they tend to forget what is really important. There would be little point in a woman's giving up colas and continuing to smoke two packs of cigarettes a day, for example. The Health Strategies feature, "How to Keep a Pregnancy Safe," sums up the risk factors most important to avoid during pregnancy.

Environmental Hazards Hazards from environmental contaminants are severe. The problem of environmental contamination is enormous, and it affects everyone. Thus it is given an entire chapter (Chapter 24) of this book. A woman who fears that she may have been exposed to an environmental danger should call a hotline to find out what to do. Even ordinary household chemicals, such as insecticides or cleaning fluids, should be used with extreme care.

Like chemicals, radiation of certain kinds can harm cells. Radiation passes through cells and disrupts their genetic material. One way a fetus might be exposed to such radiation is

Chapter 20, Section 6

The following quiz will help you assess your students' understanding of the material covered in this section of the chapter. You might use the quiz as an oral exercise, which will lead into a class discussion of the topics covered. Or, you might use it as a paper/pencil

quiz to evaluate your students individually.

Like the Quick Quiz, the Section Review can also be used as an assessment tool to spark class discussion or as an individual student evaluation. It can also be used as a review in preparation for this quiz.

1. A scar obtained during childhood is an example of a congenital abnormality. (False)
2. Genetic counselors can predict the likeli-

Spina bifida

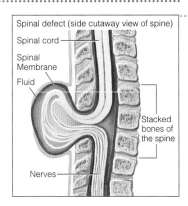
Spinal defect (side cutaway view of spine)
Spinal cord
Spinal Membrane
Fluid
Stacked bones of the spine
Nerves

Figure 20–9 Spina Bifida—A Neural Tube Defect. Normally, the bony spine fully encases the spinal cord, which is easily injured. In spina bifida, the bones of the spine never fully close around the cord. In the serious form shown here, membranes and fluid have bulged through the gap, and nerves are exposed. This leads to some loss of movement and, often, to mental retardation.

Braxton hicks
True Labor

through X rays. If an X-ray examination becomes necessary, the woman who knows or suspects that she is pregnant should inform all medical personnel. Diseases such as rubella and compounds in spoiled foods also can harm a fetus.

The harmful agents discussed here are only a few of thousands that we are exposed to every day. However, the odds of being affected by them are small. The body can tolerate small doses and repairs damage quickly, especially when it is well nourished. Parents who have nourished themselves well, who have avoided drugs and alcohol, who have obtained medical care, and who have been reasonably careful around chemicals and other harmful factors can look forward with happy anticipation to the next step of parenting—childbirth.

KEY POINTS *Pregnant women should avoid drugs, including alcohol and tobacco. They should use care around chemicals and other harmful agents.*

SECTION 7 Review

Answer the following questions on a sheet of paper.

Learning the Vocabulary

The vocabulary terms for this section are *congenital, birth defects, genetic counselor, Down syndrome, PKU (phenylketonuria), amniocentesis, spina bifida, neural tube defects,* and *sudden infant death syndrome (SIDS).*

1. Outline an article about birth defects. Use each term above in your outline.

Learning the Facts

2. Identify some causes of abnormalities in pregnancy outcome.
3. Why shouldn't pregnant women smoke?

Making Life Choices

4. What can you do to encourage parents to keep pregnancies safe?

MINI Glossary

spina (SPY-nah or SPEE-nah) **bifida** (BIFF-ih-duh): a birth defect often involving gaps in the bones of the spine, leaving the spinal cord unprotected in those spots. The cord may bulge and protrude through the gaps in the spinal column.

neural (NER-uhl) **tube defects:** a group of birth defects caused by interruption of normal development of the neural tube, the tissue from which the brain and spinal cord form. The term *neural* refers to nerve tissues.

sudden infant death syndrome (SIDS): the unexpected and unexplained death of an apparently well infant; the most common cause of death of infants between the second week and the end of the first year of life; also called *crib death.*

ASSESS

EVALUATE

SECTION 6 Review Answers

1. Answers will vary
2. genetic inheritance; exposure to harmful chemicals or radiation before or during the development of the fetus; accidents during childbirth; severe nutrient imbalances; exposure to excessive heat (p. 563)
3. Smoking limits the delivery of oxygen and nutrients to the growing fetus, resulting in retarded development and complications at birth. (p. 564)
4. Answers will vary.

WORKSHEETS

A reproducible quiz for Section 6 is provided in the Teacher's Resource Box.

CLOSE

Have the students construct charts listing inherited problems, problems not genetic in nature, and problems due to chemicals. Assign each student one of the topic areas. Students are to find at least one specific disorder associated with that type of problem and prepare an informational chart regarding that disorder. Display the chart in the classroom. Allow time for the students to view the charts and record notes on every disorder charted.

hood of birth defects. (True)
3. Down syndrome and PKU are both untreatable congenital abnormalities. (False)
4. An overdose of vitamin A during pregnancy can be harmful to the health of the developing fetus. (True)
5. A diet lacking in fruit and vegetables is likely to be lacking the essential vitamin folate. (True)
6. Alcohol is not known to cause birth

defects. (False)
7. Smoking during pregnancy will reduce the size of the fetus. (True)
8. Sudden infant death syndrome (SIDS) may be linked to second-hand smoke. (True)
9. Pregnant women should give up all forms of caffeine. (False)
10. Insecticides, radiation, and compounds in spoiled foods are forms of environmental hazards. (True)

565

SECTION 7

FOCUS

OUTCOMES

In this section the student will learn about:

1. The events and procedures of childbirth.

2. Different types of birth.

FOCUS ACTIVITY

Show the class a childbirth film. Local prenatal clinics, health departments, and childbirth class instructors at local hospitals have films readily available. There are many from which to choose. Have the students take notes during the film and write a brief explanation of the childbirth process.

TEACH & APPLY

LEARNING WITH VISUALS

Using charts and models of childbirth, which can be purchased or borrowed from health agencies, describe the steps of the birth process. Be sure to name specific body parts that are involved.

TRANSPARENCIES The transparency "Stages of Childbirth" is provided in the Transparency Acetate Binder.

SECTION 7

Childbirth

If you could look into a pregnant woman's uterus just before birth, you might notice that the fetus seems to be breathing. It is practicing, readying its fully formed lungs for the endless succession of breaths that will support life for some 70 or more years to come. The fetus wakes up, smiles, kicks, rolls over, stretches, sleeps, and dreams. It may suck its thumb. Its tiny hands may grasp the umbilical cord. The pregnant woman is well aware of these activities. When the fetus kicks, she knows it. It is she who is kicked. When the fetus hiccups, its mother feels tiny, rhythmic movements.

As the time for birth nears, conditions become cramped in the fetus's tiny quarters. Its head then turns downward and fits snugly into the mother's pelvis, an event called **lightening**. The mother feels relief from the pressure on her cramped stomach, heart, and lungs. She can breathe and eat more easily.

Near term, the mother may perceive mild contractions of her uterus and think that **labor** has begun. Termed **false labor** by some, mild contractions are common throughout later pregnancy. A more descriptive name might be "warm-up contractions," because they indicate that the muscular uterus is practicing for the hard work of the birth that will follow. Labor bears an appropriate name. It is the hardest of all physical efforts. Once labor has begun, the woman cannot rest until it is finished.

Labor and Delivery   Labor begins as the woman's hormones cause the muscles of her uterus to contract powerfully and rhythmically. Thereafter, labor proceeds by stages. In the first one, the **dilation stage**, the cervix dilates until the baby's head can pass through it. In this stage, the contractions become more and more powerful and closer and closer together.

Then a transition occurs, bringing on the still more powerful contractions of the **expulsion stage**. In this stage, the baby's head starts to emerge from the birth canal (**crowning**), the amniotic sac breaks (if it has not broken already), and the baby is born. Sometimes the birth attendant (physician or midwife) makes a small cut, an **episiotomy**, in the vaginal wall to prevent tearing of tissue during birth. The final stage of labor, the **placental stage**, consists of several final contractions that expel the placenta, or **afterbirth**.

Cesarean Delivery   Nearly all babies dive into the world head-first. Rarely, a **breech birth** occurs. In a breech birth, the baby is born feet or buttocks first, the head last. About half of these few cases pose no extra problems. In some cases, the attendant may decide to call for a surgical birth, or **cesarean section**. The physician then cuts through the mother's abdomen and lifts the baby and placenta out.

A baby who is too large to pass safely through the mother's pelvis may also be delivered by cesarean section. If other problems arise during labor—such as signs that the baby is being stressed, or the mother is bleeding excessively—a cesarean birth may be chosen as the safest way to deliver the child. Cesarean sections are relatively safe for both mothers and babies. However, recovery for mothers involves more healing and takes longer.

The birth of a baby marks the start of a new life for the whole family.

QUICK QUIZ

Chapter 20, Section 7

The following quiz will help you assess your students' understanding of the material covered in this section of the chapter. You might use the quiz as an oral exercise, which will lead into a class discussion of the topics covered. Or, you might use it as a paper/pencil

quiz to evaluate your students individually.

Like the Quick Quiz, the Section Review can also be used as an assessment tool to spark class discussion or as an individual student evaluation. It can also be used as a review in preparation for this quiz.

1. When a fetus turns downwards in the womb in preparation for birth, it is called lightening. (True)

2. The mild contractions of the uterus in

Changes after Delivery With the birth of her infant, the mother normally loses all the weight of the fetus, the placenta, and the associated fluids. She is left with the body fat she gained during pregnancy. Breastfeeding can draw on these fat stores and help the woman lose weight. Without breastfeeding, many women lose these pounds within a few weeks or months, but it may take more effort to do so.

Some women feel depressed after giving birth, feel like crying, or are unable to sleep. Such discomforts may result from the sharp changes in hormone levels that occur after birth or from simple exhaustion caused by the baby, who doesn't yet sleep for long stretches. New fathers, too, sometimes experience this **postpartum depression**, or "the blues." Spending a few weeks quietly alone with family sometimes helps to ease the adjustments.

The time after childbirth brings changes for everyone in the household. Not only is there a new baby to care for. There are also new roles to play. Suddenly, a woman is a mother, a man is a father. All these changes seemingly happen overnight. Everyone may be a bit uncertain in playing the parts at first.

Slowly, though, a new routine sets in. The new ways become as comfortable as the old ones were. However, what routine is best? Now that you have children, what do you do with them?

 KEY POINTS *Childbirth progresses in stages. It may be preceded by false labor. Some women experience depression after giving birth.* Latent active transisirent

Answer the following questions on a sheet of paper.

Learning the Vocabulary

The vocabulary terms for this section are *lightening, labor, false labor, dilation stage, expulsion stage, crowning, episiotomy, placental stage, afterbirth, breech birth, cesarean section,* and *postpartum depression.*

1. Match each of the following phrases with the appropriate term from above:
 a. warm-up contractions that many women experience before the birth process
 b. a surgical cut made during childbirth when the vagina cannot stretch enough without tearing to allow the baby to pass
 c. the emotional depression a new mother or father experiences after the birth of an infant

Learning the Facts

2. What activities does the fetus do before birth?
3. Describe the stages of labor.
4. Present the reasons why a cesarean section may be necessary.

Making Life Choices

5. Beau and Molly are having their first child and are quite concerned. The doctor thinks the baby is too big to be delivered vaginally. The doctor suggests a cesarean section. What should Beau and Molly do?

Mini Glossary

lightening: the sensation a pregnant woman experiences when the fetus settles into the birth position.

labor: contractions of the uterus strong enough to push the fetus through the vagina for delivery.

false labor: warm-up contractions that many women experience before the birth process.

dilation stage: the stage of childbirth during which the cervix is opening.

expulsion stage: the stage of childbirth during which the uterine contractions push the infant through the birth canal.

crowning: the moment in which the top (crown) of the baby's head is first seen.

episiotomy (eh-PEEZ-ee-OT-oh-me): a surgical cut made in the vagina during childbirth when the vagina cannot stretch enough without tearing to allow the baby to pass.

placental stage: the final stage of childbirth, in which the placenta is expelled.

afterbirth: the placenta and membranes expelled after the birth of the child.

breech birth: a birth in which the infant is born in a position other than the normal headfirst position.

cesarean (si-ZAIR-ee-un) **section:** surgical childbirth, in which the infant is taken through a cut in the woman's abdomen.

postpartum depression: the emotional depression a new mother or father experiences after the birth of an infant.

ASSESS

EVALUATE

Without the benefit of notes, models, or drawings, have the students list the stages of childbirth in the correct order, and give brief explanations of each step.

SECTION 7 Review Answers

1. a. false labor **b.** episiotomy **c.** postpartum depression
2. See the first paragraph on page 566.
3. *dilation stage*—the cervix dilates until the baby's head can pass through it; *expulsion stage*—the baby's head starts to emerge from the birth canal, the amniotic sac breaks, and the baby is born; *placental stage*—several final contractions that expel the placenta (p. 566)
4. a breech birth, a baby who is too large to pass safely through the mother's pelvis, signs that the baby is being distressed, the mother is bleeding excessively (p. 566)
5. Answers may vary

CLOSE

Have the students create a series of drawings to illustrate the birth process. Encourage them to label the body parts and record information about each step in the procedure to describe the process completely.

preparation for birth are often called false labor. (True)
3. Labor is begun by the voluntary contraction of the woman's uterus. (False)
4. The dilation stage of labor is followed by the expulsion stage, in which crowning and the breaking of the amniotic sac usually occur. (True)
5. Episiotomy is the last stage of labor. (False)
6. During the placental stage the placenta is expelled from the woman's body. (True)
7. In a breech birth, the baby is born head first. (False)
8. A cesarean section is a surgical procedure in which the baby is removed through the mother's abdomen. (True)
9. Breastfeeding may speed weight loss after a pregnancy. (True)
10. The depression that some women experience after giving birth is called postpartum depression. (True)

SECTION 8

FOCUS

OUTCOMES

In this section the student will learn to:

1. Debate the issues of breastfeeding versus formula feeding.
2. Identify positive parenting strategies.
3. Develop personal plans for being positive parents.

FOCUS ACTIVITY

Have students list as many positive parenting skills and negative parenting skills as they can in two minutes. Discuss the skills that they listed.

TEACH & APPLY

DEBATE

Have the students, under your direction, discuss the advantages and disadvantages of breastfeeding and formula feeding. Then divide the class into two teams: one for breastfeeding, and one for formula feeding. Have the groups study their issues and be prepared to debate the opposing group. Allow time in class for the debate. Use the handout, "Breast Milk Versus Formula," in the Teacher's Resource Box as reinforcement of the advantages of breastfeeding and formula feeding.

SECTION 8

The Elements of Parenting

Parenting is a skill that can be learned. While it is true that almost everyone has had a model to follow—that of their own parents—most people would do well to learn more about the needs of children. Doing what comes naturally may not always be best for the child. One of the first parenting decisions a couple is called upon to make is how to feed their newborn.

Breastfeeding or Formula Feeding?

In most cases, the best food for an infant is the mother's own milk. Of course, a woman can choose freely between feeding breast milk or formula. Both will support growth of the infant equally well. However, breast milk

 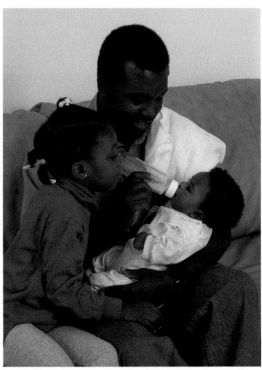

Both breast milk and infant formula are nourishing foods for growing babies but experts recommend breastfeeding whenever possible.

Ability Levels

On Level

High school health education classes have the unique opportunity to impact a significant portion of the population by influencing the health decisions and lifestyle choices of future adults. Thus, health education is one of the most important courses offered in a secondary education curriculum. Many school administrators undermine this concept by asserting that anyone can teach health. Don't be misled; research has shown that the individual classroom teacher is the most important variable for quality learning to result. A dynamic health offers additional benefits. Especially if the infant is premature, if the family has little economic support, or if other factors act to the baby's disadvantage, then breastfeeding is the best choice for the first four to six months of life.

The earliest form of breast milk, **colostrum**, protects the infant against diseases. Glands in the mother's breasts transfer immunity factors such as antibodies from the mother's blood to the colostrum. Later breast milk contains immunity factors, too, but the milk of the first few months is richest in them.

Just a few women should not breastfeed their babies. For example, if a woman abuses drugs, the drugs will usually be secreted in her breast milk. Drug addicts, including alcohol abusers, are capable of taking such high doses that their infants will become addicted through the breast milk. (Most prescription drugs, however, do not reach nursing infants in large enough quantities to harm them.) Also, women who test positive for the AIDS virus should not breastfeed uninfected babies, because the virus can be passed to the infant through breast milk.

 Breastfeeding offers some unique advantages to most babies, but formula supports growth as well as breast milk. Some women should not breastfeed because of drug abuse or infection.

Meeting Children's Needs

Parenting is not a one-way process. It is not just adult people acting on little ones. Children contribute to it, too. Children participate in their own development from early on. They make conscious choices and take advantage of opportunities presented to them. Their own choices, to a great extent, determine the adults they will become.

A parent's job is to support a child's development. This includes providing for all of their physical, emotional, and social needs.

Physical Needs Parents must, above all, meet their children's physical needs. From infancy until they are financially able to stand alone, children need food, clothing, play activities, school equipment, the company of other children, transportation to wherever these resources are, and health care. Parenting manuals offer details on these topics.

Every child needs healthy food and physical activity throughout growth. The role of food is easily explained. Infants and children need nutrients, from which they build their bodies. However, it has been shown that food, even nutritious food, without love is not enough. Given touching and attention, children grow better than they would otherwise.

Physical activity is also important. Children don't get enough exercise just by being children. In fact, the children of today are less fit, fatter, and more disease-prone than at any time in the past. Young children need physical activity. It is up to adults to give them opportunities for it.

Emotional and Social Needs As for a child's emotional and social needs, look at Erickson's scheme of the development of children in Chapter 3. This scheme is also a statement of the tasks for parents. Parents are supposed to help their children develop trust, autonomy, initiative, and industry. In other words, parents are supposed to nurture and shape the person who will someday be an adult.

Possibly the single most important task for the parent is to instill in the child a strong sense of self-esteem. As earlier chapters showed, the feeling that "I am OK, I am worthwhile" helps an individual to be effective in every

> **66** *The commonest fallacy among women is that simply having children makes one a mother—which is as absurd as believing that having a piano makes one a musician.* **99**
>
> Sydney Harris
> (1917–1986)
> American journalist and editor

Glossary

- - **colostrum** (co-LAHS-trum): a milk-like substance rich in antibodies; the breast milk made during the first few days after birth.

GROUP ACTIVITY

Divide the class into groups and assign each group one year of child development. One group takes birth to one year, one takes one to two years, and so on, as far as you deem necessary to assign all the groups a different stage. Have the groups decide on and prepare a chart of positive parenting skills for that stage of development. Encourage the class to consult some outside medical professionals and parents, and to do some research to gather additional information. Have them relate the specific parenting skills to certain developmental characteristics that occur at that stage. Refer them to Chapter 3. Have the groups pass their completed charts to the other groups. They should analyze and critique each other's charts until each group has had a chance to view each chart.

GROUP ACTIVITY

Have the groups from the previous activity assemble the parenting skills from their research and classmates' evaluations into a parenting skills pamphlet. Have each group type a concise list. Assign jobs within each group for publication of this pamphlet (designing a cover, assembling, printing, editing, and circulating). The class should culminate this activity by publishing and circulating their parenting skills pamphlet.

education teacher who is positive, encouraging, and knowledgeable can have a tremendous impact on the environment and attitude of the entire school.

One of the best methods for reinforcing an idea or illustrating a concept is to tell a story. Even if students do not long remember their teacher, they will likely remember a good

story. An instructor's knowledge and experience can be crafted into a story to illustrate a point in class. Telling a story about going to Lamaze classes, racing to the hospital at midnight, or experiencing the birth of a first child, can be far more meaningful than reading about childbirth in a textbook.

GUEST SPEAKER

Invite someone who teaches parenting classes, or works in the sheriff's office or for social services, to talk about child abuse cases. The speaker can include topics such as causes of abuse, intervention strategies by the county or local sheriff's office, and how learning good parenting skills can help prevent some types of abuse.

GROUP PROJECT

Divide the class into groups of three or four students. Have each group design a poster to promote the reporting of child abuse. A Child Abuse Hotline number for reporting should be displayed. Check with your local agencies for the current and local numbers.

FAST FACTS

Every two minutes someone abuses a child. Every two hours a child dies from abuse.

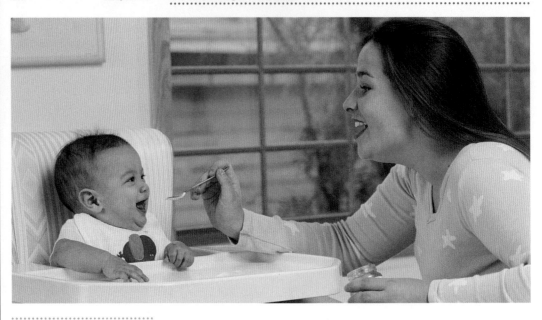

Nutritious foods help grow a healthy baby.

area of life. These include relationships with others, work, play, and contributions to society. Also vital is to place limits on behavior—that is, **discipline**. Having reasonable limits makes children feel safe.

Many people have grown up in less-than-ideal family circumstances. Parents whose own childhoods included physical, sexual, or psychological **child abuse** tend to become abusive themselves. This behavior becomes especially likely whenever their own needs are not met. People frustrated by life may discipline with anger, and may unknowingly inflict **shaken baby syndrome** on young children. Babysitters may do this, too, unless they are warned never to shake a baby. Chapter 19 provided details about dysfunctional families—the kind in which child abuse takes place.

Child abuse is illegal, of course. You can help prevent it. If you ever encounter a suspected case of sexual or other abuse of a child, believe the child. The majority of children's reports of such situations are truthful. Seek expert help, support, and counseling for the child and for the abuser. You can report child abuse without giving your name. Check the "Abuse Registry" in the front of your phone book for a toll-free number.

Some common threads draw together all the theories of child development. Children are not miniature adults. That is, they think and reason in ways unique to children. Children develop in known stages. Each child proceeds through those stages at his or her own pace. The process depends partly on the child's own genetic tendencies and partly on the environment furnished by adults.

 KEY POINTS *Parents must provide for their children's physical, emotional, and social needs. Perhaps the most important aspect of parenting is to foster children's self-esteem. Child abuse is illegal.*

QUICK QUIZ

Chapter 20, Section 8

The following quiz will help you assess your students' understanding of the material covered in this section of the chapter. You might use the quiz as an oral exercise, which will lead into a class discussion of the topics covered. Or, you might use it as a paper/pencil

quiz to evaluate your students individually.

Like the Quick Quiz, the Section Review can also be used as an assessment tool to spark class discussion or as an individual student evaluation. It can also be used as a review in preparation for this quiz.

1. Parenting skills are natural and cannot be learned. (False)
2. Colostrum is a form of breast milk which helps protect the infant against infection

Outdoor play benefits everyone.

Answers to FACT or FICTION

Here are the answers to the questions at the start of the chapter.

1. **True.**
2. **False.** Nonpregnant women may miss periods because of other factors, and a pregnant woman may have a menstrual period.
3. **True.**
4. **False.** Physical activity during pregnancy may reduce discomfort and help to ensure a quick recovery from childbirth.
5. **False.** A pregnant woman should not "eat for two," or she will gain unneeded fat.
6. **True.**

SECTION 8 Review

Answer the following questions on a sheet of paper.

Learning the Vocabulary

The vocabulary terms in this section are *colostrum, discipline, child abuse,* and *shaken baby syndrome.*
Fill in each blank with the correct answer.

1. _____ is a substance produced by the breasts before they begin producing milk.
2. Verbal, psychological, physical, or sexual assault on a child is called _____.
3. _____ is the shaping of behavior by way of rewards and/or punishments.

Learning the Facts

4. Why is breastfeeding a baby in the first few months after birth important to the baby's health?
5. What is possibly the single most important task for the parent?
6. How can you prevent child abuse?

Making Life Choices

7. Your best friend, Brianna, has been psychologically abused all her life. After reading this section, what action would you take to help your friend? Why would you take that action?

MINI Glossary

discipline: the shaping of behavior by way of rewards and/or punishments.

child abuse: verbal, psychological, physical, or sexual assault on a child. Child abuse was also defined in Chapter 19.

shaken baby syndrome: a collection of symptoms resulting from violent shaking of an infant or young child. It is the most common cause of mortality and long-term disability resulting from intentional head injury.

ASSESS

EVALUATE

SECTION 8 Review Answers

1. colostrum
2. child abuse
3. discipline
4. Glands in the mother's breasts transfer immunity factors such as antibodies from the mother's blood to colostrum, the earliest form of breast milk. These immunity factors are then transferred to the baby. (p. 569)
5. to instill in the child a strong sense of self-esteem (p. 569)
6. If you should confront a suspected case of child abuse, believe the child and seek expert help, support, and counseling for the abuser and the child. (p. 570)
7. Answers will vary.

WORKSHEETS A reproducible quiz for Section 8 is provided in the Teacher's Resource Box.

CLOSE

Review with students the parents' responsibilities of meeting a child's needs. Make sure they understand the gravity of the situation. If possible, invite a social worker to class to discuss the importance of fulfilling a child's needs as he or she grows.

and diseases. (True)
3. Women who have AIDS, who abuse alcohol, or who use drugs should not breastfeed their babies. (True)
4. Children do not actively contribute to their own development. (False)
5. Parenting includes providing for a child's emotional and social, as well as physical, needs. (True)
6. Touching and attention improve a child's growth. (True)
7. Children are naturally active and do not need to be provided with physical activities. (False)
8. A parent's primary task is to instill self-esteem in her/his child. (True)
9. Moderate discipline restricts children and causes them to feel insecure. (False)
10. A child's development depends both on genetic tendencies and on the environment. (True)

Straight
Talk

You may want to tell your students that of the leading causes of mental retardation, FAS is the only one that is preventable. The surgeon general has issued a statement that pregnant women should drink absolutely no alcohol. Containers of beer, wine, or liquor must now carry the warning. "Women should not drink alcoholic beverages during pregnancy because of the risk of birth defects."

Guest Speaker

Invite a physician or a registered nurse who works in the infant intensive care unit to come and talk to the class. The speaker should cover the kinds of problems that alcohol causes in babies. Perhaps the speaker could also supply statistics as to the percentage of infants with teen mothers who are born with fetal alcohol syndrome.

Straight Talk

Drinking during Pregnancy

Drinking alcohol during pregnancy can cause **fetal alcohol syndrome** (**FAS**). The fetal brain is delicate, and its normal development depends on a steady supply of glucose and oxygen. Alcohol reduces the blood flow to the fetal brain and so reduces the brain's supplies of these vital substances. In addition, alcohol itself crosses the placenta freely and directly damages the brain.

About 1 in every 750 children born in the United States is a victim of FAS. Three times as many babies are not diagnosed with FAS, but are born with minor damage from alcohol that cannot be seen until later. The mothers of these children drank, but not enough to cause the visible, obvious effects of FAS.

What are the symptoms of fetal alcohol syndrome?

At its most severe, FAS involves:

- ▶ Retarded physical growth, both before and after birth.
- ▶ Damage to the brain and nerves, with mental retardation, poor coordination, and hyperactivity.
- ▶ Abnormalities of the face and skull.
- ▶ Many major birth defects (defects in major organ systems—heart, ears, genitals, and urinary system).

In cases of less severe damage, **fetal alcohol effect (FAE)**, the symptoms are subtle—hidden under a normal-looking exterior. Parents of such babies may not suspect any defects, yet they may exist. They can

be disastrous: learning disabilities, abnormal behaviors, walking problems, other coordination problems, and more.

How much alcohol does a woman have to drink to cause FAS?

Clearly, 3 ounces of alcohol (the amount of alcohol in six beers or six hard-liquor drinks) a day is too much. However, as few as two drinks a day can cause the damage of FAS. The most severe damage is likely to be done in the first month, even before the woman is sure she is pregnant. Even if the woman stops drinking immediately after she learns that she is pregnant, it may be too late to prevent all the damage.

Women who drink two drinks a day are also more likely to have spontaneous abortions (miscarriages), perhaps because alcohol poisons the fetus. In one study, women who drank as little as two drinks *a week* were found to have more miscarriages than nondrinkers. Thus, in some cases, it appears that very small amounts of alcohol can endanger fetuses.

What about the timing? Why is the first month so crucial?

Oxygen is critical to the development of the fetus's central nervous system. A sudden dose of alcohol can halt the delivery of oxygen to the developing fetus. During the first month of pregnancy, even a few minutes of alcohol exposure and oxygen lack can cause major damage to the rapidly growing brain.

The effects of FAS are severe and lifelong. A person who was exposed to alcohol before birth may respond differently to alcohol in adulthood. That person may also respond differently to some drugs. Learning disabilities also last a lifetime. They are

572

enrichment....

Alcohol is only one of many drugs that can affect a developing fetus. The nicotine in cigarettes can reduce blood flow to the fetus by restricting the capillaries in the mother's body. The burning cigarette itself increases carbon monoxide levels in the mother's blood, further restricting oxygen delivery to the fetus.

Smoking during pregnancy can cause the placenta to separate from the womb too soon, causing a miscarriage. Malformation of the fetus's heart and other organs is also a possibility, which again, could lead to miscarriage.

Many common drugs such as tranquilizers, anticonvulsants, and even antibiotics can seriously affect the developing fetus. Aspirin, which is an anticoagulant, has been linked to blood disorders in fetuses.

Alcohol, drugs, and other environmental factors can harm developing infants.

caused by even low levels of alcohol intake. Not every learning disability is caused by alcohol in pregnancy, but no doubt some are. Some experiments even show ill effects from alcohol consumed *before* pregnancy occurred. The *Journal of the American Medical Association* advises women to stop drinking as soon as they *plan* to become pregnant.

It is important to know, though, that if a woman has drunk heavily during the first two thirds of her pregnancy, she can still prevent some damage by stopping heavy drinking during the last third.

 Do any authorities say that a few drinks during pregnancy are not harmful? No drinking at all seems extreme.

The answer is no. The authorities are all on one side—against drinking. On the other side, there was one opinion, but it has been changed. The American Council on Science and Health (ACSH) expressed the view, at first, that adult women who drank only a little during pregnancy should not be made to feel guilty. Recently, though, the ACSH has changed that opinion. It now says this:

Probably an occasional glass of beer or wine is tolerable in pregnancy . . . provided that one drink does not lead to another. Total prohibition of drinking is an unacceptable rule for many people. Nevertheless, we believe that many pregnant women will prefer to give up drinking for the duration of pregnancy.

 Is that the position of this book?

Yes, it is. It is a personal choice, but if we had it to make, we would choose the healthy baby.

MINI Glossary

fetal alcohol syndrome (FAS): a cluster of birth defects, including permanent mental and physical retardation and facial abnormalities, seen in children born to mothers who abuse alcohol during pregnancy. Also defined in Chapter 13.

fetal alcohol effect (FAE): a subtle version of FAS, with hidden defects including learning disabilities, behavioral abnormalities, and motor impairments.

573

The effects of illegal drugs have become fairly common knowledge in recent years. Mothers addicted to cocaine or heroine give birth to infants who are similarly addicted. The infants go through withdrawal, which can be life threatening. Babies born to cocaine addicts are often premature, extremely fragile, and jittery. They tend to have lower birth weight, smaller head circumference, and shorter body length than babies not exposed to cocaine.

You might have students do further research on children who are exposed to drugs in the womb. Their research should include answers to questions such as these: Is their learning impaired? If so, to what extent? How do these children function in school? What, if anything, are schools doing to help these children?

VOCABULARY

1. a. embryo **b.** implantation
c. morning sickness
d. Down syndrome
e. breech birth
2. a. Gestation **b.** umbilical
cord **c.** Low birth weight
d. PKU (phenylketonuria)
e. Crowning
3. a. colostrum **b.** afterbirth
c. lightening **d.** conception

RECALL

SECTION 1

1. They are more likely to lead troubled lives. (p. 546)

SECTION 2

2. How would it affect my life if I had a child to raise? (p. 548)

SECTION 3

3. It may embed itself in the prepared uterine lining, beginning a pregnancy. (p. 551)
4. It shrinks in the two weeks following ovulation and is eventually shed. (p. 551)
5. four to five days on the average (p. 552)
6. sexual intercourse while an ovum is present in the woman's body (p. 552)
7. 12 to 24 hours (p. 552)

SECTION 4

8. Nutrition affects the ova and sperm, and good nutrition supports the hormone balance needed for conception. (p. 554)

CHAPTER 20 Review

false labor
dilation stage
expulsion stage
crowning
episiotomy
placental stage
afterbirth
breech birth
cesarean section

postpartum depression
colostrum
discipline
child abuse
shaken baby syndrome
fetal alcohol syndrome (FAS)
fetal alcohol effect (FAE)

Summarizing the Chapter

Your ability to respond correctly to the following statements ensures your understanding of the main concepts in the chapter.

1. List the consequences and risks of teen pregnancy for the mother, father, and child.
2. Describe the phases of the menstrual cycle and how conception occurs.
3. Describe the signs of pregnancy and the tests used to confirm it.
4. Describe the development of the fertilized egg from conception to birth.
5. Discuss why early prenatal care and a healthy lifestyle are important to the development of the unborn baby.
6. Identify birth defects and other problems that may occur during pregnancy.
7. Describe the birth process.
8. Discuss the responsibilities of being a parent.

Learning the Vocabulary

conception
menstrual cycle
sperm
ova
ovulation
fertilization
implantation
fertility awareness method
gestation
zygote
embryo
fetus
placenta
amniotic sac
umbilical cord
critical periods
spontaneous abortion or miscarriage

lactation
morning sickness
high-risk pregnancy
prenatal care
low-birthweight
premature
small for date
congenital
birth defects
genetic counselor
Down syndrome
PKU (phenylketonuria)
amniocentesis
spina bifida
neural tube defects
sudden infant death syndrome (SIDS)
lightening
labor

Answer the following questions on a separate sheet of paper.

1. *Matching*—Match each of the following phrases with the appropriate vocabulary term from the list above:
  a. the developing infant during the second through the eighth week after conception
  b. lodging of a fertilized ovum in the wall of the uterus
  c. the nausea a pregnant woman may suffer at any time of the day
  d. an inherited condition of physical deformities and mental retardation
  e. a birth in which the infant is born in a position other than the normal head-first position
  f. milk-like substance rich in antibodies, made in the mother's breasts during the first few days after birth
  g. the placenta and membranes expelled after the birth of the child
  h. the sensation a pregnant woman experiences when the fetus settles into the birth position
  i. union of an ovum and a sperm that starts a new individual

2. a. _____ is the period from conception to birth.
  b. The rope-like structure through which the fetus's veins and arteries reach the placenta is called the _____.
  c. _____ is a birthweight of less than 5½ pounds, used as a predictor of poor health in the newborn infant.
  d. A congenital disease causing severe brain damage with mental retardation if left untreated is called _____.
  e. _____ is the moment during childbirth in which the top of the baby's head is first seen.

574

SECTION 5

9. hormones, nutrients, large proteins, and other needed items (p. 557)
10. The fetus would be left with no source of nutrients or oxygen. (p. 557)
11. the brain and central nervous system (p. 558)
12. imperfect embryos from becoming full-term infants (p. 558)
13. most types of physical activity, as long as the abdomen is protected (p. 559)
14. The number of the infant's brain cells can be reduced and every other body organ and system can be impaired. (p. 560)
15. 25 to 35 pounds (p. 560)

Recalling Important Facts and Ideas

Section 1

1. How might the child of teenage parents be affected later in life?

Section 2

2. What question should be asked before a couple decides to have a baby?

Section 3

3. What happens to the egg in the woman's body after it is fertilized?

4. Explain what happens to the uterine lining when the egg is not fertilized.

5. How long does menstruation last?

6. What must happen for conception to occur?

7. How long does the female's ovum live?

Section 4

8. Why is it important for parents to be well nourished before they start a pregnancy?

Section 5

9. What does the placenta pump into the fetal bloodstream?

10. Explain what happens to the fetus if the placenta breaks down.

11. Which body systems reach maturity first in the developing fetus?

12. What does spontaneous abortion or miscarriage often prevent?

13. What kind of physical activity is best for a pregnant woman?

14. Describe the effects of malnutrition during pregnancy.

15. What is the recommended weight gain for a pregnant woman?

Section 6

16. What are some factors known to damage developing fetuses?

Section 7

17. Describe what the doctor does when a woman has a cesarean section.

18. Why do people say that labor bears an appropriate name?

Section 8

19. Under what conditions should women not breastfeed their babies?

20. In what ways must parents provide for their children's physical needs?

Straight Talk

21. Describe the symptoms of fetal alcohol syndrome.

22. Explain why the first month of pregnancy is so critical to the development of the fetus.

Critical Thinking

1. Reread the Straight Talk section on page 572 entitled "Drinking during Pregnancy." Notice how critical the first month of pregnancy is. Note that most women do not even know they are pregnant in the first month. What can be done to help women who drink alcohol when they might be pregnant? Why do you think so many babies are born with fetal alcohol syndrome? How can we educate women about this problem? What can we do to help the infants born with fetal alcohol syndrome?

Activities

1. Call an adoption agency and ask them how long it would take to adopt a baby. Ask about babies from all ethnic groups. Which babies are the quickest to be adopted and why? Which babies take the longest to be adopted?

2. Interview your parents about your birth. What type of birth was it? Was your father present for your birth? Describe how the labor process was for your mother.

3. Write a one-page essay on your philosophy of rearing children. What things would you definitely do? What things would you definitely not do? Be sure to tell why you would or would not do the things you list.

Making Decisions about Health

1. Autumn and Jason have been married for only six months and don't feel they're ready to have a baby. They use no contraceptives and try to time sexual intercourse so that they avoid the "dangerous" time of the month, but neither is certain of exactly when that time is. So far, Autumn hasn't gotten pregnant.

   a. What is your opinion of the way Jason and Autumn are dealing with their situation? Why do you feel as you do?

   b. What do you think the outcome of this situation might eventually be and why?

575

SECTION 8

19. if a woman takes drugs, abuses alcohol, or tests positive for the AIDS virus (p. 569)

20. food, clothing, play activities, school equipment, the company of other children, transportation to wherever these resources are, and health care (p. 569)

STRAIGHT TALK

21. retarded physical growth, before and after birth; damage to the brain and nerves, with mental retardation, poor coordination, and hyperactivity; abnormalities of the face and skull; many more major birth defects (defects in the major organ systems—heart, ears, genitals, and urinary system) (p. 572)

22. Oxygen is critical to the development of the fetus's central nervous system, which occurs during the first month of development. Even a few minutes of alcohol exposure and oxygen deprivation at this crucial time can cause major damage to the rapidly growing brain. (p. 572)

SECTION 6

16. Answers will vary; could include: radiation, chemicals, smoking, alcohol, drugs, environmental contaminants, compounds in spoiled food, large doses of Vitamins A, B_6, C, and D. (pp. 563–565)

SECTION 7

17. makes an incision through the mother's abdomen and lifts the baby and placenta out (p. 566)

18. It is the hardest of all physical efforts, and the woman cannot rest until it is finished. (p. 566)

OUTCOMES

Chapter 21 is 18 pages long and divided into four sections. It begins by making a distinction between sex and sexuality and explaining the differences and the much broader meaning of these terms. Chapter 21 also introduces students to sexual activities, sexual myths, and sexual orientation. Students have the opportunity to explore their own attitudes and feelings as they study these topics.

ACTIVITIES TO INTRODUCE THE CHAPTER

1. Have students list every place from which they get sexual information. Have them rank the list in two ways: from most to least reliable and from most to least accessible. The list might include: friends, magazines, parents, teachers, books, TV, movies, church, and so on. Compare the students' lists and their rankings.

2. Another possibility for an introductory activity is for the students to brainstorm, either as a class or in small groups, 101 ways to show love without having sex.

3. Have each student interview a parent, grandparent, or friend about dating customs when he or she was the student's age. As a class, develop a list of interview questions to be used. Share these interviews as oral reports or make a class book of interviews. This is a good long-term project and can be effective to strengthen school/community ties.

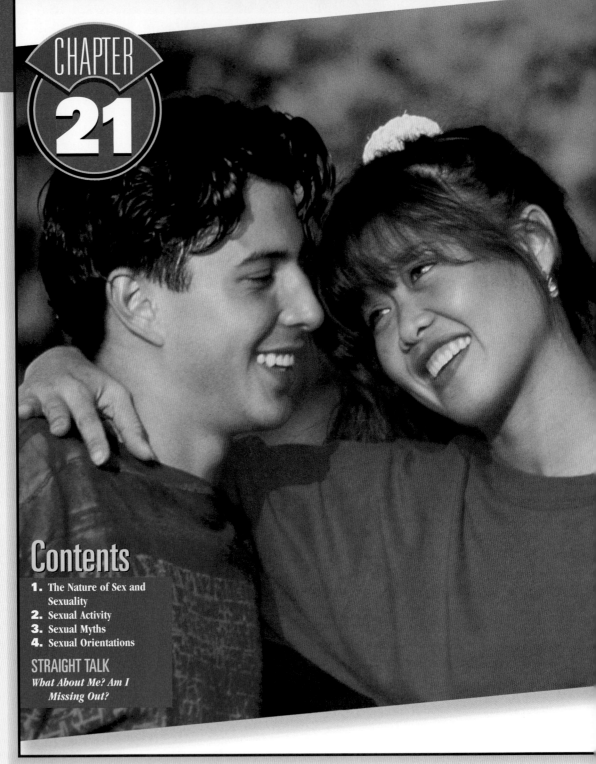

CHAPTER 21

Contents

STRAIGHT TALK
What About Me? Am I Missing Out?

NOT Enough Time?

The following are some suggestions to help you make sure you cover the key topics in the chapter if you have limited time. (Refer to the daily lesson plans in your Teacher's Resource Box for additional suggestions.)

DAY 1 Have students read Sections 1 and 2 prior to class. During class have students complete the Activity to Introduce the Chapter

Understanding Sexuality

FACT or FICTION

What do you think? Are the following statements true or false? If you think they are false, then say what is true.

1. The term *sexuality* refers to sexual activity—primarily sexual intercourse.
2. Activities such as touching, hugging, and kissing can be emotionally satisfying, as well as physically satisfying.
3. At puberty hormones produced by the body create a drive for reproduction.
4. The most important sex organs—the organs that control sexual behavior—are the penis and the clitoris.
5. Aphrodisiacs are not really able to enhance or restore people's sexual desires and abilities.
6. Homosexuals are all alike in terms of their lifestyles.

(Answers on page 588)

Introduction

What is **sex** for? What is **sexuality** all about? Sex and sexuality are such interesting subjects, and so personally important, that people seldom back off far enough to look at them from a scientific point of view. It's worth a minute to think about this, though, for sex and sexuality play important roles in all of nature.

BULLETIN BOARD IDEAS

To go along with number 3 under Activities to Introduce the Chapter, have each student bring in photographs of their parents, grandparents, and other family members when they were dating. Display the photographs prominently in the classroom.

Answers to FACT or FICTION

1. **False.** Sexuality is part of a person's personality from birth to death, with or without sexual activity.
2. **True.**
3. **True.**
4. **False.** The brain, not the penis and clitoris, is the most important sex organ.
5. **True.**
6. **False.** If you tried to identify "the" homosexual lifestyle, you could not do it.

on page 576, the Discussion activity on page 582, and the Quick Quiz on pages 582–583.

DAY 2 Have students read Sections 3 and 4 prior to class. During class complete the following activities: Discussion on page 585,

Learning with Visuals on page 587, and the Quiz Quizzes on pages 586–587 and 588–589 if time allows.

SECTION 1

FOCUS

OUTCOMES

In this section students will learn:

1. The meaning and purpose of *sex* and *sexuality*.

2. The means through which the human genetic code is passed from parents to children.

FOCUS ACTIVITY

Have students describe themselves in a list of attributes or *traits* (hair and eye color, height, artistic abilities, and so on). Then have them describe both their parents and their grandparents on both sides. Compare the lists to find traits that may have been transferred down through the generations.

TEACH & APPLY

TEACHER SUPPORT

Key Passage

Ask students to describe the purpose of sex. (It guarantees that living things will reproduce and that they will mix to create new combinations.) Ask students if they think these results of sex are positive. You may want to tell them to consider what the world would be like if living things were reproduced by cloning, which does not create different combinations. Would the world be a better or worse place to live?

SECTION 1

The Nature of Sex and Sexuality

Sex plays two major roles in nature. First, it ensures that living things reproduce their kind—that pine trees produce more pine trees; that eagles produce more eagles; and that human beings produce more human beings. Second, sex ensures that the hereditary materials individuals carry (the genes) are repeatedly shuffled and dealt out in different combinations in every new individual.

Human Genetic Inheritance

Here's how this shuffling of the genes works. You have, in the cells of your body, genes from your mother and genes from your father, for every characteristic that makes you you. Your genes govern surface traits such as your eye color, skin color, and hair color. They also direct deep-down traits, such as your musical ability (or lack of it), your friendliness or competitiveness, and many other things about you.

The potential to develop these traits was passed on to you at the moment when you were conceived. Half of them came from your father and half from your mother. The mixture determined what sort of person you turned out to be. Of course your life experiences contribute to how you turn out, too, but many limits on what you can become are set by your genes.

If it comes time for you to take part in creating a new individual, you will pass on half of this new person's traits—but they won't be your mother's half, or your father's half. They will be a mixture. You may pass on the potential to develop your mother's brown eyes and love of learning, and your father's strong hands and sense of rhythm. Your partner will also pass on a mixed set of traits, some from each parent. The child you produce will end up with a new combination never before seen in a human being. The child may, for example, have brown eyes from your mother, a sense of rhythm from your father, special mathematics ability from your partner's mother, and skill at sports from your partner's father.

Every new child is a brand-new individual, carrying a combination of traits never tried before, thanks to sexual reproduction. Sex, in short, provides a way to mix inherited traits into new combinations in every generation. Each living thing, whether it is a pine tree, an eagle, or a human being, has a unique chance to try a new way of living and thriving in an ever-changing world.

For sex to work, every individual must reduce his or her genetic material by half and then have the opportunity to get together with another indi-

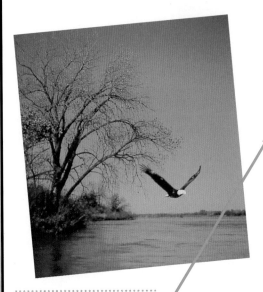

Most living things, including eagles and trees, reproduce their kind using sexual reproduction.

For Your Information

Conception was discussed in Chapter 20 of the textbook.

HEALTHY PEOPLE 2000

Increase to at least 85 percent the proportion of people aged 10 through 18 who have discussed human sexuality, including values surrounding sexuality, with their parents and/or have received information through another parentally endorsed source, such as youth, school, or religious programs.

Parents are the first and most important educators of their children in matters related to sexual behavior. From them, children receive their first lessons in sexual morality and appropriate sexual conduct, including lessons about the meaning of mutual respect, love, and marital fidelity.

Children also learn about sexuality from other sources, their schools, their peers, and the mass media. Most young people consider their parents their most important source of vidual and combine halves. That is exactly what takes place when sexual reproduction occurs. The male contributes half of his genes in a sperm. The female contributes half of hers in an egg. The sperm and egg combine, and a new individual begins to develop. (The same process does occur in eagles, and it is only slightly different in pine trees. In pine trees, it is pollen, not sperm, that carries genes from one individual to another.)

Every type of living thing survives on earth only so long as it can reproduce. For that reason, the sex drive is very strong—it must be to ensure that reproduction will take place. That is why each person's sexuality has such an influence on the person's life. The attraction between the sexes is a deep-down, basic, instinctual attraction that leads to the continuation of life. It is also linked with the expression of one of the highest forms of human emotional and spiritual development—committed, mature love.

 Sex ensures that living things reproduce, and that new combinations of genetic material emerge in every generation. Two parents each donate half of their own genetic material to create a new individual.

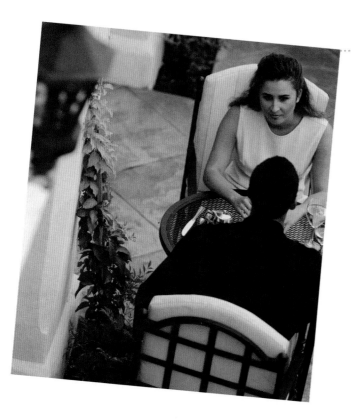

Sexual attraction motivates the expression of love.

MINI
Glossary

sex: a general term used to mean both gender and sexual intercourse.

sexuality: the quality of being sexual. Sexuality is part of the total person: physical, emotional, social, intellectual, and spiritual. Sexuality is part of who people are.

BACKGROUND INFORMATION

If students do not see the difference between the terms *sex* and *sexuality,* refer them to the definitions in the Mini Glossary. You could also tell them that sexuality is broader and more complex than sex. Sexuality involves not only sex, but what we do sexually and who we are sexually.

WORKSHEETS The Teacher's Resource Box contains a four-page questionnaire entitled "Attitudes About Sexuality," which will help students determine their own thoughts and feelings about sexuality.

DISCUSSION

Ask students to discuss what they think makes a person attractive. Are these traits always physical? Which of these traits would attract students to want to get to know a person better?

information about sexuality. Friends are the second most important, school courses rank third, with television considered the fourth most important source.

School-based sex education has been shown to increase knowledge about issues surrounding sexuality, but has not been shown to result in lower rates of sexual intercourse or pregnancy. Research consistently shows that family support, family guidance, and family structure have a significant effect on sexual activity. One of the strongest predictors of adolescent sexual attitudes and behavior is the marital status of the parents. Adolescents living with both parents have the least permissive attitudes toward nonmarital sex, followed by those living with a parent who has remarried.

ASSESS

EVALUATE

A reproducible quiz for Section 1 is provided in the Teacher's Resource Box.

SECTION 1 Review Answers

1. a. sexuality
    b. sex

2. It ensures that living things reproduce their kind, and it ensures that the hereditary materials individuals carry are repeatedly shuffled and dealt out in different combinations in every new individual. (p. 578)

3. surface traits, such as eye color, skin color, and hair color; and deep-down traits, such as friendliness, musical ability, or competitiveness (p. 578)

4. half (p. 578)

5. Answers will vary.

CLOSE

Have students pick two of their favorite celebrities (sports, entertainment, and so on) and then combine their traits for possible offspring. Make sure that students work with not only physical attributes but also social and psychological traits.

Reproducible vocabulary worksheets are provided in the Teacher's Resource Box.

Human Sexuality

Sexuality is a part of a person's total personality from birth to death, with or without sexual activity. The way you walk, think, and feel, and the ways you talk to and touch others, all are affected by your sexuality. Sexuality affects the young, the old, people with disabilities, all races, all sizes—all people.

Your sexuality is greatly influenced by the way you feel about yourself. This means that your thoughts, feelings, values, and self-concept are all part of your sexuality.

In this text you have already learned a great deal about human sexuality. In Chapter 3 you learned about the sexual maturation called puberty that takes place during your teen years. In that chapter you also learned about gender roles and gender identity. In Chapter 18 you learned about love relationships and the many sexual pressures that accompany those relationships and that exist in today's society. In Chapter 20 you learned about conception and pregnancy.

In this part of the text you will learn about sexual behaviors, ranging from a person's first physical sexual feelings to sexual intercourse. You will also learn about sexual myths and problems. Finally, you will learn about sexual orientations.

For Your Information

Committed, mature love was described in Chapter 18.

KEY POINTS *Sexuality remains part of who people are from birth to death. It affects many facets of life.*

> "We are shaped and fashioned by what we love."
>
> Johann Goethe
> (1749–1832)
> German poet and dramatist

SECTION 1 Review

Answer the following questions on a sheet of paper.

Learning the Vocabulary

The vocabulary terms in this section are *sex* and *sexuality*.

1. Match each of the following phrases with the appropriate term.
    a. the quality of being sexual
    b. a general term used to mean both gender and sexual intercourse

Learning the Facts

2. What are the two major roles sex plays in nature?

3. What two types of traits do genes govern?

4. How much of your genetic material was contributed by each of your parents?

Making Life Choices

5. Think of a friend or relative whose parents you know. List all of the characteristics (both physical traits and nonphysical traits) that you think your friend received from his or her mother. List all of the characteristics that you think your friend received from his or her father. Are the lists fairly equal? If not, are there more traits that appear to come from either the father or the mother? Why do you think this might be the case?

QUICK QUIZ

Chapter 21, Section 1

The following quiz will help you assess your students' understanding of the material covered in this section of the chapter. You might use the quiz as an oral exercise, or, you might use it as a paper-pencil quiz to evaluate your students individually.

Like the Quick Quiz, the Section Review can also be used as an assessment tool to spark class discussion or as an individual student evaluation. It can also be used as a review in preparation for this quiz.

1. Sex ensures the reproduction of living things and the unique combination of one individual's hereditary materials with another's. (True)

2. Your genes determine your physical characteristics but not your emotional tendencies. (False)

SECTION 2

Sexual Activity

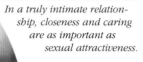

As you know from reading Chapter 20, people who have developed a healthy intimate relationship frequently decide to commit to each other. An important form of commitment between two people is marriage. Sex can add fulfillment to marriage.

Touching, hugging, and kissing are pleasurable activities physically. These activities may also satisfy emotional needs, and therefore can be emotionally fulfilling. It is normal and natural in a committed relationship for these activities to sometimes lead to **sexual intercourse**. It's also normal and natural for people to wait for a relationship to develop into a committed, loving one before initiating sexual activity. This chapter's Straight Talk section makes the point that most teenagers know and appreciate this fact, and most wait to have sexual intercourse. Let's now look at how sexual feelings and desires develop and the sexual activities that result when the time is right.

In a truly intimate relationship, closeness and caring are as important as sexual attractiveness.

The First Sexual Feelings

For most people the first sexual relationship is with themselves. At an early age boys and girls begin to flirt with themselves in the mirror, enjoying their own attractiveness. They also enjoy physical sensations, such as rubbing lotions onto the skin, sunbathing, and swimming. These are the natural healthy beginnings of sexual feelings and activities.

When young people reach puberty, the hormones produced by their bodies set up a drive for reproduction. This drive, or sexual tension, can become intense at times. People may need to release it.

One way the body provides for this release is through **wet dreams**. Almost all adolescent boys, and many girls, experience such dreams from time to time. The **orgasm** that occurs during a wet dream is the body's normal reflex for releasing sexual tension.

Eventually children's natural playfulness and curiosity lead them to explore their genitals. This may lead to **masturbation**, an activity that may continue in adulthood.

Many people are opposed to masturbation. They believe it is wrong and harmful. In the past, people were even told that masturbation caused pim-

MINI Glossary

sexual intercourse: the reproductive act between the sexes. The term *intercourse* means communication of any kind—talking, for example. Sexual intercourse between human beings is termed *coitus* (CO-ih-tus). Between animals it is termed *copulation* (cop-you-LAY-shun).

wet dreams: dreams during which orgasm occurs; a normal release for the sexual drive; in boys, these are also called *nocturnal emissions*.

orgasm: a series of muscular contractions of the sex organs, with ejaculation in the male; it typically occurs after a period of sexual stimulation.

masturbation: stimulating one's own genitals, usually until orgasm occurs.

3. Your personality is partially determined by your life experiences. (True)
4. No individual has an entirely unique set of genes. (False)
5. During sexual reproduction a male and female combine exactly half of their genetic material to create a new individual. (True)
6. The sex drive must be very strong in order to ensure reproduction of the species. (True)

7. Sexual attraction can be both the expression of both an instinctual drive and a high form of human emotional development. (True)
8. Sexuality does not affect the way a person thinks or feels. (False)
9. Values are not a part of a person's sexuality. (False)
10. Your sexuality remains an active part of your personality throughout your life. (True)

SECTION 2

FOCUS

OUTCOMES

In this section students will learn:

1. Typical reactions to early sexual feelings.
2. The four phases of sexual response.

FOCUS ACTIVITY

In small, gender-segregated groups, have students list the attributes they most desire in a person they might date. After allowing time for the lists to develop, post the lists on the wall or copy them onto the board. Lead a discussion about the similarities and differences. Commonly, boys' lists will contain more physical attributes and the girls' lists will contain more personality traits. Ask students what they would add to or subtract from the lists if they represented the person they planned to marry.

TEACH & APPLY

LEARNING WITH VISUALS

Cut out a large variety of magazine photographs of attractive, well-dressed men and women. Try to get as wide a variety of looks as possible. Have students rank the photographs from most attractive to least attractive. See if boys as a group and girls as a group can guess the order the other group will choose. Discuss the fact that different people have different opinions about what constitutes an attractive person.

581

DISCUSSION

Have students brainstorm a variety of activities for dating couples that encourage affection, but not sexual intimacy. Discuss the concept that some dates are more likely than others to lead to sexual activity. (watching a video when parents aren't home as opposed to a walk-in movie, and so on)

LEARNING WITH VISUALS

Show students as many photographs as you are able to gather of people throughout history. Be sure the people are considered (by historical standards) attractive. Old school yearbook pictures can add humor to this activity. Discuss how standards for attractiveness change as society changes. Ask the students what they believe influences our society's opinion of beauty.

INTERDISCIPLINARY ACTIVITY: HISTORY

Have students research and write a paper in which they compare the sexual and dating customs of the past to current customs. They could choose to go back 25, 50, 100, or 200 years. Have them state how they think the differences have hurt or improved society, and how sexual myths have influenced both past and current dating customs.

LEARNING WITH VISUALS

Have a group of students consult community centers, local newspapers, outdoor clubs, religious or social organizations, and so on to make a bulletin board calendar of safe and enjoyable social activities for teenagers. Have a different group update the board monthly.

ples, warts, excessive hair growth, and many other terrible things. Of course these beliefs are all myths—none of them are true.

It is fairly common for adolescent boys and girls to be troubled and confused about the desire to masturbate. Some may feel guilty and ashamed because it's something they feel they must hide. They may feel that their parents and adults do not approve.

Most medical experts believe, however, that masturbation can be useful, partly because it does not involve other people. For young people, and for people without partners, it provides a way to release sexual tension without risking pregnancy or diseases. The release of sexual tension can help people avoid sexual relationships that they would later regret.

 KEY POINTS   *In a sense, most people's first sexual relationships are with themselves. Natural playfulness often leads to masturbation, which is a way to satisfy a biological drive without involving other people.*

Sexual Intercourse

Sexual intercourse is, in a physical sense, a simple act. It is also complex, though, because the two people who engage in it bring to it their moods, ideas, self-concepts, feelings about their relationship, and everything else that makes them unique. This section is about the physical events of sexual intercourse.

Sexual stimulation results in **erection** (stiffening) of the penis in males. Fluid moves down the man's urethra, neutralizing the acid left there by urine and creating a safe environment for sperm. Females experience **engorgement** (swelling) of the clitoris and surrounding tissues, and a tipping upward of the uterus. Lubricating fluids begin to flow within the vagina.

During the early phase of the man's erection, a drop or so of fluid leaves the penis. This fluid may contain live sperm that can begin a pregnancy. Sperm can easily travel, even from the outside of the vagina, into the uterus. To prevent pregnancy, this early drop of fluid, along with any semen, must be prevented from touching the vagina.

 KEY POINTS   *Sexual stimulation leads to male erection and female engorgement, with fluid being secreted from both the penis and the vagina.*

The Stages of the Sexual Response

The mystery of the sexual response lies in the human brain. The brain—not the penis or clitoris—is the master sex organ. The brain is the commander of the events described in the next few paragraphs. Among the organs that respond to the brain's instructions are the clitoris and vagina, and the penis.

The four phases of the sexual response for both partners are **excitement**, **plateau**, orgasm (already described), and **resolution**. Each phase may differ from person to person and may vary in the same person from time to time.

Excitement   The excitement phase may begin even before physical contact occurs—people are said to be "in the mood" for sexual contact. A loving couple may kiss and then touch one another in ways that stimulate

For Your Information

Chapter 3 introduced a set of refusal skills as useful tools for handling all sorts of peer-pressure situations, including sexual pressures.

Chapter 21, Section 2

The following quiz will help you assess your students' understanding of the material covered in this section of the chapter. You might use the quiz as an oral exercise, which will lead into a class discussion of the topics covered. Or, you might use it as a paper-pencil quiz to evaluate your students individually.

Like the Quick Quiz, the Section Review can also be used as an assessment tool to spark class discussion or as an individual student evaluation. It can also be used as a review in preparation for this quiz.

1. Physical touching can satisfy emotional as well as physical needs. (True)

2. A majority of individuals prefer to develop a committed, intimate relationship before initiating sexual activity. (True)

both. This activity, frequently called **foreplay**, leads to erection in the male and engorgement in the female. During this time, the couple can enjoy the emotions of tenderness, love, and gratitude, as well as feelings of sexual pleasure.

Plateau   If sexual stimulation continues, the partners move into the plateau phase. In this phase the lower third of the vagina constricts, the uterus tilts forward, and the penis enlarges further. The clitoris withdraws under its foreskin as it becomes more sensitive.

Orgasm   With more stimulation, orgasm occurs. Orgasm is a reflex—an involuntary response that follows stimulation of the genitals. In women, orgasm involves involuntary rhythmic contractions of the uterus, the outer portion of the vagina, and the surrounding muscles. In men, it involves **ejaculation** of semen through rhythmic contractions of the penile muscles. Orgasm lasts just a few seconds. Sexual intercourse usually ends with the man's orgasm. The woman's orgasm can occur prior to, along with, or after the man's.

Resolution   In the resolution stage following orgasm, the physical changes of arousal reverse. Tensed muscles relax. Congested blood vessels and swollen tissues return to normal.

 KEY POINTS   *The sexual response is experienced in the reproductive organs but is controlled by the brain. The four stages of the sexual response are excitement, plateau, orgasm, and resolution.*

SECTION 2 Review

Answer the following questions on a sheet of paper.

Learning the Vocabulary

The vocabulary terms in this section are *sexual intercourse, wet dreams, orgasm, masturbation, erection, engorgement, excitement, plateau, resolution, foreplay,* and *ejaculation.*

1. Match each of the following phrases with the appropriate term:
  a. swelling; with reference to the sexual response, the sex organs' filling with blood preparatory to orgasm
  b. in sexual intercourse, the stage of relaxation that follows orgasm
  c. dreams during which orgasm occurs

Learning the Facts

2. When young people reach puberty, what effects do the hormones produced by their bodies bring about?
3. What do medical experts believe about masturbation?
4. What organs respond to the brain's instructions during the sexual response?
5. What are the four phases of the sexual response?
6. What happens to the uterus in the plateau phase?

Making Life Choices

7. Make a list of nonsexual ways sexual tension can be released.

MINI Glossary

erection: the state of a normally soft tissue when it fills with blood and becomes firm. Both the penis and clitoris can become erect.

engorgement: swelling; with reference to the sexual response, the sex organs' filling with blood preparatory to orgasm.

excitement: as used to describe a stage of sexual intercourse, the early stage.

plateau: literally, a high, flat place. In sexual intercourse, the plateau phase is the period of intense physical pleasure preceding orgasm.

resolution: in sexual intercourse, the stage of relaxation that follows orgasm.

foreplay: an activity in which each partner gives pleasure to the other prior to intercourse.

ejaculation: the expelling of semen from the penis, brought about by the involuntary muscular contractions of orgasm.

3. A person begins to develop his/her sexuality long before puberty. (True)
4. Girls do not experience wet dreams. (False)
5. Orgasms that occur during wet dreams are a natural reflex for releasing sexual tension. (True)
6. Masturbation allows people to satisfy their sexual drives without risking pregnancy or disease. (True)
7. Pregnancy cannot be caused by sperm that touches only the outside of the vagina. (False)
8. Females experience engorgement of the clitoris as a result of sexual stimulation. (True)
9. The brain controls the body's sexual response. (True)
10. Excitement, plateau, orgasm, and resolution are the four stages of sexual response. (True)

SECTION 3

FOCUS

OUTCOMES

In this section students will learn:

1. Some sexual myths.
2. How self-esteem relates to sexuality.

FOCUS ACTIVITY

Lead a discussion to define the word *myth*. List on the board common myths, not necessarily related to sex. Discuss why myths occur and if they are ever dangerous, such as myths saying you cannot get pregnant the first time you have sex, and beer is not as addicting as whiskey.

TEACH & APPLY

BACKGROUND INFORMATION

The common expression to represent sexual attraction, that there is "chemistry" between two people, may turn out to be true. Science has discovered that human beings, like many other species, produce odor chemicals, called *pheromones,* that are recognized by others. Pheromones produce a sensation of recognition, not a true smell. For example, pheromones are produced on the skin around a woman's nipples which helps infants to readily recognize their mothers' breasts. Adults of both genders produce pheromones around the mouth, which are exchanged during kissing.

For **Y**our **I**nformation

A healthy sexuality depends on high self-esteem. Chapter 2 of the text describes self-esteem in detail.

SECTION 3

Sexual Myths

People hold many false ideas about sexuality. For example, some people believe that people of certain physical types, considered attractive by society, are the most desirable people. Although social custom may define certain people as pleasing to look at, it is self-esteem, not physical makeup, that determines sexuality. A healthy sexuality also cannot be established by wearing the latest fashions or an expensive brand of cologne. The people with the healthiest sexuality are those with the highest self-esteem. People considered physically attractive may turn out to have high self-esteem, of course, but you can't tell by appearances.

　Probably the most widely held and destructive myths concern body measurements. One myth says that a man with a large penis makes the best lover. This is false from two points of view. First, most women experience most sexual stimulation in the clitoris, an external organ. A longer penis, therefore, is not more stimulating to a woman. Second, the brain controls the sexual response. Therefore, what a woman *thinks* about a man is at least as important as any physical aspect of intercourse.

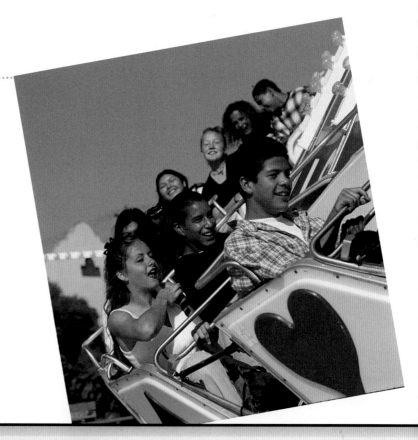

People with a healthy sexuality have high self-esteem.

special needs

Intra-personal

This chapter presents the facts regarding sex and sexuality. It will be important for students to sort through the feelings that arise as they study this material. To give them an opportunity to deal with feelings and to make personal decisions regarding sexuality and sexual

behavior, you may want to initiate this activity.

　As you begin, ask students to keep a personal journal. This will be for their own use, not to be read or graded. Encourage them to record their reactions to material and information presented. They should also record questions that may arise, especially if they are embarrassed to ask the question in class. That way, they can go back, find the question, and

Pills and Potions

Consumer SKILLS

The idea of a potion to increase sexual desire—an **aphrodisiac**—has always intrigued people. In a fairy tale, a sprinkling of magic powder can make a princess suddenly notice an overlooked suitor. In real life, no secret compound, no exotic ingredient, and no food or nutrient can enhance or restore sexual desire.

So-called aphrodisiacs do not work, and they may be dangerous. Many are strong stimulants, hormones, or depressants. According to the Food and Drug Administration, all claims for aphrodisiacs are false, misleading, or unsupported by scientific evidence.

Chances are that if the sexual response fails, the body is signaling a need for attention. Some causes of reduced sexual response include use of alcohol, drugs, or tobacco; excess worry or depression; or lack of communication between partners. Thought, time, and energy can often solve such problems. However, money spent on products cannot do so.

Critical Thinking

1. Aphrodisiacs come in all forms, from the dangerous drug called "Spanish fly" to ground-up horns of the endangered rhinoceros. Why are none of these available in drugstores?
2. If a person should fail to respond to a loved partner sexually, what are some factors that might be influencing the response?
3. What should the person do about the factors named in response to Question 2?

A related myth is that a woman with large breasts is more sexual than a woman with small breasts. Actually, a woman's breast size doesn't affect sexual responsiveness. Also, as is true for women, a man's response to a woman has much more to do with her attitudes and emotional makeup than with her physical attributes.

Another widely believed sexual myth comes from a common story line in movies, television shows, magazines, and novels. The story goes like this: two strangers' eyes meet; they dazzle one another in some mysterious way; biology takes over; and they have sexual intercourse, which leads to marriage. This myth leads people to believe that sexual intercourse with virtual strangers is the usual and healthy path to commitment. Research reveals the truth: most people who eventually marry meet as friends or co-workers—at school, at a private party, at work, at church, or at other shared activities. They may feel an attraction, but they use their brains, not biology. They wait and gradually get to know each other before they allow sex or marriage to enter the picture. In contrast, couples who have sexual intercourse right away usually part soon after.

A particularly destructive idea is that once a person has had sexual intercourse, that person is committed to having intercourse again. In reality, a person who is no longer a **virgin** can choose abstinence just as a virgin can. The person has every right to do so. Fear of pregnancy or diseases can

MINI Glossary

aphrodisiac (af-roh-DEEZ-ee-ack): a substance reputed to excite sexual desire. Actually, no known substance does this, but many claim the products they sell do so.

virgin: a term applied to people before their first occasion of sexual intercourse.

ask it of an adult they feel comfortable with, hopefully a parent. You may want to give students an opportunity to reflect and write for the last few minutes of each class session.

Encourage students to think about what they are learning, to apply it to themselves. Help them realize that thinking things through and making decisions before they are in a situation gives them control, rather than leaving

themselves vulnerable in the "heat of the moment." You may also want to focus on the responsibility associated with sexual activity by assisting students in thinking about possible results when "it just happens." Students may want to keep the journal and use it to record feelings and questions whenever they arise, not just for the purposes of the class, but as a real-life tool.

Consumer SKILLS

Answers to Critical Thinking

1. They don't work, and many are dangerous.
2. use of alcohol, drugs and tobacco; excess worry or depression; lack of communication
3. communicate with partner and try to remedy them; use thought, time, and energy.

GROUP PROJECT

Have students make "Myth Buster" books. Each student writes three to seven myths about sex along with the truth in a small booklet. Appropriate illustrations may be included.

The Teacher's Resource Box contains a handout entitled "Effects of Drugs on Sexual Functioning."

DISCUSSION

Have students describe the nicest person they know and write all the reasons that person is nice; or, have them describe the nicest character they see on TV and list all the reasons that character is nice. Have students describe the physical features of a sexy person of the same gender as the nice person. Discuss which person is preferable as a friend. Ask if their feelings are influenced by who might see them with this friend. Are there times when looks count more than personality? When and why?

585

Consumer SKILLS
CHAPTER 21: Understanding Sexuality

ASSESS

EVALUATE

Ask students to list at least three common myths about sexuality. Give them bonus points for each additional myth.

A reproducible quiz for Section 3 is provided in the Teacher's Resource Box.

SECTION 3 Review Answers

1. Answers will vary.
2. saying no (abstinence) (p. 586)
3. It is a technique used to pressure a person into having sexual intercourse by saying it is unhealthy. (p. 586)
4. communication (p. 586)
5. Answers will vary.

CLOSE

Write 12 vocabulary terms relating to the first three sections on the board. Number the words. Have student volunteers roll dice and define the word that corresponds to the number they rolled. As the game progresses, words must be used correctly in a sentence, spelled, or used as the basis of a question you develop. Here is a sample word list:

1. sexuality, 2. wet dreams,
3. masturbation, 4. erection,
5. myth, 6. foreplay, 7. virgin,
8. sex, 9. dysfunction,
10. aphrodisiac, 11. sexual orientation, 12. orgasm.

come into play at any time. The person may change moral or religious beliefs, or may simply decide to wait for the right person to come along. For many different reasons, saying no is always an option.

Another myth is that orgasm must occur for a woman to become pregnant. As mentioned, the fluid released from a man's penis before orgasm often contains sufficient sperm to initiate a pregnancy. The muscular contractions that occur during a woman's orgasm may help to speed sperm along her reproductive tract, but sperm are fully capable of swimming up the tract without this help. The truth is, whenever sexual intercourse occurs, with or without orgasm, pregnancy can follow.

Some people try to pressure others into having intercourse by claiming ill effects from sexual arousal. Is it unhealthy to become sexually aroused and then not proceed to orgasm? No, it isn't harmful, although it may be frustrating. Sometimes it is even useful. For example, if a couple is experiencing **sexual dysfunction**—an inability to perform certain sexual activities—a counselor may advise that they try to excite one another but avoid orgasm. This can work to intensify their desire for each other and help them learn alternative methods for giving and receiving pleasure.

People sometimes say that to have good sexual technique, a person must have had many sex partners. Actually, each individual has needs that differ from those of others. It is easy to learn bad habits from other people that must be unlearned later. In **monogamous**, committed relationships, people have a lifetime to explore and provide for their partners' likes and dislikes. Communication is the true key to satisfying sexual relations.

Another myth discussed in this section concerns the idea that a product might increase sexual appetite. The Consumer Skills feature on the preceding page shows that this idea is simpleminded.

 KEY POINTS *People hold many false ideas about sexuality. It is self-esteem, not physical makeup, that determines sexuality.*

SECTION 3 Review

Answer the following questions on a sheet of paper.

Learning the Vocabulary

The vocabulary terms in this section are *aphrodisiac, virgin, sexual dysfunction,* and *monogamous.*

1. Write a sentence using each of the vocabulary terms.

Learning the Facts

2. What is always an option regarding sexual intercourse?

3. Why do people believe that it is harmful to be sexually aroused and not have sexual intercourse?
4. What is the true key to satisfying sexual relations?

Making Life Choices

5. There are many myths about sexual intercourse and sexuality in general. How can education change these myths? How would you go about changing these myths?

Chapter 21, Section 3

The following quiz will help you assess your students' understanding of the material covered in this section of the chapter. You might use the quiz as an oral exercise, or, you might use it as a paper-pencil quiz to evaluate your students individually.

Like the Quick Quiz, the Section Review can

also be used as an assessment tool to spark class discussion or as an individual student evaluation. It can also be used as a review in preparation for this quiz.

*If students have difficulty with the concepts covered in the Quick Quiz and the Section Review, you might suggest they review the material using the S*urvey, *Q*uestion, *R*ead, *R*ecite, *R*eview *(SQ3R) study method, which is described in detail in the introduction to the Teacher's Wraparound Edition.*

SECTION 4

Sexual Orientations

Most people are sexually attracted to members of the opposite sex. These people are **heterosexual**. Some people, however, are attracted to members of the same sex. These people are **homosexual**—that is, they are **gay** or **lesbian**.

In the United States, many people have strong feelings, both positive and negative, about homosexuality. Religious teachings often speak against it. Because homosexual men were among the first groups to suffer high risks of the fatal disease AIDS, people may even fear homosexuality. In fact, the irrational fear of homosexuals has a name: **homophobia**. In some societies and in some groups of our society, however, homosexuality is seen as an accepted difference in some people's sexual orientation.

Evidence about the origins of homosexuality is just now being gathered. Physical brain differences between homosexual and heterosexual men have been observed. Whether these differences are responsible for homosexuality, however, has not been proved. Hormones may also play a role in the shaping of a person's sexuality, especially in early human development.

MINI Glossary

sexual dysfunction: impaired responses of sexual excitement or orgasm due to psychological, interpersonal, physical, environmental, or cultural causes; formerly called *impotence* in men and *frigidity* in women.

monogamous: having sexual relations with one partner only, excluding all others. These relationships are usually long-term relationships.

heterosexual: feeling sexual desire for persons of the other sex.

homosexual: feeling sexual desire for persons of the same sex.

gay: a general term referring to homosexuality, but often referring to homosexual men.

lesbian: a term referring to homosexual women.

homophobia: an irrational fear and hatred of homosexuals, usually based on the fear of developing AIDS or of becoming homosexual.

Everyone needs to feel accepted by a community.

1. Self-esteem determines a healthy sexuality. (True)
2. Most women experience most sexual stimulation in the clitoris. (True)
3. Women receive greater sexual stimulation from a larger penis. (False)
4. A woman's breast size indicates her sexual responsiveness. (False)
5. Sexual stimulation is an emotional as well as physical response. (True)
6. Sexual intercourse leads to emotional intimacy and commitment. (False)
7. You are free to refuse sexual intercourse at any time, whether you have agreed to sex or not. (True)
8. Orgasm must occur in order for a woman to become pregnant. (False)
9. People who have had many partners develop a good sexual technique. (False)
10. Satisfying sexual relations depend on a person's ability to communicate. (True)

SECTION 4

FOCUS

OUTCOMES

In this section students will learn:

1. The meaning of sexual orientation.
2. To evaluate their own feelings about homosexuality.

FOCUS ACTIVITY

Have students write anonymous answers to the following questions. Should homosexuals be allowed to: Adopt children? Join the military? Teach? Become members of the clergy? Serve as police officers? Marry? Discuss how enforcement of these laws would affect heterosexuals.

TEACH & APPLY

LEARNING WITH VISUALS

Get magazine photos of attractive and unattractive men, women, boys, girls, and adults of all ages. Write a general biography for each photo. Include good and bad personality traits, education, family, age, and a name. Have students choose:

1. Who they would like to date.
2. Who they would like for a friend.
3. Who they would like as a teacher.

After they have chosen, tell them the sexual orientation for each photo. Be sure to have gays, lesbians, bisexuals, asexuals, and heterosexuals. Ask the students if they would choose differently knowing the sexual orientation for each individual.

ASSESS

EVALUATE

Have students write two things they have learned in this section on a piece of paper. On the same paper, have them write any questions they might still have after studying the material. Be sure to get the answers for any questions they might ask.

SECTION 4 Review Answers

1. **a.** homophobia
   b. homosexual
   c. heterosexual
2. It is associated with gay men because they were the first to have the disease, causing more fear of homosexuals. (p. 587)
3. hormones, brain differences (p. 587)
4. No, homosexuals may be uncommitted or monogamous, secretive or open. They come from all walks of life. (p. 588)
5. Answers will vary.

CLOSE

Invite a psychologist to come to class to discuss the topic of homosexuality. Before the speaker's visit, have students write out questions they would like the speaker to answer. Be sure to read the questions yourself to screen out any that may be inappropriate. A local college or university that offers human sexuality courses would be a source for obtaining a qualified speaker.

Answers to FACT or FICTION Here are the answers to the questions at the start of Part A.

1. **False.** Sexuality is part of a person's total personality from birth to death, with or without sexual activity.
2. **True.**
3. **True.**
4. **False.** The brain, not the penis and clitoris, is the most important sex organ.
5. **True.**
6. **False.** If you tried to identify "the" homosexual lifestyle, you could not do it.

Whether people are born homosexual or whether the orientation develops from environmental influences is not known. In any case, the American Psychiatric Association no longer considers homosexuality as an emotional illness to be "cured" by therapy.

Along with other false ideas, many stereotypes surround homosexuality. One such stereotype is that homosexual people are all alike in terms of their lifestyles. If you tried to identify "the" homosexual lifestyle, however, you could not do it. Homosexual people may be uncommitted or monogamous, secretive or open. They may be lawyers, dentists, grocers, accountants, sales clerks, or anything else.

Everyone needs to feel accepted by a community. Homosexual people are no different from others in this regard. Homosexuals sometimes form communities to provide the identity and support they need.

People can also be **bisexual**, a term that refers to experiencing sexual desires for members of both sexes. Some other people are **asexual**, meaning that they do not feel sexual desire for people of either gender. Bisexuality is not the same as feeling warm toward members of both sexes and expressing affection for them by hugging, kissing, or patting on the back. Most people's expressions of such feelings do not imply bisexuality. In early adolescence, it is common for young heterosexuals to share early sexual experiences with same-sex peers. This does not indicate sexual orientation.

KEY POINTS *People may be heterosexual, homosexual, bisexual, or asexual. Regardless of sexual orientation, people need to belong to a community.*

SECTION 4 Review

Answer the following questions on a separate sheet of paper.

Learning the Vocabulary

The vocabulary terms in this section are *heterosexual, homosexual, gay, lesbian, homophobia, bisexual,* and *asexual.*

1. Match each of the following phrases with the appropriate term.
   a. an irrational fear and hatred of homosexuals
   b. feeling sexual desire for persons of the same sex
   c. feeling sexual desire for persons of the opposite sex

Learning the Facts

2. What contributions has the disease AIDS made to the fear known as homophobia?
3. What factors may play a role in the development of sexuality?
4. Is it possible to identify "the" homosexual lifestyle? Why or why not?

Making Life Choices

5. Reread the Consumer Skills feature in this section. In real life are there such compounds as those mentioned? Why do you think people believe that there are aphrodisiacs?

MINI Glossary

bisexual: being sexually oriented to members of both sexes.

asexual: having no sexual inclinations.

QUICK QUIZ

Chapter 21, Section 4

The following quiz will help you assess your students' understanding of the material covered in this section of the chapter. You might use the quiz as an oral exercise, which will lead into a class discussion of the topics covered. Or, you might use it as a paper-pencil quiz to evaluate your students individually.

Like the Quick Quiz, the Section Review can also be used as an assessment tool to spark class discussion or as an individual student evaluation. It can also be used as a review in preparation for this quiz.

1. People who are attracted to the opposite sex are called heterosexual. (True)
2. People who are attracted exclusively to members of the same sex are called bisexual. (False)
3. Homophobia is an irrational fear of

What About Me? Am I Missing Out?

 Young people hear all sorts of messages about sex. The voices of parents, teachers, and others saying it's best to wait can easily be lost in the great roar of sexual messages from other sources. These days, three quarters of the television shows airing during family TV viewing time talk about or depict sexual behavior. Magazines, books, advertisements, and movies imply or outright suggest that almost everyone is sexually active. Teenagers who forgo sexual activity are often left wondering if they are missing out on what life has to offer.

 That's true. Sometimes I wonder why, if sex is so bad, every magazine I pick up or movie I see is so full of sex. Of course I know that the stories are made up, but they reflect how real-life sexual situations work, don't they?

Actually, research about real people and their sexuality tells a much different story from the ones told by the media. Most people in this society are careful in their choices concerning sexual behavior, while people on TV seem unthinking in the choices they make. The overwhelming majority of real adults are faithful to one partner, do not have sex with strangers or casual acquaintances, and have more important things to think about most of the time. The story lines of books and movies frequently concern unfaithful spouses, and characters whose daily lives seem ruled by sex.

It isn't unusual for young people to be misled to believe that people are thinking about sex all of the time and engaging in sex most of the time. A fact to keep in mind about the media, though, is that sexual topics increase the sales of books, magazines, and movie tickets. If sex sells products and makes people tune in, then the bottom line for advertising and television execu-

tives is to keep the cash flowing. They don't think about the messages they might be sending to young people.

 What about love? The characters in stories usually see each other across a room, meet, fall madly in love, become sexually involved, and live happily ever after. Isn't love all that matters?

Love is certainly desirable in a lasting relationship. However, it is important to accept and remember the distinction that was made between love and infatuation in the textbook in Chapter 18. From your description, it sounds as though the characters meet, fall madly into *infatuation*, and become sexually active right away. Rarely does true, mature love follow such an encounter. More often, when the partners get to know each other better, the infatuation quickly fades, and the partners feel embarrassed or just plain lose interest in one another.

Whether or not they are aware of it, people who are looking for a relationship assess every new acquaintance in terms of potential for a partnership. Four areas seem most important in this regard. People most often want mates who are similar to themselves in age, race, education, and social status. The more similar to themselves the new acquaintance seems to be, the more likely they are to assess the new relationship as positive.

I'm not convinced that love doesn't follow sexual intercourse. What about stories of people who are very different from one another, but who have sex and fall in love?

What you describe may happen occasionally, but many such stories are the product of the entertainment industry and do not reflect what happens most often. A study of the longevity of relationships showed a clear connection between waiting to have sexual

Discussion
Have students brainstorm on the topic of using sex to sell products. Can they think of any examples where the advertising firm has used either sex or sexual situations to "keep the cash flowing"? Share examples in class and compare the ways in which different advertisers use sex. Another activity could be to compare like products, some using sex to sell their products and some not. Which ads do the students think are more effective?

Comprehension Check
Prepare a handout with the following questions to be answered by each student in complete sentences.

1. Why would a person ask someone he or she loves to do something against that person's personal values?

2. Why would a male think he was "owed" something because he spent money for a date?

3. What are two dangers of sexual activity with a person you are dating?

4. Give one emotional reason to practice abstinence.

5. Give one physical reason to practice abstinence.

---

homosexuals and homosexuality. (True)

4. The specific causes of sexual orientation have not been determined. (True)

5. It has been scientifically proven that a person's sexuality is determined by their genetic heritage. (False)

6. Stereotypes about homosexual lifestyles are false. (True)

7. Homosexual communities can offer support and a sense of identity to their individual members. (True)

8. It is common during early adolescence for young heterosexuals to share sexual experiences with members of the same sex. (True)

9. A person who expresses affection towards members of both sexes by hugging or kissing should be considered bisexual. (False)

10. People who do not experience sexual desire for members of either gender are called asexual. (True)

Plan a panel discussion on problems associated with teen pregnancy. Discuss the project with your principal before making arrangements for it.

Get your list of panelists approved by the principal as well.

Panel members might include:

- a middle aged woman who was a teen mother
- a high school drop-out
- the school counselor
- a social worker
- a minister
- a mother
- a father
- a student
- the teacher in charge of the program for pregnant students

Ask the panel to discuss these points:

- the incidence of teen pregnancy in your town
- problems associated with teen pregnancy
  —for the teen mother
  —for the teen father
  —for the teens' families
  —for society
- prevention of teen pregnancy
- resources for pregnant teens
- questions prepared in advance by class

Role Playing

Create some scenarios of your own to show students the most effective ways to say no to partners who are pressuring in various situations (study dates, going to a movie, and so on). Refer back to page 582 (Discussion) for suggestions for safe dates to avoid pressure situations.

intercourse and relationships that last. Among couples who first met at school and eventually married, 70 percent had waited at least one year before having sexual intercourse. In contrast, between 55 and 80 percent of couples who had sexual intercourse within one month had broken up before a second month had passed. Clearly, relationships sometimes do survive early sexual intercourse, but most times, they do not. The authors of the study conclude that their numbers lend strong support to the idea that lasting love grows gradually through friendship at first, with deepening commitment over time.

It's worth repeating here what Chapter 18 made clear. If it's love you're after, you have the best chance of getting it by waiting to have sex. Sexual activity begun too early can short-circuit the natural progression of a relationship.

 My friends all talk about sex and act like it's cool. I'm afraid to say that I'm not doing it. Actually, I don't really want to. But I'm afraid that if my friends find out, they'll think that I'm not popular.

This is a common problem, and it may seem unsolvable at first. However, experts suggest that you tell your friends the truth. You may be surprised to find out that your friends feel the same way or that they understand your point of view. Very commonly, teenagers will say they've had sexual intercourse when they haven't, just to sound important or grown-up. They may have the same fears that you have, but may talk about sex to put up a smoke screen. As often as not, locker-room talk is just talk designed to create an image.

It helps to remember that sex isn't a contest. No reward awaits the person who begins earliest or has the most partners. The truth is that fewer teenagers are having sex. More young people are waiting longer, too. For them, the pressures of having sexual intercourse are too great. They don't have time to worry about pregnancy and diseases, or just plain getting caught. Time spent planning their futures, applying to colleges, practicing music, and participating in sports is more important. Their motto seems to be, "Not me, not now."

 I was once in an uncomfortable situation where I wanted to say no to a date, but I couldn't think fast enough and ended up making the person angry. How can I handle the situation next time?

Making a smart decision is difficult, especially under pressure from a date who is trying to influ-

ence you. The best attitude is one of confidence in yourself. Let it shine through as you deliver your message. It also helps to keep thinking about the consequences, ranging from a lost opportunity for a real relationship to an unwanted pregnancy or a life-threatening disease, such as AIDS.

When you speak to your partner under pressure, stay calm but sound convincing. Calmly express your high regard for yourself by choosing your own behaviors, without angering or insulting others in the process.

 That sounds like it's "easier said than done."

As with almost every other worthwhile thing, effective communication of your wishes takes effort. You must be honest and sound firm. State clearly that your mind is made up. Give only short answers to direct questions, because there is nothing to discuss. Speak convincingly, show that you are in control, maintain eye contact, and use a steady voice.

Here are some example situations and responses that may help you practice your responses during uncomfortable situations related to sex.

Situation:

While at a party with friends, your boyfriend of a few months says, "It's hot and crowded here. Let's leave and find someplace quieter and less crowded so we can talk."

Response:

"Yes, it's crowded, but the back deck isn't so bad. Let's go there and talk."
"Oh, I see my friend over there. I'd like to introduce you to her."
"I'm thirsty. Let's go over there and get a soda."

Situation:

While on a date with someone you really like, your date challenges you to prove your affection by having sex.

Response:

"I do like you, but I don't have to prove it by having sex. I can make my own choices, and I don't choose to show my feelings for you in that way."

590

HEALTHY PEOPLE 2000

Reduce the proportion of adolescents who have engaged in sexual intercourse to no more than 15 percent by age 15 and no more than 40 percent by age 17.
One in ten young women aged 19 and younger become pregnant each year, and approximately 40 percent will experience at least one pregnancy before age 20. Initiation

of sexual activity at a young age is a primary risk factor for unintended pregnancy. By age 21, approximately one in five young people have acquired a sexually transmitted disease. Because only some teenagers are sexually active, this amounts to a rate of at least 25 percent among those who are. Sexually transmitted diseases can have profound long term consequences, including infertility and cancer. HIV infection, also one of the sexually trans-

Try to think of other situations that may occur, and practice some responses you could use in those situations. That way, you'll be prepared to handle the real thing.

 I'd like some help in carrying out my plan to postpone sexual activity. I just don't know who to turn to.

It's much easier to delay sexual activity when you have the support of people who are important to you. Talk with friends about your decision to refrain from sexual activity. (You may have to joke around about it at first.) Eventually, though, they should grow to respect your decision and support you in it. Who knows? They may be glad to have a leader to show them the way.

If you can, also talk to your parents about your decision, and ask them for their support. Sometimes you may need for them to "rescue" you from situations that are getting out of control. If they know what's going on ahead of time, they'll be likely to help out. Chapter 18 in the textbook offered many other tips on keeping a lid on sexual activity. See pages 501 to 503.

Remember that there's more to life than sex. Develop your skills at school and at home. Enjoy outdoor play. Fill your days with the company of positive people who support you as you become the person you were meant to be. These years are yours alone. Don't let pressure to have sex too early sidetrack you from having the life that you want and deserve.

For Your Information

"Not Me, Not Now" is the motto of an educational TV campaign for and by teenagers in Monroe County, New York. Teens lend support to the idea that sex and pregnancy interfere with future plans.

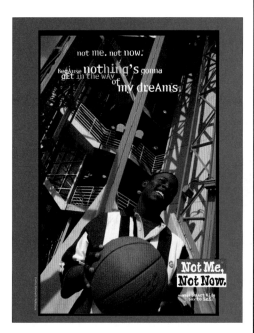

591

Divide the class into groups. Have students role play some of the pressure situations described in the Straight Talk. Have them present their answer to the situation. Afterwards, have the class discuss what they would do differently if they were in the situation.

CNN® You can update your coverage of health and fitness topics, as well as spark lively classroom discussion and deeper understanding, by using the **CNN Health and Fitness Updates.** These video updates are produced by Turner Educational Services, using the resources of CNN, the world's first 24-hour, all-news network.

With the introduction of the **CNN Health and Fitness Updates,** West Educational Publishing is proud to be the exclusive partner of CNN for textbook/video integration in high school fitness. By making use of the **CNN Health and Fitness Updates** you can bring the power of CNN, the network known for providing in-depth, live coverage and analysis of breaking news events, to your health class.

For assistance in using and incorporating the **CNN Health and Fitness Updates** into your classroom presentations, see the *Classroom Guide to the CNN Health and Fitness Updates.* The **CNN Health and Fitness Updates** are available with West Educational Publishing's *Health: Making Life Choices.*

mitted diseases, is incurable and deadly.

Sexual relationships among teenagers are often characterized by extreme impermanence. As a result, 58 percent of sexually active young women aged 15 through 19 have had two or more sexual partners and seven percent have had 10 or more partners. According to the most recent data from the National Survey of Family Growth, three quarters of young women have had sexual inter-

course by their twentieth birthday. Teenagers report that social pressure is the chief reason why their peers do not wait until they are older to have sexual intercourse. Sexual activity at young ages is more common among young people from low socioeconomic status families, and among adolescents who smoke, use alcohol or other drugs, or have evidence of delinquency.

ANSWERS TO CHAPTER 21 REVIEW

VOCABULARY

1. a. excitement
   b. aphrodisiac
   c. sexuality
2. a. Sex
   b. foreplay
   c. sexual dysfunction
   d. ejaculation
   e. masturbation
   f. bisexual
3. Answers will vary.

RECALL SECTION 1

1. It ensures that all living things reproduce their kind. It also ensures that the hereditary material individuals carry is repeatedly shuffled and dealt out in different combinations. (p. 578)
2. your thoughts, feelings, values, and self-concept (p. 580)

Summarizing the Chapter

Your ability to respond correctly to the following statements ensures your understanding of the main concepts in the chapter.

1. Identify the stages of the sexual response.
2. List and describe examples of sexual myths.
3. Describe various sexual orientations.

Learning the Vocabulary

sex	ejaculation
sexuality	aphrodisiac
sexual intercourse	virgin
wet dreams	sexual dysfunction
orgasm	monogamous
masturbation	heterosexual
erection	homosexual
engorgement	gay
excitement	lesbian
plateau	homophobia
resolution	bisexual
foreplay	asexual

Answer the following questions on a sheet of paper.

1. **Matching**—*Match each of the following phrases with the appropriate vocabulary term from the list above:*
   a. as used to describe a stage of sexual intercourse, the early stage
   b. a substance reputed (falsely) to excite sexual desire
   c. the quality of being sexual, part of the total person
   d. the expelling of semen from the penis
   e. stimulating one's own genitals, usually until orgasm occurs
   f. being sexually oriented to members of both sexes
2. a. _____ is a term used to mean both gender and sexual intercourse.
   b. An activity which gives each partner pleasure before intercourse is called _____.
   c. A problem formerly referred to as impotence in men or frigidity in women is now called _____.
3. Write a paragraph using at least ten of the vocabulary terms. Underline each vocabulary term that you use.

Recalling Important Facts and Ideas

Section 1
1. What two major roles does sex play in nature?
2. What factors have influenced your sexuality?

Section 2
3. What is an important form of commitment?
4. Why is sexual intercourse considered a complex act?
5. What is the master sex organ?

Section 3
6. Describe two myths concerning sexuality.
7. What determines sexuality?

Section 4
8. List at least two false statements about homosexuality.

Critical Thinking

1. Read the Straight Talk on pages 589-591. Why are topics about sex and sexual behavior so popular on television, in the movies, and in other media? Does the media usually depict what research on real people finds? Why or why not?
2. Think about the steps for making decisions that were discussed in Chaper 2. (Name the problem, describe it specifically, brainstorm, think about each solution, choose a solution and act on it, and evaluate the outcome.) How could these steps be helpful if someone is faced with a situation in which they are being pressured to have sex?

Activities

1. Aphrodisiacs are growing in popularity. Make posters showing various aphrodisiacs and claims for each. Write a statement to prove these claims are not true. Post these around your school.

592

2. Put together a booklet with the following phone numbers: an AIDS hot line, a local planned parenthood organization, a teen talk number, and a crisis pregnancy center. Make these available for everyone at your school to use.

3. Interview your parents or grandparents about dating customs when they were your age. Develop a list of questions with the members of your class. What are the similarities? What are the differences between the dating customs of your grandparents' era and today's customs? Share these interviews as oral reports.

4. What are your rights in a relationship? Do you have the right to make your own decisions? Do you have the right to say no? Make a list of the rights you believe you should have in a relationship. (Remember that the other person would have the same rights.) Work together with the rest of your class to compile a classroom list of relationship rights.

5. Work in groups of four or five classmates to develop a list of ways to say *no* when a relationship is about to go too far for one or both of the partners. Develop role plays that use the *no* answers your group came up with. Then,

make a list of alternative activities for the couple so that the situation can be avoided in the future.

6. Make a list of all the qualities you would like to have in a partner in a relationship. Put a + by those qualities the person must have. Put a - by the qualities you would like the person to have but could do without. How realistic is your list? Does anyone exist who has all of the qualities you listed? Remember that perfection is not something you're going to find in a partner, any more than your partner will find it in you.

Making Decisions about Health

1. Lisa has been in a relationship for several weeks, and the question of sexual intimacy has been raised. She is sexually inexperienced, and even though she cares for the other person and feels a sexual attraction, she has been taught that sex before marriage is wrong. Lisa feels confused, because part of her wants a sexual relationship, but the other part fears that sexual intimacy will lead to loss of respect or rejection. What should Lisa do at this point?

SECTION 2

3. marriage (p. 581)

4. Because the two people who engage in it bring to it their moods, ideas, self-concepts, feelings about their relationship, and everything else that makes them unique. (p. 582)

5. the brain (p. 582)

SECTION 3

6. Answers will vary; could include: a man with a large penis makes a better lover, a woman's breast size makes her more or less sexual, and the idea that certain products can increase sexual appetite. (pp. 584–586)

7. It is self-esteem, not physical make-up, that determines sexuality. The people with the healthiest sexuality are those with the highest self-esteem. (p. 584)

SECTION 4

8. Answers will vary; could include: homosexuals are all alike, AIDS is only a homosexual disease. (p. 588)

593

KEY POINTS

Chapter 22 is 30 pages long and divided into five sections. This chapter examines the important choice students make between abstinence and becoming sexually active. It looks at all the contraceptives available, explains how they work, and evaluates their effectiveness. Decisions that must be made if a teenager becomes pregnant are also explored.

ACTIVITY TO INTRODUCE THE CHAPTER

Don't tell students you will be discussing abstinence, just start with this activity.

Ask students to give examples of the attributes the ideal contraceptive would have. Students will come up with qualities such as: either sex could use it, prevents STDs, 100 percent effective, free, readily available, biodegradable, no side effects, easy to use, and so on. Write all of their responses on the board. Once the list has been completed, ask students if any one method can do all of these things. The students' immediate response is usually a firm "NO!" Ask them to think again, and quite quickly they realize abstinence is the answer. Discuss.

CHAPTER 22

Contents

STRAIGHT TALK
Why People Don't Use Contraception

NOT Enough Time?

Following are some suggestions to help you make sure you cover the key topics in this chapter if you have limited time. (Refer to the daily lesson plans in your Teacher's Resource Box for additional suggestions.)

DAY 1   Assign the chapter to be read before class. During class, complete the Focus Activity on page 596 and the last Discussion activity on page 597.

Preventing Pregnancy and Sexually Transmitted Diseases

Make a bulletin board display of all the various methods of contraception (photographs of each possibility are the best choice). Under each method, list the pros and cons of use (effectiveness, prescription, ease of use, ability to stop the spread of STDs, and so on). On another board, have a listing of all of the STDs that a person can contract during sexual activity. List underneath them the manner in which they are transmitted and the short- and long-term effects of the condition. Allow students to look over these boards during the discussion of the chapter.

What do you think? Are the following statements true or false? If you think they are false, then say what is true.

1. Most people have trouble getting pregnant.
2. Couples who openly discuss contraception can become closer and can strengthen their relationship.
3. People who first obtain all the facts can find the perfect contraceptive method.
4. Condoms used with spermicides can be as effective as oral contraceptives in preventing pregnancy.
5. Condoms are as effective as abstinence in preventing sexually transmitted diseases.
6. If a woman is not taking the Pill, this means she isn't using birth control.
7. If sexually active couples who do not wish to have a child would begin using contraception now, the majority of abortions would be prevented.

(Answers on page 616)

Introduction

Sexual intercourse, one of the main topics of the previous chapter can lead to pregnancy. For married couples who are ready to bear and raise children together, pregnancy is a happy event. It can strengthen the couple's relationship, enhance their spiritual beliefs, and promote their personal growth. For couples who are not yet ready to raise and support children, however, pregnancy can be a disaster.

In this part of the unit you will learn how people can prevent pregnancy until the time is right. You will also learn that the choice of birth control method can dramatically affect the risk of acquiring a sexually transmitted disease (STD). The knowledge you gain here could possibly prevent a lifetime of regrets.

Of course, the only guarantee that a pregnancy will not occur is total abstinence from sexual intercourse. People who are sexually active, however, and who choose to use reliable birth control, can be pretty sure of preventing pregnancy. While none of these methods offer abstinence's 100 percent effectiveness, sexually active couples can count on these methods to prevent most pregnancies.

Answers to FACT or FICTION

1. **False.** For healthy, sexually active heterosexual couples, pregnancy occurs easily.
2. **True.**
3. **False.** No contraceptive method is perfect. To obtain the advantages of one method, the person must be willing to put up with its disadvantages.
4. **True.**
5. **False.** Condoms are prone to failure, but abstinence always prevents sexually transmitted diseases.
6. **False.** A woman who isn't taking the Pill may be using another form of birth control, such as condoms or a diaphragm. The term *birth control* refers to all contraceptive methods, including the Pill.
7. **True.**

DAY 2 Discuss the different contraceptives, their effectiveness, and how they work from the information given in Section 2. Choose activities from the section that best fit your students' needs for understanding.

DAY 3 Begin discussion of Section 3 with the Focus Activity on page 612. Use the Close activity on page 613 to complete the discussion of Section 3. Complete the Discussion activity on page 615 for Section 4 and the Discussion activity on page 617 for Section 5.

SECTION 1

FOCUS

OUTCOMES

In this section students will learn that:

1. Pregnancy is the rule, not the exception, for sexually active people using no contraception.
2. Whether or not a person uses contraception is a personal choice.
3. Professional help may be needed to decide which method is best.

FOCUS ACTIVITY

Have students imagine that a couple is going to engage in sex for the first time. In small groups, ask students to brainstorm what will determine whether or not the couple will use reliable contraception. Each group can report back one or two of its ideas.

TEACH & APPLY

BACKGROUND INFORMATION

Make sure the students realize that the fact that they are studying this information does not mean that they are being advised to use contraception. The text has stressed, from page 1, the need for each person to make his or her own choices; the purpose of the text is to provide information to help people make wiser, more informed choices. This text has also presented a strong case for abstinence in several chapters prior to this one.

> " The management of fertility is one of the most important functions of adulthood. "
>
> Germaine Greer,
> (1939–)
> Author

SECTION 1 — Choosing Contraception and STD Protection

Teenagers often think that pregnancy is difficult to achieve. For healthy, sexually active heterosexual couples, though, pregnancy occurs easily. Most people have no trouble starting a pregnancy. Ninety percent of sexually active couples who use no birth control become pregnant within one year. As Figure 22–1 shows, pregnancy is the rule—not the exception—for sexually active people using no **contraception**.

Among sexually active teenagers, fewer than half report that they always use contraception. Teenagers also contract STDs at an alarming rate, exceeding the rate of any other age group. While the odds of pregnancy from unprotected sexual intercourse are high, the odds of contracting an STD are much higher.

Not all people see contraception in the same way. Some people's religious beliefs forbid its use. Other people would like everyone worldwide who is sexually active to use it. This chapter does not argue for or against contraception. It takes the position that the choice is personal, and it presents the facts people need to make informed choices.

Contraception is not for women only. It is a shared human responsibility that accompanies sexual intercourse. No one should ever assume that a partner will take care of protecting against pregnancy or STDs. According to the American Academy of Pediatrics, condoms are not optional for sexually active, unmarried teens.

Close to a million teens become pregnant each year, but three times that many teens contract an STD each year. Condoms, therefore, are a must for STD prevention among sexually active teens. This holds true even when other birth control methods, such as pills, are used to prevent pregnancy. Two contraceptive agents—latex condoms with the spermicide nonoxynol-9, and female condoms with the same spermicide applied—provide the best protection against some STDs.

Figure 22–1 The Odds of Pregnancy Are High

Among ten sexually active couples using no contraception,

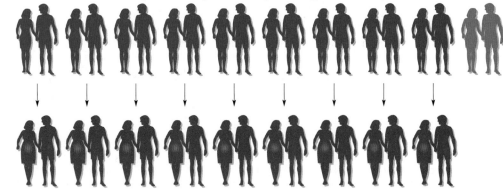

Nine become pregnant within one year.

HEALTHY PEOPLE 2000

Reduce pregnancies among girls aged 17 and younger to no more than 50 per 1,000 adolescents.

Few situations are as life-changing for a young woman and her family as an unintended, out-of-wedlock pregnancy. The manner in which she, her family, and her partner resolve the crisis may have life-long consequences for the people involved and for the broader community.

This objective targets reductions in pregnancies among all adolescents under age 18, with the assumption that such pregnancies are unintended pregnancies among unmarried teens. In 1981, an estimated 84 percent of pregnancies among young women under age 20 were unintended. Further, 96 percent of abortions among women aged 19 and younger are to unmarried women.

Honest talk about contraception leads to both wise planning and closeness.

The couple should discuss the topic openly. Being concerned about contraception shows a strong commitment to the partner's well-being. Open discussions about contraception not only help the couple find a suitable method, but also tend to bring them closer together and strengthen their relationship.

 KEY POINTS   *Whether or not to use contraception is a personal choice to be made by each sexually active person who does not want to have a child.*

Where to Get Help

Before choosing a method of contraception, a young person is wise to seek advice from a parent. Expert advice from a physician, physician's assistant, or nurse practitioner is also helpful. The professional will check for health problems, provide education, and, if one is needed, write a prescription. Student health centers, county health departments, and family planning centers often have reliable printed information sheets. Many provide other contraceptive services at a reasonable cost. Special-help clinics are sometimes available to teenagers.

Religious organizations may also provide counseling services. They may address topics of sexuality, pregnancy, and other issues, as well as contraception.

If you choose to seek outside help, make an advance appointment. Remember that such agencies are made up of individuals, and not every counselor is the right one for every person. If you should feel uncomfortable with one counselor, ask to see someone else. If you don't get the information you are seeking from one type of center, go to another.

Remember, too, that no contraceptive method is perfect. Along with the advantages a method presents, disadvantages are also a certainty. People must be willing to compromise.

MINI Glossary

contraception: any method of preventing conception (the union of the male sperm and the female ovum). The term *birth control* is often used to mean the same thing, but technically, birth control includes abortion.

Recent research suggests that the higher frequency of poor health outcomes among adolescents who give birth do not stem from intrinsic medical risk, but from socioeconomic and behavioral factors, such as low income, low levels of education, and poor nutritional patterns. Thus, while it may be possible to control these factors and demonstrate that healthy teens can have healthy pregnancies, some of the factors that may predispose a young woman to become pregnant also place her and her baby at risk for poor health outcomes. The negative effects of unintended adolescent pregnancy include induced abortions (43 percent of pregnancies among young women aged 15 through 17 end in abortion), emotional and psychological disruption, social and economic effects on the adolescent and her child, and economic consequences for society at large.

The handout, "Community Resources," in the Teacher's Resource Box provides guidelines to help students locate and organize information regarding counseling services available in their community.

COMPREHENSION CHECK

Ask the following questions to check that students are able to read and understand the information provided in Figure 22–2.

a. Are any pregnancy prevention methods as safe or safer than canoeing? (Yes) If so, which ones? (IUDs, diaphragms, condoms, spermicides, fertility awareness methods, and sterilization of men)

b. Of the pregnancy prevention methods listed, which is the most dangerous? (smoker using birth control pills)

ASSESS

EVALUATE

A reproducible quiz for Section 1 is provided in the Teacher's Resource Box.

Before choosing a method of contraception, seek accurate information.

Figure 22–2 Risks of Contraception in Perspective

Activity	Chance of Death in a Year
For all men and women:	
Motorcycling	1 in 1,000
Automobile driving	1 in 6,000
Playing football	1 in 25,000
Canoeing	1 in 100,000
For women aged 15 to 44 years:	
Using tampons	1 in 350,000
Having sexual intercourse (risk of death from pelvic inflammatory disease)	1 in 50,000
Going through pregnancy and giving birth	1 in 14,300
Preventing pregnancy:	
Using birth control pills	
Nonsmoker	1 in 63,000
Smoker	1 in 16,000
Using intrauterine devices (IUDs)	1 in 100,000
Using diaphragms, condoms, or spermicides	None
Using fertility awareness methods	None
Undergoing sterilization:	
Women	1 in 67,000
Men	1 in 300,000
Terminating pregnancy:	
Illegal abortion	1 in 3,000
Legal abortion	
Before 9 wk	1 in 500,000
Between 9 and 12 wk	1 in 67,000
Between 13 and 15 wk	1 in 23,000
After 15 wk	1 in 8,700

Source: R. A. Hatcher and coauthors, *Contraceptive Technology* (1990–1992): 146. Used with permission.

 No contraceptive method is perfect. Many people need professional help to find the one that will be best for them.

Two Kinds of Effectiveness

One of the most important aspects of a contraceptive method to consider is its **effectiveness**. For example, you may hear an expert say that the effectiveness of a contraceptive method is 98.5 percent. Later, you may hear another trusted source say it is only 92 percent effective. Both may be right. The two numbers are different because they are obtained by two different types of scientific studies.

The first expert just mentioned is quoting studies that answer the question, How well does this method work in 100 *couples who use it perfectly* for one year? These studies are run in laboratories that permit no mistakes. When this contraceptive method is used perfectly, then its **laboratory effectiveness** is 98.5 percent.

The second expert is quoting studies of what happens in real life. These studies answer the question, How many *typical users* out of 100 become pregnant while using the contraceptive method for one year? The **user effectiveness** is 92 percent. In real life, 8 women out of 100 become pregnant, because in real life people make mistakes. This chap-

Chapter 22, Section 1

The following quiz will help you assess your students' understanding of the material covered in this section of the chapter. You might use the quiz as an oral exercise, which will lead into a class discussion of the topics covered. Or, you might use it as a paper/pencil

quiz to evaluate your students individually.

1. Total abstinence from sexual intercourse is the only way to guarantee that a pregnancy will not occur. (True)

2. Pregnancy is difficult to achieve. (False)

3. Teenagers contract sexual diseases at a higher rate than any other age group. (True)

4. Condoms are essential in preventing the spread of sexually transmitted diseases.

ter lists both kinds of effectiveness ratings whenever possible. Giving only one might be misleading.

 KEY POINTS *The effectiveness rating of a contraceptive method depends on how it was studied. Laboratory studies measure effectiveness when the method is used perfectly, but real users make mistakes.*

Side Effects

The side effects of contraceptive methods can also be misleading. Some lists of side effects are long and sound threatening. Keep in mind, though, that a drug company has to report every side effect, even if it occurs in only one of a million users. Before you start to worry about the dangers of contraception, remember that carrying and delivering a baby pose risks that are far greater than those of using any contraceptive method except one (the Pill, for a woman who smokes). In fact, driving down the street is much more likely to injure your health than is using contraception. Figure 22–2 compares some other risks with those of contraception.

 KEY POINTS *Contraceptive methods carry risks, but most are far lower than the risks of carrying a pregnancy to term.*

SECTION 1 Review

Answer the following questions on a sheet of paper.

Learning the Vocabulary

The vocabulary terms in this section are *contraception, effectiveness, laboratory effectiveness,* and *user effectiveness.* Fill in the blank with the correct term.

1. The _____ of a contraceptive method is a measure of the percentage of *typical* female users who are protected from pregnancy in a year's time.
2. The _____ is the percentage of women protected from pregnancy in a year's time if they use a contraceptive method *perfectly.*
3. How well a contraceptive method or device prevents pregnancy is, in general, called its _____.

4. _____ is any method used to prevent conception.

Learning the Facts

5. What happens in a relationship in which the couple openly communicates about contraception?
6. Where can a young person go to get advice about contraceptives?
7. What must drug companies do about the side effects of products they sell?

Making Life Choices

8. Look at Figure 22–2, "Risks of Contraception in Perspective." What are the risks of dying within one year for a person riding a motorcycle? For a person going through pregnancy? For a person using contraception? Are you surprised at the results? What does this tell you about the risk of death from contraceptives?

MINI Glossary

effectiveness: how well a contraceptive method or device prevents pregnancy, expressed as a percentage. The **laboratory effectiveness** is the percentage of women protected from pregnancy in a year's time under ideal laboratory conditions. The **user effectiveness** is the percentage of typical female users who are protected.

SECTION 1 Review Answers

1. user effectiveness
2. laboratory effectiveness
3. effectiveness
4. Contraception
5. helps the couple find a suitable method of contraception and draws them closer together, strengthening their relationship (p. 597)
6. parent, physician, physician's assistant, student health-care centers, county health departments, family planning centers, religious organizations (p. 597)
7. must report every side effect, even if it has affected only one in a million users. (p. 599)
8. 1 in 1,000; 1 in 14,300; remaining answers may vary (p. 598)

CLOSE

Tell students 1 million teenagers become pregnant each year. That is 1 in every 10 American teenage girls. Other countries that are similar to the United States in standard of living and education don't have the high pregnancy rates we do. Only 1 in 30 Swedish teens and fewer than 1 in 20 English, Canadian, or French teens becomes pregnant. Ask students why they think this is so.

WORKSHEETS Reproducible vocabulary worksheets are provided in the Teacher's Resource Box.

(True)
5. Birth control pills reduce the risk of contracting a sexually transmitted disease. (False)
6. Student health centers and family planning clinics can provide information about various methods of birth control. (True)
7. Laboratory studies test the product's effectiveness when it is used perfectly. (True)

8. User effectiveness is usually higher than laboratory effectiveness. (False)
9. A drug company must report every potential side effect of a birth control medication, no matter how unlikely its occurrence. (True)
10. The risks of pregnancy are almost always greater than the health risks involved in taking contraceptives. (True)

SECTION
2

FOCUS

OUTCOMES

In this section students will learn:

1. The advantages of abstinence and how it compares to the standard methods of contraception.

2. To name and describe standard methods of contraception.

3. To describe side effects of different contraceptive methods.

FOCUS ACTIVITY

TEACHER SUPPORT

Key Passage

Explain to students that abstinence means different things to different people. Give examples of expressions of affection: holding hands, hugging, dry mouth kissing, French kissing, above-the-waist petting, below-the-waist petting, and so on. Hand an index card to each student and have students write expressions of affection between a couple that, in their opinions, can be considered abstinent. Tell students not to put their names on the cards and that the cards will be collected, shuffled, and read. Give students five minutes to write their responses. Read the students' responses to the class. Discuss. Also ask why different people define abstinence differently.

SECTION
2

The Standard Contraceptive Methods

As you read about each contraceptive method, you may notice that some are given more space than others. This is not because they are better methods, but because they are more complex in their actions. Effectiveness and safety are the main factors to consider for each one.

Abstinence

The safest, most effective contraceptive method to consider is **abstinence**. These days, young people from New York to California, from the Midwest to the southern states—in fact, teens from all over the United States—are choosing abstinence more often than ever before. Part of the reason is to avoid pregnancy. Also, teens are more aware these days of the threats they face from AIDS, herpes, and other sexually transmitted diseases.

When used correctly, abstinence is the most effective contraceptive—100 percent effective, in fact. To use abstinence correctly, though, a couple must remember that a pregnancy can begin if even a single drop of fluid from the penis is deposited near the opening of a woman's vagina. Sperm from this fluid can swim into the vagina and up through the uterus to find a waiting ovum. Therefore, to be 100 percent effective in preventing pregnancy, abstinence must include preventing any contact at all between the man's penis and the woman's vagina.

Another enormous benefit of abstinence is its 100 percent effectiveness against sexually transmitted diseases—effectiveness far above that of the latex condom, the next best choice for disease prevention. Again, proper use of the method is essential. Diseases can be transmitted by any contact between penis and vagina.

The decision to abstain from sexual intercourse can take courage and willpower in the face of internal and external pressures to look sexy and act sexy. Most people who succeed, however, say it is worth the effort. They say they can best focus on their own growth and pursue their own goals without the demands of a sexually intimate relationship. Finally, when they become ready to make a lifelong commitment, they have grown in character and self-esteem and are well able to become partners. At that point, another method of contraception may be needed. The Health Strategies section on this page, "Avoiding Pregnancy," lists abstinence and other ways to avoid pregnancy or to reduce the risk of becoming pregnant.

KEY POINTS *Abstinence is the only contraceptive method that is 100 percent effective against both pregnancy and sexually transmitted diseases.*

Health Strategies

Avoiding Pregnancy

People can completely protect themselves from pregnancy by:

1. Practicing sexual abstinence.

People can reduce their risks of becoming pregnant by using:

1. Oral contraceptives (prescription).
2. Hormone implants and injections (prescription).
3. Intrauterine devices (IUDs) (prescription).
4. Vaginal spermicides (over-the-counter).
5. Diaphragms (prescription).
6. Cervical caps (prescription).
7. Male condoms (over-the-counter).
8. Female condoms (over-the-counter).
9. The rhythm method.
10. Sterilization (surgical procedure).

HEALTHY PEOPLE 2000

Increase to at least 40 percent the proportion of sexually active adolescents aged 17 and younger who have abstained from sexual activity for the previous 3 months.

Many factors are strongly associated with sexual activity before marriage, including characteristics such as puberty, age, race, and socioeconomic status, religiousness, intelligence and academic achievement, and dating behavior; family characteristics such as family background and parental support and control; and the influence of peers. When young adolescent girls begin having sexual intercourse, it is generally infrequent and unpredictable. Some adolescents who have had recent intercourse view the event as atypical behavior which they are unlikely to repeat.

Oral Contraceptives

Many women choose **oral contraceptives**, popularly known as "the Pill." The Pill is the most popular non-surgical method of contraception. One type of oral contraceptive, the **combination pill**, uses synthetic versions of the female reproductive hormones **estrogen** and **progesterone** to prevent pregnancy. (The laboratory-made progesterone is called **progestin**.) Another type of pill, the **progestin-only pill**, contains only progestin. Figure 22–3 shows some packets of typical pills. Each packet contains a month's supply.

Figure 22–3 *Oral Contraceptives*

Oral contraceptive effectiveness:
Combination pills, laboratory rating = 99.5 percent.
Combination pill, user effectiveness = 98 percent.
Progestin-only pill, laboratory rating = 99 percent.
Progestin-only pill, user effectiveness = 95 percent.

For Your Information

Some people mistakenly believe the Pill to be the only form of birth control. Of course, the Pill is just one choice among many.

Combination Pills The estrogen present in combination pills prevents pregnancy by stopping ovulation. Pills vary in the amounts of hormone they contain. Most packets of pills deliver hormones for 21 days of the menstrual cycle, and then provide seven inactive pills to help the woman stay on schedule during menstruation. A woman may still ovulate during her first month on such pills. Therefore, she should use a backup method of contraception during this time.

Progestin-only Pill The progestin-only pill, as the name says, contains no estrogen—only progestin. Unlike combination pills, which suppress ovulation, the progestin-only pill mostly affects the uterus itself. Progestin thickens the mucus surrounding the uterine opening (cervix), so that sperm cannot penetrate. Progestin may also deactivate sperm cells. Progestin also interrupts the normal preparation of the uterine lining so that a fertilized egg may not implant.

Correct Use of Oral Contraceptives Pill users may have difficulty remembering to take the pills. The effectiveness of the Pill, as with any type of contraception, depends on regular and correct use. If a woman forgets to take her pill for a day or more, she should take the missed pill as soon as she remembers it, get back on her pill schedule, and use a backup method of contraception for the remainder of that pill cycle.

Morning-After Pill Women can also use the Pill as an emergency backup method of birth control. The so-called morning-after pill consists of a larger-than-normal dose of regular pills, taken on the day or two following unprotected intercourse. The method requires a physician's prescription to get the dosage right. The effectiveness rating for this method is not yet known.

Side Effects of Oral Contraceptives The side effects of oral contraceptives range from common, bothersome symptoms to rare, life-threatening

Glossary

abstinence: refraining completely from sexual relations with other people: also called celibacy.

oral contraceptives: pills that prevent pregnancy by stopping ovulation or by changing conditions in the uterus; often called *birth control pills* or *the Pill.*

combination pill: an oral contraceptive that contains progestin and synthetic estrogen.

estrogen: a hormone that, in females, regulates the ovulatory cycle.

progesterone: a hormone secreted in females during that portion of the menstrual cycle in which the uterine lining builds up.

progestin: a synthetic version of progesterone used in contraceptives.

progestin-only pill: an oral contraceptive containing only progestin. Another name is the *minipill.*

TEACH & APPLY

BACKGROUND INFORMATION

Some students may not realize this category of contraceptives is called *oral* contraceptives because it refers to the mouth. Tell students that oral contraceptives are those that are taken orally, through the mouth.

COMPREHENSION CHECK

You may want to refer back to the Chapter 20 discussion of ovulation before they read the explanation of how oral contraceptives work.

BACKGROUND INFORMATION

Give students the following history of "the Pill."

In 1934, progesterone was isolated in the laboratory. Researchers knew from previous experiments that ovulation did not happen in animals when progesterone levels were at their highest. The reason was that progesterone would create the illusion of a false pregnancy and no ovulation occurs during pregnancy. This was proven when it was given to animals and did inhibit ovulation.

In 1954, Carl Djerassi was successful in synthesizing progesterone. The man-made hormone was more potent than naturally occurring progesterones, so it could be used in very small amounts.

Three other researchers, Gregory Pincus (often called the "father of the Pill"), J. Rock, and C.R. Garcia were doing research to develop a more effective contraceptive. They tested hundreds of different compounds on animals until they found out what would work best.

(continued on next page)

Negative consequences of nonmarital sexual intercourse can include elevated risk of acquiring a sexually transmitted disease and suffering impaired fertility as a result of sexually transmitted infections. Therefore, abstaining from further nonmarital sexual intercourse protects adolescents from a variety of risks to health.

Peers of the same gender are a major influence on adolescent attitudes about sexual activity. The proportion of their same-sex peers that teenagers believe are sexually active and how sexually active they believe them to be are powerful predictors of sexual experience among adolescent boys and girls. However, individual behavior and attitudes are more closely related to what adolescents think their friends are doing than what they are actually doing.

conditions. The *number* of side effects is high, but remember that most side effects are rare. Among the more common, less serious side effects are tenderness of the breasts, emotional depression or fatigue, nausea or vomiting, skin conditions, weight gain or loss, stopping of menstruation, unexpected vaginal bleeding, and a tendency to develop vaginal yeast infections. More rare are high levels of sugar and fat in the blood, an impaired sex drive, headaches, and fluid retention. Among the most rare and serious side effects are diseases of the heart, kidney, liver, or gallbladder; benign tumors of the uterus; and blood clots that can lodge in vital organs and cause death.

Early symptoms almost always warn a pill user who is developing any of the serious medical conditions. A woman taking oral contraceptives should call her physician if she has:

▶ Abdominal pain.
▶ Chest pain.
▶ Breathlessness.
▶ Headaches.
▶ Blurred vision or loss of vision.
▶ Leg pain.

These symptoms may warn that a serious condition is developing.

Not all side effects are negative. For example, oral contraceptives can help to regulate irregular menstrual periods and relieve excessive menstrual cramping. Oral contraceptives have also been linked to reduced risks of certain cancers.

You may read reports that link oral contraceptives to a risk of cervical cancer, but factors other than the Pill may be the cause. Pill users often have intercourse at young ages, have many sex partners, and are unlikely to use condoms. They are therefore often exposed to the sexually transmitted virus human papilloma virus (HPV), which causes a type of cervical cancer. The Pill alone provides no protection from STDs. People relying on the Pill for pregnancy protection should still use condoms to prevent STDs.

A very dangerous combination is smoking and using the Pill. Together, they greatly increase the risk of heart attack or stroke. Chapter 14 presented a graph showing this effect (see Figure 14–4 on page 382).

The progestin-only pill produces fewer and less severe side effects than the combination pill, so women sometimes switch to it. Of course, the progestin-only pill has possible side effects of its own, including menstrual disorders and, less often, headaches. Also, it is less effective in preventing pregnancy.

Most women who use the Pill experience no side effects at all. Others who experience minor symptoms at first may find that they disappear after about three months. Sometimes a switch from one brand to another can bring relief (the woman can ask her physician).

It is important to be aware that depression, a relatively common side effect, may take some time to develop. The user therefore may not realize that it comes from oral contraceptive use. When moodiness, sadness, or irritability is not explained by life events and does not improve after several months, Pill users should suspect the pills and ask their physicians for another type.

A woman who thinks she may be pregnant should not take the Pill, because it increases the risks of birth defects. In fact, a woman using oral contraceptives who decides to become pregnant should switch to another

(continued from previous page)

In 1956 the trio tested their new contraceptive on women in Puerto Rico. It was so effective that within a short time, "the Pill" became popular worldwide. Ask students what the development of the Pill has meant to people everywhere. What impact has it had on the earth's environment?

BACKGROUND INFORMATION

Tell students that taking pills is not the only way to introduce progestins into the body. Some contraception devices, such as IUDs or vaginal rings, release the drug directly into the uterus or vagina. Women can also receive a shot of progestins that lasts for three months. The shot, called *Depo-Provera,* was approved by the FDA in late 1992 and was first available in the United States in January of 1993. Depo-Provera, Norplant, and slow-release implants of progestin are discussed on page 603.

COMPREHENSION CHECK

Ask students the difference between the user effectiveness of the progestin-only pill versus the combination pill (see Figure 22–3 on page 601). (95 percent to 98 percent) In a group of 100 women, how many more will become pregnant using the progestin-only pill as compared to the combination pill? (3 more—5 in 100 for the progestin-only pill as opposed to 2 in 100 with the combination pill)

For **Y**our **I**nformation

HPV and other sexually transmitted diseases are discussed in Chapter 16.

❝*Contraceptives should be used on every conceivable occasion.*❞

Spike Milligan
(1918–)
British actor and author

special needs

Interpersonal, Linguistic, Spatial, Logical-mathematical

The information presented in this chapter is important to students now, but it may actually be more useful to some of them at a later date. To help them summarize the information in a pamphlet that they can take home for further reference, you may decide to incorporate this activity into the study of this chapter. The overall topic of the pamphlet will be the same as the chapter title: "Preventing Pregnancy and Sexually Transmitted Diseases."

Divide the class into several groups and assign one of the following topics to each group: Where to Get Help, Effectiveness and Side Effects, Standard Contraceptive Methods, Methods Not Recommended, Sterilization, Abortion, and Adoption. Each group will be responsible for developing one section of the pamphlet.

method of contraception for at least two months (some health-care providers suggest six months to a year) before becoming pregnant.

 Oral contraceptives are highly effective in preventing pregnancy, but they must be used correctly. Side effects range from minor to severe. The most severe side effects are rare.

Hormone Implants and Injections

Progestin, the synthetic hormone of oral contraceptives, can also be delivered by slow-release capsules implanted under the skin. The product **Norplant** (shown in Figure 22–4) consists of tubes of progestin. In a simple surgical procedure, a physician implants six thin capsules (each the size of a matchstick) under the skin of a woman's upper arm. Norplant works by slowly releasing progestin for up to five years. Its effectiveness is about the same as the laboratory effectiveness of progestin-only pills.

The convenience of Norplant leads teens who choose this method of contraception to stay with it. A study of young Norplant users and oral contraceptive users found that not one of the Norplant users became pregnant. A full fourth of the oral contraceptive users became pregnant, however, because they forgot to take some pills or ran out of them. The girls who quit using Norplant did so because they experienced some of its side effects, such as menstrual irregularities, mood swings, weight gain, headaches, dizziness, and nervousness. In the rare cases where pregnancy occurs when Norplant is in place, the capsules must be removed. Norplant is not thought to cause birth defects in such pregnancies.

A woman who makes a one-time decision to use Norplant is provided excellent protection against pregnancy. This doesn't mean that worry-free sex can follow, however. Norplant offers no protection against STDs. People who are not in a committed, long-term monogamous relationship with an uninfected partner must still use condoms to prevent diseases.

As an alternative to implants, women can receive a shot of progestin (called **Depo-Provera**) that lasts for three months. Women using this method also need to use condoms for STD prevention.

 Norplant delivers progestin for up to five years from capsules implanted under the skin.

Intrauterine Device (IUD)

Many women choose an **intrauterine device**, or **IUD**, for contraception (see Figure 22–5a). The IUD is a small plastic or plastic and metal object that a physician inserts into a woman's uterus. A tiny nylon thread hangs from the IUD through the cervix into the vagina. So long as the thread is there, the woman can know that the IUD is in place.

The IUD is best suited for women who have had at least one child; are in a stable, mutually monogamous relationship (such as marriage); and have no history of pelvic inflammatory disease (PID). Teens are usually *not* the best candidates for IUD use.

The way an IUD prevents pregnancy is not fully known. One theory is that the IUD makes the uterus hostile to sperm. Another is that it prevents implantation. One available IUD contains the hormone progesterone, which it releases into the uterus.

Figure 22–4 Norplant

Norplant effectiveness:
  Laboratory rating = 99.96 percent.
  User effectiveness = 98 to 99 percent.

Glossary

- **Norplant:** a trade name for a surgical hormone delivery system that provides continuous release of progestin, thereby preventing pregnancy for up to five years.
- **Depo-Provera** (DEE-po pro-VAIR-uh): a trade name for an injectable form of progestin.
- **intrauterine device (IUD):** a device inserted into the uterus to prevent conception or implantation.

Each section of the pamphlet should include a summary of the information from the text as well as any other information you feel is important. Students should also research contacts and sources in your local area where they can get information or assistance and those names and phone numbers could be included. The groups should lay out their information in an interesting and easy-to-read format, using graphics where possible and feasible.

When all the sections have been completed, arrange them into a pamphlet. This can then be duplicated so that each student has a copy for his or her own use. You may also want to provide several copies to be added to your school library or media center and several copies to be given to the school counselors.

COMPREHENSION CHECK

Have students compare the laboratory rating to the user effectiveness rating for the oral contraceptive, implant, and IUD methods. Ask what the difference is between the two ratings for each of those contraceptives. (1.5 percent to 4 percent difference) Now ask what the difference is between laboratory and user effectiveness for vaginal spermicides. (16 percent to 18 percent difference)

LEARNING WITH VISUALS

After students have learned about all the different contraceptives described in this section, do this activity.

Tell students they will be doing some artwork for the health room and should think about one or two other people with whom they would like to work. Explain that they will be asked to design a poster that is an accurate and convincing advertisement to sell a method of birth control.

Have students bring posterboard to create the advertisements. Have students bring markers, colored pencils, crayons, or any medium they choose to work with from home. The students will need to have some class time to get their ideas together. Pick a day that the posters can be created in class. Allow enough time at the end of class for the students to show and explain their posters. Display the posters on the health-room walls.

IUD effectiveness:
  Laboratory rating = 98.5 percent.
  User effectiveness = 97 percent.

Figure 22–5a An IUD

Figure 22–5b IUD

For **Y**our **I**nformation

Figure 22–11 lists other facts and concerns about IUD use.

Pelvic inflammatory disease (PID), which can lead to sterility, has been associated with IUD use. PID may occur if, during insertion of the device, bacteria are introduced into the uterus. Also, a woman with an IUD may fail to use condoms to prevent STDs, and STDs often cause PID. An IUD may prevent pregnancy (Figure 22–5b), but it has no stopping effect on STDs.

KEY POINTS   *IUDs are devices inserted into the uterus to prevent pregnancy. An IUD is best used by a woman who has had a child, is in a stable, monogamous relationship (such as marriage), and has no history of PID. IUDs do not protect against STDs.*

Figure 22-6 Vaginal Spermicides

Spermicide (foams, creams, gels, sheets, and suppositories) effectiveness:
  Laboratory rating = 95 to 97 percent.
  User effectiveness = 79 percent.

Vaginal Spermicides

The spermicides are sperm-killing or sperm-immobilizing products that can be inserted into the vagina just before intercourse. They are available over the counter in the forms shown in Figure 22–6—foams, creams, gels, sheets, or suppositories. These contraceptives are **barrier methods**—they place a physical and chemical barrier between sperm and ovum at the opening of the uterus.

Most spermicides do not last long—only half an hour or so—and therefore must be inserted just prior to each occasion of sexual intercourse. Also, spermicides, when used alone, often fail to prevent pregnancy. When pregnancy is not an acceptable outcome, spermicides must be used with other forms of contraception, such as the diaphragm or condoms.

CRITICAL THINKING

After students have read the information about the diaphragm and the cervical cap, ask them to name at least two advantages of the cap over the diaphragm. (more durable, requires less spermicide, no additional applications) There is, however, at least one disadvantage. Ask them to name it. (has a user

The killing action of spermicides also kills some of the pathogens that cause STDs. Spermicides alone do not kill all viruses, however. The viruses that cause AIDS and herpes are unaffected by spermicides. Latex condoms used with spermicide, then, are an obvious choice for preventing both pregnancy and STDs.

 Spermicides can kill or stop sperm. They also kill some forms of pathogens that cause STDs.

Diaphragm

The **diaphragm**, another barrier method, is a circular metal spring or ring fitted with a shallow cup of thin rubber that the user fills with spermicidal cream or jelly. The device is folded into the vagina. Once inside, it springs open to cover the cervix. The diaphragm is shown in Figure 22–7. The diaphragm holds spermicide snugly against the entrance of the cervix and bars sperm from entering the uterus. The diaphragm also puts up a barrier to some STD bacteria that may otherwise invade the uterus. The diaphragm provides no protection against viruses that cause STDs, however, so condoms are still essential.

To work properly, a diaphragm must be the right size for each woman, and must be custom fitted. (Some people may be tempted to borrow a diaphragm "just to try it" before going in to be fitted by a health-care professional. This is a mistake, because the likelihood that a borrowed diaphragm will fit properly is slim indeed.) A woman must be refitted if she gains or loses 10 pounds or if she has a child.

The user of a diaphragm can insert it up to six hours before intercourse. If two hours or so have passed before the intercourse occurs, however, the user should apply another dose of spermicide. In this case, the user must remove the diaphragm, apply the spermicide, and reinsert the diaphragm.

After intercourse, the woman should leave the diaphragm in place for at least six hours and then remove it when convenient, within 24 hours. The diaphragm slips out of the vagina easily when pulled downward by its spring edge. To repeat intercourse within the six-hour period during which the diaphragm must remain in place, the woman can simply insert an application of spermicide into the vagina.

The user should store her diaphragm with care and check it often for holes or other defects by holding it up to a light. It has a limited life span.

A few years ago, a disposable diaphragm-shaped sponge was available over the counter. The Food and Drug Administration found problems with it, causing the maker to take it off the market.

 The diaphragm is a barrier device that blocks sperm from entering the uterus. The diaphragm is ineffective in preventing many sexually transmitted infections.

Cervical Cap

The **cervical cap**, shown in Figure 22–8a, is a flexible, cuplike device about an inch and a half in diameter that covers the woman's cervix. Like the diaphragm, it must fit perfectly to prevent the passage of sperm into the uterus (Figure 22–8b). A health-care provider chooses the size to fit the user.

Figure 22–7 Diaphragm with Spermicide

Diaphragm with spermicide effectiveness:
  Laboratory rating = 98 percent.
  User effectiveness = 82 to 86 percent.

MINI
Glossary

barrier methods: contraceptive methods that physically or chemically obstruct the travel of sperm toward the ovum. These devices do not alter body processes with drugs or devices.

diaphragm: a dome that fits over the cervix and holds spermicidal cream or jelly against the uterine entrance to block the passage of sperm.

cervical cap: a rubber cap that fits over the cervix, used with spermicide to prevent conception.

effectiveness of 73 percent to 92 percent as compared to 82 percent to 88 percent for the diaphragm) The 92 percent is better than the 86 percent, but of more concern is the low of 73 percent.

(continued on next page)

(continued from previous page)

woman does get pregnant, she has two choices—*To Have the Baby* or *Abort It.* Put these choices under *Pregnancy.*

If a person gets an STD, it may be *Curable,* or it may be *Incurable.* Put these two terms under *STD.* If the STD can be cured, the person can be *Completely Healthy* or have *Permanent Problems,* like sterility. Put these two possibilities under *Curable.* If they cannot be cured, as is the case with herpes or AIDS, they may have the STD for *The Rest of Their Life* or *Die from It.* Put these risks under *Incurable.*

If a girl decides to *Have Her Baby,* she has three choices—she can *Marry the Father, Raise the Baby by Herself,* or *Give the Baby Up for Adoption.* Write these three choices under *Have Her Baby* on the board.

DISCUSSION

You may want to discuss with students some major drawbacks to the use of condoms. One of the chief drawbacks is that the condom must be put on after the man has been aroused but before he enters the woman. This necessary interruption in lovemaking is the major reason for users neglecting or "forgetting" to put condoms on. Another drawback is that some men complain that sensation is dulled by the condom. The use of condoms made by animal tissue will help remedy this problem, but as the text states, the animal tissue condoms, such as the lambskin condom, will not prevent STDs.

Cervical cap with spermicide effectiveness:
Laboratory rating = 98 percent.
User effectiveness = 73 to 92 percent.

Figure 22–8a *Cervical Cap with Spermicide*

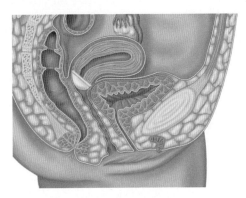

Figure 22-8b *Cervical Cap*

Like the diaphragm, the cap is used with spermicide and left in place before and after intercourse.

In a very few instances, the dangerous bacterial poisoning known as toxic shock syndrome (TSS) has been associated with diaphragm and cervical cap use. Teenage girls are its most frequent victims. (More often, as discussed in Chapter 10, toxic shock syndrome has been associated with the use of superabsorbent tampons.) Because of the risk of toxic shock syndrome, it may be wise to avoid using a diaphragm or cap during the menstrual period and always to remove it after no more than 24 hours. The early warning signs of TSS are listed on page 277 in Chapter 10.

 KEY POINTS *The cervical cap fits tightly over the cervix to prevent passage of sperm into the uterus. Toxic shock syndrome has been associated with diaphragm and cervical cap use during menstruation.*

Male Condom

Up to this point, only women's methods of contraception have been discussed. Use of a **male condom** is the only method, aside from sterilization, available to men. The condom is a disposable, thin sheath of latex (a type of rubber) or processed lamb tissue. The condom is rolled onto the erect penis before intercourse.

Condoms are shown in Figure 22–9. There are many varieties, shapes, and colors of condoms, but those designed to prevent pregnancy all work the same way. Semen collects in the tip of the condom and is discarded with it.

The choice of latex condoms for contraception is valid for two reasons. First, latex condoms offer protection against sexually transmitted diseases, such as AIDS. As mentioned, even teens who use another form of contraception against pregnancy must use condoms as well. The Pill, IUD, and

enrichment

You might want to share the following information about condom use from the *University of California at Berkeley Wellness Letter* with your students.

Condom breakage is more common than most people realize. According to a study of 98 males who use condoms, 50 percent said they had had a condom break. Of those 50 percent, 30 percent had failed to tell their partners of the breakage at least one time.

other methods may prevent pregnancy, but they leave people open to sexually transmitted diseases.

The other reason that latex condoms are a wise choice for contraception is that they are superior at preventing pregnancy. Condoms with spermicide added, if used correctly, can provide pregnancy protection rivaling that of the Pill.

When applying a condom, the user should leave it rolled up as it comes from the wrapper and place it loosely on the tip of the erect penis. The condom is gently and slowly unrolled down to the base of the penis, while the thumb and index finger of one hand hold the condom's tip to create a reservoir for the semen. The condom should not be stretched tightly over the tip of the penis—it could break during intercourse. A condom will slip off a penis that is not fully erect. A man who uses a condom must withdraw from the vagina immediately after ejaculation. Never reuse a condom. Use a new one each time.

The condom must be in place before any contact occurs between the penis and the vagina, to contain the drops of sperm-containing fluid released from the penis before intercourse begins. If the condom is applied too late, its effectiveness drops dramatically. Condoms vary in quality. Cheap ones may break easily. The stronger, more expensive ones are recommended.

Some condoms are coated with lubricating jelly or powder on the outside to reduce friction in the vagina. Products that provide extra lubrication are sold especially for this purpose. A warning is in order here. Using petroleum jelly (Vaseline) or any oil-containing ("moisturizing") lotion for lubrication can weaken the condom and make it break during intercourse. Instructions for the proper storage of condoms are presented in the next section.

Figure 22–9 *Male Condoms*

Condom effectiveness:
Condom, laboratory rating = 98 percent.
Condom, user effectiveness = 88 percent.
Condom with spermicide = same as combination pill—98 to 99.5 percent.

 KEY POINTS *Condoms are the only contraceptive method available for use by men, aside from sterilization. Latex condoms with spermicide can prevent pregnancies and often prevent the transmission of many STDs.*

Condoms and STDs

Abstinence, and restricting sexual activity to contact only with a mutually monogamous, uninfected partner, are the only ways to be 100 percent sure of preventing STDs. Beyond these methods, experts say that using condoms provides the best protection against AIDS and other STD infections. However, even those experts say that condoms are not perfect for the task. Condoms may be good, but the question "How good?" is important.

MINI Glossary

male condom: a sheath worn over the penis during intercourse to contain the semen, to prevent pregnancy, and/or to reduce the risks of sexually transmitted diseases. Condoms are also called *rubbers*.

They gave the following reasons for failing to tell:

- They didn't want to interrupt intercourse.
- They didn't want to take responsibility for the break.
- They didn't want their partner to become anxious about the break.

If a partner doesn't know about a condom breaking, they won't be likely to seek medical testing for pregnancy or sexually transmitted diseases.

GROUP ACTIVITY

Prepare enough envelopes before class so that there is one for each student. Let's assume that you have 30 students. If so, leave 27 envelopes blank. Then, on the inside flap of one envelope, in small letters, write the initials *C W* (chlamydia and warts). On a second envelope write the letter *H* (herpes), and on a third *G* (gonorrhea). If you have 30 students, these three envelopes with initials representing the common STDs will represent a one in ten risk of the students contracting an STD.

Without telling the class this is an STD exercise, tell them each person is going to get one envelope. Without letting anyone else see, tell students to look at the inside flap of their envelopes when they receive them. If they see any initials, they are to commit them to memory. Then they are to exchange envelopes with another person in the class. If they had initials on the first envelope, they now write them on the new envelopes they have just received. Whether they had initials on the first envelope or not, have them "pretend" to write something on their envelopes so no one else will know who has the initialed envelopes. Tell students they will exchange envelopes three times. Each time they exchange, they will add any initials they received on any exchange, (unless, of course, the envelope they got already has that initial on it). Go over the directions again to make sure students understand and then hand out the envelopes and do the exchanges.

Now tell students that the initials stand for chlamydia, warts, herpes and gonorrhea. Passing the envelopes three times equates to having three different

Judging Effectiveness   Some types of condoms are definitely better than others. Latex condoms manufactured with spermicide applied to them, properly used, are the most effective. The types made of natural skin and lambskin are the least effective. These have pores, as all skin does. The pores are large enough to permit bacteria and viruses to pass through them. Latex condoms have no pores, and therefore provide a barrier against microbes.

Even latex condoms do not provide perfect protection, however. While most people who use them will be protected against STDs most of the time, a certain number of individuals who use condoms, and use them correctly, still become infected with STDs. Just as they may fail to prevent pregnancy occasionally, condoms sometimes fail to prevent STDs, including AIDS.

A woman can become pregnant only a few days of each month, when she is fertile. To perfectly prevent pregnancy, condoms need only work perfectly on fertile days. A condom failure occurring on an unfertile day does not produce pregnancy. That same failure, however, allows the transmission of an STD, because both partners are susceptible to infection every day.

This is not to say that condoms are not worth using. In fact, just the opposite is true. Barring abstinence, condoms are still the best protection now available against all forms of STDs. They protect far more often than they fail.

It is important to understand condom failure in order to prevent its occurrence. Occasionally, but not often, condoms come defective from the manufacturer. Ninety-five percent of the time, new condoms are in good condition and perform as they were intended. The other 5 percent of the time, however, they burst, tear, or leak, exposing the partners to each other's secretions during intercourse.

Even a perfect condom that does not break may allow secretions to leak over the top. If STD-causing organisms are in a person's secretions, they can infect that person's partner.

Many varieties of condoms purchased from vending machines are of notoriously low quality, and may be old and brittle. Condoms from drug stores have an expiration date printed on the package, usually abbreviated *EXP*. Beyond that date, using the condoms is risky. Also, the package should say that the condoms can prevent diseases. Some condoms are just novelties and are useless for disease prevention. Also, look for the words *latex* and *nonoxynol-9*.

Testing each condom before sale is not practical. Manufacturers do spot-check batches of condoms and report the results of these tests to the Food and Drug Administration. If any batches prove defective, they are recalled from sale. Defective batches still slip through. However, by far the major cause of condom failure lies with improper storage, handling, and use by people, not with the condoms themselves.

Storing Condoms   Heat and light break condoms down. Thus they should be stored in a dark, cool place, such as a closet or drawer. Glove compartments of cars get too hot. Wallets, purses, and pockets offer little protection from keys, pens, and other sharp objects.

Opening condom packages also requires special care. Use fingers to tear the package open. Don't use teeth, fingernails, scissors, or other sharp objects that may damage the condom. Once the package is open, inspect the condom. If the material sticks to itself or is gummy or brittle, discard it.

Remember that condoms—even perfect ones—are only a second line of defense against STDs and pregnancy. A person's first and best defenses

HEALTHY PEOPLE 2000

Increase to at least 90 percent the proportion of sexually active, unmarried people aged 19 and younger who use contraception, especially combined method contraception that both effectively prevents pregnancy and provides barrier protection against disease.

The only certain way to prevent teenage pregnancy is through abstinence from sexual intercourse. Abstinence also provides absolute protection from sexually transmitted diseases, including AIDS. Mutually faithful monogamy with an uninfected partner will also protect people from sexually transmitted diseases. However, for sexually active teenagers who will not postpone sexual activity and who do not wish to become pregnant or infected with are abstinence from sexual intercourse or, in the case of STD prevention, mutual monogamy with an uninfected partner. No one should be lulled into trusting condoms completely, for they are not completely trustworthy.

 KEY POINTS *Abstinence and restricting sexual activity to a mutually monogamous, uninfected partner are the only 100 percent sure ways of preventing STDs. Condoms offer the next best protection against STDs, but condoms are not perfect. Latex condoms with spermicide are most effective against STDs.*

Female Condom

Women need to protect themselves from sexually transmitted diseases, even if their partners refuse to use condoms. To give women control of their own protection, researchers have invented the **female condom**. The device is a disposable tubular sack six and a half inches in length (shown in Figure 22–10). The material from which it is made resembles the plastic of sandwich bags, but is stronger. Flexible plastic rings at each end of the tube hold it in place in the vagina. One ring, at the closed end of the sack, fits over the cervix. The other ring remains outside the vagina to anchor the device in place and to cover parts of the female genital area (to cut down on contact with semen).

To use the device successfully, the woman must be sure that both rings are snugly in place before any contact occurs between penis and vagina. If the internal ring slipped out of place, no extra risk would result, because semen would still not escape from the pouch. Extra risk would occur if the external ring slipped into the vagina. Semen would easily spill over the edges of the condom into the vagina. The female condom is packaged with a lubricant. Using it with spermicide may boost its effectiveness in preventing pregnancy and some STDs.

....
Figure 22–10 Female Condom

Female condom effectiveness:
Laboratory rating = 88 percent.
User effectiveness = 80 percent.

 KEY POINTS *The female condom provides protection from pregnancy and gives women control of their own protection against some STDs.*

Fertility Awareness Method

The **fertility awareness method**, also called the *rhythm method*, involves neither drugs nor devices. If used perfectly, the method could be up to 95 percent effective (actual user effectiveness in typical couples is much

MINI Glossary

female condom: a soft, thin plastic tube with two end rings—one to fit over the cervix and one to serve as an anchor outside the entrance to the vagina; also called a *vaginal pouch*.

fertility awareness method: a method of charting ovulation. It involves tracking menstrual periods, body temperature, and types of cervical mucus. Also called *rhythm method*.

a sexually transmitted disease, consistent use of dual methods of contraception is the most effective means of reducing rates of pregnancy and sexually transmitted diseases.

Eighty-four percent of teenage pregnancies in 1981 were unintended and less than 5 percent of abortions to women aged 19 and younger occur among married women. Only one third of teenagers who have had sexual intercourse say that they use contraceptives all the time. Low-income teenagers are the least likely to use contraceptives consistently. Sexually active teenagers who have talked about sex, pregnancy, and contraception with their parents appear to be more likely than other teenagers to use birth control all the time. Adolescents with a stronger appreciation of the consequences if they or their partner becomes pregnant are also more likely to use contraceptives consistently.

sexual partners. Tell the class they started with the national average of one in ten teens being infected with an STD. Ask how many people now have initials on their envelopes. Discuss.

BACKGROUND INFORMATION

You may want to tell students that the rhythm method is one of the several *fertility awareness methods*. All of these methods require education, training, and planning. Other types of fertility awareness methods are the basal body temperature (BBT) method, the mucus (also called the Billings or ovulation) method, and the sympto-thermal method.

GROUP ACTIVITY

Divide the class into groups of three for this class project. Tell students that on a given day each group will present for the class how one method of contraception works. They must do the research and develop any props they might need. The presentation should be three to five minutes long. There will, however, be an interesting twist in the presentations. All the chairs will be pushed back against the walls and a large uterus with fallopian tubes and ovaries will be outlined on the floor in rope or yarn. Students will walk through these outlines. The teacher can provide a softball with white crepe paper streamers attached to represent the sperm and a large balloon or small beach ball to represent the egg. Students are encouraged to design and construct the contraceptive device they will be explaining out of paper, cardboard, cloth, foil, plastic, and so on. The design will be used in conjunction with the floor diagram. Grade students on their creativity and the accuracy of their presentations.

LEARNING WITH VISUALS

Use the questions below to get the students involved in Figure 22–11. But first, you may want to have them do a simple evaluation of these methods. Have them number a sheet of paper from 1 to 13. Then, for each of the 13 methods listed, have them write yes or no to indicate whether or not that method would be acceptable to them. Some students might prefer to keep their evaluations private, others might be willing to discuss their choices. Here are the questions:

a. Of the 13 methods listed, which is the most effective if used properly? (abstinence) Which is the most effective in typical users? (male sterilization)

b. Excluding abstinence and sterilization, what is the most effective method in typical users? (Norplant)

c. What is the least effective method in typical users? (cervical cap with spermicide)

d. Which method provides the best protection against STDs? (abstinence)

e. Which methods, other than abstinence, provide the best protection against STDs? (male condoms with spermicides and female condoms)

ASSESS

EVALUATE

A reproducible quiz for Section 2 is provided in the Teacher's Resource Box.

CHAPTER 22: Preventing Pregnancy and Sexually Transmitted Diseases

Figure 22–11 *Standard Contraceptive Methods Compared for Effectiveness*

Method	Effectiveness if Used Perfectly (%)	Effectiveness In Typical Users (%)	Factors to Consider
Abstinence	100	Unknown[a]	Abstinence must be used consistently and perfectly, or effectiveness drops to 0%. Only method that provides 100% protection against sexually transmitted diseases (STDs).
Oral contraceptives: Combination pill Progestin-only pill	99.5 99	98 95	Users who find it easy to take pills regularly use the method most successfully. No protection against STDs.
Norplant	99.96	98 to 99	Implant may be slightly visible. Long-term use is recommended. No protection against STDs.
Intrauterine device (IUD)	98.5	97	The device can be expelled without the user's awareness. Pregnancy may occur with the device in place. No protection against STDs.
Vaginal spermicides	95 to 97	79	Users who follow directions exactly use the method most successfully. Slight protection against STDs.
Diaphragm with spermicide	98	82 to 86	Successful use requires proper fit and following instructions. Slight protection against STDs.
Cervical cap with spermicide	98	73 to 92	Successful use requires proper fit and following instructions exactly. Slight protection against STDs.
Male condom	98	88	High-quality condoms are most protective. Some protection from STDs. Improper use makes failure likely.
Male condom with spermicide	99.5	98	Users must follow directions exactly. Good protection from some STDs. Poor-quality condoms make failure likely.
Female condom	88[b]	80[b]	High cost. Still proving effectiveness. Good protection against some STDs.
Fertility awareness method	80 to 95	80	Ovulation is unpredictable. A high degree of training, skill, and dedication is required.
Male sterilization	99.85	99.85	Successful, except if the user has intercourse before sperm are absent from semen or if ends of tubes grow together (very unlikely).
Female sterilization	99.7	99.7	Pregnancy is likely only if ends of tubes grow together (very unlikely).

[a]Unknown for those who allow contact between penis and vagina; otherwise provides perfect protection.
[b]Based on preliminary data.

QUICK QUIZ

Chapter 22, Section 2

The following quiz will help you assess your students' understanding of the material covered in this section of the chapter. You might use the quiz as an oral exercise, which will lead into a class discussion of the topics covered. Or, you might use it as a paper/pencil quiz to evaluate your students individually.

Like the Quick Quiz, the Section Review can also be used as an assessment tool to spark class discussion or as an individual student evaluation. It can also be used as a review in preparation for this quiz.

1. Smokers who use the Pill greatly increase their risk of heart attack and stroke. (True)

2. Norplant is surgically implanted under the skin and can prevent pregnancy for lower—only about 80 percent). The woman is taught to track the menstrual cycle and to observe body signs of ovulation, such as body temperature and mucus secretions. She can then refrain from having intercourse during the few days right after she has produced a fresh ovum.

The fertility awareness method requires no use of equipment during intercourse. It is available to anyone. However, people who wish to use it must first be trained by health professionals, because its use is complicated. Even the most technical references warn that merely reading about this method is not enough training to ensure that people can use it successfully to prevent conception. People who choose to use it, then, must go to a professional for help in getting started.

All of the methods discussed so far are effective against pregnancy to some degree. Figure 22–11 on the opposite page sums up facts concerning each method's effectiveness.

 The fertility awareness method is complex to use, but it requires no drugs or devices.

F or **Y** our **I** nformation
The fertility awareness method can be especially helpful to people trying to conceive a child.

SECTION 2 Review Answers

1. a. estrogen
   b. cervical cap
   c. Norplant
2. See pages 601–602 for possible answers.
3. with the surgical implantation of six tubes of progestin in the woman's upper arm that slowly release the progestin for up to five years (p. 603)
4. foams, creams, gels, sheets, suppositories (p. 604)
5. Answers will vary.
6. Answers will vary.

CLOSE

Although many students memorize facts for a test on contraception, they may not be able to explain how a contraceptive is used correctly or what it does to prevent pregnancy.

Before class, prepare slips of paper, each having one contraceptive method on it. You will need to have two or three slips with the same method to accommodate a class of 30 students. Fold the slips and put them in a box. Have each student draw out one. The assignment is to describe on paper how the method picked works and how it is correctly used. You may want to put a diagram of the male and female reproductive systems on the board or on an overhead projector to aid students. Collect the papers and check for understanding.

Answer the following questions on a sheet of paper.

Learning the Vocabulary

The vocabulary terms in this section are *abstinence, oral contraceptives, combination pill, estrogen, progesterone, progestin, progestin-only pill, Norplant, Depo-Provera, intrauterine device (IUD), barrier methods, diaphragm, cervical cap, male condom, female condom,* and *fertility awareness method.*

1. Match each of the following phrases with the appropriate term:
   a. a hormone that regulates the ovulatory cycle
   b. a rubber cap that fits over the cervix
   c. a trade name for a surgical hormone delivery system that provides continuous release of progestin, thereby preventing pregnancy for up to five years

Learning the Facts

2. List the side effects of taking the Pill.
3. How does Norplant work?
4. Name the different types of spermicides available.

Making Life Choices

5. Look at Figure 22–11, "Standard Contraceptive Methods Compared for Effectiveness." Explain why there is such a difference between effectiveness rates for typical users and effectiveness rates for people using the methods perfectly. Which methods show the largest differences in percentages? What factors contribute to the large differences?
6. Review Figure 22–11 again. This time, score each method on "control"—that is, to what extent partners could control the method if they chose to use it. (A man can control condom use; a woman can control pill use.)

up to five years. (True)
3. Intrauterine device (IUD) is a form of birth control that is recommended for teenagers. (False)
4. Spermicides frequently fail to prevent pregnancy when used without another form of contraception. (True)
5. Diaphragms protect the wearer from sexually transmitted disease viruses. (False)
6. Diaphragms and cervical caps have been associated with toxic shock syndrome.

(True)
7. Using Vaseline or a moisturizer on a condom for lubrication can cause the condom to break during intercourse. (True)
8. All condoms are equally effective. (False)
9. Condoms should not be stored in wallets, purses, or pockets. (True)
10. The fertility awareness method involves neither drugs nor devices, but has a low user effectiveness rate. (True)

SECTION 3

FOCUS

OUTCOMES

In this section students will learn:

1. To name several contraceptive methods that aren't effective.

2. To describe why those methods don't work.

FOCUS ACTIVITY

Ask students why someone might use one of the ineffective contraceptive methods. After students give their responses, reemphasize the importance of the responsibility a person must take with regard to when that person will decide to engage in sexual intercourse.

TEACH & APPLY

DISCUSSION

Brainstorm with the class about the myths they have heard about contraception. Make a list on the board. Students will respond with statements such as, "You can't get pregnant the first time you have sex," "You can't get pregnant if you drink ice water after sex," "A male won't be able to get a girl pregnant if he sits in a hot or cold bath before sex," "You can't get pregnant if you have sex standing up," "A girl can't get pregnant during her period," "A male can't get someone pregnant if he wears a rubber band around his penis during sex," and so on.

Discuss with students why these myths are untrue. Why do students think the myths persist? Why do some people still believe them?

CHAPTER 22: Preventing Pregnancy and Sexually Transmitted Diseases

SECTION 3

Methods Not Recommended for Contraception

People have many false notions about contraception and may recommend methods other than the effective ones just described.

Douches   Women throughout history have attempted to wash out or kill sperm after intercourse by using **douches** of fluids such as vinegar or carbonated beverages. Douches of hazardous chemicals, such as turpentine, are extremely damaging to tissues and do not prevent pregnancy. Most douches available over the counter are not intended for contraception. Using them does not prevent pregnancy. In fact, they may even help the sperm along, because a stream of fluid can wash sperm into the cervix as easily as it can wash them out. Douches cannot prevent or cure STDs, either.

Condom Misuse and Alternatives   Some people have tried to save money on condoms by reusing them or using replacements for them. Once used, a condom is weakened and likely to rupture if used again. Even simply unrolling a new condom before applying it will weaken it and make it likely to break. Covering the penis with plastic kitchen wrap, sandwich bags, or other items is unlikely to prevent semen from spilling into the vagina. Pregnancy and STD transmission can easily occur.

Condoms require special handling if they are to protect against pregnancy and STDs.

enrichment....

Sterilization (see pages 614–615) has long been a form of birth control. For instance, thousands of years ago rulers would castrate (sterilize by removal of the testicles) men to put in charge of their harems. These men were called eunuchs. Castration is never used for sterilization purposes in this country today.

It has recently been brought to the attention of the world that Sweden, in the mid-1900s,

Breastfeeding Women have also thought, wrongly, that as long as they were breastfeeding their babies, they could not become pregnant. It is true that during lactation (milk production), many women are less likely to ovulate. However, there is no way an individual woman can know for sure. Lactation does reduce the total number of children born in a population, but it is not reliable as a contraceptive method for any one woman.

Withdrawal Method A method somewhat better than those just named is the **withdrawal method**, also known as *coitus interruptus*. It is just what it sounds like—the man withdraws his penis from the vagina before he ejaculates, taking care that his semen is not deposited in, at, or near the vagina.

Two built-in errors of the method make withdrawal unreliable. First, the man finds it difficult to withdraw his penis when he is near ejaculation. Second, even if he is able to withdraw before ejaculation, live sperm in the fluid from the penis may already have entered the vagina and may fertilize an ovum. Withdrawal may be better than no method at all, but it still allows one woman out of five to become pregnant in one year of use. It is not recommended by health-care providers for people who are serious about birth control. It offers no protection against STDs.

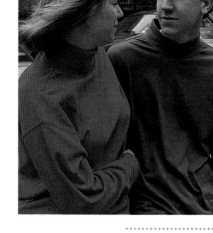

Some contraceptive methods are better than others, and some are almost useless.

 Methods not recommended for contraception include using douches, relying on lactation, or withdrawal.

 Review

Answer the following questions on a sheet of paper.

Learning the Vocabulary

The vocabulary terms in this section are *douches* and *withdrawal method* (*coitus interruptus*).

1. Write a sentence using each of the vocabulary terms.

Learning the Facts

2. How can using douches help a woman to become pregnant?

3. If lactation reduces the number of children born in a population, why can't a woman use it successfully to prevent conception?

4. Why is the withdrawal method of birth control considered nearly worthless?

Making Life Choices

Anna and Rico are engaged to be married. They don't want to have children right away, so they are looking at methods of contraception. Explain the types of contraception that are *not* recommended.

 Glossary

douches: preparations sold to cleanse the vagina.

withdrawal method (coitus interruptus): a technique in sexual intercourse of withdrawing the penis from the vagina just prior to ejaculation. It is not recommended for preventing pregnancy and is useless against STDs.

EVALUATE

Review with students the forms of contraception that don't work by having them list all of them on a piece of paper. Have the students also explain why they are ineffective. Collect their papers and check for understanding.

Section 3 Review Answers

1. Answers will vary.
2. A stream of fluid can help wash the sperm into the cervix as easily as it can wash them out. (p. 612)
3. A women cannot be sure she hasn't ovulated. (p. 613)
4. The man finds it difficult to withdraw from the vagina before ejaculation and live sperm in the fluid from the penis will already have entered the vagina and may fertilize the ovum. (p. 613)
5. Answers will vary.

 A reproducible quiz for Section 3 is provided in the Teacher's Resource Box.

CLOSE

Ask students the following questions: If a sexually active teen decides not to use a contraceptive device or uses a nonrecommended form of birth control, what conclusions might be drawn about him or her? What might be some of the outcomes of the decision? Answers will vary. List them on the board and discuss.

wrote laws that forced the sterilization of some women. The women subjected to the sterilization were considered to be inferior in some way. In many cases this meant women with learning disabilities or women who were of mixed ethnic heritage.

In modern times, sterilization has been enforced in some countries for various reasons. For example, in China, men and women are sometimes forcefully sterilized to prevent them having more than one child and is thus used as a form of population control.

SECTION 4

FOCUS

OUTCOME

In this section students will learn about:

1. The permanent methods of birth control—vasectomy and tubal ligation.

FOCUS ACTIVITY

Ask students why someone would choose sterilization as a form of contraception. What would a person need to consider before having the surgery done? Discuss.

TEACH & APPLY

BACKGROUND INFORMATION

Explain to students that a large supply of sperm is stored in the male reproductive tract. This is the reason a man can still cause a pregnancy for about six weeks after a vasectomy. A sample of the man's semen would need to be examined under a microscope to determine for sure that he could have intercourse without causing a pregnancy.

The tubal ligation is done with a small incision below the woman's navel and another off to one side slightly above the pubic hair. A lighted viewing scope is put into one opening so the doctor can view the tubes. The instrument that does the work on the tubes is put in the other opening. There are many variations to this procedure. For example, the tubes can be cut and tied, burned in half, or clipped with a device to seal them shut.

SECTION 4

Sterilization

Surgical **sterilization** is a highly effective contraceptive method—in most cases, close to 100 percent effective. Each year, millions of people choose sterilization, and the number is increasing. In fact, sterilization is the leading contraceptive method in the world.

Once chosen, sterilization puts an end to fertility for life. People choosing sterilization should be sure they will want to bear no children in the future. No one can count on being able to reverse the procedure later. Only a small number of reversal procedures work to restore fertility. Most often, attempts at reversal fail. (In rare cases, fertility is restored without efforts to reverse the sterilization. The ends of the tubes that were surgically cut find each other and grow back together, restoring fertility.) The simplest and most common sterilization procedures are **vasectomy** in men and **tubal ligation** in women.

Vasectomy

In vasectomy, a surgeon makes one or two tiny cuts in the scrotum. The surgeon then severs and seals the tubes (each of which is called a **vas deferens**) through which the sperm travel to become part of the semen. Figure 22–12 shows how this is done. The procedure takes about half an hour and may be performed under local anesthesia in a physician's office. The incisions are so tiny that vasectomies are called "Band-Aid surgery."

The vasectomized man continues to produce sperm. However, they are reduced in number, and they are absorbed by the body rather than being released into the semen. The fluid of semen is still present in ejaculation. Only the tiny portion made up by sperm cells is missing. The difference is not noticeable. The sperm do not build up or cause any unusual feelings or symptoms. A vasectomy interrupts only the delivery of sperm. It has no effect on the production of the male hormone testosterone or on sexual desire or activity.

A man is not sterile immediately after a vasectomy, because living sperm are still in storage. Usually it takes some weeks to clear them out. Once the sperm are absent from the semen, the chance of pregnancy is practically zero.

Vasectomy is a low-cost, one-time procedure. It permits the man to resume normal activity within a day or so and sexual activity within a few days. Pain is minimal, and side effects are rare.

Figure 22–12   Vasectomy

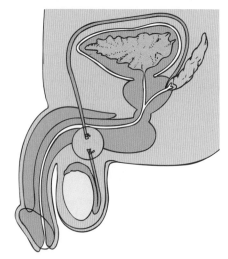

Vasectomy effectiveness:
Laboratory rating = 99.85 percent.
User effectiveness = 99.85 percent.

 KEY POINTS *In vasectomy, a surgeon cuts and seals off each vas deferens in a man to produce sterility.*

Chapter 22, Section 4

*The following quiz will help you assess your students' understanding of the material covered in this section of the chapter. You might use the quiz as an oral exercise, which will lead into a class discussion of the topics cov-*ered. Or, you might use it as a paper/pencil quiz to evaluate your students individually.

Like the Quick Quiz, the Section Review can also be used as an assessment tool to spark class discussion or as an individual student evaluation. It can also be used as a review in preparation for this quiz.

1. Sterilization is almost one hundred percent effective. (True)

Tubal Ligation

For a tubal ligation, a surgeon cuts and seals off the fallopian tubes, which conduct ova from the ovaries to the uterus. Sperm traveling up the tubes arrive at a dead end and cannot fertilize the ovum a woman might have produced.

To have the surgery performed, a woman may check into a hospital or clinic in the morning and check out that afternoon. The operation is performed with either a regional or general anesthetic. Commonly referred to as "tying the tubes," the surgery involves small incisions in the woman's abdomen through which the surgeon cuts the fallopian tubes and seals their ends. Any number of surgical methods accomplish the same objective: permanent blockage of the tubes to prevent ova and sperm from meeting.

The procedure is slightly more involved than a vasectomy, because the surgeon must cut through abdominal muscle. Still, it leaves only a tiny scar on the abdomen; in the navel; or in cases of surgery through the upper vaginal wall, in the vagina. Figure 22–13 shows the abdominal operation. The woman's hormones and her sex drive remain normal. After the surgery, the woman continues to menstruate and ovulate as before. The ripe ovum is released, but the body reabsorbs it.

Although tubal ligation is more costly than vasectomy, it is still less expensive than the costs of years of many other contraceptive methods. Most women tolerate the surgery well and recover quickly with little discomfort.

Figure 22–13 Tubal Ligation

Tubal ligation effectiveness:
Laboratory rating = 99.7 percent.
User effectiveness = 99.7 percent.

KEY POINTS *In tubal ligation, a surgeon cuts and seals off a woman's fallopian tubes, making her sterile.*

SECTION 4 Review

Answer the following questions on a sheet of paper.

Learning the Vocabulary

The vocabulary terms in this section are *sterilization, vasectomy, tubal ligation,* and *vas deferens.*

1. Match each of the following phrases with the appropriate vocabulary term.
   a. surgical cutting and sealing off of the tubes in a man through which sperm travel
   b. the process of permanently interrupting a person's ability to bear children
   c. surgical cutting and sealing off of the tubes in a woman in which sperm and ova meet

Learning the Facts

2. How many people choose sterilization each year?
3. What does a vasectomy interrupt?
4. What happens to the ova after a tubal ligation?

Making Life Choices

5. Malcolm and Denise have three children. They have decided not to have any more. They have decided that one of them should become sterile. What arguments do you have for Malcolm to get a vasectomy? What arguments do you have for Denise to get a tubal ligation?

MINI Glossary

sterilization: the process of permanently interrupting a person's ability to bear children, usually by surgically severing and sealing the vas deferens or the fallopian tubes.

vasectomy: surgical cutting and sealing off of each vas deferens to sterilize a man.

tubal ligation (lye-GAY-shun): surgical cutting and sealing off of the fallopian tubes to sterilize women.

vas deferens (plural, **vasa deferentia**): one of the two tubes that conduct sperm from the testicles toward the penis.

DISCUSSION

Ask students if they think it would be wise for teenagers to choose sterilization. Do they know any who have? Students should realize that this would not be a wise choice for most of them. They have no way of knowing whether or not they will want to have families. Even though they may think they know now that they will not want to have children later in life, they should be aware of the fact that they will mature and change a great deal in the next 20 to 30 years.

ASSESS

EVALUATE

SECTION 4 Review Answers

1. a. vasectomy
   b. sterilization
   c. tubal ligation
2. millions (p. 614)
3. the route that sperm take to become part of the semen. (p. 614)
4. it is absorbed into the body (p. 615)
5. Answers will vary.

CLOSE

Ask students why they think these methods of permanent contraception aren't used around the world more, given the problems of overpopulation, pollution, and starvation. Discuss the impact of overpopulation on future generations.

2. Sterilization is the leading method of contraception. (True)
3. Sterilization is usually reversible. (False)
4. The most common sterilization procedures are vasectomy in men and tubal ligation in women. (True)
5. Vasectomy is performed by severing the vas deferens located in the scrotum. (True)
6. Vasectomy is considered a major surgery. (False)
7. Vasectomy has no effect on sexual performance or the production of testosterone. (True)
8. Tubal ligation is performed by sealing the fallopian tubes. (True)
9. Menstruation ceases after tubal ligation. (False)
10. Tubal ligation is more involved and more costly than a vasectomy. (True)

615

FOCUS

OUTCOMES

In this section students will learn:

1. The difficult choices that must be made when contraception fails.

2. To describe the problems that may accompany adoption and abortion.

FOCUS ACTIVITY

Before class, prepare five or six scenarios involving teen couples in which the girl is pregnant or use the handout "Pregnancy Scenarios" provided in the Teacher's Resource Box. Use different ages, financial and educational backgrounds, parents' beliefs, and life plans the couple had before becoming pregnant.

Put students into groups of four. Distribute the scenarios, one to each group. More than one group can have the same scenario. Tell each group to decide what would be the best decision for each couple regarding their pregnancy. Should the couple marry, give the baby up for adoption, have an abortion, or should the mother or father raise the baby alone? Ask each group to report back to the class by reading its teen pregnancy story and telling the class why it made the decision it did.

FAST FACTS

The Center for Disease Control reports that a majority of U.S. high school students have sex. One out of every four sexually active teens does not use an effective birth control method.

Here are the answers to the questions at the start of the chapter.

1. False. For healthy, sexually active heterosexual couples, pregnancy occurs easily.

2. True.

3. False. No contraceptive method is perfect. To obtain the advantages of one method, a person must be willing to put up with its disadvantages.

4. True.

5. False. Condoms are prone to failure, but abstinence always prevents sexually transmitted diseases.

6. False. A woman who isn't taking the Pill may be using another form of birth control, such as condoms or a diaphragm. The term *birth control* refers to all contraceptive methods, including the Pill.

7. True.

Contraceptive Failure

U nwanted pregnancies are not unusual, even when couples are using contraception. All contraceptive methods, with one exception, can fail. A method's failure rate is expressed as an impersonal statistic. In human terms, however, it means that a number of couples are facing unwanted pregnancies despite efforts to prevent them. The one fail-proof exception is, of course, abstinence.

As an illustration of the human reality of contraceptive failure, let's say that a certain method is 97 percent effective. Also assume that the whole adult, fertile female population of the United States—close to 100 million women—were all using this method and using it correctly. Every single year of their reproductive lives, 3 million of these women would still become pregnant.

Actually, over 4 million women in the United States alone face unwanted pregnancies each year. Considering that each woman's fertility lasts 30 years or more, it is clear that nearly every woman may face an unwanted pregnancy sometime during her life. She and her partner may have failed to use contraception or may have used it incorrectly. She may have used contraception, but it may have failed to work. She may be the victim of rape, incest, or other sexual abuse. She may be young or old, poor or rich, a student, a professional, a blue-collar worker, or a homemaker.

Deciding about Abortion

Each woman facing an unwanted pregnancy also faces the decision of whether or not to continue her pregnancy. For some, the choice is really no choice. They have decided a course of action in advance. It may be that a woman's religious beliefs forbid **abortion**, or that she has decided to continue every pregnancy to birth for any number of reasons. She may have decided never to carry to birth any but a wanted pregnancy, and so chooses abortion. Abortion is not a method of contraception. *Contraception* means "to prevent conception." Abortion interrupts a pregnancy that is already under way.

Young people who are risking pregnancy are wise to do some thinking in advance. Otherwise, a woman who becomes pregnant unexpectedly has to think fast and answer the question on the spot. With the help of counselors, parents, or religious teachers, each person can make a right decision.

A woman who suspects that she is pregnant should obtain a pregnancy test. She must choose carefully where to go for the test. Heated battles rage between groups that support legal abortion and groups that oppose it. Both groups include extremists who may worsen a pregnant woman's stress and make the situation harder. A woman may encounter unwelcome pressure if she is tested for pregnancy by the wrong agency.

Some possible choices are a physician's office; the local health department, which will offer free or low-cost tests without accompanying advice;

CRITICAL THINKING

Bring a regular broom to school. Ask for a student volunteer to balance the broom on one finger. Ask the student first to try and balance the broom, looking just at the bottom of it, where it rests on the finger. The class will observe that the student has quite a bit of difficulty doing it this way. Now have the student try it again, looking at the top of the broom. The student should be able to balance it with much less difficulty. Now make the analogy that a person who makes their decisions looking only at today may experience problems because of disregard for future con-an abortion clinic, which will assist and support a woman in obtaining an abortion if she is pregnant; and a religious organization, which will help support a woman in carrying her pregnancy to term and assist with adoption if she chooses it. A choice to continue the pregnancy brings other choices: whether to keep the baby or give it up for adoption.

Chapter 2 said that in making decisions, a person must weigh feelings, judgments, and values. In the case of an unwanted pregnancy, all of these may well conflict with one another. Objective counseling can be a great help in deciding how to handle an unplanned pregnancy. A teenager who faces an unwanted pregnancy may have a strong family support system, and so may benefit from seeking the family's help early on.

Whatever choice is made, the woman must act promptly. Delays increase a woman's risks, whether she ultimately has an abortion or continues her pregnancy. If she chooses abortion, the longer she waits, the riskier the procedures become. If she continues the pregnancy, the longer prenatal care is delayed, the greater the danger to her health and to that of her fetus.

 KEY POINTS *When unplanned pregnancy occurs, the choice of where to go for help should be made carefully. Action to obtain abortion or prenatal care must be swift.*

Abortion Procedures

Abortion methods vary according to the length of the pregnancy. Surgical abortions performed early in pregnancy require little anesthesia and carry minimal risk to the woman's health. They are routine for the medical staff. In vacuum aspiration, suction is applied to empty the uterus of the early tissues of pregnancy, including the embryo and the tissues that would form a placenta. (These structures were described in Chapter 20). Another way that early pregnancies can be ended nonsurgically is by taking a pill—RU 486. Normally, the hormone progesterone maintains pregnancy. The RU 486 drug interferes with the action of progesterone and brings on menstruation and loss of the pregnancy. RU 486 gained tentative approval for use in the United States at the time of this writing.

Between 13 and about 16 weeks of pregnancy, more direct methods must be used to scrape or vacuum the uterus. These involve anesthesia, and so increase the risk to the woman. The scraping, but not vacuuming, of the uterus is also used for medical purposes other than abortion.

For abortions after 13 weeks' gestation, some medical methods can be used. Hormones can be administered, the woman goes into labor, and abortion results.

The physical risks of abortion are much lower today than in the past. The procedures still carry some risk, however, and the risks increase as the pregnancy goes on. Generally, abortion during the first three months is only slightly riskier than contraception. Early abortions have no effect on the woman's ability to carry future pregnancies. Some question remains about whether late abortions have long-term effects on fertility and on the outcomes of future pregnancies.

MINI Glossary

abortion: a procedure to end a pregnancy before the fetus can live outside the uterus.

sequences of their actions. A person who looks ahead and projects into the future the actions they take today will usually avoid making mistakes about major life choices.

You could also stress that a person who has sex today may be thinking of his or her desires at the moment, and not thinking that nine months later a baby will drastically

change his or her life. A person who thinks about the possibility of pregnancy resulting from sex may decide not to engage in it at all until after he or she marries.

TEACH & APPLY

WORKSHEETS The Teacher's Resource Box contains a handout called "Conflicting Views on Abortion," which provides "pro-life" and "pro-choice" views on abortion side by side. If you intend to discuss abortion, use the handout to stimulate the students' thinking and to encourage their participation in a discussion. You could, for example, ask them to pick the viewpoints that they most identify with and have them explain their reasoning.

DISCUSSION

Put *Abortion* on one side of the board and *Adoption* on the other. Divide each side of the board into two parts. Label one section *Pros* and one *Cons* for each of the two sides.

Have students brainstorm the pro and con aspects of each choice and write their responses in the appropriate place. Discuss.

GROUP ACTIVITY

Divide the class into small groups to research the cost and items needed for a single mother and newborn living on Welfare. Have groups report to the class on monthly expenses and brainstorm possible solutions for meeting the expenses. The handout "Sample Welfare Expenses" is provided in the Teacher's Resource Box.

ASSESS

EVALUATE

Have students write their feelings about the following statement: "Why might abstinence be a better choice than risking pregnancy while still in high school?" Collect papers and check for understanding.

Review Answers

1. Answers will vary.
2. 4 million (p. 616)
3. local health department, abortion clinic, a religious organization, physician's office (pp. 616–617)
4. Early abortions are believed not to affect later fertility and carry little risk to the health of the woman, while later abortions are a higher risk to the woman's health and future fertility. (p. 617)
5. religious teaching; group counseling; medical care before, during, and after the birth; adoption services; maternity and infant clothing; day care (p. 618)
6. Answers will vary.

CLOSE

Make sure that students understand that both adoption and abortion are possible choices for unwanted pregnancies, but neither of them is a form of birth control.

 KEY POINTS *Early abortions carry little risk and can be performed through vacuum aspiration. Later abortions are riskier and can be accomplished through the administration of hormones or by surgical means.*

Adoption

Women who choose to carry their unwanted pregnancies to term often need help. Agencies are available to provide for them. Women may need to find sources of help for problems such as abandonment by family or the father of the child, lack of access to medical treatment, low income, lack of emotional support, and many other problems.

Agencies that provide resources for such women are often associated with organizations calling themselves *pro-life* or *right-to-life*. They hold strong moral convictions against abortion, and they support women in unwanted pregnancies. They usually include religious teaching in their counseling. Such groups can be especially helpful when a woman wants to continue a pregnancy but needs support in doing so. Services vary from place to place. They can include free pregnancy testing; group counseling; medical care before, during, and after the birth; housing; adoption services; maternity and infant clothing; and day care.

Whether a woman chooses abortion or continues with her pregnancy, she urgently needs to use a means of contraception afterward. Otherwise, she may be faced with the same hard choices all over again—a common occurrence.

 KEY POINTS *Several kinds of organizations provide for the needs of women who carry unplanned pregnancies to term.*

 Review

Answer the following questions on a sheet of paper.

Learning the Vocabulary

The vocabulary term in this section is *abortion*.

1. Write a sentence using the vocabulary term.

Learning the Facts

2. How many unwanted pregnancies occur in the United States each year?

3. Name possible places a woman can get a pregnancy test or help with her decision about an unwanted pregnancy.

4. What is said about the risks of abortions that occur early in pregnancy and abortions that occur later in pregnancy?

5. How do agencies help support a woman who is having a baby that she will give up for adoption?

Making Life Choices

6. Kerri became pregnant in the ninth grade. Kerri didn't know what to do. Explain Kerri's options.

 QUICK QUIZ

Chapter 22, Section 5

The following quiz will help you assess your students' understanding of the material covered in this section of the chapter. You might use the quiz as an oral exercise, which will lead into a class discussion of the topics covered. Or, you might use it as a paper/pencil quiz to evaluate your students individually.

1. Unwanted pregnancies are extremely unusual in couples that are using contraception. (False)
2. Nearly every woman may face an unwanted pregnancy during her life. (True)
3. Abortion is a method of birth control. (False)
4. It is wise for a woman to think about abortion before she becomes sexually active. (True)

Straight Talk

Why People Don't Use Contraception

Many people consciously choose not to use contraception. They may have moral, religious, or personal reasons for this choice. They may want a pregnancy. However, enormous numbers of teenage girls face unwanted pregnancies each year that end in unwanted births or abortions. Most of these unplanned pregnancies are not the result of a conscious choice, but of simple failure to use contraception.

 Why do people take such chances?

Fear and emotional immaturity are two powerful reasons. People in their teen years, especially, may fear discovery and the disapproval of their parents. They may be too embarrassed to purchase condoms or to seek the help of parents or professionals in obtaining contraceptives. Some may lack information about contraception, or even fail to realize that sexual intercourse leads to pregnancy.

Emotional immaturity can also prevent people from dealing with contraception. An immature mind often rejects sexuality as part of the person's self-image. The assumption seems to be that sex is great, but nice people don't plan for it—it "just happens."

People who think this way pretend to lead a lifestyle in keeping with traditional values, while still having sexual intercourse on impulse, now and then. Using contraception makes a statement—that the person is sexually active. So does pregnancy, but an immature mind is unable to think far enough ahead to make this connection. Psychologists would call this a failure to "own" one's sexual identity—that is, a failure to accept, and take responsibility for, being sexual.

Young people who confuse sexual activity with love are less likely to use contraception. They trust "love" to be in control, and simply hope for the best. Another group failing to use contraception is made up of people who seem prone to taking chances and risks of all sorts. Such people may smoke tobacco, drink alcohol, take illegal drugs, or commit crimes—and they often engage in risky sexual behaviors. Scientists are trying to figure out why all of these behaviors seem to "go together" in some people. The answers they seek may help to identify such people early on, during childhood, when behaviors are most easily influenced.

 Aren't the mass communication media also partly responsible for many teenagers' unwanted pregnancies?

Some people think so, yes. The media push sex in every form but do not educate. Seldom do couples on TV or in movies pause in their passion to use contraception. When such scenes do occur, they are usually humorous ones that make using contraception seem foolish and unromantic.

As mentioned in the previous Straight Talk section, children and adolescents view television programs during the "family hour," from eight to nine o'clock in the evening. During that hour, sexual scenes are presented almost nonstop. Fewer than one in ten of such scenes, however, include any hint of the real-life risks that go with sexual activity, such as unplanned pregnancy and STDs. Parents might hope that such scenes just "pass over the heads" of young children. However, very few children fail to notice the sexual suggestions, jokes, or behaviors portrayed there, and most children are made uncomfortable by them.

619

5. A pregnant woman may encounter unwelcome pressure from both pro- and anti-abortion groups. (True)

6. Delaying both abortion and prenatal care greatly increases health risks. (True)

7. Surgical abortions performed early in pregnancy involve major risks to the woman's health. (False)

8. The RU 486 is a drug which ends early pregnancy nonsurgically and has tentative approval for use in the United States. (True)

9. Abortions performed after 13 weeks' gestation pose significantly greater risk to the woman's health. (True)

10. Many agencies that provide adoption resources for women also provide counseling. (True)

Four reasons for using contraception are given in this *Straight Talk* (in answer to the question "Does anyone know what makes people decide to use contraception?"). Have students read the paragraph, close their books, and write the four reasons in their own words. Do students agree that all of these reasons would make it more likely that a couple would use contraception? Which reasons do they think would be most likely to cause teenagers to use contraception? Who might people turn to for information and help in making the decision to use contraception?

Straight Talk

Why People Don't Use Contraception (continued)

Magazines also use sexy images to sell everything from automobiles to zebra-striped underclothes—everything, that is, except contraception. Neither do the T.V. networks advertise contraception, although such advertisement is legal.

The media provide poor sexual role models. The couples shown are not in control of their sexuality. They also are not responsible for it.

 Has anyone asked teenagers how they feel about contraception?

The attitudes of sexually active teenagers, when studied, seems sensible enough. They often say that they should postpone sex or use contraception. However, many teens' behaviors are like those of their poor media role models—out of line with their own knowledge and values.

Fewer than half of sexually active teenagers say they used contraception the last time they had intercourse. The other half seem to think that the rules do not apply to them, or they are too embarrassed to obtain contraceptives, or their partners resist using condoms. (See Figure 22–14 for tips on handling a hesitant partner.) These teens seem to act as though getting pregnant or catching an STD is as likely as the sky's falling, and that they are equally helpless to prevent any of them.

 Does anyone know what makes people decide to use contraception?

Four things have been observed. The more a woman owns her own sexuality, the more likely she is to use contraception. The more a couple cares about each other, the more likely they are to protect each other with contraception. The older and more sexually experienced they are, the more likely they are to use it. And the more they see pregnancy prevention as a shared responsibility, the more they will use it.

 That sounds like the kind of relationship everyone would like. Do only older partners have such supportive relationships?

Not always, but the four characteristics mentioned often come along with maturity. A mature woman has had time to get to know herself and so may be able to accept her own sexuality as part of her life. Also, people in a committed, mature love relationship didn't get there overnight. They gave their love plenty of time to grow naturally without complicating its development with early sexual intimacy.

Genuine concern for the partner is also a mark of maturity. Also, as couples make decisions about when or whether to have a child together, each partner *wants* to share responsibility for achieving that family goal. Without the shared psychological intimacy of a mature love, sexuality is more likely to be self-centered, and contraception is more likely to be ignored.

 Some people I know just don't seem to think about the price they'll pay should pregnancy occur, and so they don't use contraception.

That's a common attitude. They may think, "If I have a baby, I'm sure someone will take care of it. The father will marry me; or the mother will take care of it; or my parents will help; or I'll be an adult, then, so somehow it'll be OK." In fact, teenagers may believe that pregnancy must be all right or else it wouldn't happen. Some think pregnancy is a ticket away from an unhappy home life.

They have no idea of the enormous burden they'll carry when they alone have responsibility for a child during all its years of dependency. Some even have to carry the responsibility for the child's children—early childbearing runs in families.

620

CRITICAL THINKING

Write the following sentence on the board or on an overhead transparency: People having sexual intercourse but using no means of contraception are acting as if they wish to have a child.

This sentence is a strong statement of the importance of abstinence and/or the use of contraception. You might want to remind stu-

dents of the ways in which a baby changes the parents' lives. The following questions are from the Life Choice Inventory on page 549. You might want to discuss them again with your students.

- How will having a child affect your schooling or career?
- During the hours you can't take care of the child, who will do it?
- If your partner is unable to carry the

I've also heard some people say they think contraception lowers the sex drive or hinders performance. Is that true?

No, contraception does not reduce the sex drive or performance in people of either gender. In reality, the opposite is often true. With fear of pregnancy removed, people often feel more free to enjoy sexual intercourse.

Sometimes a sexual partner may be resistant to using condoms. Convincing the partner may require being honest and firm. To give in to not using condoms means risking disease or pregnancy, yet a person may fear that insisting on using protection may strain the relationship. Figure 22–14 offers some responses to use when a partner resists using condoms. Should these responses or others like them fail to convince the person, it may be time to rethink the relationship.

 Does sex education help teenagers make the right choices? And if so, who should be responsible for it?

Yes, it can help. Ideally, parents should be the primary sex educators. However, they sometimes fail to provide the needed information.

To make sure that all children have the information they need, society tries to provide these facts through the schools. In places where meaningful sex education is provided along with wholehearted community support, the numbers of teenage pregnancies drop. Most places in the United States, though, fail to provide such education and support, and so are seeing increased numbers of teenage pregnancies.

Sex education is only part of the solution, though. Research shows that when parents have discussed sex with their teens, those teens are least likely among peers to engage in sexual intercourse early in life and are most likely to use contraceptives later on. Individual families and society as a whole must take responsibility.

Right now, our society promotes the sex act itself without promoting a responsible attitude toward it. If society's mixed messages continue, we should not be surprised to see teen pregnancies become an even greater problem in the future.

Figure 22–14 *How to Get a Partner to Agree to Use Condoms*

Partner:	"It won't feel the same."
Response:	"You won't feel anything if you won't use a condom."
Partner:	"I don't have any condoms with me."
Response:	"I do. Here, choose one."
Partner:	"I *know* that I don't have a disease. I haven't had sex in two months."
Response:	"Thanks for telling me. I probably don't either, but one of us could have an infection and not know it."
Partner:	"Condoms aren't natural."
Response:	"STDs *are* natural, but they aren't all that great."

Source: Adapted from R. A. Hatcher and coauthors, *Contraceptive Technology* (New York: Irvington Publishers, 1994).

621

responsibility of parenthood, how will you carry it by yourself?

• How will having a child affect your relationship with others?
• Where will you be able to get help when you need to get away?
• Will you be willing to give up much of your free time to devote yourself to the needs of a child?
• Are you willing and able to pay for proper prenatal and newborn care?

• Are you willing and able to invest your money for years in the well-being of your child?
• How well would you be able to adjust to raising a less-than-perfect child?
• Are you willing to make a new baby the center of attention?
• Have you ever vented anger or frustration on pets or children in the past?

ANSWERS TO CHAPTER 22 REVIEW

VOCABULARY

1. Effectiveness is how well a contraceptive prevents pregnancy, expressed as a percentage. The laboratory effectiveness is the percentage of women protected from pregnancy in a year's time under ideal laboratory conditions. The user effectiveness is the percentage of typical women users who are protected.

2. a. abortion **b.** vas deferens **c.** intrauterine device (IUD) **d.** male condom **e.** progestin **f.** diaphragm **g.** fertility awareness **h.** progesterone

3. a. female condom **b.** vasectomy **c.** Oral contraceptives **d.** tubal ligation **e.** barrier methods

4. Answers will vary.

RECALL
SECTION 1

1. both members of a sexually active couple—a shared responsibility (p. 596)
2. effectiveness (p. 598)

SECTION 2

3. to avoid pregnancy and the threat of AIDS, herpes, and other sexually transmitted diseases. (p. 600)

CHAPTER 22 Review

Summarizing the Chapter

Your ability to respond correctly to the following statements ensures your understanding of the main concepts in the chapter.

1. Discuss the risks of using contraceptives.
2. List all of the contraceptive methods, and state the effectiveness rate of each.
3. Identify which methods of contraception also help prevent sexually transmitted diseases.
4. Explain how to use each method of contraception.
5. Identify the methods not recommended for contraception.
6. Identify the two methods of sterilization, and describe how they work.
7. List the options available to women who have unwanted/unplanned pregnancies.

Learning the Vocabulary

contraception
effectiveness
laboratory effectiveness
user effectiveness
abstinence
oral contraceptives
combination pill
estrogen
progesterone
progestin
progestin-only pill
Norplant
Depo-Provera
intrauterine device (IUD)
barrier methods

diaphragm
cervical cap
male condom
female condom
fertility awareness
  method
douches
withdrawal method
  (coitus interruptus)
sterilization
vasectomy
tubal ligation
vas deferens
abortion

Answer the following questions on a separate sheet of paper.

1. Explain the differences between effectiveness, laboratory effectiveness, and user effectiveness.

2. *Matching*—Match each of the following phrases with the appropriate vocabulary term from the list above:
  a. procedure to end a pregnancy before the fetus can live outside the uterus
  b. tubes that conduct sperm toward the penis
  c. a device inserted into the uterus to prevent conception
  d. a sheath worn over the penis during intercourse to contain the semen
  e. a synthetic version of progesterone
  f. a dome that fits over the cervix and holds spermicidal cream or jelly against the uterine entrance
  g. a method of contraception that involves tracking the menstrual cycle and observing signs of ovulation
  h. a female hormone secreted during that portion of the menstrual cycle in which the uterine lining builds up

3. a. A _____ is a soft, thin plastic tube with two end rings—one to fit over the cervix and one to serve as an anchor outside the entrance to the vagina.
  b. A surgical procedure that cuts the tubes that conduct sperm from the testicles toward the penis is called a _____.
  c. _____ are pills taken by mouth which contain synthetic hormones that prevent pregnancy by stopping ovulation.
  d. A surgical procedure that cuts the tubes that conduct the ova from the ovaries towards the uterus is called a _____.
  e. Contraceptive methods that physically or chemically obstruct the travel of sperm towards the ovum are called _____.

4. Write a paragraph using at least ten of the vocabulary terms. Underline each vocabulary term that you use.

Recalling Important Facts and Ideas

Section 1

1. Who is responsible for contraception?
2. What is one of the most important facts to consider about a contraceptive method?

Section 2

3. Why are teens all over the United States choosing abstinence more often than before?
4. What is the only 100% effective method to avoid pregnancy?

---

4. abstinence (p. 600)
5. one month (p. 601)
6. the Pill (oral contraceptives) (p. 601)
7. The progestin-only pill contains no estrogen, only progestin, and affects the uterus itself. The progestin thickens the mucus surrounding the uterine opening so that sperm cannot penetrate. Progestin can also deactivate sperm cells and interrupt the

normal preparation of the uterine lining. (p. 601)

8. abdominal pain, chest pain, breathlessness, headaches, blurred vision or loss of vision, leg pain (p. 602)
9. condoms (p. 602)
10. It increases the risks of birth defects. It is suggested that a woman switch to another method of contraception for at least two

5. When a woman begins using the Pill, for how long should she use a backup method of birth control?
6. What is the most popular nonsurgical method of birth control?
7. Explain the differences between the progestin-only pill and the combination pill.
8. What symptoms should prompt a woman to call her physician if she is on the Pill?
9. What should be used to prevent STDs when the Pill is being used for contraception?
10. Why should a woman who may be pregnant stop taking the Pill?
11. Who are the best candidates for intrauterine devices?
12. What must a woman do for a diaphragm to work properly?
13. The diaphragm must be left in place for how long after intercourse?
14. What is one danger of using a diaphragm or cervical cap during menstruation?
15. Why should a person choose latex condoms over other condoms?
16. Why shouldn't Vaseline or moisturizing lotion be used on condoms?
17. Why is the female condom effective?
18. What should a woman do before using the fertility awareness method of birth control?

Section 3
19. Describe several ineffective methods of birth control.

Section 4
20. How long after a vasectomy does it take a man to become free of sperm?

Section 5
21. Abortion is not a method of contraception. What is it?
22. What kinds of services are offered by agencies that help women carry unwanted pregnancies to term?

Critical Thinking
1. Read the Straight Talk, "Why People Don't Use Contraception." What is said about maturity and those who don't use contraceptives? How do the media push sex? Which couples are likely to use contraceptives? Does sex education help? How?

2. Maria and Joe have been dating steadily for one year. They plan to be married after graduating from high school in six months. They have not been sexually active thus far and talk about whether to remain virgins until marriage. Joe had an illness as an infant, and his doctor told him he is probably sterile. Joe believes that "no harm would be done" by having sex before marriage, Maria will not become pregnant. Maria has concerns about premarital sex based on her family and religious values. What is your opinion about what they should do?

3. Suppose you had the ability and resources to invent the ideal method of birth control. What would it be? How would it differ from what is already available? Would men or women be responsible for using it? What would be the advantages of this new method?

Activities
1. Contact an abortion clinic and ask how many abortions were performed there in the past year. Report your findings to the class.
2. Contact a family planning office and ask them to describe the services offered.
3. Contact a crisis pregnancy center and ask about the services offered.

Making Decisions about Health
1. Kelly tried the Pill, but it gave her headaches. The IUD she tried gave her cramps. Gels and diaphragms or condoms were too inconvenient. Her monthly cycle is erratic, so natural family planning is out. Now what? What other choices do you think Kelly has? If you were Kelly, what would you do? Why?
2. Jody has never taken time to learn much about birth control. Now when his wife assures him that she'll take care of it, he feels a bit uneasy—will she really take care of it? She's so forgetful. With his heavy schedule at school and a new job, the last thing he needs right now is to become a father. What options do you think Jody has in this situation? If you were in Jody's situation, what would you do? Why?

16. They can break down the latex in condoms, increasing the risk of pregnancy and STDs. (p. 607)
17. It gives women control over their own protection. When used with spermicide it is highly effective for preventing pregnancy and some STDs. (p. 609)
18. be trained by a health professional to track the menstrual cycle and to observe body signs of ovulation (p. 611)

SECTION 3

19. the withdrawal method, using other replacement materials for condoms, douching, after intercourse, relying on breastfeeding to prevent ovulation (pp. 612–613)

SECTION 4

20. several weeks (p. 614)

SECTION 5

21. a procedure to end a pregnancy (p. 616)
22. free pregnancy testing; group counseling; medical care before, during and after the birth; housing; adoption services; maternity and infant clothing; and day care (p. 618)

months prior to becoming pregnant. (pp. 602–603)
11. women who have had at least one child, those in monogamous relationships (such as marriage), have no history of pelvic inflammation disease (PID) (p. 603)
12. have a custom-fitted diaphragm, apply spermicide two hours before intercourse, leave the diaphragm in place for at least six hours after intercourse, apply new

spermicide for repeated intercourse (p. 605)
13. at least six hours (p. 605)
14. The dangerous bacterial poisoning known as toxic shock syndrome can occur. (p. 606)
15. Latex condoms offer some protection against sexually transmitted diseases and they are superior over lambskin condoms in preventing pregnancy. (p. 608)

KEY POINTS

Chapter 23 is 20 pages long and divided into three sections. This chapter discusses aging and dying. Students are introduced to the concept of successful aging and the idea of planning to age successfully. The different aspects of dying and death are also discussed. Students are informed about the different ways to prepare for death. The Straight Talk in this chapter deals with grief.

ACTIVITY TO INTRODUCE THE CHAPTER

The following activities can help you and your students get an idea what it's like to experience some of the physical limitations that can accompany aging.

1. *Stroke/Paralysis Exercise:* Try to write your name, using the opposite hand from the one you normally use. Put a ping-pong ball in your mouth, and try and talk with someone.

2. *Loss of Hearing Exercise:* Stuff an earplug into the outer part of each ear. On top of that, put on a pair of earmuffs or a stereo headset. Have someone go into another room and try and carry on a conversation. Now try and listen to the television, radio, or stereo with the sound turned low.

3. *Impaired Vision Exercise:* Put on goggles or scratched eyeglasses. Try to read, watch television, walk outdoors, or ride in a car (with someone else driving).

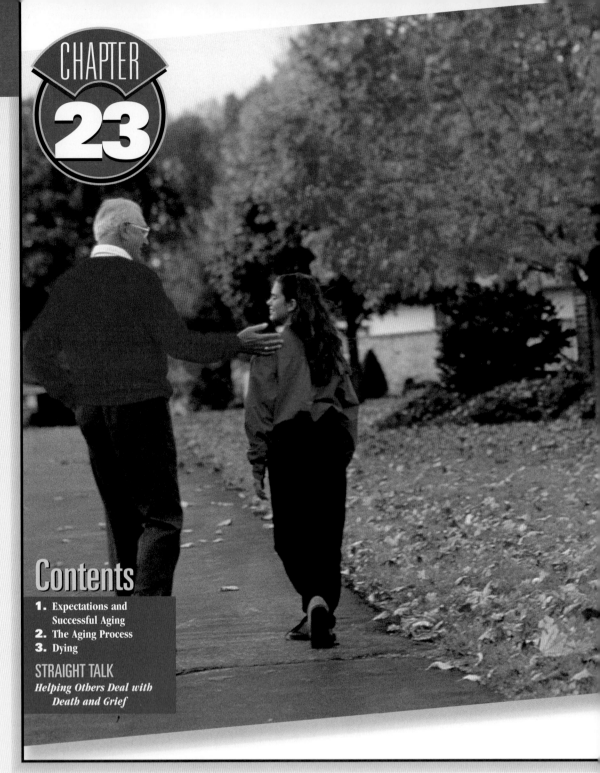

CHAPTER 23

Contents

NOT Enough Time?

Following are some suggestions to help you make sure you cover the key topics if you have limited time. (Refer to the daily lesson plans in your Teacher's Resource Box for additional suggestions.)

DAY 1 Assign Section 1 to be read prior to class. During class have students complete the Focus Activity and Discussion on page 626.

Mature Life, Aging, and Death

What do you think? Are the following statements true or false? If you think they are false, then say what is true.

1. The happiest people are those who have experienced the fewest tragedies.
2. The human life span has increased steadily over the past 100 years.
3. People should expect to lose their sexuality at around 50 years of age.
4. Most people's incomes are reduced at retirement.
5. Most people can expect to spend their later years in nursing homes.

(Answers on page 638)

Introduction

Why study aging when you are still under 20? Because you are setting your course now for the kind of older person you will become—that's why. An old expression says it this way: "As the twig is bent, so grows the tree." As the master of your "twig" (your young life), how will you bend it to grow into your "tree" (your later life)? While you are still young, how well can you develop your understanding of older people?

DAY 2 Assign Section 2 to be read prior to class. During class have students complete the Enrichment activity on page 630 and the Discussion activity on page 631. If time allows, do the Group Activity on page 633.

DAY 3 Assign Section 3 and the Straight Talk to be read prior to class. During class have students do one or more of the following activities: Focus Activity on page 637, Close activity on page 639, and the second Background Information activity on page 640.

BULLETIN BOARD IDEAS

Have the students bring in photographs of their grandparents and great-grandparents (if possible). Arrange the bulletin board in order of the age of the subject of the photograph. Discuss with the class any similarities or differences between individuals of approximately the same age.

CHAPTER PROJECT

Assign students to interview five people over the age of 40, with at least two of the interviewees over 60. As a class, prepare a questionnaire for the students to use in the interview. The students should be seeking information on lifestyle: Is the person doing anything to slow down the aging process? What do they like most and least about their current age, and why? Collect the interviews and have the students discuss their findings. As the discussion draws to a close, ask students if their views on aging changed. If so, how and why?

Answers to FACT or FICTION

1. **False.** The happiest people are those who have lived through at least one major life tragedy.
2. **False.** The human life span has not changed, but the average life expectancy has increased steadily over past years.
3. **False.** People remain sexual beings throughout life.
4. **True.**
5. **False.** Only a fraction of older people live in nursing homes.

SECTION 1

FOCUS

OUTCOMES

In this section students will learn the:

1. Correlation between one's views of "old age," and how one actually lives out these views.
2. Similarities and differences in classmates' views of aging.

Vocabulary worksheets are provided in the Teacher's Resource Box.

FOCUS ACTIVITY

Ask students, before they begin to read this chapter, to express their opinions of older people. Do they enjoy being with older people? Do they think that older people tend to have different views than their own on most issues? If so, can they provide some examples?

TEACH & APPLY

DISCUSSION

Have the students brainstorm words and thoughts that come to mind when you say the words *aging, death,* and *dying.* Count the positive responses and the negative responses. Are their ideas about these concepts primarily negative or positive? If they are negative, ask them what they can do to change these feelings.

SECTION 1

Expectations and Successful Aging

The quality of life in the future tends to become what people expect it to become. Physical health makes a difference, and so does financial security. However, people's expectations also contribute more to their futures than most people realize.

Expectations

Are you aware of how you expect your later life to be? Most people, without realizing it, believe in a stereotype—largely negative—of what it is like to be old. Then, later, they become that way.

Most people want their later lives to be successful. Some say they want to be like those who have made great intellectual and artistic achievements in their 70s and 80s. They claim they want to model themselves after older people they admire. Such older people are vibrant and happy. They can offer unique wisdom and perspective, having experienced more life than anyone else.

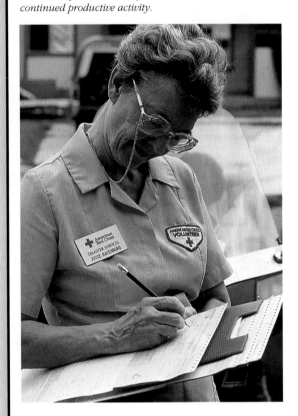

A mature life can be one of continued productive activity.

 KEY POINTS *The views people hold on aging can affect the way they live in their later years.*

Successful Aging

A 90-year-old man visited his physician, seeking relief from the pain in his left knee. Unable to find a cause for the ache, the physician said, "For heaven's sake, at your age, you have to expect such problems." The mature man replied, "Look here, Doc, my right knee is also 90, and it doesn't hurt."

The physician's attitude reflects how most people view growing old. They think disability and disease are inevitable consequences of aging. In contrast, the older man's remark suggests that elderly people may have a different view of old age. They often think that the advanced years can still be lively.

Most people in their later years are self-sufficient, physically active, socially involved, and clear thinking. Most are fully participating members of society, and report themselves to be happy and healthy. Such people tend to think positively throughout their lives. They do not believe in a rigid definition of success. Rather, they define success by their own values and live accordingly. They work not toward power and wealth but

special needs

Interpersonal

The elderly face many stereotypes as they move through normal developmental processes. The term ageism is used to identify prejudices facing senior citizens. Ask students to describe what aging means. Check for negative and positive descriptors that indicate an aging stereotype. Examples include:

- Negative: weak, frail
- Positive: patient, caring

Divide the class into groups. Ask one student to serve as the discussion facilitator and another to be the group recorder. If time allows, have each group discuss and answer each of the following questions. If time is short, assign one or two questions to each group. To conclude, have groups present their findings to the class.

toward meaningful goals. They feel their lives have purpose. Those who age successfully display these characteristics:

► Their lives have meaning and direction.
► They handle life's events in their own, sometimes unusual, ways.
► They rarely feel cheated by life.
► They have attained several long-term goals.
► They are pleased with their own growth and development.
► They love and are loved by others.
► They have many friends.
► They are cheerful.
► They can take criticism.
► They have no major fears.

What is more, the people who are enjoying life the most are likely to be beyond their 20s, and to have lived through the fears and anxieties of youth. Many of the happiest people have lived through at least one major life tragedy. Being well educated is a factor in their happiness, as is having enough money to cover life's basic needs. They also know how to balance spontaneity with planning so that their lives are neither rigid nor aimless. They strike a balance between helping others and a healthy commitment to meeting their own needs. All of these traits, taken together, define successful aging.

In short, if you want to be happy when you are old, begin practicing happiness now. If you want to strive for a long life, preserve your health to support it. It can be done. More people than ever before are living full, healthy lives in their advanced years. This chapter describes the aging process and offers insight into how to grow old gracefully.

66 *All would live long, but none would be old.* **99**

Benjamin Franklin
(1706–1790)
American statesman
and philosopher

KEY POINTS *Many people in their later years live interesting and fulfilling lives. They practiced by living well in their earlier years.*

SECTION 1 Review

Answer the following questions on a sheet of paper.

Learning the Facts

1. What are three factors that will contribute to the quality of your future, perhaps more than you realize?
2. Identify characteristics of older people who some say they want to be like.
3. How do most people view growing old?

4. List five of the ten characteristics that people who age successfully display.
5. If you want to be happy when you are old, what must you begin doing now?

Making Life Choices

6. Aging is a process that starts early in life. What are some things you can do at your age to make the aging process easier? Do you have a negative attitude about the aging process? If so, how can you change your attitude about aging?

ASSESS

EVALUATE

SECTION 1 Review Answers

1. physical health, financial security, expectations (p. 626)
2. those making great intellectual and artistic achievements in their 70s and 80s; vibrant, happy, and offer unique wisdom and perspective (p. 626)
3. disability and disease are inevitable (p. 626)
4. Answers will vary. (p. 627)
5. practice happiness, and preserve your health (p. 627)
6. Answers will vary.

WORKSHEETS

A reproducible quiz for Section 1 is provided in the Teacher's Resource Box.

CLOSE

Have students list the characteristics of people who age successfully. If they miss any, make sure to add them to the list.

1. Does "development" continue after age 60 or is this final period of life marked only by "decline"? Give examples.
2. What does your community do to promote full and active lives for the elderly?
3. What jobs are available for the elderly?
4. Have elderly relatives, neighbors, or friends had a positive impact on your life? How?
5. What are the advantages and disadvantages of mandatory retirement?

6. What can you do to make a difference in the life of the elderly?

You may want to take your class on a trip to a senior center or nursing home to conduct interviews with the elderly. Understanding that we all have the same feelings and needs will help students plan for their own "retirement years."

SECTION

2

The Aging Process

Although many people believe that aging starts around 40 or 45, aging really begins early in life. Until about age 20, aging takes the form of growth and maturing. After growth is completed, aging brings about the gradual loss of youthful appearance and condition. Inside the body, the organs and cells age, too.

Within the different body organs, cells have different aging patterns and life spans. Some blood cells live only three days or so. Most nerve cells last for the person's lifetime. In a healthy older person, each cell lives on to the end of its normal life span in much the same fashion as in the person's younger years. As the person ages, though, the cells lose some of their function, they collect products not found in younger people's cells, and their cells lose some of their ability to reproduce.

KEY POINTS *Each cell in the body has its own aging pattern. Aging of the whole body begins at maturity, about age 20.*

Life Span and Life Expectancy

The human **life span** is the *maximum* possible length of life that people can reach, conditions being ideal. A person's **life expectancy** is the *average* length of life predicted by statistics. The human life span is in the neighborhood of 100 years or more. Many people, however, do not live this long, owing to disease or accidents. Today, the life expectancy for men in the United States is about 73 years; for women, about 79 years. Another term referring to length of life is **longevity**—the actual length of life observed in an individual. Some people are blessed with extraordinary longevity, perhaps thanks to their genetic inheritance combined with the events of their lives.

People are living longer today than ever before, but the human life span (maximum) has not changed. What has changed over the past 100 years is the life expectancy (average), mainly for two reasons. First, the rate of deaths from diseases and accidents among the very young has declined. Thus there are fewer young deaths to bring the average down. Second, medical advances are prolonging adults' lives so that they more nearly reach their maximum.

Many strategies have been proposed to extend the lengths of human lives, and many do not work. A scientific review of some 200 research studies concluded that none of the proposed strategies had any life-extending effect. This chapter's

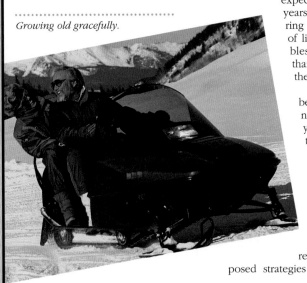

Growing old gracefully.

FOCUS

OUTCOMES

In this section students will learn the:

1. Strategies necessary for successful aging.
2. Terminology associated with old age.
3. Differences between senility that is preventable and senility that is not preventable.

FOCUS ACTIVITY

With books closed, ask the students to list the names of people over the age of 50 who have aged successfully. These people can be famous or not. Ask for some examples from their list and write these on the board. Now ask the students to list the characteristics these people have that led to their successful aging. Again, ask for examples and write these on the board. Ask the students to open their books to page 631 and compare their list to the list, Growing Old Gracefully in Figure 23–2. Choose a few items to discuss, such as numbers 1, 2, and 4. Ask students to give examples and explanations. Ask if they agree with this list. In closing, stress that these 22 characteristics might tell us something about our own lifestyles and goals in life.

CRITICAL THINKING

Research indicates that exercise and proper diet play a significant role in the aging process. While young people believe they will live forever, they need to understand:

1. that they will grow old.

2. that their lifestyles will affect both the quality and quantity of life.
3. the physiology of aging.

This activity involves two parts:

1. Have students interview someone age 40 or older who has exercised faithfully over the years. The focus should be on how

Longevity Frauds

Consumer SKILLS

People have tried everything imaginable to delay or reverse aging. Years ago, the Spaniards sailed to the New World in search of the legendary Fountain of Youth. Today, people rush to buy products, based on "new scientific breakthroughs," that promise to restore youth or even to prevent death.

The motivation behind these efforts is always the same: people want miracles. Whenever many people desire something that is impossible to have, someone steps in with empty promises and useless products and wins a growing bank account for the effort.

Frauds that plague the elderly are not limited to longevity hypes. Older people are targets of many other schemes. Why are the elderly the targets for such deception? First, many of them have ready access to money—retirement funds, pensions, insurance policies, and paid-up mortgages. Second, as people age, they

experience more symptoms and may be frustrated by the medical profession's inability to help or unwillingness to take them seriously. They seek help where it is offered, proven or not. Also, as people get older, they may develop a "what have I got to lose" attitude about trying products that claim to prolong life or improve health. Money seems less important than even the slightest chance of better health or longer life. Even brilliant, sophisticated people let themselves be bamboozled by longevity frauds.

Critical Thinking

1. Why are people so open to promises of miracles concerning aging?
2. Why are older people so often the targets of scams?
3. Based on what you've learned in other Consumer Skills features, how can you detect a longevity fraud when one is offered?

Consumer Skills feature helps to explain why people are fooled into buying products that promise to delay or reverse aging. Strategies that do help slow aging have more to do with lifestyle and less to do with pills and shots.

 KEY POINTS *The human life span has not changed, but life expectancy has increased. Longevity frauds are numerous.*

How to Age Gracefully

No magic can keep a person young forever. No matter what you do to prevent it, your body will age. You can, however, do quite a bit to slow the process of aging and maximize your wellness and enjoyment of life.

One of the most important things to do is to maintain appropriate body weight. Obesity shortens life. Aside from that, other keys to health maintenance in the later years involve all of the principles of this book's chapters: sound nutrition, including an ample water intake; adequate sleep; regular physical activity; and avoidance of alcohol, tobacco, and other drug abuse.

Much of the quality of the later years depends on the daily choices a person makes in youth and on the habits that become fixed as a result of those choices. Figure 23–1 on the next page shows a sampling of changes

MINI Glossary

life span: the maximum years of life a human being can live.

life expectancy: the average number of years lived by people in a given society.

longevity: an individual's length of life.

---

exercise and proper diet have:
a. made the person's life more productive.
b. helped the person maintain himself or herself physically (overall wellness).
2. Create four posters representing four age groups: age 18, 35, 50, and 65. Using photographs, drawings, pictures, and/or statements, create profiles of two different

people at each age:
a. one living a sedentary lifestyle.
b. another living an active lifestyle.

Emphasis and focus should be on the aging process and how it should be viewed.

COMPREHENSION CHECK

Tell students that there are 29 changes listed in Figure 23–1, Changes with Age: Preventable versus Unavoidable. Ask them how many of these changes they can help slow down or prevent. (17) How many can they not prevent? (12) Ask them if they disagree with any of these. As a more extensive follow-up activity, you may want to ask students to list behaviors that they could practice or avoid in order to slow or prevent the changes that have check marks in the middle column. (Keep the list to review or add to at the end of the chapter to help students personalize this information and review their present lifestyle.) For example, smoking, excessive alcohol consumption, and other drug abuse ages the skin.

BACKGROUND INFORMATION

You may want to point out to students the possibility of the human life span increasing in the years to come. People who are 100 years old today were born in the 1890s. Have students think about the difficulties those people may have had to deal with in terms of living conditions, lack of medicines, and lack of knowledge regarding such things as nutrition and disease. Then have the students think about the conditions in which today's newborns will grow up and mature with regard to those same areas. It could be that the life span will increase simply due to these changes and conditions.

Change with Aging	You Probably Can Slow or Prevent These Changes by Exercising, Maintaining Other Good Health Habits, and Planning Ahead:	You Probably Cannot Prevent These Changes:
Appearance		
Graying of hair		✔
Balding		✔
Drying and wrinkling of skin	✔	
Nervous System		
Impairment of near vision		✔
Some loss of hearing		✔
Reduced taste and smell		✔
Reduced touch sensitivity		✔
Slowed reactions (reflexes)		✔
Slowed mental function		✔
Mental confusion	✔	
Cardiovascular System		
Increased blood pressure	✔	
Increased resting heart rate	✔	
Decreased oxygen consumption	✔	
Body Composition/Metabolism		
Increased body fatness	✔	
Raised blood cholesterol	✔	
Slowed energy metabolism	✔	
Other Physical Characteristics		
Menopause (women)		✔
Loss of fertility (men)		✔
Loss of elasticity in joints		✔
Loss of flexibility in joints	✔	
Loss of teeth; gum disease	✔	
Bone loss	✔	
Accident/Disease Proneness		
Accidents	✔	
Inherited diseases		✔
Lifestyle diseases	✔	
Psychological/Other		
Reduced self-esteem	✔	
Loss of interest in work	✔	
Depression, loneliness	✔	
Reduced financial status	✔	

Figure 23–1 Changes with Age: Preventable versus Unavoidable

that happen with age. The figure shows that some of these changes can be prevented by continued exercise and other health-supporting habits, and that some changes will occur no matter how hard you try to prevent them. Figure 23–2 provides further suggestions.

KEY POINTS *Some changes of aging are preventable by choosing wise lifestyle habits throughout life.*

enrichment...

Give each student two index cards and a marker. On one card ask the student to answer the following question: "At what age does old age begin?" The students should be instructed to write their answers on the cards and include enough reasons to fill the whole card.

On the other card, ask the students to answer the next question with the words "positive" or "negative." Question: "When you think of growing old and passing the age you put down on the first card, do you think of it in a positive or negative way?" Give each student two pieces of double-sided tape. They are to put the tape on the backs of the cards and then put them on one of the following, which you have prepared beforehand.

a. Two poster boards—one with the words "Old age begins at . . ." and the

1. Maintain appropriate body weight.
2. Obtain regular and adequate sleep throughout life.
3. Consciously practice your stress-management skills.
4. Limit your time in the sun, or use sunscreen protection.
5. For women, see your physician about estrogen replacement to fight osteoporosis.
6. Do not smoke. If you do smoke, quit.
7. Expect to enjoy sexual activity with your husband or wife, and learn new ways of enhancing it.
8. Maintain physical fitness. Change activities to suit changing abilities and tastes.
9. Protect your eyes against excessive sunlight.
10. Be aware that your brain's and nerves' reactions are slowing down. Plan to compensate by being more careful.
11. Use alcohol only moderately, if at all. Use drugs only as prescribed. Ask your physician about potential interactions of prescribed medicines with other drugs.
12. Take care to prevent accidents. Seek medical attention if impairment from a fall seems to last too long.
13. Expect good vision and hearing throughout life. Obtain glasses and hearing aids, if necessary.
14. Maintain adequate nutrition.
15. Be alert to confusion as a disease symptom, and seek diagnosis. Do not live with an unidentified disease.
16. Stay interested in life, make new friends, and adopt new activities—control depression.
17. Drink eight glasses a day of water or other liquids, even if you aren't thirsty.
18. Practice your mental skills. Keep on solving math problems, reading, following directions, writing, imagining, and creating.
19. For adult children of aging parents: provide or obtain the needed care and stimulation for your parents.
20. Make financial plans early to ensure your security.
21. Accept change. Work at recovering from losses; practice making new friends.
22. Cultivate spiritual health. Assess your values, and make your life meaningful.

Figure 23–2 Growing Old Gracefully

Dealing with Physical Changes

Knowledge helps people deal with the changes that come with age. It is comforting to realize that some negative changes of aging are accompanied by positive ones that help compensate for lost abilities. For example, although older people are less able than younger people to recover from stress physically, older people are more able psychologically. Older people have learned how to "bounce back" from setbacks. Perhaps this is because they have seen more of life and have learned to adjust to unexpected turns of events. Another example: the immune system becomes less efficient at fighting off disease once it takes hold, but older people get infections less often than younger people do. Perhaps this is because they have developed immunity against many diseases.

Menopause and Male Menopause   In women, the later years bring **menopause**, in which monthly ovulation becomes irregular and finally

MINI Glossary

menopause: the years of stopping ovulation and menstruation in a woman.

DISCUSSION

Take a class poll on the following statements. Have students indicate whether they agree or disagree with each one. Allow volunteers to share their opinions.

1. Television accurately portrays how elderly people behave and look.
2. People over the age of 65 should not be allowed to drive.
3. Older people are boring.
4. Elderly people are unable to make important decisions.
5. It's stimulating to talk with elderly people.
6. Most elderly people are forgetful.
7. Elderly people should be able to work until they no longer want to do so.
8. Most elderly people should be in nursing homes.
9. Younger people can benefit from the experience of the elderly.
10. Elderly people are no longer productive members of society.

After discussing the students' feelings, ask them why they think they feel the way they do about the elderly. Ask them if they have any suggestions for getting to know an elderly person better and finding out what he or she is really like.

other "Old age is a —— thought."
b. A bulletin board or wall section prepared with those two statements.
c. The chalkboard prepared with those statements.

Once the students have put both cards under the appropriate statements, discuss the results using the following questions and statements as guidelines:

1. What is the range of ages at which old age begins? Why do you think our views are so varied?

2. Count the number of positives and negatives in answer to the second question. What could these answers possibly tell us? Why did some of you say "negative?" Why "positive?" Is it possible that those of us who said "positive" may not fear getting older and those of us who said "negative" do fear old age? What is there to fear? What is there to look forward to?

ceases. As the supply of the hormone estrogen dwindles, menstruation also stops. Reduced estrogen also causes the periodic feelings of warmth some women call **hot flashes**. Hot flashes are related to the dilation of the blood vessels in the skin.

A major surge of bone loss (osteoporosis) takes place at the beginning of menopause. Women whose calcium intakes and physical activity levels have been insufficient to build up the bones before menopause may lose bone material rapidly and become crippled with osteoporosis within a few years (see Chapter 7). To prevent further bone loss, as well as to prevent some of the other effects of menopause, physicians often prescribe estrogen replacement therapy. In the younger years, though, the best prevention is an abundant calcium intake from food, together with plenty of physical activity to cement the calcium into place in the bones.

Menopause sets in early in women who smoke. So does osteoporosis. This may be because smoking suppresses production of the hormone estrogen or because the ingredients of tobacco are directly toxic to the ovaries. Chapter 14 gave abundant reasons for abstaining from smoking; add these to them.

The **male menopause** is experienced as a gradual decline of fertility rather than as the abrupt end experienced by women. In fact, some men still have the ability to make sperm into their 80s. Testosterone production gradually decreases, as does sperm production. Hormones and testicular functioning may decrease, as may the desire for sexual activity.

Physical Activity   As people age, their physical abilities do change. Older muscles do not build up as quickly as younger ones do, so it takes longer and harder work to gain condition. Balanced against that, older muscles lose condition at a slower rate than young muscles do. Once fit, an older person who has to take a break from physical activity will maintain condition longer. However, he or she still should resume exercising as soon as possible.

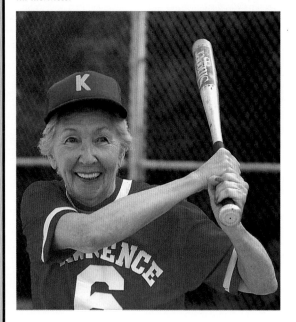

Physical activity promotes mental alertness.

The more physically active people are, the less likely they are to die of heart and lung diseases. This does not mean for sure that physical activity prolongs life. However, it does enhance the quality of life and helps keep you from dying before your time.

An older person's reflexes are slowed. The joints may be less flexible than a younger person's. A painful condition affecting the joints, **arthritis**, is to some extent unavoidable in older people. Weight control and moderate activity, however, help people to withstand its worst effects. Aspirin helps quell the pain of arthritis. Fad diets do not help.

The fact that continued physical activity helps fend off arthritis is another reminder that people should stay active all their lives. Sometimes a pain that an older person believes to be arthritis may instead be a normal ache caused by joint stiffness from years of inactivity. Older people need not exercise the same way younger people do, though. Activities should be adjusted to fit the body's changing abilities. A former

HEALTHY PEOPLE 2000

Life expectancy has increased dramatically since 1900 and people who reach the age of 65 can expect to live well into their eighties. The most important aspect of health promotion among older people is to maintain health and functional independence. Although it is commonly believed that health problems in old age are inevitable, many are in fact preventable or can be controlled.

The leading causes of death among people aged 65 and older include heart disease, cancer, stroke, chronic obstructive pulmonary disease, pneumonia and influenza. Although

Abuse of drugs. This includes alcohol abuse and the misuse or incompatibility of prescription drugs. The effects of alcohol and drugs can sometimes resemble those of strokes and seizures.

Accidents. Falls can cause skull fractures (concussions) or bleeding that puts pressure on the brain, which surgery can relieve.

Dehydration. The thirst signal may become faint. As a result, an older person may not drink enough to meet fluid needs. One of the major symptoms of dehydration is confusion.

Depression. Depression can slow down the mind in old people, as in the young.

Disease states. Diseases present different symptoms in older people than in younger ones. Tuberculosis, diabetes, and even heart attacks can all begin with confusion, rather than with fever or pain.

Disuse of mental skills. People do lose what they don't use. Practicing mental skills brings them back.

Malnutrition. Taste enjoyment, digestive secretions, and appetite diminish. Older people eat less, yet nutrient needs remain the same.

Poor vision and hearing. Both can cause confusion. Both can be corrected or compensated for.

Figure 23–3 Preventable Causes of Mental Confusion in Older People

Olympic gold medal gymnast may hike and bike in later years. A once-bone-bruising football player may jog and play a little golf. Wise advice to the older person: "Regular physical activity is important, but go easy on yourself."

 KEY POINTS *Knowing in advance what physical changes are unpreventable with aging can help people to cope as the changes take place. Compensations accompany these changes. The knowledge that this is so eases acceptance of aging.*

Dealing with Mental Changes

Some changes take place in the brain and nervous system as people age. Research has discovered declines in these areas: reasoning skill, recall (memory), speed, and senses. These declines, however, are offset by increased wisdom and judgment. People can also adopt strategies to compensate for these declines, such as learning to write things down so that they will not forget or allowing more time for certain tasks.

Senility and Depression   The mental confusion called **senility** is many times avoidable. Mental confusion in older people has many different causes—and most are preventable. Only one, brain disease itself, is not. The preventable causes of mental confusion are listed in Figure 23–3. If an older person becomes confused, try correcting these possible causes before jumping to the conclusion that senility has set in.

Depression, especially, often causes the symptoms of senility. The story is told of a woman who invited her mother to live with her while the older

Glossary

hot flashes: sudden waves of feeling hot all over, a symptom related to dilation of blood vessels in the skin, which is common during the transition into menopause.

male menopause: the gradual decline in male fertility due to advancing age.

arthritis: a painful inflammation of the joints caused by infection, body chemistry, injury, or other causes; usually results in altered joint structure and loss of function.

senility: a general term meaning weakness of mind and body occurring in old age.

health problems such as osteoporosis, arthritis, incontinence, dementia, and visual or hearing impairments, are not common causes of death, they have a significant effect on the quality of life. Even in later life, changing certain risk behaviors into healthy ones can improve health and reduce the likelihood of disability. Improvements in diet and nutrition,

reductions in tobacco use, and weight control can enhance the health of older people. Physical activity is a key ingredient to healthy aging.

In addition to primary prevention, strong social support and regular primary care services are important aspects of risk reduction for older adults.

BACKGROUND INFORMATION

Mental confusion among older patients is often caused by over-medication. Many older people take several types of long-term medications, and some use more than a dozen different drugs. Interactions among drugs, as well as overdoses of some drugs, can cause a host of complications, including mental confusion. People in their advanced years should request that their health-care providers monitor their use of mixtures of prescription drugs.

GROUP ACTIVITY

Write the following ingredients for successful aging on sheets of paper before class (one sentence on each sheet):

1. Many of the happiest people have lived through at least one major life tragedy.
2. Being well educated is a factor in happiness.
3. Having enough money for life's basic needs is essential.

Write the following sentence on posterboard: "If you want to be happy when you are old, begin practicing happiness now."

Divide the class into three groups. Give each group a piece of paper with one of the ingredients on it. Ask the students to take five minutes to brainstorm why this is such an important ingredient. Have them write their ideas on the paper. As a class, discuss the importance of each ingredient, based on students' brainstorming. Ask if everyone agrees with them. Would they add others? Then hold up the posterboard and read the statement aloud. Have students think about it and ask themselves if they practice the ingredients. Do they practice happiness?

Teen Views

Here are some questions that will help promote classroom discussion of the issues raised in the Teen Views comments:

a. Do the students have grandparents who tell lots of stories about the "good old days"? Are there any favorites that students could relate to the class?

b. Do students think that older people are interesting? Do teens often take senior citizens for granted? Do some teens fail to give older people the proper respect?

BACKGROUND INFORMATION

The Alliance for Aging research estimates that it costs the nation $90 billion to treat people with Alzheimer's, which affects at least 2 million and possibly 4 million Americans.

Teen Views

What Makes Your Favorite Senior Citizen Your Favorite?

My grandfather is a retired navy ship-man with the energy of a teenager. The jokes he tells with a dev-ilish grin on his face always make us laugh until we cry, and he has the best war stories. You learn a lot about life by listening to him talk. But above all else, he cares so much about me.
Erin Tanaka, 16,
Wilson High School, CA

My favorite senior citizen is an incredibly supportive fan of high school sports. He has been attending sporting events at Billings schools for many years and has touched the lives of many young people. He is such a special person and means a great deal to me. He has been at almost every basketball, volley-ball, and softball game I've par-ticipated in within the last two years. He has led a very inter-esting life and carries many spe-cial memories with him. His children and grandchildren don't live near him; but I am glad he has become an important mem-ber of many families here. I hope every child who doesn't have grandparents living close, finds a special senior citizen to spend time with and learn from. He constantly tells me how much children mean to him and how he loves to watch our games. I am very glad he has us. I just wish he knew exactly how much

we love having him at our games, in our lives, and in our hearts. He is extremely dear to me—as a fan, a friend, and a grandparent.
Shannon Beddow, 16,
West High School, MT

My favorite senior citizen is my favorite because they respect me for who I am. They have lived a long time and "have been there, done that," so I can ask advice and they know exactly what I'm talking about. It may not be very up to date, but I can relate it to my life. They can also give you good remedies to sicknesses instead of just using the pre-scribed medicines.
Hannah Gleason, 15,
Manzano High School, NM

woman waited for a place in a nursing home. The mother, who lived alone, had all the classic signs of senility—mental confusion, inability to make deci-sions, forgetting simple tasks—so the family decided she needed institutional care. However, after several weeks in her daughter's home—eating meals with the family and enjoying social stimulation—she became her old self again and was able to return to her home. This story has been repeated with many variations and serves to remind us that factors other than senility cause confusion. What harm could there be in first trying home life, regular meals, and plenty of tender, loving care?

   Alzheimer's Disease One unpreventable cause of confusion is **Alzheimer's disease**. The condition appears most often in people over 65 and is a major cause of death in that age group. It afflicts 30 percent of all those over 85. It starts as the loss of memory, then becomes an inability to

COOPERATIVE LEARNING

The following activity is a great way to review the vocabulary words for Chapter 23 or any other chapter. It is a fun way for students to learn not only the words but also how these words relate to each other. The activity is a game in which people draw out images and others try to guess what the word or phrase

is. By doing this, students are able to use their creativity in finding ways of describing a meaning or situation without talking.

   You can do this activity in several different ways, either by putting students in small groups and having them play their own game or by putting them in groups and having the group act as one and the entire class plays one game. If you choose to have each individ-ual group play their own game, you may want perform everyday functions, and then leads to the total inability to care for oneself. In the brain, the nerve pathways become tangled and blocked, cutting off the memory functions. Once it sets in, Alzheimer's disease is irreversible and progresses from mild confusion to disability and death in a period of months or years. The person suffering from it usually requires a level of care beyond what family members can provide. The causes are still unknown, and no cure is in sight.

 KEY POINTS *Losses of mental sharpness in aging are offset by gains in wisdom and judgment. Brain disease such as Alzheimer's disease is an unavoidable cause of senility, but most other causes are preventable.*

Preparing for Social and Other Changes

Besides physical and mental changes, people who are aging also face financial and social losses. Being aware of this and preparing for it will enable people to weather losses successfully.

Financial planning is essential. Nearly everyone suffers a loss of income in the retirement years. It is important to have set aside enough money for retirement—to have the home paid for or adequate income to pay the rent. It is also crucial to have insurance to cover unexpected medical and other expenses.

Another way to prepare is to plan for alternative living arrangements, should it become too difficult to care for the present home. A nursing home is not the only choice and usually is not the best one. Fewer than a third of older adults spend any time in a nursing home. Of those, most spend only about a year there. Rather than leave it to their children to decide for them where they will live, older adults usually decide for themselves.

Financial preparation and deciding where to live will not, however, prevent emotional and social losses, which may be many. Old friends may die or move away. Children may move away also and may be too busy to write or call. Status in the community is often lost upon retiring.

Loss of control of the environment also occurs. For example, a person may find that the home that was to be a haven in retirement now sits in the middle of a high-crime area, or that the familiar shops and fruit stands have closed. A person can develop a feeling of deep loneliness as the familiar environment shifts.

A loss of identity may accompany retirement or the death of a spouse. A working person can say, "I'm a farmer, a nurse, a manager," but what can a retired person say? A part of the person's identity is gone.

You may think it's unnecessary for a person of 15 or 18 to confront the problems of loneliness and loss in later life, but such is not the case. Emotional and social health in the later years is affected by what happens during youth. To be happy when you are old, you need to practice happiness when you are young. Losses occur when you are young, too. Learn to grieve over them and move on. Practice refilling your life with new loves, new activities, new enthusiasms. Maintain a strong social support system. Keep reaching out. Create a web of support so that as relationships are lost, others are gained.

MINI Glossary

Alzheimer's disease: a brain disease of some older people that brings mental confusion; inability to function; and in the final stage, death.

to divide the groups up into ability levels so that your more advanced students can challenge themselves more and your other students can have more success.

In playing the game, have one student draw a card (prepared in advance by you), which has one of the vocabulary words written on it. Then have them go to the board and draw a description of the word. They cannot write down any words or talk during

the time they are at the board. The students who are still in their seats try to guess the word. Continue the activity having each student draw until all of the vocabulary words have been used up. Offer extra credit for those groups or those students who guess the most vocabulary words correctly.

SECTION 2 Review Answers

1. Answers will vary.
2. Principles include: appropriate body weight; sound nutrition, including ample water intake; adequate sleep; regular physical activity; avoidance of alcohol, tobacco, and other drug use (p. 629)
3. have an abundant calcium intake from food, together with plenty of physical activity (p. 632)
4. Answers will vary.

WORKSHEETS A reproducible quiz for Section 2 is provided in the Teacher's Resource Box.

CLOSE

Have students develop a service project for a local nursing home or for local senior citizens. They may want to join the local Humane Society for their "adopt a pet" days at the nursing homes, develop a pen pal system for the elderly with no relatives or visitors, plan a holiday party for the elderly, or hold a spring clean-up day for senior citizens who need help with their yards and windows. These activity days should prove to be very successful and give the students a wonderful sense of worth and accomplishment.

To be young at heart is to be young where it counts.

Continue your education forever. New information exercises the mind. Cultivate spiritual health, too. Think about the meaning of life—both yours and that of others. Find ways to contribute your gifts, to leave something of value to those you care for. Keep working at projects that are meaningful to you. Growing is not for children only. It is a lifelong engagement.

"I've spent my whole life becoming who I am. Was it worth it?" A message of this chapter is that what a person becomes later in life is, to a large extent, whatever that person chooses to become today. The way a person deals with life's final challenge—death—is often also a matter of choice.

 KEY POINTS *A person must plan for changes in financial support, living arrangements, and social support in the later years. You are becoming now what you will be in old age.*

SECTION 2 Review

Answer the following questions on a sheet of paper.

Learning the Vocabulary

The vocabulary terms in this section are *life span, life expectancy, longevity, menopause, hot flashes, male menopause, arthritis, senility,* and *Alzheimer's disease.*

1. Write a sentence using each of the vocabulary terms above.

Learning the Facts

2. List key principles of maintaining health in the later years.
3. What might teenage women do to avoid osteoporosis later in life?

Making Life Choices

4. Describe any experiences you've had with people who are senile. What strategies can you recommend to make similar situations as comfortable as possible for everyone involved?

Chapter 23, Section 2

The following quiz will help you assess your students' understanding of the material covered in this section of the chapter. You might use the quiz as an oral exercise, which will lead into a class discussion of the topics covered. Or, you might use it as a paper/pencil

quiz to evaluate your students individually.

Like the Quick Quiz, the Section Review can also be used as an assessment tool to spark class discussion or as an individual student evaluation. It can also be used as a review in preparation for this quiz.

1. The human life span is the average length of life predicted by statistics. (False)
2. Life expectancy has decreased in the past

SECTION 3

Dying

Imagine you were told today that you had only a few weeks to live. What would you do? Would you change the way you live? Would you take any practical or financial steps? Are there emotional issues you'd wish to work out with parents, brothers or sisters, or friends? What ideas would you pass on to others who will follow you?

Now imagine that someone close to you has only weeks to live. How will you spend your time with that person? What will you say? The value of asking these questions is that they help you realize that time in life is limited—not only for you but for every other person. Knowing this can help people to spend their time today wisely.

Fear of Death

Many people cannot stand to think of death. It is natural to fear death. All creatures strive to live. To express your fear and think about death is healthy. To flee and hide from reality is unhealthy.

Consider this view: death gives meaning to life! If you knew that you had only a few weeks left to live, wouldn't that knowledge give you a keen sense of how precious life is? Many people, on learning they are soon to die, report that they have started enjoying their days as never before. Sunsets are more beautiful. Jokes are funnier. Friends are dearer. Especially, the way they spend their time becomes more important. They try to make the most of every moment.

A narrow brush with death gives people this same sense of life's values. Many people, on having near-death experiences, say their lives are totally changed afterward. One man reports that he was planning a career in law until he almost died in an accident. "I realized I wanted more than anything to work with disadvantaged children," he says, "so I gave up the law, and now I'm doing what I really love." A woman who had a similar experience decided the opposite. She quit teaching as a career and worked her way through law school for the very same reason. Given only one life to live, practicing law was what she chose to do. Others have chosen not careers but changed attitudes toward life.

Death gives you a task—to make something worthwhile of your life. Like everyone alive on earth today, you have a deadline to meet. Whatever you want to accomplish in life, you must accomplish it before you die. Death has inspired towering works of art. People who face death pass on ideas and traditions to those who follow, for it encourages them to make a heritage for their children. Death acts as a reminder to not wait until tomorrow to do what you wish to do today.

This doesn't mean people must rush through life being busy. One of life's great pleasures is to savor each present moment. Even simple things, when you stop taking them for granted, bring great rewards. An orange sunset, the twinkle of a friend's smile, a breath of scented spring breeze, or the surprise of discovery in a child's eyes can be experienced fully only when

> *I remember my youth and the feeling that will never come back any more—the feeling that I could last forever, outlast the sea, the earth, and all men.*
>
> Joseph Conrad
> (1857–1924)
> British novelist

SECTION 3

FOCUS

OUTCOMES

In this section students will learn:

1. The lessons death can teach us about life.
2. Important steps that should be taken in preparation for death.
3. Classmates' views on death issues.
4. The definition of euthanasia and the legal implications surrounding this term.
5. Some guidelines for dealing with a friend who is dying.

FOCUS ACTIVITY

You may want to discuss with students their fears of death. If you think such a discussion would have a positive effect with your students, ask them to examine their fears. What are they afraid of, exactly? Tell them that some people are afraid of the uncertainty of the afterlife—they fear what may await them. Some people fear that everything will end. Others fear the particular process of death; for example, a person with a painful, terminal illness fears the manner in which death will occur rather than death itself. Can they put their fear into words? A good way to get them to express these fears is through a private written assignment, turned in anonymously. The issues could then be brought up at the next session.

one hundred years. (False)

3. Menstruation ceases at menopause. (True)
4. Osteoporosis becomes a serious health risk for women after menopause. (True)
5. Male menopause is experienced as an abrupt decrease in fertility. (False)
6. Maintaining physical activity can help an older person avoid heart and lung disease, as well as excessive arthritis. (True)
7. Though reasoning skill, memory, and speed decline in a person's later years, wisdom and judgment have increased. (True)
8. Senility is an unavoidable aspect of growing older. (False)
9. Alzheimer's disease is an unpreventable illness that causes mental confusion and many other symptoms. (True)
10. Loss of social status and identity can be consequences of retiring. (True)

TEACH & APPLY

BACKGROUND INFORMATION

As enrichment, you may want to tell students something about what happens when a person dies without a will. The state distributes that person's property according to its laws and often the family loses much of the property. Typically, much more of the estate goes for taxes than is necessary. Without a will, the assets go not to the people the deceased would have chosen, but to the people the state chooses.

TEACHER SUPPORT

Key Passage

WORKSHEETS

The Teacher's Resource Box contains an example of a living will. You may want to check to see if these documents are legal in your state before you distribute this to your students. Also, make sure the students understand the distinction between a living will and a more traditional will. Make sure that they understand that the living will deals exclusively with situations that result from a person being alive but unable to make decisions for himself or herself.

GUEST SPEAKER

Invite a speaker from Hospice, a gerontologist, or a physician to speak to the class about some of the problems related to aging.

Answers to FACT or FICTION

Here are the answers to the questions at the start of the chapter.

1. **False.** The happiest people are those who have lived through at least one major life tragedy.
2. **False.** The human life span has not changed, but the life expectancy has increased steadily over past years.
3. **False.** People remain sexual beings throughout life.
4. **True.**
5. **False.** Only a fraction of older people live in nursing homes.

If you lose consciousness, a living will can let others know how to care for you.

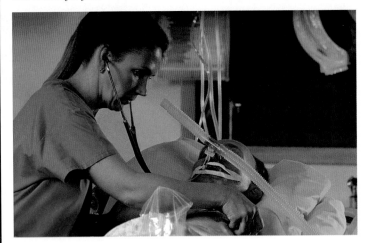

we know that our experiences of them are numbered. Acknowledging death helps people cherish their lives rather than simply pass through them.

To get over the fear of death completely may be impossible. However, people fear most the things they are unprepared to face. If you prepare for death, you will fear it less.

KEY POINTS *Fear of death is natural, but it need not be destructive. It can be channeled to give more meaning to life.*

Preparation for Death

Even young people should prepare for death in a few ways. For one thing, each young person should make a will, and start thinking about life insurance. When someone dies without having made a will, the state divides up the person's property according to its laws, and often the family loses much of it.

You may not think you have any property worth mentioning, but still, don't postpone this step for too long. Your belongings may consist of nothing more than a bicycle and a backpack, but they are your estate. Make an informal will, to be sure that the people you care about receive what you want them to have. This can be a simple letter, carried in your wallet or given to your parent or guardian to keep for you. A good time to make a formal will is when you first marry or become a parent.

Another preparation worth the effort is to decide what you want done if you lose consciousness. In that case, other people will have to decide what will happen to you. You can make your wishes known ahead of time in a **living will**. Such a document states exactly how you want to be treated, should you become unable to decide for yourself. Some people wish to instruct their families to use no **life-support systems** after **brain death** has occurred. They may even instruct their families to "pull the plug" if life-support measures have been started. Other people who fear that relatives won't have their best interests at heart may request the opposite—that *every* measure be taken to save their lives, regardless of chances for recovery. If you have feelings one way or the other, put them in a living will. Not all states recognize the living will as a legal document, however. In such places a person must name a **proxy**, who then can make decisions concerning medical treatments to prolong life.

You may not have complete control over what happens in all cases. Questions about **euthanasia** or **physician-assisted suicide**, for example, are still being debated by medical and legal professionals. If you want to die, should you be allowed to? If someone you love

QUICK QUIZ

Chapter 23, Section 3

The following quiz will help you assess your students' understanding of the material covered in this section of the chapter. You might use the quiz as an oral exercise, or, you might use it as a paper/pencil quiz to evaluate your students individually.

Like the Quick Quiz, the Section Review can also be used as an assessment tool to spark class discussion or as an individual student evaluation. It can also be used as a review in preparation for this quiz.

1. It is healthy to avoid thinking about the reality of death. (False)
2. Recognizing the inevitability of death can help you learn to cherish life. (True)
3. Fear of death is always destructive. (False)

wants to die, should you let him or her? Should you help a person stay alive as long as possible? Decisions of all these kinds are faced daily.

A familiar case is that of the person who has a fatal illness, is unconscious, has no hope of recovery, and requires machines to stay alive. One argument is to do everything possible to prolong that person's life, on the theory that where there is life, there is hope. Another opinion holds that to support life with no hope of recovery is to prolong the suffering of the dying. Clearly, it helps if the person has earlier made a living will. Most states now honor such wills, although each state places some restrictions on them.

Another choice you may make someday is whether to die in a hospital or elsewhere. Given the choice, many people prefer not to go to the hospital. They would rather die at home, using a **hospice** for support. A hospice is an agency that assists people with **terminal illnesses** and their families. The purpose is to allow a dying person to choose to stay at home—and, if appropriate, to die there—while staff people from the hospice help the family to care for the person and to deal with their grief.

Hospice services are provided by a team of physicians, nurses, and a psychiatrist or psychologist. Often social workers, members of the clergy, and trained volunteers assist as well. The hospice has a twofold mission: to control the dying person's pain and distressing symptoms, and to support the client and family psychologically and socially. Care for the family continues beyond the person's death into the grieving period.

 KEY POINTS *Preparation for death includes making a will, taking out insurance, making a living will, and learning about hospice services in your area.*

SECTION 3 Review

Answer the following questions on a sheet of paper.

Learning the Vocabulary

The vocabulary terms in this section are *living will, life-support systems, brain death, proxy, euthanasia, physician-assisted suicide, hospice,* and *terminal illnesses.*

1. Match the following phrases with the appropriate terms:
   a. a support system for dying people and their families
   b. illnesses that are expected to end in death
   c. a term used to refer to mechanical means of supporting life

   d. allowing a person to die

Learning the Facts
2. Why is it natural to fear death?
3. How do near-death experiences change people's lives?
4. Describe ways in which people should prepare for their death.

Making Life Choices
5. Raul's parents are in their mid-40s. Raul wants to talk to them about their will, but death is a subject that is seldom discussed. How can Raul help his parents understand the importance of a living will? What can he say to them without hurting their feelings? How can he help make it easier for his family to talk about death?

MINI Glossary

living will: a will that declares a person's wishes regarding treatment, should the person become unable to make decisions (for example, in the event of brain death).

life-support systems: a term used to refer to mechanical means of supporting life, such as feedings given into a central vein or machines that force air into the lungs (artificial respirators).

brain death: irreversible, total loss of higher brain functions, reflected in a flat line brainwave pattern, as opposed to the wavy pattern made by an active brain.

proxy: a person authorized to act for another.

euthanasia (you-than-AY-zee-uh): allowing a person to die by choosing not to employ life-support equipment such as artificial respirators, or the removal of life-support equipment from a patient who has no hope of recovery. Both may be legal in some cases.

physician-assisted suicide: suicide of an ill person by way of lethal drugs or other means provided by a physician; not legal in most states.

hospice (HOS-pis): a support system for dying people and their families, which helps the family let the person die at home with dignity and in comfort.

terminal illnesses: illnesses that are expected to end in death.

ASSESS

EVALUATE

SECTION 3 Review Answers

1. a. hospice **b.** terminal illnesses **c.** life-support systems **d.** euthanasia
2. All creatures strive to live. (p. 637)
3. Life becomes more precious to them, and they enjoy it more, making the most out of every moment. (p. 637)
4. make a will, provide for spouses and children with life insurance, make a living will detailing what to do in the instance of brain death or terminal illness (p. 638)
5. Answers will vary.

CLOSE

Have students imagine that after a routine examination by their physician, they have been informed that they have only a short time (perhaps a week) to live. What "loose ends" in their lives would they try and tie up? What unfinished business would they finish?

On a sheet of paper, ask students to write a letter to themselves, telling what they hope to accomplish in the next year. They are to put the letter in an envelope, self-address it, and stamp it. Tell them they will receive the letter in one year to see if they have made the most of their time or have wasted it. (You will have to remember to mail the letters back to the students in one year.)

4. Every young person should write up an informal will. (True)
5. A living will is an informal document describing what you would like done with your property in case of death. (False)
6. A proxy can decide whether or not to keep you on a life-support system. (True)
7. A person has the right to request euthanasia or physician-assisted suicide. (False)

8. A hospice assists people with terminal illnesses who prefer to stay at home rather than in a hospital. (True)
9. People generally recover from terminal illnesses. (False)
10. A living will can help to lift responsibility from your loved ones when difficult questions about life-support are required. (True)

Background Information

The Teacher's Resource Box contains an information sheet that provides you with additional descriptions of what people go through during each of these stages of grief.

Background Information

As enrichment, tell the students that people can handle grief better when they take action: They have grief work to do. Our culture has some traditions that help people come to terms with their grief after a death. These include: arranging for care for the body, writing obituaries, notifying friends and family, conducting the funeral ceremony, thanking donors, and disposing of possessions. If people avoid these activities, they may suffer grief reactions or later maladjustment. Also point out that many people make the mistake of being attentive only immediately after the death. The sense of loss really sinks in for most bereaved families after about a week has passed. People can better help grieving families if they spread the care out so that it doesn't stop after ten days.

Have students list ways they could lend support to family or friends that have lost a loved one.

Helping Others Deal with Death and Grief

Grief in response to a death or other loss is hard to deal with, especially for young people. Still, grief cannot be avoided. Those who know something about it are best prepared to deal with it and to help others do the same.

 Grief is just awful pain, isn't it? What more is there to know about it?

Grief is painful at first. However, it moves through several stages and ends with acceptance. Knowing what these stages are can help you manage grief. You can say to yourself, "What I am feeling is natural. This anger (or depression) is part of my grief." It still hurts, but understanding what you are going through can give you some feeling of control. That helps make it bearable.

The stages of grief and acceptance of death are:

▶ Denial—"No, it can't be!"
▶ Anger—"It's not fair! It's too soon!"
▶ Bargaining—"I'll do anything; just don't let this happen."
▶ Depression—"There is no hope; I just want to be alone."
▶ Acceptance—"I am ready, now. It's all right."

It helps to know that you will feel these emotions, sometimes over and over again, in the process of accepting death—your own or someone else's. Not everyone goes through all the stages, however, and they don't always come in the order shown here.

 I have a friend who is dying, and I think I must be feeling grief already.

Of course you are grieving. Your friend is, too. People grieve not only at death but at all kinds of losses, and at the news that losses are to come.

 The news that my friend is going to die is a shock to me. I find myself avoiding my friend.

Yes, that is not an uncommon reaction. We can be so shocked at the news that a death is coming that we feel we can't deal with it at all. It is natural to feel like avoiding your friend. This may help you postpone your feelings of pain, but it won't take the pain away. Furthermore, it certainly won't help your friend. Nothing you say can embarrass you, or hurt your friendship, or damage your self-esteem as badly as avoiding your friend until it is too late to help.

 But I don't know what to say, and it frightens me how bad my friend is hurting.

You don't have to say smart things. Just be there. Even saying nothing is all right. This can show your friend you care, even though you can't take away the pain.

Don't say, "I know how you feel," though—that is, unless you really do. If you have never been in the same situation that your friend is in, a better thing to say is, "Yes, it must be hard," or "I can't imagine how you must be feeling." Don't look for positive things to say, either. Bad news is bad news. Don't refuse to listen to your friend's real feelings.

CRITICAL THINKING

Engage students in discussion by asking them why a person would or should go to a funeral. Sometimes students are able to list most of these points; if not, you can mention or list them yourself.

A person goes to a funeral . . .

1. to honor the person who has died and to say goodbye to that person
2. to offer support to family and friends

One of the most helpful things you can do is to give your friend a chance to talk. Anyone who is facing death has many thoughts and feelings that need expression. Listen. Let your friend share feelings of anger, frustration, or guilt. Let your friend tell you what to do to help.

 Sometimes I forget the situation, and start to have fun. Then I remember, and I feel guilty.

One of the most important things for you to do is to take care of your own needs, and one of your needs is to be happy. Don't feel that you have to show grief all the time. In the strictest sense, much as you love your friend, the problem that someone is dying is not your problem. You are alive. You have the right to experience joy and happiness even at such a time.

 How can I help the family of a friend who has died?

Each person has different needs. It is especially important to pay attention to children in a grieving family, because they often feel lost and left out. Often, too, they don't understand what's happening, and they have irrational fears. Your attention can help them feel better.

One member of the family seems to be grieving forever. How can I make him stop?

Grief has no time limit. Many think that it takes about a year to get over someone's death. There is some truth to that, because a year permits every occasion (religious holidays, birthdays, and anniversaries) to pass, once, without the person. Still, grief can spring to the heart years after a loss and be felt as keenly as if the person had died just yesterday.

Don't set limits on anyone's recovery time. Also, don't feel you must grieve longer than your feelings say to. Everyone has a personal timetable for recovery. If you are ready to move on, do so.

A person who doesn't seem able to pull out of grief at all, for a very long time, may need help. Perhaps you can suggest that the person see a grief counselor—a professional who helps people to say their goodbyes and go on.

 Once the family has adjusted to the loss, should we all try to forget the person who has died?

No, not at all. The very opposite is usually true. After someone close has died, the memory is still very much alive. It helps a family member to know that others are thinking of the person, too. Bring back and share memories: "Sis would have enjoyed this," or "I thought of your mom today." Remarks like these let the grieving person know that you, too, remember and miss the one who is gone.

When you arrive at the point of accepting a death, you may find you have gained a deeper serenity than you knew before, and a deeper joy in life.

641

3. to receive support for themselves

Tell students that it is important to know what to say to a grieving person. If someone does not know what to say and says nothing, that silence may be incorrectly interpreted. The grief-stricken person may feel that they are being shunned or ignored. Tell students that saying "I'm sorry," is always appropriate. A person's presence and support is most important to the grieving person. Be willing to hug someone or hold a hand.

VOCABULARY

1. a. brain death **b.** life span **c.** senility **d.** hospice **e.** longevity **f.** hot flashes **g.** terminal illnesses

2. a. Menopause **b.** life expectancy **c.** Alzheimer's disease **d.** living will

3. Answers will vary.

RECALL

SECTION 1

1. Answers will vary; could include: self sufficient, physically active, socially involved, clear thinking, fully participating members of society, happy, and healthy. (p. 626)

SECTION 2

2. gradual loss of youthful appearance and condition, aging of cells and organs (p. 628)

3. rate of death from diseases and accidents among the very young has declined; medical advances are prolonging adults' lives so that they more nearly reach their maximum (p. 628)

4. maintain appropriate weight, sound nutrition, including water intake; adequate sleep; regular physical activity; avoidance of alcohol, tobacco, and other drug abuse. (p. 631)

5. Smoking causes early onset of menopause because it suppresses production of the hormone estrogen or because the ingredients of tobacco are directly toxic to the ovaries. (p. 632)

CHAPTER 23 Review

Summarizing the Chapter

Your ability to respond correctly to the following statements ensures your understanding of the main concepts in the chapter.

1. List characteristics of people who age successfully.
2. Discuss some healthful behaviors to follow in planning for good health in old age.
3. Describe the physical changes that occur during the aging process.
4. Describe the mental changes that may occur as people age.
5. List ways that people can prepare for death.
6. Describe the stages a person goes through in accepting death.
7. Discuss some ways to help a grieving person.

Learning the Vocabulary

life span	living will
life expectancy	life-support systems
longevity	brain death
menopause	proxy
hot flashes	euthanasia
male menopause	physician-assisted suicide
arthritis	hospice
senility	terminal illnesses
Alzheimer's disease	

Answer the following questions on a separate sheet of paper.

1. *Matching*—Match each of the following phrases with the appropriate vocabulary term or phrase from the list above:
  a. irreversible, total loss of higher brain functions
  b. maximum years of life a human being can live
  c. general term meaning weakness of mind and body occurring in old age

d. a support system for dying people and their families
e. an individual's length of life
f. sudden waves of feeling hot all over
g. illnesses that are expected to end in death
2. a. _____ is the time in a woman's life when ovulation and menstruation cease.
  b. The number of years an individual can expect to live, based on hereditary and other factors, is called _____.
  c. _____ is a brain disease of some older people that brings mental confusion, inability to function, and in the final state, death.
  d. A _____ is a will that declares a person's wishes regarding treatment in case the person becomes unable to decide for himself or herself.
3. Write a paragraph using as many of the vocabulary terms as you can. Underline each term that you use.

Recalling Important Facts and Ideas

Section 1
1. List some characteristics that describe most people who are in their later years.

Section 2
2. After growth is completed, what does aging bring about?
3. What two things have affected life expectancy?
4. Describe strategies to help slow the aging process.
5. What effect does smoking have on menopause in women?
6. Describe what happens during menopause and male menopause.
7. How can physical activity enhance the quality of your life?
8. List the areas in the brain and nervous system that are affected by aging.
9. Discuss the preventable causes of mental confusion in older people.
10. Describe how Alzheimer's disease progresses in an older person's brain.
11. Why is financial planning so essential for people who are aging?
12. Describe why it is important to maintain a strong support system.
13. Discuss why it is important to continue your education forever.

642

6. Menopause causes ovulation to diminish and finally stop and causes menstruation to cease; male menopause causes male fertility to gradually decline. (p. 632)

7. The more people exercise, the less likely they are to die of heart and lung diseases and more likely they are to fend off arthritis. (p. 632)

8. reasoning skill, recall (memory), speed, and senses (p. 633)

9. Preventable causes of mental confusion include abuse of drugs (including alcohol abuse, as well as misuse or incompatibility of prescription drugs); accidents (surgery can often relieve skull fractures or bleeding that puts pressure on the brain, caused

14. How can we view death in a healthy way?

15. What changes occur in many people who learn that they will die soon?

16. How does death act as a reminder to us?

Straight Talk

17. List and identify the stages of grief.

18. How long should a person grieve?

19. Why is it important to talk about someone who has died?

Critical Thinking

1. Figure 23–1 on page 630 gives you a list of preventable vs. unavoidable changes with age. You cannot do anything about the unavoidable changes of aging, but you can do something about the preventable changes. What can you do to prevent these changes? Are you practicing these behaviors now? Are your parents and grandparents doing things to prevent or delay some of the changes that come with aging?

2. At what age do you think it is appropriate to make out a will? When are you going to make out a will? Are you going to make a living will? What are some of the problems relatives of a person who has lost consciousness face when a living will has not been written?

3. After reading the Straight Talk section, "Helping Others Deal with Death and Grief," on pages 640–641, do you feel you are better prepared to face the loss of a friend? How about a family member? What have you learned about dealing with death? Do you have a grief therapist in your area? What will you do to help others deal with grief?

Activities

1. Visit a nursing home in your area and adopt a grandparent. Visit and talk with the person for an hour at least once a week for five weeks. Write a report about your experience.

2. Create a pamphlet about grief and the stages one goes through when dealing with grief. Make sure you have addresses and phone numbers of professionals in your area who deal with grief.

3. Have a class debate on euthanasia. Do you think terminally ill patients should have the right to die? What would you want your family to do if you were terminally ill?

4. Make a list of things you need to do to prepare for your funeral.

5. Watch television for an hour and write down all the commercials that deal with aging and the elderly. What are the products' claims? Do you think the claims are fraudulent?

6. Find a current magazine or newspaper article about the process of aging or some aspect of this topic. (Examples: The effects of alcohol and/or tobacco on the aging process, advancements on slowing down the aging process, and so on.) In the article, underline five to ten major points that are made. Using what you underlined in the article and items from Figure 23–2 in this chapter, "Growing Old Gracefully," compile a list of facts about aging. Then, using the Fact or Fiction feature and other information you can gather, make a list of fallacies about aging. Develop your lists into a poster that can be displayed in the classroom.

Making Decisions about Health

1. Gladys and Sylvia are seniors in high school and are best friends. They have talked about everything together for as long as they can remember. On her way home from school one day, Gladys was in a terrible car accident. She was in a coma and was put on a respirator. The girls had talked about death several times and agreed that they never wanted to be kept alive by a machine. Sylvia went to the hospital every day and talked to Gladys with no change ever taking place. Sylvia told Gladys' parents of their discussion about life-support systems. Sylvia suggested letting Gladys die peacefully. Gladys' parents didn't agree. They felt that as long as Gladys' heart was beating they had a chance for a miracle. They have been keeping Gladys alive for the past six months.

How would you feel if you were Sylvia knowing your best friend didn't want to live like this? What action would you take if you were Sylvia? Why would you take that action? What could Gladys have done to avoid this situation completely?

oneself. In the brain, the nerve pathways become tangled and blocked, cutting off the memory functions. (pp. 634–635)

11. Nearly everyone suffers a loss of income in the retirement years. There must be enough money set aide to pay for rent and have insurance to cover medical and other expenses. (p. 635)

12. to create a web of support so that as relationships are lost, others are gained (p. 635)

13. New information exercises the mind. (p. 636)

SECTION 3

14. by thinking about death and expressing our fears (p. 637)

15. they start enjoying life as they never have before; the way they spend their time becomes more important, trying to make the most of every moment. (p. 637)

16. Death reminds us to not wait until tomorrow to do what we wish to do today. (p. 637)

STRAIGHT TALK

17. Denial—"No, it can't be." Anger—"It's not fair! It's too soon!" Bargaining—"I'll do anything; just don't let this happen." Depression—"There is no hope; I just want to be alone." Acceptance—"I am ready, now. It's all right." (p. 640)

18. at least a year, but the grief could remain in the heart forever (p. 641)

19. It helps a family member know that others are thinking of the person. It lets the grieving person know that you, too, remember and miss the one who is gone. (p. 641)

by accidents); dehydration (older people do not sense thirst as easily, and a major symptom of dehydration is confusion); depression (causes slowing of the mind); disease states (tuberculosis, diabetes, and even heart attacks can all begin with confusion); disuse of mental skills (people lose what they don't use); malnutrition (older people eat less because taste enjoyment, digestive secretions, and appetite diminish as nutrition needs stay the same); and poor vision and hearing (both cause confusion). (pp. 633–635)

10. It starts as memory loss, then becomes an inability to perform everyday functions, and leads to the total inability to care for

	OUTCOMES	FEATURES
CHAPTER 24 — **Accident and Injury Prevention**	• Describe how being a defensive driver can reduce your risk of accidents. • Explain how to reduce the risk of accidents during swimming, boating, biking and play, as well as at home. • List specific guidelines for preventing fires and burns. • Describe how to prepare for natural disasters. • List the safety precautions for child care.	*Health Strategies:* How to Avoid Alcohol-Related Driving Accidents (page 650) *Health Strategies:* Water Rescue Techniques (page 652) *Health Strategies:* Points for Baby-Sitters (page 662) *Life Choice Inventory:* How Safety Conscious Are You? (page 648) *Straight Talk:* Fire Prevention and Escape (page 664)
CHAPTER 25 — **Emergency Measures**	• Identify the priorities in responding to an emergency. • Give steps in identifying and treating shock. • Describe and act out how to call for help in an emergency. • Explain the steps in CPR. • Describe how to respond to severe bleeding. • Describe what to do when either an adult or child is choking or not breathing. • Describe types of burns and their treatment. • Describe how to treat hypothermia and frostbite. • List the symptoms of hyperthermia (heat exhaustion and heat stroke) and describe how to treat hyperthermia. • List the symptoms of poisoning. • Describe how to splint a broken bone.	*Health Strategies:* Reducing Disease Risks (page 672) *Health Strategies:* First Aid for Shock (page 674) *Health Strategies:* Summary of Emergency Actions (page 676) *Health Strategies:* Splinting a Broken Bone (page 694) *Life Choice Inventory:* How Well Prepared for Emergencies Are You? (page 690) *Straight Talk:* Herbs and Folk Remedies (page 695)

TEACHING SUPPORT

Vocabulary: Learning Key Terms
Study Outline
Reading Cloze
Reteaching: Responses to a Natural Disaster
Enrichment: Accident Prevention, Baby-Sitting Safety, Ask the Professional, Teenagers and Car Accidents

Career Brief: Firefighting Occupations
Life Choice Inventory: How Safety Conscious Are You?
Handouts: Household Fire Safety Checklist
Quizzes: Sections 1–6
Tests: Chapter 24 Test A, Chapter 24 Test B

Vocabulary: Learning Key Terms, Crossword Puzzle, Fill in the Blank
Study Outline
Reading Cloze
Reteaching: First Actions First; Airway, Breathing, Circulation, Severe Bleeding, Shock; Down to Basics and Beyond
Enrichment: Investigation of Alternative Healing Methods, Help! There's Been an Accident

Career Brief: Emergency Medical Technicians
Life Choice Inventory: How Well Prepared for Emergencies Are You?
Handouts: Selected First Aid Measures, Snakebite Kits: No Substitute for Knowledge
Quizzes: Sections 1–6
Tests: Chapter 25 Test A, Chapter 25 Test B

MULTIMEDIA SUPPORT

- Health Video Library
- CNN Health and Fitness Update Videos
- Westest
- Student Review Software
- Diet Analysis Software
- Nutrition CD-ROM

LESSON PLANNING

You will find detailed daily lesson plans for both **traditional scheduling** and **block scheduling** in you Teacher's Resource Box. Other suggested scheduling formats can be found in the supplemental Lesson Plannng guide.

KEY POINTS

Chapter 24 is 24 pages long and divided into six sections. Briefly, this chapter introduces students to the concept of accident and injury prevention in various aspects of daily living. The chapter also introduces students to some key concepts and skills necessary in certain life-threatening situations.

ACTIVITY TO INTRODUCE THE CHAPTER

Borrow or purchase from your local chapter of the American Red Cross the video entitled "The American Red Cross Emergency Test," hosted by John Ritter. This video comes with official video test score cards to use for student responses as they watch the video. The video addresses all the topics discussed in this chapter plus others. Discuss the statement, "Accidents are almost always a result of human error." Before you show the video, tell students that after it's finished you will be asking for examples from the video that support this statement.

BULLETIN BOARD IDEAS

Prepare a bulletin board to list emergency and safety agencies and their phone numbers (some possibilities are listed at the end of this activity). Have the students choose, or you can assign students to either visit or call one of the following agencies to find out what educational safety programs are available in your community. Match as closely as possible each section in this

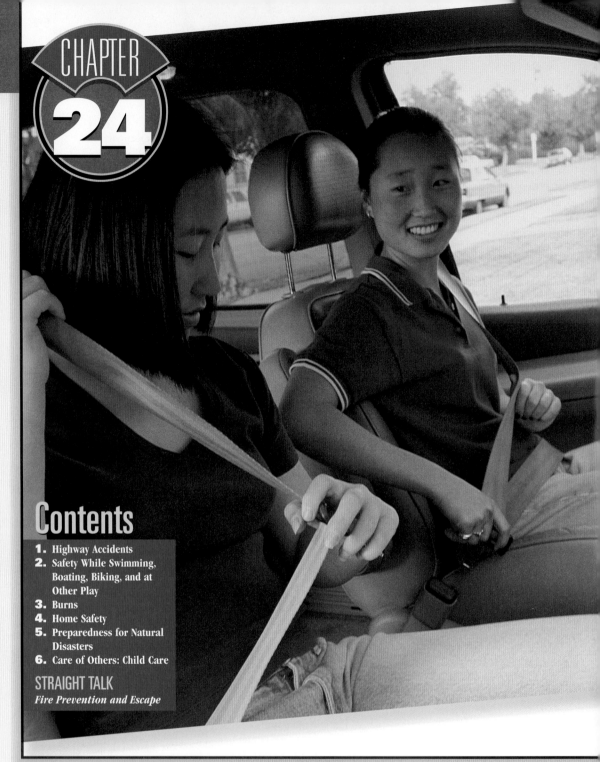

CHAPTER 24

Contents

1. Highway Accidents
2. Safety While Swimming, Boating, Biking, and at Other Play
3. Burns
4. Home Safety
5. Preparedness for Natural Disasters
6. Care of Others: Child Care

STRAIGHT TALK
Fire Prevention and Escape

NOT Enough Time?

Following are some suggestions to help you make sure you cover the key topics in this chapter if you have limited time. (Refer to the daily lesson plans in your Teacher's Resource Box for additional suggestions.)

DAY 1 Assign students to read the chapter prior to class. During class do Focus Activity 2 on page 646 to promote awareness and to stimulate thought about safety in students' own activities.

DAY 2 Because this chapter is so diverse, select one or two sections to emphasize

FOCUS

OUTCOMES

In this section students will learn that:

1. With car accidents causing nearly one half of all accidents, defensive driving is the key to saving lives.

2. Driving skills, knowledge, and judgment are dependent on driver attitude for preventing automobile accidents.

3. Responsible driving precautions are necessary for preventing automobile accidents.

FOCUS ACTIVITIES

1. Write the term "accident prone" on the board. Ask students to define the term. Ask them to identify some behaviors of an accident-prone person and list them on the board. Students should then identify which behaviors could be changed and what cautious behaviors could be substituted for the accident-prone behaviors. Discuss.

2. Invite a guest speaker from the local AAA Safety Division or city/state Motor Vehicle Safety Commission to present statistics on auto accidents, injuries, and fatalities in your area. An alternative would be to ask these agencies to supply you with current local statistics to present yourself. Ask students to write down the statistic that they find to be most surprising and explain why. Discuss the statistics in class.

Highway Accidents

Nearly half of the accidents that take place are car accidents. Good drivers do not usually cause them, but they do have them—because some accidents are unpreventable. Until you have had an accident, it is hard to believe that such a thing is possible. Remember, though, that accidents are not deliberate. You do not see them coming; you do not expect them; you do not have time to avoid them. Just think about the last time you cut yourself even slightly. You did not mean to. The trouble was, you did not see that it was about to happen. The control was not all in your hands.

The Likelihood of a Collision

A lot of people buried in cemeteries had only one car accident in their lives. Knowledge and skill are not enough to prevent car accidents. An equally important aspect of the driver is attitude. Consider the attitudes of two different drivers. Attitude 1 is, "I never have accidents. I'm in control." A person with attitude 1 simply goes out and drives, unaware of potential hazards. Attitude 2 is, "The control is not all in my hands. I need to be aware of other drivers and watch for possible accidents about to happen." A person with attitude 2 drives defensively.

Figure 24–1 Lives Lost among People under 19 Years Old to Various Causes, United States

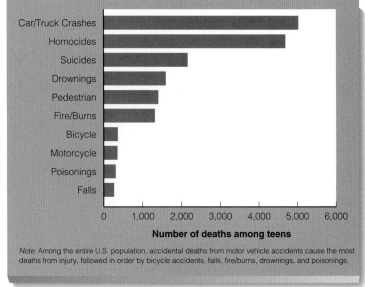

Note: Among the entire U.S. population, accidental deaths from motor vehicle accidents cause the most deaths from injury, followed in order by bicycle accidents, falls, fire/burns, drownings, and poisonings.

Source: Data from F. P. Rivara and D. C. Grossman, Prevention of traumatic deaths to children in the United States: How far have we come and where do we need to go? *Pediatrics* 97 (1996): 791–797; data for general population from F. P. Rivara, D. C. Grossman, and P. Cummings, Injury Prevention, *New England Journal of Medicine*, 337 (1997): 543–548.

HEALTHY PEOPLE 2000

. . . .

Increase use of occupant protection systems, such as safety belts, inflatable restraints, and child safety seats, to at least 85 percent of motor vehicle occupants.

Achievement of the 85-percent use goal will depend on a number of factors, including the design of occupant protection systems provided by auto makers in coming years and the number of States with mandatory safety belt use laws. Beginning with the 1990 models, automobile manufacturers are required to equip all of their passenger cars with automatic crash protection. Most of the manufacturers are providing automatic safety belts and some are offering air bag systems to meet the new Federal requirement. The restraint sys-

Accidents will happen.

For a person to move from attitude 1 to attitude 2, no more is required than to translate statistics into real-life events. Is that car you see coming from the right going to run through that intersection in front of you? No, it's not. How about the next car? No, it's not, either. In fact, the chances are only 1 in 10,000 that you will be going through an intersection just as a car drives out in front of you.

How long will it be before a car does run in front of you just as you are driving through an intersection? If you pass through enough intersections (say, ten a day), then it will take 1,000 days, on the average, for you to encounter this event. A thousand days is three years. Thus if you accumulate a total of 30 years' driving experience in your life, it is almost inevitable that ten times in your life a car will unexpectedly pull out in front of you as you pass through an intersection. That it will happen once is virtually certain. You cannot know when, but it will occur.

You can probably avoid collisions if you approach every intersection, all your driving life, with the thought that a car may suddenly pull out in front of you. With that in mind, you will slow down, you will be ready to turn or hit the brake, and you will be planning ahead to avoid colliding with the cars next to you and behind you. That is the spirit of defensive driving as it applies to one of hundreds of driving situations. Defensive driving saves thousands of lives each year. It can save yours.

Knowledge and skill are not enough to prevent accidents.

 KEY POINTS *It is a certainty that every driver will encounter other drivers who are careless. Defensive driving saves lives.*

The Defensive Driving Attitude

The instructor of a defensive driving course warns the pupils: "At the end of this course, you'll have an exam. It's a long exam. It's a tough exam. If you miss any one question, you'll fail it." Then, on the last day, the instructor doesn't give an exam on paper. Instead, he or she explains, "The exam is outside this room. You will start taking it when you get back in your car to drive home. It will go on for the rest of your life. Every time you get

66 *Danger for danger's sake is senseless.* 99

Leigh Hunt
(1784–1859)
British writer

tems themselves will need to be constantly improved to keep abreast of advancing technology and to make them convenient and comfortable to use.

Based on current usage rates for automatic and manual belt systems, achievement of this objective is not unreasonable. However, the 17 States without mandatory belt use laws in 1989 will need to enact such laws, and several States with weak laws will need to strengthen them. The law enforcement community and the public at large must be convinced that these laws are important enough to warrant vigorous enforcement and public acceptance of that enforcement. In addition, the correct use of belts for all automobile occupants, including occupants of heavy trucks, should be promoted.

A reproducible copy of the Life Choice Inventory is provided in the Teacher's Resource Box.

How Safety-Conscious Are You?

Answer true or false to these questions to find out whether you are now doing all you reasonably should do to prevent accidents, or whether you have room for improvement in this respect. Record your answers on a separate piece of paper. Then determine your score as instructed below. Your answers to the Life Choice Inventory are personal and private. Share them with others only if you are comfortable doing so.

1. I have taken a first-aid course (or I have made plans to take one).
2. I have taken a driver's education course (or I plan to take one before I begin to drive).
3. When driving, I always slow down when approaching an intersection (or I am sure I will do this when I begin to drive).
4. I always buckle my safety belt when driving or riding in a car.
5. I never drink or use drugs and then drive (or I am sure I would never do this).
6. I cross the street at crosswalks only; I do not jaywalk.
7. I keep my home (room) in order, with no objects or cords on the floor that might trip people.
8. I use a stepladder for climbing and reaching.
9. I keep a fire extinguisher where I can get to it in case of fire, and I know how to use it.
10. I know how I would escape from my bedroom in case of fire.
11. I never smoke in bed (or I do not smoke).
12. I dispose of my trash regularly.
13. I have my community's emergency phone numbers right by the phone.
14. I can swim (or I have made plans to learn to swim).
15. I obey all safety rules around water and boats.
16. I read and heed all label directions on containers of chemicals and drugs.
17. Children are not likely to hurt themselves in my home (room).
18. I maintain all electrical equipment as instructed; I replace old cords and plugs or have them replaced by a qualified person.
19. I know how to avoid back injury when lifting an object, and I practice what I know.
20. I keep containers of drinkable water available where I live.
21. I am on guard against the risks of aggression by strangers and people I know.
22. I know and abide by the rules for safe care of children.
23. I know how to perform the Heimlich Maneuver.

SCORING

Give yourself 1 point for each true answer.
20–23: You are a safety-conscious person.
16–19: You have a few more refinements to make on your choices.
11–15: You have a lot of room for improvement.
10 or below: You need to make major efforts to improve your safety awareness and behavior.

Encourage the students to take the questions in the Life Choice Inventory seriously. They should stop and think about the ways in which they typically confront the type of situations mentioned before they answer. If they do this, their scores should be a fairly good indicator of whether or not they are conscious of safety and acting in a cautious manner. Discuss the scores in class. What is the range from high to low? What is the average? Would anyone like to change his or her level of safety consciousness?

DISCUSSION

Collect newspaper articles detailing all types of vehicle accidents (automobile, bicycle, motorcycle, and so on) and ask students to choose one, read it, and write an analysis as to cause(s). They should also suggest possible ways the accidents could have been prevented. An alternative would be to obtain some copies of old accident reports from police or insurance companies and do the same activity. Develop a folder of articles for these types of accidents, which can be shared with classes in the future.

HEALTHY PEOPLE 2000

Reduce deaths caused by motor vehicle crashes to no more than 1.9 per 100 million vehicle miles traveled and 16.8 per 100,000 people.

Motor vehicle-related fatalities accounts for about half of all unintentional injury deaths and are the leading cause of work-related injury deaths. Approximately 46,000 people die each year and more than 3.5 million are injured. Society loses nearly $75 billion annually as the result of motor vehicle crashes.

This objective includes rates for deaths per 100,000 population and deaths per million VMT. Population-based rates can misrepresent the impact of highway safety measures on the road, you'll be taking this exam. And if you miss one question, you fail it."

Knowledge Driver's education courses reduce accidents. As a result, automobile insurance rates are lower for drivers who have had driver's education courses.

Judgment and Attitude Judgment is also essential to driving safety. In fact, it is just as important as skill. Driving skill is the person's ability to control the vehicle under all road conditions. Driving judgment is the driver's ability to recognize a potential accident and to know how to avoid it. The use of both skill and judgment, the Red Cross points out, depends on the driver's *attitude*. Part of the defensive driving attitude is self-defense against injury.

Safety Belts Defensive drivers buckle their lap belts (not just their shoulder belts) whenever driving and insist that passengers do the same. Some people claim that safety belts injure people in accidents. They sometimes do, but far more often, they save lives. The safest people are as motivated as the person (call her Susan) who says she cannot even repark her car without first buckling her safety belt. Buckling up becomes an effortless, unconscious action.

Susan explains that a driving instructor told her, "Think of your unprotected body flying through the air at 50 miles an hour and suddenly hitting a stationary car dashboard. When you are driving at 50 miles an hour, both your car and your body are moving *independently* at that speed. If the car hits something and stops, you'll keep flying at 50 miles an hour until *you* hit something." A safety belt slows a person's momentum as the car's momentum decreases. It distributes the force of the impact across the body's strongest parts. Also, it keeps the driver behind the wheel and in control, able to prevent further collisions. Being thrown from the vehicle is not an advantage in a collision. Rather, it increases the chances of death 25 times. Safety belts keep you inside and safe.

Head Restraints and Air Bags Two other pieces of safety equipment are important: **head restraints** to prevent whiplash injury, and **air bags** to cushion the body's impact with the dashboard, a common cause of injury. For further protection, move the driver's and front passenger's seats as far from the dash as possible, without limiting the driver's control of the car.

Air bags, while life-saving to adults and older children, can pose a hazard for infants and small children. In less than a blink of an eye, air bags inflate with a blast that can injure the neck of an infant or child in its path. Infants in front- or rear-facing car seats in the front seat are in harm's way, as are small

Air bags: one reason why children should always ride buckled into the back seat.

MINI
Glossary

head restraints: high seatbacks or other devices attached to seats in cars at head level. A head restraint prevents the person's head from snapping back too far when the body is thrown backward. This prevents neck and spinal cord injuries.

air bags: inflatable pillows, designed to inflate upon impact, stored in the center of the steering wheel of a car or in the dashboard.

because they do not measure exposure to crash risk. As the number of miles driven increases, the risk of a crash increases. Therefore, the VMT-based death rate provides a more accurate measure of motor vehicle safety. Population rates, however, are important in describing motor vehicle crash injury as a public health problem, particularly for the high-risk groups, such as young adults, for

whom VMT rates are not available. Deaths from off-road vehicle (all-terrain vehicles, trail bikes, snowmobiles) crashes are not included in this objective because the hazards encountered on these vehicles are very different from those of on-road vehicles. Furthermore, because registration of off-road vehicles or their riders is not uniformly required, data on VMT or number of users are not routinely available.

DISCUSSION

Ask students if they have ever seen any of the driving behaviors described in item number 2 in the Health Strategies on this page. Ask them to recount the situation, then ask if they reported that driver to the police. Why or why not?

CLASS ACTIVITY

Ask students if any of the automobiles owned by members of their families are in need of repair. Are any of the items mentioned in the bulleted list on this page faulty? Ask students to imagine a situation in which this faulty part could cause an accident that might otherwise be prevented. If students are not sure of the condition of their family automobiles, have them check out these parts and report back to the class. You might also want to have the students do some research to determine the cost of fixing various problems and have them compare the costs to the potential damage should an accident occur.

ASSESS

EVALUATE

A reproducible quiz for Section 1 is provided in the Teacher's Resource Box.

Toddlers and children over 1 year of age should be protected as shown.

Until infants weigh at least 20 pounds, or are 1 year of age, they should ride in the back seat and face the rear of the car.

Health Strategies

How to Avoid Alcohol-Related Driving Accidents

Alcohol and drugs are involved in the great majority of serious accidents each year. To protect yourself:

1. Don't get into a car with anyone who has been drinking.
2. If driving yourself, watch out for any other driver who:
   - ▶ Drives very slowly or fast.
   - ▶ Stops without an apparent reason.
   - ▶ Swerves, weaves, or straddles the center line.
   - ▶ Just misses hitting other vehicles or objects.
   - ▶ Drives into oncoming traffic.
   - ▶ Turns abruptly or illegally.
   - ▶ Fails to obey traffic signs and signals or is slow to obey.
   - ▶ Drives with a window down in cold weather.
   - ▶ Drives with headlights off after dark.
3. If such a driver is in front of you, stay a safe distance behind.
4. If you are in front, get off the road as soon as possible.
5. To help protect others, note the license number if you can. Report it to the police as soon as possible.

children in the front, even when buckled into safety belts. Always buckle infants into rear-facing car seats in the back seat, and buckle other children into the back seat, too.

Other Concerns   Using a cellular telephone while driving is a bad idea. Phone use has quadrupled the rate of crashes, according to one study.

If you have automatic self-closing shoulder belts, make sure that you and your passengers buckle their lap belts. Shoulder belts without lap belts can injure people badly.

The responsible driver also:

- ▶ Keeps the vehicle in good condition—tires, windshield wipers, horn, lights, brakes, wheel alignment, and steering mechanism.
- ▶ Wipes or washes all windows clean before starting the car.
- ▶ Wears glasses, if needed.
- ▶ Adjusts driving to different driving conditions.
- ▶ Obeys traffic signs and all regulations.
- ▶ Watches for pedestrians and bicyclists.
- ▶ Does not drive after drinking alcohol or after taking drugs that cause drowsiness, or when emotional, anxious, distracted, irritated, or tired.

This last item is especially important. Half of all fatal driving accidents involve alcohol. Many others involve other mind-altering drugs. The most important steps you can take to protect yourself against car accidents are never to ride with a driver who has been drinking, and never to get behind the wheel if you have been drinking yourself.

Keep in mind that being tired, angry, or upset can impair your driving, too. The more urgently you want to get where you are going, the more important it is for you to control your temper and resist pushing yourself. If you lose

QUICK QUIZ

Chapter 24, Section 1

The following quiz will help you assess your students' understanding of the material covered in this section of the chapter. You might use the quiz as an oral exercise, which will lead into a class discussion of the topics covered. Or, you might use it as a paper/pencil

quiz to evaluate your students individually.

If students have difficulty with the concepts covered in the Quick Quiz and the Section Review, you might suggest they review the material using the Survey, Question, Read, Recite, Review (SQ3R) study method, which is described in detail in the introduction to this Teacher's Wraparound Edition.

1. Injury is a major public health problem. (True)

patience with other drivers, use stress-reducing techniques to calm down (see Chapter 4 for details). If you are tired, admit it. Stop and rest. Beyond this, the suggestions made in the Health Strategies section, "How to Avoid Alcohol-Related Driving Accidents," on page 650 can help you avoid becoming a victim of someone else's drunk driving.

In a letter to columnist Ann Landers (January 3, 1992), a professional driver offers three changes in driving habits that he believes would save lives:

1. Look over your shoulder when changing lanes. Don't rely on mirrors.
2. Keep a safe distance from the car in front of you. If you can read the license plate, you are too close.
3. After a red light turns green, pause for a good five seconds before proceeding. "I have seen too many cars zip right through those lights at 60 miles an hour," he says.

All of these statements about attitude apply equally to motorcyclists. In addition, motorcyclists must use safety techniques specific to them (the highway patrol offers courses in these). They should wear helmets, whether or not they are required by law to do so.

 Driver attitude is important in preventing collisions. Defensive drivers take precautions against injuries by wearing safety belts. They take precautions against accidents by attending to the condition of the vehicle, and of the driver.

SECTION 1 Review

Answer the following questions on a sheet of paper.

Learning the Vocabulary

The vocabulary terms in this section are *head restraints* and *air bags*.

1. _____ prevent a person's head from snapping back too far when the body is thrown backward in a car.
2. _____ are stored in the center of the car's steering wheel and inflate on impact.
3. Write a sentence using each vocabulary term.

Learning the Facts

4. What is the number-one killer of young people?
5. Why are driving skill and driving judgment essential?

6. Why should lap belts always be used when shoulder belts are used?

Making Life Choices

7. Answer the following questions that apply to driving regulations:
   a. Do you think that every licensed driver should be required to take a driving test every few years? Why, or why not?
   b. Do you think that people convicted of drunk driving should lose their licenses permanently on the first offense? Why, or why not?
   c. What do you think are the most common reasons why people do not wear safety belts? Should every state in our nation have a mandatory seatbelt law for all drivers and passengers? Why, or why not?

SECTION 1 Review Answers

1. Head restraints
2. Airbags
3. Answers will vary.
4. accidents and injuries (p. 646)
5. *Driving skill* is the person's ability to control the vehicle under all road conditions, and *driving judgment* is the driver's ability to recognize a potential accident and know how to avoid it. (p. 649)
6. Shoulder belts used without lap belts can injure people. Shoulder belts used in conjunction with lap belts distribute the force of an accident across the body's strongest parts. They also keep the driver behind the wheel. (p. 649)
7. Answers will vary.

CLOSE

Before going on to the next lesson, students should be able to answer the following:

a. Name the four necessary aspects of defensive driving.
b. List four responsibilities of a driver in preventing accidents.
c. Identify four guidelines for recognizing driving under the influence of alcohol or drugs.
d. Name two safety precautions taken in the manufacture of an automobile to ensure driver protection.
e. Name four things that affect insurance rates for teenagers.

2. Diseases claim more young lives than preventable accidents. (False)
3. Good drivers don't have car accidents. (False)
4. A defensive attitude behind the wheel can help to prevent accidents. (True)
5. Defensive driving involves planning ahead to avoid collisions. (True)
6. Your attitude as a driver has no effect on your judgment or driving skill. (False)
7. A safety belt distributes the force of an

impact across the body's strongest parts. (True)
8. Being thrown from a vehicle during a collision can decrease your chances of severe injury. (False)
9. Using a cellular phone while driving may quadruple your likelihood of having an accident. (True)
10. Half of all fatal accidents involve alcohol. (True)

SECTION 2

FOCUS

OUTCOME

In this section students will learn that:

1. Training, skills, and knowledge of safety rules can prevent most accidents during swimming, boating, biking, and other play activities.

FOCUS ACTIVITY

As a class, have students identify recreational and outdoor activities in which they participate. Divide the class into groups and assign one of the activities to each group. Have each group list the following about its activity: **1.** hazards, **2.** precautions, **3.** regulations or rules (established or understood) that promote safety within the activity, and **4.** prevention education available. Encourage them to illustrate the activity and this information. Give each group a large (3 foot × 4 foot) piece of chart paper on which to work. Ask students in each group to develop an original safety slogan for the recreational activity of their group. The slogans should be short and easy to remember. They must be able to support each slogan by explaining why it's important. Display the posters in the classroom.

TEACH & APPLY

FAST FACTS

1,200 children in the United States drown annually. Most drown in swimming pools.

Health Strategies

Water Rescue Techniques

Even if you cannot swim, you can assist a swimmer who is nearby and in trouble. Just remember to throw, tow, or row to get the person to safety. Use these guidelines:

1. If the swimmer is near a dock or in a pool:
  ▶ Lie flat on the dock or pool edge. Extend an arm, leg, shirt, fishing pole, oar, or other object. Pull the victim within reach of the edge. Most pools have long cleaning tools around that work well. If a life-saving cushion or float is nearby, aim carefully, and throw it to the victim.

2. If the troubled swimmer is farther away than you can reach:
  ▶ Wade into the water up to your waist. Extend an object, push a float or board, or throw a rope where the victim can reach it.

3. If the victim fell from a boat, or you are in a boat:
  ▶ Allow the victim to hang onto the boat or to an object you hold out.

4. If the victim is too weak to hold on:
  ▶ Pull the victim into the boat carefully to avoid worsening any injuries.

5. If the victim fell through ice:
  ▶ Push a ladder or other long object, tied with a rope at the bottom rung and secured, out to the victim. You might also use ropes, poles, sticks, or a human chain to reach the person.
  ▶ If the victim is too weak to hold on, a rescuer can crawl along the ladder to help.

special needs

Spatial

To review and reiterate the many safety rules and precautions itemized in this chapter without overwhelming your students, you may wish to use the follow activity. Visual images may make it easier for many learners to incorporate the things they study into long-term

---

SECTION 2

Safety While Swimming, Boating, Biking, and at Other Play

For teens, drowning is a major cause of accidental death in this country. Most drownings occur when someone who can't swim falls into the water—often from a boat. Surprisingly, people who can't swim often put themselves in situations in which they may drown. Then they do drown. To reduce the risk of drowning:

▶ Learn to swim.
▶ Never swim alone or let others do so.
▶ Choose swimming places with care.
▶ Protect pools with fences.
▶ Use extra caution around moving water (rivers, canals, creeks, etc.). It is much more powerful than it looks.
▶ Supply boats with personal flotation devices (PFDs). Nonswimmers should always wear PFDs the proper size to fit them, when on a boat.
▶ Ease into the water when it is cold.
▶ Never play rough in or near the water.
▶ Swim only when you feel well.
▶ Do not swim if you have been drinking alcohol or using other drugs.

Precautions for Swimmers   When diving, never dive where obstructions might lurk or where you don't know the depth. Ease in feet first the first time, anyway. Do not overestimate your ability. Do not dive too deep.

It is also wise to have a boat accompany you on a distance swim. Get out of the water when lightning threatens. Even if you are in a boat, go to shore quickly in a storm. Except in emergencies, rely on your own swimming ability, not on inner tubes or floats.

If you see someone in trouble in the water, help by using the techniques described in "Water Rescue Techniques," the Health Strategies feature on this page. Only a trained lifeguard should attempt rescue by swimming out to the victim. A drowning person can easily overpower a novice and drown them both.

You may have heard that you should not swim until an hour after eating, to prevent stomach cramps. It is not necessarily dangerous to swim with a full stomach, especially if you exercise lightly. However, if you swim hard after eating, you may indeed experience cramps. They are just as likely to occur in your legs or arms as in your stomach. The rea-

memory, and then to retrieve it for real-life use. Because these lessons include accident and injury prevention information, graphic representations may be helpful.

Divide the class into groups, one for each of the following areas: car safety (Section 1), water safety (Section 2), sports activity safety (Section 2), fire safety (Section 3), home safety (Section 4), preparedness (Section 5), and child care (Section 6). Each group will be

Moving water is more powerful than it looks; use caution and safety equipment when venturing out upon it.

son may be that digestion requires energy and oxygen, which are taken from the hard-working muscles. You need not stay out of the lake altogether after a picnic. Just take it easy while your stomach is full.

Boating Safety   To ensure safe boating pleasure:

▶ Do not operate boating equipment if using alcohol or other drugs.
▶ Know your boat and the rules of the waterway.
▶ Make sure there are enough Coast Guard–approved flotation devices for everyone. Do not rely on inner tubes or toys as flotation devices.
▶ Load the boat reasonably.
▶ Keep your weight low in the boat. Sit, don't stand.
▶ Tell people on shore where you are going and when to expect you back.
▶ If the boat overturns or fills with water, hang onto it (it will probably still float).
▶ If the weather threatens, skip the trip.

Don't dive where obstructions might lurk.

Biking, Roller Blading, and Skateboarding   Of course, accidents also happen when people are moving fast on land—biking, roller blading, skateboarding, running, and the like. Probably the most important guideline for accident prevention is to wear good shoes. Not only do they protect the feet; they also give stability to the whole body. A second guideline is to use proper gear: the right-size bike, roller blades, or skateboard in good condition, and so on. Helmets are also recommended for biking, roller blading, and skateboarding. Keep in mind that no one ever has an accident on purpose. It is the unlikely, unexpected event—the one you can't control—against which you are safeguarding yourself.

Avoiding Back Injury   Finally, protect your back. Lift *nothing* by bending over, not even a feather. Your own upper body is heavy. Whenever you bend over, your lower back muscles must hoist its weight. To avoid back injury while lifting something, the Red Cross says:

responsible for summarizing the information in the chapter for their topic as well as doing any further research that may be needed. They may need to have library or computer on-line time to access the Internet or an electronic encyclopedia to complete their research.

When they have completed their written report, students should prepare a poster or display to depict the safety rules/suggestions that they have learned. Graphically representing this information will allow students of the ability levels to gain a clearer understanding. You may want to contact elementary and/or junior high schools in the area and offer to lend them the displays for a safety week exhibit.

ASSESS

EVALUATE

SECTION 2 Review Answers

1. Answers will vary; could include at least five from the list on page 652.
2. Push a ladder or other long object out to the victim; use ropes, poles, sticks, or a human chain to reach the person; if the victim is too weak to hold on, a rescuer can crawl along the ladder to help. (p. 652)
3. Cramps occur when digestion takes oxygen from the hard-working muscles. (p. 653)
4. It puts the entire weight of the upper body on the lower back muscles. (p. 653)
5. Answers will vary.

A reproducible quiz for Section 2 is provided in the Teacher's Resource Box.

CLOSE

Collect newspaper articles about various recreational accidents. Ask students to pick one and identify the following:

1. the hazard; **2.** the unsafe act, habit or behavior; **3.** the attitude; **4.** the prevention.

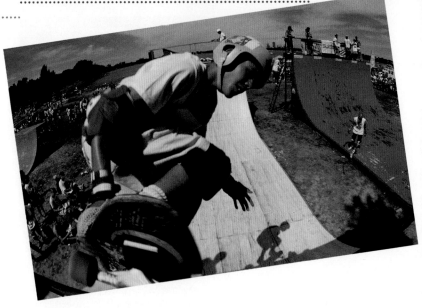

When moving fast on land, protect yourself from potential injury as best you can by wearing safety gear and using common sense.

▶ Plant the feet firmly and slightly apart. Keep your head up.
▶ Squat—do not lean—forward, keeping the back as straight as possible, and get a firm grip on the object.
▶ Lift slowly, pushing up with the strong thigh and leg muscles.
▶ Do not jerk the object upward or twist your body as you lift.
▶ To lower an object, reverse this procedure.

KEY POINTS *The first rule for water safety is "learn to swim." The next is "never swim alone." When active on land, wear shoes, use proper gear, and use your body with care.*

SECTION 2 Review

Answer the following questions on a sheet of paper.

Learning the Facts

1. List five ways to reduce the risks of drowning.
2. How might a victim who has fallen through ice be rescued?
3. Why might cramps develop if a person swims hard after eating?
4. Why shouldn't you lift anything by bending over?

Making Life Choices

5. Describe three instances in which you or someone you know have had accidents on bicycles. Describe the causes of the accidents. What factors were common to these accidents? Develop some guidelines for cyclists that would help prevent or lessen injuries from accidents.

QUICK QUIZ

Chapter 24, Section 2

The following quiz will help you assess your students' understanding of the material covered in this section of the chapter. You might use the quiz as an oral exercise, which will lead into a class discussion of the topics covered. Or, you might use it as a paper/pencil

quiz to evaluate your students individually.

*If students have difficulty with the concepts covered in the Quick Quiz and the Section Review, you might suggest they review the material using the **S**urvey, **Q**uestion, **R**ead, **R**ecite, **R**eview (SQ3R) study method, which is described in detail in the introduction to this Teacher's Wraparound Edition.*

1. Easing into cold water can reduce your risk of drowning. (True)

SECTION 3

Burns

Among teenagers and children, fires and burns rank third, behind motor vehicle deaths and drownings, as a cause of accidental death. Many of those who die are children. The majority of the deaths occur in fires at home. Fire prevention and escape is the topic of this chapter's Straight Talk section. The next chapter offers basic tips for assisting burn victims. A course in first aid can give you more.

A special class of burns—chemical burns—damages eyes, skin, and lungs without fire. Read the labels of sprays, products that contain gases, and compounds that can burn your skin or hurt your eyes. Follow directions.

Other specifics to prevent fires and burns:

► Install fire extinguishers near danger spots.
► Keep a garden hose near a faucet.
► Use chemical fire extinguishers—never water—on electrical fires. Baking soda will safely smother a grease fire, so keep a box handy in the kitchen. (See Figure 24–2 on the next page).
► Change heating-and-cooling system filters on schedule, and maintain heating systems.
► Dispose of trash immediately.
► Hang clothes well away from stoves or fireplaces.
► Store matches in a metal container and out of the reach of children.
► Be careful with hot tap water; it can cause scalds that require hospitalization. Turn down the temperature setting of the water heater to 120 degrees Fahrenheit, if possible. This will help save energy, too.
► Do not allow anyone to smoke in bed. Provide adequate ashtrays to smokers, or ask them to smoke outside.
► Install home fire detectors. The local fire department can help you choose the right types and decide on their placement.

Keep a safe home, and know what to do in emergencies.

Finally, if a fire starts, what will you do? Think now, because you need to know ahead of time what moves to make. The Straight Talk section tells you how to plan your way out of burning buildings. One thing to carry in your head at all times is the emergency telephone number for most parts of the United States: 911. You'd be smart to memorize the fire department number if it's not 911.

 KEY POINTS *Many lives are lost to fires each year. Home fires are preventable through cautious handling of equipment and chemicals.*

SECTION 3

FOCUS

OUTCOMES

In this section students will learn:

1. Prevention is the key to reducing deaths and injuries due to fires.
2. What to do in the case of fire or burns.

FOCUS ACTIVITY

Bring to class a number of newspaper articles about fires; brush fires, house fires, and business fires. Divide the class into groups. Give one article to each group. Have the groups read the articles to determine whether authorities found a cause for the fire. Then have groups brainstorm ways the fires could have been prevented.

TEACH & APPLY

LEARNING WITH VISUALS

Tell students that rows 1 and 2 from Figure 24–2 on page 656 are different symbols that represent the same thing. If these symbols appear on the fire extinguisher, it is okay to use the extinguisher for the type of fire described. The symbols in the last row mean that the extinguisher should not be used for the types of fire described. Ask them which three symbols they would look for if a grease fire occurred in their kitchen. (the middle column) An electrical fire? (the right column) An ordinary fire? (the left column)

2. You should be especially careful to check for obstructions before diving into water. (True)
3. Boaters do not have to worry about lightening. (False)
4. You should always attempt to swim out to save a drowning person. (False)
5. You should never operate boating equipment after consuming alcohol or other drugs. (True)
6. It is unsafe to swim less than one hour after eating. (False)
7. Heavy swimming exertion immediately after eating can cause cramps. (True)
8. An inner tube or blow-up toy can substitute as a flotation device. (False)
9. Good shoes protect your feet and give stability to the entire body. (True)
10. You should bend over when attempting to lift a heavy object. (False)

ASSESS

EVALUATE

Review Answers

1. fires and burns (p. 655)
2. Answers will vary; could include at least four from the list on page 655.
3. 120 degrees F (p. 655)
4. 911 (p. 655)
5. Answers will vary.

A reproducible quiz for Section 3 is provided in the Teacher's Resource Box.

CLOSE

Have students identify the three classes of fire extinguishers and either draw the symbols for each one's use(s) or name the use(s) for each one. Discuss where the fire extinguishers are located around the school facility.

ORDINARY A COMBUSTIBLES

FLAMMABLE B LIQUIDS

ELECTRICAL C EQUIPMENT

If you see these symbols on a fire extinguisher...

or

or

or

Class A (paper, wood, cloth)

Class B (flammable liquids, greases)

Class C (electrical fires)

follow these instructions:

Use the extinguisher on an ordinary fire of paper, wood, or cloth.

Use the extinguisher on a flammable liquid or grease fire.

Use the extinguisher on an electrical fire.

If you see these symbols on a fire extinguisher...

follow these instructions:

Do NOT use the extinguisher on an ordinary fire of paper, wood, or cloth.

Do NOT use the extinguisher on a flammable liquid or grease fire.

Do NOT use the extinguisher on an electrical fire.

Figure 24–2 Types of Fire Extinguishers and Fires.

Review

Answer the following questions on a sheet of paper.

Learning the Facts

1. What is the third leading cause of accidental death among children and teenagers?
2. Give four recommendations on how to prevent fires and burns.
3. The water heater in your home should not exceed what temperature?
4. What is the emergency help telephone number for most parts of the United States?

Making Life Choices

5. Develop a fire escape plan for your home. Figure out two ways to get outside from every room. Designate a place outside where you will all meet, so that you can be sure everyone is out. Advance planning is your only effective weapon.

COOPERATIVE LEARNING

Statistics show that most people will be involved in an accident in their home at some time of their life. Whether its from a fall, a fire, or a natural disaster, most people are likely to find themselves in a situation that threatens their well being. There may be few things that people can do to prevent all accidents from happening, but with careful plan-ning and preparation, they can prevent some accidents or lessen the effects of accidents and prevent even more devastating injuries. Statistics also show that people who have pre-pared plans for dealing with accidents or situations lessen the injuries caused by the accident. In some cases they have eliminated the injury all together.

Divide your class into groups of three or four. Begin by having each member of the group write out an individual safety checklist

SECTION 4

Home Safety

Falls cause many accidental deaths. Statistics demonstrate that for each person, sooner or later, one accidental fall will likely be a devastating one. The same attitude that prevents driving accidents works for falls. Anticipation and defensive action against falls can prevent them.

Most falls happen at home. To prevent slips and trips:

- ▶ Wipe up spills.
- ▶ Use nonslip floor wax.
- ▶ Secure small rugs. Do not use them at tops and bottoms of staircases.
- ▶ Clean up snow in walking areas. Use sand or salt on icy spots.
- ▶ Keep a safety mat in the bathtub, and install handholds on the wall.
- ▶ Be careful in wet grass, especially with a power mower.
- ▶ Repair torn and frayed carpet promptly.
- ▶ Keep walking areas clear and the yard picked up.
- ▶ Keep stairs and hallways well lighted—install handrails.

To prevent falls that occur when climbing or reaching:

- ▶ Use a sturdy ladder. Do not use makeshift piles of furniture or boxes.
- ▶ Inspect the ladder before you use it.
- ▶ Never paint a ladder. Paint hides structural defects.
- ▶ Move the ladder instead of reaching to the side from the top of it. Climb down, move the ladder, and climb up again.
- ▶ Lean a straight ladder at an angle to the wall, not straight up. The bottom should be placed away from the wall one-quarter of the distance from the base of the ladder to its contact point.
- ▶ Place both feet of the ladder firmly on level, nonslippery ground, and have someone steady the ladder as you climb.
- ▶ Keep your hands free to grip the ladder as you climb. Wear your tools in a tool belt.
- ▶ Keep your body weight centered.
- ▶ Face the ladder when climbing down.
- ▶ Hire an expert for high jobs, especially roof jobs or those where power wires are nearby.

Special notes for special age groups: falls are the leading cause of accidental death and injury to older people, so be aware that balance declines with age. Sudden motions affect balance the most—especially motions involving the head, which is heavy and can pull the whole body off center. Slow down, and move with grace. For the other special age group, infants, falls from tables and bassinets are a frequent cause of injury. Falls into buckets of water, toilets, swimming pools, or other bodies of water can cause death by drowning. Do not look away from an infant in such a place, even for a moment.

Handholds in the bathtub or shower can help prevent falls.

and emergency plan for their own home. For the individual checklist, have students make a list of all possible hazards that exist at their home and what needs to be done to correct the situation. Examples may include: keeping stairways clear of objects, adding a fire extinguisher, putting a nonslip mat in the bathtub, and keeping all sharp objects and poison out of reach of children. Have individuals write and diagram an evacuation plan for their home including an escape route, detailed locations of fire extinguishers, and a designated meeting place for all members to go to after leaving the house. Checklists should also include a list of phone numbers of emergency and nonemergency personnel in case they are needed.

After individuals have completed their checklists, have them compare their own list with members of their group. Have individuals make any changes to their checklists or emergency plans that seem necessary.

SECTION 4

FOCUS

OUTCOMES

In this section students will learn:

1. Several ways to prevent slips, trips, and falls when reaching and climbing.
2. Several ways to prevent work and leisure-time accidents.

FOCUS ACTIVITY

Have students find articles that indicate situations where precautions were not taken at home and a preventable injury in the form of a fall or careless use of tools, toys, guns, or other items occurred. Have the students pair up and discuss the articles. They should decide what could have prevented the accidents. Keep a file of these articles for future classes.

TEACH & APPLY

FAST FACTS

From the years 1982 to 1991, 44 children were crushed to death by automatic garage doors, according to the U.S. Consumer Product Safety Commission.

DISCUSSION

Ask students if they think that posting a list of precautions, such as the one here in the book, somewhere in their home would help to prevent accidents. Where would they post the list? Have students customize a list of home safety precautions to post in their homes.

DISCUSSION

Ask students to think for a few minutes about accidents, other than the falls (discussed previously) that have occurred in their homes. What were the causes of these accidents? Could they have been prevented? What will family members do to prevent a recurrence of this type of accident?

ASSESS

EVALUATE

Review Answers

1. Answers will vary; could include at least three from the list on page 657.
2. Answers will vary; could include at least four from the list on page 657.
3. falls (p. 657)
4. Answers will vary; could include at least three from the list on page 658.
5. Answers will vary.
6. Answers will vary.

CLOSE

Ask students to add items to the list of work and leisure-time precautions found in this section that would further help to reduce accidents, injuries, and possible death. For extra credit, have students make posters to illustrate these ideas and display them in your room or hallway.

Other accidents can arise from the careless use of tools, toys, guns, and other devices. Again, most such accidents occur in the home. Work and leisure-time accidents add significantly to the number of deaths and injuries. To prevent them:

- ▶ Use sharp objects only for their intended purpose, handle them with care, and keep them out of the reach of children.
- ▶ Mark large glass windows and doors so that everyone can see that they are not walk-through spaces.
- ▶ Follow the manufacturer's instructions carefully when using equipment.
- ▶ Unplug electric cords when equipment is not in use.
- ▶ Do not use electric appliances, such as hair dryers, around water, including full bathroom basins, tubs, and other sinks.
- ▶ Clean up spills promptly to prevent slipping.
- ▶ Sweep up broken glass promptly. Discard cracked china and glassware. Use nonbreakable dishes and containers around tile and cement surfaces.
- ▶ Remove nails from boards in storage.
- ▶ Learn and obey all firearm safety rules.
- ▶ Keep guns and ammunition in separate places, each protected by lock and key.
- ▶ Never load a gun until you are ready to shoot it. Assume that all guns you handle are loaded, even when you know they are not. Do not misuse blank cartridges. They can cause serious injury and even death.

 KEY POINTS *Falls and other accidents at home claim many lives each year. Most of these accidents can be prevented through awareness and a few precautions.*

 SECTION 4 Review

Answer the following questions on a sheet of paper.

Learning the Facts
1. Give three recommendations for preventing slips and trips.
2. List four ways to prevent falls that occur when climbing or reaching.
3. What is the leading cause of accidental death for older people?
4. Name three recommendations for avoiding work and leisure-time accidents.

Making Life Choices
5. Look over the lists in this section that specify how to prevent slips, trips, and falls. Which safety precautions do you most often ignore? Discuss why you do not follow these safety tips.
6. Falls are the leading cause of accidental death and injury to elderly people. If your grandmother were going to move into your home, what changes would you make to ensure her safety?

QUICK QUIZ

Chapter 24, Section 4

The following quiz will help you assess your students' understanding of the material covered in this section of the chapter. You might use the quiz as an oral exercise, which will lead into a class discussion of the topics covered. Or, you might use it as a paper/pencil quiz to evaluate your students individually.

Like the Quick Quiz, the Section Review can also be used as an assessment tool to spark class discussion or as an individual student evaluation. It can also be used as a review in preparation for this quiz.

1. Many accidental falls can be avoided by wiping up spills, using safety mats, and keeping walkways clear and well lighted. (True)

SECTION 5

Preparedness for Natural Disasters

Natural disasters such as hurricanes, floods, earthquakes, tornadoes, and the like are, for the most part, beyond people's ability to avoid. However, there is much people can do to prepare for them. Imagine yourself stuck in your house or in a car, unable to leave the area, having to cope for several days without outside help. What would you wish you had done beforehand? What would you wish you had with you?

Water is the first thing that should come to mind. Store some fresh, drinkable water in clean, closed containers now, in the building where you live. Store water in the car, too, if you have one. Store enough to sustain you for at least a day or so. Then, think of shoes. Suppose you had to walk a long distance to get help. Sandals or high-heeled shoes would get old fast. Store good shoes where you may need them.

Other equipment you should have ready:

▶ A portable radio, in case the power goes down.
▶ Extra batteries, in case the radio goes dead. (Alkaline batteries last the longest.)
▶ A working flashlight and batteries; also candles and matches, in case the lights go out.
▶ An adjustable wrench to turn off the electrical main switch and the gas line. (Learn how to do this in advance.)
▶ A first-aid kit, in case someone gets hurt.
▶ Canned food and a can opener, in case you aren't able to cook.

You can get by in good shape under many emergency situations with just these few simple supplies. On the other hand, you can be miserable, and your life can even be threatened, without the needed items. Remember, the time to stock up on them is now, ahead of time.

Different geographic areas are prone to different events. Learn the preparedness

There is much you can do to prepare for natural disasters.

SECTION 5

FOCUS

OUTCOME

In this section students will learn:

1. How to prepare for natural disasters.

FOCUS ACTIVITY

List the following disasters on the board and have students name precautions for each:

1. lightning **2.** flood **3.** hurricane **4.** tornado **5.** blizzard **6.** earthquake

TEACH & APPLY

LEARNING WITH VISUALS

Before beginning this section, collect periodical articles and identify library resources on each of the natural disasters addressed. Have the periodical articles available in the classroom and request the library resources be loaned to you for use in your classroom. Make a copy of a world map for each student. Using your resources, have the students place symbols on their maps (in at least 20 locations) for natural disasters common in different parts of the world.

2. A safety mat can reduce the danger of slipping in the bathtub. (True)
3. It is safe to reach sideways from the top of a sturdy ladder. (False)
4. You should always inspect a ladder before using it. (True)
5. You should always keep your hands free when climbing a ladder, and ask someone to steady the ladder from the ground. (True)
6. You should lean a straight ladder as close to the wall as possible. (False)
7. Balance declines with age. (True)
8. You should never look away from an infant who is near any body of water. (True)
9. You should keep electrical objects plugged in when not in use. (False)
10. You should always keep guns and ammunitions in the same place. (False)

ASSESS

EVALUATE

SECTION 5 Review Answers

1. Answers will vary; could include hurricanes, floods, earthquakes, and tornadoes. (p. 659)
2. Answers will vary; could include water, sturdy walking shoes, extra fuses, portable radio, extra batteries, working flashlight and batteries, candles and matches, and so on. (p. 659)
3. under sturdy furniture (p. 660)
4. stay indoors, away from water and all electrical and metal objects (p. 660)
5. Answers will vary.

WORKSHEETS

A reproducible quiz for Section 5 is provided in the Teacher's Resource Box.

CLOSE

Have students find out from a variety of local resources (civil defense, fire department, and so on) how different areas of their community would be evacuated if the necessity arose. To receive extra credit, students should obtain a street map of their community and clearly mark the evacuation routes. Display one in your classroom and post others throughout your school.

Prepare for disasters likely to hit your area.

Have on hand water to drink and good shoes to walk in.

routines for those that are likely to strike your area. Here are a few additional rules:

▶ Obey instructions. If told to leave an area, do so.
▶ In an earthquake, get under a sturdy desk, table, or other furniture, if you can. Do not run outside, where objects may fall on you.
▶ In storms, stay indoors. When lightning is nearby, keep away from water, plumbing, other metal objects, and all electrical outlets. Do not use the telephone.
▶ If rising water is a problem or if your home has structural damage from an earthquake, turn off the main power switch. Let an electrician check your home before turning on the power again.
▶ Afterwards, be aware that electrical power lines may be damaged or down. Keep well away from them.

KEY POINTS *The person who has stored water, good shoes, a radio, candles, a first-aid kit, and food is best prepared for a natural disaster.*

SECTION 5 Review

Answer the following questions on a sheet of paper.

Learning the Facts
1. Give three examples of natural disasters.
2. List six types of equipment you should have available in the event of a natural disaster.
3. In the event of an earthquake, where should you seek safety?
4. What are some precautions you should take during a lightning storm?

Making Life Choices
5. Develop a fictitious situation in which you have to prepare for a natural disaster. Describe the situation you are facing and exactly how you will prepare for it in order to ensure your safety. Discuss the damage that the disaster may cause and how you plan to survive its aftermath.

Focusing ON Self-Esteem

In addition to providing a safe physical environment, care givers must also provide safe emotional environments. You might want to share the following with these students who provide care for younger children.

The kinds of messages a child receives from adults impact the child's self-esteem. Positive messages are esteem-building. It is estimated that children need four positive messages for every negative message, just to "stay even." Conditional messages refer to the

SECTION 6

Care of Others: Child Care

SECTION 6

"**T**aking care of children is a matter of plain common sense. Everyone knows how to do it." Many people think this is so, but it is not. Love and enjoyment of children may come naturally. However, to deliver competent child care, you also have to do some formal learning. Safety precautions are a part of child care.

Home Safety   Keeping a safe home is a major part of the responsible care of children. Whether you care for younger sisters and brothers, baby-sit, or have children of your own, you should check the home, yard, garage, storage areas, basement, and play areas for hazards to the children's safety. Ask yourself these questions:

1. Are all areas free of hazards that could cause falls, as described in Section 4 of this chapter?
2. Are all areas well defended against fire, as described in Section 3?
3. If there is a pool or other body of water nearby, is it fenced off, so that the children cannot play there unsupervised or accidentally fall in?
4. Are all areas neat and free of trash and bottles?

Fix any areas that are not safe.

Teenagers and others who care for children should learn how to handle emergencies.

child's behavior; unconditional messages refer to the child's worth as an individual. "I love you" is a positive, unconditional message. "I like the way you put your toys away" is a positive, conditional message. Negative messages should be conditional, that is, focus on behavior. An example of a negative, condi-

tional message is "I want you to stop throwing blocks." Negative, unconditional messages should be avoided. Statements like "Can't you ever do anything right?" attack the child's worth as an individual and are damaging to self-esteem.

FOCUS

OUTCOMES

In this section students will learn:

1. Safety precautions for the home and play areas of children.
2. Safety tips when accepting responsibility for someone else's children.

FOCUS ACTIVITY

Have students visit the home of a neighbor who has small children (with ages ranging from six months to three years if possible). Have each student interview the parent(s) to find out what precautions they have taken in their homes and play areas to ensure the safety and well-being of the child. Ask students to share their findings in groups of three or four and make some suggestions to help improve the safety of the homes and play areas they observed. If possible, have students take the suggestions they have made for the homes and play area back to the families involved.

TEACH & APPLY

GROUP PROJECT

Have students develop safety slogans to put around various places in the home and/or play area to help remind parents and child care providers of safety precautions. If time permits, make up slogans and distribute them to young families in your community.

DISCUSSION

Ask students to evaluate their baby-sitting with regard to the pointers listed in the Health Strategies on this page. Do they practice these strategies all of the time, most of the time, occasionally, or never? Are any of these unreasonable? If so, why?

TEACHER SUPPORT

Key Passage

Ask students how many are responsible for younger children from time to time, either in paid baby-sitting situations or in taking care of younger siblings. In these situations, do they feel that they are as protective as they should be of the safety of the children? How often do they check on the children? Have any accidents or injuries ever occurred while they were responsible for the children? How did they react?

ASSESS

EVALUATE

A reproducible quiz for Section 6 is provided in the Teacher's Resource Box.

When adults focus on safety, children can be free to enjoy their play.

Health Strategies

Pointers for Baby-Sitters

Before accepting responsibility for someone else's children:

1. Find out where the parents will be and how you can reach them if you need them. Write down the phone number(s) or address(es).
2. Write down one or more neighbors' names and numbers.
3. Write down the telephone numbers of:
   ▶ The family doctor or pediatrician.
   ▶ The police department or sheriff.
   ▶ The fire department.
   The parents might also show you where they keep these numbers.
4. Ask if it's safe to go outside.
5. Know how to lock the door(s). Chain them, if you can. Secure all windows.
6. Let no one in unless told in advance that they're coming. Politely tell unexpected visitors (through a locked door) to return a little later or the next day.
7. Keep an awake child in view at all times. Check a sleeping child frequently (every 15 minutes).

Toy Safety Pay special attention to children's toys:

▶ Make sure that children do not play with sticks, or with toys or other objects that may break if the children fall. This warning applies to bottles, glasses, and even some plastic toys.
▶ Do not allow children to play with fireworks.
▶ Make sure children do not play with or around television sets, electrical devices in the kitchen and bathroom, fans, power tools, household cleaning equipment, sewing machines, lawn tools, and other dangerous objects.
▶ Do not allow children to play with any guns, including pellet guns, BB guns, and toy guns that look real.

Even if the home and toys are safe, children should not be left to play without your watchful attention. Their own judgment cannot keep them from harm. You must do so.

Prevention of Choking When feeding children, be aware that they can easily choke on food. (So can you, actually, so consider taking these precautions for yourself as well.) To prevent choking, cut meat into small pieces. Let children take only small forkfuls of any food.

QUICK QUIZ

Chapter 24, Section 6

The following quiz will help you assess your students' understanding of the material covered in this section of the chapter. You might use the quiz as an oral exercise, which will lead into a class discussion of the topics covered. Or, you might use it as a paper/pencil quiz to evaluate your students individually.

If students have difficulty with the concepts covered in the Quick Quiz and the Section Review, you might suggest they review the material using the **S***urvey,* **Q***uestion,* **R***ead,* **R***ecite,* **R***eview (SQ3R) study method, which is described in detail in the introduction to this Teacher's Wraparound Edition.*

1. Common sense is the only thing you need to safely care for children. (False)

Don't let them speak or laugh with food in their mouths. Make sure they chew each bite thoroughly before attempting to swallow. Take particular care with round pieces of food such as hot dogs, grapes or cherry tomatoes. Teach children to bite them with their front teeth to crush them. For small children, cut food (even grapes and hot dogs) into tiny pieces. Peanuts should be split open. Popcorn should not be served to small children at all, because it is light enough to be carried by the breath and round enough to lodge in the throat.

Learn the Heimlich Maneuver (abdominal thrust maneuver). If a child does choke, use the maneuver to dislodge the particle from the throat. The next chapter gives a basic description of the maneuver, but you can best learn it in a first-aid course.

When you are baby-sitting, some additional precautions are in order. See the Health Strategies section, "Pointers for Baby-Sitters."

Choking poses a real threat: young children easily choke on food.

 Competent care of children includes attention to their safety. The home and toys must be safe. The person who is responsible must keep a watchful eye on children.

SECTION 6 Review

Answer the following questions on a sheet of paper.

Learning the Facts

1. List four precautions you should follow when caring for children in your home.

2. How can children be kept from choking?

3. Name five precautions baby-sitters should take.

Making Life Choices

4. In your mind, make a safety inspection of your home. Picture yourself walking from room to room. Evaluate each specific area in terms of potential safety hazards that may exist for infants and small children. List all the safety hazards you discovered. Describe how each can best be remedied.

Answers to FACT or FICTION

Here are the answers to the questions at the start of the chapter.

1. False. One out of every three, not ten, people suffers an injury each year.
2. True.
3. False. Skill is important, but attitude is equally important in preventing accidents on the road.
4. True.
5. True.
6. True.
7. False. To deliver competent child care, you have to do some formal learning.

---

2. When checking an area for child safety, you should look for fire, fall, and water hazards. (True)

3. All toys are safe for children. (False)

4. Children should never be allowed to play with or near electrical devices, including the television. (True)

5. It is safe to leave children unattended after checking carefully for hazards. (False)

6. Trash, bottles, and breakable objects are safety hazards for children. (True)

7. Children should only be allowed to eat small mouthfuls of food. (True)

8. Children should be taught not to speak with food in their mouths and to chew thoroughly before they swallow. (True)

9. Small children are able to swallow round pieces of food without danger. (False)

10. Small children should not be allowed to eat popcorn. (True)

SECTION 6 Review Answers

1. Answers will vary; could include: check the home, yard, garage, storage areas, basement, and play areas for hazards. (pp. 661–662)

2. cut meat into small pieces, insist children take only small forkfuls of any food, do not allow speaking or laughing with food in their mouths, make sure children chew each bite thoroughly before swallowing, and teach children to bite round pieces of food (grapes, hot dogs, and cherry tomatoes) with their front teeth to crush them. (pp. 662–663)

3. Answers will vary. Refer to the Health Strategies on page 662.

4. Answers will vary.

CLOSE

Have students take a visual trip around the classroom. Have students look for the various safety problems discussed in the chapter. If a young child were to enter the classroom, what would be some hazards that could endanger the child's safety? Discuss this as a class and point out ways the classroom could be made safe.

Reproducible Study Outline and Reading Cloze worksheets for Chapter 24 are provided in the Teacher's Resource Box.

Reproducible Chapter Tests A and B are also provided in the Teacher's Resource Box.

The Teacher's Resource Box contains an extensive checklist that requires students to evaluate their households in terms of fire safety. You may want to distribute and have the students complete the checklist before they read the Straight Talk.

Background Information

Fire and flame cause many child and adolescent deaths each year in the United States. Eighty percent of fire and burn deaths are from home fires. Cigarettes are the leading preventable cause of home fires. Many other fires can be prevented by proper use of smoke detectors. Smoke detectors decrease the risk of fire and burn fatality by 71 percent. For about the price of two movie tickets, a family can dramatically decrease its fire and burn fatality risk. More expensive, but almost infallible, are residential sprinkler systems that are activated when fire breaks out.

Fire Prevention and Escape

Fires and burns are a leading cause of accidental death in the United States. It is worth studying the guidelines offered here on fire prevention, before a time comes when you need them.

That's fine with me. It never hurts to review precautions.

Good. That attitude may save your life. Many fires are caused by children's and adults' careless use of fire. Many fires are also caused by smoking in bed. To prevent these fires:

▶ Don't smoke. If you do, quit. *Or. . .*
▶ Dispose of cigarettes and matches safely. Never assume they are out when they might not be.
▶ Keep matches and lighters out of the reach of children.
▶ Do not smoke in bed. If you do, sooner or later (by the laws of chance) it is virtually certain that you will fall asleep while doing so.

Drinking alcohol and taking other drugs that make people drowsy is particularly hazardous in combination with smoking.

Other fires are caused by cooking and heating equipment. Take these precautions:

▶ Keep cooking and heating equipment clean and in good repair.
▶ If a gas pilot light or a burner on the stove or oven goes out, ventilate the area before lighting a burner. Do not turn electric switches on or off before the area is ventilated, as switches make a tiny spark when used.
▶ Turn pot handles on the stove so that you won't knock them when you walk by. Make sure that children cannot reach them.
▶ Keep the cords of electric cookware on the counter, not dangling.
▶ Keep portable space heaters out of indoor traffic lanes. Turn them off before going to bed. Keep flammable materials away from space heaters.
▶ Keep cloth (curtains, pot holders, your own loose clothing) and other flammable materials away from cooking surfaces and fires.

Still other fires are caused by liquids. Be sure to:

▶ Use flammable liquids only as directed.
▶ Store surplus quantities of flammable liquids outside, in containers designed to hold in fumes as well as fluid.

Also, buy fire-retardant clothes for children. Be especially careful to buy fire-retardant pajamas, nightgowns, and robes.

What if a fire starts? What should I do?

First of all, whenever you go into an unfamiliar building, imagine it going up in flames while you are in it, and plan your escape. Locate the exits, fire escapes, extinguishers, and stairways. (Never use an elevator in a fire.)

enrichment...

In addition to the information in the text you may want to give students a few more guidelines for anticipating and preparing for a house fire:

• Everyone in the family should have a responsibility.
• Older children should look out for younger ones.
• Rehearsals should be conducted in the dark.

Most importantly, make an escape plan for your home. Figure out two ways to get outside from every room. Involve everyone. Make plans to ensure that people with disabilities can get out. Rehearse. Have a fire drill or two. Designate a place to meet outside, so that you can be sure everyone is out.

Picture the fire actually burning in your home. Think through how a fire would spread from one place to another and how you would fight it. Put a fire extinguisher here and another here. Should a fire start, you'll have only about 30 seconds in which to put out the blaze. After that time is up, you must leave.

Remove all trash, so fire will not spread across it. Install an outdoor faucet on all sides of the building, and keep hoses nearby. Advance planning is the only effective weapon. Wishes are of no use in emergencies.

 ### How about installing fire alarms in homes?

By all means do. Maintain them, too. Often, by the time people feel the heat or smell the smoke of a fire, it is too late to get out. Most people die in fires because they are unable to breathe, not because they are burned. Once you hear the alarm, you generally have about three minutes to escape.

The fire alarms most recommended for homes are smoke detectors. They should first be placed in sleeping areas. Additional detectors can be placed in other areas.

Install fire extinguishers, too, but do not put them where the fire is most likely to be. Put them where you can most likely get to them in case of fire. Learn how to use them. Using water on an electrical or chemical fire can do more harm than good (see Figure 24–2 on page 656).

 ### OK, let's say a fire has started. Now what?

Because most fatal home fires happen when the occupants are asleep, it is best to sleep with the bedroom door closed. Smoke can be deadly.

If you are alerted to a fire:

1. Roll out of bed, staying low. Heat rises and may overcome you if you stand up.
2. Crawl quickly to the door. Black smoke may interfere with vision—crawl anyway.
3. Feel the door for heat. If it's cool, open it carefully, but stand behind it. Be ready to slam it shut if smoke or heat rush in. If the door is hot, don't open it. Go some other way.
4. Crawl out quickly. Close doors behind you.
5. Don't go back for pets or possessions—lives have been lost over parakeets and pictures.
6. Don't use elevators during fires; use stairs. If trapped on an upper floor, wrap yourself in a blanket, cover your head, hang out a window, and yell. Don't jump unless you absolutely must.
7. Meet your family as prearranged.
8. Call the fire department from a neighbor's phone.

If your clothes catch fire, do not run. Stop, drop, and roll. To help someone else whose clothes have caught on fire, force the same motion if you can. Then smother the person's flaming clothes with a coat or blanket.

665

- Make sure the plan is realistic and doable. Don't assume anything (that a small child can climb out a window, for example). Practice it to make sure.

- Adults can be hard to wake-up. Children should try to wake the adults but then leave by themselves if they can't arouse the adults.

VOCABULARY

1. Head restraints
2. airbags
3. Answers will vary.

RECALL

SECTION 1

1. 1 out of 3 (p. 645)
2. A defensive driver knows accidents are likely and takes precautions against them. (p. 646)
3. It slows the person's momentum and distributes the force of the impact across the body's strongest parts. It also keeps the driver behind the wheel. (p. 649)
4. Answers will vary. Refer to the Health Strategies on "How to Avoid Alcohol-Related Driving Accidents" on page 650.
5. a. Look over your shoulder when changing lanes. Don't rely on mirrors. **b.** Keep a safe distance from the car in front of you. **c.** Pause five seconds after a red light turns green before proceeding to ensure that no cars are still going through the intersection. (p. 651)

SECTION 2

6. Answers will vary; could include: never dive where obstructions might lurk or where you don't know the depth; don't overestimate your ability; and do not dive too deep. (p. 652)

CHAPTER 24 Review

Summarizing the Chapter

Your ability to respond correctly to the following statements ensures your understanding of the main concepts in the chapter.

1. Describe how being a defensive driver can reduce your risk of accidents.
2. Explain how to reduce the risk of accidents during swimming, boating, biking and play, as well as at home.
3. List specific guidelines for preventing fires and burns.
4. Describe how to prepare for natural disasters.
5. List the safety precautions for child care.

Learning the Vocabulary

head restraints   air bags

Answer the following questions on a separate sheet of paper.

1. _____ are high seat backs or devices attached to seats in cars, intended to prevent neck and spinal cord injury.
2. Inflatable pillows known as _____ are stored in the steering wheels of cars and are designed to inflate on impact.
3. Write a paragraph using the vocabulary terms from the list above. Underline each term.

Recalling Important Facts and Ideas

Section 1

1. What are the chances that someone you know will suffer an injury this year?
2. Describe the attitude of a defensive driver.
3. Explain why safety belts should be worn by all occupants in a car.
4. What are some ways to avoid alcohol-related accidents?

5. Name three changes in driving habits that could save lives.

Section 2

6. List three safety precautions for diving.
7. If you cannot swim, how can you assist a swimmer who is in trouble?
8. List three tips for safe boating.

Section 3

9. What product should be used to smother a grease fire?
10. List the three classes of fire extinguishers and the type of fire each is used for.

Section 4

11. Why are falls the leading cause of accidental death and injury for older people?
12. What are the most common types of falls experienced by infants?
13. Give two firearm safety precautions.

Section 5

14. List at least 5 items you should have on hand to be prepared for natural disasters.

Section 6

15. When baby-sitting, what phone numbers should you be sure to have in your possession before the parents leave?

Straight Talk

16. How can house fires be prevented?
17. What should you do if your clothes catch on fire?

Critical Thinking

1. Imagine the governor of your state has just signed a law stating that all cars must have a device installed that will prevent them from going over 55 mph. Do you agree with this law? Why, or why not? Do you believe it will lower the accident rate? What are the advantages and disadvantages of this law? If you had the power to do so, and money were not a factor, what would you choose as ideal safety features for automobiles?
2. Describe an emergency situation that you personally experienced or witnessed. Comment on how it felt to be at the scene. Do you ever worry about what to do or whether you would panic in an emergency? Why, or why not? Injuries and deaths during emergencies frequently occur because people panic. How can

666

7. Answers will vary. Refer to the Health Strategies on "Water Rescue Techniques" on page 652.

8. Answers will vary; could include: do not operate boating equipment if using alcohol or other drugs; know your boat and rules of the waterway; make sure there are feelings of panic be reduced? What would help people feel calm in an emergency?

3. Why do people take unnecessary risks? Discuss why people behave in unsafe ways when they *know* better. Why do you think most of us think, "It won't happen to me"?

4. Discuss an unnecessary risk you took with your own safety. Describe what you could have done to lessen the risk.

Activities

1. Investigate the different first aid and lifesaving courses that are available in your community this year. Make a poster and list the dates, locations, and any fees for these courses.

2. Using library resources, research disasters that have occurred in your state. Write a brief summary of your findings.

3. Develop a bicycle safety pamphlet. Include illustrations of specific bicycle parts that should be checked periodically, illustrations of hand signals, and information on safety gear. Describe safety precautions to be taken in various traffic and weather conditions.

4. Obtain and read a new car brochure from an automobile dealer in your community. Describe the safety features built into the car. Rate the automobile strictly from a safety viewpoint. Discuss any features you think need to be added to make the car safer. Write a one-page report on your investigation and include the brochure.

5. Interview the fire marshall in your area about the most serious problems the fire department faces. Ask what students can do to help promote fire safety. Hand in an audio tape of your interview.

6. Hand in a list of seven sources of medical help that could be called in the event of an accident. Include the phone number of each source named.

7. Imagine you are a state legislator who is responsible for establishing laws to curtail drinking and driving. Discuss the laws you would propose regarding: suspending and revoking drivers' licenses, plea bargaining, jail sentences, community service, and fines.

8. Investigate the safety belt laws in your state. What are the laws about securing small children? What is the weight or age a small child must reach before being allowed to use the same safety belt as an adult? Are the laws different for front-seat and back-seat passengers? Are there any fines for not wearing a safety belt or for not securing a small child in a car seat? If so, what are they? Write a brief report on your findings.

9. Create a photo essay on accident prevention tips. Use your photographs to portray five basic safety rules that are general enough to apply to most types of accidents and emergencies covered in the chapter.

10. Develop eight original safety slogans for bumper stickers. Design each bumper sticker. Include illustrations on the stickers if you choose.

11. Investigate new safety features that have been introduced into automobile designs in the last 20 years. Make a poster that illustrates these features.

12. Meet with the school nurse to find out what the most common accidents and injuries are at school. List them and identify ways these accidents could be prevented.

13. Bring to class an article from the newspaper about a situation where precautions were not taken at home and a preventable injury (a fall, careless use of tools, toys, guns, or other items) occurred. Work with a partner and discuss both articles. Decide what could or should have been done to prevent the accident. Write a one-page essay explaining what could have been done and why you think the way you do.

Making Decisions about Health

Describe how each of the following situations could best be handled:

1. Your car breaks down on a deserted road at night and you are alone.
2. One of the children you are baby-sitting for has just fallen and received a cut that may require stitches.
3. You are in your home when an earthquake hits.
4. Your friend who is drunk offers you a ride home.
5. The smoke detector in your home has just gone off and woken you from a sound sleep.

SECTION 3

9. baking soda (p. 655)
10. Class A, ordinary fire of paper, wood or cloth; Class B, flammable liquid (gases); Class C, electrical equipment (see Figure 22–2). (p. 656)

SECTION 4

11. balance declines with age (p. 657)
12. falls from tables and bassinets (p. 657)
13. Answers will vary; could include: learn and obey all firearm safety rules; keep guns and ammunition in separate places; and never load a gun until you are ready to fire it. (p. 658)

SECTION 5

14. Answers will vary. Refer to the bulleted list on page 659.

SECTION 6

15. Phone numbers of where the parents will be, one or more neighbors, family doctor or pediatrician, police department or sheriff, and the fire department. (p. 662)

STRAIGHT TALK

16. Answers will vary. Refer to Straight Talk on "Fire Prevention and Escape" starting on page 664.
17. stop, drop, and roll. (p. 665)

enough Coast Guard–approved flotation devices for everyone; load the boat reasonably; keep your weight low in the boat; tell someone on shore where you are going and when to expect you back; if the boat upsets or fills with water, hang on to it; and if the weather is threatening, skip the trip. (p. 653)

KEY POINTS

Chapter 25 is 32 pages long and divided into six sections. This chapter introduces students to first-aid skills and techniques to be used in emergencies. The chapter emphasizes the importance of knowing what emergency measures to use to help protect and possibly save lives. It is recommended that before you begin this chapter, you become a certified instructor in CPR and first aid through the American Red Cross or the American Heart Association.

ACTIVITY TO INTRODUCE THE CHAPTER

Call your community's department responsible for fire and rescue. Ask to have rescue personnel come to your school in their truck to show students their equipment for CPR and first-aid emergencies. Ask the emergency medical technicians to explain to students the nature of their work, the most frequent type of call they respond to, what their response time is, how citizens contact their local fire and rescue, and how well the community deals with the emergency situations before rescue arrives.

Have students each write one question on an index card. Give the cards to the EMTs when they arrive so that all students' questions can be answered.

After the rescue personnel have finished their presentation, have students summarize the presentation by listing five new ideas they learned and writing one paragraph about the importance of knowing CPR and first aid.

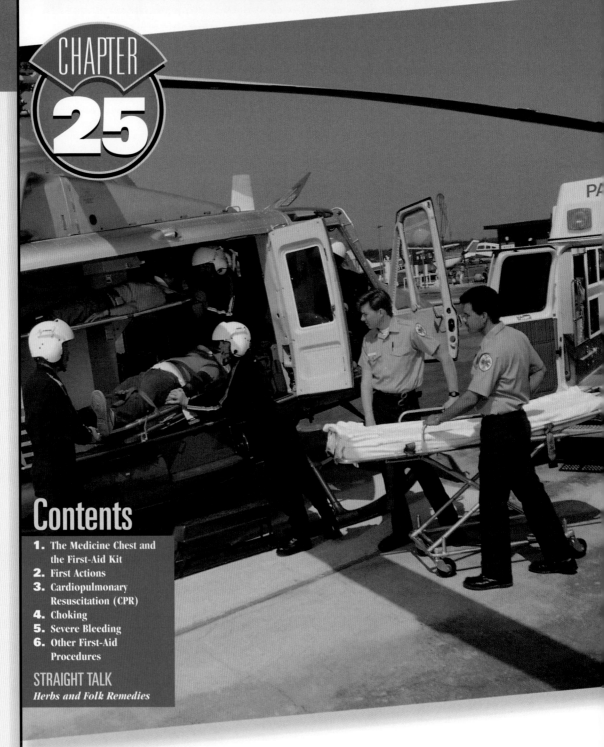

CHAPTER 25

Contents

NOT Enough Time?

Following are some suggestions to help you make sure that you cover the key topics in this chapter if you have limited time. (Refer to the daily lesson plans in your Teacher's Resource Box for additional suggestions.)

DAY 1 On Day 1 read aloud Chapter 25 as a class. Pick several students to read the various sections. At the end of each section, discuss the key points.

Emergency Measures

FACT or FICTION

What do you think? Are the following statements true or false? If you think they are false, then say what is true.

1. To be of real help in an emergency, a person needs mainly to keep a level head and use common sense.
2. Disposable rubber gloves are one of the most important self-protective items to have in a first-aid kit.
3. The first thing to do in an emergency is to move the victim away from the scene to prevent further upset.
4. A person in a state of shock is experiencing a normal and common emotional reaction that will soon pass on its own.
5. A person who is choking typically makes no sound at all.
6. The first thing to do for a person who has a bleeding wound is to apply a tourniquet.
7. A light sunburn is a first-degree burn.
8. One of the best things to do when frostbite sets in is to rub the affected body part.
9. The best way to determine if a victim has broken any bones is to lift each limb and move it at its joints.

(Answers on page 692)

Introduction

In an emergency, fast, effective action can save a life, perhaps your own. Many people die needlessly after accidents each year because no one nearby knows how to help effectively. This chapter presents some basic emergency measures. However, understand that reading alone cannot adequately prepare you to be of real help in an emergency. Also, attempts to help without the right knowledge can many times do more harm than good.

Take a class from a qualified instructor who teaches **first aid**. This chapter's task is to make you aware that emergencies do arise, and that your actions can make a difference. The Life Choice Inventory will show you the basics you need in order to be really helpful in emergencies.

First and most important is to know how to call for help in emergencies. A single call to the number 911 will, in most communities, connect you right away with a **dispatcher**.

The dispatcher can, with one call, send out a team of people who can help. These people, plus poison control centers and hospital emergency room personnel, are all known as the **emergency medical service (EMS)**.

Answers to

FACT or FICTION

1. **False.** To be of real help, and not make things worse, the helper needs to apply training gained through a class in first aid from a qualified instructor.
2. **True.**
3. **False.** The first thing to do in an emergency is to inspect the scene to determine what happened. Move the victim only if the scene presents immediate danger.
4. **False.** A person in a state of shock is experiencing a *physical* reaction to injury. Shock is a dangerous condition, and first-aid treatment is recommended.
5. **True.**
6. **False.** You should not use a tourniquet to control bleeding. A tourniquet almost always kills the limb to which it is applied.
7. **True.**
8. **False.** Frostbitten parts should be handled gently to prevent tissue destruction.
9. **False.** The best way to determine if a victim has broken any bones is to ask the person to move each joint. Forcing limbs with broken bones to move can worsen a break.

DAY 2 On Day 2 do the Activity to Introduce the Chapter on page 668, inviting rescue personnel with their truck to the school to share with your class how they respond to emergency cases.

DAY 3 On Day 3 have students score themselves using the Life Choice Inventory, "How Well Prepared for Emergencies Are You?" found on page 669. Students may then determine how well prepared they would be in responding to a medical emergency.

SECTION 1

FOCUS

OUTCOMES

In this section students will learn:

1. What standard supplies should be stocked in the home medicine chest and portable first-aid kit.
2. That rubber gloves and a face shield are useful devices for self-protection against the risk of contracting AIDS and other communicable diseases.

FOCUS ACTIVITY

Divide your class into four groups and assign each group one of the four categories of supplies found in Figure 25–1. Tell students to brainstorm possible substitutes for each item in their group's category. Discuss.

TEACH & APPLY

DISCUSSION

Ask students if there is one place in their homes where medical and first-aid supplies are stored. Without checking at home first, can students name which of the items listed on this page are contained in their medicine chests? After discussing this in class, have students inspect their home medicine chests and use Figure 25–1 to determine whether they have the standard supplies recommended. Discuss their results.

Figure 25–1 *Standard Supplies for the Medicine Chest*

SECTION 1

The Medicine Chest and the First-Aid Kit

To best offer emergency treatment, you need the right supplies and the right training. The equipment of a well-stocked home medicine chest is listed in Figure 25–1. On trips, take along a first-aid kit, so that the supplies will go wherever you go. The items marked with an asterisk (*) in

Items marked with an asterisk (*) should be included in a first-aid kit kept in the car.

Item	Purpose
For Disease Prevention	
*Disposable rubber gloves	To protect you from disease when you assist a bleeding person
*Antiseptic Hand Cleaners	To remove infectious organisms from your hands
Bandages and Dressings	
*Ace bandages, 3-inch	To wrap and hold sterile dressings or splints in place
*Rolled white gauze bandages, 2- and 3-inch widths	To wrap and hold sterile dressings or splints in place
*Ready-to-apply sterile first-aid dressings, individually packaged, various sizes	To apply directly to open wounds or burns
*Triangular bandages, 36 x 36 inches	To fold diagonally, as slings for fractured or broken arms or shoulders; To hold dressings in place; to make into folded compresses
*Rolls of sticky tape, 2- and 3-inch widths	To be cut to size for simple wounds
*Band-Aids, various widths and shapes	To cover minor cuts and scrapes
Medicines	
Aspirin or aspirin substitute[a]	To relieve pain
*Antiseptic cream or petroleum jelly	To prevent bandages from sticking to minor wounds; to reduce chance of infection by some disease-causing organisms.
*Liquid antiseptic	To cleanse skin surfaces in cases of minor wounds
Calamine lotion	To relieve itching from insect bites or exposure to skin irritants
Syrup of ipecac[b]	To induce vomiting in certain cases of poisoning if told to do so
Activated charcoal[b]	To treat certain cases of poisoning if told to do so
Miscellaneous	
*Adhesive tape	To fasten bandages or dressings
*Large safety pins	To fasten bandages or slings
Tweezers	To remove splinters or insect stingers
*Blunt-tipped scissors	To cut lengths of bandages, adhesive tape, and the like
Thermometer(s)	To take rectal or oral temperature
Hypoallergenic soap	To cleanse wounds
*Absorbent cotton, paper tissues	To wipe and cleanse wounds
*Chemically activated cold pack	To prevent or reduce swelling
*Small flashlight (and extra batteries)	To improve visibility after dark

[a]Reye's syndrome is a rare and potentially life threatening condition linked to aspirin use associated with chicken pox or flu. Children and teenagers should never take aspirin. They should be treated with an aspirin substitute such as acetaminophen.
[b]You should have these supplies on hand so that when you call for help in an emergency, you can use them as directed.

Ability Levels

Assign each student to assemble a medicine kit for their car, bicycle, or backback, using the list of standard supplies for the medicine chest in this chapter. Have the students put their medicine kit in a convenient receptacle such as a plastic box or coffee can, appropri-ately labeled. Have each student write a list of the contents and use of each item it contains. It may include the following items:

- disposable rubber gloves
- antiseptic hand cleaners
- Ace bandages
- rolled white gauze bandages

Figure 25–1 are all a traveling first-aid kit need contain. A first-aid course will teach you to use the equipment properly.

The risk of contracting an infectious disease makes it important to follow the procedures in the Health Strategies section "Reducing Disease Risks" on page 672 and to have self-protective items in your first-aid kit. The two most useful devices are shown in Figure 25–2. Disposable rubber gloves will protect you from exposure to the blood or body fluids of anyone who might have a disease. A good soap-and-water washing before and after administering first aid removes disease-causing organisms from your hands. When an accident occurs out of reach of soap and water, waterless antiseptic hand cleansers can do the same thing. Use them before giving aid, to protect the victim's wounds from the germs on your hands. Use them afterward, too, to kill any germs from a victim's blood or body fluids.

If you don't have the supplies named in Figures 25–1 and 25–2, find substitutes. For example, if you have no gauze to cover wounds or burns, substitute freshly laundered clothing. A standard reference, such as the American Red Cross publication *Standard First Aid*, will help remind you of what to do in emergencies. Keep one close at hand.

KEY POINTS *To help in emergencies, a person must have access to basic first-aid supplies or make substitutes from materials at hand.*

***Figure 25–2** Products for Preventing the Spread of Diseases During First Aid*

Use disposable rubber gloves to avoid contact with blood or body fluids.

Use waterless antiseptic hand cleaners to kill germs before and after giving care.

SECTION 1 Review

Learning the Vocabulary

The vocabulary terms in this section are *first aid, dispatcher,* and *emergency medical service (EMS).*

1. Write a sentence using each vocabulary term.

Learning the Facts

2. What is the first and most important thing to do in an emergency?

3. What do you need to have to best offer emergency treatment?

4. What are two items needed in your first-aid kits that will help reduce the chance of contracting an infectious disease?

Making Life Choices

5. Look at Figure 25–1. Do you have a first-aid kit at home? If not, why not? If so, does it have all the items listed in Figure 25–1? Do you have first-aid kits in your car(s)?

MINI Glossary

first aid: literally, "help given first"—medical help given immediately in an emergency, before the victim is transported to a hospital or treatment center.

dispatcher: a person who answers calls and relays messages to the proper helping service.

emergency medical service (EMS): a team of people who are trained to respond in emergencies, and who can be contacted through a single dispatcher.

- ready-to-apply sterile first aid dressings, various packages
- triangular bandages
- adhesive tape
- Band-Aids, various widths and shapes
- antiseptic cream
- petroleum jelly
- liquid antiseptic
- large safety pins
- blunt-tipped scissors
- absorbent cotton, paper tissues

- chemically activated cold pack
- small flashlight (and extra batteries)

Note:
- Avoid packing products with expiration dates. Soap and water are good cleaning agents for minor wounds.
- Petroleum jelly is not likely to produce allergic reactions.
- Don't use hydrogen peroxide to clean wounds—it can cause scarring.

FOCUS

OUTCOMES

In this section students will learn:

1. The necessity for making assessments when an emergency strikes.

2. The three action steps to take in sequence when dealing with an emergency.

FOCUS ACTIVITY

To get students thinking critically and to raise their interest, open class with a dramatic scene planned ahead of time with the cooperation of student volunteers. An example could be: a student is passed out on the floor, broken plastic is scattered around to represent broken glass, water is on the floor, and an electric cord is lying across the victim (student), who is cut and bleeding. Ask students observing the scene to list on a piece of paper all the actions *you* take as you enter and deal with this "emergency." Display both correct and incorrect actions as you proceed through the three action steps identified in this section of the chapter. (Give them about five minutes to observe this scene.) Ask students to look over their lists and mark each action observed with either a Y (yes) for those actions they view as being correct or an N (no) for those actions they view as incorrect. Initiate a discussion in which students share what they observed about your actions. Ask, "What should I have done that you did not see me do?" Next, ask the students to read Section 2, "First Actions" and

For Your Information

Call for help, then proceed. Calls to 911 are free, even from pay phones.

Health Strategies

Reducing Disease Risks

To minimize your contact with someone else's blood or other body fluids:

► Place a barrier between you and the fluid, such as rubber gloves, plastic wrap, or plastic bags.

► Keep your hands away from your own face or any other opening on your body during and after giving treatments.

► Wash your hands with soap and water after providing treatment. Wash under nails gently with a soft brush.

special needs

Linguistic or Bodily-kinesthetic

Some of your students may think that emergencies only happen to other people. To assist your students in internalizing the emergency procedures learned in this chapter, you may want to use one of the following activities.

First Actions

When emergency strikes, what should you do? Take a moment to think clearly and take these three actions:

Step 1. Survey the scene for safety and information, and inspect the victim swiftly (two to four minutes). Help only if there are immediate threats to life.

Step 2. Phone for help (two to three minutes).

Step 3. Inspect the victim more closely (two to five minutes).

The sections that follow describe each of these three actions.

Step 1: Survey of Scene and Victims (2 to 4 Minutes)

In surveying the scene quickly, you should ask yourself:

► Is it safe?
► What has happened?
► Are there victims? How many?

Get someone to call for help right away if you can.

As for yourself, first and foremost, don't rush in. Look around. Is it safe? Are hazards present, such as fire, fumes, fast traffic, live electrical wires, or fast-moving water? If the hazards are extreme, do not attempt rescue. Placing yourself in harm's way serves no one. Don't let haste or a false sense of bravery make you a victim.

As you survey the scene, survey the people around you. Might there be other victims nearby? Who can help by controlling crowds, or by directing traffic? Ask them to do whatever is needed.

Do Not Move Most Victims Do not move anyone. Assume that every accident victim has an injured neck or spine. Further injury to the spinal cord can cause permanent paralysis or death. Tell the injured person not to move.

The only exception to this rule is if you must move someone away from fire, water, poisonous gas, or other dangers to save a life *and* if you can do so safely.

If you must move someone, and can do so safely, keep on assuming that the spine may be injured. Move the person the shortest possible distance. Keep the head and body in line. If possible, pull from the head end, with your hands under the shoulders and the head resting on your arms. Pull the person in a straight line.

If the person is floating in water face down, you must move the person a little. (Remember, don't risk your own life.) If you can walk in and stand while you do it, roll the person face up as a unit. Then pull the person out of the water just enough to permit you to start giving breathing help.

1. Ask students to think back on experiences they have had that involved an emergency situation of some sort. Ask them to write a short narrative explaining the situation and also detailing their reactions and feelings regarding the emergency. They might also write about how the emergency should have been handled based on the information they have learned in this chapter. If

In an emergency call 911.

Determining Who to Help First   If several people are injured, help first the one who seems to need your help most, and can benefit from it. Most urgent is to help those with the life-threatening A, B, C, and S conditions described on the next page.

Talking to the Victim   First, speak to the person. Reassure: "I am here to help you." Get information: "What happened?" Caution: "Please don't try to move until help arrives."

The responses to what you say will tell you things you must report when you call for help. A victim who can answer you is conscious. An inappropriate answer may suggest injury to the head.

If the victim cannot speak, look around quickly for clues. For example, should you find an unconscious person lying near a tipped canoe in shallow water, you might suspect that the person had inhaled water or sustained a blow to the head. On finding a crying child lying near a bicycle, you might suspect broken bones, and so on.

Say who you are. If the victim can talk, you must ask for permission to help. If you have been trained by a professional instructor, say so. However, you cannot make the claim of being trained in first aid after simply reading a chapter such as this one.

Life-Threatening Conditions   In inspecting each victim, you are looking for the four life-threatening conditions shown in Figure 25–3, and for three other conditions that you may need to report when you call for help. The four life-threatening conditions you must look for are:

A Airway—is it blocked?
B Breathing—has it stopped?
C Circulation—has the heartbeat stopped?
S Severe bleeding—is blood pulsing or welling up from a wound?

The other three things to notice are:

▶ Is the person conscious?
▶ Does the person have a neck or spinal injury?
▶ Is the person in shock?

For A, B, C, and S, you must give help right away. Courses that teach **CPR**, or **cardiopulmonary resuscitation**, explain how to approach the

For **Y**our **I**nformation
Before giving first aid to a conscious person, you *must* ask for permission from that person.

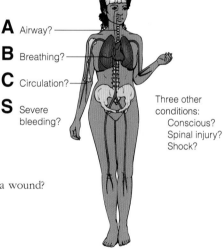

A Airway?

B Breathing?

C Circulation?

S Severe bleeding?

Three other conditions:
Conscious?
Spinal injury?
Shock?

Figure 25–3 *The Primary Survey: A, B, C, S*

"Step 1: Survey the Scene and the Victims," beginning on page 672. Allow them about five minutes for reading. Now, ask them again what was right or wrong with your actions. Repeat this for each of the three action steps discussed on pages 672–677. (Read and react; assessing the previously enacted scene.)

TEACH & APPLY

COMPREHENSION CHECK

A great deal of information is provided to the students early in the chapter. After students have read the explanations in Step 1, have them close their books and, as a group, see how many of the procedures they can remember. Some key points are:

a. Get someone to call for help.
b. Assess the danger—don't put yourself in jeopardy.
c. Determine if someone else can help.
d. Avoid moving the injured party or move the person as little as possible.
e. Help the person who needs it most, first.
f. Get information from the patient, if possible.
g. Look for clues to what happened.

CLASS ACTIVITY

To review the three steps to take when emergency strikes, have the students list the three major steps on the board. Have the students give more detailed instructions on what to do in an emergency under each step. Have all students participate until the list is complete.

they have not had an experience with an emergency firsthand, you may want to have them interview someone who has had to deal with an emergency. They can then write a short report based on that information.

2. Using situations students have experienced, ask students to role play. You may want to have them first dramatize a situa-

tion as it actually happened. Then discuss the emergency and alternative courses of action. Finally, ask the students to dramatize how the situation could have been handled more effectively based on the things they have learned as they studied this chapter.

TEACHER SUPPORT

Key Passage

You may want to give students some additional information at this point about shock. Tell them that the state of shock may develop rapidly or may be delayed until hours after the event. Shock occurs to some degree after every injury; it may be so slight as not to be noticed or so serious that it results in death even though the injuries received ordinarily would not prove fatal. Some of the major causes of shock are severe loss of blood, intense pain, severe injury, burns, anxiety, poisonous gases, surgical operations, extremes of heat or cold, electrical shock, allergic reactions, bites and stings of poisonous snakes or insects, poisons taken internally, certain illnesses, emotional stress, and intense emotion.

BACKGROUND INFORMATION

Have students investigate the Good Samaritan laws in your state. (A Good Samaritan law is one that protects people who help others in emergencies from being sued for accidentally doing the wrong thing or not doing the right thing.)

Get a copy of your state's Good Samaritan laws, read it for your students, and discuss the degree of protection afforded to the rescuer. Ask students for examples of what might constitute gross negligence or willful misconduct.

first three of these conditions. Often you can rule them out, but if you can't, you must check for these immediate threats to life. Concentrate, and do not let anyone interrupt you. Inspect the victims, allowing just a minute or two for each. Follow these steps.

Airway and Breathing To check for a blocked airway and for breathing, place your ear and cheek close to the victim's mouth and nose. Look, listen, and use the sensitive skin of your cheek to feel for breathing, as shown in Figure 25–4. Chest movements alone don't mean breathing is occurring. They may just be muscle spasms that mimic breathing.

Circulation At the same time, determine if the person's heart is beating. Take the **carotid pulse**, also depicted in Figure 25–4. To be sure you'll be able to find it in an emergency, practice on yourself right now.

Severe Bleeding The spurting of blood from a large artery can reduce the body's supply of blood dangerously in just seconds. Respond quickly to stop it as instructed on page 686.

Calling for Help While providing care, keep shouting for help if no one has called yet. If no one responds, then wait to call until after you have controlled airway, breathing, circulation, and severe bleeding the best you can.

Next Conditions to Note When the vital four conditions are controlled, check or review three other things. Then go make your call. To review, here are the three:

▶ Is the victim conscious?
▶ Are neck and other spinal injuries a possibility?
▶ Is the victim in shock?

You have checked to see if the person is conscious. You have surveyed the scene and determined what has happened, so you have some idea whether neck or other spinal injuries have occurred. Also check for **shock**.

In shock, the circulation is disrupted. Shock has many causes, but it presents one danger: it can cause death. It is very common in accident victims. It can come on fast, or in stages. At first, blood flow to the brain may diminish, causing loss of consciousness. Blood supply to other vital organs may also fail, and the heart itself may fail.

The signs and symptoms of shock are shown in Figure 25–5. It demands professional emergency treatment. Call for help. After you've called, take the steps listed in the Health Strategies section "First Aid for Shock." The first aid is simple and should be offered to all accident victims. Other injuries, such as broken bones, can wait.

Health Strategies

First Aid for Shock

To reduce the risk of shock:

▶ Lay the person flat to ease circulation. Elevate only those body parts that have been treated for bleeding. The feet may be raised slightly by resting them on a folded blanket or other object if there is no chest bleeding.

▶ Loosen any tight clothing, particularly collars, belts, and waistbands.

▶ Help the person maintain normal body temperature. For example, if the person appears overly cool or chilled, try to cover the person with blankets.

▶ Normally it is best to give *no* food or liquids to people in shock. However, if the victim is conscious and has no abdominal or head injuries, and if help is not likely to arrive within an hour, you may want to give very small amounts of room-temperature fluids every 15 minutes. If salt is available, add ⅛ teaspoon or less to each half glass of fluid.

 KEY POINTS *The first action in an emergency is to survey the scene to determine whether or not it is safe, what may have happened, and who is available to help. The first inspection of a victim serves to identify and treat for the four life-threatening conditions—(A) blocked airway, (B) failure to breathe, (C) no circulation, and (S) severe bleeding. Give help for these and call for help. Inspect for consciousness, spinal injuries, and shock.*

COOPERATIVE LEARNING

Divide the class into small groups. Give each group either a type of potential accident (burn, cut, food poisoning, and so on) or a location in the house (kitchen, bathroom, and so on). Have each group use this assignment to compile a list of potential household accidents that could occur. Possibilities for types

of accidents include, in addition to those listed above, lead poisoning (from water, faucets, pipes, dishes, paint), falls, and chemical poisoning (from household cleaning products, medications, and so on). Encourage students to think through the various careless actions which can lead to accidents, such as spilling boiling liquids, leaving handles sticking out so children can pull pans of hot food off the stove and onto themselves, carelessly

Figure 25–4 Airway, Breathing, and Circulation. Look, listen, and feel: Look *at the person's chest for the rise and fall of breathing.* Listen *for breathing.* Feel *with your cheek for moving air.* Feel *for the carotid pulse.*

Touch the Adam's apple lightly, using two fingers.

Slide your fingers into the groove next to the Adam's apple. You should feel a pulse (the carotid pulse).

In an infant, look for a pulse in the arm.

Figure 25–5 Signs and Symptoms of Shock

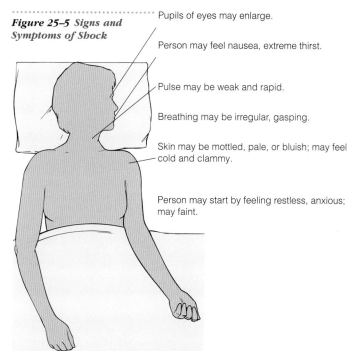

Pupils of eyes may enlarge.

Person may feel nausea, extreme thirst.

Pulse may be weak and rapid.

Breathing may be irregular, gasping.

Skin may be mottled, pale, or bluish; may feel cold and clammy.

Person may start by feeling restless, anxious; may faint.

MINI Glossary

CPR (cardiopulmonary resuscitation): a technique of maintaining blood and oxygen flow through the body of a person whose heart and breathing have stopped.

carotid (ca-ROT-id) **pulse:** the pulse in either of the carotid arteries, the main arteries next to the airway (and "Adam's apple") in the front of the neck.

shock: failure or disruption of the blood circulation, a life-threatening reaction to accidents and injuries.

opening something steam-filled from the microwave oven, keeping blow dryers or electric curling irons with damaged cords, using electrical appliances near the bathtub, and using unsafe methods of getting to high shelves.

When each group has compiled a list of several household accidents, have the groups exchange their lists. Each group is then to go through its new list and write out ways to pre-

vent each accident. Encourage students to provide multiple solutions to each accident-prone situation. When the groups have completed their work, have them share their solutions with the class. Discuss the answers. Complete the discussion with a review of the first aid procedures which would be involved with each of the potential accidents discussed.

BACKGROUND INFORMATION

At this point, you may want to refer students back to Chapter 17 for a quick review of the cardiovascular system. Then tell them that cardiopulmonary resuscitation is a lifesaving technical procedure that requires exactness and good physical coordination. Simple textbook knowledge on how to administer CPR is not enough. Correct practice at frequent intervals is required. A mannequin—not a healthy person—should be used during CPR practice sessions. Training in a formal course of instruction is offered and certified by either the American Heart Association or the American National Red Cross.

GROUP ACTIVITY

Have students move into groups of two or three. After looking over Figure 25–4, have them take turns being the victim and the rescuer. Make sure that they check through the ABC's thoroughly (Airway, Breathing, and Circulation). Remind them that their quick and practiced actions could be the difference between life and death for an unconscious victim. On the first turn it may be helpful to work on the steps together (Look, Listen, and Feel).

CLASS ACTIVITY

Have the students list the signs and symptoms of shock on the board. Have them explain how to reduce the risk of shock, using the information from the Health Strategies as reinforcement.

GUEST SPEAKER

Invite a Red Cross or American Heart Association volunteer/instructor to visit your class to talk to your students about taking a CPR course. Ask the speaker to include the following:

1. locations where classes are offered
2. times when classes meet
3. which courses are offered
4. which certifications can be earned
5. number of hours of training required for certifications
6. age requirements
7. validity periods for certifications
8. cost for taking a course
9. which courses are needed for jobs in day care and lifeguarding

ROLE PLAYING

Tell students, "Pretend you are a rescuer in an accident. Create a scenario and write the report you would give on the phone to rescue personnel when calling in the accident." Students should include the six areas to report listed under "Step 2: Calling for Help," on this page.

ASSESS

EVALUATE

A reproducible quiz for Section 2 is provided in the Teacher's Resource Box.

FAST FACTS

Some people have been saved after as many as eight hours of artificial respiration.

Step 2: Calling for Help (2 to 3 Minutes)

When you call for help, you must report:

▶ Your name.
▶ Where you are.
▶ The telephone number you are calling from.
▶ What has happened.
▶ How many victims there are.
▶ How each is hurt.

In a serious emergency, it is urgent that someone call for help at the earliest possible moment. If you are the only one available and you have been trained in first-aid techniques, give first aid first, then call.

The key to making an effective call is to be prepared to give the needed information. If you send someone else to make the call, be sure that person knows all the needed information.

Here is an example of a poor accident report: "I'm somewhere downtown, and I've just seen an accident. It's awful. Please come quickly." (Click.)

Here is an example of a useful report: "This is Kevin White. I'm at the intersection of Adams and Congress Streets, at the pay phone. The number here is 625-4949. A truck has hit a car head-on, and two people were thrown out of the car. One is bleeding, not badly, but I think he's going into shock. He's very pale, his hands are cold, and he seems confused. The other one is trapped under the car. He's unconscious but breathing OK. Before losing consciousness, he said he had no feeling in his legs. The truck driver is OK. I have a first-aid kit with me, but I haven't been trained in first aid. What do you want me to do?"

From the second report, the dispatcher knows how many ambulances and what personnel and equipment to send. The caller kept a level head and gathered all the necessary information before calling.

 Call emergency services. Provide accurate information.

Step 3: Secondary Survey of Victims (2 to 5 Minutes)

The secondary survey is a head-to-toe survey, and should be swift. You have checked for life-threatening conditions, have controlled the ones you can, and have called for help. Now you are inspecting the victim for less severe, but still serious, injuries. Such injuries may require first aid to prevent their getting worse.

The best way to start is to ask the victim about pain. Injured areas usually hurt (although spinal injuries may not). Pain in breathing indicates a problem in the

Health Strategies

Summary of Emergency Actions

A helper should first take these actions in the order listed:

▶ Survey the scene for any danger, such as traffic or toxic gases. Take action to evade danger.
▶ Don't help if you are likely to lose your life or be severely injured yourself.
▶ Assume each victim's neck is broken. Do not move anyone at all, except to escape immediate danger.
▶ Check quickly for life-threatening conditions: (A) blocked airway, (B) no breathing, (C) no circulation, (S) severe bleeding.
▶ If any of these are present, quickly take appropriate steps to correct them.
▶ Call or have someone else call emergency services for help.
▶ Check or recheck for consciousness, spinal injuries, and shock.
▶ Inspect the victim again to identify other injuries.
▶ Do nothing to worsen injuries and do not rush recovery.
▶ Provide first aid for each condition.
▶ Maintain the victim's temperature and comfort.

Chapter 25, Section 2

The following quiz will help you assess your students' understanding of the material covered in this section of the chapter. You might use the quiz as an oral exercise, which will lead into a class discussion of the topics covered. Or, you might use it as a paper/pencil

quiz to evaluate your students individually.

1. The first thing you should do in an emergency is to start treating the victim. (False)
2. You should always check the scene for safety hazards before trying to help. (True)
3. You should always try to move an injured person away from the scene of an accident. (False)
4. You should make a quick inspection of

chest or abdomen. Don't touch or move the painful part, except to provide the needed aid.

Conduct a rapid inspection, not more than five minutes in duration. Start with the head and work downward. Look for bumps, bruises, blood, or any odd formations or positions of body parts. Repeat: if you suspect head, neck, or back injuries, do not move the person at all except to get out of immediate danger.

Healthy limbs move freely. If you do not suspect neck or back injuries, ask the person to *slowly* move each joint. For example, a person with a broken collar bone would not be able to shrug the shoulders. Do not lift or try to move the joints for the victim. You may dislocate the ends of a broken bone or worsen other injuries in doing so.

During this close inspection of the victim, keep the person lying quietly until you are certain no serious injury exists. Meanwhile, help defend the person's body temperature. Provide blankets, if necessary. Help the victim rest comfortably. Treat all conditions according to the instructions in the following sections. Always stay aware of the person's breathing and heartbeat.

The Health Strategies section on the previous page, "Summary of Emergency Actions," reviews the first actions to take in emergencies as described so far. The three next sections return to the A, B, C life-threatening conditions to give details of treatment. Later sections discuss aid for the S condition, and another: choking.

> **66** *A timid person is frightened before a danger, and a coward during the time, and a courageous person afterwards.* **99**
>
> John Paul Richter
> (1763–1825)
> German writer

KEY POINTS *A close inspection of the victim can reveal injuries that require treatment to prevent further damage.*

SECTION 2 Review

Learning the Vocabulary

The vocabulary terms in this section are *CPR (cardiopulmonary resuscitation), carotid pulse,* and *shock.*

1. Match each of the following phrases with the vocabulary term from above:
  a. the heartbeat in the main arteries in the front of the neck
  b. techniques of maintaining blood and oxygen flow through the body of a person whose heart has stopped
  c. life-threatening reaction to injuries

Learning the Facts

2. What should you always assume about an accident victim?
3. What are the four life-threatening conditions to look for when calling for help?
4. What information should you report when you call for help?

Making Life Choices

5. Reread the Health Strategies section entitled "Summary of Emergency Actions." Why is it important to follow these steps in order? How can you encourage other people to learn these steps?

the scene of an accident and the victims before phoning for help. (True)
5. The four life-threatening conditions you should look for in an injured person are blocked air passage, difficulty breathing, stopped heartbeat, and severe bleeding. (True)
6. Shock is very common in accident victims, and does not require emergency medical treatment. (False)
7. When calling for help, you should give

as much information as you can and be as specific as possible. (True)
8. In your secondary survey of the victims, you should look for bumps, bruises, odd positioning of body parts, and bleeding. (True)
9. You should move the victim's joints when checking for broken bones. (False)
10. You should keep the victim lying quietly until you are absolutely certain no serious injury exists. (True)

SECTION 2 Review Answers

1. a. carotid pulse
  b. CPR (cardiopulmonary resuscitation)
  c. shock
2. that every accident victim has an injured neck or spine (p. 672)
3. blocked airway, no breathing, no circulation, severe bleeding (p. 673)
4. your name, where you are, the telephone number you are calling from, what has happened, how many victims there are, how each is hurt (p. 676)
5. Answers will vary.

CLOSE

Before going on to the next section, students should be able to answer these questions:

1. List three emergency action steps, in proper sequence, when dealing with an emergency situation.
2. For each of the three steps, explain why you take the step, and how you carry it out.
3. List three possible risk categories for the rescuer when giving aid in an emergency situation.
4. State the rule regarding moving a victim.
5. State the only exception to the rule regarding moving a victim.
6. How do you check the person for a clear airway, breathing, and circulation? Discuss the answers to these questions in class.

SECTION 3

FOCUS

OUTCOMES

In this section students will learn:

1. What to do to deliver air to a person who has stopped breathing.

2. That CPR is a life-sustaining technique when a victim is not breathing and has no pulse.

3. Everyone can and should be trained by a certified instructor before attempting to perform CPR.

FOCUS ACTIVITY

A heart attack victim often needs CPR to save his or her life. To help students recognize a heart attack in progress, review the warning signs of a heart attack and stroke from Chapter 17 (page 462). **1.** Ask students to name as many symptoms as they can remember. **2.** List the symptoms on the board as they are identified. End this activity by having a student find the heart attack and stroke symptoms in Chapter 17 for the purpose of checking to see that none have been overlooked.

COMPREHENSION CHECK

Have the students write summaries of the details of CPR techniques for A, B, C emergencies. Be sure they include descriptions of preparing to give breathing assistance, opening the airway, and rescue breathing. Ask for a few volunteers to read their summaries aloud as a way to review the correct answers.

SECTION 3
Cardiopulmonary Resuscitation (CPR)

Someone who has stopped breathing and who has no pulse needs help fast. CPR combines breathing and heartbeat assistance that can sustain life until EMS help arrives. This section describes CPR techniques appropriate for A, B, C emergencies—airway, breathing, and circulation.

A: Opening the Airway

If breathing stops, restoring it is urgent. Within five minutes after breathing stops, death occurs in over 50 percent of people. Almost all others die within ten minutes. Many emergencies can stop a person's breathing: allergic reactions, burns, drug overdoses, poisoning, and others.

A first step to restoring breathing is opening the airway. Don't move the person unless you have to, for access. If you move the person, keep the spine straight. Position the person, and clear the mouth as shown in Figure 25–6.

Even now, the airway may be collapsed shut. Open it without disturbing the neck bones as shown in Figure 25–7.

KEY POINTS *When breathing stops, restoring it is urgent. Opening the airway is the first step to restoring breathing.*

B: Breathing Assistance

To learn to properly perform the rescue breathing method described here, a person should obtain first-aid training and practice on a model of a victim. Several hazards make the procedure risky for untrained people to try:

Figure 25–6 Preparing to Give Breathing Assistance

1. If you must roll the person over, keep the spine straight as shown.

2. Use a finger. Be careful. Don't push anything down the throat. Sweep out anything you find in the mouth.

HEALTHY PEOPLE 2000

Reduce nonfatal spinal cord injuries so that hospitalizations for this condition are no more than 5 per 100,000 people.

Spinal cord injuries are catastrophic health events resulting in enormous human and economic costs. Estimates of spinal cord injury in the United States range from 2.8 to 5 per 100,000 people. Approximately 40 percent of spinal cord injuries are fatal, but data on spinal cord injuries in people dying prior to receiving treatment are inadequate. Males sustain about 80 percent of spinal cord injuries. Adolescents and young adults (aged 15 through 24) are at highest risk of spinal cord injuries, which result in lifelong needs for

▶ If you blow air into the stomach, it may cause vomiting. This can block the airway and make breathing impossible.

▶ If you try to move the head of someone with a neck injury, it may cause permanent paralysis.

▶ You have to know when to stop giving assistance. When a victim begins to breathe spontaneously (on his or her own) but weakly, continued efforts on your part using a different rhythm may shut down the victim's spontaneous breathing.

▶ If you force air into a drowning person's lungs when the person is struggling to cough up water, you may push water into the lungs.

▶ The procedures for helping adults can harm infants.

The details are too numerous to cover adequately in this chapter, but too important to skip. For these reasons, the next two figures (see page 680) show how to give breathing assistance to an adult (Figure 25–8), or to a child or infant (Figure 25–9). You are urged to take a first-aid course, though, to master the techniques. You will be better prepared to save a life if you do.

Figure 25–7 *Opening the Airway*

If head and neck are flat on the ground, the tongue can block the airway.

Tongue is blocking airway.

Tongue is out of the way and airway is open.

Hold the forehead, lift the chin, and the tongue will move out of the way.

Alternative: Open the jaw without moving the neck, as shown.

Infant: Tilt the head back. The force of your breath will open the airway.

special services and reduced potential for employment.

Motor vehicle crashes are the primary cause of spinal cord injuries in the United States, accounting for about 50 percent of the cases. Falls are the second leading cause, followed by diving. In some urban settings, firearms and assaults are the major causes.

Some spinal cord injuries occur after con-

tact with the health care system. Appropriate handling of injured persons by medical care personnel will reduce the incidence of these injuries. Proper handling will also avoid more severe injury to those already injured. Increasing the awareness of emergency medical service personnel and others should be a priority for training programs and other injury prevention programs.

DISCUSSION

Tell students to guard against the following common mistakes made while administering rescue breathing:

a. failure to give two full breaths initially

b. failure to allow the victim to exhale between breaths; the lungs must deflate fully

c. giving too many or too few breaths

d. not keeping an adult's head tilted back far enough or tilting an infant's or child's head too far.

e. failure to form an adequate seal around the victim's mouth and/or nose

f. failure to pinch the nostrils tightly closed

The rescuer should continue resuscitation efforts until one of the following occurs:

a. effective, spontaneous circulation and respiration have been restored

b. resuscitation efforts have been transferred to another responsible and trained person

c. the rescuer is exhausted and unable to continue

Ask students to tell how rescue breathing for adults differs from rescue breathing for children. How is the procedure the same for both? Emphasize the ways the treatment of infants and children is unique.

Figure 25–8 Rescue Breathing for an Adult

Keep holding the airway open. Pinch the victim's nose closed. Cover the mouth with your mouth. Blow air into the lungs. You can feel it go down. Let it come out. Blow again. About 12 breaths per minute is fine for an adult. Make each breath long and strong, about 1½ seconds.

After two breaths, back off. Has breathing started? Look, listen, and feel for about five seconds. If no breathing, check for a pulse: use two fingers. Feel for the carotid artery in the groove of the neck, next to the Adam's apple. If there's a pulse, give another full breath, wait five seconds, give another, and listen for breathing. Repeat this sequence until breathing starts. If there's NO pulse, try to restart the heart: go to "Six Steps to Chest Compression" in Figure 25–10 on page 682.

Figure 25–9 Rescue Breathing for a Child or Infant

Keep your finger under the chin, lifting slightly. This will help to keep a seal between your lips and the child's face. Put your mouth over the child's mouth and nose. Give small, slow, gentle breaths. Blow just enough air to make the chest rise. Release, and let the breath be exhaled. Each breath should take 1½ seconds.

After two breaths, back off. Has breathing started? Good. If no breathing, check for a pulse. If there's a pulse, give two more breaths, and listen again for breathing. Keep repeating this sequence. If there's NO pulse, try to restart the heart. Go on to Figure 25–10 on page 682.

Pursuing wellness

As students learn what to do in the event of an accident, encourage them to consider important ways to avoid injury in the event of an accident. Have the class brainstorm ways in which they can live more safely.

The following information may get the list started.

• Wear seat belts—they save lives.

• Air bags have been a subject of concern recently, but they do save lives. The effectiveness of air bags can be increased by use of lap and shoulder belts. In addition, tilt the steering wheel down (this aims the

POINTS *For a person who has stopped breathing, deliver air to the lungs by using the standard breathing assistance method.*

C: Circulation—Chest Compressions

When a victim's heart stops beating, breathing also ceases. During the first critical few minutes, chest compression and breathing assistance are essential. However, it takes professional trainers to properly teach the method. Practice on medical models is part of the training. An untrained person who attempts chest compressions may even stop a heart that is already beating, thus placing the victim in severe danger.

A properly trained helper can assist a person whose heart has stopped. After the helper has:

▶ determined the person is unconscious,
▶ called EMS,
▶ opened the airway and listened for breathing,
▶ if no breathing, has administered 2 breaths,
▶ checked for a pulse,
▶ determined no pulse exists,

then the helper may begin chest compressions as instructed below.

Starting Chest Compressions While breathing assistance keeps oxygen flowing into the lungs, chest compressions keep the blood circulating to the brain and heart. This combination allows critical organs to live until professional help arrives. The brain begins to die within just a few minutes after circulation ceases, so start CPR quickly—don't wait:

Warning: a beating but weakened heart can be stopped by chest compression. Be sure no heartbeat is present before administering chest compressions.

When you are sure, follow the steps outlined in Figure 25–10. Give 15 chest compressions and two breaths per cycle. Repeat the cycle three more times (four in all) before stopping once again to check for breathing and pulse.

For **Y**our **I**nformation

Strive for 80 to 100 chest compressions per minute. This pace allows blood to fill the heart's chambers between beats and provides enough blood flow to maintain life.

Breathing assistance keeps oxygen flowing to the lungs; chest compressions circulate blood to the brain and heart.

air bag toward the chest, not the face) and sit at least 10 inches away from the steering wheel. If the car has a passenger-side air bag, have the passenger move the seat back as far as possible. Children should not ride in the front seat of a car equipped with a passenger-side air bag.
• Whenever possible, children under 13 should ride in the back seat of a car, even if the car is not equipped with an air bag.
• Wear a helmet when bicycling or in-line skating. Of the 27 percent of bicycle owners who own helmets, only 17.6 percent usually wear them, even though helmets reduce the risk of brain injury in an accident by nearly 90 percent!

1. Kneeling at victim's side, locate lower edge of rib cage. Follow it up to the notched center.

2. Place your middle finger in the notch, index finger above on breastbone.

3. Press heel of other hand above index finger on breastbone.

Avoid pressing on this part of the breastbone (the xiphoid process)—it breaks easily

4. Place heel of hand used to find notch on top of other hand. Hold fingers slightly upward, off the victim's chest.

5. Align your shoulder over heel of bottom hand, elbow straight.

6. Press down to compress victim's chest, and release compression in a smooth series of motions. Do not lift your hand away from chest. Repeat 15 compressions and 2 breaths 4 times per minute. All together, the chest compressions and breaths take about one minute.

Figure 25–10 CPR for Adults: Six Steps to Chest Compression

For infants and children, you must be much gentler, and the pace must be faster. Figure 25–11 shows the key differences.

To learn the proper timing of chest compressions it helps to know that, for an adult, 15 compressions should take about ten seconds. Practice this: Try counting aloud, "one-up-two-up . . . ," while pushing down on the count, and letting up on the "up." Use a stopwatch to time yourself, or have a partner time you. You should reach the count of 15 as the time reaches ten seconds.

QUICK QUIZ

Chapter 25, Section 3

The following quiz will help you assess your students' understanding of the material covered in this section of the chapter. You might use the quiz as an oral exercise, which will lead into a class discussion of the topics covered. Or, you might use it as a paper/pencil quiz to evaluate your students individually.

Like the Quick Quiz, the Section Review can also be used as an assessment tool to spark class discussion or as an individual student evaluation. It can also be used as a review in preparation for this quiz.

1. Cardiopulmonary resuscitation can assist a person's breathing and heartbeat until medical help arrives. (True)

2. A person is almost certain to die within ten minutes after his/her breathing has stopped. (True)

INFANT

CHILD

Figure 25–11 CPR for Infants and Children

Position two fingers as shown, on the child's breastbone, about a finger's width below the nipples. Do compressions and give breaths at a rapid pace: 1, 2, 3, 4, 5 compressions, 1 breath; 5 and 1; 5 and 1; 20 times a minute. At each compression push the chest down 1/2 to 1 inch. Keep repeating until heartbeat and breathing resume.

Move two fingers' width above the notch of the ribs, and place the heel of the hand on the breastbone as shown. Keep fingers up (don't touch ribs). Do 5 compressions and give 1 breath, 12 times a minute. Make each compression 1 to 1 1/2 inches deep. Keep repeating until heartbeat and breathing resume.

If the heart resumes beating, check the breathing. If breathing resumes, monitor both heartbeat and breathing until help arrives.

KEY POINTS *For victims of heart attack or other heart-stopping events, CPR may be the only means of keeping them alive. Learning to perform it correctly and safely requires training by professionals.*

SECTION 3 Review

Learning the Facts

1. What happens to people who have stopped breathing after five minutes? What happens after 10 minutes?

2. List the emergencies that may stop a person's breathing.

3. What does CPR actually do for the victim?

4. What should you be sure of before giving chest compressions?

Making Life Choices

5. Identify the hazards in giving breathing assistance without being trained. Are you trained in breathing assistance? What would you do if you had to perform breathing assistance on a family member?

3. You should begin CPR by blowing air into the victim's stomach. (False)

4. Accidentally moving the head of a person with a neck injury can cause permanent paralysis. (True)

5. You should continue CPR even when it seems that the victim is beginning to breathe on his/her own. (False)

6. Improper CPR can actually force water down into a drowning person's lungs. (True)

7. Infants and adults require the same CPR procedures. (False)

8. An untrained person attempting to give CPR may cause serious injury to the victim. (True)

9. Chest compressions keep blood circulating to the brain and heart, allowing critical organs to live. (True)

10. CPR should never be attempted by anyone who has not received proper training. (True)

SECTION 4

FOCUS

OUTCOME

In this section the student will learn:

1. How to clear a blocked airway when a person is choking using the Heimlich maneuver.

FOCUS ACTIVITY

At the beginning of class, inform students they will be studying the Heimlich maneuver. Tell them you are going to make five different distress gestures, which they are to observe. With each gesture, they should try to guess what message you are trying to convey. Let them guess after each gesture. (examples: throwing your hands in the air and waving them around; a coughing or vomiting type of noise; just pointing to your face or head area) One of the gestures that you give should be the universal sign for choking, placing your hands at your throat. Discuss why this gesture is the best.

TEACH & APPLY

COMPREHENSION CHECK

Emphasize with students that they are not to punch the victim. They should place their fists firmly against the victim's abdomen before thrusting. Also make sure that all students know the location of the abdomen. They must start the movement below the rib cage.

SECTION 4

Choking

Eating hastily, taking large bites of solid foods, talking, laughing, or breathing hard while eating can invite choking. Choking occurs when food enters and sticks in the air passage to the lungs instead of being swallowed into the stomach. Everyone should learn to give and recognize the universal distress signal for choking shown in Figure 25–12.

The Heimlich Maneuver

When someone is choking, you must perform the **Heimlich Maneuver (abdominal thrust maneuver)** immediately. Take these steps:

1. First, ask, "Can you make any sound at all?"

If the victim makes a sound, air is moving over the vocal cords, which means that some air can get into the lungs. In this case, the person can try bending over, coughing, and other self-help maneuvers before you intervene. Don't hit the victim on the back while the victim is standing or sitting erect. If you do, the particle caught in the throat may lodge deeper in the air passage.

If the victim cannot make a sound, this means the airway is blocked. Your next moves are to:

2. Shout for help.
3. Perform the Heimlich Maneuver as shown in Figure 25–13.

Position the person. Place your fist above the navel (belly button) as shown. Grasp your fist with your other hand. Then thrust inward and upward four or five times in rapid succession to propel the obstacle out of the throat.

If the person is large or unconscious, you can perform the maneuver while the victim remains lying on his or her back. Kneel astride the thighs, and place your fist below the rib cage. Press on your fist with your other hand, quickly and firmly, upward, four times. Be sure to make contact with your fist before the thrust—don't punch, but press suddenly.

If it is you who is choking, you can act as your own rescuer by thrusting your fist into your own abdomen, or thrusting your body forward forcefully against a firmly placed object—the back of a chair, side of a table, or edge of a sink or stove.

Often, the Heimlich Maneuver is all it takes to save a life. One student who rescued his mother this way reports that her first words, as soon as she could speak, were: "Teach this to everyone else in the family, right now." He did.

Figure 25–12 Universal Distress Signal for Choking. *A person giving this signal has a blocked airway and needs help right away.*

CRITICAL THINKING

Discuss home safety with your class and prepare, as a class, a home safety evaluation checklist. Have students use the checklist to conduct a home safety evaluation and grade their home on the level of safety they find on their inspection. Encourage them to review the checklist with their parents and work with them to correct any potential dangers they have found. The following may provide ideas for building the evaluation checklist. As you build the list, be sure to have students suggest possible improvements or corrections to potentially unsafe conditions.

Are dangerous household chemicals or medicines stored where they could be found and swallowed by children? Are there danger-

For a person who can stand:

For yourself:

Stand behind the person. Ball up your fist. Rotate your thumb toward the person's stomach. Grasp your fist with your other hand, and position it against the abdomen, just below the rib cage. Squeeze rapidly, inward and upward—one, two, three, four times in rapid succession. The object is to propel air upwards out of the lungs and eject the article from the throat. Repeat, if necessary.

Use the back of a chair or the edge of a table to push against, and perform the same maneuver.

Figure 25–13 Unblocking the Airway with the Heimlich Maneuver

 KEY POINTS *If a person is choking, use the Heimlich Maneuver. This technique can dislodge a particle that is caught in the throat and is blocking breathing.*

SECTION 4 Review

Learning the Vocabulary

The vocabulary term in this section is *Heimlich Maneuver (abdominal thrust maneuver)*.

1. Write a sentence using the vocabulary term.

Learning the Facts

2. List some actions that may cause a person to choke.

3. Describe the action you would take if you were choking and by yourself.

4. Identify the hazard in hitting a choking victim on the back while the person is standing or sitting erect.

Making Life Choices

5. What would you do if a student in the school cafeteria began to choke?

MINI Glossary

Heimlich (HIME-lick) **Maneuver (abdominal thrust maneuver):** a technique of dislodging a particle that is blocking a person's airway. The Heimlich Maneuver is named for the physician who invented it.

ous or hazardous materials stored in the garage or basement? Are railings safe or can a child's head be caught between? What precautions are taken to prevent the spread of bacteria in the preparation of food? Is the house equipped with a fire detector, and is it working properly? How many fire extinguishers are there? Do people know how to use them? Does the home have a carbon-monoxide detector, and is it working properly? Are any electrical cords damaged, and are bare wires exposed? Are outlets overloaded? Does the family have a plan for how to escape the house in the event of a fire? Is everyone in the family aware of escape routes? Is everyone aware of what to do during an earthquake, tornado or other disaster?

FOCUS

OUTCOME

In this section students will learn that:

1. Direct pressure to the wound and elevating the limb controls severe bleeding.

FOCUS ACTIVITY

Have a volunteer student pretend to be bleeding. Demonstrate the proper methods to stop bleeding.

TEACH & APPLY

COMPREHENSION CHECK

Impress upon students the importance of controlling external bleeding. This is second only to the maintenance of air passages and the restoration of breathing.

ASSESS

EVALUATE

Review Answers

1. when arteries and veins have been severed
2. promptly treat the wound
3. Have someone call for help, use direct pressure, elevate the wound

CLOSE

Ask students to describe the best way to stop severe bleeding.

Severe Bleeding

Bleeding can be life-threatening when arteries or veins have been severed in an injury. If you can't see a wound because of clothing, cut or tear away the clothing. In severe bleeding, the blood will be welling or pulsing out of the wound, and the amount of blood will seem dramatically great.

In almost all cases, bleeding can be controlled by continuous, direct pressure. Figure 25–14 shows an example of how to apply pressure on a bleeding wound. *Don't* use a tourniquet (a tight band around a limb) to control bleeding. A tourniquet almost always kills the limb to which it is applied and should be used rarely, if ever. Also, don't try to apply pressure at "pressure points," unless you have been trained in the technique. Constricting an artery at a pressure point can damage the healthy tissue normally fed by that artery, and should be used only in cases of severe hemorrhage where direct pressure will not stop the flow.

Elevate the injured part to encourage blood to drain back into the body and to slow the blood flow from it. After bleeding stops, prompt treatment of wounds will be necessary to prevent infection.

Use sterile gauze or a clean folded cloth to cover the wound. Wear gloves. Use your hand to apply pressure. Bleeding should stop or slow to oozing in under 30 minutes.

Figure 25–14 *Using Direct Pressure to Control Bleeding*

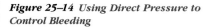 **KEY POINTS** *To stop severe bleeding, use direct pressure.*

 Review

Learning the Facts
1. When is bleeding life-threatening?
2. What should you do after you control bleeding?

Making Life Choices
3. As you're walking home you come across a child who has fallen from a bike. A puddle of blood is beginning to form under the child's arm. What will you do?

CRITICAL THINKING

Have students brainstorm a list of potential outdoor dangers that could be encountered by a hiker in the woods. Possible answers will include tick bites, spider bites, other insect bites, stings, and poison plants.

Bring to class photographs of poison ivy, poison oak, and poison sumac plants and help students learn how to identify these. Recognizing these plants is a basic step to preventing poisoning. Discuss other methods of preventing exposure to these plants. Suggestions may include wearing long pants and long sleeves when hiking, avoiding underbrush, and staying on paths or trails.

Other First-Aid Procedures

The first-aid measures described so far are basic to many emergencies. However, there is much more to know about treating injuries and burns, normalizing temperature, dealing with poisonings, and other specifics. The sections that follow provide a few more basic techniques.

Classifying and Treating Wounds

Wounds are of four types: scrapes, tears, cuts, and punctures. Each can be mild or serious. If they are mild, the most important step is to wash them well with soap and water, then keep them clean.

If a wound is deeper than the outer layers of the skin, it is serious. Serious wounds should be evaluated by a health-care professional after the first-aid treatments are provided. Medical treatment is a must for any wound that has spurted blood, even if first aid has controlled it. Medical treatment is also necessary for any wound that may have involved muscles, tendons, ligaments, or nerves; any bite wound (animal or human); any heavily contaminated wound; or any wound that contains soil or object fragments. Objects sticking into the flesh should be left in place when possible until medical help can be obtained.

A concern in providing first aid to bleeding victims is your own safety. Some serious diseases can be transmitted to you through contact with an infected person's body fluids—blood, vomit, feces, or urine. This doesn't mean you should not help a wounded person, but it does mean that you should take measures to protect yourself from contact with the victim's body fluids. See the Health Strategies section "Reducing Disease Risks" earlier in the chapter.

 Treat minor wounds to prevent infection. Major wounds need professional care. Protect yourself from contact with the victim's blood and other body fluids.

Burns

Burns are classified by the depth of tissue injury. Proper help for a burn victim depends on whether the burn is of the first, second, or third degree. First-degree burns injure just the top layers of skin and appear as redness, with mild swelling and pain. They heal rapidly. A light sunburn and a mild scald are examples.

Second-degree burns involve deeper tissue damage. They appear red or mottled, develop blisters, swell considerably, and are wet at the surface. A deep sunburn, a flash burn from burning fluid, or a burn from contact with very hot liquid is likely to be a second-degree burn.

Third-degree burns involve deep tissue destruction and have a white or charred appearance. Sometimes third-degree burns will appear to be second degree at first. Flames, ignited clothing, prolonged contact with hot fluids or objects, or electricity can all cause third-degree burns.

If a person is exposed to any of these poisonous plants, there are basic steps which can be taken. First of all, the exposed area should be thoroughly cleansed, immediately, with soap and water. Any clothing which came into contact with the poisonous plants should be carefully removed and washed. If absorption of the poison has already begun and a rash or weeping sores has developed, a paste of baking soda and water applied to the area several times a day can help reduce discomfort. Lotions such as Calamine can soothe the affected area, and Benadryl may help dry up the sores. If the sores worsen or spread, or are on the face, consult a physician.

FOCUS

OUTCOMES

In this section students will learn:

1. How to classify first-, second-, and third-degree burns.
2. The signs, symptoms, and first aid for victims of temperature extremes—hypothermia and hyperthermia.
3. The signs, symptoms, and treatments of poisoning.
4. What a fracture consists of and the two types of fractures that can occur.

FOCUS ACTIVITY

Have students brainstorm all of the remedies that they have heard for the injuries and illnesses that are described in this section (wounds, burns, hyper- and hypothermia, poisoning, broken bones). Have any of the students tried these remedies? Were they successful? Have the students look ahead to see the remedies and treatments that are presented in this section. Do these treatments seem more useful?

 Handout—Selected First-Aid Measures. The Teacher's Resource Box contains a handout that lists the types of wounds and treatment for both minor and serious wounds for each type. You may want to distribute the handout at this time.

TEACH & APPLY

LEARNING WITH VISUALS

Obtain posters and pamphlets that relate to sunburn from your local Cancer Society. Display these in the classroom and discuss the sayings highlighted in them. Continue the discussion by asking the following questions:

1. What degree of burn is a sunburn?
2. What causes a sunburn? What are some ways to prevent a sunburn from occurring?
3. How should you decide what suntan lotion to buy? What should you look for on the bottle of suntan lotion?

COMPREHENSION CHECK

After reading the information on burns, have the students make two columns on a piece of paper and label one column DO'S and the other column DON'TS. Have students go back through the text and list all the DO'S of caring for burns in general, not the specific degree of burns. They should then list all the DON'TS. (example: do monitor breathing; don't remove burned clothing) Have students add to their own papers the items shared by the class that were not on their lists.

DISCUSSION

As a class, discuss precautions that can be taken around the home to prevent burns from happening to family members. Students may relate any specific incidents that occurred to them or their family members, describing what happened and what, if anything, could have been done to prevent the burns from occurring.

Figure 25–15 Standard Treatments for Burns

To treat first-degree burns:
- Dip the burned part in cool water, or apply gauze soaked in cool water.
- Then, if exposure to anything unclean is likely, layer dry gauze over the wet gauze to create a barrier to bacteria.
- Never apply grease of any kind to any burn.

To treat second-degree burns:
- Treat as described above for first-degree burns, and seek medical treatment. Do not break blisters, remove tissue, or use antiseptic spray, cream, or any other product.
- Elevate burned part.

To treat third-degree burns:
- Elevate the burned part, especially the limbs.
- Cover the burn with many layers of dry, sterile gauze.
- Do not apply water unless the area is still burning.
- An ice pack wrapped in a dry towel may be applied on top of the gauze for pain relief.
- Treat for shock, and arrange transportation to an emergency medical facility.
- Do not attempt to remove clothing or debris from the burn.

One key thing to remember about burns is that the skin regulates the body's temperature. When skin is burned, the body can lose heat and grow very cold, very fast. That's why covering a burn victim can be important—but don't cover a person whose clothing is still smoldering. Let the surface reach a neutral temperature, then cover.

Another key: burns on the face may mean that the airway is burned. Look for singed facial hair (eyebrows, mustache). A facial burn may lead to swelling and a blocked airway. Monitor breathing closely in a person who is burned. Figure 25–15 shows the standard treatments for first-, second-, and third-degree burns.

Never put water on a burn that is caused by a dry powder. Just brush the powder off. A powder may react with water and burn the victim further.

KEY POINTS *Burns require first aid according to their severity. Defend the victim's body temperature.*

Pursuing wellness

- Since improper handling of even a minor eye injury could lead to permanent damage, eye injuries are best treated by specialists. Only superficial foreign bodies should be removed, and then always using thoroughly cleansed hands and sterile materials.

- Tearing is the body's attempt to remove foreign particles, but rubbing the eye can cause damage by scratching the delicate eye tissue or perhaps lodging the particle more deeply in the eye. Under no circumstances should the eye be rubbed.

- If a particle is loose in the eye, flush the eye with clean water, holding the eyelids apart. Sometimes, a particle lodged under

Temperature Extremes

For the body tissues to function normally, they must be kept at normal temperature—close to 98.6 degrees Fahrenheit. A person whose internal body parts lose heat is at serious risk and needs help fast. Similarly, internal body parts must not be overheated. This, too, poses a serious threat. While **hypothermia** and **hyperthermia** can threaten life when allowed to advance unchecked, some simple first-aid measures can, when administered quickly, be life-saving. In cases of temperature extremes, call the emergency services immediately. Then proceed as described here.

Hypothermia   Hypothermia, or abnormally low internal body temperature, develops when the body loses heat to the environment faster than it can generate heat. Exposure to low temperatures, high winds, and high humidity makes anyone likely to develop hypothermia. However, people who are ill or elderly can grow cold internally even in a room as warm as 65 degrees Fahrenheit. The temperature of the surroundings does not have to be anywhere near freezing for the condition to occur. Thousands of older people probably die of hypothermia each year.

A person with hypothermia may have stiff muscles, with some shivering or trembling; dizziness; weakness; cold skin; problems with coordination; and slowed breathing and heart rate. As hypothermia progresses, the person

Covering a burn victim can help maintain proper body temperature.

MINI Glossary

hypothermia (*hypo* means "too low"; *thermia* means "temperature"): a condition of too little body heat with abnormally low internal body temperature.

hyperthermia (*hyper* means "too high"; *thermia* means "temperature"): a condition of too much body heat with abnormally high internal body temperature.

the upper eyelid can be removed by drawing the upper eyelid over the lower eyelid so that the lower lashes wipe the inside of the upper lid. Remember, however, that this method can also introduce particles into the eye. The eyelashes can be gripped to turn back the upper or lower eyelid and expose particles caught there, which can be carefully removed with a

corner of sterile gauze.
• If something is embedded in an eye, it should only be treated by a doctor or eye specialist. The best course of action is to apply a loose bandage to *both* eyes. This will help prevent the injured eye from moving. Keep the victim lying down and transport him or her in that position.

COMPREHENSION CHECK

On the board list as many activities as possible that could cause hypothermia. Once the activities have been listed, have the students pick five of them and write down five precautions that could be taken while involved in each one to prevent hypothermia from occurring.

FAST FACTS

In an average year about 175 Americans die from summer heat and too much sun.

CNN® You can update your coverage of health and fitness topics, as well as spark lively classroom discussion and deeper understanding, by using the **CNN Health and Fitness Updates.** These video updates are produced by Turner Educational Services, using the resources of CNN, the world's first 24-hour, all-news network.

With the introduction of the **CNN Health and Fitness Updates,** West Educational Publishing is proud to be the exclusive partner of CNN for textbook/video integration in high school fitness. By making use of the **CNN Health and Fitness Updates** you can bring the power of CNN, the network known for providing in-depth, live coverage and analysis of breaking news events, to your health class.

For assistance in using and incorporating **CNN Health and Fitness Updates** into your classroom presentations, see the *Classroom Guide to the CNN Health and Fitness Updates.* The **CNN Health and Fitness Updates** are available with West Educational Publishing's *Health: Making Life Choices.*

How Well Prepared for Emergencies Are You?

On a separate piece of paper, answer each question true or false to see how well prepared you are for emergencies. Your answers to the Life Choice Inventory are personal and private. Share them with others only if you are comfortable doing so.

1. I have a well-stocked medicine chest (or my family does).
2. I carry a first-aid kit in my car (or my family does).
3. My (my family's) emergency supplies include waterless antiseptic hand cleansers and gloves to protect us from exposure to blood.
4. I own an up-to-date first-aid manual, and I can put my hands on it when I need it.
5. I have taken a first-aid course.
6. I know how to give CPR (cardiopulmonary resuscitation).
7. I know how to perform the Heimlich Maneuver.
8. On the scene of an accident, I know what to do first, second, third, and fourth.
9. I know the emergency telephone number for my area.
10. I know how to determine whether I should attempt a rescue or whether the attempt might threaten my own life.

SCORING

Give yourself 1 point for each true answer.

8–10: Excellent. You are well prepared for emergencies.
6–7: Good. You are better prepared than average, but you may want to fill in the gaps in your knowledge.
4–5: Fair. You are on your way to becoming a competent manager of emergencies. Learn more.
Below 4: Poor. You have much to learn. A good way to begin is to read this chapter.

Have the students number from 1 to 10 on a sheet of paper and answer true or false to each of the ten items in the inventory. Some of the questions will need to be answered at home or after students have had an opportunity to talk to their parents about a few of the items. Discuss the results of the inventory in class. What actions do the students plan to take? An alternative approach is to have students exchange their papers after doing the inventory and then have the student grading each paper make recommendations for improvement. Ask more advanced students also to supply a rationale for their recommendations.

COMPREHENSION CHECK

Write the word *frostbite* on the board. Under it make two columns, DO'S and DON'TS. Fill each column with the do's and don'ts of treating a victim of frostbite.

---

may become confused and drowsy, may lose muscle coordination, and may stop shivering.

If you suspect hypothermia, call for help immediately. While waiting for help, move the person to a warm place, taking care to prevent injury. Do not handle the person roughly (the heart is weak when the body is cold). Do not attempt to rewarm the person with hot baths, electric blankets, or hot-water bottles. Do, though, offer warm food or drink to victims who are conscious. If the person is unconscious, don't force anything—fluids or food. Do not raise the feet or legs, for the blood there is cooler than in other parts of the body and can further chill the body's core. Do wrap the person in available covering such as blankets, towels, pillows, scarves, or newspapers.

Frostbite   Another risk of exposure to cold is **frostbite**. A child busily making a snowman or a teen skiing down a powdered slope may not be aware of frostbite's dangers as they set in. However, the later effects of frostbite—painful injury to the fingers, toes, ears, cheeks, or nose, and possible loss of function—are severe. Some frostbite injuries are so severe as to require surgical removal of the injured part.

CRITICAL THINKING

First Aid Practice

People who practice for a variety of emergency situations are better able to help another person or themselves when in need. During a real emergency there is no time to learn how to apply first aid, so people need practice with mock accidents. Remind students that even though they have practiced, real situations are more difficult and confusing; they need to continue to practice on their own to stay prepared.

Divide your class into groups of three or four students. Have one student be the victim in the group and have the other students administer first aid to a mock injury. Switch victims with every situation. Let the students use their book or give them a list of steps to take in administering the first aid. Make sure

Frostbite can sneak up on those too busy to notice.

Frostbite sets in when ice crystals form in body tissues. The crystals freeze the body part and cut off its circulation. Also, ice crystals form as sharp, jagged daggers that easily puncture delicate cell membranes as the ice crystals grow larger. Once their membranes are punctured, cells spill out their internal contents, collapse, and die.

Frostbite's symptoms include color changes in the skin, usually to white, gray, or blue. The part may feel numb, so the person may have no warning that injury is setting in. Pain can be severe, however, when warmth restores feeling to the previously numb parts.

One of the worst things to do when frostbite sets in is to rub the affected body part. Rubbing saws the ice crystals back and forth, jabbing the membranes of neighboring cells and killing them, too. To prevent this unnecessary destruction of tissue, always handle frostbitten parts gently. Remove wet or tight clothing. Cover the affected parts with dry, sterile dressing. Don't pack the area in snow or cold water. The affected tissues need to be gently warmed, so that the ice crystals will slowly melt.

Transport the victim to a hospital. If that is impossible, treat the frostbite as best you can. Move the victim in from the cold. Soak the injured part in comfortably warm (100 degrees Fahrenheit), not hot, water. (If the water is too hot, or if the body part thaws and refreezes, it will die.) Loosely bandage the part by wrapping it lightly with gauze, and seek medical help.

MINI Glossary

frostbite: the formation of ice crystals in body parts exposed to temperatures below freezing; freezing of body parts, especially toes and fingers, and nose and other face parts.

BACKGROUND INFORMATION

Frostbite, like burns, is classified into categories. There are three categories measured by the extent of tissue damage:

1. *Incipient first-degree frostbite.* That is injury to surface skin. Somewhat like a sunburn, the affected part will show redness, swelling, burning, and tingling without formation of blisters. There is usually no tissue loss.

2. *Superficial second-degree frostbite.* This is similar to first-degree frostbite in appearance. Blisters occur minutes to hours after the cold injury. Undue redness of the skin on rewarming and swelling may occur.

3. *Deep third-degree frostbite.* This involves damage to deep tissues. Much of the frozen part is lost, possibly all of it. Usually no blisters or swelling occur.

DISCUSSION

Choose a student to read aloud the symptoms of heat exhaustion and another to read aloud the symptoms of heat stroke. Once the symptoms have been read, discuss the differences between the conditions and the treatments for both.

---

that all groups cover several different situations, such as burns of various severities and types (electrical, sun, chemical, frost bite, hypothermia, choking, bleeding injuries (minor and severe), rescue breathing, and CPR situations.

After they have completed each step in the care of the injured person, tell them what to do next. Example: If a group has an unconscious victim lying on the floor and students

have checked breathing and pulse rate, tell them the outcome (whether they find a pulse or not; whether the person is breathing or not). If they miss any steps, do not let them continue until they complete the step. Make sure they understand what they are to do next. This activity may take more than one class period.

BACKGROUND INFORMATION

Treatment for hyperthermia is varied. Students may try sponging the victim's bare skin with cool water, applying cool packs, or placing the victim in a tub of cool water until the temperature is sufficiently lowered. They also can try fanning the victim to create a cooling draft, or moving the person into an air-conditioned space.

CLASS DISCUSSION

Compare and contrast hyperthermia and hypothermia, and their treatments.

GROUP ACTIVITY

Bring in magazines or have students bring in magazines from home. Have students go through the magazines and make collages with pictures of items that can cause poisoning. Display these collages in the room. As the posters are displayed, point out any unusual or noteworthy sources that students found.

FAST FACTS

Approximately 90 percent of all poisonings involve children.

Here are the answers to the questions at the start of the chapter.

1. **False.** To be of real help and not make things worse, the helper needs to apply training gained through a class in first aid from a qualified instructor.
2. **True.**
3. **False.** The first thing to do in an emergency is to inspect the scene to determine what happened. Move the victim only if the scene presents immediate danger.
4. **False.** A person in a state of shock is experiencing a *physical* reaction to injury. Shock is a dangerous condition, and first-aid treatment is recommended.
5. **True.**
6. **False.** You should not use a tourniquet to control bleeding. A tourniquet almost always kills the limb to which it is applied.
7. **True.**
8. **False.** Frostbitten parts should be handled gently to prevent tissue destruction.
9. **False.** The best way to determine if a victim has broken any bones is to ask the person to move each joint. Forcing limbs with broken bones to move can worsen a break.

Figure 25–16 Symptoms of Hyperthermia

Hyperthermia Hyperthermia is likely whenever people are exposed to high temperatures with high humidity. You need not be active to experience it—you need only be hot. Athletes and exercisers aren't the only ones prone to hyperthermia. Babies, old people, those taking certain medications, and the overweight are especially likely to tolerate heat poorly. Figure 25–16 below describes the symptoms of the two dangerous stages of hyperthermia—heat exhaustion and heat stroke. (You learned in Chapter 9 about heat cramps, heat exhaustion, and heat stroke, but a review is given here.)

An overheated person who receives no help may sicken as the body tries to defend itself against the high temperature. In the early stages, the body struggles to cool itself through heavy sweating. Should exposure to the hot conditions continue, though, the body may sweat so much that it begins to run out of fluid with which to make more sweat. As the body loses fluid, it stops sweating, and thereby loses its only defense against overheating further. Then, like an overheating car radiator, the body temperature climbs to the point of damaging all systems, especially the brain.

To prevent damage or death from heat injuries, first call for emergency help. Then cool the person's body by fanning. Apply cold, wet wraps such as wet towels or clothing. Offer the conscious victim a small amount—about half a cup—of plain cool water to drink every 15 minutes or so. Between drinks, lay the person down and treat for shock.

KEY POINTS *First aid for hypothermia consists of calling for help and allowing the person's body to slowly regain its proper temperature. First aid for frostbite consists of slowly warming the parts and seeking help. First aid for hyperthermia consists of calling for help, cooling the person, offering fluids, and treating for shock.*

Poisonings, Bites, and Stings

Any adverse effect on the body from a chemical substance is considered poisoning, from an overdose of drugs to the inhalation of fumes from household products. Poisonings pose difficult problems for those administering first aid, because they vary in symptoms and treatments according to

	Hyperthermia (Heat Exhaustion)	Severe Hyperthermia (Heat Stroke)
Skin	Cool, moist, pale or red	Dry, hot, red
Sweating	Heavy sweating	No sweating
Body temperature	Normal or below normal	Very high, possibly to 106 degrees Fahrenheit
Pulse	Faster than normal	Fast and weak
Breathing	Possible deep breathing	Fast, shallow breathing
Other	Dizziness and weakness, headache, nausea	Mental confusion, loss of consciousness, brain damage, death

enrichment

Dog and cat bites are the most common animal bites among humans, but bites by other humans place third. Since the human mouth harbors a number of species of bacteria, human bites are more likely to become infected than are dog bites. Herpes viruses and

hepatitis B and C can be transmitted through human bites. Some of the more dangerous human bites occur during fights, when one person strikes another in the mouth and the hand is lacerated by the other person's teeth.

Rabies is a potential danger with animal bites, particularly bites from wild animals. Rabies, if not treated, is fatal, and is passed the substance involved. Poisons can enter the body by being eaten or drunk, breathed in, absorbed through the skin, or injected.

What to Do for Poisonings The most common household poisonings involve overdoses of aspirin or other over-the-counter pain relievers, eaten by children or taken by mistake by adults. A person who has eaten poison may display any of the symptoms shown in Figure 25–17. In such a case, give nothing by mouth. Quickly call the emergency services. Then call the poison control center (the number is on the front page of your telephone book). Describe the poisoning.

If the poison involved is an illegal drug, do *not* try to protect the victim by concealing information. Legal penalties are small when compared with loss of life. Don't hesitate—call. If possible, read aloud over the phone, from the poison container, the information on its label. Follow the instructions given by the poison control experts.

If a poison has been taken by injection, the person may need breathing assistance. It may also be necessary to treat for shock.

Bites and Stings Bites and stings present a special case of poisoning. Insect bites and stings are especially common. These can be extremely threatening to those who are allergic to them.

The primary threat from most insect bites and stings is allergic reaction to the **venom**, which can set in within seconds of the sting. Call emergency services immediately if the person has a red, flushed, or swelling face or trouble breathing. Be ready to administer breathing assistance until help arrives.

For ordinary stings in nonallergic people, quickly remove any remaining stinger by scraping it out. The longer the stinger remains in the skin, the more venom enters the flesh, so work quickly. Most stinging insects leave no stinger.

Few people are bitten by snakes in the United States each year, and only a handful of those suffer lasting effects or are killed by such bites. Most people receive help promptly. The majority of snakebites occur near home. Most snakebites need no first-aid treatment. However, the victim should be kept calm and still, and receive medical help within 30 minutes, just to be sure. Never cut or suck on a snakebite. Never use a snakebite kit that requires cutting into the flesh to treat a bite. Use a kit that applies suction only.

 KEY POINTS *Poisonings demand immediate help. Call a poison control center, and follow directions. Allergic reactions to stings may lead to breathing failure; obtain help quickly. Snakebites require medical attention.*

Figure 25–17 Symptoms of Poisoning

Symptoms of Poisoning:
- Burns or injury to tongue or lip area (if the poison was taken by mouth).
- Difficulty breathing.
- Pain in the chest or abdomen; diarrhea, nausea, vomiting.
- Sweating.
- The person may have seizures or lose consciousness.

MINI Glossary

venom: poison from a living creature, such as a snake or scorpion.

through the saliva of the diseased animal. Wild animals behaving oddly, such as nocturnal animals active during the day or wild animals which do not avoid people, should be regarded with suspicion. Wild animals should not be petted or fed. If someone is bitten by a wild animal, it is important to get them away from the animal without trying to catch it.

However, if possible, remember what the animal looked like and where it was seen so that authorities can capture it for observation.

There are four kinds of poisonous snakes in the United States (rattlesnake, water moccasin, copperhead, and coral snake), and rattlesnake bites are the most common.

BACKGROUND INFORMATION

Tell the students that when in doubt, treat a sprain or a strain like a break as far as the first-aid procedure is concerned.

ASSESS

EVALUATE

SECTION 6 Review Answers

1. hypothermia
2. Venom
3. fracture
4. when a wound has spurted blood; involves muscles, tendons, ligaments, or nerves; any bite wound; any heavily contaminated wound, or any wound that contains soil or object fragments (p. 687)
5. deep tissue destruction, white or charred appearance (p. 687)
6. changes in the skin's color (to white, gray, or blue), numbness in the affected area (p. 691)
7. eaten or drunk, breathed in, absorbed through the skin, or injected (p. 693)
8. Answers will vary. (p. 688)

CLOSE

Divide the class into groups of five. Ask group members to describe a scene from a television show in which someone was injured. Each group should produce a two-paragraph report describing the incident and what rescue personnel did to treat the victim. Groups can then share their findings with the class.

Health Strategies

Splinting a Broken Bone

When a bone is broken:

▶ Treat the limb in the position in which you found it—don't move it.
▶ Place a stick, board, or other such unbendable object (a splint) against the limb. Usually, support an arm from below, a leg from the side.
▶ If possible, place the splint so that it holds the joints still, too, both above and below the break.
▶ Tie the splint snugly to the limb in several places, leaving the broken area untied. Don't tie it too tightly. A tight splint may cut off circulation.
▶ Elevate the part, if possible.
▶ Cover exposed bone with moist, sterile dressing.

MINI Glossary

fracture: a break in a bone. An *open fracture* is a break with a wound in the overlying tissues. A *closed fracture* is a break or crack with no visible wound.

splint: a stick or board used to support a broken bone to keep its separated parts from moving until it can be set.

Broken Bones

A person with a **fracture** (a break in a bone) needs medical treatment. A break in a bone that does not penetrate the skin is called a "closed" break. Open breaks, where the bone end has punctured the skin, may bleed. In the case of an open break, control the bleeding. Remember to use rubber gloves or materials to protect your hands from the blood.

Neither you nor the injured person may be able to tell whether an injury is a broken bone, a sprain, or a strain. For this reason, the Red Cross suggests, "When in doubt, splint." In other words, if you suspect a fracture, tie a **splint** to the injured part while waiting for emergency help. The Health Strategies section on this page, "Splinting a Broken Bone," tells how to do this. Also, if any part of the bone is exposed to the air, keep it moist. Don't try to put it back in place. Just cover it with moist, sterile, or clean dressing.

Splinting techniques vary with injury location, and a first-aid course teaches many splinting techniques. No matter the location, though, the main task remains to keep the injured bone still to prevent further damage.

KEY POINTS *If you suspect that a bone may be broken, apply a splint to keep the part still and prevent further damage.*

SECTION 6 Review

Learning the Vocabulary

The vocabulary terms in this section are *hypothermia, hyperthermia, frostbite, venom, fracture,* and *splint.* Fill in the blank with the correct answer.

1. If a person has too little body heat, it is called _____.
2. _____ is a poison from a living creature.
3. A break in a bone is called a _____.

Learning the Facts

4. When is medical treatment necessary for wounds?

5. Describe characteristics of a third-degree burn.
6. What are the symptoms of frostbite?
7. How can poisons enter the body?

Making Life Choices

8. Look at Figure 25–15 on page 688, "Standard Treatments for Burns." Describe the differences in treatments for the different degrees of burns. Why is it important to know the treatments? What could happen to a person who is treated incorrectly?

QUICK QUIZ

Chapter 25, Section 6

The following quiz will help you assess your students' understanding of the material covered in this section of the chapter. You might use the quiz as an oral exercise, which will lead into a class discussion of the topics covered. Or, you might use it as a paper/pencil quiz to evaluate your students individually.

Like the Quick Quiz, the Section Review can also be used as an assessment tool to spark class discussion or as an individual student evaluation. It can also be used as a review in preparation for this quiz.

1. Medical treatment is necessary for any cut that has spurted blood, that involves injury to the ligament or muscle, or that may be contaminated. (True)
2. When giving first aid, you should try to

Herbs and Folk Remedies

From earliest times, ancient people treated their coughs, aches, infections, sleeplessness, wounds, burns, and other ills with tissues from the plants and animals that surrounded them. Even today there is no question that many wild plants and animals contain compounds that act as drugs.

Today, many of these same **herbs** and other "remedies" are for sale on store shelves. People may wonder if **"folk medicine"** might offer safer or more "natural" remedies for curing human ills than drugs made in the chemist's laboratory. Even if some do work, the products may not be safe. For this reason, some warnings are in order: See Figure 25–18 on the next page.

 All those warnings make me afraid to think about trying folk medicines. Why do people bother with them?

There are probably as many reasons as there are users. Some people want to return to the olden days. Other people grew up in families that used herbs as medicines and feel comfortable in using them. Still others claim to believe that herbs are safer than refined drugs because they're "natural."

 Aren't natural things safe?

The word *natural* doesn't mean harmless—far from it. The natural herbs **hemlock** and **belladonna** are two infamous and deadly poisons. The herb **sassafras** contains a cancer-causing chemical. The herb **ma huang**, sold to induce weight loss, contains a stimulant drug, ephedrine, associated with several deaths in the United States. Other herbs, such as **witch hazel**, are harmless but also useless.

 What about the herb ginseng? How does it rate as a medicine?

The herb **ginseng** is the root of a wild, slow-growing plant. It is so highly prized for its proved and imaginary drug effects that it has been hunted and gathered almost to extinction. In a scientific study, ginseng worked against inflammation (the swelling, heat, and redness of injuries) more effectively than the medical drug hydrocortisone. In another study, ginseng changed people's blood chemistries in a way that reduced their risks of heart disease. Ginseng has a wake-up effect like that of caffeine, too.

Even if ginseng itself is useful in some cases, the products called ginseng for sale on store shelves are rarely effective. Unfortunately, ginseng products vary so widely in contents that there's no guessing at their effects. Also, real ginseng may cause negative side effects. Insomnia, nervousness, confusion, and depression make up a group of symptoms called the **ginseng abuse syndrome**. Ginseng makes a poor drug, because its negative effects occur at about the same dose levels as its drug effects.

 Do any herbs work, that aren't too dangerous to try?

You know of one already—caffeine. Three others are **aloe**, **chamomile**, and **echinacea**. People have used aloe plants for thousands of years to treat burns and skin injuries. Experienced cooks may keep potted aloe plants on kitchen windowsills. For minor kitchen burns and cuts, they pluck a leaf and apply the gel that oozes out. It relieves pain, and some scientists think it makes minor wounds heal faster. On the other hand, aloe may delay or complicate the healing of severely damaged skin.

695

---

avoid contact with the victim's body fluids. (True)
3. A mild sunburn is an example of a second-degree burn. (False)
4. A person suffering from burns is very vulnerable to changes in body temperature. (True)
5. Hypothermia is caused by exposure to extreme heat. (False)
6. Some of the symptoms of hypothermia are stiff muscles, dizziness, and slowed breathing and heart rate. (True)
7. You should treat frostbite by vigorously rubbing the affected body part. (False)
8. Heat exhaustion and heat stroke are forms of hyperthermia. (True)
9. Poisoning can be caused by food, insect bites, over-the-counter medication, and illegal drugs. (True)
10. If you suspect that a bone is broken, you should apply a splint in order to prevent further damage. (True)

Discussion

Ask students if they have ever tried any of these home remedies. Did they work? If they haven't tried them, would they be willing to try them the next time they have one of these problems? Have volunteers report to the class periodically on the effectiveness of these folk remedies.

Comprehension Check

Ask students to write a brief essay expressing their opinions of folk medicines as they compare to commercial medicines. In their papers they should state whether or not they would ever use folk remedies and give reasons for their opinions. If they would use folk medicines, they should cite the personal experiences of successful use of the medicines or experiences of people they know who have had success with these remedies. Have students read their papers in class.

Herbs and Folk Remedies (continued)

As for chamomile, it contains a drug that relieves digestive and menstrual cramping. Whether tea brewed from chamomile flowers has these effects is unknown. This is because the drug doesn't dissolve in water, and only a little of it ends up in a cup of tea. Perhaps the effects of drinking the tea may build up over time.

After thousands of years' use, reports of negative side effects from chamomile tea are almost unknown, except for one: the flowers can cause allergy in people who are sensitive to pollen. If you have hay fever, stay away from chamomile and other herbs as well.

The popular herb echinacea is gaining recognition as a treatment for colds, flu, and related infections. Studies show echinacea may help to fight infection by increasing the number of immune cells in the blood. More studies are needed, however, to determine echinacea's effectiveness. Because echinacea can affect the immune system, people with immune disorders such as arthritis, should not use it.

What about other folk remedies?

Among the thousands of claims made for herbs and potions, a few more folk remedies are worth mentioning. One is the hormone **melatonin**, which is thought to influence the body's day and night cycles. It is marketed with promises of reducing jet lag, the ill feelings that follow adjustment to different time zones. Also, some people who have trouble sleeping say it helps them get to sleep.

> **Warning 1:** Even if an herb is known to contain an effective drug, people cannot be sure that the products they buy contain the drug they hope to receive. All plants, including herbs, vary from batch to batch, from strain to strain, and from season to season. Also, people make mistakes in using herbs. A man confused **foxglove** (from which the potent heart medicine digoxin is extracted) with **comfrey** (an herb popular for making tea). Upon drinking about a quart of foxglove tea over several days, the man was poisoned with digoxin. Comfrey itself is poisonous when used regularly, but foxglove is even more so.

> **Warning 2:** Different people react differently to the drugs in herbs, just as they do to other drugs. Children and people with certain medical conditions are most sensitive and should not be given any folk medicines.

> **Warning 3:** False claims are common. Many products claim to promote health, but few do in truth.

> **Warning 4:** Harmful side effects are common. A product that contains useful compounds is likely to contain some harmful ones as well. Some 700 plants have caused serious illnesses or deaths in this part of the world.

Figure 25–18 Warnings About Herbal Medicines

696

•multicultural issues•

Students may be interested in further information on herbal medicines. In the United States, if the product label does not make any medicinal claims, it is not regulated by the FDA. In addition, under the Dietary Supplement Health and Education Act of 1994, the government must prove that a product is harmful before it can be removed from the market. Since herbal medicines are not regulated by the FDA, there are no industry-wide standards for quality, concentration, or dosage.

Herbal remedies are widely used in some European nations. In Germany, a variety of herbal remedies are actually registered with

A kitchen product, meat tenderizer (the kind without seasoning), contains papain, a chemical that breaks down proteins. The stinging venoms of bees and jellyfish are made of protein. Some people find that meat tenderizer kills the pain and reduces the swelling of these stings. To treat a sting, remove the stinger, if any, and apply ice. Then spread a paste of tenderizer to destroy the painful protein in the venom. Applying vinegar may work, too.

Some other accurate folksy tips include these:

► Sugar, if allowed to dissolve and trickle down the throat, can interfere with the nerve signals that cause hiccups.
► A gargle of warm saltwater can soothe a sore throat and may kill more germs than commercial mouthwashes can.
► A mixture of lemon and honey can soothe a sore throat and may quiet a minor cough.

While these treatments are safe to try, stay away from most other folk remedies. They often are more harmful than helpful. At the very least, they are a waste of money.

Glossary

herbs: nonwoody plants or plant parts valued for their flavor, aroma, or medicinal qualities.

folk medicine: the use of herbs and other natural substances in the treatment of disease as practiced among people of various regions.

hemlock: any part of the hemlock plant, which causes severe pain, convulsions, and death within 15 minutes.

belladonna: any part of the deadly nightshade plant; a deadly poison.

sassafras: root bark from the sassafras tree, once used in beverages but now banned as an ingredient in foods or beverages because it contains cancer-causing chemicals.

ma huang: an herbal preparation sold with promises of weight loss and increased energy, but that contains ephedrine, a dangerous heart stimulant.

witch hazel: leaves or bark of a witch hazel tree; not proved to have healing powers.

ginseng (JIN-seng): a plant containing chemicals that have drug effects.

ginseng abuse syndrome: a group of symptoms associated with the overuse of ginseng, including high blood pressure, insomnia, nervousness, confusion, and depression.

aloe: a tropical plant with widely claimed, but mostly unproved, medical value.

chamomile: a plant with flowers that may provide some limited medical value in soothing intestinal and stomach discomforts.

echinacea: an herb popular for its assumed "anti-infectious" properties and as an all-purpose remedy, especially for colds and allergy. Also called *cone flower.*

melatonin: a hormone of a gland of the brain, believed to help regulate the body's daily rhythms. Claims for life extension or enhancement of sexual prowess are without merit. Proof of melatonin's safety or effectiveness is lacking.

foxglove: a plant that contains a substance used in the heart medicine digoxin.

comfrey: leaves and roots of the comfrey plant; believed, but not proved, to have drug effects. Comfrey contains cancer-causing chemicals.

697

Discussion
Ask students if any special medicines or treatments are used in their families. Does someone in the family prepare home remedies? Ask them to describe any of these special treatments. Ask other students if they would try these remedies.

Class Activity
Ask students to look on containers at home that have a potentially poisonous material in them. The students need to find what is poisonous in the container and write a one-page report on what symbol is used to represent poisonous materials, whether any antidotes are listed on the container, and any other warning information stated on the label. Report the findings to the class.

Reproducible Study Outline and Reading Cloze worksheets for Chapter 25 are provided in the Teacher's Resource Box.

Reproducible Chapter Tests A and B are also provided in the Teacher's Resource Box.

the German government. The responsible department of the government does not research the claims of various herbal remedies but does review evidence to determine safety and usefulness and to provide information on the parts of plants to be used, how to use them, active chemicals in them, and possible side effects. In addition, herbal remedies must meet certain manufacturing standards, and dangerous products, such as comfrey and coltsfoot, are banned. German doctors routinely prescribe registered herbal remedies, which are paid for by the government health insurance.

VOCABULARY

1. a. dispatcher **b.** frostbite **c.** splint **d.** carotid pulse **e.** Heimlich maneuver **f.** first aid **g.** hypothermia
2. a. shock **b.** Venom **c.** fracture **d.** emergency medical service
3. Answers will vary.

RECALL

SECTION 1

1. disposable rubber gloves and waterless antiseptic hand cleaners (p. 671)

SECTION 2

2. Answers may vary; could include fire, fumes, fast traffic, live electrical wires, fast-moving water. (p. 672)
3. by checking each victim for blocked airways, no breathing, no circulation, and severe bleeding, and helping the person who needs immediate help (p. 673)
4. Place your ear and cheek close to the victim's mouth and nose. Look, listen, and use the sensitive skin of your cheek to feel for breathing. (p. 674)
5. Blood flow to the brain and other vital organs is diminished, causing loss of consciousness. Blood supply to other vital organs, including the heart, may fail as well. (p. 674)
6. less severe, but serious injuries (p. 676)

CHAPTER 25 Review

Summarizing the Chapter

Your ability to respond correctly to the following statements ensures your understanding of the main concepts in the chapter.

1. Identify the priorities in responding to an emergency.
2. Give steps in identifying and treating shock.
3. Describe and act out how to call for help in an emergency.
4. Explain the steps in CPR.
5. Describe how to respond to severe bleeding.
6. Describe what to do when either an adult or child is choking or not breathing.
7. Describe types of burns and their treatment.
8. Describe how to treat hypothermia and frostbite.
9. List the symptoms of hyperthermia (heat exhaustion and heat stroke) and describe how to treat hyperthermia.
10. List the symptoms of poisoning.
11. Describe how to splint a broken bone.

Learning the Vocabulary

first aid	splint
dispatcher	herbs
emergency medical service (EMS)	folk medicine
	hemlock
CPR (cardiopulmonary resuscitation)	belladonna
	sassafras
carotid pulse	ma huang
shock	witch hazel
Heimlich Maneuver (abdominal thrust maneuver)	ginseng
	ginseng abuse syndrome
	aloe
hypothermia	chamomile
hyperthermia	echinacea
frostbite	melatonin
venom	foxglove
fracture	comfrey

Answer the following questions on a separate sheet of paper.

1. *Matching*—Match each of the following phrases with the appropriate vocabulary term from the list above:
  a. person who answers calls and relays messages to the proper helping service
  b. formation of ice crystals in body parts exposed to temperatures below freezing
  c. a stick or board to support a broken bone
  d. the heartbeat in main arteries next to the airway in the front of the neck
  e. a technique of dislodging a particle that is blocking a person's airway
  f. medical help given immediately in an emergency
  g. a condition of too little body heat with abnormally low internal body temperature
2. a. A life-threatening reaction to accidents and injuries is called _____.
  b. _____ is a poison from a living creature such as a snake or scorpion.
  c. A break in a bone is called a _____.
  d. The _____ is a team of people who are trained to respond in emergencies, and who can be contacted through a single dispatcher.
3. Write a paragraph using at least ten of the vocabulary terms. Underline each vocabulary term that you use.

Recalling Important Facts and Ideas

Section 1

1. What are the two most important self-protective items to keep in a first aid kit?

Section 2

2. What are common hazards present when you survey an accident scene?
3. How do you decide who needs treatment first when there are several victims?
4. Describe how you should check a victim's airway.
5. What happens to the blood and other vital organs of a person who goes into shock?
6. When you do a secondary survey of a victim, what are you looking for?

Section 3

7. How long does it take for a person to die when oxygen is cut off?
8. What is one problem that occurs when an untrained person attempts CPR?

698

SECTION 3

7. 50 percent die within five minutes, almost all others die within ten minutes. (p. 678)
8. They may stop a heart that is already beating, placing the victim in severe danger. (p. 681)

SECTION 4

9. clutch the throat area with both hands while the mouth is open (p. 684)

10. intervene only after the victim has tried self-help maneuvers without success (p. 684)
11. shout for help and perform the Heimlich maneuver (p. 684)

SECTION 5

12. A tourniquet almost always kills the limb to which it is applied. (p. 686)

Section 4

9. Explain the universal distress signal for choking.
10. If a person is choking but can make a sound, what should a rescuer do?
11. If a person is choking but cannot make a sound, what should a rescuer do?

Section 5

12. Why shouldn't a tourniquet be used to control bleeding?

Section 6

13. How are burns classified?
14. Describe what a second degree burn looks like.
15. What should you be concerned about when a person has a facial burn?
16. What temperature should the body be for tissues to function normally?
17. What are symptoms of hypothermia?
18. What is the treatment for hypothermia?
19. What shouldn't you do when treating for frostbite?
20. What is the most common cause of poisoning?

Critical Thinking

1. After taking the Life Choice Inventory on page 690, how do you feel about your results? What can and will you do to improve your score? If you are already in the excellent range, what will you do to stay in the excellent range?

Activities

1. Make a video of how to perform the Heimlich Maneuver and show it to the rest of the school.
2. Visit a local hospital. Ask the emergency room personnel how many people have died in the last month. Out of that number how many have died because no CPR was performed on them? Give an oral report to your class.
3. Make posters on the ABC's of first aid. Put them up around your school.
4. Make a pamphlet that explains different types of wounds, burns, and broken bones. Explain the first-aid procedures necessary for treating these problems.
5. Question your family members on the procedures to follow in first-aid situations. Explain to them the importance of knowing how to perform first aid. Encourage them to take a class in first aid and emergency procedures.

6. Interview your principal and see how prepared the school is in case of an emergency. How many teachers are certified in first aid? How many are certified in CPR? Write a report on your findings.
7. Make up a play that explains what to have in a first-aid kit, and what the items are for. Show this play to the children at local elementary schools.
8. Check to see if you have a first-aid kit at home. Bring it to class and describe the items that are in the kit and what they are used for. Also describe the items that are missing and why they are needed. If you don't have a kit at home describe the items you would put in one and what their purposes are.
9. Contact the local office of the Red Cross or American Heart Association. Ask for information about CPR classes. Use the following list as guidelines.

   ▶ Locations where classes are offered
   ▶ Times when classes meet
   ▶ Which courses are offered
   ▶ Which certifications can be earned
   ▶ Number of hours of training required for certifications
   ▶ Age requirements
   ▶ Validity periods for certifications
   ▶ Cost for taking a course
   ▶ Which courses are needed for jobs in day care and life guarding

   Share the information you gather with the rest of your class.

Making Decisions about Health

1. You are at your neighbor's house baby-sitting. About halfway through the evening one of the kids, Katherine, feels very sick. You feel her forehead and she is burning up. The other two kids, Webster and Jimmy, are fine. What would you do in this situation? How will you take care of Katherine and keep the other two kids supervised?
2. You are backpacking on your family vacation, and your mother has slipped off the trail and stumbled down a large embankment. When you go to help her, all her vital signs are good. You think she may be going into shock, though. What action will you take? Why will you take such action?

699

SECTION 6

13. by the depth of tissue injury (p. 687)
14. red and mottled, with blisters, considerable swelling, wet at the surface (p. 687)
15. that the airway is burned (p. 688)
16. 98.6 degrees F (p. 689)
17. stiff muscles, with some shivering or trembling; dizziness; weakness; cold skin; problems with coordination; slowed breathing and heart rate; confusion and drowsiness (p. 689)

18. warm food or drink; not raising the feet; wrapping the person in blankets, towels, pillows, scarves, or newspapers (p. 690)
19. rub the affected body parts, pack affected parts in snow or cold water (p. 691)
20. overdose of aspirin or other over-the-counter pain relievers, eaten by children or taken by mistake by adults (p. 693)

UNIT 8 PLANNING GUIDE

OUTCOMES	FEATURES

CHAPTER 26

The Environment and Your Health

- Describe how the environment affects your body's health.
- List and identify the global environmental problems in the late 1990s.
- Explain how our lifestyle choices affect the environment and our health.
- Discuss how we can help our environment while shopping.
- Describe how we can conserve energy and water in our homes.
- Describe the environmental problems associated with waste disposal.
- Discuss the impact of hunger on the environment.

Life Choice Inventory: How Well Do You Care for the Environment? (page 704)

Straight Talk: Personal Strategy—Voluntary Simplicity (page 726)

Teen Views: Should You Be Doing More to Protect Our Environment? If So, What Should You Be Doing? (page 717)

CHAPTER 27

The Consumer and the Health-Care System

- Discuss the benefits of managed care plans such as health maintenance organizations (HMOs).
- Describe three broad areas of health insurance.
- Identify ways to select a medical care facility.
- Identify reasons why health-care insurance costs are on the rise.
- Discuss the problems and advantages associated with our health-care system.
- Describe the services of health-care providers.
- Discuss how to choose a health-care provider.
- Define alternative therapy.

Health Strategies: Selecting and Using Medical Care Facilities (page 734)

Health Strategies: Hints for Emergency Room Visits (page 736)

Health Strategies: Choosing a Health-Care Provider (page 742)

Consumer Skills: Genuine and Fake Credentials (page 743)

Straight Talk: Health Claims and Quackery (page 746)

TEACHING SUPPORT

Vocabulary: Learning Key Terms, Crossword Puzzle, Fill in the Blank
Study Outline
Reading Cloze
Reteaching: You and Your Environment, Helping the Environment
Enrichment: Environmental Problems, Caring for the Environment, Protecting the Environment, Clean Up the Environment: A Group Project
Career Brief: Foresters and Conservation Scientists
Life Choice Inventory: How Well Do You Care for the Environment?
Handouts: Living a Simpler Lifestyle; Lifestyle Choices Affect the Environment and Health; Sound Intensities and their Effects; Some Ways

to Reduce, Reuse, and Recycle; Home Appliances and Global Warming; Energy Used by Appliances; Using Nontoxic Products in the Home; U.S. Public Health Service Objectives for the Nation
Quizzes: Sections 1–6
Tests: Chapter 26 Test A, Chapter 26 Test B
Transparencies: All Things Connected; Accumulation of Toxic compounds at the Top of the Food Chain; Hazardous Wastes in the United States; Radiation Levels of Chernobyl Nuclear Accident, 1986; The Rate of Loss of the World's Rain Forests; Population Growth

Vocabulary: Learning Key Terms, Crossword Puzzle
Study Outline
Reading Cloze
Reteaching: How Will I Pay for My Health Care?, Making an Informed Decision about Your Physician
Enrichment: Fee (Fi Fo Fum), Who Can Help?, Health-Care Expectations—What's Your Opinion?
Career Brief: Insurance Agents and Brokers

Handouts: Health Care Delivery—Past and Present/Future, Guidelines for Chapter Project, Advertising of Drugs
Quizzes: Sections 1–3
Tests: Chapter 27 Test A, Chapter 27 Test B

MULTIMEDIA SUPPORT

- Health Video Library
- CNN Health and Fitness Update Videos
- Westest
- Student Review Software
- Diet Analysis Software
- Nutrition CD-ROM

LESSON PLANNING

You will find detailed daily lesson plans for both **traditional scheduling** and **block scheduling** in you Teacher's Resource Box. Other suggested scheduling formats can be found in the supplemental Lesson Plannng guide.

KEY POINTS

Chapter 26 is 30 pages long and divided into six sections. Chapter 26 focuses on developing student empathy regarding global environmental issues and student involvement in implementing environmentally sound practices into daily life. Students become informed about local environmental issues, realize that one person or a small group can make a difference, and create and carry out action plans. Activities encourage students to lead simpler lives and persuade others to do the same, thereby consuming less energy and fewer resources.

ACTIVITY TO INTRODUCE THE CHAPTER

Ask students to list all of the products that they used this morning to get ready for school. Ask if they created any waste. If so, could this waste be recycled? Tell students that not only do people need to be aware of the items they purchase that cause waste, they also need to recognize that some wastes can be recycled.

CHAPTER 26

Contents

1. You and the Environment: A Single System
2. Human Impacts on the Earth
3. Shopping
4. Energy Use in the Home
5. Water Use, Trash, and Garbage
6. Hunger and the Environment

STRAIGHT TALK
*Personal Strategy—
Voluntary Simplicity*

NOT Enough Time?

Following are some suggestions to help you make sure you cover the key topics in this chapter if you have limited time. (Refer to the daily lesson plans in your Teacher's Resource Box for additional suggestions.)

DAY 1   Complete the Activity to Introduce the Chapter on page 700 and the Focus Activity on page 702. Have students complete the Life Choice Inventory on page 704. Assign students to read Sections 1 and 2 for homework.

DAY 2   Begin class with the Key Passage on page 706. Read and discuss with students.

The Environment and Your Health

What do you think? Are the following statements true or false? If you think they are false, then say what is true.

1. Small groups of people can change the world.
2. All products that people buy are harmful to the environment.
3. Local products cost less than the same products shipped in from far away.
4. All-electric homes pollute the environment less than homes that use gas or oil for heating and appliances.
5. The average electric range is one of the most energy-guzzling home appliances.
6. If U.S. consumers used less energy, this would help solve the world's hunger problem.

(Answers on page 724)

Introduction

A healthy **environment** supports personal health. A damaged environment erodes it. Consider your needs. Ideally, wherever you lived and worked—inner city, farm, or wilderness—the air would be clean; the water, pure; the food, nourishing and safe; the scenery and sounds, enjoyable; the space, open for play; and all other elements, both seen and unseen, in harmony together. It is unrealistic, of course, to think that everyone in today's world can enjoy such a life. It is also untrue that such perfect conditions are necessary to health. It is true, however, that people will survive only so long as we maintain our environment so that it can sustain us.

We and our environment are really part of a single system. Our environment supplies the materials our bodies are made of. It also provides forms of energy (especially light and heat energy) that make our lives possible. Materials and energy constantly flow into and through us, and we alter the environment just by being here.

BULLETIN BOARD IDEAS

Have students bring in a variety of waste products and packaging that can be recycled, as well as some that cannot. Have students help you sort through the items and place each in its proper pile for recycling. Have students find locations of places that will accept each type of item to be recycled. Then have students highlight these places on a map of your community, using different colors of highlighter for each type of recyclable material. Make a key below the map that shows the colors on the map and which materials correspond. Display the map where it can be easily seen by all students.

Answers to FACT or FICTION

1. **True.**
2. **False.** Products are beneficial to the environment if they help *relieve* pollution or displace other products that pollute.
3. **False.** Local products may cost more, but they may be a good choice for environmental reasons.
4. **False.** Fossil fuels are burned to produce electricity.
5. **False.** Refrigerators, hot water heaters, and air conditioners use more energy, because they are on all the time.
6. **True.**

Do the Learning with Visuals activity on page 708 and close with the Evaluate activity on page 710.

DAY 3 Have students read Sections 3 and 4 prior to class. Have students complete the Focus Activity on page 711. Then do the Group Activity on page 713. Close with the Evaluate activity on page 719.

DAY 4 Have students read Sections 5 and 6 prior to class. During class do a selection of the following activities: the second Discussion activity on page 720, the Close activity on page 721, Focus Activity 2 on page 722, and the Evaluate activity on page 724.

SECTION 1

FOCUS

OUTCOME

In this section students will learn that:

1. Their behavior affects the earth's air, water, and living things.

FOCUS ACTIVITY

Have students brainstorm ways the environment can affect our health. Discuss students' answers and use their responses to introduce topics that will be covered in this chapter.

TEACH & APPLY

BACKGROUND INFORMATION

Make sure students understand the meaning of the sentence beginning the second paragraph of the introduction, "We and our environment are really part of a single system." First ask them to define *environment* in a way that suggests that they are separate from the environment. Then ask them to explain how a person and his or her environment are part of a single system. (environment supplies material making up the body; environment provides energy; materials and energy flow through our bodies from the environment and back to the environment)

SECTION 1

You and the Environment: A Single System

Just as your environment affects your body's health each day, you also affect the environment each day. Each day of your life, you breathe its air, eat its food, and leave your wastes in it. Many of your activites involve choices—what you eat, how you dispose of your waste, and so forth. To make your choices consciously, you can learn which ones leave the earth better or worse off each day.

It is in your interest to learn this, partly because of the environment's impact on you. For example:

▶ If the air is clean, your lungs can be healthy. If the air is polluted, you and your family may suffer chronic lung diseases.

▶ If the water is pure, you can drink it without fear. If the water is polluted, it can bring with it all manner of harmful chemicals, including many that cause cancer.

▶ If the soil is free of poisons, it will grow food that will sustain you. If it is contaminated, the food may be unwholesome. Some contaminated soil cannot even support plant life, or any kind of living things.

Some pollution you can see for yourself. . .

Chapter 26, Section 1

The following quiz will help you assess your students' understanding of the material covered in this section of the chapter. You might use the quiz as an oral exercise, which will lead into a class discussion of the topics covered. Or, you might use it as a paper/pencil

quiz to evaluate your students individually.

1. The state of the environment has a direct effect on your personal health. (True)

2. The way our clothes and foods are produced is linked to poverty, disease and hunger in many different parts of the world. (True)

3. The choices of U.S. consumers do not have a significant impact on the environment. (False)

Vast changes are taking place in your environment today. You may not recognize these changes. Once your eyes are open, however, you will see them all around you. When you have become conscious of how your own choices affect the environment, you will also see the effects of the choices of others—and not only the choices of individuals but also those of groups, including industry, agriculture, and government.

You have the right to a healthy environment—the right to clean air, pure water, and safe food. Together with your neighbors, you can demand that other people respect that right. As large as the world's environmental problems may be, they are all caused by people's choices. They can also only be solved by people's choices.

The sections that follow show you, first, how human behaviors are affecting the earth. They then explain how you can shape your behaviors for the better in several areas—in your shopping choices, your home energy use, and others. The Life Choice Inventory on the next page gives you a starting point. It allows you to see how aware you already are of your responsibilities toward the earth.

 KEY POINTS *All things are connected. Human behaviors affect the world's air, water, and living things. In turn, the air, water, and all life on earth affect human health.*

. . . but even air and water that appear clean often contain invisible pollutants.

 SECTION 1 Review

Answer the following questions on a sheet of paper.

Learning the Vocabulary

The vocabulary word in this section is *environment*.

1. Write a sentence using the vocabulary word.

Learning the Facts

2. What does your environment do to your personal health?

3. What is the cause of the world's environmental problems and what can solve them?

Making Life Choices

4. Take the Life Choice Inventory that accompanies this section. Which environmentally aware choices do you make each day? Which habits do you need to change? Explain your answers.

 MINI Glossary

environment: everything "outside" the living organism—air, water, soil, other organisms, and forms of radiation.

 SECTION 1 Review Answers

1. Answers will vary.
2. Answers will vary. (p. 702)
3. The choices people make cause the problems, and the choices people make can solve the problems. (p. 703)
4. Answers will vary.

CLOSE

Walk with students around your school campus. After returning to the classroom, have students make two lists: one list will include choices people at the school have made to benefit the environment (example: recycling bin for aluminum cans); the second list will include choices people have made that will damage the environment (example: litter on the ground instead of in the trash cans). Encourage students to keep their lists and use the information they gain in this chapter to develop ideas that will help change the damaging choices into beneficial choices.

4. Fifteen children die of malnutrition every 30 seconds. (True)
5. The greenhouse effect is the result of an increase in the amount of carbon dioxide in the atmosphere. (True)
6. The accelerating of fossil fuels has resulted in an increased depletion of the ozone layer. (True)
7. Deforestation and desertification have recently begun to decrease. (False)
8. A single individual's environmentally conscious behavior may help to make many other people become aware of the consequences of their actions. (True)
9. The Kyoto Protocol is an international treaty designed to improve the environment. (True)
10. Sustainable choices are often healthier for the individual as well as for the environment. (True)

A reproducible copy of the Life Choice Inventory is provided in the Teacher's Resource Box.

Comprehension Check

Before students begin the inventory, have them read the scoring directions. They need to go through the list of suggestions in the inventory twice. It might help to have them make two columns on a sheet of paper, one entitled, "I am aware of this," and another entitled "I practice this habit." They should then put check marks in the appropriate columns for each number. When they are finished, check marks in the first column count one point and check marks in the second column count two points. Compare scores in class.

GUEST SPEAKER

Have either a city official who deals with the environmental controls of the city or a lawyer who specializes in environmental law come into class to discuss the laws that attempt to provide us with a clean and natural environment. Allow students to ask questions.

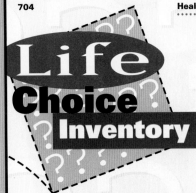

How Well Do You Care for the Environment?

The following questions are selected and adapted from a conservation action checklist subtitled "65 Things You Can Do to Help Save Tropical Forests and Other Natural Resources." On your own paper, record your answers and calculate your score as described.

Keep a copy of these suggestions in a place where you will be sure to see them once every month. Every time you read the list, try to adopt another conservation habit. If everyone does these things, it will significantly help our planet's health and, in turn, your own health. Your answers to the Life Choice Inventory are personal and private. Share them with others only if you are comfortable doing so.

In your home, do you:

1. Recycle everything you can: newspapers, cans, glass bottles and jars, scrap metal, used oil, etc.?
2. Use cold water in the washer whenever possible?
3. Avoid using appliances (such as electric can openers) to do things you can do by hand?
4. Reuse brown paper bags to line your trash? Reuse bread bags, butter tubs, etc.?
5. Store food in reusable containers rather than plastic wrap or aluminum foil?

In your yard, do you:

6. Pull weeds instead of using herbicides?
7. Fertilize with manure and compost, rather than with chemical fertilizers?
8. Compost your leaves and yard debris, rather than burning them?
9. Take extra plastic and rubber pots back to the nursery?

On vacation, do you:

10. Turn down the heat and turn off the hot water heater before you leave?
11. Carry reusable cups, dishes, and flatware (and use them)?
12. Dispose of trash in trash containers (never litter)?
13. Buy no souvenirs made from wild or endangered animals?
14. Stay on roads and trails, and not trample dunes and fragile undergrowth?

About your car, do you:

15. Keep your car tuned up for maximum fuel efficiency?
16. Use public transit whenever possible?
17. Ride your bike or walk whenever possible?
18. Plan to replace your car with a more fuel-efficient model when you can?
19. Recycle your engine oil?

At school or work, do you:

20. Recycle paper whenever possible?
21. Use scrap paper for notes to yourself and others?
22. Print or copy on both sides of the paper?
23. Reuse large envelopes and file folders?
24. Use the stairs instead of the elevator whenever you can?

Focusing ON Self-Esteem

When we protect the environment, we feel better about ourselves and that raises self-esteem. So, how can your students start feeling better about themselves and the environment? Offer the following ways to handle the trash, and ask students to brainstorm ways they can begin. What are students already doing to change the way they treat the natural environment? Are there ways they can encourage their family members to get on the environmental "bandwagon"?

1. Reduce the quantity of waste produced.
2. Reuse items.
3. Recycle. Recycling reduces landfill impact,

When you're buying, do you:

25. Buy as little plastic and foam packaging as possible?
26. Buy permanent, rather than disposable, products?
27. Buy paper rather than plastic, if you must buy disposable products?
28. Buy fresh produce grown locally?
29. Buy in bulk to avoid unnecessary packaging?

In other areas, do you:

30. Volunteer your time to conservation projects?
31. Encourage your family, friends, and neighbors to save resources, too?
32. Write letters to support conservation issues?

SCORING

First, give yourself 4 points for answering this quiz:_____
Then, give yourself 1 point each for all the habits you know people should adopt. This is to give you credit for your awareness, even if you haven't acted on it, yet (total possible points = 32): _____

Finally, give yourself 2 more points for each habit you have adopted—or honestly would if you could (total possible points = 64): _____
Total score:
1 to 25: You are a beginner in stewardship of the earth. Try to improve.
26 to 50: You are well on your way. Few consumers do even as well as this, yet.
51 to 75: Excellent. Pat yourself on the back, and keep on improving.
76 to 100: Outstanding. You are a shining example for others to follow.

Source: Adapted from *Conservation Action Checklist,* produced by the Washington Park Zoo, Portland, Oregon, and available from Conservation International, 1015 18th St. NW, Suite 1000, Washington, D.C. 20036; 1-800-406-2306. (Web site:http://www.conservation.org). Call or write for copies of the original or for more information.

For your health's sake, take care of your environment.

reduces pollution, and reuses natural resources.
4. Compost. Composting also reduces the need for landfills, produces fertile humus, and reuses natural resources.
5. Recover energy from waste. Each ton of solid waste is equivalent to the energy in 70 gallons of gasoline.
6. Trash the landfills. Landfills are unattrac-

tive, they use valuable land resources, they pollute air and water, and they burn natural resources. Find new solutions to the trash problem.

Think Creatively!

SECTION 2

FOCUS

OUTCOMES

In this section students will learn:

1. How the environment affects their health.
2. To describe the major global environmental problems of the 1990s.

FOCUS ACTIVITY

Have students name as many environmental problems as possible. They should name global problems, not just local ones. Discuss.

TEACH & APPLY

TEACHER SUPPORT

Key Passage

Emphasize that each person's choices make a difference in our environment. Tell the students that some of the choices are small. For example, a motorist who sits for ten minutes in a traffic jam could keep the car running or turn it off so that it would pollute the air a little less. Then there are big choices. For example, a hospital administrator might choose for the sake of profit to have disease-carrying refuse dumped into the nearest river rather than disposing of it properly. All these choices make a difference.

For Your Information

Three rules of the environment:

1. Nothing ever goes away. Substances thrown away, flushed, drained, or even burned are still with us and find their way back into our soil, water, and air.
2. Everything we use or consume costs the environment something to produce or run.
3. All things are connected. People and the environment are part of one system.

For Your Information

▶ The average molecule of food eaten in this country travels 1,300 miles before the consumer swallows it.
▶ To drive a semitrailer 1,300 miles requires about 250 gallons of gas.
▶ 250 gallons of gas burned as fuel releases 2½ tons of carbon dioxide. Carbon dioxide accumulation in the atmosphere is warming up the globe.
▶ The consumer who drinks a typical can of diet soda obtains from it 1 calorie of food energy. To manufacture the can, however, costs 800 calories in fuel, pollutes the soil at the mining site with toxic materials, and uses more water than the soda that ends up in the can.

SECTION 2

Human Impacts on the Earth

Most people buy and use goods and services without thinking about the effects these products have on our environment. Seldom do they ask such questions as, "What is the cost of this product or service in electricity, gasoline, water, and **pollution**?" or "How does my choice of this product or service affect the global environment?" However, the ways our clothes, foods, and toys are produced do affect the global environment. They are even linked to poverty, hunger, and disease of populations on the other side of the world. If we realized the impacts of our choices, we might choose differently—yet still enjoy our lives just as much as we do now.

Impacts of U.S. Consumption

The production of goods for U.S. consumers is one of the globe's biggest businesses. It involves huge manufacturing efforts that use water and fuel; huge tracts of land to produce raw materials; huge amounts of packaging materials and fuel to make goods ready for market; a huge transportation network—in short, enormous consumption of resources and production of pollution. Today's consumers, becoming aware of the environmental impacts of their choices and eager to become conscious choosers, are fascinated by facts like those in the margin.

Choices that are far less harmful to the environment are possible. For example, Floridians need not eat carrots that have been shipped in from California. They can eat carrots grown in Florida (and Californians can eat carrots grown in California). In place of five or six diet sodas in aluminum cans, the consumer might pour drinks of soda from one large plastic bottle. Both cans and plastic bottles are recyclable, but producing and recycling the large bottles costs less environmentally.

Many other examples of environmental impacts will appear in this chapter. In every case, the purpose is to make you aware of your alternatives. A choice one person makes, one time, of local carrots or a plastic bottle may be insignificant in the scheme of things. However, several benefits come out of such choices. For one, a single person's awareness and example, shared with others, is shared again, and so it multiplies. For another, an action taken one time is likely to happen a second and third time, so that a habit is formed.

 KEY POINTS *The United States consumes vast amounts of the world's resources. Choices of U.S. consumers powerfully influence the environment.*

Global Environmental Problems

A sense of individual control is needed for people to take action. Today's global environmental problems can easily seem so overwhelming to single individuals as to make them feel passive and hopeless. At the present time, all of the following trends are taking place at once:

▶ *Hunger, poverty, and population growth.* Millions of people are starving. Fifteen children die of malnutrition every 30 seconds, but 75 children are born in that same 30 seconds.

HEALTHY PEOPLE 2000

Reduce human exposure to toxic agents by confining total pounds of toxic agents released into the air, water, and soil each year to no more than:

0.24 billion pounds of those toxic agents included on the Department of Health and Human Services list of carcinogens.

2.6 billion pounds of those toxic agents included on the Agency for Toxic Substances and Disease Registry list of the most toxic chemicals.

According to EPA, toxic pollutants are one of today's most serious emerging problems. Toxic substances are found in all environmental media. Despite low concentrations, toxic chemicals emitted into the air by human activities may have serious short-term and long-

- ▶ *Losses of land to produce food.* Land to produce food is becoming more salty, eroding, and being paved over.
- ▶ *Accelerating **fossil fuel** use.* Fuel use is accelerating, along with pollution of air, soil, and water; **ozone** depletion; and global warming.
- ▶ *Increasing **air pollution**.* Air quality is diminishing all over the globe. Acids in the air are causing **acid rain**.
- ▶ *Global warming*, *droughts, and floods.* Atmospheric levels of heat-trapping carbon dioxide are now 26 percent higher than before the age of industry, and they are continuing to climb. As a result, a massive warming trend, known as the **greenhouse effect**, is taking place. This is changing the climate, causing both droughts and floods, destroying crops, and forcing people from their homes.
- ▶ *Ozone loss from the outer atmosphere.* The outer atmosphere's protective **ozone layer** is growing thinner. This is permitting harmful radiation from the sun to damage crops and ecosystems and to cause cancers in people.
- ▶ *Water shortages.* The world's supplies of freshwater are dwindling and becoming polluted.
- ▶ *Deforestation and desertification.* Forests are shrinking. Deserts are growing. By the year 2000, *new* deserts worldwide will cover an area 1½ times the size of the United States.
- ▶ *Ocean and lake pollution.* Ocean and lake pollution is killing fish. Overfishing is depleting the numbers of those that remain. Pollution is making them unsafe to eat.
- ▶ *Extinctions of species.* Vast extinctions of animals and plants are taking place—a minimum of 140 species *a day*. Some 20 percent more of those species remaining are expected to die out in the next ten years. Extinction is forever. Many kinds of whales, birds, giant mammals, colorful butterflies, and thousands of others will never again be seen in the universe.

Despite the magnitude of these disasters, there is much that people can do to help slow, stop, and even reverse these processes and restore a livable world. On some fronts people can act as individuals. Each of us can choose what products to buy, what foods to eat, and the like. On other fronts people can act in groups. Groups can lobby legislators to write laws that protect the environment, demand that the laws be enforced, and insist that corporations and governments honor their principles. According to a famous activist (Margaret Mead), you should "never doubt that a small group of thoughtful, committed people can change the world. Indeed," she says, "it is the only thing that ever has."

Once aware of their impacts, if people choose to change their actions, two kinds of **ripple effect** can follow. One is the ripple effect that takes place in each person's own mind, as one level of awareness leads to another. First, a person learns how to improve the immediate surroundings. Soon, however, the person learns how to reach much farther. The other kind of ripple effect is the effect on people who hear and see what the person is doing. A word of awareness dropped into another's ear may start a ripple there that grows into a wave. Students often start such waves as they learn of current events and start trying to change them.

Governments can change things, too, and their degree of commitment to doing so matters greatly. Recently, 150 nations signed a treaty known as

MINI
Glossary

pollution: contamination of the environment with anything that impairs its ability to support life.

fossil fuel: coal, oil, and natural gas, which all come from the fossilized remains of plant life of earlier times.

ozone: a substance created when certain types of energy, such as the sun's ultra-violet rays, react with oxygen. When this reaction takes place high above the earth in the outer atmosphere, the ozone absorbs the most dangerous UV rays.

air pollution: contamination of the air with gases or particles not normally found there.

acid rain: rain that carries acid air pollutants; it harms the plants and damages the soil on which it falls.

global warming: warming of the planet, a trend that threatens life on earth.

greenhouse effect: the heat-trapping effect of the glass in a greenhouse. The same effect is caused by gases that are accumulating in the earth's outer atmosphere, which are trapping the sun's heat and warming the planet.

ozone layer: a layer of ozone in the earth's outer atmosphere that protects living things on earth from harmful ultraviolet radiation from the sun.

ripple effect: the effect seen when a pebble is thrown into a pond and waves radiate out from it. The term is used to describe how one person's actions may affect many other people, and how their actions will affect still other people.

term effects on human health. More than 300 chemicals released by manufacturers and others into the air, soil, and water are tracked by the EPA Toxic Chemical Release Inventory. Once released, these toxic substances are available for human intake. Persistent substances may accumulate in the environment and in the food chain.

Once toxic contaminants are emitted, people may be exposed to them in a variety of ways. The most common exposure is through inhalation. Indirect exposure may occur after airborne particles fall to earth and are taken up by crops, animals, or fish that we consume. Particles may also contaminate the water we drink. Through these routes, some toxins accumulate over time and become highly concentrated in human fatty tissue and breast milk.

LEARNING WITH VISUALS

The purpose of Figure 26–1 is to help students see that all the major environmental problems are interconnected. The problems identified in the ten circles are roughly equivalent to the list of ten environmental problems that students studied on the preceding pages in this chapter. Each numbered arrow is explained in a key on the opposite page. You may make many different kinds of assignments using this illustration, but first make sure that students appreciate the main point—that each problem contributes to the worsening of the other problems. Students should begin to realize, as the text stated earlier, that if one problem is solved it will help solve all of the others. Among the different activities you could have students do are the following:

a. Have them pick a number, any number, follow that arrow, and then guess without looking at the key how the one problem affects the other. After writing down one or two guesses, students could look at the key.

b. The class could read through the entire list of impacts from 1 to 43 in order, with each student reading a different number.

c. Students could be divided into ten groups, one for each type of problem. Each group would be assigned to develop a poster for that problem. They would also then create an original way of presenting each of the impacts originating from their circle.

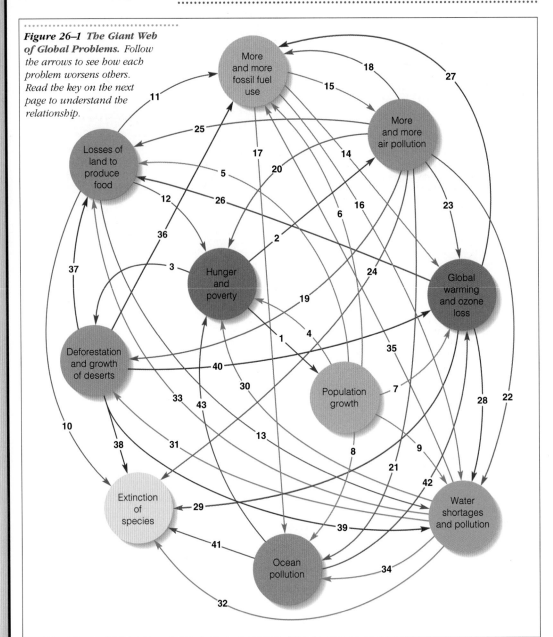

Figure 26–1 The Giant Web of Global Problems. *Follow the arrows to see how each problem worsens others. Read the key on the next page to understand the relationship.*

COOPERATIVE LEARNING

Saving the Environment

The following activity will help students understand the importance of protecting our environment as well as the reasons why we need to protect our environment. They will gain an understanding of how taking steps to protect the environment will benefit them both physically and financially. By protecting our environment we can better assure that we will have clear air to breath, clean water to drink, an abundance of food to eat, and we will be free of infectious disease and protected against sun related cancers. Financially, people will save on the costs of food, electricity, and other items if they learn to conserve, recycle, and reuse goods that they get from the environment.

Divide your class into groups of three or four students. Supply them with poster board

KEY:

1. Hunger and poverty make people fear their children will die, so they bear as many children as they can. This is explained later.
2. Poor people burn wood for fuel.
3. Landless people cut and burn trees to establish farmland.
4. The more mouths to feed, the worse the poverty becomes.
5. Growing cities take up the land of former farms.
6. Growing populations use more and more gas, coal, and oil for homes, cars, and factories.
7. The more people, the more cattle, which release the methane that contributes to both global warming and ozone loss. Also, the more people, the more air conditioners and refrigerators, which leak ozone-destroying refrigerants.
8. Growing populations pollute waterways and the ocean with sewage, garbage, fertilizers, and pesticides.
9. Growing populations need more water to drink, to grow their food, and to support their mining and manufacturing. The more people, the more human waste and agricultural and industrial pollution.
10. Land losses lead to losses of habitats. Then species die out.
11. As farmland is paved over, new farms try to use land with poorer soil. This requires more tractors (which use fossil fuels) and more fertilizer (which is made from fossil fuels).
12. As land suitable to produce food diminishes, food shortages intensify.
13. New farmland on poor soil demands irrigation, which uses up water, salts the land, and pollutes waterways.
14. The more gas, coal, and oil are burned, the more they release global-warming gases and pollutants that destroy outer-atmosphere ozone.
15. The more gas, coal, and oil are burned, the more air pollutants they release.
16. Fuels (and fertilizers made from them) pollute rivers and groundwater.
17. The transportation of fossil fuels in ocean-going tankers leads to oil spills.
18. As outdoor air becomes impossible to breathe, people use more air conditioners and purifiers, demanding more fuel to run them.
19. Air pollution deprives plants of needed sunlight.
20. Air pollution worsens living and working conditions and destroys health.
21. Rain falling through polluted air washes the pollutants into the ocean.
22. Air pollution pollutes the rain. This pollutes both surface water and groundwater.
23. Many air pollutants rise to the outer atmosphere, trapping heat and destroying ozone.
24. Air pollution degrades the conditions for life.
25. Air pollution falls in rain and ruins land.
26. As the ocean warms, it expands, and land masses shrink.
27. The warmer the climate, the more people use air conditioning and refrigeration.
28. Droughts cause water shortages. Floods wash pollution into water supplies.
29. A warmer climate threatens plant and animal life. Ozone loss means that harmful radiation from the sun will damage living things.
30. Water shortages and pollution force people from their homes.
31. Water shortages cause fields and forests to dry up and die.
32. Water shortages and pollution wipe out plants and animals.
33. Water shortages dry up land. Polluted water ruins soil.
34. Polluted rivers pollute the ocean.
35. To transport water over long distances, to desalt ocean water, and to purify polluted water for reuse, more and more energy is required.
36. With less wood to rely on, people turn to fossil fuels to burn for energy and to make plastics.
37. As deserts grow, land areas suitable for farming shrink.
38. Losses of once-forested or fertile lands rob species of needed habitat.
39. Deforested lands and dried-up wetlands cannot absorb and hold pollutants. Instead, pollutants run into rivers and lakes.
40. The more tropical forests are burned, the more global-warming gases trap earth's heat, and the fewer trees remain to remove these gases from the air.
41. Even though the ocean is very large and its species very numerous, pollution can destroy the conditions necessary for life.
42. Ocean pollution is beginning to kill ocean algae, which help control the planet's temperature.
43. Ocean pollution kills ocean life, leading to losses of fisheries.

and permanent markers. Instruct the students to create several posters that promote steps that can be taken to protect the environment. Examples may include reasons to recycle paper, aluminum, plastic, and glass. The posters should list all the benefits of recycling to both the individual and society. After groups have completed their posters, have them displayed in various locations throughout the halls of the school.

Also have students make arrangements with teachers in the school to place recycling bins for aluminum cans, paper, plastic, and glass in every classroom. Make sure that you have a plan to have those students empty the recycling bins on a regular basis.

Completing this activity will not only give your class the knowledge of the importance of protecting the environment, but it also gets the entire student body involved.

d. Another possibility would be to have each student in the class represent one of the 43 factors. Designate ten areas in the classroom, one for each of the ten major problems. Have each student begin in the area from which his arrow originates. Students would state the sentence of their numbers and then walk to the area affected. Number 1 would be followed by number 2, and so on.

GROUP ACTIVITY

Divide students into groups. Have each group create a way to teach environmental awareness to elementary school children. Give students different topics, such as energy use, reducing solid wastes, keeping air and water clean, recycling, and using toxic chemicals. Have the groups develop an educational program around their topics to teach to small children. Assess student knowledge by watching them present their educational programs to the class. Pick the best programs and take those students on a field trip to a neighboring elementary school to present the programs to the children.

GROUP PROJECT

Have the students think of and carry out community service projects aimed at protecting or cleaning up the local environment. Some examples of projects might include cleaning up around a lake or pond, picking up and recycling aluminum cans, educating consumers about how their choices affect the environment, or becoming involved in a demonstration or movement surrounding a local environmental issue.

710
CHAPTER 26: The Environment and
Your Health

ASSESS

EVALUATE

To assess how much the students learned from this section, ask them to tell you ways in which humans have a negative effect on their environment. What could be done in a sustainable way to change each of these negative effects?

SECTION 2 Review Answers

1. Air pollution
2. ozone layer
3. Fossil fuel
4. It involves manufacturing efforts involving water and fuel; huge tracts of land to produce raw materials; huge amounts of packaging materials and fuels; a huge transportation network; and production of pollution. (p. 706)
5. Producing and recycling the large bottles costs less environmentally. (p. 706)
6. One kind of ripple effect takes place in each person's own mind, as one level of awareness leads to another. The other kind of ripple effect is the effect on people who hear and see what the person is doing. The awareness may lead to changes. (p. 707)
7. Answers will vary.

CLOSE

Bring in an item from the grocery store. Have students write the steps involved in getting this item to the shelf of the store for purchase. Have them tell how these steps affected our environment.

the **Kyoto Protocol**. The treaty calls for reducing the kinds of pollution, particularly carbon dioxide gas, known to speed up global warming. As a result, by 2012 both industry and private citizens across the globe must change their habits to reduce pollution. The treaty also rewards countries that maintain forests, because trees absorb ozone-destroying carbon dioxide gas. Forests are also beneficial to the biological species of the world, and benefit people in other ways that are explained later.

The global problems that need to be solved are all related. Their causes overlap, and so do their solutions. That means that any action a person takes to help solve one problem will help solve many others. Figure 26–1 on page 708 shows a few of the many links among today's global environmental problems, to which U.S. consumers unknowingly contribute.

The task for consumers is to become aware of their impacts, and to find **sustainable** ways of doing things. These are ways of living that use up resources at a rate that nature, forestry, or agriculture can replace. They are ways of living that pollute the earth at a rate that nature or human cleanup efforts can keep up with.

One of the nicest things about sustainable choices is that they often benefit the health of the human body while also benefiting the environment. Bicycling instead of driving not only keeps the rider fit, but also reduces pollution. Eating a diet of mostly foods from plants benefits health, too. People's health depends upon healthy surroundings, for the two are closely connected.

KEY POINTS *Human impacts are damaging the earth's land, air, water, oceans, climate, and outer atmosphere. This endangers people's health. Alternatives are possible and require that people find sustainable ways of doing things.*

MINI Glossary

Kyoto Protocol (kee-OH-toe pro-toe-call): An agreement signed by many of the world's leaders in 1997, that spells out the degree of reduction in carbon dioxide emission required of each nation by the year 2012. *Kyoto* is a city in Japan where the leaders met to write the agreement. *Protocol* means the first draft of an agreement.

sustainable: a term used to describe the use of resources at such a rate that the earth can keep on replacing them—for example, a rate of cutting trees no faster than new ones grow. Also, *sustainable* describes the production of pollutants at a rate that the environment or human cleanup efforts can handle, so that there is no net accumulation of pollution.

SECTION 2 Review

Answer the following questions on a sheet of paper.

Learning the Vocabulary

The vocabulary terms in this section are *pollution, fossil fuel, ozone, air pollution, acid rain, global warming, greenhouse effect, ozone layer, ripple effect, Kyoto Protocol,* and *sustainable*. Fill in the blanks with the correct answer.

1. _____ is the contamination of the air with gases or particles not normally found there.
2. The outer atmosphere that protects living things on earth from harmful ultraviolet radiation from the sun is called the _____.
3. _____ is any resource such as coal, oil, or natural gas, burned to provide energy.

Learning the Facts

4. What is involved in the production of goods for U.S. consumers?
5. Why is it better to buy large plastic bottles of soda instead of cans?
6. Describe how the ripple effect works.

Making Life Choices

7. Study Figure 26–1 on the previous pages. Choose one environmental problem, and describe how it contributes to others and how others contribute to it. Explain how, if you helped solve one problem, you would be helping solve all the others.

enrichment

In some areas of the United States, food banks are dehydrating their excess foods. This allows for a much longer shelf life for the foods. You might use the following activity to introduce your students to dehydrated foods.

Locate a variety of dehydrated food products. Have students look carefully at the packaging. Have them read the labels to determine nutrient content of the foods. Compare labels of dehydrated foods with labels of similar canned or frozen products. Is there a

SECTION 3

Shopping

Shopping involves trips to stores, choices of goods once you are at the store, package choices, and choices of bags in which to carry things home. Let's consider the shopping trips first.

Shopping without a car can be a pleasure.

Shopping Trips

In 1998, more than 500 million cars were in use around the world. Every year, 19 million more cars are being added. Motor vehicles are the world's single largest source of air pollution. They harm people with lung problems, children, and the elderly; reduce crop yields; cause acid rain; damage forests; and produce major amounts of the global-warming gas carbon dioxide. Transporting oil to provide gasoline for cars is a major cause of oil spills that harm ocean life.

Alternatives to the use of private cars are carpools, mass transit, walking, bicycling, and even skateboarding or roller blading, where practical. It will help if cities combine homes, workplaces, and retail stores in neighborhoods and provide sidewalks and bike paths to make walking and biking feasible.

It also helps when shoppers get organized, make lists, and limit shopping trips to once each week. Some share rides to the mall, or take turns shopping for one another. It is a pleasure to shop at neighborhood stores, and walk or bicycle to get there. When choosing a car, look for the most fuel-efficient model you can find.

On each trip, by the way, take along your own shopping bags—either retail bags you received with other purchases or canvas or net bags you can reuse indefinitely. They save pollution in another way, as shown later.

 KEY POINTS *Automobiles are the world's single largest cause of air pollution. Future societies need to find ways of reducing or eliminating car use.*

Products to Choose: Green Products

From the point of view of the environment, the ideal product is a truly "green" product. A product is "green"—that is, most environmentally harmless—if it earns a yes answer to each of the questions in the margin on page 712.

On Question 2, you may wonder why recyclable is second best. The reason is that only about half of recyclable material is saved during recycling.

For Your Information

Over 30 years, a typical shopper who drives 5 miles to the store each day in a car getting 25 miles to the gallon:

▶ Uses up 4,000 gallons of gasoline.

▶ Uses up one car just for shopping.

▶ Releases about 70,000 pounds (30 tons) of carbon dioxide into the air (each gallon of gas releases 16 pounds of carbon dioxide).

▶ Spends over $4,000 on gasoline just for shopping.

Another shopper who drives just 1 mile to the store each day in a car getting 50 miles to the gallon, over 30 years:

▶ Uses 63 gallons of gas.

▶ Releases just over 1,000 pounds of carbon dioxide into the air.

▶ Spends just $63 for gas to take the same number of shopping trips.

---

significant difference in the nutritive value of the foods? How is the preparation of dehydrated food different from preparing other food? What dehydrated foods do your students' families use on a regular basis? As a demonstration or as part of a student lab, prepare one or more dishes using dehydrated food. Provide time for sampling the foods. How do the students like the products? Do they detect any difference between dehydrated foods and fresh, frozen, or canned items?

SECTION 3

FOCUS

OUTCOMES

In this section students will learn the:

1. Ways we can help our environment while shopping.

2. Tips for selecting products that are environmentally safe.

3. Impact of environmental problems on living things and the food chain.

FOCUS ACTIVITY

Have students name ways in which our choices of what to buy can have an effect on our environment. Write all their ideas on the board. Discuss which decisions have the greatest impact.

TEACH & APPLY

GROUP ACTIVITY

Have students create a list of items that their parents routinely buy at the grocery store. Next to each item, have them write what feature of the item to check for or substitute for in order to make that choice more environmentally sound. In doing their analysis, students should consider, among other things, packaging, energy used in transporting or manufacturing the item, and energy used to store the item.

BACKGROUND INFORMATION

Point out to students that many products labeled "green" or "recyclable" are actually neither. Many plastic items fall into this category. Plastic containers of all sorts are now printed with recycle symbols. Recycling centers, however, may be able to handle only beverage containers. The other plastics, even though they bear the symbol, are actually throwaway types. Another scam is the recycle label on paper products that actually contain no paper that has been through human hands. Real recycled paper is *postconsumer* paper.

LEARNING WITH VISUALS

Have each student evaluate his or her family's use of the products listed in Figure 26–2. Have them use a grading system, such as a 1 to 10, with 10 being very good. Have students write a sentence or two summarizing the family's use of the product.

The transparency "Accumulation of Toxic Compounds at the Top of the Food Chain" is provided in the Transparency Acetate Binder.

GROUP PROJECT

Bring labels of products to class and have students help you decide which of the products could be labeled as "green" products. Then have students go to the store and find at least ten products that are "green" products. "Green" products must meet all of the eight requirements listed in For Your Information on this page.

These cleansers clean as well as their toxic alternatives such as chlorine bleach or products in aerosol cans, and they do no damage to the environment. They cost less than the toxic kind, too.

For Your Information

A green product gets a yes answer to each of these questions.

1. Is it designed to meet reasonable human needs without being frivolous?
2. Is it durable and reusable (best)? If not, then is it **recyclable** or **biodegradable** (second best)? If it is **disposable**, avoid it.
3. Does it release only safe substances—no **persistent** toxins—into the environment during production? During use? When it is thrown away?
4. Does it consume minimal energy and resources during production, use, and disposal?
5. Is it made from recycled materials or renewable resources?
6. If manufactured, is it manufactured in a way that preserves the environment?
7. Is it minimally packaged?
8. Is it responsibly packaged? (Does the packaging material fit the same criteria as the product?)

The other half becomes waste. If the material is recycled again, another half is lost, and so on. We need to do much better than that.

Unfortunately, many products are labeled "green" that really are not. Beware of misleading "green" labels on products. Figure 26–2 lists products that truly benefit the earth.

Many of the products we use in our homes contain or release toxins. If used as directed, these products may not harm us. However, their manufacture may pollute the environment. Furthermore, when we dispose of them or their containers, they may again cause harm.

A prime example is chlorine bleach. It works well as a disinfectant, because it kills living cells. That same quality, however, makes it deadly when it goes down the drain. Where strong chlorine concentrations run into waterways, they kill all life—from tiny creatures at the bottom of the **food chain** on up to fish and fish-eating birds. (Figure 26–3 shows the workings of a food chain.) Also, chlorine combines with naturally occurring ammonia to produce deadly **dioxins**.

People can learn to do without chlorine. Norway has banned its production and use altogether. Other nations are following suit. People can also do without aerosol cans (the propellants destroy ozone and pollute the air), strong cleansers, polishes, insecticides, and many other products.

Figure 26–2 Products to Benefit the Earth

Each of the products recommended benefits the environment:

- Compact fluorescent lightbulbs (because they last longer and use much less electricity than ordinary bulbs).
- Cloth or net shopping bags (because both paper and plastic bags at the grocery store pollute both before and after use).
- Cloth diapers, dishcloths, napkins, and towels to replace the throwaway types.
- Dishes, cups, glasses, and tableware to replace the disposable versions. (Yes, it costs fuel and hot water to wash them, but not as much as the fuel and water it costs to keep manufacturing and shipping disposables.)
- Flow-reducing showerheads and other devices that help you save water and the fuel to heat it.
- Energy-efficient appliances (if you must have them at all).
- Haircuts, rather than permanent waves and coloring (since cutting hair means a pollution-free job for somebody, while perms and colorings involve chemicals, containers, fuel, and pollution).
- A good-quality bicycle (to use in place of a car).
- Recycled paper products with a high post-consumer (paper used by a consumer and then recycled) waste content (rather than paper made from new trees).
- Secondhand items (garage-sale items, used clothing, and the like).

HEALTHY PEOPLE 2000

Establish programs for recyclable materials and household hazardous waste in at least 75 percent of counties.

Recycling is a process involving separation of reusable material from the waste stream, collection (before or after separation), processing, marketing, and reuse of materials as the raw material for products which may or may not be similar to the original. Materials currently recovered for their value as reusable materials include used motor oil, newspapers, corrugated boxes, office papers, mixed papers, ferrous metals, glass containers, aluminum cans, plastic soft drink and milk containers, and lead-acid automobile batteries.

Hazardous chemicals are frequently present in small amounts in products commonly found in American households. If toxic materials are discarded with other trash, they can contribute to air and drinking water contami-

Figure 26–3 How a Food Chain Works.
A person who eats many fish may consume about 100 pounds of fish in a year. These fish will, in turn, have consumed a few tons of plant-eating fish in the course of their lifetimes. The plant eaters, in their lifetimes, will have consumed several tons of the tiniest organisms. If these bottom-level organisms have become contaminated with toxic chemicals, these chemicals become more concentrated in the bodies of the fish that consume them. One person may ingest the same amount of the contaminant as was present in the original several tons of bottom-level organisms. If strong chemical agents, such as chlorine, kill off the bottom-level population, organisms at all other levels either starve or move to a healthier environment.

Level 4
A 150-pound person

Level 3
100 pounds of fish

Level 2
A few tons of plant-eating fish

Level 1 Several tons of tiny organisms

KEY POINTS *To benefit the environment, buy only products that you need, that produce little pollution, and that are responsibly packaged. Refuse nonrecyclables and disposables. Many cleansers are unnecessarily toxic. Nontoxic alternatives are available and cost less.*

Foods

Like nutritionists, environmentalists urge people to eat low on the meat-producing food chain. That is, center the diet on plant foods rather than on meats and other products from animals, especially grain-eating animals.

The health benefits of a diet high in grains and vegetables, and low in meats and fats, are well known and were presented in earlier chapters. Eating less meat makes sense environmentally, too. Growing meat animals by feeding them grain uses more land than does growing grain to feed directly to people. Meat animals also use more water; pollute waterways more; and in general, destroy more native vegetation and wildlife than most plants (there are significant exceptions, however). Furthermore, more fossil fuels are needed just to grow the feed for animals—to run tractors, harvest grain, and

nation, either by leaching out of landfills, or if incinerated, as toxic gas or ash. For example, phenol, a colorless or white solid, is used in household cleaners as a disinfectant. Repeated exposure to low levels of phenol in drinking water has been linked with diarrhea and mouth sores in humans; eating very large amounts has resulted in death. Effects on human health due to breathing phenol are unknown; exposure of animals to high levels of phenol in air for a few minutes is irritating

to the lungs, and repeated exposure for several days causes muscle tremors and loss of coordination. Exposure to high levels of phenol for several weeks results in paralysis and severe injury to the heart, kidneys, liver, and lungs, followed by death in some cases.

Special community collection of household toxic waste would help to ensure that such wastes are disposed of correctly, thus reducing the risk of air and ground and surface water contamination.

MINI Glossary

recyclable: made of material that can be used over again.

biodegradable: able to decompose; able to be converted by living organisms into harmless waste products that can be used over again to build or grow new things.

disposable: a description of any product that is intended to be used once and then thrown away.

persistent: the opposite of biodegradable—unable to decompose or to be converted by living organisms into harmless wastes.

food chain: the sequence in which living things depend on other living things for food. Algae are near the bottom and human beings at the top of the food chain.

dioxins: deadly pollutants formed when chlorine bleach reacts with other compounds.

INTERDISCIPLINARY ACTIVITY: SCIENCE

TRANSPARENCIES The transparency "Accumulation of Toxic Compounds at the Top of the Food Chain" can be used for this activity.

Through science classes, students should learn about the different parts of the food chain and how they relate to each other. In health, expand the relationship to include pollution and poisoning. Help students realize that the ways people live or affect the earth have an effect on all other living things. Chemicals used by humans can accumulate in the food chain and become concentrated by the time they reach the carnivores. Have students draw a diagram that shows how the toxins at the first level (producers—tiny organisms) can affect humans at the top.

GROUP ACTIVITY

Have students make a list of products they know to be harmful to the environment. Beside each product have students list the way in which the product negatively impacts the environment. Have each student interview ten friends to see how many people use each of these products and whether or not these students know how the product is bad for the environment. If they don't, students should explain. Discuss student responses to interviews. Discuss the positive impact that your students can have on the environment by educating those people with whom they have just made contact. Count the number of students in your classes and multiply that number by ten to show what kind of an impact student activities can generate.

713

transport it. The growing of feed pollutes the environment with fertilizers and pesticides. Wastes from the animals themselves pollute it further.

It also makes sense, as far as possible, to avoid buying canned beef products of any kind—soups, stews, chili, corned beef, or even beef-flavored pet food. Much canned beef comes from land that was part of the tropical rain forest only a few years ago. The rain forests are the earth's most threatened **ecosystems**. They are home to many tribes of native people and many species of plants and animals that are in danger of being wiped out. To cut the forest and convert it to beef ranches is an unsustainable practice. Rain forest soil wears out within only a few years when used this way. To keep growing beef, ranchers exploiting such land have to keep clearing more land. However, the forest can't grow back on the ruined soil. Each pound of beef produced this way costs the loss of 200 square feet of rain forest—permanently.

Buy products that support the sustaining of the rain forest. When consumers buy Brazil nuts, cashews, or fruits harvested from the rain forest, they are helping to preserve the rain forest for its long-range economic value. As long as the people who live in the forest can sell its renewable products, they will preserve the forest along with their own ways of life.

In general, though, buy foods grown as close to home as possible. Locally grown foods may cost more, but they have traveled the shortest distance to the market, and so have required little fossil fuel for packaging, labeling, refrigeration, transportation, and marketing.

 KEY POINTS *Eat more plant foods and fewer meats. Buy locally grown foods when possible.*

Packages

The products we buy come in a multitude of packages—cans, shrink-wrap, foam trays, waxed cardboard, clay-coated cardboard, plastic bottles, glass jars, and dozens of others. It costs energy and resources to make packages, and it may cost land or pollution to dispose of them, too. In general, the packages that are best for the environment are *no* packages. Next best are minimal, reusable, or recyclable ones.

Carry everything home in a nonpolluting, nonwasteful way. This applies not only to food but also to clothing, books, household items, cosmetics, and everything else you shop for. Reject one-time-use paper or plastic bags that have to be thrown away. Every 700 paper bags not used represent one 15- to 20-year-old tree that need not be cut down.

Paper is made from a renewable resource—trees. However, trees are being cut in this country faster than they are being grown. Environmentalists fear that the nation's forests are not being managed sustainably. Furthermore, in the making of paper, pulp mills use chemicals that contaminate waterways with pollutants in quantities so large and so destructive that they have destroyed whole bays and fisheries.

Plastic bags, like most plastics, are a petroleum product. This means in most cases that the oil used to make the plastic bags has had to be transported here from the Middle East at a great cost in fuel, oil spills, and military readiness. Furthermore, when thrown away, plastics last for years or decades. They create masses of refuse that clog landfills. Some plastics are labeled "degradable," but few really do degrade fully to pure, simple com-

> ❝ *The twentieth century will be remembered chiefly, not as an age of political conflicts and technical inventions, but as an age in which human society dared to think of the health of the whole human race as a practical objective.* ❞
>
> Arnold Toynbee
> (1889–1975)
> British historian

Chapter 26, Section 3

The following quiz will help you assess your students' understanding of the material covered in this section of the chapter. You might use the quiz as an oral exercise, which will lead into a class discussion of the topics covered. Or, you might use it as a paper/pencil quiz to evaluate your students individually.

Like the Quick Quiz, the Section Review can also be used as an assessment tool to spark class discussion or as an individual student evaluation. It can also be used as a review in preparation for this quiz.

1. Motor vehicles are the world's single largest source of air pollution. (True)

2. Carpools, mass transit, walking, and biking are feasible alternatives to the use of pounds that nature can recycle. Some degrade only if exposed to sun and air—not when buried under other trash, and they almost always end up buried. Some plastics are recyclable. This makes them highly preferable to other plastics, but still not perfect, since recycling is only partially efficient.

The best choice, then, is to carry reusable shopping bags to the store and refuse all others. Failing in this, ask for plastic bags if they are recyclable—and then be sure to recycle them. The third choice is paper bags, and last is nonrecyclable plastic.

Permanent bags are infinitely reusable and leave the earth less burdened with litter.

 KEY POINTS *Reject unnecessary packaging, including paper and plastic bags. Carry your own reusable shopping bags.*

SECTION 3 Review

Answer the following questions on a sheet of paper.

Learning the Vocabulary

The vocabulary terms in this section are *recyclable, biodegradable, disposable, persistent, food chain, dioxins,* and *ecosystems.*

1. Match each of the following phrases with the appropriate term from above:
   a. products that are intended to be used once and then thrown away
   b. deadly pollutants formed when chlorine bleach reacts with other compounds
   c. made of material that can be used over again

Learning the Facts

2. How does pollution from automobiles harm people's health and their environment?
3. What are the effects of chlorine bleach on our environment?
4. How does eating less meat make sense environmentally?

Making Life Choices

5. Figure 26–2 on page 712 presents a list of products to benefit the earth. What can you do to replace products that you use at home with these products?

MINI
Glossary

ecosystems: systems of land, plants, and animals that have existed together for thousands or millions of years and that are interdependent.

private cars. (True)
3. 100% of recyclable material is saved during recycling. (False)
4. A "green" product is environmentally harmless. (True)
5. Toxic cleansers such as chlorine harm the environment but are indispensable in the household. (False)
6. Responsible consumers buy only what they need, and avoid nonrecyclables and disposables. (True)

7. Canned beef is an example of a "green" product. (False)
8. An environmentally conscious person will buy foods grown close to their home, even though they cost more. (True)
9. The rainforests are the world's most rapidly diminishing ecosystem. (True)
10. Most plastic bags degrade quickly into compounds that nature can recycle. (False)

ASSESS

EVALUATE

Have students list at least three activities or products whose use requires money and energy that is not necessary. The papers should point out that simple ways are more cost effective and more environmentally sound.

SECTION 3 Review Answers

1. a. disposable **b.** dioxins **c.** recyclable
2. Answers will vary: could include lung problems, harm to children and the elderly, reduced crop yields, etc. (p. 711)
3. Concentrated amounts in waterways kill tiny creatures on up to large fish and fish-eating birds. When it combines with naturally occurring ammonia, deadly dioxins are produced. (p. 712)
4. Since meat production uses so much more land and natural resources than production of grain, it is smart to eat less of it. Meat production also causes the depletion of rain forests, because the trees are cut down to provide grazing areas for cattle. (p. 714)
5. Answers will vary.

CLOSE

Start a discussion with a statement such as: "People are more important than the environment or a bunch of trees. If we save trees, then people will die of starvation."

715

FOCUS

OUTCOMES

In this section students will learn the:

1. Ways to conserve energy in the home.
2. Alternatives to traditional energy sources and energy-using appliances.

FOCUS ACTIVITY

Ask students to brainstorm a list of appliances they use in the morning when getting ready for school. Go through this list and have students decide what items they could live without or use less of for the benefit of the environment.

TEACH & APPLY

DISCUSSION

Have students think of a time that the electricity went out in their homes. Ask students what they had to go without during that time and what they did for entertainment. Tell them that before electricity was discovered, people did everything they needed to do in different ways. Find out whether students think they could live with fewer appliances. Ask them how they would prepare for another "lights out" if they knew in advance that it would happen. Have them imagine what life might be like if energy were rationed and people had to use less energy.

SECTION 4

Energy Use in the Home

Home energy use has many environmental implications. A naive consumer might respond to such a statement by saying, "I don't use any fossil fuels in my home. My home is all electric." However, electricity, of course, is most often generated by burning fossil fuels, too—only at the power plant, rather than at the site of use. An all-electric home produces air pollutants and global-warming gases just as if the homeowner were burning fossil fuels at home.

Cooking Methods

An example of an environmentally sound way to prepare foods is the Asian way. Asian cooks cut foods into bite-sized pieces, and then stir-fry them fast in small amounts of oil. This uses little fuel, so it pollutes only a little.

Other than stir-frying, two ways to cook foods quickly are to use the pressure cooker or the microwave oven. The pressure cooker can tenderize pounds of meat in half the normal cooking time, or cook a potful of potatoes in five minutes. The microwave can cook small portions quickly or warm whole plates of leftovers (which saves using several burners on the stove and washing up the pots afterward).

The conventional oven, in contrast, is a fuel waster, especially when the entire oven is heated just to bake a potato. Instead, when using the oven, cook many items on both racks, using all the heated space. Don't peek often. Each door opening drops the oven temperature by 25 to 50 degrees Fahrenheit.

Microwave cooking is quick and efficient and saves energy.

enrichment

Have students brainstorm strategies for protecting the environment. List their ideas on the board. Have each student copy the list and then use the list to interview ten friends or family members. The students will ask which strategies each person uses, what other strategies they might use, and how involved that person is in the various strategies.

Have the students share their findings, and compile a master list of the most used tips. Discuss why some are more used than others.

Should You Be Doing More To Protect Our Environment? If so, What Should You Be Doing?

I think we should be careful of our environment, but we should focus more on the lives of young teens who throw their lives away everyday. We worry more about the environment than living, breathing people. Let's save our future of people, then we can worry about our surroundings.
Josh MacDonald, 14,
Manzano High School, NM

Yes, I think that everyone should be doing more. I see many kids throw their lunch bags away on the lawns or parking lot, as if they don't care about anything or respect others. My grandfather always taught me to put garbage where it belongs, and to respect and enjoy nature by taking care of it. And I have seen the devastating effects of lack of care. Almost everytime I go hiking into the mountains I come back with a garbage bag full of other people's junk. Why can't people think of the future and clean up after themselves? It only takes a little effort to make a big difference.
Elichai J. Fowler, 19
West High School, MT

I think I should be doing more for the environment. I already recycle newspaper through the local pickup, and put my note paper in the collection bins at school, but I don't go out of my way to recycle aluminum cans, which aren't picked up with the plastic and newspaper. After all, I have to live here for another fifty-odd years; I want to have a good home planet for myself and my nieces and nephews.
Katye Blackwell, 14,
Northeastern High School, NC

I think that I try pretty hard to protect our environment but there are things that I could do more of. I could recycle more and help pick up litter. I could ride my bike or walk to places that are close, rather than drive. I could use fewer products that aren't biodegradable. I do not have to be an eco-maniac to help out.
Emilee Owen, 15,
Manzano High School, NM

I should probably be doing more to protect my environment because I am not very aware of the environment. I should be recycling more and doing more community service projects to reduce litter. I should help people be more aware also so they can protect the environment. I help a little bit by walking everywhere and hardly ever riding in the car. In some ways I am very conscious of what waste products I use. For example, I would never use styrofoam and I cut up all my plastic six pack holders. Most of all I *don't* smoke.
Hannah Gleason, 15,
Manzano High School, NM

Yes! We need to keep the water clean for us and any organisms on Earth. Keeping the parks, schools, libraries, and national monuments clean will help us greatly. We need to keep our planet clean, because if it goes, so do we.
Andrea Sisneras, 15,
Manzano High School, NM

I am most concerned with air pollution, because air is our most important resource. Chemicals from our automobiles and factories effect the changes in the earth's climate causing the greenhouse effect. We must all help by carpooling, recycling, and conserving water. Remember—earth is the only planet we have.
Zeenat Shah, 15,
Robert E. Lee High School, TX

Lack of concern bothers me most. Unless other people start worrying about and trying to help our environment, the problems facing us will multiply. Too many people don't believe that one person can make a difference. Other people take the environment for granted. Mother Nature has a lot to take care of; it's time we learned to clean up the messes we have made.
Michelle Porter, 15,
Orange Park High School, FL

Follow-Up
Following are some questions you may want to use to encourage discussion of the ideas expressed by the students in the Teen Views feature:

a. How can the students encourage their peers to recycle more? Are they willing to confront litter-bugs and others who leave recyclables on the ground with their environmentally unsafe ways? Could they start or join a community action group dealing with recycling in their area?

b. How many students recycle? Do they do it faithfully or sporadically?

c. Do students think that we should be worried about our children and grandchildren, or should each generation take care of itself?

d. Do students know the air quality in their area? If the quality is poor, what are the major causes of this and what can they do about it?

e. Do students agree with Michelle Porter that most people are not as concerned as they should be about the environment? What can be done?

Then ask students, "What needs to be done before the majority of the people will start to be environmentally conscious? How can these people be reached?" Discuss why students often "make waves" first and make them the biggest. (because today's adults did not grow up with any awareness of environmental problems, they are not as educated about environmental problems as are today's young people, and today's adults will not live long enough to be affected as much as today's youth by the results of environmental problems)

GROUP ACTIVITY

Call a local distributor and find out the cost of installing photovoltaic panels and how much money would be saved on the monthly electric bill. Set up an activity for students to complete in which they calculate the savings over time and find out how much time might pass before the cost of the panels would be reimbursed in the form of energy savings.

GUEST SPEAKER

Invite someone from a local energy company to speak to the class about how students can make their homes more energy efficient. Ask about alternative sources of energy, how well they work, and the cost of installation and regular use.

BACKGROUND INFORMATION

For enrichment, you may want to give students another example of how they can save energy in the home. For example, there are several measures they can use to save water-heating energy. They can set the heater at 120 degrees Fahrenheit, no hotter; they can put on a timer; they can wrap it in a blanket; and wrap the pipes carrying the hot water. They can also install heat-trapping devices at the inlets to keep heat from creeping along the lines when the water is standing. When buying a hot-water heater, people can choose smaller, instant-type heaters, gas rather than electric, and solar heaters.

For Your Information

The most energy-guzzling home appliances:

▶ Refrigerators (because they run all the time).
▶ Hot-water heaters (these run many hours per day).
▶ Heaters and air conditioners (these also run many hours per day).

Choose for energy efficiency when choosing these appliances. You'll save money and reduce pollution, too.

For Your Information

This book was written in an office that the authors converted to run on solar PV panels. They keep their lunches in a DC refrigerator there.

On the stove top, use flat-bottomed pots that fit the burners, with close-fitting lids. That way, each burner will donate all its heat to cooking something, not just to heating the kitchen (and the planet). Turn electric burners and all ovens off before food is fully cooked. Let the cooking finish as the stove cools.

KEY POINTS *Cutting foods up and cooking fast are energy-efficient ways to cook foods. Pressure-cooking and microwaving also save energy.*

Power Tools and Appliances

A tour around the home reveals many appliances, large and small, that people use to cook, to clean, to heat and cool their homes, and to entertain themselves. All of these appliances run on energy from fossil fuels, with pollution and global warming as by-products.

The fewer appliances you use and the shorter the times you use them, the better for the environment. Realizing this, many consumers today are returning to "old-fashioned" ways of doing things. They dry clothes on a clothesline in the sun; trim yard greenery with hand tools; and rake the refuse with rakes rather than using electric clothes dryers, weed whackers, hedge trimmers, and leaf blowers.

These practices save only small amounts of energy. Refraining from buying power tools and appliances in the first place also saves the energy it would have cost to manufacture, transport, package, advertise, and market them.

People who use solar energy reduce their demand for energy from more polluting sources. More than 20,000 U.S. families are now using solar energy to meet most of their homes' electricity needs. In an **active solar** home, the sun's light strikes **photovoltaic (PV) panels** on the roof. These convert the light energy to electrical energy, which is stored in a battery. Having a battery permits the use of a DC (direct current) refrigerator, rather than an AC (alternating current) refrigerator. No fossil fuel is used to run a DC refrigerator operated this way. Sunlight is free, reliable, and pollution-free.

Photovoltaic panels capture the sun's energy and convert it into electrical power.

Chapter 26, Section 4

The following quiz will help you assess your students' understanding of the material covered in this section of the chapter. You might use the quiz as an oral exercise, or, you might use it as a paper/pencil quiz to evaluate your students individually.

Like the Quick Quiz, the Section Review can also be used as an assessment tool to spark class discussion or as an individual student evaluation. It can also be used as a review in preparation for this quiz.

1. Using a pressure cooker or a microwave is environmentally preferable to using a conventional oven. (True)
2. When using the oven, you should open it as infrequently as possible. (True)

The high initial cost of PV panels, the battery, and the DC refrigerator prevents most people from considering them. For those who can afford to get started, it becomes possible to meet most of a home's electrical needs with solar energy, thus reducing utility bills to only a few dollars a month. The savings in utilities pay back the initial investment within about 7 years. From that point on, energy is virtually free—compliments of the sun.

The highest priorities for the human race to save the planet are to convert to solar energy, get off automobiles, use land and wealth so as to relieve poverty, and stop multiplying. To take these steps demands "reduced consumption of resources by the rich to make room for higher living standards for the poor."

 Use appliances efficiently, replace them when possible with energy-efficient models, and start converting to solar energy.

Lights

An ordinary 75-watt incandescent lightbulb burns for about 2,500 hours, gives off considerable heat, and demands fuel whose carbon dioxide output amounts to 200 pounds or so over the lifetime of the bulb. Energy- and pollution-conscious people are replacing these lightbulbs with 22-watt, high-efficiency compact fluorescent (CF) bulbs such as those shown in Figure 26–4. One CF bulb can match the light output of the incandescent bulb it replaces, but it uses one-fourth the energy to do so. The CF bulbs also last ten or more times as long. Each CF bulb used in place of a succession of "regular" lightbulbs keeps a ton of carbon dioxide out of the air.

 Replace incandescent lightbulbs with compact fluorescent (CF) bulbs to save energy.

Figure 26–4 Energy-Efficient Lightbulbs Can Replace Incandescent Bulbs. A typical compact fluorescent bulb costs more than an ordinary bulb, but lasts many times longer and uses much less electricity, making it the more economical choice.

SECTION 4 Review

Answer the following questions on a sheet of paper.

Learning the Vocabulary
The vocabulary terms in this section are *active solar* and *photovoltaic (PV) panels.*

1. Write a sentence using each of the vocabulary terms.

Learning the Facts
2. List three ways to save energy while cooking.

3. Name three "old-fashioned" ways of doing things that are better for the environment.
4. What three household appliances use the most energy?

Making Life Choices
5. This section deals with conserving energy at home. Do your parents follow these procedures? If not, how can you persuade your parents to conserve energy at home? What arguments can you make for energy conservation?

MINI Glossary

active solar: using photovoltaic panels to generate electricity from sunlight. (A passive solar home is one that is built to take advantage of the available sun and shade so as to minimize heating and cooling costs.)

photovoltaic (PV) panels: panels that convert light (photons) into electricity (volts).

ASSESS

EVALUATE

Have students go to an appliance store for information on energy-saving appliances and fixtures. Have students do a cost evaluation, explaining the cost of installing the newer model as compared to the cost of installing a traditional model. Emphasize the importance of finding out how much energy will be saved monthly and how soon a person can expect to see those savings above and beyond the difference in the installation costs. Have students ask how popular these energy-saving appliances are, if they are growing in popularity, and why or why not?

SECTION 4 Review Answers

1. Answers will vary.
2. Cutting foods up and stir-frying in small amounts of oil, using pressure cookers, and using microwaves (p. 716)
3. dry clothes on a clothesline, trim yard greenery with hand tools, use a rake instead of a power blower (p. 718)
4. refrigerators, hot-water heaters, air conditioners, and heaters (p. 718)
5. Answers will vary.

CLOSE

Ask students to list the different types of energy and tell why each is important in our attempts to conserve energy sources or make posters with environmental slogans to be displayed around the school.

3. Home electricity does not produce air pollutants or global-warming gases. (False)
4. All home electric appliances run on fossil fuels. (True)
5. "Old-fashioned" methods, such as drying clothes in the sun, can save energy around the home. (True)
6. Solar equipment is widely used because it is inexpensive. (False)
7. An active solar home uses photovoltaic panels to convert light energy into electrical energy. (True)
8. Solar energy causes some pollution to the environment. (False)
9. Rich countries like the United States will have to reduce consumption in order for the living standards of poorer nations to improve. (True)
10. Compact fluorescent bulbs can massively reduce the amount of carbon dioxide polluting the air. (True)

SECTION 5

FOCUS

OUTCOME

In this section students will learn the:

1. Environmental problems associated with waste disposal.

FOCUS ACTIVITY

Have students list ways to cut down on water usage in their homes. Suggest that students keep these tips in mind and perhaps make water-saving notes to be placed by each faucet in their homes.

TEACH & APPLY

DISCUSSION

The second paragraph of this section gives several suggestions for conserving water. Ask students how many they currently use. Which ones could they use if they are not using them already?

DISCUSSION

Have students tell you in what type of containers they carry their lunches. Multiply the percentages of the types of containers in your class by the entire student body to represent how much energy might be wasted each day in one school in the form of containers. Discuss how habits could be changed to save energy.

SECTION 5

Water Use, Trash, and Garbage

Where water is abundant and inexpensive, people use it freely. It is really not free, though. Major expenses may not be visible on water bills, but are paid for by people's tax money. These expenses include water purification, monitoring, and cleanup.

Conscious of water's true worth, people become more inclined to conserve it. There are many ways to do so. A running faucet uses as much as 3 to 5 gallons of water a minute. Therefore, leaky faucets must be repaired immediately. Just at the bathroom sink, you can save many gallons by turning the faucet off while brushing your teeth. You can run the faucet only when actually filling a glass or rinsing your toothbrush, and turn it off between times. You can install a water-saving washer on the faucet to deliver a pleasant stream of water with a reduced flow per minute. For dishes, a dishwasher uses less water than does washing dishes by hand (just load it

Compost is a natural, recycled fertilizer.

Chapter 26, Section 5

The following quiz will help you assess your students' understanding of the material covered in this section of the chapter. You might use the quiz as an oral exercise, or, you might use it as a paper/pencil quiz to evaluate your students individually.

Like the Quick Quiz, the Section Review can also be used as an assessment tool to spark class discussion or as an individual student evaluation. It can also be used as a review in preparation for this quiz.

1. There are many costs associated with water that are not visible on your water bill. (True)

2. You can save gallons of water simply by turning off the faucet when you brush full, for maximum efficiency). You can also reuse clean water. After boiling an egg, for example, let the water cool, and then water the houseplants with it.

As for trash, an average American household of four people produces about 100 pounds a week. National concern has focused on this issue, for the nation is running out of landfill space in which to dispose of all this trash. However, landfill space is not the only problem associated with trash. Every item thrown away is a resource lost—an aluminum can that could be used to make a new aluminum can; a plastic bottle that could become part of a beautiful carpet.

Recycled trash is a national treasure. As it is now, however, about 70 percent of all the metal mined in the United States is used only once and then discarded. The aluminum thrown away every three months could rebuild the entire U.S. air fleet. The ideal community recycles everything—paper, cardboard, glass, cans, plastic—and permits no materials to be sold that cannot be recycled.

As for garbage—that is, vegetable scraps, fruit peelings, and leftover plant-based foods—it is a special material. It is biodegradable, like the leaves and grass cuttings people rake up in their yards. All of these materials can be piled up together with some soil and allowed to decompose naturally. They will form **compost**, a rich, crumbly material that can be used, as it is in nature, to fertilize growing things. Natural fertilizers such as compost and manure are preferable, environmentally, to synthetic fertilizers on both a large and small scale. They require no mining; they recycle natural materials rather than wasting them; and they add needed texture, as well as nutrients, to the soil. Some communities, recognizing this, conduct composting programs to recycle people's yard debris. Some homeowners maintain their own composting piles.

 KEY POINTS *Save water by using water-conserving habits and devices. To the greatest extent possible, recycle trash and compost plant scraps.*

F or **Y** our **I** nformation

The authors' office floor is covered with a luxurious wall-to-wall carpet made of recycled plastic soda and ketchup bottles—45 bottles per square yard.

SECTION 5 Review

Answer the following questions on a sheet of paper.

Learning the Vocabulary

The vocabulary term in this section is *compost.*

1. Write a sentence using the vocabulary term.

Learning the Facts

2. How much water can you save by turning the water off while brushing your teeth?

3. How much trash is produced per week by an average American household of four?

4. What is said about all metal mined in the United States?

5. Describe what the ideal community recycles.

Making Life Choices

6. Landfills are a national concern. People are producing more trash each year, and our nation is running out of landfill space. What do you think should be done about this problem?

MINI
Glossary

compost: rotted vegetable matter, used as fertilizer.

your teeth. (True)

3. You can conserve water washing dishes by hand instead of using a dishwasher. (False)

4. Leaky faucets are a major waste of water and must be repaired immediately. (True)

5. The United States is currently creating more trash than we can dispose of in our landfills. (True)

6. The majority of metal mined in the United States is currently being recycled. (False)

7. An ideal community would recycle 100% of its materials. (True)

8. Vegetable scraps and other plant-based garbage are biodegradable. (True)

9. Synthetic fertilizers are environmentally preferable to composts. (False)

10. You can form your own compost pile using biodegradable refuse from your home. (True)

FOCUS

OUTCOME

In this section students will learn the:

1. Impact of hunger on the environment.

FOCUS ACTIVITIES

1. Ask students to answer this question: "How might a person who is living comfortably come to be one of the homeless or suffer from hunger? Are hungry people to blame for their situation? Why or why not?"

2. Ask students: "What can you do to decrease the number of hungry people in your neighborhood? What would your first step be?"

TEACH & APPLY

GROUP PROJECT

Have students set up and run a food pantry at school. If this is not possible, have students lead a food drive to collect for a local community pantry. Have competition between classes to see which class can donate the most food or run a campuswide food campaign. Have students make posters advertising the food drive to hang in the halls.

GROUP ACTIVITY

In groups, have the students research countries that have the biggest problems with hunger and starvation. Assign a different country to each group. Have one group research hunger in

> **❝** There is no finer investment for any community than putting milk into babies. Healthy citizens are the greatest asset any country can have. **❞**
>
> Winston Churchill
> (1874–1965)
> British statesman; Prime Minister

For Your Information

The text quote comes from L. Schwartz-Nobel, *Starving in the Shadow of Plenty* (New York: Putnam, 1981), pp. 35–36.

SECTION 6

Hunger and the Environment

As the 20th century was drawing to a close, four in every ten of the world's people were experiencing the chronic, painful hunger that arises when no food is available. Many, many more lacked the vitamins and minerals needed to support health and growth. At the same time, the population was continuing to grow, and the world's reserves of stored food had dropped to lower levels than ever before.

Hunger is terrible. A Boston writer describes it this way:

I've had no income and I've paid no rent for many months. My landlord let me stay. He felt sorry for me because I had no money. The Friday before Christmas he gave me ten dollars. For days I had nothing but water. I knew I needed food; I tried to go out but I was too weak to walk to the store. I felt as if I were dying. I saw the mailman and told him I thought I was starving. He brought me food and then made some phone calls and that's when they began delivering these lunches. But I had already lost so much weight that five meals a week are not enough to keep me going.

I just pray to God I can survive. I keep praying I can have the will to save some of my food so I can divide it up and make it last. It's hard to save because I am so hungry that I want to eat it right away. On Friday, I held over two peas from the lunch. I ate one pea on Saturday morning. Then I got into bed with the taste of food in my mouth and I waited as long as I could. Later on in the day I ate the other pea.

Today I saved the container that the mashed potatoes were in and tonight, before bed, I'll lick the sides of the container.

When there are bones I keep them. I know this is going to be hard for you to believe and I am almost ashamed to tell you, but these days I boil the bones till they're soft and then I eat them. Today there were no bones.

The Extent of Hunger and Starvation

Some 20 million people in the United States—12 million children and 8 million adults—are chronically hungry. U.S. hunger reaches into all segments of society. Not only the disadvantaged—migrant workers, unemployed minorities, and some elderly—are hungry. Also displaced farm families and former blue-collar and white-collar workers forced out of their trades and professions into minimum-wage jobs suffer from hunger. A minority of the poor in America are on welfare. Most are working people. The most compelling single reason for their hunger is poverty.

Hundreds of millions of people around the globe are also suffering from hunger. About 250 million are children of preschool age, and 10 million of these are drastically underweight. Half a million children go blind every year because of vitamin deficiencies.

COOPERATIVE LEARNING

Where can a person or a family in your community obtain food if they need help? Divide the class into small cooperative learning groups. Have each group begin the investigation by compiling a list of possible reasons why a person might need help. *Reasons might include loss of job, unexpected disaster such as fire, hurricane, or tornado, huge medical bills.* Then, have the students list places where peo-

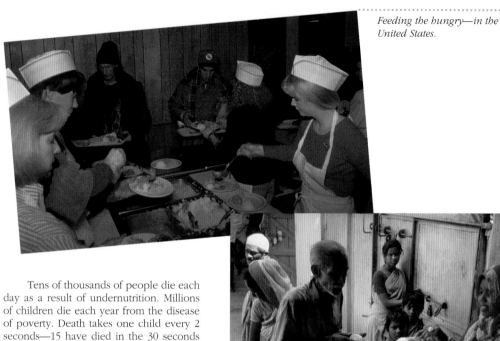

Feeding the hungry—in the United States.

Tens of thousands of people die each day as a result of undernutrition. Millions of children die each year from the disease of poverty. Death takes one child every 2 seconds—15 have died in the 30 seconds it may take you to read this paragraph. Poverty, infection, and malnutrition are the killers that cut life short in dozens of developing countries.

Of the world's 5 billion population, 1 billion people have no land and no possessions at all. They survive on less than $1 a day each, they lack water that is safe to drink, and they cannot read or write. The average U.S. housecat eats twice as much protein every day as one of these people, and the yearly cost of keeping that cat is greater than these people's annual income.

Feeding the hungry—in a developing country.

 KEY POINTS *Poverty is extreme for 1 billion of the world's 5 billion people. It is a major cause of disease, starvation, and death.*

The Environment and Poverty

The giant web of Figure 26–1 on pages 708 and 709 showed that many environmental causes contribute to poverty and hunger. Population growth contributes, for the more mouths there are to feed, the worse poverty and hunger become. As more people need homes, the land best suited for producing food may be taken to build houses. Pollution caused by more and more fossil fuel use worsens the health problems and misery of the poor.

ple might obtain food for little or no money. *Possible food sources include the Salvation Army, local churches, food banks, state and local government agencies.* Assign each group to talk with one of these community groups to find out exactly how one goes about obtaining assistance. Encourage the students to write out the questions they need answered before they visit the agency. Ask each group to write a report summarizing their investigation. Have them share their findings orally with the rest of the class.

the United States. Have each group share its report orally in class. Require that they begin their presentations with the answers to the following questions: "What event or series of events caused this problem? What is being done, if anything, in these countries to solve this problem?"

DISCUSSION

Have students write a short paragraph describing all the things in their lives that improve the quality of life and are taken for granted. Pick something to which a person who is poor, homeless, or hungry would probably not have access. Compare lists in class and discuss what other possibilities could be included.

COMPREHENSION CHECK

Paragraphs from the beginning of Section 6 to the key point contain numerous facts and examples about the terrible worldwide problems resulting from hunger and poverty. Have students reread this information and pick one fact or example that makes the greatest impression on them. Have each student state which piece of information he or she picked and why.

BACKGROUND INFORMATION

For enrichment, you might want to tell your students that in the mid-1800s the world population was a billion people, in 1880 it was two billion, and in 1930 it was four billion. Now the world's population is over five billion. If growth remains at its present rate, in less than 50 years it will be ten billion people—the maximum the world can support.

DISCUSSION

Before students read the part of Section 6 entitled "Poverty, Hunger, and Overpopulation," ask them if they think couples in poverty would be more likely or less likely to have large families. Ask for reasons for their opinions. They will probably be surprised that poverty and hunger actually encourage larger families.

The transparency "Population Growth" is provided in the Transparency Acetate Binder. It shows the growth of the world's population from 1950 to 1990 and the projected growth up to the year 2150.

ASSESS

EVALUATE

Refer to the handout "Living a Simpler Lifestyle" in the Teacher's Resource Box. Have students use tips from this chart to make a poster complete with pictures, either drawn or from magazines, that illustrate these tips. Tell them to hang the posters in their homes so their families will have a constant reminder of how to live simpler lives that require less energy consumption. Have each student outline a plan for his/her family to follow that meets these guidelines. The plan should include how the students will educate family members about the need to live simple lives.

Here are the answers to the questions at the start of the chapter.

1. **True.**
2. **False.** Products are beneficial to the environment if they help *relieve* pollution or displace other products that pollute.
3. **False.** Local products may cost more, but they may be good choices for environmental reasons.
4. **False.** Fossil fuels are burned to produce electricity.
5. **False.** Refrigerators, hot water heaters, and heaters and air conditioners use more energy, because they are on all the time.
6. **True.**

Water shortages force the poor from their homes, too, and create further hardship. The world's poorest people live in the world's most damaged and harmful environments.

KEY POINTS *Environmental degradation not only causes hunger directly but contributes indirectly by worsening the effect of poverty.*

Poverty, Hunger, and Overpopulation

Strange as it may seem, poverty and hunger encourage people to bear more children. A family in poverty depends on its children to farm the land for food, to haul water, and to make the adults secure in their old age. To complicate things, poverty costs many young lives, so parents must bear many children to ensure that a few will survive to adulthood. Children represent the "social security of the poor."

Reducing Population   To help reduce population growth, it is first necessary to help relieve poverty and hunger. When people have better access to health care and education, the death rate falls. As more family members survive, families become willing to risk having smaller numbers of children. Then the birth rate falls.

The Present Threat   At present, however, the world's population is continuing to grow. This is threatening the world's capacity to produce adequate food in the future. The activities of billions of human beings on the earth's limited surface are seriously and adversely affecting the planet. We are wiping out many varieties of plant life, heating up the climate, using up fresh water supplies, and destroying the protective ozone layer that shields life

Public health programs provide many children with the food they need.

Chapter 26, Section 6

The following quiz will help you assess your students' understanding of the material covered in this section of the chapter. You might use the quiz as an oral exercise, which will lead into a class discussion of the topics covered. Or, you might use it as a paper/pencil

quiz to evaluate your students individually.

*If students have difficulty with the concepts covered in the Quick Quiz and the Section Review, you might suggest they review the material using the **S**urvey, **Q**uestion, **R**ead, **R**ecite, **R**eview (SQ3R) study method, which is described in detail in the introduction to this Teacher's Wraparound Edition.*

1. Hunger has reached epidemic proportions worldwide. (True) from the sun's damaging rays. In short, human beings are overstraining the earth's ability to support life.

Population control is one of the world's most pressing needs. Until the nations of the world solve the population problem, they can neither succeed in supporting the lives of people already born, nor remedy the planet's galloping destruction. To resolve the population problem, they must remedy the poverty problems. Of the 92 million people being added to the population each year, 88 million are being added in the poorest areas of the world. Population growth worsens environmental damage, poverty, and hunger. Economics and population increases are interdependent.

Conclusion U.S. consumers could help substantially to slow and reverse the downward trends described here by altering their choices. If we were willing to use fewer goods, devour fewer resources, create less pollution, and consume less energy, this would go a long way toward remedying global environmental problems. It would also help solve the hunger problem—indirectly, but it would help a lot.

Many other steps to resolve these problems are needed at many levels. To find out how you can fight against hunger and poverty, write to some of the organizations listed in Figure 26–5.

To many people, the preservation of the health of the earth matters not just for people's sake, but for the sake of wildlife as well. The earth's preservation is a moral responsibility. It concerns us at a deep, spiritual level. Native Americans have traditionally known:

> *This we know. The Earth does not belong to man; man belongs to the Earth. This we know. All things are connected like the blood which unites one family. All things are connected. Whatever befalls the Earth befalls the sons of the Earth. Man did not weave the web of life, he is merely a strand in it. Whatever he does to the web, he does to himself.*
> —*Chief Seattle, 1854*

KEY POINTS *All things are connected.*

Bread for the World
802 Rhode Island Ave. NE
Washington, DC 20018

Food Research and Action Center
1875 Connecticut Ave. NW,
Suite 540
Washington, DC 20009

Institute for Food and Development Policy
398 60th St.
Oakland, CA 94618

Interfaith Impact for Justice and Peace
110 Maryland Ave. NE,
Box 63
Washington, DC 20002

Oxfam America
115 Broadway
Boston, MA 02116

Seeds
P.O. Box 6170
Waco, TX 76706

Figure 26–5 Hunger Relief Organizations You Can Join

SECTION 6 Review

Answer the following questions on a sheet of paper.

Learning the Facts
1. How many people in the United States are chronically hungry?
2. List at least four environmental causes that contribute to poverty and hunger.

3. Why do the poor bear so many children?

Making Life Choices
4. This section described how we as U.S. consumers could slow and reverse the downward trends of global environmental problems. What are the steps to resolve these problems? Would the steps also help solve the hunger problems? Explain your answer.

For **Y**our **I**nformation

Three steps to environmental correction:

1. *Recognition.* People must first recognize that a problem exists.
2. *Outrage.* People must put their foot down and refuse to accept the unacceptable.
3. *Advocacy.* People must join together to make the necessary changes.

SECTION 6 Review Answers

1. 20 million (p. 722)
2. Answers will vary; could include: population growth, pollution, water shortages, used-up land, heating up the climate, and wiping out many varieties of plant life. (p. 723)
3. to have more workers to help support the family; children are "Social Security for the poor" (p. 724)
4. Answers will vary.

A reproducible quiz for Section 6 is provided in the Teacher's Resource Box.

CLOSE

1. Have students brainstorm a list of ways they can help alleviate local problems of hunger. Discuss with students ways that they would go about accomplishing these tasks.
2. Have students draw an illustration showing poverty and starvation as they imagine it. Tell them that their artwork should represent some of the feelings the people living in that situation might be experiencing.

2. Most poor people in the United States are on welfare. (False)
3. Only disadvantaged and unemployed people suffer from hunger in the United States. (False)
4. Poverty is the greatest cause of hunger in the United States. (True)
5. One-fifth of the world's population survive on less than $1 per day. (True)
6. Population growth does not directly contribute to poverty. (False)
7. Environmental degradation worsens the effect of poverty. (True)
8. Population cannot be reduced without first relieving poverty and hunger. (True)
9. Population control is one of the world's most pressing concerns. (True)
10. Your actions as an individual consumer are not connected to world poverty. (False)

Straight Talk

Discussion

Ask students if they can think of any examples in their own lives that demonstrate how the ripple effect works. Perhaps one or two students at school began wearing a certain type of gym shoe or other article of clothing, leading to a majority of students in this school eventually wearing the same clothing. What other examples can they think of?

Background Information

Increasing the average fuel economy in American automobiles from 28 miles per gallon to 40 miles per gallon could save 2.4 million barrels of oil a day and prevent 440 million tons of carbon dioxide from entering the atmosphere each year.

Group Project

Have students design an energy-efficient way of living, from the layout of their homes to the appliances and tools used within. Have them create a plan on graph paper of the house structure they would build, showing energy-saving features. Have them write about the energy uses in the home and internal features and appliances that save energy.

Personal Strategy—Voluntary Simplicity

The problems of the environment and the world's growing population may appear so great that they seem solvable only by political leaders. However, consider this: you can change the world. Perhaps most fitting for a book about personal choices is to describe some of the things one person can do. After all, a society is the sum of its people. As we go, so goes our world.

I'm just a kid. I can't have any effect on the way the world goes. In fact, when I think about it, I feel overwhelmed, depressed, and pessimistic.

Thoughtful people of all ages feel just as you do at times and are tempted to give up. Optimism is important, though, and many people are working to develop it. They know that optimism gives them energy and makes their efforts to shape the world's future more effective.

How do I go about developing optimism?

By living your own life. Don't try to solve all the world's problems. Mentally draw a small circle around yourself. Work to better yourself through education, spiritual growth, and physical health. Work, too, to better the small world within the circle around yourself.

That sounds simple enough, but I don't see how it will help anything. In fact, it almost sounds selfish.

It will help, though. Every move you make

leaves the world a better or worse place. Your actions have a ripple effect, often far beyond what you may think. Tending to the lives nearest you, including your own, is your first responsibility. Many great religious teachings express that value.

Your second responsibility is to make sure you can answer yes to the following question: If everyone lived as I do, would the young children of today grow up in a better world?

Those who study the future are convinced that the hope of the world lies in everyone's adopting a simple lifestyle. Many experts agree that the simplification of our lives can benefit all of the world's people.

Are you saying that everybody needs to live in poverty? I can't see how my being poor would help anyone. Besides, wealthy people would never agree.

No, the suggestion is not that everyone become poor. It is said that poverty is repressive, and simplicity is liberating. Poverty gives people a sense of helplessness, but simplicity gives them creativity. In other words, to become poor would solve nothing. Poverty hinders personal growth, but simplicity opens the way to it. You are also right that few people would willingly give up their wealth, even if it would help. What *is* suggested has nothing to do with wealth. It is a lifestyle—a commitment to live more simply in view of the world's limited resources.

Think in terms of *elegance*, not poverty. Streamlined things, that have no unnecessary frills, are elegant. Life is, too. Don't carry extra baggage around. It only burdens you.

726

special needs

Logical-mathematical, Spatial, Musical

This chapter teaches students that just as the environment affects our physical health on a daily basis, so do we affect the environment every day. The Straight Talk feature deals with some of the feelings teens have about being able to make a difference. This activity gives students a chance to use their creative

strengths to develop an idea for recycling, wise energy use, or simplifying their lifestyle. Applying suggestions to a real project will help students internalize what they have learned and transfer learning to everyday life.

Artistic or scientifically inclined students could be asked to devise/invent a new use for a commonly found, usually discarded object. You may want to sponsor an exhibit of the items developed to give other students an

What does living a life of voluntary simplicity involve?

Such a life involves a thousand small decisions, like the ones that were presented in the chapter. The chapter described ways to reduce consumption of goods, energy and water use, and the throwing away of trash and garbage. Everything you do, you can do simply, with little cost or even a benefit to the earth, or you can do it complexly, with a high cost and no benefit. Together, all the things you do add up to your personal style.

To live simply, it isn't necessary to make every choice the chapter suggested. Some choices may not be right for you. Some choices may be your own original ones, and they may be better ideas than anyone else has yet dreamed up.

Voluntary is a key word, just as *simplicity* is. Each individual must look within to discover a personal sense of what actions are appropriate. Each person needs to find a balance—a path, suitable for that individual, that leads between the extremes of poverty and self-indulgence.

I'm not ready to apply the ideas in the chapter, yet. I still have to gain my education and prepare for life. I'll wait and begin to live simply when I'm ready.

Some of the chapter ideas may have to wait. However, you have already begun your life, and in some ways it is already beneficial to the earth. Improving yourself is the first step toward improving the world—remember the ripple effect. Learn all you can. Work on your education, and on your emotional and spiritual growth. You will then be better equipped to participate in the world community.

Do you really think that if everyone made choices like these, it would help the state of the world?

Yes. Every agency that has studied the future has reached the same conclusion: voluntary simplicity can work. It does not mean living primitively. Most people prefer beauty and ease to ugliness and discomfort. Voluntary simplicity does mean seeking a life free of distractions, clutter, and self-importance—a life that includes self-discipline. The words of an old poem speak to this idea, and they are fitting here:

Beyond a wholesome discipline, be gentle with yourself. You are a child of the universe, no less than the trees and the stars; you have a right to be here. And whether or not it is clear to you, no doubt the universe is unfolding as it should. Therefore be at peace with God, whatever you conceive him to be, and whatever your labors and aspirations . . . keep peace with your soul. Desiderata, *found in Old St. Paul's Church, Baltimore, dated 1692, author unknown. Although it has not been proven, some authorities believe that Max Ehrmann wrote the* Desiderata *in 1948.*

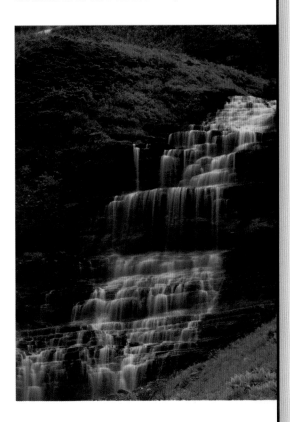

opportunity to begin thinking about ways they can make a positive impact toward beginning to solve global problems. Another option would be to have artistic students create a coloring book with recycling and energy-wise information to be copied (on recycled paper, of course!) and distributed to younger brothers and sisters or children at nearby elementary schools.

Students with creative writing, speaking, or musical skills could author a short musical presentation dramatizing ways children and teens can help to improve the environment. New words, based on information and ideas learned in this chapter, can be written to familiar tunes. You may want to have your students give a presentation for a school assembly or contact elementary schools to arrange to present your program and recycling exhibit.

VOCABULARY

1. a. pollution **b.** global warming **c.** compost **d.** food chain **e.** ecosystems **f.** persistent **g.** sustainable **h.** biodegradable **i.** environment
2. a. Photovoltaic (PV) panels **b.** ripple effect **c.** greenhouse effect **d.** acid rain **e.** Active solar
3. Answers will vary.

RECALL

SECTION 1

1. You can get sick, and possibly get cancer. (p. 702)

SECTION 2

2. hunger, poverty, and population growth; losses of land to produce food; accelerating fossil fuel use; increasing air pollution; global warming, droughts, and floods; ozone loss from the outer atmosphere; water shortages; deforestation and desertification; ocean and lake pollution; extinction of species; see pages 706–707 for descriptions
3. Individually choose what products to buy and what foods to eat. Groups can lobby legislators to write laws that protect the environment, demand that the laws be enforced, and insist that corporations and governments honor their principles. (p. 707)

CHAPTER 26 Review

Summarizing the Chapter

Your ability to respond correctly to the following statements ensures your understanding of the main concepts in the chapter.

1. Describe how the environment affects your body's health.
2. List and identify the global environmental problems in the late 1990s.
3. Explain how our lifestyle choices affect the environment and our health.
4. Discuss how we can help our environment while shopping.
5. Describe how we can conserve energy and water in our homes.
6. Describe the environmental problems associated with waste disposal.
7. Discuss the impact of hunger on the environment.

Learning the Vocabulary

environment	sustainable
pollution	recyclable
fossil fuel	biodegradable
ozone	disposable
air pollution	persistent
acid rain	food chain
global warming	dioxins
greenhouse effect	ecosystems
ozone layer	active solar
ripple effect	photovoltaic (PV) panels
Kyoto Protocol	compost

Answer the following questions on a separate sheet of paper.

1. *Matching*—Match each of the following phrases with the appropriate vocabulary term from the list above:
  a. contamination of the environment with anything that impairs its ability to support life

728

b. warming of the planet, which threatens life on earth
c. rotted vegetable matter, used as fertilizer
d. the sequence in which living things depend on other living things for food
2. a. _____ are panels that convert light into electricity.
  b. The term used to describe how one person's actions may affect many other people is the _____.
  c. The _____ is the heat-trapping effect of the glass in a greenhouse.
  d. Rain that carries acid air pollutants, which harms plant life and endangers the soil is called _____.
  e. _____ is the use of photovoltaic panels to generate electricity from sunlight.
  f. systems of land, plants, and animals that have existed together for thousands or millions of years and that are interdependent
  g. The opposite of biodegradable—unable to decompose is _____.
  h. _____ is the use of resources at such a rate that the earth can keep on replacing them.
  i. _____ means able to be converted by living organisms into harmless waste products that can be used over again to build or grow new things.
  j. The _____ is everything "outside" the living organism—air, water, soil, other organisms.
3. Write a paragraph using at least ten of the vocabulary terms listed. Underline each vocabulary term that you use.

Recalling Important Facts and Ideas

Section 1
1. What can happen to your body when the water you drink is polluted?

Section 2
2. List and briefly describe ten global environmental problems.
3. How can you help slow, stop, or even reverse the global environmental problems?
4. Describe how sustainable choices you make are beneficial to the environment and also to your health.

Section 3
5. What is the single largest source of air pollution?

4. Sustainable choices help to keep the level of pollution down so that the environment can recover from its effects and replace natural resources. The choices most bene- ficial to the environment also benefit health. People's health greatly depends on the health of their surroundings. (p. 710)

6. How often should you shop? What other tips are given about shopping?
7. How long do plastics last?

Section 4

8. How many families are now using solar energy?
9. What keeps most people from using PV panels, a battery, and a DC refrigerator?
10. Among kitchen appliances, which is the biggest energy user?
11. What can you do to save energy while using lightbulbs?

Section 5

12. What can a recycled plastic water bottle become?
13. What materials can be piled up together with some soil and decompose naturally?
14. Describe why natural fertilizers are better for the environment than synthetic fertilizers.

Section 6

15. How many children go blind each year from vitamin deficiencies?
16. In what ways are we overstraining the earth's ability to support life?

Critical Thinking

1. Read the Straight Talk section on page 726, "Personal Strategy—Voluntary Simplicity." What suggestions are given about our lives? How can you simplify your life? What will happen to our environment if nobody changes?

Activities

1. Visit a local health-care clinic. Find out how many people have come in due to hunger. What health problems do victims of hunger have? Share your findings with the rest of the class in an oral report.
2. Contact a Hunger Relief Organization in your area. What will your donations actually do for hungry people? How much money goes directly to the people who need it for food? How much money goes to the organization that is helping?

3. Make posters on ways we can recycle products in our homes. Post these around school.
4. Write an editorial in your school newspaper about how our lifestyle choices affect our environment and our health. In your editorial, challenge students to change habits to help the environment and their health.
5. Design a pamphlet that explains how to use non-toxic products to clean our homes. Make copies available to all students.
6. Interview your parents on how they are helping the environment by recycling. Ask them how they are recycling their trash and garbage. What else are they doing to help the environment?
7. Visit the local waste-water treatment plant. How does the plant dispose of waste products? Write a one-page report about your trip and the process the plant goes through each day.
8. Make a video about the ten different global environmental problems described in this chapter. For each problem listed, come up with a solution. Share your work with the rest of the class.
9. Make up a play on ways to help our environment. Show this play to children at a local elementary school.
10. Watch television for an hour and write down all the products that are being advertised. Which of these products are designed, manufactured, and packaged with the most concern for the environment? How? Rank the products from best to worst for the environment.

Making Decisions about Health

1. Hunger is a major problem in the world. What can you do about the hunger problem? Will you concentrate your efforts on the United States or on other countries? Why?
2. Garbage is a major problem for our environment. Recycling can help control this problem. How could you make everyone in the world recycle? What laws would you pass? How would you enforce these laws?

SECTION 4

8. more than 20,000 families (p. 718)
9. the high initial cost (p. 719)
10. refrigerator (p. 718)
11. use high-efficiency compact fluorescent bulbs (p. 719)

SECTION 5

12. part of a beautiful carpet (p. 721)
13. vegetable scraps, fruit peelings, leftover plant-based foods, leaves and grass cuttings (p. 721)
14. they require no mining; they recycle natural materials; and they add needed texture and nutrients to the soil (p. 721)

SECTION 6

15. half a million (p. 722)
16. Answers will vary; could include: wiping out many varieties of plant life, heating up the climate, using up freshwater supplies, and destroying the protective ozone layer that shields life from the sun's damaging rays. (p. 724)

SECTION 3

5. Motor vehicles (p. 711)
6. once each week. Answers may vary; could include: share rides to the mall, take turns shopping for one another, shop at neighborhood stores, walk or use a bicycle, choose the most fuel-efficient model of car. (p. 711)
7. for years or decades, creating masses of refuse that clog landfills (p. 714)

KEY POINTS

Chapter 27 is 20 pages long and divided into three sections. This chapter introduces the concept of the individual as a consumer within the health-care system. The importance of understanding methods of paying for health care is explained. Medicare, Medicaid, HMOs, and different kinds of insurance are compared. The costs of health care are affected by the increasing number of lawsuits, the expense of malpractice insurance, and problems in the health-care system. There are many health-care resources available in your community and it is important to learn how to access and choose them appropriately. Students will learn about career options in the field of health care as well as how to detect and report fraudulent advertising practices. For additional information on careers in health care, see Appendix A.

ACTIVITY TO INTRODUCE THE CHAPTER

Have students look in the Yellow Pages of the local phone book for listings of various medical services and health-care providers. Have students make a list of the categories as represented by the headings in the local phone book under which medical information/services can be found. Then have them place check marks by the services their families have used.

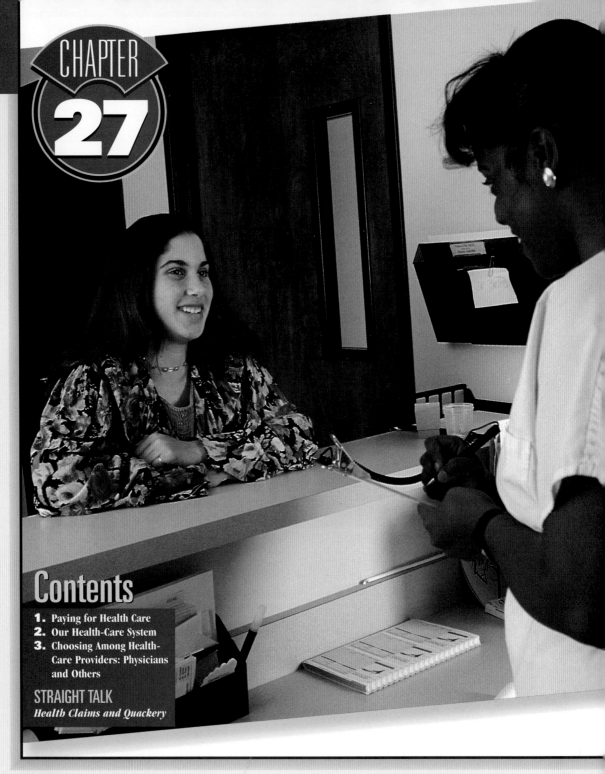

CHAPTER 27

Contents

1. Paying for Health Care
2. Our Health-Care System
3. Choosing Among Health-Care Providers: Physicians and Others

STRAIGHT TALK
Health Claims and Quackery

NOT Enough Time?

Following are some suggestions to help you make sure that you cover the key topics in this chapter if you have limited time. (Refer to the daily lesson plans in your Teacher's Resource Box for additional suggestions.)

DAY 1   On the day prior to beginning Chapter 27, ask students to read the chapter so they will be ready to discuss it in class. On

The Consumer and the Health-Care System

FACT or FICTION

What do you think? Are the following statements true or false? If you think they are false, then say what is true.

1. HMO stands for home medical operation—minor surgery that people can perform for themselves.
2. If you have medical and surgical insurance, you are probably covered for the costs of most medical treatments you might need.
3. Some operations are often recommended when they are not necessary, so it pays to get a second opinion before having surgery.
4. The worst problem of the United States' health-care system is a lack of new technology.
5. Anyone can adopt the title "doctor," but there are penalties for falsely claiming to be a medical doctor (M.D.) with a degree from a particular school.

(Answers on page 744)

Introduction

No doubt you have been a consumer of the **health-care system**. Virtually everyone who attends public school must be immunized, and many teens have been treated for bouts of flu or broken bones. When you need the health-care system, nothing else can take its place. At present, your parents, your guardians, or other adults probably attempt to get you the treatment you need at a cost your family can afford. By the time you leave home, though, you will need to know how to find your own way around in the system. This chapter invites you to learn to use the health-care system to best support your health.

BULLETIN BOARD IDEAS

List as many health-care providers as you can on a bulletin board where everyone can see. Discuss with the students why there are so many options for health care. You might suggest that students bring in pictures of their doctors or health-care providers to put faces to the types of providers. (See Appendix A.)

Answers to FACT or FICTION

1. **False.** HMO stands for *health maintenance organization*. People should not perform surgery on themselves.
2. **False.** You may need as many as five different kinds of insurance. Even then, specific medical needs might not be covered.
3. **True.**
4. **False.** The high cost of health care in the United States is the worst problem.
5. **True.**

FAST FACTS

Over a typical two-year period, at least 25 percent of the U.S. population goes without health insurance for at least one month, according to the U.S. Census Bureau. Young adults between the ages of 18 and 21 were the age group most likely to lack insurance.

Day 1, start with the Activity to Introduce the Chapter. Review payment options and availability of resources in your community. Evaluate with the Quick Quizzes on pages 732–733 and 738–739.

DAY 2 On Day 2 begin with the Focus Activity on page 740. Then review Section 3. Discuss health resources in your community. Close the class with the Close activity on page 745.

SECTION
1

FOCUS

OUTCOMES

In this section students will learn:

1. Three different approaches to paying for health care: no insurance, insurance, and managed care.
2. How services are paid for under each option.
3. Advantages of each option.

FOCUS ACTIVITY

Write on the board: "Everyone needs health insurance because it is cheaper than 'paying as you go' health care." Ask students whether they agree or disagree and why.

TEACH & APPLY

TEACHER SUPPORT

Key Passage

Ask students to compare HMO plans to insurance. Students should see that belonging to an HMO is much the same as buying insurance. You pay premiums for your insurance whether you receive any benefits or not. You pay a monthly fee to the HMO whether you use it or not. Most insurance policies do not cover wellcare, but HMO plans usually do. Insurance policies usually cover hospital expenses; HMO plans usually do not.

SECTION 1

Paying for Health Care

L et us suppose you are going to have three problems this year. For one thing, you are going to get a severe sore throat that, unless promptly treated, will develop into a major, whole-body infection. Second, you are going to break your arm. Third, you are developing a heart condition (even though you may be young), but you will not have any symptoms for 15 years.

How these events will affect your health and your wallet depends on the choices you have already made. Consider three possibilities.

No Plan   First, suppose you have chosen the unprepared approach: you have no insurance, you have no personal health-care provider, and you have no health-care plan. When your sore throat strikes, you try to live with it. Then it becomes so painful that you have to go to the hospital emergency room. There, you have to pay $100 in advance, are given some medicine, and are dismissed. You are still so sick that you lose a week of classes or work. When you break your arm, you again rush to the hospital and find that they will not even set your arm in a cast until you have again paid in advance—this time, $500. Total cost of treatment for the year: $600, a week of missed classes or work, and failure to detect your advancing heart condition.

Insurance and Private Physician Plan   The second approach, the insurance approach, makes the story different. You are paying, say, $50 a month for insurance. Now you get your sore throat. You let it get really painful, as before. You then go to the hospital. This time, however, you present your insurance card and are treated without question. The same thing happens when you break your arm: you are admitted and treated right away. After both events, the bills may be simply paid for you. If you must pay up front, you will soon have your money (or most of it) back. Total cost to you: still $600 for the year. However, this time you have 12 equal payments, called **premiums**, of $50 rather than two surprise lump sums to pay. You still miss a week of classes or work, and no one detects your heart condition.

A private physician can change the story even more. If you have insurance and a private physician to consult for your sore throat, you may seek help from this person immediately. Prompt treatment spares you the pain of a bad throat, as well as the loss of a week's classes or work. No change occurs concerning your broken arm—you pay $500 as before, and get it back later. However, one other thing happens that is to your benefit. Your health-care provider gives you a routine physical examination, detects your heart trouble, and starts treating you for it, adding years to your life.

Your insurance does not cover your physical examination, so you are out about $100 for that. However, the future benefits of freedom from heart disease outweigh that price by far. Insurance does pay for the rest, so your costs are $600 for insurance, $100 for your exam, and no loss of a productive week. You even may be able to lower your cost by using a walk-in medical clinic or a community health center. Here a staff physician can treat your sore throat, and may even detect your heart problem.

Managed Care Plan   Still another option is to join a **managed care** plan, such as a **health maintenance organization (HMO)**. The HMO

When you need the health-care system, nothing else can take its place.

QUICK QUIZ

Chapter 27, Section 1

The following quiz will help you assess your students' understanding of the material covered in this section of the chapter. You might use the quiz as an oral exercise, which will lead into a class discussion of the topics covered. Or, you might use it as a paper/pencil quiz to evaluate your students individually.

1. A person with no health plan is responsible for 100 percent of her/his medical bills. (True)
2. People who have an insurance must pay a monthly premium which may be greater or less than the cost of their monthly medical bills. (True)
3. A person with insurance and a private physician plan receives a free routine physical examination. (False)
4. You may be able to lower your medical

charges you a fee each month that is slightly higher than insurance—say, $75 ($900 for the year). For this you receive many services without paying extra for them. The routine physical examination to catch your heart disease is usually paid for by the plan.

As a member of an HMO, you do not hesitate to get prompt treatment, because it doesn't cost you anything extra. Therefore, when your sore throat hits, you do not lose a week to illness. When you break your arm, although you still go to the hospital for treatment, the HMO pays most of the fees. Because your HMO wants to avoid costly treatment of diseases later in life, it encourages your physical exam and pays for it.

The key difference between a managed care plan and other health-care providers is in how they are paid. An HMO offers a **prepayment plan**. Other health-care providers charge for each service as you receive it. Their method of payment is described as a **fee-for-service system**.

Managed care plans have come into criticism lately, partly because some unethical profit-minded managers delay or deny care for patients who need it. The industry has responded by developing a quality "report card" for grading how well a plan meets the medical needs of clients. Consumers who know what to look for in a plan can make informed choices among providers. A first step is to ask several participating clients and physicians how they feel about the plan. If they aren't satisfied, chances are that you won't be, either.

Comparison of Choices   In summary, of the three approaches to health care, the unprepared approach is most risky. The insurance approach is safer but doesn't offer the benefits of preventive care. It also doesn't tell you where to go or whom to see in emergencies. You have to figure that out for yourself. The managed care approach provides a map to the health-care system. It guides you along its paths as your needs arise.

 KEY POINTS *People who have no medical insurance must pay at each illness. Those with insurance pay in advance, and only a limited amount. Members of managed care plans also pay in advance, and then receive treatment at little or no extra cost through the plan providers.*

SECTION 1 Review

Answer the following questions on a sheet of paper.

Learning the Vocabulary

The vocabulary terms in this section are *health-care system, premiums, managed care, health maintenance organization (HMO), prepayment plan,* and *fee-for-service system.*

1. Use each of the vocabulary terms above in a sentence.

Learning the Facts

2. What are the three health-care approaches listed in this section?
3. List three benefits of a managed care plan.

Making Life Choices

4. Your family has just moved to a little town from a big city. Your family used to belong to an HMO, but the little town does not have one. How are you going to provide for your medical care? How will you choose the best care?

MINI Glossary

health-care system: the total of all health-care providers and medical treatment facilities that work together to provide medical care to the population.

premiums: regular payments made to an insurance company to cover the costs of unforeseen events such as medical emergencies.

managed care: a system of providing health care based on a prepaid basis. By emphasizing preventive care, controlling physician charges, and screening requests for expensive tests and procedures, managed care plans control costs of providing care.

health maintenance organization (HMO): a group of physicians who practice together and who treat people's health problems under a prepayment plan.

prepayment plan: a system of paying for health care in which the clients pay a fixed fee every month, regardless of how many services they receive.

fee-for-service system: a system of paying for health care in which clients pay individual fees for the services they receive.

ASSESS

EVALUATE

 A reproducible quiz for Section 1 is provided in the Teacher's Resource Box.

SECTION 1 Review Answers

1. Answers will vary.
2. no insurance, insurance, and managed care (p. 732)
3. Answers may vary, but should include: receiving medical services without paying extra for them; routine physical exam is usually part of the plan; and you don't hesitate to get prompt treatment. (p. 733)
4. Answers will vary.

CLOSE

Invite guest speakers, such as a health-insurance agent, an HMO representative, and someone who does not believe it is wise to buy health coverage. Have the speakers explain the different types of coverage, costs, exemptions, and so on. Then have students compare the different options and give reasons for the choices they would make.

 Reproducible vocabulary worksheets are provided in the Teacher's Resource Box.

costs by using a walk-in medical clinic or a community health center. (True)
5. Routine physical examinations may help to prevent major diseases from developing. (True)
6. A health maintenance organization (HMO) provides minimal health coverage at reduced rates. (False)
7. A managed care plan will usually provide a routine physical examination for no extra fee, but has a higher monthly fee. (True)
8. An HMO operates on a fee-for-service system. (False)
9. A person on a prepayment plan pays for his/her medical services in advance, but pays only a limited amount. (True)
10. The availability of preventive care is a major benefit of an HMO. (True)

SECTION 2

FOCUS

OUTCOMES

In this section students will learn:

1. About various types of insurance coverage.
2. Ways to reduce health-care costs by carefully selecting the appropriate care provider or service.
3. That there are many problems with the health-care system in this country.

FOCUS ACTIVITY

Write on the board: "Think of the times when your family has used health insurance to help with health care costs. Be ready to share with the class." Have students volunteer their stories.

TEACH & APPLY

BACKGROUND INFORMATION

You may want to give students additional information about how to evaluate an insurance policy for health care. First they should ask how much the deductible is, and whether or not the policy covers the following: inhospital and outpatient costs, diagnostic tests, second opinions, medicines, prevention, education, ambulance service, and psychological counseling.

SECTION 2

Our Health-Care System

Medical care isn't cheap. A serious illness may easily require treatments costing more than the average family makes in a year. The insurance system is devised to help people avoid being wiped out financially by serious illness.

Health Insurance

"I'm sorry, but your insurance policy doesn't cover this. Pay in advance please." People can avoid the pain of this situation only if they use some know-how in shopping for health insurance. The five types of insurance related to people's personal health care are:

1. **Hospitalization insurance.**
2. **Surgical insurance.**
3. **Medical insurance.**
4. **Major medical insurance.**
5. **Disability insurance.**

The different kinds of insurance cover each of these: accidents, hospitalization, surgery, physician services, medicines, pregnancy, and disabilities that might prevent your working. Policies differ. Read them, and think about your needs. For example, if you are planning to start a family soon, be sure your insurance covers those costs.

If you have a healthy lifestyle, you may be charged lower insurance rates than others. Nonsmokers, people of normal weight, nonusers of alcohol, or regular exercisers are more likely to stay healthy. Insurance companies know that they are more likely to have to pay large medical bills for people who smoke, who are obese, who use alcohol, who fail to exercise, who don't wear safety belts, and whose blood cholesterol and blood pressure are high.

Special groups of people may be covered by **Medicare** and **Medicaid**. Medicare pays hospital expenses for senior citizens who also receive Social Security benefits. Medicaid is medical insurance provided for those who receive public assistance (welfare).

No matter how much insurance you have, you cannot be sure of covering every circumstance. Clients of insurance companies and their families pay all costs not covered by insurance, so insurance is not a substitute for careful financial planning.

 KEY POINTS *Insurance can pay for the costs of accidents, hospitalization, surgery, health-care provider services, medicines, and disabilities. It does not cover everything, and it is no substitute for careful financial planning.*

Health Strategies

Selecting and Using Medical Care Facilities

When selecting and using medical care facilities:

1. Know what facilities are available and what their specialties are.
2. Avoid emergency room visits.
3. Get a second or third opinion.
4. Consider alternatives to hospital tests and surgery.
5. Use the hospital on weekdays; avoid weekends.
6. Ask about each facility's policy on payment.
7. Find out the physician's and hospital's ways of handling insurance claims. They may file the claims, or you may have to.
8. Protest if the bill is in error.
9. Be willing to go out of state, if necessary, for specialized medical care.

COOPERATIVE LEARNING

Health care is one of the biggest concerns for people in the United States today. Politicians make it an issue during their campaigns for public office. Employers are finding it harder and harder to provide insurance benefits to their employees because of the rising costs of health care, and many families are now going without any medical insurance because of the high costs. Many people also go without health-care services because they cannot afford them or because they are confused by what services and programs are available. The following activity will help students gain a better understanding of how the health system works, what problems the system faces, and what programs will be available to them.

Divide the class into groups of three. In each group, one member will have a text book open, one member will have notebook

Malpractice Insurance

Insurance can be abused. The chief insurance abuse driving the cost of medical care higher is the abuse of **malpractice insurance**. Malpractice insurance is not for you. It is for your health-care provider. If a physician is sued for providing improper care, and loses the case, the insurance will pay the cost.

Only a few physicians hurt clients on purpose or by foolish errors. However, almost all feel they must protect themselves with malpractice insurance. The premiums can amount to a large percentage of a physician's yearly income. This forces physicians to raise their fees. You, the physician's client, end up paying extra to cover the costs.

 KEY POINTS *Malpractice insurance is costly and helps drive up the costs of health care.*

Medical Resources in the Community

A goal of the health-care system is to meet the needs of people within their own communities. Many agencies—both government-run and private, voluntary types—work together to achieve this goal. The federal government runs programs to provide many functions that everyone needs, such as the law-enforcing functions of the Food and Drug Administration (FDA). The FDA is a watchdog agency that checks up on the manufacturers of foods and drugs. Figure 27–1 on the next page briefly describes a few of the many resources working together to meet the nation's health needs.

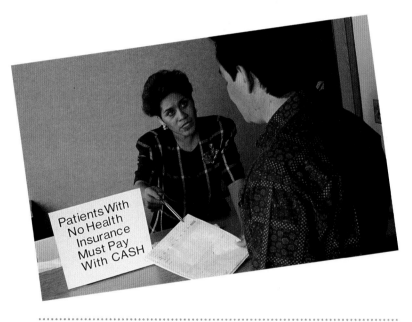

Without health insurance coverage, serious illness may bring financial ruin.

MINI Glossary

hospitalization insurance: insurance to pay the cost of a hospital stay. See also *Medicare* and *Medicaid*.

surgical insurance: insurance to pay the surgeon's fees. See also *Medicaid*.

medical insurance: insurance to pay physicians' fees, lab fees, and fees for prescription medications.

major medical insurance: insurance to pay high bills not covered by other insurance.

disability insurance: insurance to replace lost income if a person should be unable to work due to a long illness.

Medicare: hospitalization insurance for people who are receiving Social Security.

Medicaid: hospitalization and surgical insurance available for people who qualify as needy.

malpractice insurance: insurance that protects providers of health care against lawsuits by people claiming to have been harmed by a health-care provider.

---

paper and a pen or pencil, and one member will be the questioner. To make sure that all members participate equally, have them switch roles in the group after they finish each section of the chapter.

To begin, the person with the book reads Section 1 to the other group members. While he or she is reading, the person with the paper and pen or pencil is to write down the important points, as well as any questions the questioner may ask. The questioner is to pose

questions for the group members to discuss. After the group has finished one chapter section, have students switch roles before reading and discussing the next chapter section. After the entire chapter has been covered, have all the groups discuss their views of the health-care system and what problems and advantages our health-care system has. Conclude by having each group share their views with the class.

DISCUSSION

Ask students if they think the fact that people live longer increases or decreases the cost of health insurance. Students might think that people are living longer and must be healthier, causing insurance rates to go down. Just the opposite is true, however. Because people live longer they need care for longer periods of time later in life.

GROUP ACTIVITY

Divide the class into groups of three to five. Using various health-plan options and case study examples, have students choose the plan that would work best for the scenario. Example: Mr. G has been to his physician for the following services: yearly checkup—$75; flu shot—$25; office visit for bronchitis—$35. He also broke his leg falling from a ladder while painting his house and had to go to the emergency room— $700 (includes X-rays $150, cast $150, doctor's fees $300, miscellaneous medicines for pain and swelling, $100). Develop other scenarios to fit the insurance information available. Have students defend or explain why they chose the plan they did.

BACKGROUND INFORMATION

As enrichment, give students a list of several different types of health-care facilities and their primary functions:

a. Birthing center—place to give birth in a homelike atmosphere.

b. Convalescent home—place other than a hospital to recover from illness or surgery.

(continued on next page)

(continued from previous page)

c. Extended care center—similar to a convalescent home but with more medical and nursing services.
d. Health center—serves the routine health-care needs of a special group.
e. Nursing home—cares for the elderly who can no longer live independently; a residential rather than a medical facility.
f. Teaching hospital—place where students can learn their professions.
g. Trauma center—for treating extreme emergency cases.
h. Walk-in emergency center—for emergency care similar to the emergency room in a hospital.

DISCUSSION

State: "It is important to plan financially for medical costs. Examining various insurance plans is a good way to do this. Examine your health-care needs and options when selecting a plan for yourself and your family. Consider your income level, health status, upcoming needs, community resources, coverage options, and costs when making your decision." Then ask students to choose a plan that would be good for them as young single adults going to postsecondary school or working with no insurance coverage. Let them choose from options and plans reviewed in class.

Figure 27–1 *Sample Agencies Focusing on Improved Community Health*

These and many other agencies are dedicated to improving the health of people in the United States.

At the national level:

• Food and Drug Administration enforces laws intended to ensure pure, well-labeled food, and safe and effective drugs.
• Centers for Disease Control runs research and programs to prevent and halt disease epidemics.
• National Institutes of Health conducts research that yields national health statistics.
• Medicare and Medicaid help meet the medical needs of the elderly and low-income citizens.
• Private research groups, such as the American Heart Association and the National Safety Council, focus on discovering more about diseases, safety, and health.

At the local level:

• School clinics may provide care by nurses, first aid, pregnancy prevention, substance abuse prevention, or other services each community deems are needed for its students.
• Public Health Department provides immunizations, family planning services, maternal and child services, health worker training, addiction recovery programs, and mental illness services, among others.
• Hospitals, clinics, and physicians provide medical testing, screening, and treatments.

Health Strategies

Hints for Emergency Room Visits

When you must go to an emergency room:

1. Call your regular health-care provider first. Leave a message with the answering service stating who you are, what the problem is, and where you are going.
2. Have only one person go with you, not the whole family.
3. Take some identification and your insurance card with you.
4. Tell the person at the admissions desk if you have been there before. If you have, the personnel can find your file and skip some paperwork.
5. Know your own medical history and what medicines you are taking.

Some aspects of health care are better provided at the local level, because communities' needs differ. A large city may need to provide more services for urban low-income groups, while a farming community may have entirely different needs.

Among the private providers of health services, medical facilities have different strengths and weaknesses. When you need the services provided by such facilities, you must decide which to use. The better you know what is available ahead of time, the better you can choose one that will serve you in time of need. The Health Strategies section on page 734, "Selecting and Using Medical Care Facilities," can help you make that choice.

Smart strategies can also help you save money and needless struggles. For example, if possible, try to see a health-care professional during office hours—do not go to a hospital emergency room. Emergency rooms always cost extra. In case you must go to the emergency room, the Health Strategies section on this page, "Hints for Emergency Room Visits," offers a few suggestions to make your visit easier.

Another suggestion is to seek a **second opinion** before allowing any test or surgery. Some operations, especially **ton-**

HEALTHY PEOPLE 2000

Increase to at least 90 percent the proportion of hospitals, health maintenance organizations, and large group practices that provide patient education programs, **and to at least 90 percent the proportion of community hospitals that offer community health promotion programs addressing the priority health needs of their communities.**

Patient education services include a broad array of planned and coordinated inpatient

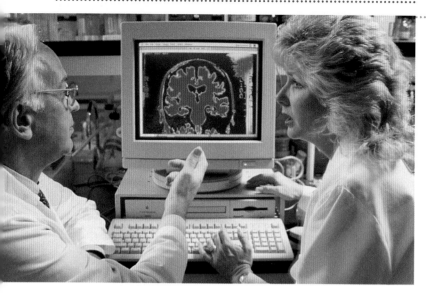

New medical technologies help to save lives, but they can raise costs of treatment enormously.

sillectomy and **hysterectomy**, are overperformed. That is, they are often recommended when they are not medically necessary. Insurance may cover the cost of a second opinion. If the two opinions differ, consider getting a third.

About payment: as many as 90 percent of most hospital bills contain errors. Read through your bills to check that you have not been overcharged. If you question any charge, ask for an itemized list of services you received, and send it to your insurance company. The insurance company may be able to get the charges reduced.

 To use health-care facilities to your advantage, compare those available, choose the ones that will serve you best, and assert your rights as to choices in treatments and reasonable costs.

Problems and Advantages of Our Health-Care System

Not all nations' health-care systems operate as the U.S. system does. For example, Canada has a national program of insurance that offers basic health care to more than 99 percent of its citizens. A problem for Canadians, however, is a lack of advanced technology. Clients with special needs must often travel to U.S. medical centers.

Galloping costs may be the worst problem in our system. There seems to be no limit on how high costs can go, and high costs prevent some people of limited means from receiving the care they need. Malpractice insurance, already mentioned, raises costs. So do the extremely high costs of modern hospital technology. Figure 27–2 on the next page makes the point that while our health-care system could use some improvement, it also has advantages appreciated by people the world over.

Mini Glossary

second opinion: a second assessment of a diagnosis and treatment plan by another health-care provider, usually on the request of a client, to double-check the validity of the original plan.

tonsillectomy: removal of the tonsils (in the throat), an operation sometimes performed needlessly.

hysterectomy: removal of the uterus, an operation performed more often than necessary.

and outpatient educational activities to "enable patients, and their families and friends, when appropriate, to make informed decisions about their health; to manage their illnesses; and to implement followup care at home." Patient education programs for diabetes, asthma, and other conditions are valued by patients and can help to improve the efficiency and effectiveness of care. Patient education programs may reduce length of hospital stay, prevent hospital readmissions, and reduce emergency room visits.

(continued from previous page)

physician's office whether their insurance will cover it and what help will be available in filing the claim. Many hospitals expect the bill to be paid immediately, with the patient being reimbursed later by the insurance company. Some will help the patient file the claim; others will not.

LEARNING WITH VISUALS

Have students read carefully Figure 27–2, "Some Problems and Advantages of Our Health-Care System." Discuss each problem area with students to ensure that they understand them. Then, have students work individually to rank the problems from 1 to 6, with 1 being the most serious problem and 6 being the least serious problem. When students have finished, use their rankings to develop a class list. Allow students to offer arguments for the ranking of individual problems. (They may have some stories to share about people they know who have had some of the problems listed here.)

You might have students work in groups to come up with solutions to some or all of the problems listed.

If time allows, have students rank the advantages from 1 to 6, with one being the most advantageous. Use students' answers to develop a class ranking. Ask students to share why they feel one advantage is preferable over another.

FAST FACTS

The United States spends more for health care than any other country in the world, yet ranks in the mid-20s in infant mortality.

Figure 27–2 Some Problems and Advantages of Our Health-Care System

The problems of our health-care system are real, but many overlook its important advantages. Here is a list of some of its problems that need solving and some of its advantages that are worth protecting.

Problems	Advantages
Insurance problems of the sick Insurance companies can cancel a policy or charge an unaffordable fee, should someone develop a disease whose treatment involves unusually high costs. (AIDS is such a disease.)	*Access to life-saving technology* The U.S. health-care system supports research and technology, and offers many new technologically advanced treatments that people from around the globe come to receive.
Malpractice suits The legal system allows too many high-dollar awards and frivolous lawsuits against physicians and hospitals, driving up health-care costs.	*Access to physicians* Patients can speak directly to physicians by phone, and make emergency appointments when illness strikes. Also, clients have time to ask questions and receive advice. In some other health-care systems, none of this is possible, because physicians see up to 100 patients a day.
Job lock Often, when a person changes jobs, that person must also change his insurance carrier. A person who becomes ill under one policy may be turned down for coverage of that illness on a new policy. Some sick people feel locked into a job for fear of losing their insurance coverage.	*Confidentiality and privacy* Anyone has the right to limit access to their medical records should they wish to keep them private. This is because they are kept in private offices, not in central computer warehouses, as in some other countries.
Uninsured citizens Some 20% of the population have no insurance, and may be denied some forms of health care. Some emergency rooms must treat them anyway, and so are taxed with serving nonpaying customers. The emergency rooms raise other prices to cover these costs, or try to recover them from tax money.	*Equitable treatment options* Treatment is available to all who can afford it. Some other systems limit treatment given to elderly or terminally ill patients.
Tax unfairness Large employers can deduct 100% of their insurance expenses from their income taxes. Self-employed and unemployed people can deduct only a fraction or no insurance expenses, and so effectively pay double for health coverage.	*Local treatment facilities* Most communities have access to most procedures, so that a diagnosis of a serious condition normally doesn't require long-distance travel for treatment. In other countries, certain hospitals perform only certain procedures, and sick people must journey many miles for treatments.
Overuse of the system People who feel they are "spending the insurance company's money" have no reason to be frugal about their health-care spending.	*Quick access to care* Once a diagnosis is made, treatment is swift. In other countries, sick people often wait months or even years for treatment, even if they need surgery and are in pain.

Part of a solution to the cost problem might be to roll back medical technology in some locations. A system of small clinics equipped simply for handling routine health care, and staffed by physician's assistants or nurse practitioners, could cost less and fill a need for basic health-care services.

Chapter 27, Section 2

The following quiz will help you assess your students' understanding of the material covered in this section of the chapter. You might use the quiz as an oral exercise, which will lead into a class discussion of the topics covered. Or, you might use it as a paper/pencil quiz to evaluate your students individually.

Like the Quick Quiz, the Section Review can also be used as an assessment tool to spark class discussion or as an individual student evaluation. It can also be used as a review in preparation for this quiz.

1. Hospitalization insurance, surgical insurance, medical insurance, major medical insurance, and disability insurance are the five types of health care insurance. (True)

2. All insurance policies are basically the

Such a community clinic might deliver women's health care or specialize in facilitating normal births, for example.

New technologies open other possibilities. New communications technology, for example, now makes possible a sort of "video clinic." An expert at, say, the University of Chicago sets up a video conference call with a clinic in Kentucky or California that has a patient with specialized problems. Over two-way video cameras, the expert and patient view and speak with each other. The expert observes tests, monitors heartbeat and other vital signs, and offers a diagnosis and a treatment plan. One day, perhaps video clinics will offer needed expertise to most small-town clinics at a reasonable cost.

The backbone of any health-care system is the people who provide health care. The next section discusses the educational qualifications of some health-care providers.

KEY POINTS *Problems in the health-care system include high costs, which limits access. Solutions to these problems include systems such as community clinics that offer basic care at a low cost and new technology.*

> **❝** *Be careful about reading health books. You could die of a misprint.* **❞**
>
> Mark Twain
> (1835–1910)
> American writer

SECTION 2 Review

Answer the following questions on a sheet of paper.

Learning the Vocabulary

The vocabulary terms in this section are *hospitalization insurance, surgical insurance, medical insurance, major medical insurance, disability insurance, Medicare, Medicaid, malpractice insurance, second opinion, tonsillectomy,* and *hysterectomy.*

1. Match each of the following phrases with the appropriate term:
   a. insurance to pay the surgeon's fee
   b. hospitalization insurance for people who are receiving Social Security
   c. insurance to protect health-care providers against lawsuits by people claiming to have been harmed by health-care providers.
2. Write a paragraph using at least five of the vocabulary terms.

Learning the Facts

3. List the five types of insurance related to your personal health.
4. Who is eligible for Medicare?
5. Describe the role of the Food and Drug Administration in helping to meet people's health needs.
6. List and describe what to do when selecting and using medical care facilities.
7. Describe a problem with Canada's health-care system.
8. What is the backbone of a health-care system?

Making Life Choices

9. Alberto was out on a bike ride when his front tire hit a rock and threw him off the bike. He landed hard on his wrist. A friend drove him to the emergency room for treatment. At the hospital, Alberto was told he had to pay $400 up front in order to receive treatment. What could Alberto have done in advance to prevent this from happening?

ASSESS

EVALUATE

A reproducible quiz for Section 2 is provided in the Teacher's Resource Box.

SECTION 2 Review Answers

1. **a.** surgical insurance **b.** Medicare **c.** malpractice insurance
2. Answers will vary.
3. hospitalization, surgical, medical, major medical, disability (p. 734)
4. those receiving Social Security benefits (p. 734)
5. They are a watchdog agency that checks up on food and drugs, making sure they are safe and accurately labeled. (p. 735)
6. For possible answers see the Health Strategies on page 734.
7. The lack of advanced technology causes many physicians to send their clients to the U.S. for special treatment. (p. 737)
8. the people who provide health care (p. 739)
9. Answers will vary.

CLOSE

Have students present oral reports from the Discussion activity on cultural beliefs (page 737). Compare in class the beliefs and practices of the different ethnic groups.

same. (False)
3. People who smoke or drink alcohol are likely to have higher insurance rates. (True)
4. Medicare is a form of medical insurance associated with welfare. (False)
5. Insurance eliminates the need for careful financial planning. (False)
6. The necessity of purchasing malpractice insurance causes physicians to raise their medical fees. (True)
7. Competent physicians do not need to purchase malpractice insurance. (False)
8. The Food and Drug Administration is an example of a private health care provider. (False)
9. Going to a hospital emergency room is less expensive than visiting a regular doctor during office hours. (False)
10. Tonsillectomies and hysterectomies are operations that are often performed unnecessarily. (True)

SECTION 3
FOCUS

OUTCOMES

In this section students will learn:

1. Factors to consider when choosing a health-care provider.

2. The training and education requirements to receive a medical degree (M.D.).

3. Who to ask and where to look for information when choosing a new health-care provider.

4. What to watch for in fraudulent products, advertising, services, and care providers.

FOCUS ACTIVITY

Write on the board: "List as many health-care jobs as you can think of in one minute." When students have finished writing ask volunteers to read their lists aloud and compile a class list with as many different jobs as time allows. Discuss the careers that students think they would enjoy. (See Appendix A.)

TEACH & APPLY

DISCUSSION

Have students research different kinds of health-care careers and report to the class. They should include information such as: training or schooling, job outlook, employment practices, working conditions, earnings, advantages, disadvantages. Have the students discuss the various careers and share which they would most like to do.

SECTION 3
Choosing Among Health-Care Providers: Physicians and Others

A person who gets sick usually will think in terms of "going to the doctor"—but what is a doctor? Anyone can be called "doctor," but not all are trained the same way, and some are even dishonest. This section attempts to sort out who's who in the health-care world. Appendix A, at the end of this book, lists these and many more health-care providers for the person who wants to sort them all out—or become one.

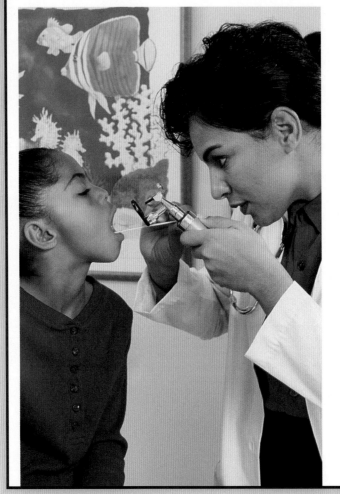

Expect a thorough physical examination from a health-care provider.

The Health-Care Provider

The health-care provider most people think of is the medical doctor, or M.D. This is as it should be, for medical school training equips the M.D. to handle many kinds of medical problems. This book refers to such a person as the *doctor* or *physician*.

Kinds of Doctors A long course of education leads to the M.D. degree and to the license to practice medicine. Another type of doctor, the osteopath (D.O.), takes the same course of training as an M.D., but in a school of osteopathy, which specializes in the muscles and skeleton.

Following four years of college, the person seeking to become a physician attends three years of medical school to learn to treat diseases. This is followed by a two-year **internship** and a one-year **residency**. Then the person must pass a state examination to receive a license to practice. Even more schooling is necessary to become a **specialist**, such as a **gynecologist** or **pediatrician**.

A physician is licensed to provide medical care under his or her own authority. Other professionals who can provide care independently are the nurse practitioner (N.P. or R.N.P.) and the physician's assistant (P.A.).

COOPERATIVE LEARNING

Assign students to cooperative learning groups to prepare a project on one of the following topics. Each group should choose one topic, gather information on it, and write a class presentation to be given orally to the rest of the class. Groups may choose from the following topics or from other topics approved by you.

1. Private versus Group Practice
2. Health Maintenance Organizations

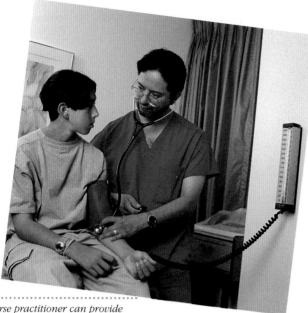

A nurse practitioner can provide some basic medical care.

Many people seek services from a chiropractor (doctor of chiropractic, or D.C.). Not everyone realizes that this person, although called "doctor," has not received the same medical training as an M.D. A chiropractor's office may resemble a physician's office, but the services are not the same. Chiropractors can relieve pain (especially from pressure on nerves). However, other medical services, such as diagnosing illnesses and prescribing treatments for them, are the exclusive domain of the M.D.

Some dishonest people, hoping to make money on people's illnesses, may only claim to have medical training. Anyone can claim the title "doctor." There are penalties only for falsely claiming to have an M.D. degree from a particular medical school. This chapter's Consumer Skills feature explores the fake **credentials** of these corrupt people.

What to Expect at an Appointment Once you have found a qualified health-care provider, call the person's office. Ask the questions listed in the Health Strategies section on the next page, "Choosing a Health-Care Provider." When you go for an appointment, it is a good idea to write down your medical questions beforehand and take them with you. Also, jot down answers as you talk to the professional.

A good health-care provider will take a thorough **history**—that is, provide a question-and-answer session about your past medical experiences. The history provides about 70 percent of the information needed for an accurate diagnosis. Time spent on providing an accurate history can save both illness and money later on.

For **Y**our **I**nformation

Appendix A lists various health-care providers and describes what they are qualified to do.

MINI Glossary

internship: a length of time spent in a medical facility as part of the training of health-care providers.

residency: a length of time spent in a medical facility as part of the M.D.'s training after the internship.

specialist: a physician with training in a specialty area beyond the medical degree requirements.

gynecologist: a specialist in the care of the female reproductive system.

pediatrician: a specialist concerned with the health care of infants and children.

credentials: (kre-DEN-shulls): official evidence of education or other qualifications of an authority; diplomas, licenses, and the like.

history (medical): an interview in which a health-care professional asks about past medical experience.

Key Passage
You may want to tell students that many people are intimidated by doctors; they believe that doctors are much smarter and better educated than they are. Therefore, when they don't understand a doctor's answer, they assume it's because they lack sufficient knowledge. Tell students that competent, concerned health-care providers want patients to know and understand any conditions or illnesses being discussed, but that they cannot clarify their explanations unless the patient asks questions. When they are patients, students should not be embarrassed if they don't understand. It's important that they ask questions.

TEACHER SUPPORT

GUEST SPEAKERS

Invite various health-care providers to participate on a panel discussion about health careers, services offered, benefits, advantages, disadvantages, wages, training, education, and so on.

CLASS ACTIVITY

Have students select a local physician or other health-care provider and research the person's credentials using the library, a physician's referral service, the American Medical Association, or the state health department for the agency that provides medical credentials in your state. Present findings to the class.

GROUP ACTIVITY

Have students identify group and private practices in your community. Then have them phone or make visits to find: hours of operation, typical costs for services, types and number of employees, payment policies, insurance policies, services available, credentials of care providers, or other information that seems appropriate for your community.

BACKGROUND INFORMATION

Do not assume that students know what a *diagnosis* is. Ask them to define it. Diagnosis means the use of scientific and skillful methods to establish the nature of a person's illness. This is done by evaluating the history of the disease process; the signs and symptoms present; and laboratory data.

GROUP ACTIVITY

Divide students into groups and give each group a phone book. Ask each group to find how many doctors are listed under each specialty. The list could include, but is not limited to, Community/Environmental Health (allergist), Drugs (pharmacist), Substance Abuse Counselor, Nutrition (registered dietitian), Diseases (family practice doctor, internist), Safety and First Aid (EMT), Growth and Development (pediatrician), Mental Health (psychiatrist, counselor), Fitness and Exercise (athletic trainer), Rehabilitation (physical therapist). The specialties will vary from community to community. Ask if there are any missing specialties so that a person would have to go to another community to access that type of care. Make a chart with the names of each specialty and the number of specialists for each. Post in the room.

Also expect a thorough **physical examination**, head to toe. The person who gives you a once-over-lightly is not starting by getting to know your physical condition very well. Expect certain tests—for example, a blood and urine analysis or a chest X-ray exam.

Expect to be told the diagnosis and the treatment options. By the time you leave the office, you should feel satisfied that you have been well examined, understood, and instructed. If this is not the case, you may want to find another health-care provider.

KEY POINTS   *Health-care providers other than physicians, physician's assistants, and nurse practitioners come in many stripes. The match between you and your health-care provider should be a satisfying one. Select this person with care. Don't accept second best. Beware of frauds.*

Health Strategies

Choosing a Health-Care Provider

When choosing a health-care provider:

1. Ask the American Medical Association or people you trust for recommendations.
2. Check the provider's credentials. Look for membership in the American College of Physicians or the American College of Surgeons.
3. Ask these questions:
   - ▶ What are the fees for office visits? Other visits?
   - ▶ Will you accept my insurance as complete payment for the care you provide?
   - ▶ What are your office hours?
   - ▶ Can I obtain advice by phone? At what times?
   - ▶ Do you recommend that I have periodic checkups? How often?
   - ▶ Who handles the calls when you are not around?
4. Try a first appointment, and notice how it goes.
5. Expect to be listened to.
6. Expect a thorough history.
7. Expect a thorough physical examination.

Alternative Therapies

Among people calling themselves "doctor" are many practitioners of **alternative therapies**. These people diagnose and treat illnesses in ways unrelated to standard medical procedures. A person seeking an alternative therapy for a headache, for example, might be advised to chew a few fresh leaves of the herb feverfew, or to receive a massage or acupuncture.

One of every three people are estimated to use an alternative therapy each year for everything from headaches to cancer. Alternative therapies cost consumers an estimated $13.7 billion of their health-care dollars every year.

The problem is that unproven alternative therapies can't be guaranteed. Nobody yet knows whether or not they work, or even if they are safe. By definition, an alternative therapy:

- ▶ Is not taught by most medical schools in the United States.
- ▶ Is not reimbursable by most health insurance providers in the United States.
- ▶ Is not well supported by scientific tests establishing safety and effectiveness.

Often, people who seek alternative therapies have come to distrust the medical system. It's easy to feel overwhelmed by impersonal tests and treatments based on technology. Many people want more personal contact, more control over both their own health and their own cures. When traditional medical therapies fail them, where else can they turn?

Some future day, some alternative therapies may well be proved useful in disease prevention and cure. Cancer radiation therapy, by example, was once considered unconventional, but now is often central to

enrichment

You might want to share with students some additional information about naturopathic medicine (see Figure 27–3 on page 744).

Naturopathic medicine has five basic principles:

1. *Utilize the healing power of nature.* Naturopathic physicians work to restore the inherent healing systems of the body and mind when they have broken down.
2. *First, do no harm.* Naturopathic physicians use noninvasive treatments, which decrease the risk of harmful side effects.

Genuine and Fake Credentials

Consumer SKILLS

Most degrees listed next to health-care providers' names are strong degrees that equip people to truly provide help to those who need it. However, **bogus** degrees complicate the picture. Not everyone who posts a doctor's diploma on the office wall has spent all those years studying and has passed all those examinations. Some organizations that call themselves colleges or universities simply sell official-looking diplomas for $50 or $75 by mail.

To find out whether a college or university is for real, a person must do some research at the library. The institution should have an address, some buildings, and a faculty consisting of people with valid degrees and credentials of their own. If you telephone and ask to speak to the dean of undergraduate studies, that person should exist. A post office box number without a street address is almost a guarantee that the degree-granting institution is a fraud. The university should also be **accredited** by a professional group (for example, the American Medical Association, for physicians).

Watch out, though. There are also bogus professional groups and bogus licenses to practice. The rule seems to be that for every true symbol of legal right to practice, there is a counterfeit that copies it.

A famous quack buster, Victor Herbert, M.D., took action to show how little knowledge some fake "institutions" require of the "graduate." He applied for diplomas from two official-sounding groups, and sent in the required fees on behalf of Charlie Herbert and Sassafras Herbert. Both are fully accredited now. (Charlie is a cat; Sassafras is a pet poodle.) If you can apply to an institution for a degree, a diploma, or a license to practice in the name of your pet cat or poodle—and get it—then you have uncovered a fraud.

Critical Thinking

1. *Why is it important for clients to be certain of their health-care providers' credentials?*
2. *If a person with a bogus degree applied for membership in a real professional group, what do you think would happen? Why?*
3. *If you were suspicious of someone's credentials, how would you check on them?*

---

the treatment of many cancers. Until they are proved, though, it's best to view these therapies and the people practicing them through a pair of "skeptical spectacles." All sorts of unscrupulous people posing as experts try to separate people from their money with claims of life-extending cure-alls. The Straight Talk section can help you sharpen your skills for detecting such quackery.

Meanwhile, keep an open mind as you read about the alternative therapies listed in Figure 27–3 on the next page. However, keep your skeptical spectacles on, too. When profits soar into the billions in any health field, quacks are never far behind.

For those who await more information on alternative therapies, there may soon be some news. The National Institutes of Health (NIH) has created

MINI Glossary

physical examination: an examination of the body to gather information about its general condition or to make a diagnosis. It normally includes observations by looking, listening, or feeling body parts and by medical test results.

---

3. *Find the cause.* The physician will find and remove the underlying cause of a disease. Causes may include diet, lifestyle, or harmful habits.
4. *Treat the whole person.* Naturopathic physicians take into account emotional, physical, dietary, genetic, environmental,

and lifestyle factors.

5. *Preventative medicine.* Patients are taught how to live a healthy life, which can help prevent major illnesses.

Consumer SKILLS

Answers to Critical Thinking

1. to make sure that the health-care provider is not a fraud
2. Answers will vary.
3. Do some library research on the institution that gave the credentials.

GROUP ACTIVITY

Have each student interview and/or shadow a health-care worker (with permission) and write a report on his/her findings. As a class, prepare the questions to use during the interview.

ROLE PLAY

Divide students into pairs to role play visiting a health-care provider. Have them brainstorm questions to ask during their appointments. Think of questions for different types of problems. Use different health situations, such as headaches, shortness of breath, blurry vision, ringing in the ears, routine or sports physical.

LEARNING WITH VISUALS

Have each student write an advertisement for a fictional health product. Students should also design a logo, label, and packaging for their products. Have students share their products with the class in the form of an advertising pitch for prospective buyers.

GROUP ACTIVITY

Have half of the class make collages of legitimate, useful health products found in magazine and newspaper advertisements. Have the other students make collages of questionable products, such as weight-loss products/gadgets, hair growth tonics, exercise gimmicks, and muscle developers. Discuss and compare the collages.

GROUP ACTIVITY

Have students visit a drugstore to compare costs and ingredients of name brand versus generic or store-brand health products. Have students share their findings in class.

ASSESS

EVALUATE

Have students role play an interview with a doctor or other health-care provider using the guidelines in the Health Strategies feature for choosing a health-care provider.

A reproducible quiz for Section 3 is provided in the Teacher's Resource Box.

FAST FACTS

In the United States there are about 20 practicing physicians per every 10,000 people. The ratio is slightly higher than in England, Canada, and Australia but considerably lower than in Italy, Germany, France, and Scandinavia.

Answers to FACT or FICTION

Here are the answers to the questions at the start of the chapter.

1. **False.** HMO stands for *health maintenance organization*. People should not perform surgery on themselves.
2. **False.** You may need as many as five different kinds of insurance. Even then, specific medical needs might not be covered.
3. **True.**
4. **False.** The high cost of health care in the United States is the worst problem.
5. **True.**

Figure 27–3 *Alternative Therapy Terms*

*acupuncture (Ak-you-PUNK-cher): a method of piercing of the skin with long, thin needles at points believed to relieve pain or illnesses.

aroma therapy: a technique that uses oil extracts from plants and flowers (usually applied by massage or baths) to enhance physical, psychological, and spiritual health.

*ayurveda (EYE-your-VAY-dah): a traditional Hindu system of herbs, diet, meditation, massage, and yoga believed to improve the body's disease-fighting capacity.

*bioelectromagnetic medicine: the use of electrical or magnetic energy to stimulate bone repair, wound healing, and tissue regeneration.

*biofeedback: the use of machines that detect and convey information about heart rate, blood pressure, brain or nerve activity, and muscle tension, to enable a person to learn how it feels to relax, and so slow the pulse and lower blood pressure.

herbal medicine: the use of plants to treat disease or improve health.

homeopathic (home-ee-OP-ah-thick) **medicine:** practices based on the theory that "like cures like"—that is, that substances that cause symptoms in healthy people can cure those symptoms when given in very dilute amounts (homeo = like; pathos = suffering).

*hypnotherapy: the use of hypnosis and the power of suggestion to change behaviors, relieve pain, and heal.

massage therapy: a method of kneading of muscles to reduce tension, help blood circulate, and improve joint mobility; believed to promote healing.

naturopathic medicine: a mixture of traditional and alternative therapies.

*These therapies are currently under study by the National Institutes of Health (NIH). The NIH endorses the use of acupuncture as effective against nausea following surgery and chemotherapy and during pregnancy and following dental surgery.

---

the Office of Alternative Medicine. Its task is "to more adequately explore unconventional medical practices." The therapies under study by the NIH are marked with an asterisk (*) in Figure 27–3.

KEY POINTS *Billions of consumer health dollars are spent seeking health from alternative medical therapies. The use of these therapies is not yet supported by science, the therapies are not taught in most medical schools, and the costs of using them are not covered by insurance. Seekers of alternative medicine must watch out for unscrupulous people practicing quackery.*

 QUICK QUIZ

Chapter 27, Section 3

The following quiz will help you assess your students' understanding of the material covered in this section of the chapter. You might use the quiz as an oral exercise, which will lead into a class discussion of the topics covered. Or, you might use it as a paper/pencil quiz to evaluate your students individually.

1. An M.D. must attend college and medical school, perform an internship and a residency, and pass a state examination before receiving her/his license. (True)
2. Nurse practitioners and physician's assistants are not licensed to provide care independently. (False)
3. Gynecologists and pediatricians are M.D.s who have received additional specialized training. (True)
4. You must have a medical degree in order

Researchers are trying to determine the effectiveness of some alternative therapies.

1. A gynecologist is a specialist of the female reproductive system, while the pediatrician specializes in the care of infants and children. (pp. 740–741)
2. That institution is approved by a professional group qualified to judge the programs offered. (p. 743)
3. written evidence of education or other qualifications of an authority (pp. 741, 743)
4. a mixture of traditional and alternative therapies (p. 744)
5. A general practitioner has ten years. A specialist has more. (p. 740)
6. They can relieve pain, but not diagnose illnesses or prescribe treatments. (p. 741)
7. Refer to the Health Strategies on page 742 for possible answers.
8. Answers will vary. (p. 743)

SECTION 3 Review

Answer the following questions on a sheet of paper.

Learning the Vocabulary

The vocabulary terms for this section are *internship, residency, specialist, gynecologist, pediatrician, credentials, history (medical), bogus, accredited, physical examination, alternative therapies, acupuncture, aroma therapy, ayurveda, bioelectromagnetic medicine, biofeedback, herbal medicine, homeopathic medicine, hypnotherapy, massage therapy,* and *naturopathic medicine.*

1. What is the difference between a gynecologist and a pediatrician?
2. What does it mean when an institution is accredited?

3. What are credentials?
4. What is naturopathic medicine?

Learning the Facts

5. Counting the years of college, internship, and residency, how long does a doctor stay in school altogether?
6. What services can chiropractors offer?
7. List six questions you should ask a physician before your visit.

Making Life Choices

8. After rereading the Consumer Skills feature in this section, "Genuine and Fake Credentials," how would you feel about being treated by a fraud? What can you do to help control this problem? What could your school do to help in this area? How about your community?

MINI Glossary

alternative therapies: approaches to medical diagnosis and treatment that are not fully accepted by the established medical community. As such, they are not widely taught at U. S. medical schools or practiced in U. S. hospitals. Also called *adjunctive, unconventional,* or *unorthodox therapies.*

bogus: fake. There are bogus doctors, bogus professional groups, bogus licenses to practice, bogus certifications, and bogus registrations.

accredited: approved; in the case of a college or university, approved by a professional group qualified to judge the program offered.

CLOSE

Remind students that there are many kinds of health-care providers, and that it is their responsibility as consumers to evaluate and select the ones who are qualified to meet their health needs. There are many ways to be a good health consumer. Ask students to summarize ideas for being smart consumers of health care.

FAST FACTS

The United States has more than its share of specialists. In developed countries other than the United States, generalists make up 50 percent to 75 percent of the medical professionals. In the United States only 30 percent of physicians are generalists.

to call yourself a doctor. (False)
5. A doctor should take your history as well as perform a thorough physical examination during your first appointment. (True)
6. Alternative therapies, such as massage and acupuncture, are unrelated to standard medical procedures. (True)
7. Alternative therapies are usually reimbursable by health insurance providers. (False)
8. Alternative therapy is well supported by

scientific evidence. (False)
9. It is necessary to exercise extreme caution when investing in an alternative therapy. (True)
10. The National Institute of Health (NIH) has recently created a division which explores unconventional medical practices. (True)

Straight
Talk

Discussion

Ask students if they regularly read articles in newspapers and in magazines about health topics. Why or why not? Have they become more interested as they've taken this course? Do they tend to believe what they read?

Discussion

Students will probably ask whether or not the newspapers and magazines they read are trustworthy sources of health information. Tell them that even the most well-known national publications should not be trusted blindly. They are in the business of selling a product and the newest, latest findings, whether tested or not, help sell newspapers and magazines. Point out that in most cases these publications are not printing fictitious information—their reports are true; it's just that there may be conflicting reports or the reports may not yet be substantiated by the scientific community.

Discussion

After discussing various health resources in the community, create possible health situations or scenarios that require use of some of the resources. Have students make charts, graphs, or lists to indicate which ones they would use. Compare choices. Have students explain or defend their choices.

Health Claims and Quackery

All through this course you have been asked to take responsibility for your own habits and choices. Once you leave the classroom, you will still be put to the test in the larger world. Unfortunately, not everyone who claims to have your health in mind has pure motivations. How can you know what to believe and to apply to your life, and what to discount?

 I like trying new health-care products, and I think people should give new methods a chance. But how can I know whom to trust?

You are wise to question sources of new products and schemes. Not all sources are equally valid, although all may claim that their statements are facts. Take, for example, advertisements in which actors, dressed as scientists or physicians, appear on television or in magazines making solemn statements about "research." When you look closely, you often find little or no evidence to back up their claims. To find the truth, you need skill in sifting the valid health information from the rubbish.

 How can I tell the difference between valid and invalid claims?

Ideally, when you first saw the claim for a product or service, you would have time to research it

thoroughly. You would find out the credentials of the person making the claim, check out the evidence on which the claim was made, ask where the evidence was published, and analyze the style in which it was stated. Remember, just being famous does not qualify a person to make a health claim. A poet's words on physical fitness may sound beautiful, but the words of a trainer of Olympic athletes are probably more accurate. A famed heart surgeon knows hearts, but a family therapist is qualified to speak on love. When someone speaks on health, size up that person's training, education, skill, credentials, and reputation in the field.

 That sounds complicated. How can I know how to judge the person making claims?

It can be complicated and time-consuming to check someone out completely. For most purposes, though, you can answer this most critical question: If the person or organization making the claim stands to profit by selling you something you would not otherwise buy, the claim is probably false. It can be as simple as that. Remember, though, that if you take shortcuts in checking credentials, you do so at your own risk. Study Figure 27–4 for some tips on how to detect health quackery. If you detect any of the red flags listed there, your best move is to hold tightly onto your wallet as you walk away.

746

enrichment...

Have each student find an article about a health-care product or health-care issue and read it at home with a parent. Have the student ask the parent for an opinion of the

information. During class ask all students to report their findings. How did parents evaluate the articles? Students should make a list of questions their parents used to evaluate the articles. Have students compare the compiled list of questions and strategies to those listed here. Now can students, as a class, develop a

Figure 27–4 Red Flags of Health Quackery

Too good to be true
Presents simple answers to complex problems; says what people want to hear.

Suspicions about food supply or medical drugs
Urges distrust of current medical methods or suspicion about food. Sells "alternatives" profiting the seller.

Testimonials
Includes histories of people claiming to have been "healed" or "made younger" by the product or treatment.

Fake credentials
Uses titles such as "doctor" or "university," but has simply created or bought the titles.

Unpublished studies
Cites studies that are not published and so cannot be evaluated.

STEP RIGHT UP! **VITE-O-MITE** WILL MAKE YOU AS **HEALTHY AS A HORSE**—GUARANTEED! FEEL **STRONGER**, **LOSE** WEIGHT, **IMPROVE** YOUR MEMORY ALL WITH THE HELP OF **VITE-O-MITE**! OH SURE, YOU MAY HAVE HEARD THAT **VITE-O-MITE** IS NOT ALL THAT WE SAY IT IS, BUT THAT'S WHAT THE FDA WANTS YOU TO THINK! **OUR DOCTORS** AND SCIENTISTS SAY IT'S THE ULTIMATE VITAMIN SUPPLEMENT. SAY NO! TO THE WEAKENED VITAMINS IN TODAY'S FOODS. **VITE-O-MITE** INCLUDES **POTENT SECRET INGREDIENTS** THAT YOU CANNOT GET WITH ANY OTHER PRODUCT! YESSIREE FOLKS. STEP RIGHT UP!

BEFORE / AFTER

DOCTOR OF SCIENCE

STUDY

VITE⊙MITE

Persecution claims:
Claims that the medical community "is after" them. Tries to convince you that physicians "want to keep you ill" so you'll keep paying for office visits.

Authority not cited
Asks you to trust that what is being said is true.

Motive: personal gain
Makes a profit from your believing the claim.

Advertisement
Has claims that look scientific but that are made by a paid advertiser. Look for the words *advertisement*, probably in tiny print, on the page.

Unreliable publication
Cites studies that are published, but in newsletters or magazines that publish misinformation.

Logic without proof
Makes a reasonable case for the claim, but offers no science to back it up.

747

more comprehensive list of evaluation questions?

1. Who is making the claim?
2. What are the person's qualifications for making such statements?
3. On what evidence is the claim based?
4. Where is that evidence published?
5. In what language style is it stated?

Have students share this list (or their more comprehensive list) with their parents.

VOCABULARY

1. **a.** bogus **b.** herbal medicine **c.** medical insurance **d.** Medicaid **e.** health-care system **f.** disability insurance **g.** internship **h.** pediatrician **i.** gynecologist
2. **a.** residency **b.** health maintenance organization **c.** specialist **d.** malpractice insurance

RECALL

SECTION 1

1. prevent illness, gives routine exams (p. 732)
2. The unprepared approach is most risky because you have no insurance, no health-care provider, and no health-care plan. (p. 732)

SECTION 2

3. people on welfare (p. 734)
4. the client (p. 734)
5. abuse of malpractice insurance as greedy people unjustly sue physicians to win huge rewards (p. 735)
6. Call your regular health-care provider—this allows

CHAPTER 27 Review

Summarizing the Chapter

Your ability to respond correctly to the following statements ensures your understanding of the main concepts in the chapter.

1. Discuss the benefits of managed care plans such as health maintenance organizations (HMOs).
2. Describe three broad areas of health insurance.
3. Identify ways to select a medical care facility.
4. Identify reasons why health-care insurance costs are on the rise.
5. Discuss the problems and advantages associated with our health-care system.
6. Describe the services of health-care providers.
7. Discuss how to choose a health-care provider.
8. Define alternative therapy.

Learning the Vocabulary

health-care system	specialist
premiums	gynecologist
managed care	pediatrician
health maintenance organization (HMO)	credentials
	history (medical)
prepayment plan	physical examination
fee-for-service system	alternative therapies
hospitalization insurance	acupuncture
surgical insurance	aroma therapy
medical insurance	ayurveda
major medical insurance	bioelectromagnetic
disability insurance	medicine
Medicare	biofeedback
Medicaid	herbal medicine
malpractice insurance	homeopathic medicine
second opinion	hypnotherapy
tonsillectomy	massage therapy
hysterectomy	naturopathic medicine
internship	bogus
residency	accredited

Answer the following questions on a separate sheet of paper.

1. **Matching**—*Match each of the following phrases with the appropriate term:*
   a. fake
   b. the use of plants to treat disease or improve health
   c. insurance to pay physicians' fees, lab fees, and fees for prescription medications
   d. hospitalization and surgical insurance available for people who qualify as needy
   e. the total of all health-care providers and medical treatment facilities that work together to provide medical care to the population
   f. insurance to replace lost income if a person should be unable to work due to a long illness
   g. a length of time spent in training in a medical facility as part of the curriculum of a health care provider
   h. a medical specialist concerned with the care of infants and children
   i. a medical specialist in the care of the female reproductive system
2. **a.** A _____ is a length of time spent in a medical facility as part of the M.D.'s training after an internship.
   b. The _____ is a system of paying for health care in which the clients pay a fixed fee every month regardless of how many services they receive.
   c. A physician with training in a specialty area beyond the medical degree requirements is called a _____.
   d. _____ protects providers of health care against lawsuits by people claiming to have been harmed by their treatments.

Recalling Important Facts and Ideas

Section 1

1. Describe what a health-care provider does beyond treatment.
2. Which of the three approaches to health care is the most risky and why?

Section 2

3. What people can receive Medicaid insurance?
4. Who must pay costs not covered by insurance?
5. What drives our insurance premiums up higher than they should be?

748

6. List five hints for emergency room visits.
7. What should you do before an operation, especially a tonsillectomy or hysterectomy, and why?
8. If you have questions about your hospital bill, what should you do?

Section 3

9. How much would it cost to purchase an official-looking physician's diploma?
10. What is the first step in selecting a health-care provider?
11. Describe what tests you should expect during a physical examination.
12. Why is it important to give the physician your medical history?

Critical Thinking

1. Marie has been looking for medical insurance. She has discovered that most insurance companies require that you have a physical examination before they sell you a policy. She is a smoker, uses alcohol, and is obese. She cannot find an insurance company that will cover her. Most premiums are too expensive for her. What can Marie do? Why is it necessary for her to have insurance? What will happen to her family if she gets sick without insurance? What can her family do? What would you do? Why would you take that action if you were in this situation?

Activities

1. Divide into groups and interview local insurance agents. Compare prices and coverage from two companies on:
   a. Medical insurance
   b. Hospitalization insurance
   c. Surgical insurance
   d. Major medical insurance
   e. Disability insurance
   Report your findings to the other groups.
2. Make a video about the different kinds of disability insurance policies available and the benefits of long-term coverage as opposed to term coverage. How do insurance companies encourage you to purchase a policy? What are some of the advertising quirks they use? Put these in your video.
3. Have a class debate on the health- and medical-care system of the United States vs. Canada's health-care system. What are some

positive and negative aspects of each? Combine the good qualities of both and make up your own health-care system.
4. Look in several magazines for articles on quackery. Cut them out and make a collage on quackery for your class. What do these articles have in common?
5. Write or call the American College of Physicians and the American College of Surgeons. Have them send you a list of all the physicians in your area who are members of their associations. Report your findings in your school newspaper.
6. Do research to find out about the following types of health-care facilities and the services they provide:

   ▶ Birthing center
   ▶ Convalescent home
   ▶ Extended care center
   ▶ Health center
   ▶ Nursing home
   ▶ Teaching hospital
   ▶ Trauma center
   ▶ Walk-in emergency center

7. Choose a health-care career and talk with someone in that career. Find out information about training or schooling, job outlook, employment practices, working conditions, earnings, advantages, and disadvantages. Share the information you gather with the rest of your class.

Making Decisions about Health

1. You have had a medical emergency and had to spend a few days in the hospital. On admitting you, the desk clerk asks for your insurance and you present your card. Now you are checking out, and you have to stop by the cashier's office. The cashier tells you that your insurance does not cover the expenses you have just incurred. You are expected to pay $1,000 in fees within the next 90 days. Describe how you would handle this situation based on this chapter.

that person's office to know who you are, what the problem is, and where you are.

Have only one person go with you. Take some identification and your insurance card. Tell the person at the admissions desk if you have been there before—this will cut down on paperwork.

Know your own medical history and what medicines you are taking. (p. 736)
7. Get a second opinion, because these surgeries are often overperformed. (p. 737)
8. Ask for an itemized list of services you received and send it to your insurance company. (p. 737)

SECTION 3

9. $50–$75 (p. 743)
10. ask the local American Medical Association or people you trust for recommendations (p. 742)
11. blood and urine analysis, chest X-ray (p. 742)
12. The medical history provides about 70 percent of the information needed for an accurate diagnosis. (p. 741)

Appendix A: Careers in Health

Do you think you might be interested in a health-related career? If so, you can use this appendix to discover some possible careers and to find out what schooling is necessary to prepare for them and other factors to consider.

Job Title/Earning Potential	Description of Responsibilities	Education, Training, and Professional Qualifications	Other Considerations
Anesthesiologist (see Physician) $180,000–$200,000	Administers anesthetic drugs to patients to prevent pain during surgical and other medical procedures. Examines patients to determine the degree of surgical risk. Keeps records before, during, and after anesthesia.	All states require licensure. Successful completion of 4 years of medical school and a residency are required before completion of specialty degree. Physicians seeking board certification from the American Board of Medical Specialists may spend up to 7 years acquiring certification after passing a final examination.	Requires ability to deal with people and to make judgments and decisions in emergencies. Requires reaching, seeing clearly up close, and seeing colors. Irregular work hours.
Athletic trainer $24,000 for schools, $55,000 for professional teams	Advises and treats athletes to maintain their physical fitness. Prescribes diets and exercises to strengthen muscles. Organizes and supervises physical examinations. Recommends massages to relieve strain and soreness. Gives first aid to injured players. Treats chronic or minor injuries. Inspects and selects equipment. Keeps medical records and files insurance reports.	1 to 2 years of community college, vocational/technical school, or apprenticeship. National Athletic Trainers Association certifies trainers after they have earned a college degree; completed a basic educational program with 800 hours of clinical experience; and passed a 3-part exam, including a written and oral test. Some states require certification and licensure.	Requires ability to take responsibility; deal with people; work under stress; make judgments and decisions; teach through explaining and demonstrating; and lift, walk, run, and stand for long periods of time. Irregular work hours, weekend work, overnight travel, and working outside often required.
Audiologist $30,000–$50,000	Diagnoses and treats patients with hearing disorders and develops treatment programs. Tests noise levels in work places and conducts hearing protection programs. Keeps records on the evaluation and progress of patients.	College with master's degree; by the year 2005, a doctoral degree may be required. State licensure.	Requires ability to take responsibility, deal with people, and make judgments and decisions. Requires use of hands and fingers, seeing up close. Regular work hours, limited travel.

Job Title/Earning Potential	Description of Responsibilities	Education, Training, and Professional Qualifications	Other Considerations
Chiropractor $40,000–$60,000	Diagnoses and treats muscular, nervous, and skeletal problems. Takes medical history; conducts physical, neurological, and orthopedic examinations; and may order laboratory tests. Manually adjusts the spinal column. May *not* diagnose or treat diseases, including cancer. Does not prescribe drugs or perform surgery.	Most states require 2 years of undergraduate, 4 years of chiropractic college. Must pass state board examination for licensure by Department of Business and Professional Regulation. Specialties: naturopathic doctor.	Requires ability to deal with people and to make judgments and decisions. Requires lifting, pushing, stooping, and standing for long periods of time, and seeing clearly up close. Irregular work hours, weekend work.
Counselor, mental health $35,000–$50,000	Emphasizes prevention and works with individuals and groups to deal with problems concerning addiction, substance abuse, parenting, marital problems, suicide, and stress management.	Most states require that counselors in private practice have state licensure. For voluntary certification by the National Academy of Certified Clinical Mental Health Counselors, candidates must have a master's degree in counseling, 2 years of post-master's degree experience, supervised clinical experience, and a passing grade on a written examination.	Requires ability to deal with people, make judgment and decisions, and work under stress. Irregular work hours, weekend work.
Dental assistant $10,000–$20,000	Works with dentist, prepares patient for treatment by dentist, takes dental histories, and assists dentist with instruments and materials during examination and treatment. Sterilizes and disinfects instruments, prepares trays for dental work, and prepares material for making impressions. May schedule appointments and order dental supplies.	1 to 2 years of community college or vocational/technical school. Entry-level position with learning on the job.	Requires ability to adapt to changing duties, deal with people, and meet strict standards. Requires standing for long periods of time, reaching, using hands and fingers, and seeing clearly up close. Regular work hours, limited travel.

Job Title/Earning Potential	Description of Responsibilities	Education, Training, and Professional Qualifications	Other Considerations
Dental/hygienist $25,000–$50,000	Works with dentist. Examines patients' teeth and gums, records presence of disease, cleans teeth, and gives fluoride treatments. Places temporary fillings; removes stitches; and exposes and develops X rays. Makes impressions of teeth and may administer local anesthetics.	1 to 2 years of college or vocational/technical school and graduation from an accredited dental hygiene school. Associate degree program is sufficient for working in a private dental office. Bachelor's or master's degree required for research, teaching, or clinical practice.	Requires ability to deal with people; make judgments and decisions; and meet strict standards with precision tools. Requires standing for long periods, reaching, using hands and fingers, talking, seeing clearly up close, and judging depth and distance. Regular work hours, limited travel.
Dentist (D.D.S. or D.M.D.) $60,000–$80,000	Diagnoses, prevents, and treats problems of the teeth and tissues of the mouth. Removes decay and fills cavities, examines X rays, straightens teeth, and repairs broken teeth. Performs corrective surgery of the gums and supporting bones to treat gum diseases. Extracts teeth and makes molds and measurements for dentures. Provides instruction in brushing, flossing, and the use of fluoride. Administers anesthetics and writes prescriptions for antibiotics and other medications.	4 years of dental school accredited by the American Dental Association's Commission on Dental Accreditation; pass a written and practical examination. All states require licensure. Dentists who want to teach or do research spend an additional 2 to 5 years in advanced dental training.	Requires ability to deal with people; work under stress; make judgments and decisions; and meet strict standards. Must be able to use hands and fingers, and see clearly up close. Regular work hours, limited travel.
Dietetic technician, registered $25,000–$30,000	Provides services related to health and nutrition under the supervision of a registered dietitian. May screen patients to identify nutritional problems, provide patient education, or develop menus and recipes. May keep computerized records of patient nutrition information.	2-year associate degree from an American Dietetics Association–approved program that combines classroom and supervised experience. Licensure requires registration by the American Dietetic Association after completion of education and internship and passing the national registration examination.	Requires ability to deal with people, make judgments and decisions, and meet strict standards. Requires standing, walking, and using hands and fingers. May require computer skills. May include rotating shift work, weekend work.

Job Title/Earning Potential	Description of Responsibilities	Education, Training, and Professional Qualifications	Other Considerations
Dietitian, registered $25,000–$45,000	Plans nutrition programs in public health, sports-related, or clinical settings. May provide nutrition advice to families. A community nutritionist may work in state or federal agencies to promote health through nutrition and to treat nutrition-related disease. A clinical dietitian helps prevent and treat illnesses by promoting healthy eating and providing medical nutrition therapy; evaluates clients' diets; and makes modifications to diets. Other dietitians supervise preparation of meals in hospitals, nursing homes, clinics, sports training centers, and schools; manage food purchases and budgets; and may teach, do research, or consult.	4-year college degree with a major in dietetics, food and nutrition, or food services systems management. Internship required. National registration by the American Dietetic Association after passing the national registration examination. Graduate degree for research, advanced clinical positions, or public health. State licensure by the Department of Business and Professional Regulation in some states.	Requires ability to adapt to many changing duties, take responsibility, deal with people, counsel and advise people, plan staff work tasks, and make judgments and decisions. Requires reaching and using hands and fingers. Rotating shift work, weekend work.
Emergency medical technician $25,000–$30,000	Responds to medical emergencies, drives specially equipped vehicles to the scene of emergencies, alerts police or fire department, gives first aid to sick or injured persons, and transports them to medical facilities. May treat bleeding, breathing problems, shock, or wounds; give care in childbirth, heart attack, poisoning, or burns. May give drugs or intravenous therapy, give oxygen, and use a defibrillator to give shocks to a stopped heart. Must follow strict guidelines for which procedures are performed. Maintains vehicles and medical and communication equipment.	High school diploma and less than 1 year of vocational or trade school. Formal basic training is 100 to 120 hours of classroom work plus 10 hours of internship in a hospital emergency room. Licensure regulated by the Department of Health and Rehabilitative Services. Related education programs: ambulance, paramedic. Specialties can include paramedic.	Requires ability to deal with people, work and drive under stress, make judgments and decisions, and meet strict standards. Requires lifting, carrying, stooping, kneeling, reaching, talking, hearing, using hands and fingers, seeing clearly up close and at a distance, safe driving, judging depth and distance, focusing eyes, and seeing color differences. Irregular work hours, weekend work. Work outside; high noise intensity; exposure to toxic or caustic chemicals and disease-causing organisms.

Job Title/Earning Potential	Description of Responsibilities	Education, Training, and Professional Qualifications	Other Considerations
Exercise and aerobics instructor $15,000–$30,000	Conducts fitness testing and recommends exercise programs. Teaches exercises for weight loss, aerobics to strengthen the heart, and resistance training for strength. Instructs participants on exercise equipment, such as weights, bicycles, and treadmills.	Employers may require certification by the American Council on Exercise or the American College of Sports Medicine, or other certifications. The Aerobics and Fitness Association of America or the YMCA offers certification.	Requires ability to adapt to many changing duties; take responsibility, deal with people, counsel and advise people, and make judgments and decisions. Requires varied physical abilities. Varied hours, weekend work.
Geneticist $30,000–$50,000	Studies inheritance and variation of characteristics in forms of life. Determines what causes specific inherited traits. Devises methods for altering or producing new traits. May perform genetic counseling.	Ph.D. degree required for college teaching, independent research, and advancement to administrative positions. A master's degree is required for applied research, management, inspection, sales, and service. A bachelor's degree is needed for nonresearch jobs.	Requires ability to adapt to many changing duties; take responsibility; make judgments and decisions; and meet strict standards. Requires reaching, using hands and fingers, and seeing clearly up close. Regular work hours, limited travel.
Geriatric aide $15,000–$25,000	Helps care for physically ill, injured, disabled, or infirm elderly persons who are confined to nursing or residential care facilities. Works under the supervision of registered nurses or physicians. Answers residents' call bells; delivers messages; serves meals; makes beds; and takes and records temperature, pulse, respiration, and blood pressure. Assists patients with bathing, dressing, feeding, and walking.	No special licensing or certification is required. Nursing homes may require inexperienced workers to complete 75 hours of training and pass a written examination within 4 months of employment.	Requires ability to work with elderly people and adapt to many changing duties. Requires standing, pulling, and lifting. Weekend work and rotating shift work.
Health services administrator $45,000–$120,000	Plans, organizes, coordinates, and supervises the delivery of health care in nursing homes, hospitals, and outpatient care facilities. Requires supervising employees and directing and advising supervisors. May be employed by home health agencies, insurance agencies, consulting firms, or regulatory agencies.	Requires a graduate degree in health services administration, nursing administration, or business administration, and may require clinical experience. All states require administrators of long-term care facilities to be licensed. A license is not required in other areas of health services management.	Requires ability to adapt to many changing duties; deal with people; and make judgments and decisions. May require travel.

Job Title/Earning Potential	Description of Responsibilities	Education, Training, and Professional Qualifications	Other Considerations
Home health aide $10,000–$15,000	Helps elderly, disabled, and ill persons to live in their own homes. Provides housekeeping services, personal care, and emotional support. Plans meals (including special diets), shops for food, and cooks. May check pulse, temperature, and respiration; help with exercises; and assist with medication routines. May accompany clients outside the home. Keeps records of services performed and of clients' condition and progress.	Currently, less than 1 year of community college or vocational/trade school. A federal law suggests at least 75 hours of classroom and practical training supervised by a registered nurse. Federally approved training and testing programs may be offered by the employing agency. Training programs may vary, depending upon state regulations.	Requires ability to adapt to many changing duties; deal with people, and make judgments and decisions. Requires lifting, carrying, pushing, pulling, reaching, using hands, talking, hearing, and seeing clearly up close. Weekend work, overnight travel.
Massage therapist $10,000–$20,000	Massages customers to stimulate blood circulation and to relax tense muscles; gives other body-conditioning treatments. Applies alcohol, lotions, or other rubbing compounds.	1 to 2 years of community college or vocational/ trade school. Licensure regulated by the Department of Business and Professional Regulation.	Requires ability to deal with people and to make judgments and decisions. Requires lifting, pushing, pulling, standing for long periods of time, reaching, and using hands and fingertips. Irregular hours, weekend work.
Medical record technician $20,000–$40,000	Keeps medical records of patients in a hospital, clinic, or doctor's office. Fills out medical and insurance forms. Uses computer to analyze data to improve patient care and control costs.	Formal training in a 2-year associate degree program offered at a community college or vocational/technical school. Most employers prefer to hire accredited record technicians, who have passed a written examination from American Health Information Management Record Association.	Requires ability to adapt to many changing duties; make judgments and decisions; and meet strict standards. Requires reaching, using hands and fingers, talking, hearing, and seeing clearly up close. Regular work hours, limited travel.
Medical secretary $20,000–$28,000	May transcribe dictation, prepare correspondence, answer telephones, schedule appointments, and organize and maintain files. May operate office equipment, maintain financial records, and handle credits and collections. May record medical histories and schedule surgeries.	No special licensing or certification is required, although certification is available and recommended. Certification for a certified professional secretary requires passing a series of examinations from the Institute for Certifying Secretaries.	Requires ability to adapt to many changing duties, take responsibility, deal with people, and make judgments and decisions. Requires knowledge of basic office skills, including word processing, spreadsheet, and database management programs. Requires talking, hearing,

Job Title/Earning Potential	Description of Responsibilities	Education, Training, and Professional Qualifications	Other Considerations
Medical technologist $25,000–$40,000	Performs chemical, biological, and microscopic tests on blood, tissue, and other body substances. Determines the presence of microorganisms; determines blood glucose or cholesterol levels. Determines blood types from samples.	Bachelor's degree with a major in medical technology or life sciences. May qualify through on-the-job experience, specialized training, or a combination of these.	Requires reaching, using hands and fingers, talking, hearing, seeing clearly up close, and seeing color differences. Requires ability to meet strict standards. Rotating shift work, weekend work.
Nurse, registered $30,000–$50,000	Cares for the sick, helps people stay well. Provides for the physical, mental, and emotional needs of patients. Observes, assesses, and records symptoms, reactions, and progress. Assists physicians during treatments and examinations, administers medications, and assists in convalescence and rehabilitation. Develops and manages nursing care plans, instructs patients and their families in proper care, and helps individuals take steps to improve or maintain their health.	All states require licensure. Licensure requirements include graduation from an accredited nursing school and passing a national licensing examination. Three educational paths lead to nursing: (1) a 2-year associate degree (A.D.N.), offered by community and junior colleges; (2) a 4-to-5-year bachelor's degree (B.S.N.) offered by colleges and universities; and (3) a 2-to-3-year diploma program, given in a hospital. Clinical nurse specialist, nurse practitioner, certified nurse midwife, or nurse anesthetist require 1 or 2 years of graduate education, leading to a certificate or master's degree.	Requires ability to take responsibility, deal with people, make judgments and decisions, and meet strict standards. Requires standing for long periods of time, reaching, using hands and fingers, talking, hearing, seeing clearly up close, walking, and seeing color differences. Rotating shift work, weekend work.
Nurse practitioner $45,000–$60,000	Diagnoses and treats health problems and chronic diseases, such as diabetes and high blood pressure. Performs patient assessments, including medical and social history and physical examinations. Orders and interprets laboratory work, and prescribes medications. Provides health maintenance care. Often works in specialized areas, such as geriatrics, family care, or pediatrics.	Registered nurses with special advanced education and training requirements. State requirements vary; may require a master's degree.	Requires ability to take responsibility, deal with people, make judgments and decisions, and meet strict standards. Requires standing for long periods, reaching, using hands and fingers, talking, hearing, seeing clearly, walking, and seeing color differences. Rotating shift work, weekend work.

Job Title/Earning Potential	Description of Responsibilities	Education, Training, and Professional Qualifications	Other Considerations
Occupational therapist $30,000–$50,000	Helps mentally, physically, developmentally, or emotionally disabled people to develop, recover, or maintain daily work skills and independence. Plans and directs educational, vocational, and recreational activities. Tests the abilities of patients, sets goals for them, and plans therapy programs. Plans activities and games. Uses computer programs. May design special adaptive equipment, teach, or consult.	Bachelor's degree in occupational therapy. Most states require licensure. For licensure, must have degree or post-baccalaureate certificate from an accredited educational program and pass a national examination given by the American Occupational Therapy Certification Board.	Requires ability to adapt to many changing duties; take responsibility; deal with people; influence people; and make judgments and decisions. Requires lifting, reaching, using hands and fingers, talking, hearing, seeing clearly up close, judging depth and distance, and focusing eyes. Regular work hours, limited travel.
Osteopath (D.O.) $50,000–$120,000	Diagnoses and treats disorders of the human body, with special emphasis on bones, muscles, and nerves. Examines patients; takes medical histories; and advises on disease prevention through exercise, hygiene, diet, and preventive health care. May perform surgery and prescribe medicines.	All states require physicians to be licensed. Licensure requirements include graduation from an accredited osteopathic school. Requires 5 years of college; a 12-month rotating internship; and up to 7 years in residency training.	Requires ability to work with people, work under stress, and make judgments and decisions. Requires pushing, pulling, using hands and fingers, talking, hearing, seeing clearly up close, judging depth and distance, and seeing color differences. Irregular hours, weekend work.
Pharmacist $40,000–$65,000	Dispenses drugs and medicines prescribed by physicians and dentists. Advises physicians and health practitioners of the selection, dosages, interactions, and side effects of medications. Advises people on the use of medicines. Keeps computerized records of the drugs that patients use to prevent harmful drug interactions. May work in drugstores, buy and sell goods, and hire and supervise staff. May prepare medicines and test drugs for purity and strength. May teach, conduct research, consult, and write and edit technical articles.	All states require licensure to practice. To be licensed, pharmacists must graduate from an accredited pharmacy program. Bachelor's degree in pharmacy is required for community pharmacies. Many hospitals prefer a Pharm.D. degree. A master's or Ph.D. degree in pharmacy is required for research. A Pharm.D., master's, or Ph.D. is necessary for administrative or college faculty positions.	Requires ability to adapt to many changing duties, make judgments and decisions, and meet strict standards. Requires standing for long periods, reaching, using hands and fingers, talking, hearing, seeing clearly up close, focusing eyes, and seeing color differences. Irregular hours, weekend work, overtime work.

Job Title/Earning Potential	Description of Responsibilities	Education, Training, and Professional Qualifications	Other Considerations
Physical therapist $30,000–$55,000	Advises and treats medical patients to improve their mobility, relieve their pain, and prevent or limit permanent physical disabilities from injuries or diseases. Evaluates patients and their medical histories; tests and measures their strength, range of motion, and ability to function; develops written treatment plans. Teaches patients to use crutches, wheelchairs, and prostheses. Documents progress and conducts periodic evaluations.	All states require licensure. Licensure requirements include graduation from an accredited physical therapy program. A person with a 4-year degree in a related field, such as genetics or biology, can enroll in a master's degree physical therapy program. A master's degree is also necessary for an administrative position, research, or teaching.	Requires ability to take responsibility, influence people and make judgments and decisions. Requires lifting, carrying, pushing, reaching, using hands and fingers, talking, hearing, and seeing clearly up close. Irregular work hours, weekend work.
Physician $100,000–$250,000	Diagnoses illnesses. Prescribes and gives treatment for injuries and disease. Examines patients and takes medical histories. Orders, performs, and interprets diagnostic tests. Advises patients on how to prevent disease through exercise, hygiene, diet, and preventive health care. May be a member of a team that coordinates care for a group of patients. May specialize in a certain field of medicine. May refer patients to other medical specialists. Usually works in offices and in hospitals, but may work with patients in nursing homes and other facilities. May also do research or teach in medical schools. May write and edit medical books.	All states require licensure. Licensure requirements include graduation from an accredited medical school, passing an examination, and between 1 and 7 years of graduate medical education. Minimum requirement for acceptance to a medical school is 3 years of college; most applicants have a bachelor's degree. Following medical school (4 years), almost all M.D.s go directly on to graduate medical education, called a residency. A few medical schools offer a combined college and medical school program that lasts 6 years instead of the customary 8 years. To teach or do research, physicians may need a master's or doctoral degree in a field such as biochemistry or microbiology.	Requires ability to deal with people, make judgments, work under stress, and stay calm through emergencies. Must stay informed of changes in medical technology and advances in medical therapies. Requires using hands and fingers, talking, hearing, seeing clearly up close, and focusing eyes. Irregular hours, weekend work, overtime work.

Job Title/Earning Potential	Description of Responsibilities	Education, Training, and Professional Qualifications	Other Considerations
Physician's assistant $30,000–$65,000	Provides routine health care services under the supervision of a physician. Takes medical histories and examines patients. Orders and interprets laboratory tests and X rays. Makes preliminary diagnoses. Treats minor injuries. Instructs and counsels patients, and orders or carries out therapy. May prescribe medications. May supervise technicians and assistants. May order medical supplies.	Almost all states require licensure. Many programs require 2 years of college and some work experience in the health-care field. Most physician's assistant programs are located in medical schools, schools of allied health, or 4-year colleges of allied health, or 4-year colleges.	Requires ability to deal with people, make judgments and decisions and meet strict standards. Requires standing for long periods, reaching, using hands and fingers, talking, seeing, hearing, seeing clearly up close, and walking. Irregular hours, weekend work, rotating shift work.
Psychologist $25,000–$65,000	Provides mental health services in private settings, hospitals, clinics, and schools. Studies human behavior and mental processes related to that behavior. Applies knowledge and techniques to human services, management, education, law, and sports. Observes, interviews, and questions patients to help solve problems.	A doctoral degree is generally required for employment as a clinical or counseling psychologist or in research. A master's degree is generally accepted in business or for psychological assistants. May teach in 2-year colleges or work as school counselors.	Requires ability to adapt to many changing duties, deal with people, and make judgments and decisions. Requires talking, hearing, and seeing clearly up close. Irregular work hours, weekend work, overnight travel.
Social worker $25,000–$35,000	Helps individuals or families with problems such as homelessness, inadequate housing, disabilities, substance abuse, unemployment, unwanted pregnancy, or lack of job skills. Provides direct counseling or information to provide assistance. May research and analyze polices and programs, identify social problems, and suggest solutions. May help raise funds or write grants to support programs.	All states require licensing, certification, or registration. A master's degree in social work (5 years) is required in the mental health field and for administrative, supervisory, or research positions. A doctorate in social work is required for teaching and research positions.	Job settings vary greatly, depending on the type of employer. Requires ability to deal with people, make judgments and decisions, and work under stress. Irregular work hours, weekend work.

Job Title/Earning Potential	Description of Responsibilities	Education, Training, and Professional Qualifications	Other Considerations
Speech therapist $40,000–$50,000	Works as part of a team that evaluates and treats patients with hearing and speech problems. Talks with patients to discuss hearing and speaking problems, and their possible causes and treatments. Examines ears. Evaluates examination and test data to determine type and amount of hearing loss. Treats hearing problems using hearing aids and other treatments. Helps patients in selecting and using hearing aids. Conducts programs to help patients improve their speaking skills.	A master's degree in audiology or speech therapy is required.	Requires ability to take responsibility, deal with people, and make judgments and decisions. Requires crouching, crawling, sitting for long periods, reaching, and using hands and fingers. Regular work hours and limited travel.
Vocational rehabilitation counselor $25,000–$55,000	Helps clients identify appropriate job goals. Helps them get education, training, and equipment needed for employment. Evaluates strengths and limitations of individuals. Provides personal and job counseling. Arranges for medical care and social services. Consults with medical and other professional personnel. May specialize in a particular disability, for example, disability from birth defects.	Agencies require a master's degree in rehabilitation counseling, counseling and guidance, or counseling psychology for rehabilitation counselor jobs. May accept applicants with a bachelor's degree in rehabilitation services, counseling, psychology, or related fields.	Requires ability to adapt to many changing duties, take responsibility, deal with people, and make judgments and decisions. Requires talking, hearing, and seeing clearly up close. Regular work hours, limited travel.

Appendix B:
Nutrition Standards

The United States has developed several sets of standards that state how much of each nutrient best supports health. The set of standards presented in Figure B–1 is the Daily Values, the same set used on food labels. Another U.S. standard specifies how much energy an average healthy person needs to consume each day to maintain a healthy weight. These values, presented in Figure B–2, are the Recommended Energy Intakes for the United States. The standards in Figure B–3 represent the triceps fatfold measurements of teenagers in this country.

Figure B–1 *Daily Values*[a]

Food Component	Amount	Nutrient	Amount	Nutrient	Amount
Protein	50 g[b]	Thiamin	1.5 mg	Calcium	1,000 mg
Fat	65 g	Riboflavin	1.7 mg	Iron	18 mg
Saturated fatty acids	20 g	Niacin	20 mg	Zinc	15 mg
Cholesterol	300 mg[c]	Biotin	300 µg	Iodine	150 µg
Total carbohydrate	300 g	Pantothenic acid	10 mg	Copper	2 mg
Fiber	25 g	Vitamin B_6	2 mg	Chromium	120 µg
Sodium	2,400 mg	Folate	400 µg	Selenium	70 µg
Potassium	3,500 mg	Vitamin B_{12}	6 µg[d]	Molybdenum	75 µg
		Vitamin C	60 mg	Manganese	2 mg
		Vitamin A	5,000 IU[e]	Chloride	3,400 mg
		Vitamin D	400 IU[e]	Magnesium	400 mg
		Vitamin E	30 IU[e]	Phosphorus	1 g
		Vitamin K	80 µg		

[a]Based on 2,000 calories a day for adults and children over 4 years old.

[b]The Daily Values for protein vary for different groups of people: children 1 to 4 years, 16 g; infants under 1 year, 14 g; pregnant women, 60 g; nursing mothers, 65 g. g = grams.

[c]mg = milligrams.

[d]µg = micrograms.

[e]Equivalent values for the three nutrients expressed as international units (IU) are vitamin A, 875 RE; vitamin D, 10 µg; vitamin E, 9 mg.

Figure B–2 *Median Heights and Weights and Recommended Energy Intakes (United States)*

Age	Weight		Height		Average Energy Allowance			
(Years)	(Kg)	(Lb)	(Cm)	(Inches)	REE[a] (Cal/Day)	Multiples of REE[b]	Cal/Kg	Cal/Day[c]
Males								
11–14	45	99	157	62	1,440	1.70	55	2,500
15–18	66	145	176	69	1,760	1.67	45	3,000
19–24	72	160	177	70	1,780	1.67	40	2,900
25–50	79	174	176	70	1,800	1.60	37	2,900
51+	77	170	173	68	1,530	1.50	30	2,300
Females								
11–14	46	101	157	62	1,310	1.67	47	2,200
15–18	55	120	163	64	1,370	1.60	40	2,200
19–24	58	128	164	65	1,350	1.60	38	2,200
25–50	63	138	163	64	1,380	1.55	36	2,200
51+	65	143	160	63	1,280	1.50	30	1,900
Pregnant (2nd and 3rd trimesters)								+300
Lactating								+500

[a]REE (resting energy expenditure) represents the energy expended by a person at rest under normal conditions.
[b]Recommended energy allowances assume light to moderate activity and were calculated by multiplying the REE by an activity factor.
[c]Average energy allowances have been rounded.
Source: Adapted with permission from *Recommended Dietary Allowances*, 10th ed., © 1989 by the National Academy of Sciences. Published by the National Academy Press, Washington, D.C.

Figure B–3 *Triceps Fatfold Standards (Millimeters) for Teenage Males and Females (Percentiles)*

	Male					Female				
Age	5th	25th	50th	75th	95th	5th	25th	50th	75th	95th
12–12.9	6	8	11	14	28	8	11	14	18	27
13–13.9	5	7	10	14	26	8	12	15	21	30
14–14.9	4	7	9	14	24	9	13	16	21	28
15–15.9	4	6	8	11	24	8	12	17	21	32
16–16.9	4	6	8	12	22	10	15	18	22	31
17–17.9	5	6	8	12	19	10	13	19	24	37
18–18.9	4	6	9	13	24	10	15	18	22	30

Source: Adapted from A.R. Frisancho, New norms of upper limb fat and muscle areas for assessment of nutritional status, *American Journal of Clinical Nutrition* 34 (1981): 2540–2545. © American Society of Clinical Nutrition.

Figure B–3 presents standards for fatfold measurements taken at the back of the arm (over the triceps muscle). Triceps fatfold measurements should be taken on the person's right arm while the person is standing (see Figure 8–1 on page 204). Here's how to take the measurement:

1. Place your fingers on the back of the person's upper arm, midway between the shoulder and the elbow.
2. Grasp, between your thumb and your forefinger, a fold of skin and fat that lies just under the skin. To be sure that you are holding only skin and fat—no muscle—have the person contract and relax the triceps muscle.
3. Place the "pinchers" of the fatfold caliper just above where your finger and thumb are holding the fatfold (the pinchers don't hurt). Let the pressure of the caliper alone close the pinchers and establish the measurement. Read the measurement and remove the caliper. Repeat this entire procedure three times. Average the two closest measures to establish the final value.
4. Compare the final value with the percentile values listed for a person of the same age and gender in Figure B–3. A value that falls at the 75th percentile means that the person's fatfold is thicker than the triceps fatfolds of 75 percent of the rest of the population. A fatfold measure that falls at the 50th percentile is in the middle—half of the population have thicker fatfolds, and half have thinner fatfolds.

A fatfold value close to the middle of the range of percentiles is considered to reflect an appropriate amount of body fat. Values much above the 75th percentile or below the 25th percentile may also be appropriate. However, a person with an extra-high or extra-low value would probably be wise to consult a physician for further evaluation.

Appendix C:
The Law and Sexuality

An unfortunate reality in our society is the all-too-frequent occurrence of sexual crimes. It may help you to know about the types of sexual crimes that occur and the penalties that result.

Following are descriptions of five general categories of sexual crimes: rape, sexual abuse of children, prostitution, deviate sexual behavior, and harassment. These descriptions provide an overview of the laws as they exist currently in the United States as a whole. As with all laws, the laws related to sexuality may vary from state to state. For specific laws in your state, contact your state's attorney general's office.

Rape

Throughout history, rape has been defined as an illegal act in which a man forces a woman to have sexual intercourse against her will. In most states today the definition of rape has been broadened to include a wide range of sexual assaults, which apply to both men and women. Rape is a felony, which means it is a serious crime, punishable by at least one year in prison.

Sexual Abuse of Children

Many different sex crimes are committed against children. Statutory rape is a rape committed against a female who is not legally old enough to agree to have sexual intercourse. In this type of rape, consent is not an issue. If the female is underage, it is rape whether she consents or not. The legal age varies from state to state (for example: Connecticut, 16; Wisconsin, 17; Texas, 17) and even within the same state, depending on circumstances.

Other types of sexual crimes against children include abduction or enticement; child pornography, which is the exploitation of children in sexual ways for financial gain; and incest (sexual relations between people who are closely related), which is a crime usually committed against children. All forceful or violent sexual attacks against children are, of course, illegal.

Prostitution

Prostitution is the act of engaging in sexual relations in exchange for money or something of value. A person can also be convicted of prostitution if he or she offers to engage in a sexual act for money or requests money for performing a sexual act. Prostitution is illegal in all states except Nevada.

Deviate Sexual Behavior

Until 1961 all states outlawed sex between members of the same sex. Since that time, however, many states have made such acts legal for consenting adults, in private. (Both heterosexual and homosexual acts committed in public are crimes.) About half the states still have laws such as the Texas law that says, "A person commits an offense if he engages in deviate sexual behavior with another individual of the same sex."

Sexual Harassment

Sexual harassment cases have received increased attention in recent years and many cities and states have written laws to prohibit this type of conduct. Sexual harassment involves unwelcome sexual advances or requests for sexual favors. These advances and requests may be combined with undesirable verbal or physical conduct of a sexual nature.

Glossary

A

abortion: a procedure to end a pregnancy before the fetus can live outside the uterus.

abstinence: refraining completely from sexual relations with other people. Also called *celibacy* (SELL-ih-ba-see).

accredited: approved; in the case of a college or university, approved by a professional group qualified to judge the program offered.

acetaminophen (ah-SEET-ah-MIN-o-fen): a drug that relieves fever and pain.

acid rain: rain that carries acid air pollutants; it harms the plants and damages the soil on which it falls.

acne: a continuing condition of inflamed skin ducts and glands, with a buildup of oils under the skin, forming pimples.

acquired immune deficiency syndrome (AIDS): a fatal, transmissible viral disease of the immune system that creates a severe immune deficiency, and that leaves people defenseless against infections and cancer.

acromegaly (ack-ro-MEG-a-lee): a disease caused by above-normal levels of human growth hormone.

active abuse: abuse involving one person's aggression against another, such as hitting or sexually abusing the victim.

active ingredients: ingredients in a medicine that produce physical effects on the body.

active solar: using photovoltaic panels to generate electricity from sunlight. (A passive solar home is one that is built to take advantage of the available sun and shade so as to minimize heating and cooling costs.)

acupuncture (AK-you-PUNK-cher): a method of piercing of the skin with long, thin needles at points believed to relieve pain or illnesses.

acute stress: a temporary bout of stress that calls forth alertness or alarm to prompt the person to deal with an event.

adapt: to change or adjust in order to accommodate new conditions.

addiction: a physical or psychological craving for higher and higher doses of a drug that leads to bodily harm, social maladjustment, or economic hardship; dependence on a substance, habit, or behavior.

adolescence: the period of growth from the beginning of puberty to full maturity. Timing of adolescence varies from person to person.

aerobic (air-ROE-bic): refers to energy-producing processes that use oxygen (aero = air).

afterbirth: the placenta and membranes expelled after the birth of the child.

aggressive: possessing the characteristic of being insulting or overly demanding to others or otherwise invading their territory; an inappropriate expression of feelings.

AIDS dementia complex: the mental disorder resulting from an attack by HIV on the brain and nerves.

air bags: inflatable pillows, designed to inflate upon impact, stored in the center of the steering wheel of a car or in the dashboard.

air pollution: contamination of the air with gases or particles not normally found there.

alarm: the first phase of the stress response, in which the person faces a challenge and starts paying attention to it.

alcohol: a class of chemical compounds. The alcohol of alcoholic beverages, *ethanol* or *ethyl alcohol*, is one member of this class.

alcohol addict (alcoholic): a person who has the full blown disease of alcoholism. This person's problems, caused by alcohol abuse, are out of control.

alcoholism: the disease characterized by loss of control over drinking and dependence on alcohol, both of which harm health, family relations, and social and work functioning.

alienation: withdrawing from others because of differences that cannot be resolved.

aloe: a tropical plant with widely claimed, but mostly unproved, medical value.

alternative therapies: approaches to medical diagnosis and treatment that are not fully accepted by the established medical community. As such, they are not widely taught at U. S. medical schools or practiced in U. S. hospitals. Also called adjunctive, unconventional, or unorthodox therapies.

Alzheimer's disease: a brain disease of some older people that brings mental confusion; inability to function; and in the final stage, death.

amino acids: simple forms of protein normally used to build tissues or, under some conditions, burned for energy.

amnesia: loss of memory.

amniocentesis (am-nee-oh-cen-TEE-sis): a test of fetal cells drawn by needle through the woman's abdomen.

amniotic (am-nee-OTT-ic) **sac:** the "bag of waters" in the uterus, in which the fetus floats.

amotivational syndrome: loss of ambition and drive; a characteristic of long-term abusers of marijuana.

amphetamines (am-FETT-ah-meenz): powerful, addictive stimulant drugs. Because they suppress appetite, they are reserved for use in cases where overfatness threatens health. Also called *speed*.

anaerobic (AN-air-ROE-bic): refers to energy-producing processes that do not use oxygen (an = without).

anemia: reduced number or size of the red blood cells; a symptom of any of many different diseases, including some nutrient deficiencies.

anesthetics (an-us-THET-icks): drugs that kill pain, with or without producing loss of consciousness.

aneurysm (AN-your-ism): the ballooning out of an artery wall at a point where it has grown weak.

angina (an-JYE-nuh or ANN-juh-nuh): pain in the heart region caused by lack of oxygen.

anorexia (an-or-EX-ee-uh) **nervosa:** a disorder of self-starvation to the extreme.

antagonist (an-TAG-uh-nist): a drug that opposes the action of another drug.

antibiotics: drugs used to fight bacterial infection.

antibodies: large protein molecules produced to fight infective or foreign tissue.

antigens: foreign substances in the body, such as viruses or bacteria, that stimulate the immune system to produce antibodies.

antihistamines: drugs that counteract inflammation caused by histamine, one of the chemicals involved in allergic reactions.

antioxidant (AN-tee-OX-ih-dant): a chemical that can stop the destructive chain reactions of free radicals. Among the nutrients, vitamins C and E, beta-carotene, and the mineral selenium are examples.

antiseptics: agents that prevent the growth of microorganisms on body surfaces and on wounds.

anxiety attack: a sudden, unexpected episode of severe anxiety with symptoms such as rapid heartbeat, sweating, dizziness, and nausea.

anxiety: an emotional state of high energy, with the stress response as the body's reaction to it.

aorta (ay-OR-tah): the largest artery in the body; it conducts freshly oxygenated blood from the heart to the tissues.

aphrodisiac (af-roh-DEEZ-ee-ack): a substance reputed to excite sexual desire. Actually, no known substance does this, but many claim the products they sell do so.

appetite: the psychological desire to eat, a learned motivation and a positive sensation that accompanies the sight, smell, or thought of food.

aroma therapy: a technique that uses oil extracts from plants and flowers (usually applied by massage or baths) to enhance physical, psychological, and spiritual health.

arteries: blood vessels that carry blood from the heart to the tissues.

arthritis: a painful inflammation of the joints caused by infection, body chemistry, injury, or other causes; usually results in altered joint structure and loss of function.

artificial heart: a pump designed to fit into the human chest cavity and perform the heart's function of pumping blood around the body.

asexual: having no sexual inclinations.

aspirin: a drug that relieves fever, pain, and inflammation.

assertive: possessing the characteristic of appropriately expressing feelings, wants, and needs while respecting those of others. Assertiveness is the key to obtaining cooperation.

asthma: difficulty breathing, with wheezing sounds from the chest caused by air rushing through narrowed air passages.

atherosclerosis (ATH-uh-roh-scler-OH-sis): the most common form of cardiovascular disease; a disease characterized by plaques along the inner walls of the arteries.

athlete's foot: a fungal infection of the feet, usually transmitted through contact with floors.

atria (singular, **atrium**): the two upper chambers of the heart—the receiving areas that pool incoming blood.

attention-deficit/hyperactivity disorder (ADHD): an inability to pay attention, often with hyperactivity and poor impulse control. ADHD is most often diagnosed in children younger than age seven. It interferes with home life, schoolwork, or other functions.

ayurveda: (EYE-your-VAY-dah): a traditional Hindu system of herbs, diet, meditation, massage, and yoga believed to improve the body's disease-fighting capacity.

B

B cells: lymphocytes that make antibodies.

bacteria (singular, **bacterium**): microscopic, single-celled organisms of varying shapes and sizes, some capable of causing disease.

balanced meal: a meal with foods to provide the right amounts of carbohydrate, fat, and protein.

barbiturates: depressant drugs that slow the activity of the central nervous system.

barrier methods: contraceptive methods that physically or chemically obstruct the travel of sperm toward the ovum. These devices do not alter body processes with drugs or devices.

basal energy: the sum total of all the energy needed to support the chemical activities of the cells and to sustain life, exclusive of voluntary activities; the largest component of a person's daily energy expenditure.

behavior modification: changing one's choices or actions by manipulating the cues that trigger the actions, the actions themselves, or the consequences of the actions.

belladonna: any part of the deadly nightshade plant; a deadly poison.

benign (be-NINE): noncancerous; not harmful; a description of a tumor that is not able to spread from one area to another.

beta-carotene (bay-tah CARE-oh-teen): an orange vegetable pigment that the body can change into the active form of vitamin A; one of the antioxidant nutrients.

binge drinker: a person who drinks four or more drinks in a short period.

binge eating: overeating to an extreme degree.

binge eating disorder (BED): repeated binge eating, but not followed by vomiting.

biodegradable: able to decompose; able to be converted by living organisms into harmless waste products that can be used over again to build or grow new things.

bioelectromagnetic medicine: the use of electrical or magnetic energy to stimulate bone repair, wound healing, and tissue regeneration.

biofeedback: the use of machines that detect and convey information about heart rate, blood pressure, brain or nerve activity, and muscle tension, to enable a person to learn how it feels to relax, and so slow the pulse and lower blood pressure; a clinical technique used to help a person learn to relax by monitoring muscle tension, heart rate, brainwave activity, or other body activities.

birth defects: physical abnormalities present from birth.

birth order: the placement of a child among his or her siblings, such as oldest, middle, or youngest child.

bisexual: being sexually oriented to members of both sexes.

blackhead: an open pimple with dark skin pigments (not dirt) in its opening.

blackouts: episodes of amnesia regarding periods of time while drinking. The person may act normal during a blackout, but later be unable to recall anything about it. Blackouts are likely to occur in the life of a person with alcoholism.

blended family: a family created by remarriage after the death or divorce of a spouse; blended families include a biological or adoptive parent and step-parent, along with the children of one or both of them.

blood: the thick, red fluid that flows through the body's blood vessels and transports gases, nutrients, wastes, and other important substances around the body. Blood also plays roles in body temperature regulation.

body composition: a component of fitness; the proportions of lean tissue as compared with fat tissue in the body.

body image: the way a person thinks his or her body looks, which may or may not be the way it actually does look.

body systems: groups of related organs that work together to perform major body functions.

bogus: fake. There are bogus doctors, bogus professional groups, bogus licenses to practice, bogus certifications, and bogus registrations.

botulin toxin: a potent poison produced by bacteria in sealed cans, plastic packs, or jars of food.

botulism: the often fatal condition of poisoning with the botulin toxin.

brain death: irreversible, total loss of higher brain functions, reflected in a flat line brainwave pattern, as opposed to the wavy pattern made by an active brain.

brand names: the names companies give to drugs; the names by which they are sold.

breathalyzer test: a test of the alcohol level in a person's breath, which reflects the blood level of alcohol.

breech birth: a birth in which the infant is born in a position other than the normal headfirst position.

bronchi (BRONK-eye): the two main airways in the lungs; branches of the windpipe (trachea). The singular form is *bronchus*.

bronchitis (bron-KITE-us): a respiratory disorder with irritation of the bronchi; thickened mucus; and deep, harsh coughing.

bubonic plague: a bacterial infection causing swollen lymph glands and pneumonia, frequently fatal.

bulimia (byoo-LEEM-ee-uh): repeated binge eating, usually followed by vomiting (also spelled bulemia).

C

caffeine: a mild stimulant of the central nervous system (brain and spinal cord) found in common foods, beverages, and medicines.

calisthenics: exercise routines for strength conditioning that use the parts of the body as weights.

calories: units used to measure energy. Calories indicate how much energy in a food can be used by the body or stored in body fat.

cancer: a disease in which abnormal cells multiply out of control, spread into surrounding tissues and other body parts, and disrupt normal functioning of one or more organs.

capillaries: the smallest blood vessels, which connect the smallest arteries with the smallest veins. Nourishment and fluid normally trapped in thick-walled arteries and veins can easily pass through the delicate walls of the capillaries.

carbohydrate: a class of nutrients made of sugars; these nutrients include sugar, starch, and fiber. All but fiber provide energy. Often referred to in the plural, *carbohydrates*.

carbon monoxide: a deadly gas; a gas formed during the burning of tobacco.

carcinogens (car-SIN-oh-gens): cancer-causing agents.

carcinomas (car-sin-OH-mahs): cancers that arise in the skin, body chamber linings, or glands.

cardiovascular disease (CVD): a general term for all diseases of the heart and blood vessels.

cardiovascular endurance: a component of fitness; the ability of the heart and lungs to sustain effort over a long time.

cardiovascular system: the system of structures that circulate blood and lymph throughout the body. Also called the *circulatory system*.

carotid (ca-ROT-id) **pulse:** the pulse in either of the carotid arteries, the main arteries next to the airway (and "Adam's apple") in the front of the neck.

cavity: a hole in a tooth caused by decay. (Tooth decay is also called dental *caries*.)

cells: the smallest units in which independent life can exist. All living things are single cells or organisms made of cells.

centenarians: people who have reached the age of 100 years or older.

cerebral thrombosis: the closing off of a vessel that feeds the brain by a stationary clot, or *thrombus*.

cervical cap: a rubber cap that fits over the cervix, used with spermicide to prevent conception.

cesarean (si-ZAIR-ee-un) **section:** surgical childbirth, in which the infant is taken through a cut in the woman's abdomen.

chambers: rooms; in the heart, large, hollow areas that receive incoming blood from the lungs and tissues and ship it out again.

chamomile: a plant with flowers that may provide some limited medical value in soothing intestinal and stomach discomforts.

chancre (SHANG-ker): a hard, painless sore; chancres develop early in syphilis infections.

chemotherapy: the administration of drugs that harm cancer cells, but that do not harm the client, or at least do not harm the client as much as the disease does.

chicken pox: a usually mild, easily transmitted viral disease causing fever, weakness, and itchy blisters.

child abuse: verbal, psychological, physical, or sexual assault on a child.

chlamydia (cla-MID-ee-uh): an infection of the reproductive tract, with or without symptoms; a frequent cause of ectopic pregnancy or failure to become pregnant.

cholera (KAH-ler-uh): a dangerous bacterial infection causing violent muscle cramps, severe vomiting and diarrhea, severe water loss, and death.

cholesterol: a type of fat made by the body from saturated fat; a minor part of fat in foods.

chromosomes: slender bodies inside the cell's nucleus, which carry the genes.

chronic: in relation to illness, this term refers to a disease or condition that develops slowly, shows little change, and lasts a long time.

chronic dieters: people who frequently diet in unhealthy ways in an attempt to lose weight.

chronic fatigue syndrome: unexplained repeated bouts of extreme fatigue that bed rest does not cure and that last at least six months; caused by a virus.

chronic obstructive lung disease (COLD): a term for several diseases that interfere with breathing. Asthma, bronchitis, and emphysema are examples of COLD.

chronic stress: unrelieved stress that continues to tax a person's resources to the point of exhaustion; stress that is damaging to health.

chronological age: age as measured in years from date of birth.

cilia: hairlike structures extending from the surface of cells that line body passageways, including the trachea and upper lungs. The cilia wave, propelling a coating of mucus along to sweep away debris.

cliques: peer groups that reject newcomers and that judge both their members and nonmembers harshly.

codeine: a narcotic drug that is commonly used for suppressing coughs.

codependent: a person who is so focused on the needs of others that the person's own needs are neglected. Also, an enabler who is a member of the family of, or has a close relationship with, a person addicted to a drug.

cold: an upper respiratory tract infection.

colostrum (co-LAHS-trum): a milklike substance rich in antibodies; the breast milk made during the first few days after birth.

combination pill: an oral contraceptive that contains progestin and synthetic estrogen.

comedogenic (coh-MEE-doh-JEN-ick): causing acne.

comfrey: leaves and roots of the comfrey plant; believed, but not proved, to have drug effects. Comfrey contains cancer-causing chemicals.

commitment: a decision adhered to for the long term; a promise kept.

communication: a two-way exchange of ideas or thoughts.

compost: rotted vegetable matter, used as fertilizer.

compulsions: irresistible impulses to perform senseless acts.

conception: the union of an ovum and a sperm that starts a new individual.

conditioning: the hundreds of small changes that cells make in response to physical activity that make the body more able to do the work at hand.

conflict: a struggle or opposition between people; especially, when people compete for something in the belief that only one can have what he or she wants, at the expense of the other.

confrontation: a showdown; an interaction in which one person expresses feelings to another. Managed aggressively, a confrontation may be a destructive fight. Managed assertively, a confrontation may be a constructive conversation in which one person makes his or her wishes known to another.

congeners (CON-jen-ers): ingredients in alcoholic beverages, other than the alcohol itself, that may irritate the nervous system.

congenital (con-JEN-ih-tal): present from birth.

connective tissues: fluid, gelatin-like, fibrous, or strap-like materials that bind, support, or protect other body tissues; tendons, cartilage, and ligaments are connective tissue.

constipation: hard, slow stools that are difficult to eliminate; often a result of too little fiber in the diet.

contraception: any method of preventing conception (the union of the male sperm and the female ovum). The term *birth control* is often used to mean the same thing, but technically, birth control includes abortion.

coping devices: nonharmful ways of dealing with stress, such as displacement or ventilation.

coronary arteries: the two arteries that supply blood to the heart muscle.

coronary artery bypass surgery: surgery to provide an alternate route for blood to reach heart tissue, bypassing a blocked coronary artery.

coronary thrombosis: the closing off of a vessel that feeds the heart muscle by a stationary clot, or *thrombus*.

cortex: the outer layer of an organ; in the brain, the outer, thinking portion—the gray matter.

CPR (cardiopulmonary resuscitation): a technique of maintaining blood and oxygen flow through the body of a person whose heart and breathing have stopped.

credentials: (kre-DEN-shulls): official evidence of education or other qualifications of an authority; diplomas, licenses, and the like.

critical periods: periods during development when a body organ is especially sensitive to harmful factors. A critical period is usually a period of rapid cell division.

critical phase: in atherosclerosis, the stage when plaques cover more than half of the inner surfaces of the arteries.

crowning: the moment in which the top (crown) of the baby's head is first seen.

cruciferous vegetables: vegetables of the cabbage family.

cults: groups of people who share intense admiration or adoration of a particular person or principle.

cuticles: the borders of hardened skin at the bases of the fingernails.

cyst (SIST): an enlarged, deep pimple.

D

date rape: sexual assault by a known person in a dating situation. Also called *acquaintance rape.*

date: to engage in social events designed to allow people to get to know each other. A double date (two couples) is a safe arrangement for early dates with people you do not know well.

day care: supervision, usually at a facility, for preschool children or elderly people who must be supervised during daytime working hours.

defense mechanisms: self-destructive ways of dealing with stress; automatic, subconscious reactions to emotional injury, such as denial, fantasy, projection, rationalization, regression, selective forgetting, or withdrawal.

deficiency (dee-FISH-en-see): too little of a nutrient in the body. Severe deficiencies cause diseases.

dehydration: loss of water. The symptoms progress rapidly from thirst to weakness to exhaustion, confusion, and even death.

delirium: a state of mental confusion, usually with hallucinations and continual movement.

denial (dee-NIGH-al): refusal to believe the facts of a circumstance—for example, to deny that a person is a problem drinker in the face of clear evidence that it is so.

dental plaque (PLAK): a buildup of sticky material on the surfaces of the teeth; a forerunner of tooth damage.

dentin: a tooth's softer, middle layer.

Depo-Provera (DEE-po pro-VAIR-uh): a trade name for an injectable form of progestin.

depression: the condition of feeling apathetic, hopeless, and withdrawn from others. A *major depression* is an emotionally crippling depressed state linked to physical causes; it may be, at the extreme, a suicidal state.

dermatologist: a physician (M.D.) who specializes in treating conditions of the skin.

designer drugs: laboratory-made drugs that closely resemble illegal drugs in chemical structure, but that are different enough to be legal until ruled illegal.

deviant: outside the normal system.

diabetes (DYE-uh-BEE-teez) **mellitus** (MEL-ih-tuss): a condition of abnormal use of glucose, usually caused by too little insulin or lack of response to insulin.

diabetic coma: a loss of consciousness due to uncontrolled diabetes, and the resulting buildup of toxic ketones in the blood.

diaphragm: a dome that fits over the cervix and holds spermicidal cream or jelly against the uterine entrance to block the passage of sperm.

diastolic (DYE-as-tol-ic) **pressure:** the blood pressure during that part of the heartbeat when the heart's ventricles are relaxing.

diet pills: medications that reduce the appetite or otherwise promote weight loss. Pills available over the counter usually contain caffeine and other drugs that cause more nervousness than weight loss. Prescription pills include amphetamines.

digestion: the breaking down of food into nutrients the body can use. The *digestive system* is a series of body organs that break foods down and absorb their nutrients. (See Chapter 6 for details of the system.)

dilation stage: the stage of childbirth during which the cervix is opening.

dioxins: deadly pollutants formed when chlorine bleach reacts with other compounds.

disability insurance: insurance to replace lost income if a person should be unable to work due to a long illness.

discipline: the shaping of behavior by way of rewards and/or punishments.

disinfectants: chemicals that kill microbes on surfaces. Bleach is a disinfectant.

dispatcher: a person who answers calls and relays messages to the proper helping service.

displacement: channeling the energy of suffering into something else— for example, using the emotional energy churned up by problems to do tasks or other familiar activities.

disposable: a description of any product that is intended to be used once and then thrown away.

diuretic (die-yoo-RETT-ick): a drug that causes the body to lose fluids; not effective for loss of body fat.

DNA (deoxyribonucleic acid): the genetic material of cells which serves as a blueprint for making all of the proteins a cell needs to make exact copies of itself.

douches (DOOSH-es): preparations sold to cleanse the vagina. Actually, vaginas clean themselves constantly with no help. Douches can wash dangerous bacteria into the reproductive tract.

Down syndrome: a congenital condition of physical deformities and mental retardation.

drink: the amount of a beverage that delivers ½ ounce of pure ethanol— 12 ounces of beer, 3 to 4 ounces of wine, 1 (10-ounce) wine cooler, or 1 ounce of 100-proof liquor.

drives: motivations that are inborn, not learned, such as hunger, thirst, fear, and need for sleep. Also known as *instincts*.

drug abuse: the deliberate taking of a drug for other than a medical purpose and in a manner that can result in damage to a person's health or ability to function.

drug addiction (dependence): a physical or psychological need for higher and higher doses of a drug.

drug misuse: the taking of a drug for its medically intended purpose, but not in the appropriate amount, frequency, strength, or manner.

drug-resistant: a term that describes microbes that have lost their sensitivity to particular drugs. For example, diseases caused by drug-resistant bacteria no longer respond to antibiotic therapy.

drugs: substances taken into the body that change one or more of the body's functions.

drug synergy: the combined action of two drugs that is greater than or different from the action of either drug alone.

drug trafficker: a person involved in the transport and sales of illegal drugs.

drug use: the taking of a drug for its medically intended purpose, and in the appropriate amount, frequency, strength, and manner.

DUI: driving under the influence (of alcohol or other mind-altering substances). See *DWI*.

duration: continuance in time; in exercise, the length of time spent in each exercise session.

DWI: driving while intoxicated with alcohol or any abusable substance— a crime by law. Intoxication is defined by blood alcohol level (a level of 0.08 percent in some states and 0.10 percent in other states).

dysfunctional family: a family with abnormal or impaired ways of coping that injure the self-esteem and emotional health of family members.

dysphoria (dis-FORE-ee-uh): unpleasant feelings that occur when endorphins are lacking; these feelings often follow drug-induced euphoria.

E

eating disorder: abnormal food intake stemming from emotional causes and related to addiction. In *anorexia nervosa*, young people starve themselves to lose weight. In *bulimia*, they binge on food, then starve or vomit.

echinacea: an herb popular for its assumed "anti-infectious" properties and as an all-purpose remedy, especially for colds and allergy. Also called *cone flower*.

ecosystems: systems of land, plants, and animals that have existed together for thousands or millions of years and that are interdependent.

ectopic pregnancy: a pregnancy that develops in one of the fallopian tubes or elsewhere outside the uterus; a dangerous condition.

effective: having the medically intended effect; part of the legal requirement for a drug.

effectiveness: how well a contraceptive method or device prevents pregnancy, expressed as a percentage. The laboratory effectiveness is the percentage of women protected from pregnancy in a year's time under ideal laboratory conditions. The **user effectiveness** is the percentage of typical female users who are protected.

ejaculation: the expelling of semen from the penis, brought about by the involuntary muscular contractions of orgasm.

elasticity: the characteristic of a tissue's being easily stretched or bent and able to return to its original size and shape.

elder abuse: verbal, psychological, physical, or sexual assault on an elderly person.

electrocardiogram: a record of the electrical activity of the heart that, if abnormal, may indicate heart disease.

electrolytes (ee-LECK-tro-lites): minerals that carry electrical charges that help maintain the body's fluid balance.

embolism: the sudden closure of a blood vessel by a traveling blood clot, or *embolus*.

embolus (EM-bow-luss): a clot that breaks loose and travels through the bloodstream. When it causes sudden closure of a blood vessel, this dangerous event is an *embolism*.

embryo (EM-bree-oh): the developing infant during the third through eighth week after conception.

emergency medical service (EMS): a team of people who are trained to respond in emergencies, and who can be contacted through a single dispatcher.

emetics (em-ETT-ics): drugs that cause vomiting.

emotion: a feeling that occurs in response to an event as experienced by an individual. Examples are love, anger, and fear.

emotional health: the state of being free of mental disturbances that limit functioning; also the state of having developed healthy perceptions and responses to other people and life events, based on thoughts, emotions, and values. Also called *mental health*.

emotional intelligence (EQ): the ability to recognize and appropriately express one's emotions in a way that enhances living.

emotional problems: patterns of behavior or thinking that cause a person to feel significant emotional pain or to be unable to function in any one or more of three important areas—social or family relations, occupation (including school performance), or use of leisure time.

emphysema (em-fih-ZEE-muh): a disease of the lungs in which many small, flexible air sacs burst and form a few large, rigid air pockets.

empty calories: a popular term referring to foods that contribute much energy (calories) but too little of the nutrients.

enable: make possible. In addiction, enabling means "helping" by trying to "save" the addicted person from the consequences of the behavior. This makes possible continued alcohol or other drug abuse. An enabler is a person who actually does harm by supporting a troubled person's continued self-destructive attitude or behavior.

enabling: misguided "helping."

enamel: a tooth's tough outer layer.

endorphins: chemicals in the brain that produce feelings of pleasure in response to a variety of activities.

energy: the capacity to do work or produce heat.

engorgement: swelling; with reference to the sexual response, the sex organs' filling with blood preparatory to orgasm.

environment: everything "outside" the living organism—air, water, soil, other organisms, and forms of radiation.

environmental tobacco smoke (ETS): the combination of exhaled mainstream smoke and sidestream smoke that enters the air and may be inhaled by other people.

ephedrine: a stimulant added to look-alikes and diet pills, and found in herbs such as ma huang; has caused heart attacks, strokes, seizures, and death, especially when combined with caffeine.

epidemic (EP-ih-DEM-ick): an infection that spreads rapidly through a population, affecting many people at the same time.

epinephrine (EP-uh-NEFF-rin): one of the stress hormones; also called *adrenaline*.

episiotomy (eh-PEEZ-ee-OT-oh-me): a surgical cut made in the vagina during childbirth when the vagina cannot stretch enough without tearing to allow the baby to pass.

erection: the state of a normally soft tissue when it fills with blood and becomes firm. Both the penis and clitoris can become erect.

ergogenic (ER-go-JEN-ick): a term that claims to mean "work-enhancing." In fact, no products enhance the ability to do work.

essential amino acids: amino acids that are needed, but cannot be made by the body; they must be eaten in foods.

estrogen: a hormone that, in females, regulates the ovulatory cycle.

ethanol (ethyl alcohol): see *alcohol*.

ethics: moral principles or values.

euphoria (you-FORE-ee-uh): a sense of great well-being and pleasure brought on by some drugs; popularly called a *high*.

euthanasia (you-than-AY-zee-uh): allowing a person to die by choosing not to employ life-support equipment such as artificial respirators, or the removal of life-support equipment from a patient who has no hope of recovery. Both may be legal in some cases.

excitement: as used to describe a stage of sexual intercourse, the early stage.

exercise physiology: the study of how the body works and changes in response to exercise. An exercise physiology laboratory has equipment to measure the components of fitness and to take other measurements.

exhaustion: a harmful third phase of the stress response, in which stress exceeds the body's ability to recover.

expulsion stage: the stage of childbirth during which the uterine contractions push the infant through the birth canal.

extended family: a family of parents, children, and other relatives, such as grandparents or aunts and uncles. The relatives may live in one household, or they may live close by and share responsibilities, such as childraising.

external pressures: regarding sexual feelings, messages from society, peers, and others that pressure people to have sexual intercourse.

F

false labor: warm-up contractions that many women experience before the birth process.

family: a group of people who are related by adoption, blood, or marriage, and are committed to each other; especially a father, mother, and their children. All blood relatives and ancestors of a family.

family identity: a unique sense of belonging together as a unit, distinct and different from other people or groups.

fat: a class of nutrients that does not mix with water. Fat is made mostly of fatty acids, which provide energy to the body. Technically referred to as *lipids*.

fatfold caliper: a pinching device that measures body fat under the skin.

fatfold test: a test of body fatness done with a *fatfold caliper*.

fat-soluble (SOL-you-bul): a chemist's term meaning "able to dissolve in fat."

fatty acids: simple forms of fat that supply energy fuel for most of the body's cells.

fee-for-service system: a system of paying for health care in which clients pay individual fees for the services they receive.

female condom: a soft, thin plastic tube with two end rings—one to fit over the cervix and one to serve as an anchor outside the entrance to the vagina; also called a *vaginal pouch*.

femininity: traits, including biological and social traits, associated with being female.

fertility awareness method: a method of charting ovulation. It involves tracking menstrual periods, body temperature, and types of cervical mucus. Also called *rhythm method*.

fertilization: the joining of an ovum and a sperm.

fetal alcohol effect (FAE): a subtle version of fetal alcohol syndrome (FAS), with hidden defects including learning disabilities, behavioral abnormalities, and motor impairments.

fetal alcohol syndrome (FAS): a cluster of birth defects, including permanent mental and physical retardation and facial abnormalities, seen in children born to mothers who abuse alcohol during pregnancy.

fetus (FEET-us): the developing infant from the ninth week after conception until birth.

feud: a bitter, continuing hostility, often involving groups of people.

fiber: indigestible substances in foods, made mostly of carbohydrate.

fibrillation (FIH-brill-AY-shun): extremely rapid contractions of the heart that lack the power needed to pump blood around the body.

fight-or-flight reaction: the body's response to immediate physical danger; the stress response. Energy is mobilized, either to mount an aggressive response against the danger, or to run away.

first aid: literally, "help given first"—medical help given immediately in an emergency, before the victim is transported to a hospital or treatment center.

fitness: the characteristics of the body that enable it to perform physical activity, to meet routine physical demands with enough reserve energy to rise to sudden challenges, and to withstand stresses of all kinds.

flexibility: a component of fitness; the ability to bend the joints without injury.

flu: short for **influenza** (in-flew-EN-za), a highly contagious respiratory infection caused by any of a variety of viruses.

folk medicine: the use of herbs and other natural substances in the treatment of disease as practiced among people of various regions.

follicles: vessel-like structures in the skin that contain the oil glands, the muscles that control hair movement (and also goose bumps), and the roots of hairs.

food chain: the sequence in which living things depend on other living things for food. Algae are near the bottom and human beings at the top of the food chain.

foreplay: an activity in which each partner gives pleasure to the other prior to intercourse.

formaldehyde: a substance related to alcohol. Formaldehyde is made by the body from alcohol and contributes to hangovers.

fossil fuel: coal, oil, and natural gas, which all come from the fossilized remains of plant life of earlier times.

foster family: a family formed when a government agency places a child in the temporary care of an adult or couple. The child's own parents may have died or for some reason cannot care for the child.

foxglove: a plant that contains a substance used in the heart medicine digoxin.

fracture: a break in a bone. An *open fracture* is a break with a wound in the overlying tissues. A *closed fracture* is a break or crack with no visible wound.

free radicals: chemicals that harm the body's tissues by starting destructive chain reactions in the molecules of the body's cells. Such reactions are believed to trigger or worsen some diseases.

frequency: the number of activity units per unit of time (for example, the number of exercise sessions per week).

frostbite: the formation of ice crystals in body parts exposed to temperatures below freezing; freezing of body parts, especially toes and fingers, and nose and other face parts.

fungi: living things that absorb and use nutrients of organisms they invade. Fungi that cause illnesses include *yeasts* and *molds*.

G

gangs: peer groups that exist largely to express aggression against other groups.

gateway drug: a drug whose abuse is likely to lead to abuse of other, more potent and dangerous drugs. Alcohol, marijuana, and tobacco are most often named as gateway drugs.

gay: a general term referring to homosexuality, but often referring to homosexual men.

gender: the classification of being male or female.

gender identity: that part of a person's self-image that is determined by the person's gender.

gender roles: roles assigned by society to people of each gender.

generic (jeh-NEHR-ick) **names:** the chemical names for drugs, as opposed to the brand names; the names everyone can use.

genes (JEENZ): the units of a cell's inheritance, which direct the making of equipment to do the cell's work.

genetic counselor: an advisor who predicts and advises on the likelihood that congenital defects will occur in a family.

genetic engineering: a science of manipulating the genes of living things to instill some desirable trait not present in the original organism. An example is a tomato given a gene to delay its rotting.

genital herpes (HER-peez): a common, incurable sexually transmitted disease caused by a virus that produces blisters. The symptoms clear up on their own, but the virus remains to cause future outbreaks.

genital warts: contagious wartlike growths on infected areas, caused by human papilloma viruses. Sometimes called *condyloma* (con-di-LOW-ma). The viruses that cause genital warts can also cause cervical cancer in women.

gestation (jes-TAY-shun): the period from conception to birth. For human beings, normal gestation lasts from 38 to 42 weeks.

ginseng (JIN-seng): a plant containing chemicals that have drug effects.

ginseng abuse syndrome: a group of symptoms associated with the overuse of ginseng, including high blood pressure, insomnia, nervousness, confusion, and depression.

gland: an organ of the body that secretes one or more hormones.

global warming: warming of the planet, a trend that threatens life on earth.

glucose: the body's blood sugar; a simple form of carbohydrate.

glycogen: the form in which the liver and muscles store glucose.

gonorrhea (gon-oh-REE-uh): a bacterial sexually transmitted disease that often advances without symptoms to spread though the body, causing problems in many organs.

grams (abbreviated **g**): units of weight in which many nutrients are measured; 28 grams equals 1 ounce.

greenhouse effect: the heat-trapping effect of the glass in a greenhouse. The same effect is caused by gases that are accumulating in the earth's outer atmosphere, which are trapping the sun's heat and warming the planet.

grieve: to feel keen emotional pain and suffering over a loss.

guilt: the normal feeling that arises from the conscience when a person acts against internal values ("I did a bad thing").

gum disease: inflammation and degeneration of the pink tissue (gums) that is attached to the teeth and helps to hold them in place.

gynecologist: a specialist in the care of the female reproductive system.

H

hallucinations: false perceptions; imagined sights, sounds, smells, or other feelings, sometimes brought on by drug abuse, sometimes by mental or physical illness.

hallucinogens (hal-LOO-sin-oh-jens): drugs that cause visions and other sensory illusions.

head lice: tiny, but visible, white parasitic insects that burrow into the skin or hairy body areas.

head restraints: high seatbacks or other devices attached to seats in cars at head level. A head restraint prevents the person's head from snapping back too far when the body is thrown backward. This prevents neck and spinal cord injuries.

health: a range of states with physical, mental, emotional, spiritual, and social components. At a minimum, *health* means freedom from physical disease, poor physical condition, social maladjustment, and other negative states. At a maximum, *health* means "wellness."

health-care system: the total of all health-care providers and medical treatment facilities that work together to provide medical care to the population.

health maintenance organization (HMO): a group of physicians who practice together and who treat people's health problems under a pre-payment plan.

heart attack: the event in which vessels that feed the heart muscle become blocked, causing tissue death.

heart disease: any disease of the heart muscle or other working parts of the heart.

heart murmur: a heart sound that reflects damaged or abnormal heart valves.

heart transplant: the surgical replacement of a diseased heart with a healthy one.

heat exhaustion: a serious stage of overheating which can lead to heat stroke.

heat stroke: a life-threatening condition that results from a buildup of body heat; can be fatal.

Heimlich (HIME-lick) **Maneuver (abdominal thrust maneuver):** a technique of dislodging a particle that is blocking a person's airway. The Heimlich Maneuver is named for the physician who invented it.

hemlock: any part of the hemlock plant, which causes severe pain, convulsions, and death within 15 minutes.

hemorrhoids: swollen, painful rectal veins; often a result of constipation.

hepatitis: a liver disease caused by any of several types of viruses transmitted by infected needles (drug use, tattoos, blood transfusions), by eating raw seafood from contaminated water, and by any contact (including sexual contact) with body secretions from infected people.

hepatitis B: a viral sexually transmitted disease that causes loss of liver function and severe liver disease. Hepatitis B is preventable, but not curable.

herbal medicine: the use of plants to treat disease or improve health.

herbs: nonwoody plants or plant parts valued for their flavor, aroma, or medicinal qualities.

heroin: a narcotic drug derived from morphine.

heterosexual: feeling sexual desire for persons of the other sex.

hierarchy: a ranking system in which each thing is placed above or below others.

high-density lipoproteins (HDLs): lipoproteins that carry fat and cholesterol away from the tissues (and from plaques) back to the liver for breakdown and removal from the body.

high-risk pregnancy: a pregnancy more likely than others to have problems, such as premature delivery (prior to the 38th week of gestation) or a low birthweight. Many factors contribute to pregnancy risks.

histamine (HIST-uh-meen): a chemical of the immune response that produces inflammation (swelling and irritation) of tissue.

history (medical): an interview in which a health-care professional asks about past medical experience.

HIV: an abbreviation for *human immunodeficiency virus*, the virus that causes AIDS.

Hodgkin's disease: a lymphoma that attacks people in early life and is treatable with radiation therapy.

homeopathic (home-ee-OP-ah-thick) **medicine:** practices based on the theory that "like cures like"—that is, that substances that cause symptoms in healthy people can cure those symptoms when given in very dilute amounts (homeo = like; pathos = suffering).

homeostasis (HOH-me-oh-STAY-sis): the maintenance of a stable body environment, achieved as body systems adapt to changing conditions.

homophobia: an irrational fear and hatred of homosexuals, usually based on the fear of developing AIDS or of becoming homosexual.

homosexual: feeling sexual desire for persons of the same sex.

hormonal system: the system of glands—organs that send and receive blood-borne chemical messages—that control body functions in cooperation with the nervous system.

hormone: a chemical that serves as a messenger. Each hormone is secreted by a gland and travels to one or more target organs, where it brings about responses.

hospice (HOS-pis): a support system for dying people and their families, which helps the family let the person die at home with dignity and in comfort.

hospital infections: infectious illnesses acquired during hospitalization.

hospitalization insurance: insurance to pay the cost of a hospital stay. See also *Medicare* and *Medicaid*.

hot flashes: sudden waves of feeling hot all over, a symptom related to dilation of blood vessels in the skin, which is common during the transition into menopause.

human growth hormone: a nonsteroid hormone produced in the body that promotes growth; taken as a drug by athletes to enhance muscle growth; also called *somatotropin*.

human papilloma virus (HPV): any of over 50 related viruses whose effects include genital warts and cervical cancer. Members of this virus family also cause skin warts, commonly found on the hands.

hunger: the physiological need to eat, experienced as a drive for obtaining food, an unpleasant sensation that demands relief.

hyperactivity: a condition of excessive activity. In children, hyperactivity is demonstrated by constant fidgeting, talking, moving, running, climbing, and so on. In adolescents and adults, hyperactivity takes the form of restless feelings and difficulty sitting still.

hypertension: high blood pressure.

hyperthermia (*hyper* means "too high"; *thermia* means "temperature"): a condition of too much body heat with abnormally high internal body temperature.

hypnotherapy: the use of hypnosis and the power of suggestion to change behaviors, relieve pain, and heal.

hypothalamus (high-po-THALL-uh-mus): a brain regulatory center.

hypothermia (*hypo* means "too low"; *thermia* means "temperature"): a condition of too little body heat with abnormally low internal body temperature.

hysterectomy: removal of the uterus, an operation performed more often than necessary.

I

ibuprofen (EYE-byoo-PRO-fen): a drug that relieves fever, pain, and inflammation.

immune system: the cells, tissues, and organs that protect the body from disease. The immune system is composed of the white blood cells, bone marrow, thymus gland, spleen, and other parts.

immunity: the body's capacity for identifying, destroying, and disposing of disease-causing agents.

immunizations: injected or oral doses of medicine that stimulate the immune system to develop the long-term ability to quickly fight off infectious diseases; also called *vaccinations*.

implantation: the lodging of a fertilized ovum in the wall of the uterus.

impulse control: the ability to wait and think before acting or speaking.

inactive ingredients: ingredients that give a medicine qualities other than medical effects. For example, oils and waxes may be mixed with a medication to be used on the skin; water, colorants, and flavors may be added to liquid medicines taken by mouth.

inert: not active.

infatuation: the state of being completely carried away by unreasoning passion or attraction; addictive love.

infectious diseases: diseases caused, and transmitted from person to person, by microorganisms or their toxins. Also called *communicable* or *contagious diseases*, or simply *infections*.

infectious mononucleosis (MON-oh-new-klee-OH-sis): a viral infection involving mononucleocytes, a type of white blood cell. The symptoms vary from mild, coldlike symptoms to high fevers, swollen glands, and spleen and liver involvement. Also called *mono*.

inflammation: pain and swelling caused by irritation.

initiator: a carcinogen, an agent required to start the formation of cancer.

insomnia (in-SOM-nee-uh): sleep abnormalities, including difficulty in falling asleep and wakefulness through the night.

insulin shock: the result of too much insulin, which causes a dangerous drop in blood glucose. Also called *hypoglycemia*.

insulin: a hormone produced by the pancreas and released in response to high blood glucose following a meal. Insulin promotes the use and storage of glucose by the body's tissues.

intensity: the degree of exertion while exercising (for example, jogging takes more exertion than walking and so is more intense).

internal pressures: regarding sexual feelings, a person's internal biological urges toward having sexual intercourse.

internship: a length of time spent in a medical facility as part of the training of health-care providers.

intimacy: being very close and familiar, as in relationships involving private and personal sharing.

intoxication: literally, a state of being poisoned; often used to mean drunkenness.

intrauterine device (IUD): a device inserted into the uterus to prevent conception or implantation.

intravenous (IV) drug abuse: the practice of using needles to inject drugs of abuse into the veins. (The word *intravenous* means "into a vein.")

irradiation: ionizing radiation applied to food to kill microorganisms and other pests. Ionizing radiation disrupts the internal molecular workings of cells, killing them.

J

jock itch: a fungal infection of the groin and inner thigh; not a sexually transmitted disease.

juvenile: a legal term meaning a person under age 18; a minor. Crimes committed by juveniles are usually punished according to the judgments of juvenile justice, and often not by adult standards.

K

Kaposi's (cap-OH-zeez) **sarcoma:** a normally rare skin cancer causing a purplish discoloration of the skin, seen commonly among people with AIDS.

keratin: the normal protein of hair and nails.

ketones: fragments formed by the tissues during incomplete use of fat for energy, and released into the blood.

ketoprofen (KEE-toe-PRO-fen): a drug that relieves fever, pain, and inflammation. Its small pill size eases swallowing for those who have trouble swallowing regular pills.

Kyoto Protocol (kee-OH-toe pro-toe-call): an agreement signed by many of the world's leaders in 1997, that spells out the degree of reduction in carbon dioxide emission required of each nation by the year 2012. *Kyoto* is a city in Japan where the leaders met to write the agreement. *Protocol* means the first draft of an agreement.

L

labor: contractions of the uterus strong enough to push the fetus through the vagina for delivery.

lactation: the production of milk by the mammary glands of the breasts for the purpose of feeding babies.

lapses: times of falling back into former habits, a normal part of both weight change and weight maintenance.

latent: temporarily unseen or inactive.

learning disorder: any of a number of nerve or brain dysfunctions that interfere with normal learning, believed to affect 2 to 3 children in each class of 30. The disorders may affect attention, memory, language, organizational skills, problem solving, social awareness, and other aspects of learning.

lesbian: a term referring to homosexual women.

lethal dose: the amount of a drug necessary to produce death.

leukemias (loo-KEE-me-ahs): cancers that arise in the blood cell–making tissues.

leukoplakia (loo-koh-PLAKE-ee-uh): whitish or grayish patches that develop in the mouths of tobacco users and that may lead to cancer.

life expectancy: the average number of years lived by people in a given society.

life management skills: the skills that help a person to realize his or her potential to be well and enjoy life. This book's Health Strategies sections give examples.

life span: the maximum years of life a human being can live.

life-support systems: a term used to refer to mechanical means of supporting life, such as feedings given into a central vein or machines that force air into the lungs (artificial respirators).

lifestyle choices: choices, made daily, of how to treat the body and mind. Examples are what to eat, when to exercise, and whether to use alcohol or other drugs.

lifestyle diseases: diseases that are made likely by neglect of the body. They cannot be passed from person to person. Examples are heart disease, cancer, and diabetes. Lifestyle choices that promote health can help prevent lifestyle diseases.

lightening: the sensation a pregnant woman experiences when the fetus settles into the birth position.

lipoproteins (LIP-oh-PRO-teens): protein and fat clusters that transport fats in the blood.

living will: a will that declares a person's wishes regarding treatment, should the person become unable to make decisions (for example, in the event of brain death).

longevity: an individual's length of life.

look-alikes: combinations of over-the-counter drugs and other chemicals packaged to look like prescription medications or illegal drugs.

love: affection, attachment, devotion.

low birthweight: a birthweight of less than 5½ pounds (2,500 grams), used as a predictor of poor health in the newborn infant.

low-density lipoproteins (LDLs): lipoproteins that carry fat and cholesterol from the liver, where they are made, to the tissues where they are used. LDLs also deposit cholesterol in arteries, forming plaques.

low-impact aerobic dance: aerobic dance in which one foot remains on the floor to prevent shock to the lower body.

LSD (lysergic acid diethylamide): a powerful hallucinogenic drug. Also called *acid*.

Lyme disease: a bacterial infection spread by tiny deer ticks.

lymph: the clear fluid that bathes each cell and transfers needed substances and wastes back and forth between the blood and the cells. Lymph also plays a role in immunity.

lymphocytes (LIM-fo-sites): white blood cells, active in immunity.

lymphomas (limf-OH-mahs): cancers that arise in organs of the immune system.

M

ma huang: an herbal preparation sold with promises of weight loss and increased energy, but that contains ephedrine, a dangerous heart stimulant.

mainstream smoke: the smoke that flows through the cigarette and into the lungs when a smoker inhales.

major medical insurance: insurance to pay high bills not covered by other insurance.

male condom: a sheath worn over the penis during intercourse to contain the semen, to prevent pregnancy, and/or to reduce the risks of sexually transmitted diseases. Condoms are also called *rubbers*.

male menopause: the gradual decline in male fertility due to advancing age.

malignancy: a dangerous cancerous growth that sheds cells into body fluids and spreads to new locations to start new cancer colonies. (The word *malignant* means "growing worse.")

malnutrition: the results in the body of poor nutrition; undernutrition, overnutrition, or any nutrient deficiency.

malpractice insurance: insurance that protects providers of health care against lawsuits by people claiming to have been harmed by a health-care provider.

mammogram: X-ray examination of the breast, a screening test for cancer.

managed care: a system of providing health care based on a prepaid basis. By emphasizing preventive care, controlling physician charges, and screening requests for expensive tests and procedures, managed care plans control costs of providing care.

marriage: the institution that joins a man and a woman by agreement for the purpose of creating and maintaining a family.

married couple: a family consisting of two married adults.

masculinity: traits, including biological and social traits, associated with being male.

massage therapy: a method of kneading of muscles to reduce tension, help blood circulation, and improve joint mobility; believed to promote healing.

masturbation: stimulating one's own genitals, usually until orgasm occurs.

mature love: a strong affection for, and an enduring, deep attachment to, a person whose character the partner knows well.

measles: a highly contagious viral disease characterized by rash, high fever, sensitivity to light, and cough and cold symptoms; preventable by immunization.

mediator: a neutral third person who helps two people in conflict to communicate more effectively.

Medicaid: hospitalization and surgical insurance available for people who qualify as needy.

medical insurance: insurance to pay physicians' fees, lab fees, and fees for prescription medications.

Medicare: hospitalization insurance for people who are receiving Social Security.

medicines: drugs used to help cure disease, lessen disease severity, relieve symptoms, prevent disease, help with diagnosis, or produce other desired effects.

melanin (MELL-eh-nin): the protective skin pigment responsible for the tan, brown, or black color of human skin; produced in abundance upon exposure to ultraviolet radiation.

melanoma: an especially dangerous cancer of the pigmented cells of the skin, related to sun exposure in people with light-colored skin.

melatonin: a hormone of a gland of the brain, believed to help regulate the body's daily rhythms. Claims for life extension or enhancement of sexual prowess are without merit. Proof of melatonin's safety or effectiveness is lacking.

menopause: the years of stopping ovulation and menstruation in a woman.

menstrual cramps: contractions of the uterus, during and a few days before menstruation, that may cause pain.

menstrual cycle: the cyclic ripening of an ovum and the preparation of the uterus for pregnancy. Also called the *ovulatory cycle.*

menstruation: the monthly shedding of the uterine lining in nonpregnant females.

mentor: a wise person who gives advice and assistance.

mescaline: the hallucinogen produced by the peyote cactus.

metastasized (meh-TASS-tuh-sized): when speaking of cancer cells, a term that means the cancer cells have migrated from one part of the body to another, and started new growths just like the original tumor.

methadone: a drug used to treat heroin addiction; it holds off withdrawal and helps people recover socially.

microbes: tiny organisms, such as bacteria, yeasts, and viruses, that are too small to be seen with the naked eye. Also called *microorganisms.*

minerals: elements of the earth needed in the diet, which perform many functions in body tissues.

moderate drinker: a person who does not drink excessively. The person doesn't behave inappropriately because of alcohol. The person's health is not harmed by alcohol over the long term.

moderation: an amount of alcohol that causes no harm to health: not more than one to two drinks a day for healthy adults.

molds: many-celled fungi, some of which cause diseases.

monogamous: having sexual relations with one partner only, excluding all others. These relationships are usually long-term relationships.

morning sickness: the nausea (upset stomach) a pregnant woman may suffer at any time of the day; thought to be related to the hormones that maintain pregnancy.

morphine: a narcotic drug that physicians prescribe as a painkiller.

motivation: the force that moves people to act. Motivation may be either instinctive (drives) or learned.

mucus (MYOO-cuss): a slippery secretion produced by cells of the body's linings that protects the surfaces of the linings.

mumps: a highly contagious viral disease that causes swelling of the salivary glands and, occasionally, of the testicles; preventable by immunization.

muscle endurance: a component of fitness; the ability of muscles to sustain an effort for a long time.

muscle strength: a component of fitness; the ability of muscles to work against resistance.

mutation (myoo-TAY-shun): a change in a cell's genetic material. Once the genetic material has changed, the change is inherited by the offspring of that cell.

myeloma: a cancer originating in the cells of the bone marrow.

N

naproxen sodium (na-PROX-en): a drug that relieves fever, pain, and inflammation. It provides longer relief from a single dose than other common pain relievers.

narcotic antagonists: drugs that oppose the actions of other drugs. The word *antagonist* means something or someone who struggles with, or opposes, another.

Narcotics Anonymous (NA): a free, self-help program of addiction recovery. It uses a 12-step program, promotes personal growth, and leads to the person's helping others to recover.

narcotics: habit-forming drugs that relieve pain and produce sleep when taken in moderate doses. Also called *opiates,* because most are derived from the opium poppy.

naturopathic medicine: a mixture of traditional and alternative therapies.

needs: urgent wants for necessary things.

nervous system: the body system of nervous tissues—organized into the brain, spinal cord, and nerves—that send and receive messages and integrate the body's activities.

neural (NER-uhl) **tube defects:** a group of birth defects caused by interruption of normal development of the neural tube, the tissue from which the brain and spinal cord form. The term *neural* refers to nerve tissues.

nicotine (NICK-oh-teen): an addictive drug present in tobacco.

night blindness: slow recovery of vision after flashes of bright light at night; an early symptom of vitamin A deficiency.

nonconformist: a person who does not share society's values and therefore behaves in unconventional ways.

nontraditional family: a group of unrelated people who live together and offer support to one another.

norepinephrine: one of the stress hormones; also called *noradrenaline.*

Norplant: a trade name for a surgical hormone delivery system that provides continuous release of progestin, thereby preventing pregnancy for up to five years.

nuclear family: a mother and father and their natural or adopted children.

nucleus: inside a cell, the structure that contains the genes.

nutrient deficiencies (dee-FISH-en-sees): too little of one or more nutrients in the diet; a form of malnutrition.

nutrients: compounds in food that the body requires for proper growth, maintenance, and functioning.

O

obesity: overfatness to the point of injuring health. Obesity is often defined as 20 percent or more above the appropriate weight for height.

obsessive-compulsive disorder: the uncontrollable need to perform repetitive acts.

opiates: a group of drugs derived from the opium poppy that relieve pain and induce sleep. Also known as *narcotics.*

opium: a narcotic drug that relieves pain and induces sleep, made from the opium poppy.

oral contraceptives: pills that prevent pregnancy by stopping ovulation or by changing conditions in the uterus; often called *birth control pills* or *the Pill.*

organs: whole units, made of tissues, that perform specific jobs.

orgasm: a series of muscular contractions of the sex organs, with ejaculation in the male; it typically occurs after a period of sexual stimulation.

osteoporosis (OS-tee-oh-por-OH-sis): a disease of gradual bone loss, which can cripple people in later life.

ostracism: rejection and exclusion from society.

ova (singular, **ovum**): the female cells of reproduction. Ova are also called eggs.

over-the-counter (OTC) drugs: drugs legally available without a prescription.

overload: an extra physical demand placed on the body.

overnutrition: too much food energy or excess nutrients to the degree of causing disease or increasing risk of disease; a form of malnutrition.

ovulation: the ripening and release of an ovum.

ozone layer: a layer of ozone in the earth's outer atmosphere that protects living things on earth from harmful ultraviolet radiation from the sun.

ozone: a substance created when certain types of energy, such as the sun's ultra-violet rays, react with oxygen. When this reaction takes place high above the earth in the outer atmosphere, the ozone absorbs the most dangerous UV rays.

P

pacemaker: a device that delivers electrical impulses to the heart to regulate the heartbeat.

Pap test: a test for cancer of the cervix (the lower part of the uterus). A few cells are removed painlessly and examined in a laboratory.

parasites: living things that depend for nourishment on the bodies of others that they inhabit.

passive abuse: abuse involving not taking needed actions, such as neglecting to provide food or shelter to a dependent victim.

passive: possessing the characteristic of not expressing feelings appropriately, of remaining silent.

pathogens: microbes that cause diseases.

PCP (phencyclidine hydrochloride): a drug of abuse; an animal tranquilizer, abused by human beings as a hallucinogen.

PCP (*Pneumocystis carinii* pneumonia): the pneumonia characteristic of AIDS.

pediatrician: a specialist concerned with the health care of infants and children.

peer groups: groups of people who are similar in age and stage of life.

peer pressure: the internal pressure one feels to behave as a peer group does, in order to gain its members' approval.

pelvic inflammatory disease (PID): an infection of the fallopian tubes and pelvic cavity in women, causing ectopic pregnancy and pregnancy failures.

perception: a meaning given to an event or occurrence based on a person's previous experience or understanding.

persistent: the opposite of biodegradable—unable to decompose or to be converted by living organisms into harmless wastes.

personality: the characteristics of a person that are apparent to others.

peyote: a cactus that produces the hallucinogen mescaline.

phobia (FOH-bee-uh): an extreme, irrational fear of an object or situation.

photovoltaic (PV) panels: panels that convert light (photons) into electricity (volts).

physical addiction: a change in the body's chemistry so that without the presence of a substance (drug), normal functioning begins to fail, and withdrawal symptoms set in; also called *physical dependence*.

physical examination: an examination of the body to gather information about its general condition or to make a diagnosis. It normally includes observations by looking, listening, or feeling body parts and by medical test results.

physician-assisted suicide: suicide of an ill person by way of lethal drugs or other means provided by a physician; not legal in most states.

physiological age: age as estimated from the body's health and probable life expectancy.

phytochemicals: chemicals in plant-based foods that are not nutrients but that have effects on the body.

pinch test: an informal way of measuring body fatness.

pinworms: small, visible, white parasitic worms that commonly infect the intestines of young children.

PKU (phenylketonuria): a congenital disease causing severe brain damage with mental retardation if left untreated; now detected and treated at birth.

placebo effect: the healing effect that faith in medicine, even inert medicine, often has.

placenta (plah-SEN-tah): an organ that develops during pregnancy; it permits exchange of materials between maternal and fetal blood.

placental stage: the final stage of childbirth, in which the placenta is expelled.

plaques (PLACKS): mounds of fat, mixed with minerals, that build up along artery walls in atherosclerosis.

plateau: literally, a high, flat place. In sexual intercourse, the plateau phase is the period of intense physical pleasure preceding orgasm.

platelets: tiny, disk-shaped bodies in the blood, important in blood clot formation.

pneumonia: a disease caused by a virus or bacterium that infects the lungs, with high fever, severe cough, and pain in the chest; especially dangerous to the very old or young.

polio (poliomyelitis): a viral infection that produces mild respiratory or digestive symptoms in most cases but that may produce permanent paralysis or death; preventable by immunization.

pollution: contamination of the environment with anything that impairs its ability to support life.

polyps: tumors that grow on a stem, resembling mushrooms. Polyps bleed easily, and some have the tendency to become malignant.

polyunsaturated: a type of unsaturated fat especially useful as a replacement for saturated fat in a heart-healthy diet.

positive self-talk: the practice of making affirming statements about oneself to oneself, helpful in building self-esteem.

post-traumatic stress disorder: a reaction to stress such as wartime suffering or rape, arising after the event is over.

postpartum depression: the emotional depression a new mother or father experiences after the birth of an infant.

premature infant: an infant born before the 38th week of gestation.

premenstrual syndrome (PMS): symptoms such as physical discomfort, moodiness, and nervousness that occur in some women each month before menstruation.

premiums: regular payments made to an insurance company to cover the costs of unforeseen events such as medical emergencies.

prenatal care: medical and health care provided during pregnancy.

prepayment plan: a system of paying for health care in which the clients pay a fixed fee every month, regardless of how many services they receive.

prescription drugs: drugs legally available only with a physician's order.

problem drinker or **alcohol abuser:** a person who suffers social, emotional, family, job-related, or other problems because of alcohol. This person is on the way to alcoholism.

prodrome: the onset of general symptoms common to many diseases, such as fever, sneezing, and coughing.

progesterone: a hormone secreted in females during that portion of the menstrual cycle in which the uterine lining builds up.

progestin-only pill: an oral contraceptive containing only progestin. Another name is the *minipill.*

progestin: a synthetic version of progesterone used in contraceptives.

progressive muscle relaxation: a technique of learning to relax by focusing on relaxing each of the body's muscle groups in turn.

progressive overload principle: the training principle that a body system, in order to improve, must be worked at frequencies, intensities, or durations that increase over time.

promoter: a substance that assists in the development of malignant tumors, but does not initiate them on its own.

proof: a measure of the percentage of alcohol in alcoholic beverages. *100 proof* means 50 percent alcohol, *90 proof* means 45 percent, and so forth.

protease inhibitors: drugs that stop the action of an enzyme which ordinarily helps HIV to reproduce. The drugs help slow HIV reproduction, but takers run an increased risk of developing diabetes.

protein: a class of nutrients that builds body tissues and supplies energy. Protein is made of amino acids. Referred to only in the singular, *protein*.

protozoa (PRO-toh-ZOH-ah): tiny, animal-like cells, some of which can cause illnesses.

proxy: a person authorized to act for another.

Prozac: the brand name of one drug of a group of drugs used to restore normal brain chemistry in people with depression.

psilocybin (sill-oh-SI-bin), **psilocin** (sill-OH-sin): two hallucinogens produced by a type of wild mushroom.

psychological addiction: a craving for something; mental dependence on a drug, habit, or behavior; also called *psychological dependence*.

psychology: the scientific study of behavior and the mind.

puberty (PYOO-ber-tee): the period of life in which a person becomes physically capable of reproduction.

pubic lice: a sexually transmitted disease caused by tiny parasites that breed in pubic hair and cause intense itching.

pulp cavity: a tooth's deepest chamber, which houses its blood vessels and nerves.

pulse rate: the number of heartbeats per minute.

pus: a mixture of fluids and white blood cells that collects around infected areas.

Q

quacks: people pretending to have medical skills, and usually having products for sale.

quality time: time spent with another, of sufficient duration to allow a meaningful exchange of ideas.

quid: a small portion of any form of smokeless tobacco.

R

rabies: a viral disease of the central nervous system that causes paralysis and death.

radiation therapy: the application of cell-destroying radiation to kill cancerous tissues.

radon (RAY-don): a gas that arises from the earth where radioactive materials are present.

range of motion: the mobility of a joint; the direction and the extent to which it bends.

recovery: a healthy third phase of the stress response, in which the body returns to normal.

recreational drug use: a term made up, to describe their drug use, by people who claim their drug taking produces no harmful social or health effects; a term not defined by the Food and Drug Administration (FDA).

rectum: the last part of the digestive tract, through which stools are eliminated.

recyclable: made of material that can be used over again.

refusal skills: a set of social strategies that enable people to competently resist the pressure by others to engage in dangerous or otherwise undesirable behaviors.

relapses: illnesses that return after being treated and almost cured. Relapses are often more severe than the original illnesses.

relaxation response: the opposite of the stress response; the normal state of the body.

REM (rapid eye movement pronounced as the syllable *rem*) **sleep:** the periods of sleep in which a person is dreaming.

resentment: anger that has built up due to failure to express it.

residency: a length of time spent in a medical facility as part of the M.D.'s training after the internship.

resistance: a force that opposes another; in fitness, the weight or other opposing force against which muscles must work.

resistance: in stress, the second phase of the stress response, in which the body mobilizes its resources to withstand the effects of the stress.

resolution: in sexual intercourse, the stage of relaxation that follows orgasm.

ripple effect: the effect seen when a pebble is thrown into a pond and waves radiate out from it. The term is used to describe how one person's actions may affect many other people, and how their actions will affect still other people.

risk factors: factors linked with a disease by association but not yet proved to be causes.

rubella: a viral disease that resembles measles but that lasts only a few days and does not cause serious complications, except in pregnancy; preventable by immunization.

S

safe: causing no undue harm; part of the legal requirement for a drug.

safer-sex strategies: behavior guidelines that reduce sexually transmitted disease risk, but that do not reduce the risk to zero.

Salmonella: a common food-borne pathogen causing digestive system infections in many people each year.

salt: a compound made of minerals that, in water, dissolve and form electrolytes.

sarcomas (sar-KOH-mahs): cancers that arise in the connective tissue cells, including bones, ligaments, and muscles.

sassafras: root bark from the sassafras tree, once used in beverages but now banned as an ingredient in foods or beverages because it contains cancer-causing chemicals.

saturated: concerning fats and health, those fats associated strongly with heart and artery disease; mainly fats from animal sources.

schizophrenia (SKITZ-oh-FREN-ee-uh): a mental illness, a condition of losing touch with reality accompanied by reduced ability to function.

sebum (SEE-bum): the skin's natural oil—actually a mixture of oils and waxes—that helps keep the skin and hair moist.

second opinion: a second assessment of a diagnosis and treatment plan by another health-care provider, usually on the request of a client, to double-check the validity of the original plan.

sedatives: drugs that have a soothing or tranquilizing effect.

sedentary: physically inactive (literally, "sitting down a lot").

self-actualization: the reaching of one's full potential; the highest attainable state in Maslow's hierarchy of needs.

self-efficacy (EFF-ih-kasee): a person's belief in his or her ability to succeed at the task at hand.

self-esteem: the value a person attaches to his or her self-image. Self-esteem is high in those who value themselves. It is a vitally important part of emotional health.

self-image: the characteristics that a person sees in himself or herself.

senility: a general term meaning weakness of mind and body occurring in old age.

set: a specific number of times to repeat a weight-training exercise.

sex: a general term used to mean both gender and sexual intercourse.

sexual dysfunction: impaired responses of sexual excitement or orgasm due to psychological, interpersonal, physical, environmental, or cultural causes; formerly called *impotence* in men and *frigidity* in women.

sexual harassment: unwanted sexual attention, often from someone in power, that makes the victim feel uncomfortable or threatened.

sexual intercourse: the reproductive act between the sexes. The term *intercourse* means communication of any kind—talking, for example. Sexual intercourse between human beings is termed coitus (CO-ih-tus). Between animals it is termed *copulation* (cop-you-LAY-shun).

sexuality: the quality of being sexual. Sexuality is part of the total person: physical, emotional, social, intellectual, and spiritual. Sexuality is part of who people are.

sexually transmitted diseases (STDs): diseases that are transmitted by way of direct sexual contact. An older name was *venereal diseases*.

shaken baby syndrome: a collection of symptoms resulting from violent shaking of an infant or young child. It is the most common cause of mortality and long-term disability resulting from intentional head injury.

shame: the extreme feeling of guilt that arises when a person internalizes mistakes ("I am a bad person because I did it").

shin splints: damage to the muscles and connective tissues of the lower front leg from stress. Such damage usually heals with rest.

shingles: a painful skin condition caused by the reemergence of the chicken pox virus in later life.

shock: failure or disruption of the blood circulation, a life-threatening reaction to accidents and injuries.

sibling rivalry: competition among sisters and brothers, often for the attention or affection of parents.

siblings: two or more people with one or more parents in common; brothers or sisters.

side effects: effects of drugs other than the desired medical effects.

sidestream smoke: the smoke that escapes into the air from the burning tip of a cigarette or cigar, or from burning pipe tobacco.

single-parent family: one parent and his or her natural or adopted children.

sinuses (SIGN-us-es): spaces in the bones of the skull.

small for date: a term used to describe an infant underdeveloped for its age, often because of malnutrition of the mother.

smallpox: a severe viral infection with skin eruptions; once often fatal, it is now believed to be wiped out world wide, thanks to immunizations.

smokeless tobacco: tobacco used for snuff or chewing rather than for smoking.

sober: free of alcohol's effects and of addiction; not drunk.

social drinker: a person who drinks only on social occasions. Depending on how alcohol affects the person's life, the person may be a moderate drinker or a problem drinker.

specialist: a physician with training in a specialty area beyond the medical degree requirements.

sperm: the male cells of reproduction.

spermicide: the compound nonoxynol-9, intended for birth control, that also kills or weakens some STD organisms.

spina (SPY-nah or SPEE-nah) **bifida** (BIFF-ih-duh): a birth defect often involving gaps in the bones of the spine, leaving the spinal cord unprotected in those spots. The cord may bulge and protrude through the gaps in the spinal column.

spine: the stack of 33 vertebrae that form the backbone and hold the spinal cord, whose nerves enter and exit through spaces between the bones.

splint: a stick or board used to support a broken bone to keep its separated parts from moving until it can be set.

spontaneous abortion, or miscarriage: the expelling of a zygote, embryo, or fetus from the uterus, not induced by medical means.

spouse abuse: verbal, psychological, physical, or sexual assault on a spouse.

starch: a carbohydrate, the main food energy source for human beings.

status: a person's standing or rank in relation to others, many times falsely based on wealth, power, or influence. While desirable to many, these characteristics do not define human worth.

step aerobics: aerobic activity in which each participant steps up and down on a stable platform called a step bench ranging from about 6 inches to 12 inches high.

stepparents: people who marry into a family after a biological parent departs through death or divorce.

stereotypes: fixed pictures of how everyone in a group is thought to be; ideas that do not recognize anyone's individuality.

sterilization: the process of permanently interrupting a person's ability to bear children, usually by surgically severing and sealing the vas deferens or the fallopian tubes.

steroids: hormones of a certain chemical type that occur naturally in the body, some of which promote muscle growth. Available as drugs, they are abused by athletes seeking a shortcut to large muscles.

stimulant: any of a wide variety of drugs, including amphetamines, caffeine, and others, that speed up the central nervous system.

stranger rape: sexual assault by a stranger. Also called *street rape.*

stress: the effect of physical and psychological demands (stressors) on a person. Stress that provides a welcome challenge is *eustress* ("good" stress, pronounced YOU-stress); stress that is perceived as negative is *distress* ("bad" stress).

stress eating: eating in response to stress, an inappropriate activity.

stress fractures: bone damage from repeated physical force that strains the place where ligament is attached to bone.

stress hormones: epinephrine and norepinephrine, secreted as part of the reaction of the nervous system to stress.

stressor: a demand placed on the body to adapt.

stress response: the response to a demand or stressor. The stress response has three phases—*alarm, resistance,* and *recovery* or *exhaustion.*

stroke: the shutting off of the blood flow to the brain by plaques, a clot, or hemorrhage.

sudden infant death syndrome (SIDS): the unexpected and unexplained death of an apparently well infant; the most common cause of death of infants between the second week and the end of the first year of life; also called *crib death.*

sudden sniffing death syndrome: sudden death, usually from heart failure, in a person who is startled while abusing inhalants. The fright often occurs upon discovery of the sniffer by an authority figure or when the drug produces a frightening hallucination.

sugars: carbohydrates found both in food and in the body.

sun block: a total block against the cancer-causing rays of the sun. A sun block has an SPF (sun protection factor) of 50 or greater. Zinc oxide is an example of a sun block.

sunscreen: a partial block against the cancer-causing rays of the sun (gamma radiation).

suntan lotion: lotion that may or may not have any sunscreen protection.

supplement: a pill, powder, liquid, or the like containing only nutrients; not a food.

support system: a network of individuals or groups with which one identifies and exchanges emotional support.

suppress: to hold back or restrain.

surgical insurance: insurance to pay the surgeon's fees. See also *Medicaid.*

sustainable: a term used to describe the use of resources at such a rate that the earth can keep on replacing them—for example, a rate of cutting trees no faster than new ones grow. Also, *sustainable* describes the produc-

tion of pollutants at a rate that the environment or human cleanup efforts can handle, so that there is no net accumulation of pollution.

syphilis: a bacterial sexually transmitted disease that, if untreated, advances from a sore (chancre) to flulike symptoms, then through a long symptomless period, and later to a final stage of irreversible brain and nerve damage, ending in death.

systolic (sis-TOL-ic) **pressure:** the blood pressure during that part of the heartbeat when the heart's ventricles are contracted and the blood is being pushed out into the arteries.

T

T cells: lymphocytes that can recognize invaders that cause illness.

target heart rate: the heartbeat rate that will condition a person's cardiovascular system—fast enough to push the heart, but not so fast as to strain it.

tars: chemicals present in (among other things) tobacco. Burning tars release many carcinogens.

tennis elbow: a painful condition of the arm and joint, usually caused by strain, as from poor form in playing tennis.

terminal illnesses: illnesses that are expected to end in death.

tetanus: a disease caused by a toxin produced by bacteria deep within a wound.

therapy: treatment that heals.

thoughts: those mental processes of which a person is always conscious.

thrill seekers: people who are especially likely to take chances in exchange for momentary excitement.

thrombus: a stationary clot. When it has grown enough to close off a blood vessel, this dangerous event is a *thrombosis.*

thymus gland: an organ of the immune system.

tissues: systems of cells working together to perform special tasks.

tolerance: in drug use, a state that develops in users of certain drugs that makes larger and larger amounts of the drugs necessary to produce the same effect.

tolerance: in relationships with others, accommodation and acceptance of differences between oneself and others; being tolerant of people's age, body shape, gender, disabilities, race, religion, views, and other differences.

tonsillectomy: removal of the tonsils (in the throat), an operation sometimes performed needlessly.

toxic shock syndrome (TSS): a type of poisoning that can occur when bacteria break down menstrual blood; often associated with use of super-absorbent tampons.

toxin: a poison.

trace minerals: minerals essential in nutrition, needed in small quantities (traces) daily. Iron and zinc are examples.

transdermal: literally, "across the skin." In a drug delivery system, a drug is placed in contact with the skin by way of an adhesive patch. The drug is absorbed across the skin and into the bloodstream.

tremors: continuous quivering or shaking.

trichomoniasis (trick-oh-mo-NEYE-uh-sis): a sexually transmitted disease caused by a parasite that can cause bladder and urethral infections.

tubal ligation (lye-GAY-shun): surgical cutting and sealing off of the fallopian tubes to sterilize women.

tuberculosis (TB): a bacterial infection of the lungs.

tumor: an abnormal mass of tissue that can live and reproduce itself, but performs no service to the body.

U

ulcers: open sores in the lining of the digestive system.

umbilical (um-BIL-ih-cul) **cord:** the ropelike structure through which the fetus's veins and arteries extend to and from the placenta.

undernutrition: too little food energy or too few nutrients to prevent disease or to promote growth; a form of malnutrition.

underweight: weight too low for health. Underweight is often defined as weight 10 percent or more below the appropriate weight for height.

unethical: against the rules of right and wrong; not in line with accepted moral standards.

unsaturated: concerning fats and health, fats less associated with heart and artery disease; mainly fats from plant sources.

upper respiratory infection: an infection of the membranes of the nasal cavities, sinuses, throat, and trachea, but not involving the lungs.

urinary tract infections (UTIs): bacterial infections of the urethra that can travel to the bladder and kidneys; not a sexually transmitted disease.

urine: fluid wastes removed from the body by the kidneys.

V

vaccine: a drug made from altered microbes or their poisons injected or given by mouth to produce immunity.

values: a person's set of rules for behavior; what the person thinks of as right and wrong, or sees as important.

valves: flaps of tissue that open and close to allow the flow of blood in one direction only. The heart's valves are located at the entrances and exits of its chambers.

variables: changeable factors that affect outcomes.

vas deferens (plural, **vasa deferentia**): one of the two tubes that conduct sperm from the testicles toward the penis.

vasectomy: surgical cutting and sealing off of each vas deferens to sterilize a man.

vegetarians: people who omit meat, fish, and poultry from their diets. Some vegetarians also omit milk products and eggs.

veins: blood vessels that carry waste-containing blood from the tissues back to the heart.

venom: poison from a living creature, such as a snake or scorpion.

ventilation: the act of verbally venting one's feelings; letting off steam by talking, crying, swearing, or laughing.

ventricles: the two lower chambers of the heart—the shipping areas that send blood on its way to the lungs or the tissues.

vertebrae (VERT-eh-bray; singular, **vertebra**): the delicate, hollow bones of the spine.

violence: brutal physical force intended to damage or injure another.

violent crime: a crime that involves threat or uses force, including assault, murder, rape, or robbery.

virgin: a term applied to people before their first occasion of sexual intercourse.

viruses: organisms that contain only genetic material and protein coats, and that are totally dependent on the cells they infect.

vitamins: essential nutrients that do not yield energy, but that are required for growth and proper functioning of the body.

voluntary activities: movements of the body under the command of the conscious mind; one component of a person's daily energy expenditure.

W

water-soluble: able to dissolve in water.

weight training: exercise routines for strength conditioning that use weights or machines to provide resistance against which the muscles can work.

wellness: maximum well-being; the top of the range of health states; the goal of the person who strives toward realizing his or her full potential physically, mentally, emotionally, spiritually, and socially.

wet dreams: dreams during which orgasm occurs; a normal release for the sexual drive; in boys, these are also called *nocturnal emissions*.

whitehead: a pimple filled with pus, caused by the plugging of oil-gland ducts with shed material from the duct lining.

will: a person's intent, which leads to action.

witch hazel: leaves or bark of a witch hazel tree; not proved to have healing powers.

withdrawal method (coitus interruptus): a technique in sexual intercourse of withdrawing the penis from the vagina just prior to ejaculation. It is not recommended for preventing pregnancy and is useless against sexually transmitted diseases.

withdrawal: the physical symptoms that occur when a drug to which a person is addicted is cleared from the body tissues.

worms: visible parasites that burrow into the blood supplies of victims.

Y

yeasts: one-celled fungi, some of which cause diseases.

yeast infection, or **candidiasis** (can-did-EYE-a-sis): an infection caused by a yeast that multiplies out of control in the vagina; not a sexually transmitted disease.

Z

zygote: the product of the union of ovum and sperm, so termed for two weeks after conception. (After that, it is called an *embryo*.)

Glosario

A

abortion - aborto: procedimiento para poner término al embarazo antes de que el feto pueda vivir fuera del útero.

abstinence - abstinencia: abstenerse totalmente de tener relaciones sexuales con otras personas, también denominado *celibato*.

accredited - acreditado: aprobado; en el caso de una universidad o instituto de estudios superiores, aprobado por un grupo profesional calificado para evaluar el currículo ofrecido.

acetaminophen (ah -SEET -ah -MIN -ofen) **- acetaminófeno**: un fármaco que alivia la fiebre y el dolor.

acid rain - lluvia ácida: una lluvia que porta contaminantes de aire ácido que perjudica a las plantas y daña el suelo donde cae.

acne - acné: una condición prolongada de inflamación de los poros y glándulas de la piel con una acumulación de aceites bajo la piel que causa granos pequeños.

acquired inmune deficiency syndrome (AIDS) - síndrome de inmunodeficiencia adquirida (SIDA): una enfermedad viral fatal transmisible del sistema inmunológico que crea una deficiencia severa de inmunidad, la cual deja a las personas sin defensas contra las infecciones y el cáncer.

acromegaly (ack -ro -MEG -a -lee) **- acromegalia:** una enfermedad causada por niveles que exceden los niveles normales de la hormona humana del crecimiento.

active abuse - abuso activo: el abuso que involucra la agresión de una persona contra la otra, tales como golpes o el abuso sexual de la víctima.

active ingredientes - ingredientes activos: los ingredientes de un fármaco que producen efectos físicos en el cuerpo.

active solar - solar activo: la utilización de paneles fotovoltágicos para generar electricidad de la luz solar. (Un hogar solar pasivo es aquel que fue construido para aprovechar la luz solar y la sombra disponible de manera de reducir los costos de calefacción y refrigeración.)

acupuncture (AK -you -PUNK -cher) **- acupuntura:** un método de inserción de agujas largas y delgadas en puntos de la piel con el objeto de aliviar el dolor o una enfermedad.

acute stress - estrés agudo: un incidente temporal de estrés que hace aflorar el estado de alerta o alarma para impulsar a la persona a enfrentar un evento.

adapt - adaptarse: cambiar o ajustarse a fin de acomodarse a nuevas condiciones.

addiction - adicción: un deseo físico o psicológico por dosis cada vez mayores de una droga que conlleva a daños corporales, desadaptación social, o penurias económicas; dependencia de una sustancia, hábito o comportamiento.

adolescence - adolescencia: el período de crecimiento entre el inicio de la pubertad y la plena madurez. El inicio de la adolescencia varía de persona a persona.

aerobic (air -ROE -bic) **- aeróbico:** se refiere a los procesos de producción de energía que utilizan oxígeno (aero = aire).

afterbirth - secundinas: la placenta y las membranas expulsadas después del nacimiento del niño (a).

aggresive - agresivo: que posee las características de ser insultante o demasiado exigente con otros o que de alguna otra manera invade su territorio; una expresión inapropiada de los sentimientos.

AIDS dementia complex - complejo de demencia por SIDA: el desorden mental resultante de un ataque de VIH sobre el cerebro y los nervios.

air bags - almohadas inflables: almohadas inflables, diseñadas para inflarse por impacto, almacenadas en el centro del volante o en el tablero de instrumentos del automóvil.

air pollution - contaminación ambiental: la contaminación del aire por gases o partículas que normalmente no se encuentran en éste.

alarm - alarma: la primera fase de la respuesta al estrés, en la cual el individuo se enfrenta a un desafío y comienza a prestarle atención.

alcohol - alcohol: una clase de compuestos químicos. El alcohol en las bebidas alcohólicas, el *etanol* o *alcohol etílico*, es un miembro de esta clase.

alcohol addict (alcoholic) - adicto al alcohol (alcohólico): una persona con la enfermedad del alcoholismo en pleno desarrollo. Los problemas de esta persona, causados por el abuso del alcohol, se encuentran fuera de control.

alcoholism - alcoholismo: una enfermedad caracterizada por una pérdida de control sobre la bebida y dependencia en el alcohol, ambos de los cuales causan daño a la salud, las relaciones familiares y el desempeño social y laboral.

alienation - enajenación mental: separarse de otros debido a diferencias que no se pueden resolver.

aloe - áloe: una planta tropical con amplias aseveraciones respecto de su valor medicinal, la mayoría de las cuales no han sido comprobadas.

alternative therapies - terapias alternativas: enfoques al diagnóstico y tratamiento médico que no son totalmente aceptados por la comunidad médica tradicional. Como tal, no son generalmente enseñadas en las escuelas de medicina de los Estados Unidos o practicadas en los hospitales estadounidenses. También denominadas terapias auxiliares, no convencionales o no ortodoxas.

Alzheimer's disease - enfermedad de Alzheimer: una enfermedad del cerebro en algunas personas ancianas que se manifiesta en confusión mental; incapacidad para actuar; y en las fases finales, la muerte.

amino acids - aminoácidos: formas simples de proteína generalmente utilizados para construir tejidos, o bajo ciertas condiciones, quemar para obtener energía.

amniocentesis (am -nee -oh -cen -TEE -sis) **- amniocentesis:** un examen de las células fetales obtenidas mediante la inserción de una aguja a través del abdomen de la mujer.

amniotic (am -nee -OTT -ic) **sac - bolsa amniótica:** la "bolsa de agua" en el útero, en el cual flota el feto.

amotivational syndrome - síndrome amotivacional: la pérdida de ambición o empuje; una característica de los que abusan de la marihuana a largo plazo.

amphetamines (am -FETT -ah -meenz) - **anfetaminas:** fármacos estimulantes poderosamente adictivos. Debido a que inhiben el apetito, están reservados para uso en casos en donde la obesidad hace peligrar la salud. También llamadas *speed* o *estimulantes*.

anaerobic (AN -air -ROE -bic) - **anaeróbico:** se refiere a procesos de producción de energía que no utilizan oxígeno (an = sin).

anemia - anemia: la reducción en el número o tamaño de los glóbulos rojos; un síntoma de varias enfermedades diferentes; incluyendo algunas deficiencias nutricionales.

anesthetics (an -us -THET -icks) **anestésicos:** fármacos que eliminan el dolor, con o sin la pérdida del conocimiento.

aneurysm (AN -your -ism) - **aneurisma:** la formación de una bolsa en la pared arterial en un punto en el cual se ha debilitado.

angina (an -JYE -nuh o ANN -juh -nuh) - **angina:** un dolor en la región del corazón causado por la falta de oxígeno.

anorexia (an -or -Exee -uh) **nervosa - anorexia nerviosa**: un desorden de autoinanición extrema.

antagonist (an -TAG -uh -nist) - **antagonista:** un fármaco que se contrapone a la acción de otro fármaco.

antibiotics - antibióticos: fármacos utilizados para combatir la infección bacteriana.

antibodies - anticuerpos: grandes moléculas de proteína producidas para combatir tejidos infectivos o extraños.

antigens - antígenos: sustancias extrañas en el cuerpo, tales como virus o bacteria, que estimulan al sistema inmunológico a producir anticuerpos.

antihistamines - antihistamínico: fármacos que contrarrestan la inflamación causada por la histamina, una de las sustancias químicas que participan en las reacciones alérgicas.

antioxidant (AN -tee -OX -ih -dant) - **antioxidante:** una sustancia química que puede detener las destructivas reacciones en cadena de los radicales libres. Entre los nutrientes, las vitaminas C y E, el betacaroteno, y el mineral selenio, son ejemplos.

antiseptics - antisépticos: agentes que impiden el crecimiento de los microorganismos en las superficies corporales y en las heridas.

anxiety attack - ataque de ansiedad: un súbito e inesperado episodio de ansiedad severa con síntomas tales como taquicardia, transpiración, mareos y nausea.

anxiety - ansiedad: un estado emocional de alta energía con una respuesta de estrés a medida que el cuerpo reacciona a éste.

aorta (ay -OR -tah) - **aorta:** la arteria más grande del cuerpo; transporta la sangre recientemente oxigenada desde el corazón a los tejidos.

aphrodisiac (af-roh-DEEZ-ee-ack) - **afrodisíaco:** una substancia que supuestamente excita el deseo sexual. En la realidad, ninguna substancia conocida lo hace, pero muchos afirman que los productos que ellos venden si lo hacen.

appetite - apetito: el deseo psicológico de comer, una motivación aprendida y una sensación positiva que se produce al ver, oler o pensar en comida.

aroma therapy - aromaterapia: una técnica que utiliza extractos de aceites provenientes de plantas y flores (generalmente aplicados por medio de masajes o baños) para aumentar la salud física, psicológica y espiritual.

arteries - arterias: los vasos sanguíneos que transportan la sangre desde el corazón a los tejidos.

arthritis - artritis: una dolorosa inflamación de las articulaciones causada por infección, el organismo, lesiones u otras causas. Generalmente resulta en una alteración de la estructura de las articulaciones y pérdida de sus funciones.

artificial heart - corazón artificial: una bomba diseñada para encajar en la cavidad pectoral del cuerpo humano y realizar la función de bombeo de la sangre a todo el cuerpo.

asexual - asexual: no tener ninguna inclinación sexual.

aspirin - aspirina: un fármaco que alivia la fiebre y la inflamación.

assertive - asertivo: que posee la característica de expresar apropiadamente sus sentimientos y necesidades mientras que respeta los de otros. La asertividad es la clave para obtener cooperación.

asthma - asma: dificultad para respirar, con emanación de sonidos de resuello provenientes del pecho causados por el paso del aire a través de conductos respiratorios que se han reducido en tamaño.

artherosclerosis (ATH -uh -roh -scler -OH -sis) - **arteriosclerosis:** la forma más común de las enfermedades cardiovasculares. Una enfermedad caracterizada por placas a lo largo de las paredes interiores de las arterias.

athlete's foot - pie de atleta: una infección fúngal de los pies, generalmente transmitida mediante el contacto con el piso.

atria (singular **atrium**) - **atria** (singular **atrio**): las dos cámaras superiores del corazón - las áreas de recepción que acopian la sangre que ingresa.

attention - deficit / hiperactivity disorder (ADHD) - transtorno por déficit de la atención / hiperactividad: la inhabilidad para prestar atención, a menudo se presenta acompañada de una hiperactividad y control deficiente de los impulsos. ADHD a menudo se diagnostica en niños menores de siete años de edad. Interfiere con la vida familiar, la escuela y otras funciones.

ayurveda (EYE -your -VAY -dah) - **ayurveda:** sistema tradicional hindú de hierbas, dieta, meditación, masaje y yoga, que según se cree, mejora la capacidad del organismo para defenderse de las enfermedades.

B

B cells - células B: los linfocitos que producen los anticuerpos.

bacteria (singular **bacterium) - bacteria** (singular **bacteria**): organismos unicelulares microscópicos de variadas formas y tamaños, algunos capaces de causar enfermedades.

balanced meal - comida balanceada: una comida con alimentos que proveen la cantidad correcta de carbohidratos, grasas y proteínas.

barbiturates - barbitúricos: fármacos depresivos que reducen la actividad del sistema nervioso central.

barrier methods - métodos de barrera: método anticonceptivo que física o químicamente obstruyen el desplazamiento de la esperma hacia el óvulo. Estos elementos no alteran los procesos corporales con fármacos o aparatos.

basal energy - energía basal: la suma total de la energía necesaria para mantener las actividades químicas de las células y para mantener la vida, excluyendo las actividades voluntarias. El principal componente de los gastos diarios de energía de una persona.

behavior modification - modificación de la conducta: un cambio de las decisiones o acciones de la persona mediante el manejo de señales que gatillan las acciones, las acciones en sí, o las consecuencias de las acciones.

belladona - belladona: cualquier parte de la mortal planta *Atropa belladona*, un veneno mortal.

benign (be -NINE) **- benigno:** no canceroso, no dañino. La descripción de un tumor que no es capaz de propagarse de un área a otra.

beta-carotene (bay -tah CARE -oh -teen) **- beta-caroteno:** un pigmento vegetal color naranja que el cuerpo puede convertir a una forma activa de la vitamina A. Uno de los nutrientes antioxidantes.

binge drinker - sobre ingesta de tragos: una persona que bebe cuatro o más bebidas alcohólicas en un período corto.

binge eating disorder (BED) - trastorno de ingesta excesiva de alimentos: ingesta repetida de grandes cantidades de alimentos, pero no seguido por vómitos.

binge eating - sobre ingesta de alimentos: comer en exceso a un grado extremo.

biodegradable - biodegradable: que se puede descomponer; capaz de ser convertido en desechos inofensivos por organismos vivientes y que puede ser reutilizado nuevamente para construir o cultivar nuevas cosas.

bioelectromagnetic medicine - medicina bioelectromagnética: la utilización de energía magnética o eléctrica para estimular la restauración ósea, el proceso de curación de las heridas y la regeneración de tejidos.

biofeedback - biorretroalimentación: el uso de máquinas que detectan y entregan información acerca del pulso, presión arterial, actividad cerebral o nerviosa y tensión muscular, para permitir a la persona a aprender como se siente estar relajado y así reducir el pulso y la presión sanguínea. Una técnica clínica utilizada para ayudar a la persona a aprender a relajarse mediante el monitoreo de su tensión muscular, pulso, actividad de las ondas cerebrales u otras actividades corporales.

birth defects - defectos de nacimiento: anormalidades físicas presentes desde el nacimiento.

birth order - orden de nacimiento: la ubicación de un niño entre sus hermanos y hermanas, tales como el mayor, el intermedio o el menor.

bisexual: atracción sexual por miembros de ambos sexos.

blackhead - puntos negros: una espinilla abierta con pigmentación oscura (no suciedad) en la abertura.

blackouts - privación del sentido: episodios de amnesia durante períodos de tiempo mientras se bebe. La persona puede actuar normalmente durante estos episodios, pero posteriormente es incapaz de recordar lo sucedido. La privación del sentido tiene probabilidades de ocurrir durante la vida de una persona que sufre de alcoholismo.

blended family - familia combinada: una familia creada por un nuevo matrimonio después del fallecimiento o divorcio de uno de los esposos. Las familias combinadas incluyen un padre o madre biológico (a) o adoptivo (a) y un padrastro o madrastra, junto con los hijos de uno o de ambos.

blood - sangre: el líquido espeso y rojo que fluye a través de los vasos sanguíneos del cuerpo y transporta gases, nutrientes, desechos y otras sustancias importantes a través del cuerpo. La sangre también cumple un papel importante en la regulación de la temperatura corporal.

body composition - composición corporal: un componente del estado físico del cuerpo. Las proporciones de tejido magro en comparación de los tejidos adiposos del cuerpo.

body image - imagen corporal: la manera en que una persona piensa que su cuerpo luce, lo cual puede o no ser la forma como realmente luce.

body systems - sistemas corporales: grupos de órganos relacionados que trabajan en conjunto para realizar las principales funciones del organismo.

bogus - falso: engañoso. Existen médicos falsos, grupos profesionales falsos, licencias para la práctica de la medicina falsas, certificados falsos y registros falsos.

botulin toxin - toxina botulínica: un veneno potente producido por bacteria en latas selladas, envases de plástico o frascos de alimentos.

botulism - botulismo: la condición, a menudo fatal, de envenenamiento por la toxina botulínica.

brain death - muerte cerebral: la pérdida total e irreversible de las funciones cerebrales superiores, reflejadas en una onda cerebral de línea plana, lo opuesto a la onda cerebral de línea ondulada producida por un cerebro activo.

brand names - nombre comercial: los nombres que las empresas dan a los fármacos. Los nombres por los cuales se venden.

breathalyzer test - prueba del alcotest: la medición del nivel de alcohol en el aliento de la persona, lo cual refleja el nivel de alcohol en la sangre.

breech birth - parto de nalgas: un parto en el cual el lactante nace en una posición diferente a la normal de cabeza primero.

bronchi (BRONK -eye) **- bronquios:** los dos conductos respiratorios principales en los pulmones. Ramificaciones de la traquea. La forma singular es *bronquio*.

bronchitis (bron -KITE -us) **- bronquitis:** un trastorno respiratorio con irritación de los bronquios, mucosa espesa y una tos profunda y ronca.

bubonic plague - peste bubónica: una infección bacteriana que ocasiona hinchazón de los nódulos linfáticos y neumonía, con frecuencia es fatal.

bulimia - bulimia: la ingesta insaciable de alimentos, generalmente seguido por vómitos.

C

caffeine - cafeína: un estimulante leve del sistema nervioso central (cerebro y médula espinal) encontrado en alimentos comunes, bebidas y medicinas.

calisthenics - calistenia: rutinas de ejercicios para acondicionamiento de la resistencia que utiliza las partes del cuerpo como pesas.

calories - calorías: la unidad utilizada para medir la energía. Las calorías indican cuanta energía de un alimento puede ser utilizado por el cuerpo o almacenado como tejido adiposo.

cancer - cáncer: una enfermedad en la cual las células anormales se multiplican sin de control, se esparcen a los tejidos vecinos y a otras partes del organismo y perturban el funcionamiento normal de uno o más órganos.

capillaries - capilares: los vasos sanguíneos más pequeños, los cuales conectan las arterias más pequeñas con las venas más pequeñas. Los nutrientes y líquidos que generalmente quedan atrapados en las gruesas paredes de las arterias y las venas pueden pasar fácilmente a través de las delicadas paredes de los capilares.

carbohydrate - carbohidrato: una clase de nutrientes compuestos por azucares. Estos nutrientes incluyen el azúcar, el almidón y la fibra. Todos menos la fibra producen energía. A menudo se les denomina en la forma plural como *carbohidratos*.

carbon monoxide - monóxido de carbono: un gas letal. Un gas creado durante al quemar tabaco.

carcinogens (car -SIN -oh -gens) **- carcinógenos:** los agentes que causan cáncer.

carcinomas (car -sin -OH -mahs) **- carcinomas:** tipos de cáncer que surgen en la piel, en el revestimiento de las cámaras del cuerpo o en las glándulas.

cardiovascular disease (CVD) - enfermedad cardiovascular: un término general utilizado para todas las enfermedades del corazón y los vasos sanguíneos.

cardiovascular endurance - resistencia cardiovascular: un componente del acondicionamiento físico. La habilidad del corazón y los pulmones para soportar el esfuerzo durante un tiempo prolongado.

cardiovascular system - sistema cardiovascular: el sistema de estructuras que hace circular la sangre y línfas a través de todo el cuerpo. También denominado el *sistema circulatorio*.

carotid (ca -ROT -id) **pulse - pulso arterial:** el pulso en cualquiera de las arterias carótidas, las arterias principales cerca del dúcto respiratorio (y "manzana de Adán") en la parte delantera del cuello.

cavity - carie: el orificio en un diente causado por la descomposición. (A la descomposición del diente también se le llama *dental caries* o *carie dental*).

cells - células: las unidades más pequeñas en las cuales puede existir la vida independiente. Todos los seres vivientes son células únicas u organismos compuestos por células.

centenarian - centenario: personas que han alcanzado la edad de 100 años o más.

cerebral thrombosis - trombosis cerebral: la obstrucción total de un vaso que alimenta el cerebro por un coágulo estacionario, o *trombo*.

cervical cap - tapa cervical: Tapa de caucho, utilizada con espermicida, que encaja sobre la cérvix para prevenir la concepción .

cesarean (si -ZAIR -ee -un) **section - parto por cesárea:** parto quirúrgico, en el cual el lactante se extrae a través de un corte realizado en el abdomen de la mujer.

chambers - cámaras: espacio: en el corazón, las grandes áreas huecas que reciben la sangre que llega de los pulmones y los tejidos y la envían hacia fuera nuevamente.

chamomile - camomila: una planta con flores que podrían dar un valor medicinal limitado para aliviar las molestias intestinales y estomacales.

chancre (SHANG -ker) **- chancro:** una lesión indolora y dura. Los chancros se desarrollan tempranamente durante las infecciones por sífilis.

chemotherapy - quimioterapia: la administración de fármacos que dañan las células del cáncer, pero que no causan daño al cliente, o que por lo menos no dañan al paciente tanto como la enfermedad.

chicken pox - varicela: una enfermedad viral generalmente leve y de fácil contagio que ocasiona fiebre, debilidad, ampollas, y picazón.

child abuse - abuso infantil: agresión verbal, física o sexual contra un niño (a).

chlamydia (cla -MID -ee -uh) **- chlamydia:** una enfermedad del tracto reproductivo, con o sin síntomas; una causa frecuente del embarazo ectópico o la inhabilidad de quedar embarazada.

cholera (KAH -ler -uh) **- cólera:** una peligrosa infección bacteriana que causa violentas contracciones musculares, vómitos severos y diarrea, deshidratación severa y la muerte.

cholesterol - colesterol: un tipo de grasa fabricado por el cuerpo de grasas saturadas. Una parte menor de la grasa en los alimentos.

chromosomes - cromosomas: cuerpos delgados dentro del núcleo de la célula, los cuales contienen los genes.

chronic - crónico: en relación a la enfermedad, este término se refiere a una enfermedad o condición que se desarrolla lentamente, muestra poco cambio y dura mucho tiempo.

chronic dieters - en dieta crónica: las personas que frecuentemente hacen dieta en forma no saludable en un intento por perder peso.

chronic fatigue syndrome - síndrome de fatiga crónica: episodios repetidos inexplicables de fatiga extrema que el reposo en cama no cura y que dura por lo menos seis meses; causado por un virus.

chronic obstructive lung disease (COLD) - enfermedad pulmonar obstructiva crónica (EPOC): un término para varias enfermedades que interfieren con la respiración. El asma, la bronquitis y el enfisema son ejemplos de EPOC.

chronic stress - estrés crónico: un estrés sin alivio que continua acaparando los recurso de una persona hasta el punto en que queda exhausto. Estrés que es dañino para la salud.

chronological age - edad cronológica: la edad medida en años desde la fecha del nacimiento.

cilia - cilios: estructuras de tipo velloso que se extienden desde la superficie de células que cubren los conductos del cuerpo, incluyendo la traquea y la parte superior de los pulmones. Los cilios ondulan, impulsando una capa de mucosa para deshacerse de las partículas de desecho.

cliques - camarillas: grupos de pares que rechazan a los recién llegados y que juzgan duramente tanto a los miembros como a los no miembros.

codeine - codeína: un fármaco narcótico utilizado comúnmente para suprimir la tos.

codependent - codependiente: una persona que está tan enfocada en las necesidades de otros que desatiende sus propias necesidades. También un facilitador que es miembro de una familia de, o tiene una relación cercana con, una persona adicta a una droga.

cold - resfrío: un infección de las vías respiratorias superiores.

colostrum (co -LAHS -trum) **- calostro:** una sustancia parecida a la leche rica en anticuerpos. La leche materna producida durante los primeros días posteriores al parto.

combination pill - píldora combinada: anticonceptivo oral que contiene progestina y estrógeno sintético.

comedogenic (coh -MEE -doh -JEN -ick) **- comedogénico:** que produce acné.

comfrey - consuelda: las hojas y raíces de la planta consuelda, la cual se considera, aunque no se ha demostrado, que tiene efectos similares a la droga. La consuelda contiene sustancias químicas que producen cáncer.

commitment - compromiso: una decisión que se mantiene a largo plazo. Una promesa que se cumple.

communication - comunicación: un intercambio de ideas o pensamientos.

compost - abono: una materia vegetal descompuesta utilizada como fertilizante.

compulsions - compulsiones: impulsos irresistibles de realizar actos sin sentido.

conception - concepción: la unión de un óvulo y un espermatozoide que genera un nuevo individuo.

conditioning - condicionamiento: los cientos de pequeños cambios que las células realizan en respuesta a la actividad física que hacen posible que el cuerpo esté más propenso a realizar la tarea que ha emprendido.

conflict - conflicto: una lucha u oposición entre personas, especialmente cuando las personas compiten por algo en la creencia que solamente una de ellas puede tener lo que él o ella desea, a costa de la otra.

confrontation - confrontación: un enfrentamiento. Una interacción en la cual una persona expresa sus sentimientos a otra. Si se maneja agresivamente, una confrontación puede ser una pelea destructiva. Si se maneja asertivamente, una confrontación puede ser una conversación constructiva en la cual una persona hace saber sus deseos a la otra.

congeners (CON -jen -ers) **- congénere:** ingredientes en las bebidas alcohólicas, aparte del alcohol en sí, que pueden irritar el sistema nervioso.

congenital (con -JEN -ih -tal) **- congénito:** presente desde el nacimiento.

connective tissues - tejidos conectivos: materiales de consistencia fluida, gelatinosa, fibrosa o de bandas que ligan, sostienen o protegen otros tejidos del organismo. Los tendones, cartílagos y ligamentos son tejidos conectivos.

constipation - constipación: heces duras y lentas que son de difícil evacuación, a menudo debido a una falta de fibra en la dieta.

contraception - contracepción: cualquier método para prevenir la concepción (la unión del esperma masculino con el óvulo femenino). El término control de la natalidad también se usa a menudo para referirse a lo mismo pero, técnicamente, el control de la natalidad incluye el aborto.

coping devices - elementos de afrontamiento: maneras no dañinas de manejar el estrés, tales como el desplazamiento o la ventilación.

coronary arteries - arterias coronarias: las dos arterias que suministran sangre al músculo del corazón.

coronary artery bypass surgery - cirugía de derivación coronaria: cirugía para proporcionar una ruta alterna para que la sangre pueda llegar a los tejidos del corazón, evitando pasar por una arteria coronaria obstruida.

coronary trombosis - trombosis coronaria: la obstrucción de un vaso que alimenta el músculo del corazón por un coágulo estacionario, o *trombo*.

cortex - corteza: la capa externa de un órgano. En el cerebro, la parte externa pensante - la materia gris.

CPR (cardiopulmonary resucitation) - RCP (resucitación cardiopulmonar): una técnica para mantener el flujo de la sangre y el oxígeno a través del cuerpo de una persona cuyo corazón y respiración se ha detenido.

credentials (kre -DEN -shulls) **- credenciales:** la evidencia oficial de educación u otras calificaciones por parte de una autoridad; diplomas, licencias, y similares.

critical periods - períodos críticos: los períodos durante el desarrollo cuando uno de los órganos del cuerpo se encuentra especialmente susceptible a factores dañinos. Un período crítico generalmente es un período de rápidas divisiones celulares.

critical phase - fase crítica: en arteriosclerosis, la etapa en la cual las placas cubren más de la mitad de las superficies internas de las arterias.

crowning - coronamiento: el momento en que la parte superior (corona) de la cabeza del bebé se ve por primera vez.

cruciferous vegetables - vegetales crucíferos: vegetales de la familia de la col.

cults - sectas: grupos de personas que comparten una intensa admiración o adoración por una persona o principio en particular.

cuticles - cutículas: los bordes de piel endurecida en la base de las uñas.

cyst (SIST) **- quiste:** una espinilla abultada y profunda.

D

date rape - violación por novio o conocido: agresión sexual por una persona conocida en una situación de una cita.

date - cita: la participación en eventos sociales diseñados para permitir que las personas se conozcan unos a otros. Una cita doble (dos parejas) es un arreglo seguro para las primeras citas con personas a las que uno no conoce bien.

day care - guardería diurna: supervisión, generalmente en un establecimiento, para niños en edad preescolar o adultos mayores que deben estar bajo supervisión durante las horas de trabajo diurnas.

defense mechanisms - mecanismos de defensa: formas autodestructivas de manejar el estrés. Reacciones automáticas y subconscientes ante el daño emocional, tales como la negación, la fantasía, la proyección, la racionalización, la regresión, el olvido selectivo o el aislamiento.

deficiency (dee -FISH -en -see) **- deficiencia:** la falta de un nutriente en el cuerpo. Las deficiencias severas causan enfermedades.

dehydration - deshidratación: la pérdida de agua. Los síntomas avanzan rápidamente desde la sed a la debilidad al agotamiento, la confusión e incluso la muerte.

delirium - delirio: un estado de confusión mental, generalmente con alucinaciones y movimiento continuo.

denial (dee -NIGH -al) **- negación:** el rechazo a creer los hechos de una circunstancias - por ejemplo, negar que una persona es un bebedor problema frente a evidencias claras de que lo es.

dental plaque (PLAK) **- placa dental:** la acumulación de un material pegajoso sobre la superficie de los dientes. Un antecesor del daño a los dientes.

dentin - dentina: la capa intermedia blanda del diente.

Depo-Provera (DEE-po pro-ValR-uh) **- Depo-Provera:** marca comercial de un tipo inyectable de progestina.

depression - depresión: la condición de sentirse apático, descorazonado y aislado de otros. Una depresión mayor es un estado depresivo emocionalmente incapacitante ligado a causas físicas. Podría ser, en un extremo, un estado suicida.

dermatologist - dermatólogo: un médico (M.D.) que se especializa en el tratamiento de enfermedades de la piel.

designer drugs - drogas de diseñador: drogas fabricadas en el laboratorio que se asemejan mucho a las drogas ilegales en su estructura química, pero que son lo suficientemente diferentes como para ser legales hasta que su uso se declare ilegal.

deviant - desviado: fuera del sistema normal.

diabetes (DYE -uh -BEE -teez) **mellitus** (MEL -ih -tuss) **- diabetes mellitus:** una condición de uso anormal de la glucosa, generalmente causado por muy poca insulina o la falta de respuesta a la insulina.

diabetic coma - coma diabético: la pérdida del conocimiento debido a una diabetes no controlada y el acumulamiento resultante de cetonas tóxicas en la sangre.

diaphragm - diafragma: domo que se coloca sobre la cérvix y contiene crema o jalea espermicida para bloquear el ingreso de la esperma.

diastolic (DYE -as -tol -ic) **pressure - presión diastólica:** la presión sanguínea durante la parte del latido del corazón cuando los ventrículos del corazón están relajados.

diet pills - pastillas para adelgazar: aquellos medicamentos que suprimen el apetito o de alguna manera promueven la pérdida de peso. Las pastillas que se venden sin receta generalmente contienen cafeína y otras drogas que causan más nerviosismo que pérdida de peso. La pastilla que se expenden con receta incluyen las anfetaminas.

digestion - digestión: el proceso por el cual el cuerpo convierte los alimentos en nutrientes que el cuerpo puede utilizar. El *sistema digestivo* es un conjunto de órganos en el cuerpo que procesan los alimentos y absorben sus nutrientes. (Vea el Capítulo 6 para detalles acerca del sistema.)

dilation stage - nivel de dilatación: la etapa durante el parto en que la cérvix se está abriendo.

dioxins - dioxinas: contaminantes letales que se forman cuando el cloro reacciona con otros compuestos.

disability insurance - seguro de invalidez: un seguro para reemplazar la pérdida de los ingresos si una persona estuviere incapacitada para trabajar debido a una larga enfermedad.

discipline - disciplina: la formación del comportamiento mediante recompensas y/o castigos.

disinfectants - desinfectantes: compuestos químicos que matan los microbios en la superficie. El cloro es un desinfectante.

dispatcher - despachador: una persona que contesta llamadas y transfiere mensajes al servicio de asistencia adecuado.

displacement - desplazamiento: la canalización de la energía del sufrimiento hacía otra cosa. Por ejemplo, usar la energía emocional ocasionada por un problema para realizar tareas u otras actividades habituales.

disposable - descartable: la descripción de cualquier producto que se utiliza una vez y luego se desecha.

diuretic (die -yoo -RETT -ick) **- diurético:** un fármaco que causa que el cuerpo pierda líquido. No es eficaz para la pérdida de la grasa del cuerpo.

DNA (deoxyribonucleic acid) - ADN (ácido desoxirribonucleico): el material genético de las células que sirve de programa para elaborar todas las proteínas que la célula necesita para efectuar copias exactas de sí misma.

douches - duchas: preparados que se venden para limpiar la vagina. En realidad, las vaginas se limpian a sí mismas constantemente sin ayuda. Las duchas pueden insertar bacterias peligrosas en el tracto reproductivo.

Down syndrome - síndrome de Down: una condición congénita de deformación física y retardo mental.

drink - bebida: la cantidad de una bebida que suministra _ onza de etanol puro. 12 onzas de cerveza, 3 a 4 onzas de vino, 1 (10 onzas) refresco en base a vino, o 1 onza de licor de 100 grados.

drives - impulsos: motivaciones que son innatas, no aprendidas, tales como el hambre, la sed, el miedo y la necesidad de dormir. También conocidos como *instintos*.

drug abuse - abuso de las drogas: la ingesta deliberada de una droga por un propósito no medicinal y de una forma que puede resultar en daños a la salud o habilidad de funcionar de una persona.

drug addiction (dependence) - drogadicción (dependencia): una necesidad física o psicológica de dosis cada vez mayores de una droga.

drug misuse - mal uso de una droga: el uso de un fármaco para el propósito medicinal para el cual fue diseñado, pero no en la dosis, frecuencia, concentración o forma adecuada.

drug-resistant - resistente a la droga: un término que describe los microbios que han perdido su sensibilidad a ciertos fármacos. Por ejemplo, las enfermedades causadas por bacteria resistente a la droga ya no responden a la terapia con antibióticos.

drugs - drogas: sustancias que cuando ingresan al cuerpo cambian una o más de las funciones del cuerpo.

drug synergy - sinergia farmacológica: la acción combinada de dos fármacos que es mayor que o diferente de la acción de cualquiera de las drogas por sí sola.

drug trafficker - narcotraficante: una persona que está involucrada en el transporte y venta de drogas ilegales.

drug use - uso de drogas: el uso de un fármaco para el propósito medicinal para el cual fue diseñado, en la dosis, frecuencia, concentración o forma adecuada.

DUI: que conduce bajo los efectos (del alcohol o de otras sustancias que alteran la mente). Ver *DWI*.

duration - duración: continuación en el tiempo. En los ejercicios, la cantidad de tiempo que se pasa en cada sesión de ejercicio.

DWI: que conduce en estado de intoxicación con alcohol u otras sustancias enervantes - por ley un crimen. La intoxicación se define por el nivel de alcohol en la sangre (un nivel de 0.08 por ciento en algunos estados y de 0.10 por ciento en otros estados).

dysfunctional family - familia disfuncional: una familia con formas de afrontamiento anormales o deterioradas que dañan la autoestima y la salud emocional de los miembros de la familia.

dysphoria (dis -FORE -ee -uh) **- disforia:** un sentimiento desagradable que ocurre cuando hay falta de endorfina. Estos sentimientos a menudo siguen a la euforia inducida por las drogas.

E

eating disorder - trastorno alimentario: la ingesta anormal de alimentos originado por causas emocionales y relacionado con la adicción. En la *anorexia nerviosa*, los jóvenes se privan de alimentos hasta la inanición para perder peso. En la *bulimia*, comen en exceso para después abstenerse totalmente de ellos o vomitar.

echinacea - equinacea: una hierba popular por sus supuestas propiedades "antiinfecciosas" y como un cúralo todo, especialmente para resfríos y alergias. También se le llama flor de cono.

ecosystems - ecosistemas: los sistemas de tierra, plantas y animales que han coexistido por miles o millones de años y que son interdependientes.

ectopic pregnancy - embarazo ectópico: un embarazo que se desarrolla en una de las trompas de Falopio o en otra parte fuera del útero. Una condición seria.

effective - eficaz: tener el efecto medicinal propuesto: parte de los requisitos legales para un fármaco.

effectiveness - efectividad: la efectividad con que un método o elemento anticonceptivo evita el embarazo, expresado en porcentajes. La eficacia de laboratorio es el porcentaje de mujeres protegidas del embarazo durante un período de un año bajo condiciones ideales de laboratorio. La eficacia del usuario es el porcentaje de mujeres típicas que han sido protegidas.

ejaculation - eyaculación: la expulsión de semen por el pene, ocasionado por las contracciones musculares involuntarias del orgasmo.

elasticity - elasticidad: la característica de un tejido para estirarse o doblarse y luego tener la capacidad de volver a su tamaño y forma original.

elder abuse - abuso del adulto mayor: la agresión verbal, física o sexual contra una persona de edad.

electrocardiogram - electrocardiograma: registro de la actividad eléctrica del corazón que, si es anormal, podría indicar enfermedades cardiacas.

electrolytes (ee -LECK -tro -lites) - **electrolitos**: minerales que transportan cargas eléctricas que ayudan a mantener el equilibrio de los fluidos del organismo.

embolism - embolismo: la obstrucción repentina de un vaso sanguíneo por un coágulo de sangre no estacionario, o *embolo*.

embolus (EM -bow -luss) - **émbolo:** un coágulo que se desprende y viaja a través de la corriente sanguínea. Cuando causa la obstrucción repentina de un vaso sanguíneo, a este peligroso evento se le denomina un *embolismo*.

embryo (EM -bree -oh) - **embrión:** el lactante en desarrollo durante la tercera a la octava semana posterior a la concepción.

emergency medical services (EMS) - servicios médicos de emergencias (SME): un equipo de personas entrenadas para responder a emergencias y que puede ser contactado a través de un solo despachador.

emetics (em -ETT -ics) - **emético:** drogas que provocan el vómito.

emotion - emoción: el sentimiento que ocurre en respuesta a un evento experimentado por un individuo. Algunos ejemplos son el amor, el enojo y el miedo.

emotional health - salud emocional: el estado de estar libre de trastornos mentales que limitan las funciones. También, el estado de haber desarrollado percepciones saludables hacia otras personas y eventos de la vida, basado en el pensamiento, las emociones y los valores. También denominado *salud mental*.

emotional intelligence (EQ) - inteligencia emocional (CE): la capacidad de reconocer y expresar apropiadamente nuestras emociones en una manera que mejora la vida.

emotional problems - problemas emocionales: los modelos de comportamiento o pensamiento que causan que una persona sienta un dolor emocional de importancia o sea incapaz de funcionar en cualquiera o más de tres áreas importantes - las relaciones sociales o familiares, el trabajo (incluyendo el desempeño escolar) o la utilización del tiempo libre.

emphysema (em -fih -ZEE -muh) - **enfisema:** una enfermedad de los pulmones en la cual muchos de los pequeños y flexibles sacos de aire se revientan y forman algunas bolsas de aire grandes y rígidas.

empty calories - calorías vacías: un término popular para designar a los alimentos que aportan mucha energía (calorías) y pocos nutrientes.

enable - facilitar: hacer posible. En la adicción significa "ayudar" para tratar de "salvar" a la persona adicta de las consecuencias de su comportamiento. Esto facilita el abuso prolongado del alcohol y de otras drogas. Un facilitador es una persona que en realidad causa un daño a la persona en dificultades al respaldar su actitud o conducta autodestructiva.

enabling - facilitar: "ayuda" mal guiada.

enamel - esmalte: la capa dura exterior del diente.

endorphins - endorfínas: los elementos químicos del cerebro que producen sentimientos de placer en respuesta a una serie de actividades.

energy - energía: la capacidad de trabajar o producir calor.

engorgement - congestionamiento: hinchazón, respecto a la respuesta sexual, el órgano sexual se inunda de sangre en preparación al orgasmo.

environment - ambiente: todo lo que queda "fuera" de los organismos vivientes - el aire, agua, suelo, otros organismos y formas de radiación.

environmental tobacco smoke (ETS) - humo ambiental de tabaco: la combinación del humo principal exhalado y el humo indirecto que ingresa al aire y que podría ser inhalado por otras personas.

ephedrine - efedrina: un estimulante que se agrega a las pastillas para adelgazar y que se encuentra en yerbas tales como el ma huang. Ha sido causa de ataques al corazón, derrames cerebrales, convulsiones y muerte, especialmente en combinación con la cafeína.

epidemic (EP -ih -DEM -ick) - **epidemia:** una infección que se esparce rápidamente a través de la población, afectando a muchas personas a la vez.

epinephrine (EP -uh -NEFF -rin) - **epinefrina:** una de las hormonas del estrés, también denominada *adrenalina*.

episiotomy (eh -PEEZ -ee -OT -oh -me) - **episiotomía:** un corte quirúrgico hecho en la vagina durante el parto cuando la vagina no puede expandirse lo suficiente sin desgarrarse para permitir el paso del bebé.

erection - erección: el estado en el cual un tejido generalmente blando, cuando se llena de sangre y se pone firme. Tanto el pene y el clítoris pueden estar erectos.

ergogenic (ER -go -JEN -ick) - **ergogénico:** término que afirma significar que "realza el trabajo". De hecho, ningún producto puede realzar la habilidad de trabajar."

essential amino acids - aminoácidos esenciales: aminoácidos necesarios pero que no pueden ser elaborados por el organismo, deben ser suministrados por los alimentos.

estrogen - estrógeno: una hormona que, en la mujer, regula el ciclo de ovulación.

ethanol (ethyl alcohol) - etanol (alcohol etílico): ver *alcohol*.

ethics - ética: los principios morales o valores.

euphoria (you -FORE -ee -uh) **- euforia:** una sensación de inmenso bienestar y placer que dan ciertas drogas; popularmente llamadas estimulantes [high].

euthanasia (you -than -AY -zee -uh) **- eutanasia:** permitir que una persona muera al elegir no utilizar equipos de soporte vital, tales como respiradores artificiales, o el retiro de los equipos de soporte vital de un paciente que no tiene esperanzas de recuperación. Ambas podrían ser legales en ciertos casos.

excitement - excitación: se utiliza para describir una fase del coito, la fase inicial.

exercise physiology - fisiología del ejercicio: el estudio del funcionamiento y los cambios experimentados por el cuerpo en respuesta al ejercicio. Un laboratorio de fisiología del ejercicio cuenta con equipos para medir los componentes del estado físico y otras mediciones.

exhaustion - agotamiento: la tercera etapa dañina de la respuesta al estrés, en la cual el estrés excede la capacidad del organismo para recuperarse.

expulsion stage - fase de expulsión: la fase, durante el parto en la cual las contracciones uterinas impulsan al lactante a través del canal del parto.

extended family - familia ampliada: una familia compuesta por los padres, hijos y otros parientes, tales como abuelos o tíos y tías. Los parientes pueden vivir en una casa o pueden vivir cerca y comparten las responsabilidades, tales como la crianza de los niños.

external pressures - presiones externas: en lo referente a los sentimientos sexuales, los mensajes provenientes de la sociedad, los pares y otros, que presiona a las personas a tener relaciones sexuales.

F

false labor - parto falso: las contracciones preliminares experimentadas por muchas mujeres antes de que se inicie el trabajo de parto.

family - familia: un grupo de personas que se relacionan entre sí por adopción, sangre o matrimonio y están comprometidas entre sí, especialmente un padre, una madre y sus hijos. Todos los parientes consanguíneos y antepasados de una familia.

family identity - identidad familiar: un sentido único de pertenecer juntos como una unidad, distintos y diferentes de otras personas o grupos.

fat - grasa: una clase de nutrientes que no se mezclan con el agua. La grasa está compuesta principalmente de ácidos grasos, los cuales suministran energía al cuerpo. Técnicamente se les denomina *lípidos*.

fatfold caliper - calibre de pliegue de grasa: un tipo de pinza que mide la grasa del cuerpo bajo la piel.

fatfold test - prueba del pliegue de grasa: una prueba de la grasa del cuerpo realizada con un *calibre de pliegue de grasa*.

fat-soluble (SOL -you -bul) **- soluble en grasa:** el término químico que significa "capaz de disolverse en grasa."

fatty acids - ácidos grasos: formas simples de grasa que suministran energía calórica a la mayoría de las células del cuerpo.

fee-for-service system - sistema de pago por visita: el sistema para el pago de los servicios de salud en el cual los clientes pagan tarifas individuales por los servicios que reciben.

female condom - condón femenino: un tubo de plástico suave y delgado con dos anillos en los extremos - uno que encaja sobre la cérvix y uno que sirve como ancla fuera de la entrada a la vagina; también se le denomina como una bolsa vaginal.

femininity - femineidad: las características, incluyendo características biológicas y sociales, asociadas con el hecho de ser mujer.

fertility awareness method - método de conciencia fértil: un método de graficar la ovulación. Involucra el seguimiento de los períodos menstruales, temperatura corporal y tipos de mucosa cervical. También se le refiere como método del calendario.

fertilization - fertilización: la unión de un óvulo con un espermatozoide.

fetal alcohol effect (FAE) - efecto de alcoholismo fetal (EAF): una versión más sutil del síndrome de alcoholismo fetal (SAF), con efectos ocultos, incluyendo discapacidad de aprendizaje, anormalidades del comportamiento y deficiencias motoras.

fetal alcohol syndrome (FAS) - síndrome de alcoholismo fetal (SAF): un grupo de defectos de nacimiento, incluyendo el retardo mental y físico permanente y las anormalidades faciales, que se observa en niños cuyas madres han abusado del alcohol durante el embarazo.

fetus (FEET -us) **- feto:** el lactante en desarrollo desde la novena semana posterior a la concepción hasta el nacimiento.

feud - enemistad: una amarga y continua hostilidad, que a menudo involucra a grupos de personas.

fiber - fibra: sustancias no digeribles en los alimentos, compuestos generalmente de carbohidratos.

fibrillation (FIH -brill -AY -shun) **- fibrilación:** contracciones extremadamente rápidas del corazón que no tienen la fuerza para bombear la sangre a lo largo del cuerpo.

fight-or-flight reaction - reacción pelear o huir: la respuesta del organismo a un peligro físico inmediato, la respuesta al estrés. La energía se moviliza, ya sea para montar una respuesta agresiva contra el peligro o para huir de éste.

first aid - primeros auxilios: en inglés, significa literalmente "ayuda brindada primero" - asistencia médica dada de inmediato en una situación de emergencia, antes que la víctima sea transportada a un hospital o centro de tratamiento.

fitness - estado físico: las características del cuerpo que le permiten realizar actividad física para satisfacer las exigencias físicas con suficiente energía de reserva para enfrentar desafíos súbitos y para soportar estrés de todo tipo.

flexibility - flexibilidad: un componente del estado físico; la habilidad de flectar las articulaciones sin sufrir daños.

flu - gripe: abreviación de **influenza** (in -flew -EN -za), una infección respiratoria altamente contagiosa causada por una variedad de virus.

folk medicine - medicina popular: el uso de hierbas y otras sustancias naturales en el tratamiento de enfermedades practicada por personas de distintas regiones.

follicles - folículos: estructuras de la piel similares a vasos que contienen las glándulas sebáceas, los músculos que controlan el movimiento del cabello (y también la piel de gallina) y las raíces del cabello.

food chain - cadena alimenticia: la secuencia en que los elementos vivientes dependen de otros elementos vivientes para alimentarse. Las algas están cerca de la base y los seres humanos en la cima de ella.

foreplay - estimulación erótica: una actividad en la cual cada pareja da placer a la otra antes del coito.

formaldehyde - formaldehído: una sustancia relacionada con el alcohol. El formaldehído es elaborado por el organismo con el alcohol y contribuye al malestar posterior al estado de ebriedad.

fossil fuel - combustible fósil: el carbón, el petróleo y el gas natural, todos provienen de los restos fosilizados de la vida vegetal de tiempos pretéritos.

foster family - familia sustituta: una familia creada cuando una agencia gubernamental coloca a un niño bajo el cuidado temporal de un adulto o una pareja. Los padres del niño pueden haber fallecido o por algún motivo no pueden cuidar del niño.

foxglove - dedalera: una planta que contiene una sustancia utilizada en digoxin, la medicina para el corazón.

fracture - fractura: una fisura en un hueso. Una *fractura abierta* es una fisura con una herida en los tejidos sobrepuestos. Una *fractura cerrada* es un quiebre o fisura sin una herida visible.

free radicals - radicales libres: sustancias químicas que causan daño a los tejidos del organismo iniciando destructivas cadenas en reacción en las moléculas de las células del organismo. Se considera que dichas reacciones gatillan o empeoran algunas enfermedades.

frequency - frecuencia: el número de unidades de actividad por unidad de tiempo (por ejemplo, el número de sesiones de ejercicio por semana).

frostbite - congelación: la formación de cristales de hielo en partes del cuerpo expuestas a temperaturas por debajo del nivel de congelación. La congelación de las partes del cuerpo, especialmente los dedos de los pies y de las manos y la nariz y otras partes de la cara.

fungi - hongos: seres vivientes que absorben y utilizan los nutrientes de los organismos que invaden. Los hongos que causan enfermedades incluyen la *levadura* y el *moho*.

G

gangs - pandillas: Grupos de pares que tienen como objetivo principal expresar su agresión hacia otros grupos.

gateway drug - droga de entrada: una droga cuyo abuso es probable que conduzca al abuso de otras drogas más potentes y peligrosas. El alcohol, la marihuana y el tabaco son las que más a menudo se nombran como drogas de entrada.

gay - homosexual: término general que se refiere a la homosexualidad, pero a menudo en referencia a hombres homosexuales.

gender - género: la clasificación de ser masculino o femenino.

gender identity - identidad de género: esa parte de la autoimagen de una persona que está determinada por el sexo de la misma.

gender roles - roles de género: los roles asignados por la sociedad a personas de cada sexo.

generic (jeh -NEHR -ick) **names - nombres genéricos:** los nombres químicos de las drogas en contraposición a los nombres de marca comercial; los nombres que todo el mundo puede usar.

genes (JEENZ) **- genes:** unidades de herencia de una célula que dirigen la elaboración del equipo que ejecuta el trabajo de una célula.

genetic counselor - consejero genético: un consejero que predice y aconseja sobre la posibilidad de la ocurrencia de defectos congénitos en una familia.

genetic engineering - ingeniería genética: la ciencia que manipula los genes de seres vivientes con el objetivo de introducir alguna característica deseable que no está presente en el organismo original. Un ejemplo es un tomate al que se le introduce un gene para retrasar la descomposición.

genital herpes (HER -peez) **- herpes genital:** una enfermedad venérea común incurable causada por un virus que produce ampollas. Los síntomas desaparecen por sí solos, pero el virus queda para causar nuevos brotes.

genital warts - verrugas genitales: formaciones contagiosas similares a las verrugas en las áreas infectadas, causadas por el virus humano papiloma. A veces se les llama *condiloma* (con -di -LOW -ma). Los virus que causan las verrugas genitales también pueden causar cáncer cervical en la mujer.

gestation (jes -TAY -shun) **- gestación:** el período comprendido desde la concepción hasta el nacimiento. En los seres humanos normalmente dura entre 38 a 42 semanas.

ginseng (JIN -seng) **- ginseng:** una planta que contiene sustancias químicas que tienen efectos enervantes.

ginseng abuse syndrome - síndrome del abuso del ginseng: el conjunto de síntomas asociados con el abuso del ginseng, incluyen presión arterial alta, insomnio, nerviosismo, confusión y depresión.

gland - glándula: un órgano del cuerpo que secreta una o más hormonas.

global warming - calentamiento global: el calentamiento del planeta, una tendencia que amenaza la vida sobre la tierra.

glucose - glucosa: el azúcar de la sangre en el cuerpo, una forma simple de carbohidrato.

glycogen - glicógeno: la forma en que el hígado y los músculos almacenan la glucosa.

gonorrea - gonorreha (gon -oh -REE -uh): una enfermedad bacteriana de transmisión sexual que a menudo avanza hasta extenderse por todo el cuerpo sin presentar síntomas, causado problemas en muchos órganos.

grams (abreviado **g**) **- gramos:** la unidad de peso con la cual se miden muchos de los nutrientes. 28 gramos equivalen a 1 onza.

greenhouse effect - efecto invernadero: el efecto de conservación del calor efectuado por el vidrio de un invernadero. El mismo efecto es ocasionado por los gases que se están acumulando en la atmósfera externa de la Tierra, los que están atrapando el calor del sol y calentando el planeta.

grieve - lamentar: sentir un profundo dolor y sufrimiento emocional por una pérdida.

guilt - culpabilidad: el sentimiento normal que surge de la conciencia cuando una persona actúa en contra de sus valores internos ("hice algo malo").

gum disease - enfermedad de las encías: inflamación y degeneración del tejido rosado (encías) que está fijado a los dientes y ayuda a mantenerlos en su lugar.

gynecologist - ginecólogo: especialista en el cuidado del sistema reproductivo femenino.

H

hallucinations - alucinaciones: falsas percepciones, imaginación de visiones, sonidos, olores, u otros sentimientos, a veces ocasionados por el abuso de las drogas, a veces por enfermedades mentales o físicas.

hallucinogens (hal -LOO -sin -oh -jens) **- alucinógenos:** drogas que pueden causar visiones y otras ilusiones sensoriales.

head lice - piojos: parásitos blancos pequeñísimos, pero visibles, que se introducen en las áreas de la piel o del cabello.

head restraints - apoyo para la cabeza: asientos con respaldos altos u otros artefactos fijados a los asientos de los automóviles al nivel de la cabeza. Los apoyos para la cabeza evitan que la cabeza de la persona se incline demasiado hacía atrás cuando el cuerpo es propulsado hacía atrás. De esa manera evita los daños a la nuca y a la médula espinal.

health - salud: rango de estados con componentes físicos, mentales, emocionales, espirituales y sociales. En su grado mínimo, significa libre de enfermedades físicas, condiciones físicas deficientes, desajuste social y otros estados negativos. En su grado máximo, significa "saludable".

health care system - sistema de atención de salud: el conjunto de todos los proveedores de atención a la salud y centros de atención médica que trabajan unidos para dar atención médica a la población.

health maintenance organization (HMO) - organización de mantenimiento de la salud: un grupo de médicos que trabajan juntos y que tratan los problemas de salud de otras personas bajo un plan de prepagos.

heart attack - ataque al corazón: el evento en el cual los vasos que alimentan el músculo del corazón se obstruyen, causando la muerte del tejido.

heart disease - enfermedad cardíaca: cualquier enfermedad del músculo del corazón o de las otras partes funcionales del corazón.

heart murmur - murmullo cardíaco: un sonido del corazón que refleja que las válvulas del corazón están dañadas o anormales.

heart transplant - transplante de corazón: el reemplazo quirúrgico de un corazón enfermo por uno saludable.

heat exhaustion - agotamiento por calor: una seria etapa del sobre calentamiento que puede resultar en un golpe de calor.

heat stroke - golpe de calor: una condición que amenaza la vida y que resulta como consecuencia de una acumulación de la temperatura corporal. Esta condición puede ser fatal.

Heimlich (HIME -lick) **Maneuver (abdominal thrust maneuver) - Maniobra de Heimlich (maniobra de expulsión abdominal):** una técnica usada para desalojar lo que obstruye el conducto de aire de una persona. La Maniobra de Heimlich lleva el nombre del médico que la inventó.

hemlock - cicuta: cualquier parte de la planta cicuta, la cual causa dolores severos, convulsiones y la muerte dentro de un plazo de 15 minutos.

hemorrhoids - hemorroides: venas rectales dolorosamente hinchadas, frecuentemente como resultado de la constipación.

hepatitis - hepatitis: una enfermedad del hígado causada por uno de varios virus transmitidos por agujas infectadas (uso de drogas, tatuajes, transfusiones de sangre), por comer mariscos crudos provenientes de aguas contaminadas y por cualquier contacto (incluyendo contacto sexual) con las secreciones corporales de personas infectadas.

hepatitis B - hepatitis B: una enfermedad viral transmisible por contacto sexual que ocasiona la pérdida de las funciones del hígado y enfermedad severa del hígado. La hepatitis B se puede prevenir pero no se puede curar.

herbal medicine - medicina de hierbas: el uso de plantas para curar enfermedades y mejorar la salud.

herbs - hierbas: plantas no leñosas o partes de plantas valorizadas por su sabor, aroma o cualidades medicinales.

heroin - heroína: una droga narcótica obtenida de la morfina.

heterosexual - heterosexual: atracción sexual por miembros del sexo opuesto.

hierarchy - jerarquía: un sistema de clasificación en el cual cada cosa está colocada sobre o debajo de otras.

high-density lipoproteins (HDLs) - lipoproteínas de alta densidad (HDL): las lipoproteínas que transportan grasa y colesterol desde los tejidos (y desde las placas) hacía el hígado para su descomposición y eliminación del organismo.

high risk pregnancy - embarazo de alto riesgo: un embarazo con mayores probabilidades que otros de sufrir complicaciones, tales como un parto prematuro (antes de la 38ª semana de gestación), o un bajo peso de nacimiento. Muchos factores contribuyen a los riesgos del embarazo.

histamine (HIST -uh -meen) **- histamina:** una sustancia química de la respuesta inmunitaria que produce inflamación (hinchazón e irritación) de los tejidos.

history (medical) - historia (médica): una entrevista en la cual un profesional de los servicios de salud interroga sobre experiencia médica en el pasado.

HIV - VIH: abreviación de *virus de inmunodeficiencia humana*, el virus que causa el SIDA.

Hodgkin's disease - enfermedad de Hodgkin: un linfoma que ataca a las personas de temprana edad y es tratable con radioterapia.

homeopathic (home -ee -OP -ah -thick) **medicine - medicina homeopática:** medicina que se practica basado en la teoría que "lo semejante cura lo semejante " - esto es, que las sustancias que causan síntomas en gente saludable pueden curar esos síntomas cuando se dan en cantidades muy diluidas (homeo = igual, pathos = sufrimiento).

homeostasis (HOH -me -oh -STAY -sis) **- homeostasis:** el mantenimiento de un medio ambiente estable dentro del organismo que se logra cuando los sistemas corpóreos se adaptan a condiciones cambiantes.

homophobia - homofobia: temor irracional y odio de los homosexuales, generalmente basado en el temor de contraer SIDA o de convertirse en homosexual.

homosexual - homosexual: atracción sexual por miembros del mismo sexo.

hormonal system - sistema hormonal: el sistema de glándulas - los órganos que envían y reciben mensajes químicos transportados por la sangre - que controlan las funciones del organismo en cooperación con el sistema nervioso.

hormone - hormona: una sustancia química que sirve como mensajero. Cada hormona es secretada por una glándula y viaja hacía uno o más órganos objetivo, donde produce respuestas.

hospice (HOS -pis) **- hospicio:** un sistema de apoyo para personas en estado terminal y a sus familias, que ayuda a la familia para que deje que la persona muera en su hogar con dignidad y comodidad.

hospital infections - infección intrahospitalaria: las enfermedades infecciosas adquiridas durante una hospitalización.

hospitalization insurance - seguro de hospitalización: seguro que paga el costo de una estadía en el hospital. Ver también *Medicare* y *Medicaid*.

hot flashes - bochornos: sensación transitoria y súbita que se siente por todo el cuerpo, un síntoma relacionado con la dilatación de los vasos sanguíneos en la piel, lo cual es común durante la transición hacia la menopausia.

human growth hormone - hormona humana del crecimiento: una hormona no esteroide producida en el cuerpo que promueve el crecimiento. Es utilizada como droga por algunos atletas para aumentar el crecimiento muscular. También denominada *somatotroprina*.

human papilloma virus (HPV) - virus del papiloma humano: cualquiera de más de 50 virus cuyos efectos incluyen las verrugas genitales y el cáncer cervical. Los miembros de esta familia de virus también pueden causar verrugas en la piel, comúnmente se encuentran en el área de las manos.

hunger - hambre: la necesidad psicológica de comer, experimentada como un impulso de obtener alimento. Una sensación desagradable que exige alivio.

hyperactivity - hiperactividad: una condición de actividad excesiva. Se manifiesta en los niños por una constante intranquilidad, conversación, movimiento, treparse, etc. En los adolescentes y adultos toma la forma de sentimientos de intranquilidad y dificultad para sentarse tranquilo.

hypertension - hipertensión: presión arterial alta.

hyperthermia - hipertermia (*hiper* significa "demasiado alto", *termia* significa "temperatura")**:** una condición de demasiado calor corporal con una temperatura corporal interna anormalmente alta.

hypothalamus (high -po -THALL -uh -mus) **- hipotálamo:** un centro regulador del cerebro.

hypnotherapy - hipnoterapia: el uso de la hipnosis y el poder de la sugestión para cambiar comportamientos, aliviar el dolor y curar.

hypothermia - hipotermia (*hipo* significa "demasiado bajo", *termia* significa "temperatura")**:** una condición de muy poco calor corporal con una temperatura corporal interna anormalmente baja.

hysterectomy - histerectomía: remoción del útero, una operación realizada con más frecuencia de lo necesario.

I

ibuprofen (EYE -byoo -PRO -fen) **- ibuprofen:** un fármaco que alivia la fiebre, el dolor y la inflamación.

inmune system - sistema inmunológico: las células, tejidos y órganos que protegen al cuerpo de las enfermedades. El sistema inmunológico está compuesto por glóbulos blancos, médula ósea, la glándula timo, el bazo y otras partes.

immunity - inmunidad: la capacidad del organismo para identificar, destruir y eliminar los agentes que causan enfermedades.

immunization - inmunización: una dosis inyectada u oral de medicina que estimula el sistema inmunológico para desarrollar la habilidad a largo plazo de combatir rápidamente las enfermedades infecciosas; también denominada *vacuna*.

implantation - implantación: la inserción de un óvulo fertilizado en la pared del útero.

impulse control - control de los impulsos: la habilidad de esperar y pensar antes de actuar o hablar.

inactive ingredients - ingredientes inactivos: los ingredientes que dan a una medicina cualidades distintas a los efectos medicinales. Por ejemplo, se pueden mezclar ceras y aceites con una medicina que será utilizada en la piel; se pueden agregar agua, colorantes y sabores a medicinas líquidas que se ingerirán por vía oral.

inert - inerte: no activo.

infatuation - infatuación: el estado de dejarse llevar completamente por una pasión o atracción irracional; amor adictivo.

infectious diseases - enfermedades infecciosas: una enfermedad causada y transmitida de persona a persona, por microorganismos o por sus toxinas. También denominadas *enfermedades contagiosas* o *transmisibles* o simplemente *infecciones*.

infectious mononucleosis (MON -oh -new -klee -OH -sis) **- mononucleosis infecciosa:** una infección viral que involucra mononucleocitos, un tipo de glóbulo blanco. Los síntomas varían desde les síntomas parecidos al resfrío a fiebres altas, glándulas inflamadas y compromiso del bazo y el hígado. También denominada *mono*.

inflamation - inflamación: el dolor e hinchazón causada por la irritación.

initiator - iniciador: un carcinógeno, agente necesario para iniciar la formación del cáncer.

insomnia (in -SOM -nee -uh) **- insomnio:** anormalidades del sueño, incluyendo dificultad para conciliar el sueño y desvelo durante la noche.

insulin shock - shock insulínico: el resultado de demasiada insulina, lo cual causa una peligrosa caída del nivel de glucosa en la sangre. También llamada *hipoglicemia*.

insulin - insulina: una hormona producida por el páncreas y liberada en respuesta a un aumento en el nivel de glucosa en la sangre después de una comida. La insulina promueve el uso y almacenaje de glucosa por los tejidos del organismo.

intensity - intensidad: el grado de esfuerzo mientras se ejecuta un ejercicio. (por ejemplo, trotar requiere más esfuerzo que caminar y por lo tanto es más intensivo).

internal pressures - presiones internas: Con respecto a los sentimientos sexuales, los impulsos biológicos internos de una persona que la impulsa a tener relaciones sexuales.

internship - internado: el período de aprendizaje pasado en un establecimiento médico como parte del entrenamiento de los que suministran los cuidados de la salud.

intimacy - intimidad: estado de cercanía o proximidad, como en las relaciones que involucra el compartir lo privado y lo personal.

intoxication - intoxicación: literalmente, se refiere al estado de envenenamiento; a menudo se usa para referirse al estado de ebriedad.

intrauterine device (IUD) – dispositivo intrauterino(DIU): elemento que se inserta en el útero para prevenir la concepción o implantación.

intravenous (IV) drug abuse - abuso de drogas intravenoso (IV): la práctica de utilizar agujas para inyectar drogas de abuso en las venas. (La palabra *intravenosa* significa "en la vena").

irradiation - irradiación: radiación ionizante aplicada a los alimentos para destruir los microorganismos y otras pestes. La radiación ionizante interrumpe el funcionamiento molecular interno de las células, y las destruye.

J

jock-itch - prurito del jockey: una infección fúngica de la ingle y el muslo interno. No es una enfermedad transmitida por contacto sexual.

juvenile - menor de edad: término legal que significa que una persona es menor de 18 años de edad; un menor de edad. Los crímenes cometidos por los menores de edad generalmente se castigan de acuerdo al fallo de la corte juvenil y a menudo no por los estándares de los adultos.

K

Kaposi's (cap -OH -zeez) **sarcoma - sarcoma de Kaposi:** una rara forma de cáncer de la piel que causa una decoloración púrpura de la piel, observado con frecuencia entre aquellas personas que padecen de SIDA:

keratin - queratina: la proteína normal del cabello y las uñas.

ketones - cetonas: fragmentos formados por los tejidos durante el uso incompleto de grasa para obtener energía, que son finalmente liberados en la sangre.

ketoprofen (KEE -toe -PRO -fen) - **ketoprofeno:** un fármaco que alivia la fiebre, el dolor y la inflamación. El tamaño pequeño de la píldora facilita la ingesta para aquellos que tienen problemas para ingerir píldoras de tamaño normal.

Kyoto Protocol (kee -OH -toe pro -toe -call) - **Protocolo de Kyoto:** acuerdo firmado por muchos de los líderes mundiales en 1997, que fija el grado de reducción de las emisiones de monóxido de carbono en cada nación para el año 2012. *Kyoto* es una ciudad en Japón en la cual los líderes se reunieron para redactar el acuerdo. *Protocolo* significa primer borrador de un acuerdo.

L

labor - trabajo de parto: las contracciones del útero de intensidad suficiente como para impulsar el feto a través de la vagina para su nacimiento.

lactation - lactación: la producción de leche por las glándulas mamarias en las mamas para el propósito de alimentar a los bebés.

lapses - lapsos: períodos de retroceso a hábitos antiguos, parte normal de los procesos de pérdida o aumento de peso y mantenimiento de este.

latent - latente: temporalmente oculto o inactivo.

learning disorder - trastorno del aprendizaje: cualquiera de una variedad de disfunciones nerviosas o cerebrales que interfieren con el aprendizaje normal, que se cree afecta a 2 de 3 niños de cada curso de 30. Los desórdenes pueden afectar la atención, memoria, lenguaje, habilidades de organización, habilidades de solución de problemas, de conciencia social y otros aspectos del aprendizaje.

lesbian - lesbiana: término utilizado para referirse a las mujeres homosexuales.

lethal dose - dosis letal: la cantidad de droga necesaria para producir la muerte.

leukemias (loo -KEE -me -ahs) - **leucemias:** tipos de cáncer que surgen en los tejidos que fabrican glóbulos rojos.

leukoplakia (loo -koh -PLAKE -ee -uh) - **leucoplaquia:** unas manchas blancuzcas o grisáceas que se desarrollan en las bocas de los consumidores de tabaco y que pueden terminar en cáncer.

life expectancy - expectativa de vida: el número promedio de años vividos por la gente en una sociedad en particular.

life management skills - habilidades para administrar la vida: las habilidades que ayudan a una persona a realizar sus potenciales de bienestar y disfrutar de la vida.

life span - duración de vida: el número máximo de años que un ser humano puede llegar a vivir.

life-support systems - sistemas de soporte vital: término utilizado para referirse a los medios mecánicos utilizados para prolongar la vida, tales como la alimentación suministrada por una vena central o máquinas que fuerzan aire a los pulmones (respiradores artificiales).

lifestyle choices - opciones de estilo de vida: las opciones tomadas diariamente sobre como tratar el cuerpo y la mente. Algunos ejemplos de estas opciones se refieren a que comer, cuando ejercitarse, y si consumir alcohol u otras drogas.

lifestyle diseases - enfermedades de estilo de vida: aquellas enfermedades que se hacen posibles por descuido del organismo. No se pueden transmitir de una persona a otra. Algunos ejemplos son las enfermedades cardíacas, el cáncer y la diabetes. Las opciones de estilo de vida que promueven la salud pueden ayudar a evitar enfermedades de estilo de vida.

lightening - liviandad: la sensación que una mujer embarazada experimenta cuando el feto se asienta en la posición de nacimiento.

lipoproteins (LIP -oh -PRO -teens) - **lipoproteínas:** grupos de proteínas y grasa que transportan grasa a la sangre.

living will - testamento vital: testamento en que se declara los deseos de una persona respecto del tratamiento en caso de que la persona se encuentre incapacitada para tomar decisiones (por ejemplo en el evento de muerte cerebral).

longevity - longevidad: la duración de vida de un individuo.

look-alikes - similares: combinaciones de fármacos de venta sin receta y otras sustancias químicas envasadas para parecer medicinas de prescripción o drogas ilegales.

love - amor: afecto, **apego, devoción.**

low birthweight - bajo peso de nacimiento: un peso al nacer de menos de 5 _ libras (2,500 gramos) se utiliza como presagio de salud deficiente para el lactante recién nacido.

low-density lipoproteins (LDLs) - lipoproteínas de baja densidad (LDL): lipoproteínas que transportan grasa y colesterol desde el hígado, donde se fabrican, a los tejidos donde se utilizan. Los LDL también depositan colesterol en las arterias, formando placas.

low-impact aerobic dance - danza aeróbica de bajo impacto: una danza aeróbica en la cual un pie se mantiene en el piso para evitar shock sobre la parte inferior del cuerpo.

LSD (lysergic acid diethylamide) - LSD: una poderosa droga alucinógena. Conocida también como *ácido*.

Lyme disease - enfermedad de Lyme: una infección bacteriana propagada por pequeñas garrapatas de venados.

lymph - linfa: el líquido transparente que baña cada célula y transfiere sustancias necesarias y desechos en una y otra dirección entre la sangre y las células. La linfa también cumple un papel en la inmunidad.

lymphocytes (LIM -fo -sites) **- linfocitos:** glóbulos blancos, que participan activamente en la inmunidad.

limphomas (limf -OH -mahs) **- linfomas:** tipo de cáncer que surge en los órganos del sistema inmunológico.

M

ma huang - mahuang: un preparado de hierbas que se vende con la promesa de que promueve la pérdida de peso y que aumenta la energía, pero que contiene efedrina, un peligroso estimulante cardíaco.

mainstream smoke - humo principal: el humo que fluye a través del cigarrillo hasta los pulmones cuando el fumador inhala.

major medical insurance - seguro de enfermedades catastróficas: un seguro para pagar cuentas onerosas que no son cubiertas por otros tipos de seguros.

male condom - condón masculino: funda que cubre el pene durante el coito para retener el semen, prevenir el embarazo, y/o reducir los riesgos de enfermedades de transmisión sexual. A los condones también se les llama preservativos.

male menopause - menopausia masculina: la reducción gradual en la fertilidad masculina debido a una edad avanzada.

malignancy - malignidad: un peligroso tumor canceroso que desprende células en los fluidos corporales y se esparce a nuevas ubicaciones para iniciar nuevas colonias cancerosas. (La palabra *malignidad* significa "empeorando").

malnutrition - malnutrición: los resultados en el organismo de una nutrición deficiente, desnutrición, sobre nutrición, o cualquier deficiencia de nutrientes.

malpractice insurance - seguro de negligencia: un seguro que protege a los prestadores de servicios de salud de las querellas presentadas por personas que afirman que han sido damnificadas por el prestador de servicios de salud.

mammogram - mamograma: radiografía de la mama, una prueba de descarte para el cáncer.

managed care - salud administrada: un sistema que ofrece servicios de salud, en base a un sistema de prepagos. Al enfatizar los cuidados preventivos, controlar los honorarios de los médicos, e investigar las solicitudes para pruebas y procedimientos costosos, se ha logrado un control de los costos de las prestaciones de servicios de salud.

marriage - matrimonio: la institución que une a un hombre y a una mujer por medio de un contrato con el propósito de crear y preservar una familia.

married couple - pareja de casados: una familia que consiste de dos adultos casados.

masculinity - masculinidad: las características, incluyendo las biológicas y sociales, asociadas con el sexo masculino.

massage therapy - terapia de masaje: un método de dar masajes a los músculos para reducir la tensión, ayudar a la circulación de la sangre, y mejorar la movilidad de las articulaciones, que se cree, promueve la curación.

masturbation - masturbación: estimulación de sus propios genitales, generalmente hasta alcanzar el orgasmo.

mature love - amor maduro: un fuerte afecto, apego profundo y perdurable hacia una persona cuyo carácter el compañero conoce bien.

measles - sarampión: una enfermedad viral altamente contagiosa caracterizada por erupciones cutáneas, fiebre alta, fotosensibilidad, tos y síntomas de resfrío. Se puede prevenir mediante la inmunización.

mediator - mediador: una tercera persona neutral que ayuda a dos personas en conflicto a comunicarse más efectivamente.

Medicaid - Medicaid: un seguro de hospitalización y de cirugía para personas que califican como necesitadas.

medical insurance - seguro de salud: Un tipo de seguro que paga los honorarios de los médicos, las tarifas de laboratorio, y los costos de las medicinas con prescripción.

Medicare - Medicare: un seguro de hospitalización para personas que reciben el Seguro Social.

medicines - medicamentos: drogas utilizadas para ayudar a curar enfermedades, disminuir la gravedad de la enfermedad, aliviar los síntomas, evitar la enfermedad, ayudar con su diagnosis, o producir otros efectos deseados.

melanin (MELL -eh -nin) **- melanina:** el pigmento protector de la piel responsable por el color bronceado, marrón o negro de la piel humana. Se produce en abundancia bajo la exposición a la radiación ultravioleta.

melanoma - melanoma: un cáncer especialmente peligroso de las células pigmentadas de la piel, relacionado con la exposición al sol por personas de piel clara.

melatonin - melatonina: hormona producida por una glándula del cerebro que se considera ayuda a regular los ritmos diarios del organismo. Las afirmaciones que alarga la vida o que aumenta el poder sexual no tienen fundamento. No existe prueba de la seguridad o efectividad de la melatonina.

menopause - menopausia: los años en que se detiene la ovulación y menstruación en la mujer.

menstrual cramps - calambres menstruales: las contracciones del útero, durante y unos días antes de la menstruación que pueden causar dolores.

menstrual cycle - ciclo menstrual: la maduración cíclica de un óvulo y la preparación del útero para el embarazo. También denominado el ciclo ovulatorio.

menstruation - menstruación: la descarga mensual del endómetro del útero en mujeres no embarazadas.

mentor - mentor: una persona sabia que da consejos y ayuda.

mescaline - mezcalina: el alucinógeno producido por el cacto peyote.

metastasized (meh -TASS -tuh -sized) **- metastizado:** al referirse a las células cancerígenas, término utilizado para indicar que las células cancerígenas han migrado desde una parte del cuerpo hacia otra y han iniciado nuevos tumores iguales al tumor original.

methadone - metadona: una droga usada para tratar la adicción a la heroína, que detiene el aislamiento y ayuda a las personas a recuperarse socialmente.

microbes - microbios: pequeños organismos, tales como bacteria, levadura y virus que son demasiado pequeños para ser observados a simple vista. También se les llama *microorganismos*.

minerals - minerales: elementos de la tierra necesarios en la dieta, que ejecutan muchas funciones en los tejidos corporales.

moderate drinker - bebedor moderado: una persona que no bebe en exceso. La persona no se comporta inapropiadamente debido al alcohol. La salud de la persona no sufre daños a largo plazo debido al alcohol.

moderation - moderación: una cantidad de alcohol que no causa daño a la salud. No más de uno o dos tragos al día para adultos saludables.

molds - mohos: hongos multicelulares, algunos de los cuales causan enfermedades.

monogamus - monógamo: tener relaciones sexuales con una sola pareja, excluyendo a todos los demás. Estas relaciones generalmente son relaciones de largo plazo.

morning sickness - nauseas matinales: las nauseas que una mujer embarazada puede experimentar en cualquier momento del día. Se piensa que están relacionadas con las hormonas que mantienen el embarazo.

morphine - morfina: una droga narcótica que los médicos prescriben como analgésico.

motivation - motivación: la fuerza que mueve a las personas a actuar. La motivación puede ser instintiva (impulsos) o aprendida.

mucus (MYOO -cuss) **- moco:** una secreción resbalosa producida por las células del revestimiento del organismo que protege la superficie del revestimiento.

mumps - paperas: una enfermedad viral altamente contagiosa que causa inflamación de las glándulas salivales y, ocasionalmente, de los testículos. Se puede prevenir mediante la inmunización.

muscle endurance - capacidad muscular: componente de un buen estado físico. La capacidad de los músculos para soportar un esfuerzo por un largo tiempo.

muscle strength - fuerza muscular: componente de un buen estado físico. La capacidad de los músculos para trabajar contra la resistencia.

mutation (myoo -TAY -shun) **- mutación:** un cambio en el material genético de la célula. Una vez que el material genético ha cambiado, el cambio es heredado por la progenie de esa célula.

myeloma - mieloma: un cáncer que se origina en las células de la médula ósea.

N

naproxen sodium (na -PROX -en) **- sodio de naproxen:** un fármaco que alivia la fiebre, el dolor y la inflamación. Suministra alivio durante un período más prolongado con una sola dosis que la mayoría de los analgésicos comunes.

narcotic antagonist - antagonista narcótico: un fármaco que se opone a la acción de otro fármaco. La palabra *antagonista* significa alguien o algo que lucha o se opone a otro.

Narcotics Anonymous (NA) - Narcóticos Anónimos (NA): un grupo de auto ayuda, libre de costo, para la recuperación de la adicción. Utiliza un programa de 12 pasos, promueve el desarrollo personal y está enfocado hacía que las personas ayuden a otras a recuperarse.

narcotics - narcóticos: drogas adictivas que alivian el dolor y producen sueño cuando se toman en dosis moderadas. También llamados *opiáceos* debido a que la mayoría se obtienen de la amapola del opio.

naturopathic medicine - medicina naturopática: una mezcla de terapias tradicionales y alternativas.

needs - necesidades: deseos urgentes de cosas necesarias.

nervous system - sistema nervioso: el sistema de tejidos nerviosos del organismo - organizado en el cerebro, la médula espinal y los nervios - que envían y reciben mensajes e integran las actividades del organismo.

neural (NER -uhl) **tube defects - defectos del tubo neural:** un grupo de defectos de nacimiento causados por la interrupción del desarrollo normal del tubo neural, el tejido del que se forma el cerebro y la médula espinal.

nicotine (NICK -oh -teen) **- nicotina:** una droga adictiva presente en el tabaco.

night blindness - ceguera nocturna: la recuperación lenta de la visión después de destellos de luz brillante. Un indicador temprano de una deficiencia de vitamina A.

nonconformist - noconformista: una persona que no comparte los valores de la sociedad y por lo tanto se comporta en forma no convencional.

nontraditional family - familia no tradicional: grupo de personas no relacionadas que viven juntas y a menudo se ofrecen apoyo unas a otras.

norepinephrine - noradrenalina: una de las hormonas del estrés.

Norplant - Norplant: marca comercial de un sistema quirúrgico de administración de hormonas que entrega una descarga continua de progestina, evitando de esa forma el embarazo durante un máximo de cinco años.

nuclear family - núcleo familiar: el padre, la madre y los hijos naturales o adoptivos.

nucleus - núcleo: en el interior de una célula, la estructura que contiene los genes.

nutrient deficiencies (dee -FISH -en -sees) **- deficiencias de nutrientes:** muy poco de uno o más nutrientes en la dieta. Una forma de la malnutrición.

nutrients - nutrientes: compuestos presentes en los alimentos que el organismo necesita para crecer, mantenerse y funcionar apropiadamente.

O

obesity - obesidad: sobrepeso al punto de ser dañino para la salud. La obesidad se define frecuentemente como un peso corporal que supera en un 20 por ciento o más el peso apropiado en relación a la altura.

obsessive-compulsive disorder - trastorno obsesivo compulsivo: la necesidad incontrolable de realizar actos repetitivos.

opiates - opiáceos: un grupo de drogas que se derivan de la amapola del opio y que alivian el dolor e induce el sueño. También conocidos como *narcóticos*.

opium - opio: una droga narcótica que alivia el dolor e induce el sueño, hecho de la amapola del opio.

oral contraceptives - contraceptivo oral: píldoras que previenen el embarazo inhibiendo la ovulación o cambiando las condiciones en el útero; a menudo referidas como píldoras anticonceptivas o la Píldora.

organs - órganos: unidades completas compuestas de tejidos que realizan tareas específicas.

orgasm - orgasmo: una serie de contracciones musculares de los órganos sexuales, con eyaculación en el hombre; ocurre típicamente después de un período de estimulación sexual.

osteoporosis (OS -tee -oh -por -OH -sis) **- osteoporosis:** una enfermedad que causa la pérdida gradual de hueso, lo cual puede incapacitar a la persona posteriormente en la vida.

ostracism - ostracismo: rechazo y exclusión de la sociedad.

ova (singular **ovum**) **- óvulos** (singular **óvulo**)**:** las células femeninas de reproducción. También se les denomina huevos.

over the counter (OTC) drugs - fármacos de venta sin receta: fármacos disponibles legalmente sin receta.

overload - sobrecarga: una exigencia física adicional puesta sobre el cuerpo.

overnutrition - sobrenutrición: ingesta excesiva de energía alimentaria o de nutrientes al grado de ocasionar enfermedad o aumento del riesgo de contraer una enfermedad, una forma de malnutrición.

ovulation - ovulación: la maduración y liberación de un óvulo.

ozone layer - capa de ozono: la capa de ozono en la atmósfera exterior de la tierra que protege a los seres vivientes de los dañinos rayos ultravioleta provenientes del sol.

ozone - ozono: una sustancia que se crea cuando ciertos tipos de energía, tales como los rayos ultravioleta del sol reaccionan con el oxígeno. Cuando tiene lugar esta reacción a una gran distancia sobre la Tierra en la atmósfera externa, el ozono absorbe la mayor parte de los rayos ultravioleta más peligrosos.

P

pacemaker - marcapasos: un aparato que suministra impulsos eléctricos al corazón para regular los latidos.

pap test - método de papanicolau: un examen para cáncer cervical (de la parte inferior del útero). Se retiran unas cuantas células, sin dolor, que se examinan en el laboratorio.

parasites - parásitos: seres vivientes que dependen de los nutrientes de los cuerpos de otros seres en los cuales habitan.

passive abuse - abuso pasivo: mal trato que involucra no tomar las acciones necesarias, como el descuido en proveer comida o amparo a una víctima dependiente.

passive - pasivo: que posee la característica de no expresar sus sentimientos apropiadamente. Que se mantiene en silencio respecto de sus sentimientos.

pathogens - patógenos: microbios que causan enfermedad.

PCP (phencyclidine hydrochloride) - PCP: droga de abuso. Un tranquilizante animal, abusado por los seres humanos como alucinógeno.

PCP (Pneumocystis carinii pneumonia) - neumonía carinii pneumocystis: la neumonía característica del SIDA.

pediatrician - pediatra: un especialista que se preocupa del cuidado de la salud de lactantes y niños.

peer groups - grupos de pares: grupos de personas similares en edad y etapa de la vida.

peer pressure - presión de pares: la presión interna que se experimenta para comportarse de la forma en que lo hace el grupo de pares, para ganarse la aprobación de sus miembros.

pelvic inflammatory disease (PIV) - enfermedad de inflamación pélvica: una infección de las trompas de Falopio y la cavidad pélvica en las mujeres, que causa embarazo ectópico y abortos.

perception - percepción: el significado dado a un evento u ocurrencia basado en la experiencia o comprensión previa del individuo.

persistent - persistente: lo opuesto de biodegradable - incapaz de ser convertido en desechos inofensivos por organismos vivientes.

personality - personalidad: las características de una persona que son evidentes para otros.

peyote - peyote: cacto que produce el alucinógeno mezcalina.

phobia (FOH -bee -uh) **- fobia:** un miedo extremo e irracional a un objeto o situación.

photovoltaic (PV) panels - paneles fotovoltaicos: paneles fotoeléctricos que convierten la luz (fotones) en electricidad (volts).

physical addiction - adicción física: un cambio en la química del organismo que hace que en la ausencia de dosis cada vez mayores de determinada sustancia (droga), su funcionamiento normal empiece a fallar y se desarrollen síntomas de aislamiento. También se le llama *dependencia física*.

physical examination - examen físico: un examen del cuerpo para recopilar información acerca de su condición general o para hacer un diagnóstico. Normalmente incluye observaciones realizadas mirando, escuchando y palpando las diferentes partes del cuerpo y por medio de los resultados de exámenes médicos.

physician-assited suicide - suicidio asistido por un médico: el suicidio de una persona enferma mediante drogas letales u otros medios suministrados por un médico. No es legal en la mayoría de los estados.

physiological age - edad fisiológica: la edad estimada de acuerdo al estado de salud del organismo y la esperanza de vida probable.

phytochemicals - fitoquímicos: productos químicos en alimentos basados en plantas que no son nutrientes pero que tienen algún efecto sobre el organismo.

pinch test - prueba del pellizco: una manera informal de medir la grasa corporal.

pinworms - lombriz intestinal: lombrices parasíticas blancas, pequeñas y visibles que comúnmente infectan los intestinos de niños de corta edad.

PKU (phenylketonuria) - fenilcetonuria: una enfermedad congénita que ocasiona daño cerebral severo con retraso mental si se deja sin tratamiento. En la actualidad se detecta y trata al nacer.

placebo effect - efecto placebo: el efecto curativo de la fe en la medicina que aún los medicamentos inertes tienen.

placenta (plah -SEN -tah) - **placenta:** un órgano que se desarrolla durante el embarazo; permite el intercambio de materiales entre la sangre de la madre y la sangre del feto.

placental stage - período placentario del parto: la etapa final del parto, en la cual se expulsa la placenta.

plaques (PLAKS) - **placas:** montículos de grasa mezclada con minerales que se acumulan a lo largo de las paredes de las arterias en la arteriosclerosis.

plateau - altiplano: literalmente, un lugar alto y llano. En el coito, esta fase es el período de placer físico intenso que precede al orgasmo.

platelets - plaquetas: pequeños cuerpos en forma de disco encontrados en la sangre, una parte importante de la formación de coágulos.

pneumonia - neumonía: una enfermedad causada por un virus o bacteria que infecta a los pulmones con fiebre alta, tos severa y dolor en el pecho. Especialmente peligroso en los muy viejos o muy jóvenes.

polio (poliomyelitis) - polio (poliomielitis): una infección viral que en la mayoría de los casos produce síntomas respiratorios o digestivos leves pero que puede producir parálisis permanente o incluso la muerte. Se puede prevenir con la inmunización.

pollution - contaminación: contaminación del medio ambiente con cualquier cosa que perjudique su habilidad de mantener la vida.

polyps - pólipos: tumores que crecen en un tallo, asemejándose a los hongos. Los pólipos sangran fácilmente y tienen la tendencia de convertirse en malignos.

polyunsaturated - poliinsaturado: tipo de grasa no saturada especialmente útil como sustituto de la grasa saturada en una dieta saludable para el corazón.

positive self-talk - autoplática positiva: la práctica de formularse aseveraciones positivas a sí mismo sobre uno mismo, que ayudan a desarrollar la auto estima.

post-traumatic stress disorder - trastorno de estrés pos traumático: una reacción al estrés que enfatiza sufrimientos tales como los ocurridos durante una guerra o violación que aparecen con posterioridad a su ocurrencia.

postpartum depression - depresión pos parto: la depresión emocional que experimenta un nuevo padre o una nueva madre después del nacimiento del lactante.

premature infant - lactante prematuro: un lactante nacido antes de la 38ª semana de gestación.

premenstrual syndrome (PMS) - síndrome premenstrual (SPM): síntomas tales como incomodidad física, mal genio y nerviosismo que experimentan algunas mujeres cada mes antes de la menstruación.

premiums - primas: pagos regulares efectuados a una compañía de seguros para cubrir los costos de acontecimientos imprevistos, como ser las emergencias médicas.

prenatal care - cuidado prenatal: los cuidados médicos y sanitarios proporcionados durante el embarazo.

prepayment plan - plan de prepago: un sistema de pago por atención de salud en la cual los clientes pagan una tarifa fija cada mes, sin importar cuantos servicios reciben.

prescription drugs - drogas de prescripción: aquellos fármacos que solamente están legalmente disponibles con la receta de un médico.

problem drinker or **alcohol abuser - bebedor problema** o **bebedor excesivo:** una persona que sufre problemas sociales, emocionales, familiares o laborales debido al alcohol. Esta persona está en camino al alcoholismo.

prodrome - pródromo: la aparición de síntomas generales comunes a muchas enfermedades, tales como fiebre, estornudos y tos.

progesterone - progesterona: hormona secretada por las mujeres durante la parte del ciclo menstrual en que el revestimiento uterino se acumula.

progestin - progestina: versión sintética de la progesterona utilizada en los anticonceptivos.

progestin-only pill - píldora de solamente progentina: anticonceptivo oral que solo contiene progestina. Otro nombre es la minipíldora.

progressive muscle relaxation - relajamiento muscular progresivo: la técnica de aprender a relajarse enfocándose en relajar los grupos de músculos del cuerpo de uno en uno.

progressive overload principle - principio de sobrecarga progresiva: el principio de entrenamiento basado en que un sistema corporal, para poder mejorar, tiene que ser trabajado en frecuencias, intensidades o duraciones que aumentan con el tiempo.

promoter - promotor: la sustancia que ayuda al desarrollo de tumores malignos, pero que no los inicia por sí sola.

proof - graduación: la medida del porcentaje de alcohol de las bebidas alcohólicas. *100 grados* significa 50 por ciento de alcohol, *90 grados* significa 45 por ciento, etc.

protease inhibitors - inhibidores de la proteasa: fármacos que detienen la acción de la enzima que generalmente ayuda a que el VIH se reproduzca. El fármaco ayuda a aminorar la reproducción del VIH, pero los que la toman corren un riesgo mayor de desarrollar diabetes.

protein - proteína: tipo de nutriente que elabora los tejidos del cuerpo y que proporciona energía. La proteína está compuesta de aminoácidos. Se le refiere solamente en el singular *proteína*.

protozoa (PRO -toh -ZOH -ah) - **protozoos:** pequeñas células de forma animal, algunas de las cuales pueden causar enfermedades.

proxy - representante: una persona autorizada para actuar a nombre de otra.

Prozac - Prozac: el nombre de marca comercial de una droga de un grupo de drogas usadas para restablecer la química normal del cerebro de una persona con depresión.

psilocybin (sill -oh -SI -bin), **psilocin** (sill -OH -sin) - **psilocibin, psilocin:** dos alucinógenos producidos por un tipo de hongo silvestre.

psychological addiction - adicción psicológica: el anhelo de algo; la dependencia mental de una droga, hábito o conducta. También se le denomina *dependencia psicológica*.

psychology - psicología: el estudio científico del comportamiento y la mente.

puberty (PYOO -ver -tee) - **pubertad:** el período de la vida en el cual la persona se vuelve físicamente capaz de reproducir.

pubic lice - piojo púbico: una enfermedad de transmisión sexual causada por pequeños parásitos que se reproducen en el vello púbico y causan una picazón intensa.

pulp cavity - cavidad de la pulpa dental: la cámara más profunda del diente, en la cual se encuentran los vasos sanguíneos y los nervios.

pulse rate - pulso: el número de latidos por minuto del corazón.

pus - pus: una mezcla de líquidos y glóbulos blancos que se juntan alrededor de zonas infectadas.

Q

quacks: las personas que pretenden tener conocimientos médicos y que generalmente tienen productos para la venta.

quality time - tiempo de calidad: el tiempo pasado con otro, de una duración suficiente que permita un intercambio significativo de ideas.

quid - mascada: una pequeña porción de cualquier forma de tabaco para mascar.

R

rabies - rabia: una enfermedad viral del sistema nervioso central que causa parálisis y muerte.

radiation therapy - radioterapia: la aplicación de radiación que destruye las células para destruir el tejido canceroso.

radon - radón: elemento gaseoso que se origina de la tierra donde se encuentran materiales radioactivos.

range of motion - arco de movilidad: la movilidad de una articulación; la dirección y la amplitud con que se puede flexionar.

recovery - recuperación: una tercera fase saludable de la respuesta al estrés durante la cual el cuerpo vuelve a su estado normal.

recreational drug use - uso de fármacos para fines recreativos: un término ideado por las personas para describir su consumo de drogas afirmando que su consumo no produce efectos nocivos para su salud o la sociedad; un término no definido por la Food and Drug Administration (FDA).

rectum - recto: la última porción del tracto digestivo, a través del cual se eliminan las deposiciones. (vea el Capítulo 6)

recyclable - reciclable: elaborado con materiales que pueden ser utilizados nuevamente.

refusal skills - técnicas de rechazo: un conjunto de estrategias sociales que permiten que las personas resistan de manera eficaz la presión de sus pares para involucrarse en conductas peligrosas o indeseables.

relapses - recidiva: enfermedades que reaparecen después de ser tratadas y prácticamente curadas. Con frecuencia las recidivas son más graves que la enfermedad original.

resolution - resolución: en el coito, la fase de relajación que sigue al orgasmo.

ripple effect - efecto de propagación el efecto que se observa cuando se arroja una piedra dentro de una laguna u se forman ondas que irradian desde el centro. El término se utiliza par explicar como las acciones de una persona pueden afectar a mucha otra gente y como sus acciones afectarán aun a más gente.

risk factors - factores de riesgo: factores relacionados con una enfermedad por asociación que aun no se ha demostrado su relación de causalidad con esta.

rubella - rubéola: una enfermedad viral que se asemeja al sarampión pero que solo dura unos pocos días y no causa complicaciones serias, excepto durante el embarazo; se puede prevenir mediante la inmunización.

S

safe - seguro: que no causa daño excesivo; parte de los requisitos legales para un fármaco.

safer-sex strategies - prácticas sexuales seguras: las pautas del comportamiento para reducir el riesgo de contraer enfermedades de transmisión sexual, pero que no reducen el riesgo a cero.

Salmonella - Salmonella: un patógeno transmitido por vía alimentaria que produce infecciones al sistema digestivo en mucha gente cada año.

sal - sal: un compuesto de minerales que disueltos en agua forman electrolitos.

sarcomas (sar -KOH -mahs) **- sarcomas:** tipos de cáncer que se producen en las células del tejido conectivo, incluyendo los huesos, ligamentos y músculos.

sassafras - sasafrás: la corteza de la raíz del árbol de sasafrás utilizado en una época en algunas bebidas pero prohibido en la actualidad como ingrediente en los alimentos y bebidas debido a que contienen sustancias químicas cancerígenas.

saturated - saturado: relativo a las grasas y la salud, aquellas grasas asociadas con las enfermedades del corazón y las arterias; principalmente las grasas de origen animal.

schizophrenia (SKITZ.oh -FREN -EE -uh) **- esquizofrenia:** una enfermedad mental, una condición de pérdida del contacto con la realidad acompañado por una capacidad reducida para funcionar.

sebum (SEE -bum) **- sebo:** la grasa natural de la piel, en esencia una mezcla de aceites y ceras, que ayuda a mantener la piel y el cabello humectados.

second opinion - segunda opinión: una segunda valoración de un diagnóstico y plan terapéutico
realizado por otro proveedor de salud, generalmente a pedido del paciente, a fin de verificar la validez del plan terapéutico inicial.

sedatives - sedantes: tipos de fármacos que poseen un efecto calmante o tranquilizante.

sedentary - sedentario: físicamente inactivo (literalmente, "pasa mucho tiempo sentado").

self-actualization - autorrealización: la máxima realización del propio potencial; el más alto estado alcanzable de acuerdo a la jerarquía de necesidades de Maslow.

self-efficacy (EFF -ih -kasee) **- autoeficacia:** la creencia de una persona en su propia capacidad para tener éxito en la tarea que ha iniciado.

self-esteem - autoestima: el valor que da una persona a su autoimagen. Es alto en aquéllos que se valoran a sí mismos. Constituye una parte de vital importancia para la salud emocional.

self-image - autoimagen: las características que una persona ve en sí misma.

senility - senilidad: un término general asociado al estado de vigor reducido de la mente y el cuerpo que ocurre con el envejecimiento.

set - conjunto: el número específico de veces que se debe repetir un ejercicio de levantamiento de pesas.

sex - sexo: un término general utilizado para referirse al género y la relación sexual.

sexual dysfunction - disfunción sexual: deterioro de la excitación sexual u orgasmo debido a causas psicológicas, interpersonales, físicas, ambientales o culturales. Antiguamente se les llamaba impotencia en los hombres y frigidez en las mujeres.

sexual harassment - acoso sexual: la atención sexual indeseada, frecuentemente por parte de alguien con poder, que hace que la víctima se sienta incómoda o amenazada.

sexual intercourse - relación sexual: el acto de reproducción entre los sexos. El término intercourse significa la comunicación de cualquier tipo - hablar, por ejemplo. La relación sexual entre los seres humanos se le denomina como coito. Entre animales se le denomina como copulación.

sexuality - sexualidad: la cualidad de ser sexual. La sexualidad es parte integrante de la persona total: física, emocional, social, intelectual y espiritual. La sexualidad es parte de lo que son las personas.

sexually transmitted diseases (STD) - enfermedades de transmisión sexual (ETS): aquellas enfermedades que son transmitidas por vía del contacto sexual directo. Se conocían anteriormente como enfermedades venéreas.

shame - vergüenza: un sentimiento extremo de culpa que se produce cuando una persona internaliza los errores ("Soy malo porque yo lo hice").

shin splints - desgarros a la espinilla: daño a los músculos y tejido conectivo de la parte anterior inferior de la pierna producida por el estrés. Tales daños pueden curarse con descanso.

shingles - herpes zoster: un trastorno doloroso de la piel causado por la recurrencia del virus de la varicela en una edad posterior.

shock - shock: la falla o interrupción de la circulación sanguínea, una reacción a accidentes y lesiones que amenaza la vida.

sibling rivalry - rivalidad entre hermanos: la competencia entre hermanos y hermanas, con frecuencia para atraer la atención o afecto de los padres.

siblings - hermanos: dos o más personas con uno o más padres en común; hermanos o hermanas.

side effects - efectos secundarios: efectos de los fármacos distintos a los efectos médicos deseados.

sidestream smoke - humo indirecto: el humo que se escapa al aire de un cigarrillo, puro o pipa encendidos.

single-parent family - familia de un solo progenitor: un progenitor y sus hijos (as) naturales o adoptados.

sinuses (SIGN -us -es) **- senos nasales:** espacios en los huesos del cráneo.

small for date - pequeño para la edad gestacional: término utilizado para describir a un lactante subdesarrollado para su edad gestacional, con frecuencia debido a la malnutrición de la madre.

smallpox - viruela: una infección viral grave con erupciones cutáneas; con frecuencia fatal en alguna época, en la actualidad se considera erradicada a nivel mundial gracias a las inmunizaciones.

smokeless tobacco - tabaco sin humo: tabaco utilizado para aspirar o masticar en lugar de fumarlo.

sober - sobrio: libre de los efectos del tabaco y de adicción a este; no embriagado

social drinker - bebedor social: persona que solo bebe en ocasiones sociales. Dependiendo de cómo el alcohol afecta su vida, la persona puede calificarse como un bebedor moderado o un bebedor problema.

specialist - especialista: un médico con estudios en un área de especialidad superiores a los requisitos para obtener el título de médico cirujano.

sperm - semen: las células masculinas de reproducción.

spermicide - espermicida: el compuesto nonoynol -9, destinado al control natal que también permite destruir o debilitar algunos organismos ETS.

spina (SPY -nah or SPEE -nah) **bifida** (BIFF -ih -duh) **- espina bífida:** un defecto de nacimiento que con frecuencia presenta huecos entre los huesos que deja al descubierto la médula espinal en aquellos puntos. La médula espinal puede abultar y sobresalir a través de los huecos en la espina dorsal.

spine - espina: conjunto de 33 vertebras que forman l a columna vertebral y sostienen la médula espinal, cuyos nervios ingresan y egresan a través de los espacios entre los huesos.

splint - férula: tablilla o pala utilizado para apoyar un hueso quebrado y evitar que sus fragmentos se muevan hasta que sane.

spontaneous abortion, or miscarriage - aborto espontáneo: la expulsión del zigoto, embrión o feto desde el útero, no inducido por medios médicos.

spouse abuse - abuso del cónyuge: la agresión verbal, psicológica, física o sexual del cónyuge.

starch - almidón: un carbohidrato, fuente principal de sustento para todo ser humano.

status - posición social: la situación o categoría de una persona en relación a otras, a menudo basada equivocadamente en la riqueza, el poder o la influencia, características que siendo deseables para algunos no definen el valor humano.

step aerobics - aeróbica con step: una actividad aeróbica en la cual cada participante sube y baja sobre una plataforma estable denominada step de alrededor de 6 a 12 pulgadas de altura.

stepparents - padrastro, madrastra: una persona que se casa integrándose una familia luego de que uno de los padres biológicos la abandona por muerte o divorcio.

stereotypes - estereotipo: la generalización sobre la forma de ser de los miembros de un grupo, ideas que no admiten la individualidad

sterilization - esterilización: proceso de interrumpir en forma permanente la habilidad de procrear de la persona, generalmente mediante el corte y sellado quirúrgico del conducto deferente o de las Trompas de Falopio.

steroids - esteroides: hormonas de un tipo químico específico que se produce en forma natural en el cuerpo, algunas de las cuales estimulan el desarrollo muscular. Disponibles en la forma de fármacos, los atletas abusan de ellas en la búsqueda del camino fácil para obtener músculos desarrollados.

stimulant - estimulantes: cualquiera de una amplia variedad de fármacos, incluyendo las anfetaminas, la cafeína y otros que aceleran el sistema nervioso central.

stranger rape - violación por extraños: la agresión sexual por un extraño. También denominada violación en la calle.

stress - estrés: el efecto de las exigencias físicas y sicológicas (factores estresantes) sobre una persona. El estrés que proporciona un desafío bienvenido se denomina *euestrés* ("estrés positivo", que se pronuncia YOU - STRESS); el estrés que se percibe como negativo se denomina *sufrimiento* (estrés negativo).

stress eating - comer por estrés: comer en respuesta al estrés, una actividad inapropiada.

stress fracture - fractura por sobrecarga: daño óseo por una fuerza física repetida que estira la unión de los ligamentos a los huesos.

stress hormones - hormonas del estrés: epinefrina y norepinefrina, secretadas como parte de la reacción del sistema nervioso al estrés.

stressor - factores estresantes: una exigencia de adaptación impuesta al cuerpo.

stress response - respuesta al estrés: la reacción ante una exigencia o factor estresante. La respuesta al estrés posee tres etapas - *alarma, resistencia, y recuperación o agotamiento*.

stroke - ataque apopléjico: la interrupción del flujo sanguíneo al cerebro por placas, un coágulo o una hemorragia.

sudden infant death syndrome (SIDS) - síndrome de muerte súbita: muerte inesperada y sin explicación de un lactante aparentemente saludable; la causa más común de muerte en los lactantes entre la segunda semana y el primer año de vida; también se le conoce como *crib death* (muerte en la cuna).

sudden sniffing death syndrome (SIDS) - síndrome de muerte súbita por inhalación: muerte repentina, generalmente por insuficiencia cardíaca, de una persona sorprendida abusando de inhalantes. El susto se produce frecuentemente al ser sorprendidos por una figura de autoridad o cuando la droga produce una alucinación aterradora.

sugars - azúcares: carbohidratos que se encuentran tanto en los alimentos como en el cuerpo.

sun block - bloqueador solar: bloqueador total de los rayos solares cancerígenos. Un bloqueador solar posee un SPF (factor de protección solar) de 50 o más. El óxido de zinc es un ejemplo de un bloqueador solar.

sunscreen - pantalla solar: bloqueador parcial de los rayos solares cancerígenos (radiación gamma).

suntan lotion - bronceador: loción que puede o no contener protección solar.

supplement - suplemento: una píldora, polvo, líquido o similar que contiene nutrientes solamente, no es un alimento.

support system - sistema de apoyo: una red de individuos o grupos con los cuales uno se identifica e intercambia apoyo emocional.

suppress - suprimir: reprimir o contener.

surgical insurance - seguro para cirugías: seguro para el pago de los honorarios de médico cirujano. Vea *Medicaid*.

sustainable - sustentable: el término utilizado para describir el uso de recursos a una velocidad tal que la tierra pueda renovarlos. Por ejemplo, una velocidad de tala de arboles no mayor a la velocidad con que crecen. *Sustentable* también describe la producción de contaminantes a una velocidad que pueda manejar el medio ambiente o los esfuerzos del hombre puedan limpiar de tal forma que no haya acumulación de contaminantes.

syphilis - sífilis: una enfermedad bacteriana de transmisión sexual que si no se trata progresa desde una lesión cutánea (chancro) a síntomas parecidos a la gripe, luego pasa por un período libre de síntomas para después pasar a una etapa final de daño cerebral o nervioso irreversible y terminar en la muerte.

systolic (sis -TOL -ic) **pressure - presión sistólica:** la presión sanguínea durante aquella parte del latido del corazón cuando los ventrículos del corazón se contraen y la sangre es impulsada dentro de las arterias.

T

T cells - células T: linfocitos que pueden reconocer a los invasores que causan enfermedades.

target heart rate - frecuencia cardíaca objetivo: la frecuencia cardíaca que condicionará el sistema cardiovascular de una persona - lo suficientemente rápido para acelerar el corazón pero no tan rápido como para sobreexcitarlo.

tar - alquitrán: sustancias químicas que se encuentran entre otras cosas en el tabaco. Al quemarse los alquitranes liberan muchos carcinógenos.

tennis elbow - codo de tenista: una lesión dolorosa del brazo y articulaciones, generalmente causada por un esfuerzo, como ser por un movimiento incorrecto al jugar tenis.

terminal illnesses - enfermedades terminales: enfermedades que se espera terminen en la muerte.

tetanus - tétanos: una enfermedad causada por una toxina elaborada por bacteria que se encuentra en la parte profunda de una herida.

therapy - terapia: tratamiento que cura.

thoughts - pensamientos: aquellos procesos mentales de los cuales una persona siempre está consciente.

thrill-seekers - buscadores de emociones: aquellas personas que son particularmente propensas a tomar riesgos a cambio de una excitación momentánea.

thrombus - trombo: un coágulo estacionario. Cuando ha crecido lo suficiente para obstruir completamente un vaso sanguíneo, este peligroso evento se denomina una *trombosis*.

thymus gland - glándula del timo: un órgano del sistema inmunológico.

tissues - tejidos: sistemas de células que trabajan unidas para realizar tareas especiales.

tolerance - tolerancia: en el consumo de drogas, el estado que se desarrolla en los usuarios de ciertas drogas que hace que se necesiten cantidades cada vez mayores de la droga para producir el mismo efecto.

tolerance - tolerancia: en las relaciones con los demás, la adaptación y aceptación de las diferencias entre uno mismo y los demás; siendo tolerante de la edad, forma del cuerpo, sexo, discapacidades, raza, religión, formas de pensar y otras diferencias de las personas. (Otro significado de tolerancia tiene que ver con la adaptación del cuerpo a medicamentos y fármacos, según se define en el Capítulo 11).

tonsillectomy - tonsilectomía: la extracción de las amígdalas (de la garganta), una operación llevada a cabo muchas veces innecesariamente

toxic shock syndrome (TSS) - síndrome del shock tóxico (SST): un tipo de envenenamiento que ocurre cuando la bacteria descompone la sangre menstrual; a menudo asociado con el uso de tampones super absorbentes.

toxin - toxina: un veneno.

Index

bones, 133, 134, 136–137, 694
botulism, 412–413, 414
boys. *See* males
brain, 27, 109, 351, 353
    as sex organ, 582, 584
    See also nervous system
brain death, 638–639
breast cancer, 481
breastfeeding, 438, 568–569, 613
breathalyzer tests, 356, 357
breech birth, 566, 567
bronchitis, 378, 379, 412
bubonic plague, 405
bulimia, 225–227
burns, 655–656, 664–665, 687–688
    chemical, 655
    degrees of, 687
bypass surgery, 463–464

C

cesarean delivery, 566, 567
caffeine, 304–305, 316, 564, 695
calcium, 191
calisthenics, 248
calories, 172, 173
    in Daily Food Guide, 165–166
    empty, 177, 216
    and energy, 207, 209
    and fats, 179–180
    teens' need for, 170
    in weight control, 215–217, 222–223
cancer, 473–485
    detection of, 480–482
    development of, 473–475
    and fiber, 175
    metastasized, 474, 475
    risk factors, 476–479
    and smoking, 377, 380, 476
    treatment of, 483–485
candidiasis, 431
capillaries, 457
car accidents, 646–651
carbohydrates, 164, 165, 171–176, 210, 256–260
carbon monoxide, 381, 384–385
carcinogens, 377, 380
carcinomas, 473
cardiovascular disease, 457–472
    and cholesterol, 178
    and emotions, 471–472
    risk reduction for, 466
    and smoking, 381, 466–467
    and stress, 89
    treatment for, 463–464
cardiovascular system, 134, 135, 144–145, 457–458
    and physical activities, 239–244
careers, 43–44

cavities, 266, 267
celibacy. *See* abstinence, sexual
cells, 132, 133, 137
    aging of, 628
centenarians, 10
cerebral thrombosis, 460
cervical cap, 605–606, 610
cervix, 601, 603, 605, 609
chamomile, 695, 696, 697
chancre, 428, 429, 430
chemotherapy, 484
chewing tobacco, 386–387
chicken pox, 402–403
child abuse, 534, 535, 536–537, 570
childbirth, 438, 566–567
children, 569–570, 581, 661–663
    adoption of, 549–550
    care of, 538, 539
chiropractors, 741
chlamydia, 421, 424
choking, 662–663, 684–685
cholera, 404
cholesterol, 178, 179, 469–471
chromosomes, 133
chronic fatigue syndrome, 403
chronic obstructive lung diseases, 379
cigar smoking, 383
cigarettes. *See* nicotine; smoking; tobacco
circulatory system. *See* cardiovascular system
circumcision, 157
cliques, 67
clitoris, 582, 583, 584
cocaine, 320–321, 325–326
codeine, 327
codependency, 123, 360, 361, 536
coitus interruptus, 613
colds, 402, 403, 410, 412
colostrum, 569
comfrey, 696, 697
commitment, 18–19, 504–506, 581
communication, 70
    in families, 522–530, 540–541
    in sexual relations, 586, 590–591
    styles of, 38, 39
compost, 721
compromise, 70
compulsions, 115
conception, 552–553
conditioning, 234–238, 248–251
condoms, 441, 443, 606–609, 612
    and disease prevention, 527, 603, 605, 610
    female, 609, 610
conflict resolution, 34–39, 507, 527, 528
confrontation, 33, 38
congeners, 352–353
conservation, 704–705, 720–721

constipation, 175
contraception, 596–621
    cervical cap as, 605–606, 610
    condoms as, 606–607, 609, 610
    diaphragm as, 605, 610
    effectiveness of, 598–599, 601, 603, 604, 608, 610
    failures of, 616
    fertility awareness method of, 609, 610, 611
    hormone implant as, 603, 610
    ineffective methods of, 612–613
    IUDs as, 603–604, 610
    oral, 596, 599, 601–602, 610
    resistance to, 619–621
    risks of, 598
    side effects of, 599, 601–602
    spermicide as, 604–605
    and STD protection, 596–597
    sterilization as, 606, 610, 614–615
    tubal ligation as, 614–615
    vasectomy as, 614
    See also abstinence
coping devices, 96–97
coronary artery, 457, 458
    bypass surgery, 463–464
coronary thrombosis, 460
cosmetics, 273, 275
counselors, 121
Cousins, Norman, 102–103
CPR (cardiopulmonary resuscitation), 673–674, 678–683
crimes, 45–47, 509–511
crowning, 566, 567
cults, 67, 70–71
cuticles, 271
cysts, 273

D

Daily Food Guide, 165–167, 170
dandruff, 271
dating, 499–500
day care, 538, 539
death, 5, 637–639
    from drug abuse, 329, 350
    from smoking, 379, 381
    of teens, 646
    from undernutrition, 723
decision making, 41–42
defense mechanisms, 97
defensive driving, 647, 649
deforestation, 707–709
dehydration, 254–255
delirium tremors, 352, 353
dementia complex, 434, 435
denial, 361
Depo-Provera, 603
depressants, 326–327

Photo Credits

xii (top) Image ©1998 PhotoDisc, Inc.; xii (middle) ©Jeff Greenberg/Rainbow; xii (bottom) David Young-Wolff/Tony Stone Images; xiii (top) ©D. Young-Wolff/PhotoEdit; xiii (bottom left) ©Alan Raphael; xiii (bottom right) Image ©1998 PhotoDisc, Inc.; xiv (top) ©Alan Raphael; xiv (middle) ©Tony Freeman/PhotoEdit; xiv (bottom) Mothers Against Drunk Driving; xv (top) American Cancer Society; xv (middle) Image ©1998 PhotoDisc, Inc.; xv (bottom) ©Lawrence Migdale/Photo Researchers, Inc.; xvi (top) ©Mary Kate Denny/PhotoEdit; xvi (middle) ©Alan Raphael; xvi (bottom left) Image ©1998 PhotoDisc, Inc.; xvi (bottom right) Robert Torrez/©Tony Stone Images; xvii (top) Digital Stock; xvii (middle) Image ©1998 PhotoDisc, Inc.; xvii (bottom) Image ©1998 PhotoDisc, Inc.; xviii (left) Image ©1998 PhotoDisc, Inc.; xviii (right) ©Myrleen Ferguson/PhotoEdit; xix (top) Image ©1998 PhotoDisc, Inc.; xix (bottom) Image ©1998 PhotoDisc, Inc.; xx (top) ©Coco McCoy/Rainbow; xx (bottom) ©Roy Morsch/The Stock Market; xxi (top) ©Jon Riley/Tony Stone Images; xxi (middle) ©Mary Kate Denny/PhotoEdit; xxi (bottom) Image ©1998 PhotoDisc, Inc.; xxii (top) David Young-Wolff/Corbis; xxii (middle) Image ©1998 PhotoDisc, Inc.; xxii (bottom) Image ©1998 PhotoDisc, Inc.;

Chapter 1 02 ©Jon Riley/Tony Stone Images; 04 Image ©1998 PhotoDisc, Inc.; 10 Kevin Horan/Tony Stone Images; 11 (left) Image ©1998 PhotoDisc, Inc.; 11 (right) Image ©1998 PhotoDisc, Inc.; 15 ©David R. Frazier Photolibrary; 18 ©Mark E. Gibson; 21 ©Tony Freeman/PhotoEdit.

Chapter 2 24 ©Myrleen Ferguson/PhotoEdit; 27 Skjold Photographs; 29 ©Frank Siteman/Rainbow; 30 ©Mark Richards/PhotoEdit; 32 Skjold Photographs; 34 Corbis-Bettmann; 35 ©Jeff Greenberg/Rainbow; 39 Image ©1998 PhotoDisc, Inc.; 42 ©Coco McCoy/Rainbow; 43 Myrleen Cate/©Tony Stone Images, Inc; 45 Frank Orel/©Tony Stone Images.

Chapter 3 50 ©D. Young-Wolff/PhotoEdit; 57 Image ©1998 PhotoDisc, Inc.; 52 ©Frank Siteman/Rainbow; 58 ©Michael Newman/PhotoEdit; 59 Los Angeles Daily News; 60 George Hall/Corbis; 67 Image ©1998 PhotoDisc, Inc.; 70 Don Milici; 73 ©Jeff Greenberg/Rainbow.

Chapter 4 78 Digital Stock; 84 ©Michael A. Keller Studios Ltd./The Stock Market; 86 Image ©1998 PhotoDisc, Inc.; 90 Robert Torrez/©Tony Stone Images; 95 ©Tony Freeman/PhotoEdit; 97 ©Jeff Greenberg/Rainbow; 98 ©Michael Newman/PhotoEdit; 100 ©Myrleen Ferguson/PhotoEdit.

Chapter 5 106 ©Mary Kate Denny/PhotoEdit; 111 ©Myrleen Ferguson/PhotoEdit; 114 ©T.J. Florian/Rainbow; 116 Jeff Greenberg/©DAvid R. Frazier Photolibrary; 118 ©Mary Kate Denny/PhotoEdit; 119 ©David Young-Wolff/PhotoEdit; 121 Corbis; 123 Mary Kate Denny/PhotoEdit; 126 Image ©1998 PhotoDisc, Inc.

Chapter 6 130 ©David R. Frazier Photolibrary.

Chapter 7 160 ©Lawrence Migdale/Photo Researchers, Inc.; 163 Image ©1998 PhotoDisc, Inc.; 164 Image ©1998 PhotoDisc, Inc.; 165 Mary Kate Denny/PhotoEdit; 166 (bottom left) Courtesy United States Department of Agriculture; 166 (bottom right) Courtesy United States Department of Agriculture; 166 (top left) Aaron Haupt/©David R. Frazier Photolibrary; 166 (top right) Courtesy United States Department of Agriculture; 167 (left) Courtesy United States Department of Agriculture; 167 (right) ©Felicia Martinez/PhotoEdit; 169 Rosemary Weller/©Tony Stone Images; 171 Image ©1998

PhotoDisc, Inc.; 173 ©Felicia Martinez/PhotoEdit; 174 David Young-Wolff/Tony Stone Images; 177 (bottom) ©Don Milici; 177 (top right) Image ©1998 PhotoDisc, Inc.; 179 ©Felicia Martinez/PhotoEdit; 180 (all) ©Ray Stanyard/PhotoEdit; 183 ©Jose L. Pelaez/The Stock Market; 186 (left to right) ©David Farr; 190 ©Felicia Martinez/PhotoEdit; 191 ©Tony Freeman/PhotoEdit; 195 ©Lawrence Migdal/Photo Researchers; 197 Dan McCoy/Rainbow.

Chapter 8 200 ©Mark E. Gibson; 202 (left) ©Tony Freeman/PhotoEdit; 202 (right) ©Myrleen Ferguson/PhotoEdit; 207 Digital Stock; 210 ©David Young-Wolff/PhotoEdit; 212 ©Myrleen Ferguson/PhotoEdit; 214 ©NIH Science Source/Photo Researchers; 217 Image ©1998 PhotoDisc, Inc.; 219 Digital Stock; 222 ©David Madison; 224 ©Mary Kate Denny/PhotoEdit; 226 ©Michael Newman/PhotoEdit.

Chapter 9 230 Digital Stock; 235 ©Lawrence Migdale/Photo Researchers, Inc.; 237 Image ©1998 PhotoDisc, Inc.; 239 (bottom) Image ©1998 PhotoDisc, Inc.; 239 (top) Digital Stock; 251 Image ©1998 PhotoDisc, Inc.; 253 ©Tony Freeman/PhotoEdit; 258 Image ©1998 PhotoDisc, Inc.; 260 ©Coco McCoy/Rainbow; 261 (all) ©Felicia Martinez/PhotoEdit.

Chapter 10 264 Image ©1998 PhotoDisc, Inc.; 267 ©Mary Kate Denny/PhotoEdit; 271 ©Jose Carillo/PhotoEdit; 272 ©Tony Freeman/PhotoEdit; 281 ©Roy Morsch/The Stock Market; 285 Image ©1998 PhotoDisc, Inc.

Chapter 11 288 ©Dana White/PhotoEdit; 290 Image ©1998 PhotoDisc, Inc.; 295 Digital Stock; 297 ©Bill Aron/PhotoEdit; 303 Image ©1998 PhotoDisc, Inc.

Chapter 12 308 ©Michael Newman/PhotoEdit; 310 Image ©1998 PhotoDisc, Inc.; 313 ©John Eastcott/Photo Researchers; 315 ©Mark Richards/PhotoEdit; 316 Image ©1998 PhotoDisc, Inc.; 319 Image ©1998 PhotoDisc, Inc.; 326 Image ©1998 PhotoDisc, Inc.; 327 ©VU/Cabisco; 331 Image ©1998 PhotoDisc, Inc.; 335 ©Mary Kate Denny/PhotoEdit; 336 (bottom) ©David K. Crow/PhotoEdit; 336 (top) ©Michael Newman/PhotoEdit.

Chapter 13 342 ©Mary Kate Denny/PhotoEdit; 344 ©David Young-Wolff/PhotoEdit; 346 ©Bill Bachmann/PhotoEdit; 349 ©Mary Kate Denny/PhotoEdit; 352 ©Richard Hutchings/Photo Researchers, Inc.; 354 ©A. Glauberman/Photo Researchers, Inc.; 356 (bottom) Digital Stock; 356 (top) Image ©1998 PhotoDisc, Inc.; 357 ©Michael Newman/Photo Edit; 359 Courtesy of Mothers Against Drunk Driving; 361 ©Larry Mulvehill/Photo Researchers, Inc.; 363 ©Mary Kate Denny/Photo Edit; 364 ©David R. Frazier Photolibrary; 367 ©Billy Barnes/PhotoEdit.

Chapter 14 370 Image ©1998 PhotoDisc, Inc.; 372 (center) for Disease Control; 373 ©Michael Newman/PhotoEdit; 375 (bottom) American Cancer Society; 375 (top) ©Michael Newman; 378 Lester V. Bergman/Corbis; 381 ©Pete Saloutos/The Stock Market; 383 Digital Stock; 385 ©Billy E. Barnes/PhotoEdit; 386 Todd Gipstein/Corbis; 387 (left) Image ©1998 PhotoDisc, Inc.; 387 (right) John Radcliffe Hospital/Science Photo Library/Photo Researchers, Inc.; 389 American Cancer Society; 392 Digital Stock.

Chapter 15 398 ©Biophoto Associates/Photo Researchers, Inc.; 401 (bottom) Oliver Meckes/Photo Researchers, Inc.; 401 (top) CNRI/Science Photo Library/Photo Researchers, Inc.; 407 ©Oscar Burriel/Science Photo Library/Photo Researchers, Inc.; 414 ©MIchael Newman/PhotoEdit.

812